Pediatric and Neonatal Tests and Procedures

Pediatric and Neonatal Tests and Procedures

▲ H. William Taeusch, M.D.
Professor of Pediatrics
University of California, San Francisco, School of Medicine
Vice Chair, Department of Pediatrics
Chief, Pediatric Service
San Francisco General Hospital Medical Center
San Francisco, California

▲ Robert O. Christiansen, M.D.
Professor of Pediatrics
Charles R. Drew University of Medicine and Science
Director, Inpatient and Critical Care Division
Martin Luther King, Jr./Charles R. Drew Medical Center
Los Angeles, California

▲ E. Stephen Buescher, M.D.
Associate Professor of Pediatrics
Center for Pediatric Research
Eastern Virginia Medical School
Children's Hospital of the King's Daughters
Norfolk, Virginia

W.B. SAUNDERS COMPANY
A Division of Harcourt Brace & Company
Philadelphia London Toronto Montreal Sydney Tokyo

W.B. SAUNDERS COMPANY
A Division of Harcourt Brace & Company

The Curtis Center
Independence Square West
Philadelphia, Pennsylvania 19106

Library of Congress Cataloging-in-Publication Data

Pediatric and neonatal tests and procedures / H. William Taeusch, Robert O. Christiansen, E. Stephen Buescher, [editors]. — 1st ed.

p. cm.

ISBN 0-7216-5159-3

1. Children—Diseases—Diagnosis. 2. Children—Diseases—Treatment. 3. Infants (Newborn)—Diseases—Diagnosis. 4. Infants (Newborn)—Diseases—Treatment. I. Taeusch, H. William. II. Christiansen, Robert O. III. Buescher, E. Stephen. [DNLM: 1. Diagnosis, Laboratory—in infancy & childhood. 2. Pediatrics—methods. 3. Physical Examination—in infancy & childhood. 4. Infant, Newborn, Diseases—diagnosis. WS 141 P3676 1996]

RJ45.P3925 1996 618.92—dc20

DNLM/DLC 95-37881

Pediatric and Neonatal Tests and Procedures ISBN 0-7216-5159-3

Printed in the United States of America

Last digit is the print number: 9 8 7 6 5 4 3 2 1

Preface

A number of years ago at our hospital book fair, George Fee, the area sales representative for W.B. Saunders Company, was asked what he believed to be the most obviously "missing" text in pediatrics. He believed that a book on tests and procedures was among the most frequently requested. That conversation resonated with us because of our frequent need to offer the same basic information to trainees in pediatrics and our inability to find a text outside of subspecialty texts that fit the bill. We generalists believed that having a readily available description of the more rare procedures done primarily by specialists would enable us to prepare our patients and their parents. Finally, we needed some information about what the results of the tests and procedures meant.

With these thoughts in mind, we worked up a table of contents for the type of book we believed would be useful to us and the trainees for whom we were responsible (medical students, interns and residents, nurses, respiratory therapists, and specialists dealing with children).

Soon thereafter, we discovered that W.B. Saunders Company had published two editions of a book on this same subject: *Pediatric Procedures*, by W.T. Hughes, and a subsequent edition by W.T. Hughes and E.S. Buescher. The book was out of print and hard to obtain, and it had become somewhat dated because of the explosion of new diagnostic approaches to the pediatric patient, but it was concise and clear and had excellent illustrations created by Dr. Buescher when he was a resident in pediatrics at Johns Hopkins University. Therefore, Dr. Christiansen and Dr. Taeusch contacted Dr. Buescher and Dr. Hughes for aid in this new venture, *Pediatric and Neonatal Tests and Procedures*.

In putting together this book, we recruited physicians who expertly carry out the tests and procedures frequently and have firm ideas about how these procedures should be done. We have not emphasized why particular tests and procedures should be done, nor have we discussed the skills and background required by those who carry out the procedures. We have detailed the more common tests and procedures and allocated less space for the more rare, but not unimportant, ones. The choice of what to include and exclude has been determined, to a large extent, by these contributing experts.

Great credit is due the many people who worked on synthesizing all the contributions into a workable whole. Two of these people are Marcia Holmes and Cathy Duran. Special thanks are also due Stephen Taeusch, who used most of a vacation filing, correcting, editing, arranging, corresponding, calling, following up, and fighting a balky computer. The editors at W.B. Saunders Company—Nellie McGrew, Judith Fletcher, and Lisette Bralow—all should receive the patience-of-the-decade award.

We hope you like the book, and we invite you to give us your comments.

H. William Taeusch
Robert O. Christiansen
E. Stephen Buescher

Contributors

Myles B. Abbott, M.D.
Clinical Professor of Pediatrics, University of California, San Francisco, School of Medicine, San Francisco, California; Attending Pediatrician, East Bay Children's Hospital, Oakland, California
Well Infant and Child Procedures

Sana Al-Jundi, M.D.
Staff Pediatric Intensivist, Children's Hospital of Orange County, Orange, California
Intra-aortic Balloon Pump; Intracranial Pressure Monitoring

Teresa Allard, Pharm.D.
Associate Professor, Division of Clinical Pharmacy, University of California, San Francisco, School of Pharmacy; Clinical Pharmacist, San Francisco General Hospital Medical Center, San Francisco, California
Management of Pain and Sedation

Sudhir K. Anand, M.D.
Professor of Pediatrics, Charles R. Drew University of Medicine and Science; Professor of Clinical Pediatrics, University of California, Los Angeles, School of Medicine; Associate Director in Patient Pediatrics, Martin Luther King, Jr./Charles R. Drew Medical Center, Los Angeles, California
Tests and Procedures for Evaluation of Renal Disorders

Nick G. Anas, M.D.
Associate Professor, Department of Pediatrics, University of California, Los Angeles, School of Medicine, Los Angeles, California; Director, Pediatric Intensive Care Unit, Children's Hospital of Orange County, Orange, California
Oxygen Saturation Monitoring; End-Tidal Carbon Dioxide Monitoring (Capnography)

Azizullah N. Ansari, M.D.
Associate Professor of Radiology and Internal Medicine, University of Southern California School of Medicine; Specialist Physician, Los Angeles County–University of Southern California Medical Center, Los Angeles, California
Diagnostic Nuclear Medicine Imaging in Pediatric Endocrinology

Ernest G. Bertha, M.D.
Assistant Professor, Eastern Virginia Medical School; Staff, Center for Pediatric Research, Children's Hospital of the King's Daughters, Norfolk, Virginia
Pediatric Toxicology Tests and Procedures

J. Warren Bradley, R.R.T.
Staff, Department of Respiratory Care, Medical University of South Carolina, Charleston, South Carolina
Ventilatory Support in Infants and Children

J. Scott Brandeburg, M.S., R.R.T.
Staff, Department of Respiratory Care, Medical University of South Carolina, Charleston, South Carolina
Ventilatory Support in Infants and Children

Yvonne Brouard, M.D., M.P.H.
Formerly, Chief Resident in Pediatrics, San Francisco General Hospital Medical Center, San Francisco, California; Associate, Alameda Pediatric Associates, Alameda, California; Attending Physician, Children's Hospital Medical Center of Northern California, Oakland, California
Outpatient Minor Surgical Procedures

E. Stephen Buescher, M.D.
Associate Professor of Pediatrics, Center for Pediatric Research, Eastern Virginia Medical School, Children's Hospital of the King's Daughters, Norfolk, Virginia
Pediatric Trauma and Musculoskeletal Procedures; Pediatric Toxicology Tests and Procedures; Central Nervous System; Pediatric Ear, Nose, and Throat Procedures and Tests; Immunology and Infectious Diseases Procedures and Tests

Neil T. Campbell, M.D.
Staff, Department of Neonatology, Royal Children's Hospital, Parkville, Victoria, Australia
Withholding or Withdrawing Active Medical Treatment in Critically Ill Infants and Children

James P. Cappon, M.D.
Assistant Professor of Pediatrics, Division of Pediatric Critical Care, University of New Mexico School of Medicine, Albuquerque, New Mexico
High-Frequency Oscillatory Ventilation

Robert O. Christiansen, M.D.
Professor of Pediatrics, Charles R. Drew University of Medicine and Science; Director, Inpatient and Critical Care Division, Martin Luther King, Jr./Charles R. Drew Medical Center, Los Angeles, California
Pediatric Endocrine Procedures

Kevin Coulter, M.D.
Associate Professor of Pediatrics, University of California, San Francisco, School of Medicine; Director, Children's Health Center, San Francisco General Hospital Medical Center, San Francisco, California
Sexual Abuse

Craig S. Derkay, M.D.
Associate Professor, Departments of Otolaryngology and Pediatrics, Eastern Virginia Medical School; Director and Chief, Department of Pediatric Otolaryngology, Children's Hospital of the King's Daughters, Norfolk, Virginia
Pediatric Ear, Nose, and Throat Procedures and Tests

Ronald A. Dieckmann, M.D., M.P.H.
Associate Clinical Professor, Departments of Pediatrics and Medicine, University of California, San Francisco, School of Medicine; Director of Pediatric Emergency Medicine, San Francisco General Hospital Medical Center, San Francisco, California
Cardiopulmonary Arrest and Resuscitation: Older Infants and Children

Ralph Downey, III, Ph.D.
Assistant Professor of Medicine and Pediatrics and Adjunct Assistant Professor of Psychology, Loma Linda University School of Medicine; Director, Loma Linda Sleep Disorders Center for Adults and Children, Loma Linda University Medical Center and Jerry L. Pettis Memorial Veterans' Hospital, Loma Linda, California
Sleep Apnea Testing Using Clinical Polysomnography

Donna Ferriero, M.D.
Associate Professor, Departments of Neurology and Pediatrics, University of California, San Francisco, School of Medicine; Director, Child Neurology Clinic, San Francisco General Hospital Medical Center, San Francisco, California
Central Nervous System

Ragini K. Fredrich, M.D.
Clinical Instructor, University of California, Los Angeles, School of Medicine; Staff Nephrologist, Pediatric Nephrology and Transplant Immunology, Cedars-Sinai Medical Center, Los Angeles, California
Tests and Procedures for Evaluation of Renal Disorders

Robert W. Frenck, Jr., M.D.
Assistant Clinical Professor of Pediatrics, Uniformed Services University of the Health Sciences, Bethesda, Maryland; Eastern Virginia Medical School, Norfolk, Virginia; Head, Pediatric Infectious Diseases, Department of Pediatrics, United States Naval Hospital, Portsmouth, Virginia
Pediatric Trauma and Musculoskeletal System Procedures

Elena Fuentes-Afflick, M.D., M.P.H.
Assistant Professor, Department of Pediatrics, University of California, San Francisco, School of Medicine, San Francisco, California
Circumcision

John German, M.D.
Assistant Clinical Professor of Surgery, University of California Irvine Medical Center; Chief, Department of Surgery, Children's Hospital of Orange County, Orange, California
Central Venous Access

Kathleen E. Gilbride, Ph.D.
Assistant Clinical Professor of Pediatrics, University of California, Los Angeles, School of Medicine, Los Angeles, California; Clinical Psychologist, Harbor-UCLA Medical Center, Torrance, California
Developmental and Psychological Assessment Procedures and Instruments

Gary Goodman, M.D.
Staff, Pediatric Intensive Care Unit, Children's Hospital of Orange County, Orange, California
Renal Replacement Therapy—Critical Care Perspective

Moses Grossman, M.D.
Professor of Pediatrics (Emeritus), University of California, San Francisco, School of Medicine; Attending Pediatrician, San Francisco General Hospital Medical Center, San Francisco, California
Well Infant and Child Procedures

David M. Habib, M.D.
Staff, Department of Pediatrics, Children's Hospital of Orange County, Orange, California
Ventilatory Support in Infants and Children

Lubna Hasanain, M.D., M.P.H.
Attending Physician, John Muir Hospital, Walnut Creek, California; Attending Physician, Alta Bates, Berkeley, California
Outpatient Minor Surgical Procedures

David A. Hicks, M.D.
Co-Director, Apnea Diagnostic Center, Children's Hospital of Orange County, Orange, California
Cystic Fibrosis—Diagnosis

Walter T. Hughes, M.D.
Professor of Pediatrics, University of Tennessee College of Medicine; Chairman, Department of Infectious Diseases, St. Jude Children's Research Hospital, Memphis, Tennessee
Fluid and Metabolic Therapy; The Eye

Elaine S. Kamil, M.D.
Associate Professor of Pediatrics, University of California, Los Angeles, School of Medicine; Associate Director, Pediatric Nephrology and Transplant Immunology, Cedars-Sinai Medical Center, Los Angeles, California
Tests and Procedures for Evaluation of Renal Disorders

John O. Leighton, R.D.M.S.
Diagnostic Ultrasound Technician, Martin Luther King, Jr./Charles R. Drew Medical Center, Los Angeles, California
Diagnostic Ultrasound Screening of Infants

Robert H. Levin, Pharm.D.
Professor of Clinical Pharmacy and Pediatrics, University of California, San Francisco, School of Medicine; Associate Director, Department of Pharmaceutical Services, San Francisco General Hospital Medical Center, San Francisco, California
Management of Pain and Sedation

Peter M. Loughnan, M.D.
Staff, Department of Neonatology, Royal Children's Hospital, Parkville, Victoria, Australia
Withholding or Withdrawing Active Medical Treatment for Critically Ill Infants and Children

Paul Lubinsky, M.D.
Clinical Instructor, Department of Pediatrics, Harbor-UCLA Medical Center, Torrance, California; Associate Director, Pediatric Intensive Care Unit, Children's Hospital of Orange County, Orange, California
Aerosols; Left Ventricular Assist Devices

Ivy Luong, Pharm.D.
Formerly, Resident, Veterans Affairs Medical Center; Staff, Department of Pediatrics, San Francisco General Hospital Medical Center, San Francisco, California
Management of Pain and Sedation

Peter N. McDougall, M.D.
Deputy Director of Neonatology, Royal Children's Hospital, Parkville, Victoria, Australia
Withholding or Withdrawing Active Medical Treatment for Critically Ill Infants and Children

David Moromisato, M.D.
Assistant Professor of Pediatrics, Division of Respiratory and Critical Care, Department of Pediatrics, Harbor-UCLA Medical Center, Torrance, California
Therapeutic Plasma Exchange

Asha Moudgil, M.D.
Staff, University of California, Los Angeles, School of Medicine; Clinical Fellow, Department of Pediatrics, Cedars-Sinai Medical Center, Los Angeles, California
Tests and Procedures for Evaluation of Renal Disorders

Bruce G. Nickerson, M.D.
Associate Clinical Professor, Department of Pediatrics, University of California, Los Angeles, School of Medicine, Los Angeles, California; Director of Pulmonary Medicine, Children's Hospital of Orange County, Orange, California
Fiberoptic Bronchoscopy

Ronald M. Perkin, M.D.
Professor and Associate Chairman, Department of Pediatrics, Loma Linda University School of Medicine; Director of Pediatric Critical Care and Inpatient Respiratory Services, Loma Linda University Children's Hospital, Loma Linda, California
Sleep Apnea Testing Using Clinical Polysomnography; Intraosseous Access and Infusion

Michael G. Regalado, M.D.
Associate Professor of Clinical Pediatrics, University of Southern California School of Medicine; Director, Developmental and Behavioral Pediatrics Program, Children's Hospital of Los Angeles, Los Angeles, California
Developmental and Psychological Assessment Procedures and Instruments

Anthony H. Repucci, M.D.
Assistant Professor of Pediatrics, Case Western Reserve University School of Medicine; Division of Pediatric Gastroenterology, MetroHealth Medical Center, Cleveland, Ohio
Pediatric Gastroenterology

Julie A. Ressler, M.D.
Radiology Resident, Martin Luther King, Jr./Charles R. Drew Medical Center, Los Angeles, California *Diagnostic Nuclear Medicine Imaging in Pediatric Endocrinology*

Katherine I. Schooley, M.D.
Director, Neonatal Services, St. Mary Desert Valley Hospital, Apple Valley, California
Endotracheal Intubation

Adam J. Schwarz, M.D.
Clinical Instructor, Department of Pediatrics, Harbor-UCLA Medical Center, Torrance, California; Fellow, Pediatric Critical Care Program, Harbor-UCLA Medical Center and Martin Luther King, Jr./Charles R. Drew Medical Center, Los Angeles, California; Children's Hospital of Orange County, Orange, California
Pulmonary Artery Catheters

Sabitha S. Sehgal, M.D.
Assistant Professor of Pediatrics, University of California, Los Angeles, School of Medicine; Staff Neonatologist, Cedars-Sinai Medical Center, Los Angeles, California
Prenatal Assessment

Sandra C. Short-Bartlett, M.D.
Neonatologist, Children's Hospital of Orange County, Orange, California
Arterial Catheterization

Susan Sniderman, M.D.
Chief of Neonatology Service, San Francisco General Hospital Medical Center, San Francisco, California
Neonatal Resuscitation

Michael E. Spieth, M.D.
Assistant Professor of Radiology,

Charles R. Drew University of Medicine and Science; Assistant Clinical Professor of Radiology and Nuclear Medicine, University of Southern California School of Medicine, Los Angeles, California
Diagnostic Nuclear Medicine Imaging in Pediatric Endocrinology

Rocky Stone, R.R.T.
Clinical Coordinator of Patient Care, Respiratory Services, Children's Hospital of Orange County, Orange, California
Chest Physical Therapy; Postural Drainage Techniques

Daniel Stromberg, M.D.
Fellow, Pediatric Cardiology, Baylor College of Medicine and Texas Children's Hospital, Houston, Texas
Electrocardiogram; Cardiac Ultrasonography (Echocardiography); Cardiac Catheterization; Patent Ductus Arteriosus

James Swift, M.D.
Clinical Instructor of Pediatrics, University of California, Los Angeles, School of Medicine, Los Angeles, California; Harbor-UCLA Medical Center, Torrance, California; Associate Intensivist, Pediatric Intensive Care Unit Center for Children, Medical City Dallas Hospital, Dallas, Texas
Thoracentesis and Thoracostomy Tubes

H. William Taeusch, M.D.
Professor of Pediatrics, University of California, San Francisco, School of Medicine; Vice Chair, Department of Pediatrics; Chief, Pediatric Service, San Francisco General Hospital Medical Center, San Francisco, California
Neonatal Resuscitation; Hematological Tests and Procedures

Daved van Stralen, M.D.
Instructor, Department of Pediatrics, Loma Linda University School of Medicine; Medical Director, Program in Emergency Medical Care, Department of Cardiopulmonary Science, Loma Linda University School of Allied Health Professions; Medical Director, Pediatric Critical Care Transport, Loma Linda University Children's Hospital, Loma Linda, California
Intraosseous Access and Infusion

Panukorn Vasinrapee, M.D.
Professor of Radiology, Charles R. Drew University of Medicine and Science; Chief, Special Imaging, Department of Radiology; Martin Luther King, Jr./Charles R. Drew Medical Center, Los Angeles, California
Diagnostic Nuclear Medicine Imaging in Pediatric Endocrinology

Sylvia Fernandez Villarreal, M.D.
Associate Clinical Professor, Department of Pediatrics, University of California, San Francisco, School of Medicine; Director, Inpatient Pediatrics, San Francisco General Hospital Medical Center, San Francisco, California
Management of Pain and Sedation

Frans J. Walther, M.D., Ph.D.
Professor of Pediatrics, University of California, Los Angeles, School of Medicine; Neonatologist, Martin Luther King, Jr./Charles R. Drew Medical Center, Los Angeles, California
Diagnostic Ultrasound Screening of Infants

Carrie Worcester, M.D.
Director, Neonatal Intensive Care Program, and Co-Director, Apnea Diagnostic Center, Children's Hospital of Orange County, Orange, California
Neonatal Extracorporeal Membrane Oxygenation

Contents

Section A

Cardiopulmonary Resuscitation

Chapter 1

Neonatal Resuscitation

H. William Taeusch and Susan Sniderman

Preparation and anticipation are keys to delivery room resuscitation. Good preparation includes written protocols outlining resuscitation practices covering personnel, equipment, and the types of deliveries requiring attendance by a pediatrician. The American Heart Association (AHA) and the American Academy of Pediatrics (AAP) have produced a detailed but straightforward approach to delivery room resuscitation. A self-teaching handbook that leads to certification in neonatal resuscitation (American Heart Association, 1994) is available.

GOALS OF RESUSCITATION

Besides the obvious saving of life, the goals of resuscitation include prevention of acute asphyxia and the sequelae of asphyxia (e.g., meconium aspiration pneumonia, persistent fetal circulation with right to left shunting, hypoxic ischemic encephalopathy, respiratory distress, air leak, intracranial hemorrhage, seizures, multi-organ failure, mental retardation, cerebral palsy). Prenatal, perinatal, or neonatal ischemia, hypoxemia, or hypercarbia represents significant injury in which insufficient gas exchange in the fetus or newborn occurs to the degree that the damaging effects persist even after gas exchange is restored. Fetal heart rate late decelerations reflect events that can vary in severity from those in which the fetus fully recovers within minutes to those in which the fetus dies.

Asphyxia is an insult of varying severity. The degree of organ damage and the potential for recovery depend not only on the severity of the initial insult but also on its duration, as well as on other factors, including perfusion, gas exchange, and defense mechanisms (e.g., antioxidants). Since asphyxia is always a secondary event, it is no more a diagnosis than is fever. For this reason asphyxia should not appear as a diagnosis on a hospital chart. This caveat does not mean that the true events of a case should be omitted or distorted, or that malpractice should not be identified and dealt with. Rather, specific diagnoses should be recorded; for example, "renal shutdown secondary to severe prenatal fetal depression associated with prolonged late decelerations secondary to abruptio placentae." Pediatricians have the right and responsibility to make diagnoses on newborns, such as "hypoxic ischemic encephalopathy." Usually, pediatricians should not make prenatal diagnoses de novo.

PERINATAL INTERVENTION

When a fetus is in distress, there are remedies other than an emergency cesarean section. Those responsible for the welfare of the newborn should not be bashful about making recommendations when obstetricians and anesthesiologists prepare for an emergency cesarean section. Anticipating the need for resuscitation (Table 1–1) is wise, as is taking the following steps to prevent needing to resuscitate the newborn: controlling diabetes and preeclampsia; preventing the gravid uterus from compressing the cava and aorta (by putting a wedge under the mother's lumbar spine while she lies supine); giving the mother oxygen, amnioinfusion (in case of suspected cord compression or oligohydramnios), or tocolytic therapy (or stopping oxytocin) for uterine hypertonicity; and using the Trendelenburg position and pushing up on the presenting fetal part during cord prolapse.

PERSONNEL AND EQUIPMENT

All deliveries should be attended by someone who has successfully completed the American Heart Association/American Academy of Pediatrics Neonatal course—Neonatal Advanced Life Support (NALS). This person may be a nurse, an obstetrician, a family medicine specialist, a pediatrician, a physician's assistant, or a respiratory therapist. Anticipatory actions should be taken by all responsible personnel. This means discussion with the parents, obstetrician, and anesthesiologist; checking the prenatal history; and ascertaining that all drugs are available and all equipment is in working order.

A clear plan should be formulated. If a difficult resuscitation is anticipated, at least two people qualified for newborn resuscitation should attend the delivery. While waiting for a high-risk delivery, personnel should do the following:

1. Decide who will manage airway and ventilation, listen to the heart, place monitor leads, provide cardiac massage, draw up medications, record events, and obtain vascular access.
2. Check the resuscitation setup. Turn on the overhead warmer and light. Turn on the oxygen, with a flow rate of 7 to 10 L/min. Occlude the mask and ensure that the bag fills to sufficient pressures (20–35 cm H_2O). Test the laryngoscope light. Choose the appropriately sized endotracheal tube, and insert and withdraw the stylet a few times. Turn on the suction and check that occluded suction is − 80 to −90 mm Hg. Turn on the cardiorespiratory monitor, blood pressure device, and O_2 saturation monitor, and ensure that all probes and leads are attached.
3. Ascertain the need for placental assessments or culture, cord blood gases, and amniotic fluid tests and cultures.

Suggested equipment for neonatal resuscitation includes the following:

- Overhead warmer with servo-controlled temperature probe
- Stethoscope (newborn)
- Suction source and suction catheters, suction bulbs
- Warmed, humidified oxygen; several sizes of masks and hand-ventilation bags
- O_2-air blender
- O_2 analyzer
- Laryngoscope and blades sizes 0 and 1, spare batteries, bulbs
- Endotracheal tubes
- Blood pressure measuring device

Table 1–1 Factors Indicating Potential Need for Delivery Room Resuscitation

Antecedents	Clinical Conditions
Interference with maternal blood and/or oxygen supply to the placenta	Maternal hypotension, respiratory insufficiency
Interference with uteroplacental circulation	Placenta previa, abruptio placentae, intrauterine growth retardation
Interference with fetoplacental circulation	Cord compression, prolapsed cord, fetal hypovolemia
Mechanical problems	Breech presentation, twins, macrosomia
Maternal medications	Neonatal depression

- Umbilical artery/vein catheters and catheterization trays
- Heart rate and respiration monitor
- O_2 saturation monitor

DELIVERY ROOM RESUSCITATION JUDGMENT

Before the birth of a fetus with severe abnormalities, sometimes the parents, pediatrician, and obstetrician agree that the infant will not be resuscitated. Obviously, infants with lethal anomalies (e.g., anencephaly) should not be resuscitated (Yellin, 1995). However, infants with multiple anomalies should be resuscitated so that the anomalies can be evaluated for possible correction. An extensive resuscitative effort is usually not made for an extremely low birth weight infant if initial ventilation and cardiac massage are unsuccessful. However, if there is doubt about whether to resuscitate and the senior physician is unavailable, errors should occur on the side of continuing life support. Nevertheless, such errors can be as catastrophic as errors of not resuscitating. The survival rate of 23-week-gestation infants is less than 10%. If the infant lives for 1 week, survival odds increase to approximately 20%. If the infant lives and is discharged, the chances for a major neurodevelopmental handicap are approximately 30%. Many physicians believe that most infants less than 24 weeks' gestation and less than 500 g birth weight are not viable, and in consultation with parents and obstetricians do not resuscitate them. However, when infants are limp and blue, they may appear smaller and less mature than when they are pink and active. Thus, it is advisable to initiate resuscitation and assess the response, until the weight and gestational age can be assessed.

INITIAL ASSESSMENT

While the newborn is being dried, a quick assessment should be done. Gross anomalies and obvious cardiopulmonary distress are immediately evident. The airway, breathing, and circulation (ABCs) are evaluated. Apgar scoring (Table 1–2) is done at 1 minute and 5 minutes traditionally, and every 5 minutes thereafter until the score is greater than 7. The Apgar score was designed to assess neonatal depression secondary to acute perinatal asphyxia; however, maternal drugs and fetal immaturity strongly affect the score as well. Currently, only extremely low scores that fail to improve by 5 minutes are of clinical interest or prognostic value. Wide variability exists in the rigor with which the scoring is performed.

Table 1–2 Apgar Scoring Values

	0	1	2
Appearance (color)	Blue or pale	Pink with acrocyanosis	Pink
Pulse	Absent	< 100	> 100
Grimace (response) to stimulation)	Absent	Minimal	Brisk
Activity (tone)	Limp	Decreased tone	Normal tone
Respirations	Absent	Irregular	Sustained

FULL-SCALE DELIVERY ROOM RESUSCITATION OF A NEWBORN

A calm, professional approach will help difficult resuscitations proceed. To solve 95% of resuscitation problems, the following initial steps should be performed:

1. Stimulate, dry, and place the infant under a heat source.
2. Suction mouth and nares briefly.
3. If the baby is cyanotic and not breathing regularly, give blow-by oxygen or several breaths of bag-and-mask ventilation. Then, assess heart rate and perfusion.

If the infant has not responded to these initial steps, personnel should be organized to perform the following functions:

- One person to manage the airway, to bag-and-mask ventilate, or to intubate, as appropriate
- One person to do external cardiac massage, if necessary; to evaluate endotracheal tube position, and to assess pulses and perfusion
- One person to draw up medications and attach monitors and a temperature probe
- One person to keep a resuscitation record

Someone should be assigned to obtain vascular access. Usually the person managing the airway should be the most experienced and should supervise the resuscitation and decide when efforts should be abandoned.

Technique of Bag-and-Mask Ventilation

A mask that covers the infant's nose and mouth without covering the eyes should be selected. Bag size should not exceed 750 ml. Self-inflating bags should have an oxygen reservoir attached. Bags should be attached to manometers to measure pressure and to supply humidified 100% oxygen at a minimum flow rate of 5 L/min. The infant is placed in a sniffing position and is suctioned. The mask is positioned over the infant's open mouth and tip of nose. The physician's left thumb and forefinger should be positioned around the mask, with the left little finger holding the infant's mandible forward. Undue pressure should not be exerted on the eyes or the occiput, nor should the infant's neck be flexed. Once there is a good seal, ventilations of 20 to 40 cm H_2O at a rate of 40 to 60 breaths/minute should be instituted. Good breath sounds bilaterally and modest chest movement should occur.

Intubation (See also Chapter 3)

The protocol for elective neonatal intubation is as follows:

- Ensure that heart rate and O_2 saturation monitors are working.
- Consider premedication with atropine and morphine (usually not possible in the delivery room).
- Wash hands and wear sterile gloves.
- Select an appropriate noncuffed endotracheal tube and adapter with a side port if surfactant administration is anticipated.
- Mark the desired "tip (of endotracheal tube)-to-lip" distance with adhesive tape.
- Clean the skin with gauze and warm water.
- Dry the skin and apply benzoin tincture to the upper lip and cheeks.
- After the benzoin dries, put an Elastoplast mustache on the top lip.
- Preoxygenate and ventilate the infant.
- Position and suction the infant.
- Insert the laryngoscope into the vallecula. Then, apply pressure caudad and approximately 30 degrees anteriorly while applying thyroid cartilage pressure with little finger of left hand.
- When the glottis is visible, insert the endotracheal tube 1 cm to 2.5 cm beyond the glottis, ascertaining the proper tip-to-lip distance.
- Ascertain that the tube is well placed.
- Pass a 4-0 silk suture through the Elastoplast mustache, avoiding the infant's skin, and suture it to the endotracheal tube plastic or the circumferential tape on the tube at the lip. Wrap the suture material around the tube about 10 times, then tie securely. Split tape ends from the upper lip can be wound around the endotracheal tube for additional security.
- Ascertain (usually via chest radiograph) that the endotracheal tip lies two thirds of the distance from the glottis to the carina.

Table 1–3 Endotracheal Tube Size Selection Based on Birth Weight Estimate

Birth Weight	Endotracheal Tube Size (mm internal diameter)	Distance from Lip to Endotracheal Tube Tip (cm)
< 1000 g	2.5	7
1000–2000 g	3.0	8
2000–4000 g	3.5	9
> 4000 g	4.0	10

The infant's little finger diameter is the first approximation for tube size. Additional suggestions for size are given in Tables 1–3 and 1–4.

Emergency endotracheal intubation is orotracheal; many centers use nasotracheal intubation after the infant is stabilized on ventilator support. Most delivery room personnel use stylets to help direct the endotracheal tube, especially after it becomes more pliable from heating to greater than 33°C under the overhead warmer. The stylet should not protrude beyond the end of the endotracheal tube. Occasionally, great difficulty is encountered in attempting to remove the stylet after the infant is intubated. This situation can be resolved by using sterile saline as a mild lubricant.

Most experts do not premedicate for intubation in the delivery room under emergency conditions, but premedication is too commonly overlooked for elective reintubations. A variety of models and mannequins are available for practicing intubation (Laerdal, Ambu).

Table 1–4 Endotracheal Tube Size Selection Based on Gestation Estimate*

Gestation	24 wk	28 wk	32 wk	36 wk	40 wk
Tube Size	2.5	2.5	3.0	3.5	4.0

*Gestation age is divided by 10 and rounded to the nearest 0.5.
From Ahmed P, Chen YW: Cliincal tip. *Contemp Pediatr,* 11:88, 1994.

Evidence for a well-positioned endotracheal tube includes the following:

- Water vapor condenses on the inside of the endotracheal tube during expiration.
- Advancement of the endotracheal tube through the glottis feels snug.
- A 'click' is felt with finger on the neck over the glottic area on intubation.
- Initial nonvocal coughing efforts occur soon after placement.
- Rapid ventilation with bag results in good bilateral breath sounds with bilateral chest movement.
- Improvement of heart rate and color occurs with continued bagging.

Listening at the adapter hub for breath sounds can be useful for those few infants who are taking regular spontaneous breaths. Other, more elaborate, auditory or visual evidence of bidirectional gas flow at the endotracheal tube inlet has been suggested (Krishel, 1992).

Evidence for incorrect placement of endotracheal tube is as follows:

- No improvement in or worsening of color and heart rate with bag-to-tube ventilation
- Audible crying
- Poor or absent breath sounds with ventilation
- Gurgles or air entry heard over stomach with slow bag inflation
- Poor chest movement with bagging
- Increasing abdominal distention with bagging
- Stomach contents coming up from the endotracheal tube
- Good breath sounds on the right but not on the left, indicating that the tube tip is in the right main stem bronchus

Capnography, the technique of measuring end-tidal partial pressure of carbon dioxide, may be useful in confirming appropriate endotracheal tube placement. Difficult neonatal intubations can be overcome with the troubleshooting methods listed in Table 1–5.

If intubation does not go well, an anesthesiologist may be able to help. Occasionally, difficult resuscitation problems require specialized intubation techniques (Fig. 1–1). Alternative techniques of intubation (e.g., digital technique) are useful for specific situations and have been adapted for routine use in some nurseries (Heller, 1994) (Fig. 1–2).

Complications

Complications of orotracheal intubation include the following:

Table 1–5 Troubleshooting Difficult Neonatal Intubations

Problem	Solution
Copious secretions obscure landmarks.	Suction vigorously. (Atropine may be of use in elective intubations).
Heart rate and O_2 saturation drop immediately on introduction of laryngoscope.	Pre-oxygenate the infant with bag-and-mask ventilation for 2 to 3 minutes. In a breathing infant, it may be helpful to tape a small oxygen-delivering catheter to the blade of the laryngoscope to maintain some oxygenation during visualization of the glottis.
Cannot ventilate well with bag and mask.	Suction the infant and reposition the infant's head. Open the mouth and reposition the mask. Ventilate with more pressure. Rarely, a small oral airway will be helpful.
Cannot visualize vocal cords or glottis.	Usually, the endotracheal tube has advanced down the esophagus and must be pulled back. The head may be repositioned in slight extension. Intermittent tracheal pressure can be applied over the cricoid cartilage to see the larynx swing down into view from a more anterior position.
Infant struggles so much that tube placement is difficult.	Reconsider the need for the tube, or consider sedation and paralysis.
Can visualize glottis but cannot pass endotracheal tube.	Flick the infant's heel to cause crying, which opens the glottis. Turn the bevel of the endotracheal tube 90 degrees so that the bevel of the endotracheal tube aligns with the glottic slit. If difficulty persists, try a smaller-sized endotracheal tube.
Endotracheal tube passes glottis but will not advance down trachea.	This situation is extremely rare. It may be associated with a congenital anomaly, and tracheostomy may be the only recourse if the infant is moribund and otherwise not able to be resuscitated.

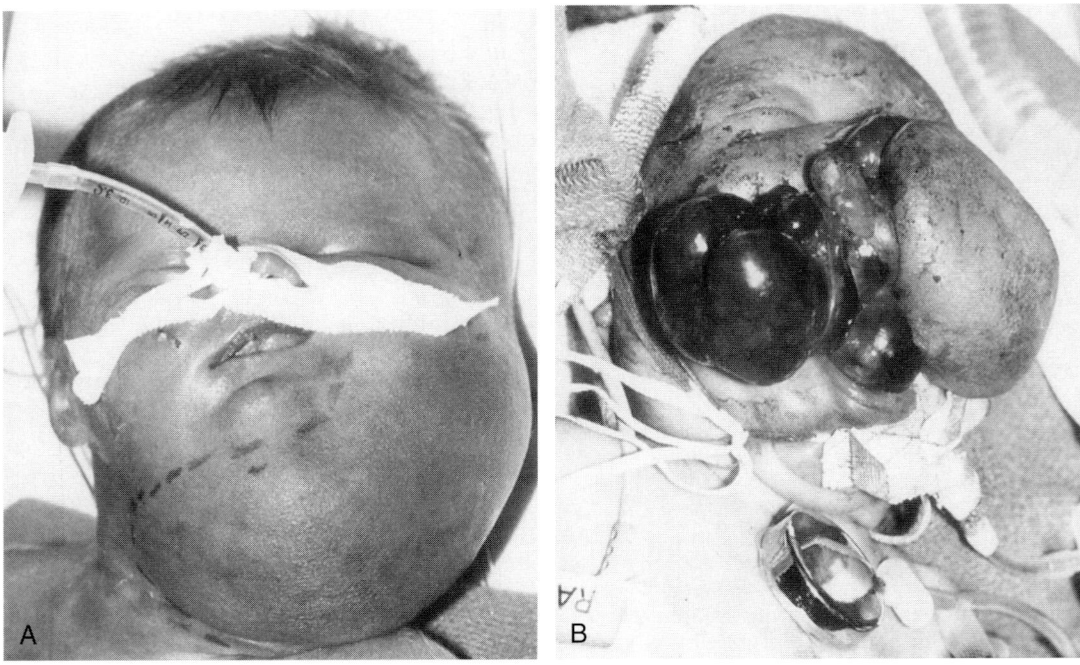

Figure 1–1 Difficult intubations. **A.** A newborn with a large cervical hemangioma. **B.** A newborn with an oropharyngeal teratoma. (From Schulman S, et al: Fetal tracheal intubation with intact uteroplacental circulation. *Anesth Analg,* 76:197, 1993.)

- Tracheal or esophageal perforation
- Laryngeal edema
- Subglottic stenosis
- Palatal groove

Cardiac Massage

Cardiac massage should be started if the infant has a heart rate below 80 to 90 beats/min unresponsive to 30 seconds of positive pressure ventilation with 100% FIO_2 (fraction of inspired oxygen). The two-handed approach encircling the infant's chest and pumping on the lower sternum with two thumbs is best in infants (Fig. 1–3). Experts disagree about whether it is better to interrupt bag-and-tube ventilation for cardiac massage. It may be best to carry out bagging and cardiac massage simultaneously. Depth of compression is 1/2 to 3/4 inch, depending on the size of the infant, and the rate should be about 120 compressions/min.

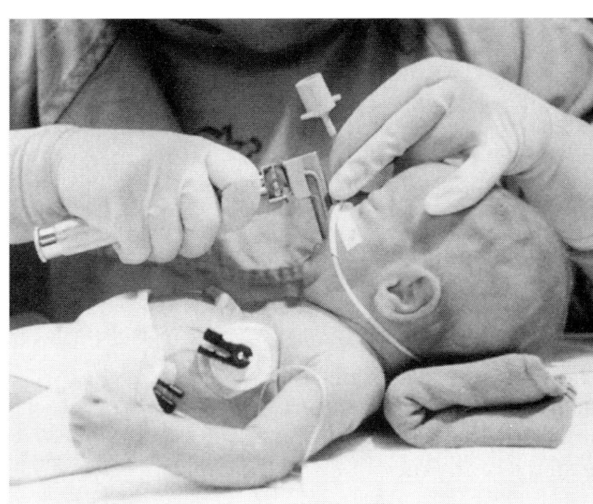

Figure 1–2 Right-sided intubation technique. This technique is useful for infants who are already attached to monitoring devices in the neonatal intensive care unit (NICU) and for whom movement is stressful and difficult. The endotracheal tube is held in the left hand; the laryngoscope is held in the right hand. This is opposite of the conventional intubation technique, which is performed at the head of the infant. (From Polak M, Fazi L: Right sided endotracheal intubation: An alternative method for neonates. *Neonatal Intensive Care,* Jan/Feb 1993, p 32.)

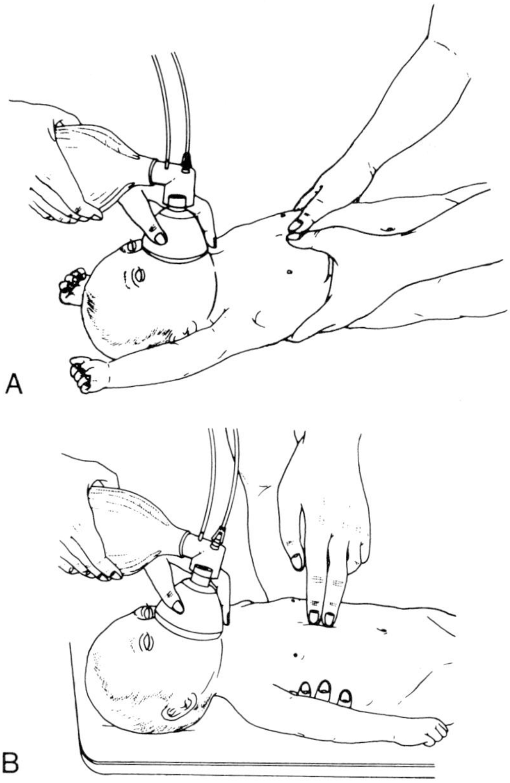

Figure 1–3 **A.** Chest compressions carried out by the preferred thumb compression technique. **B.** Two-finger method. (Reproduced with permission. © Textbook of Neonatal Resuscitation, 1987, 1990. Copyright American Heart Association.)

Drugs

A need for more than epinephrine, volume expansion, glucose, and sodium bicarbonate is extremely rare. The use of naloxone is discouraged until 10 or 15 minutes after birth because it distracts those carrying out the resuscitation from concern about establishing adequate ventilation. A newborn with normal lungs who is on narcotics should be easily managed by bag-and-mask ventilation. Calcium and atropine are rarely needed in the delivery room. For the technique of endotracheal drug administration, see Chapter 2.

Vascular Access

The most rapid vascular access is through the umbilical vein. After quick preparation of the umbilical stump with povidone-iodine, a catheter is advanced until blood return (usually 2 to 4 cm) occurs. Volume expanders and drugs can be given, and blood for laboratory testing can be drawn using this catheter. As the resuscitation proceeds (at approximately 10 minutes), placing an umbilical artery catheter to monitor blood pressure and arterial blood gases should be considered.

Defibrillation

The need for defibrillation in a newborn in the neonatal intensive care unit is rare, and it is even more rare in a newborn in the delivery room. Paddles should be approximately 4 cm in diameter and deliver 2 joules/kg initially; if there is no response, 4 joules/kg are delivered. Place the saline or electrode paste carefully between the paddles to avoid an electrical bridge that will cause burns.

INFANTS WHO FAIL TO RESPOND TO RESUSCITATION

Check Ventilation

- Is oxygen running?
- Is the tube in the proper place and patent?
- Is blood volume adequate?
- Is there a space-occupying lesion in the chest (i.e., is there pneumothorax, pleural effusion, hypoplastic lungs, diaphragmatic hernia)?

Check Cardiac Function

- Is there asystole?
- Does fibrillation exist?
- Is there electrical-mechanical dissociation?
- Is there adequate circulating blood volume?

If the heart rate remains low after bag-to-endotracheal tube ventilation, the most common reason is that the endotracheal tube is in the esophagus and needs to be replaced.

Determining When to Terminate Resuscitation

In the delivery room, resuscitative efforts usually may be stopped when no sustained heart rate can be achieved (i.e., after approximately 20 to 30 minutes) or when Apgar scores at 1 and 5 minutes are truly 0 (i.e., no heartbeat at all after resuscitative measures). Terminating resuscitation also depends on an assessment of history, prenatal and postnatal course, and physical examination.

MECONIUM

Much has been written about meconium aspiration and its consequences in the newborn period (Katz, 1992). Meconium in the lungs interferes with ventilation, may lead to air trapping and pneumothorax, and can cause an aspiration and inflammatory pneumonitis. Therefore, it should be removed from the airways as much as possible, as long as its removal does not increase insult to the newborn. The infant born through thick or particulate meconium should immediately be intubated without prior stimulation while heart rate is monitored and blow-by oxygen is provided. Generally, no more than three passes through the glottis for suctioning meconium (if each pass is productive) are made before stopping to ventilate the infant.

Removing Meconium

Removing meconium requires suction preferably by a large-bore catheter or endotracheal tube from a high-vacuum (wall) source (approximately −80 mm Hg in closed system). Suctioning meconium by mouth from the endotracheal tube is inappropriate owing to the risk of hepatitis and AIDS. Irrigation with saline to remove airway meconium has not been shown to be helpful. More research into ways of reducing harm from suctioning is needed (Segar, 1993). More sophisticated airway suctioning devices for newborns are being developed (e.g., Kurtis meconium suction device, Fig. 1–4).

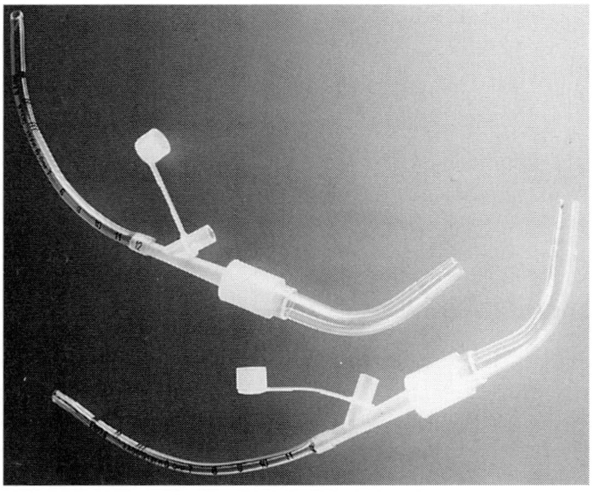

Figure 1–4 The Kurtis meconium suction device is a useful adaptation of an endotracheal tube. An integral stylet in the wall of the tube and a side port for suctioning or introducing medications are the adaptations. (Courtesy of Vital Signs, Inc., Totowa, NJ.)

Risk of Persistent Fetal Circulation

Meconium aspiration is frequently associated with high pulmonary vascular resistance and persistence of fetal circulation, with right-to-left shunting at the atrial and ductal levels. In this situation, pulmonary blood flow is diminished, and partial pressure of oxygen (PaO_2) may be very low. (The differential diagnosis, therefore, includes cyanotic congenital heart defects such as transposition and total anomalous venous drainage.) Infants older than 35 weeks' gestation, who have a negligible risk of retinopathy of prematurity, should be given generous amounts of supplemental oxygen (to maintain an O_2 saturation > 95% and a PaO_2 > 85 mm Hg) during and after suctioning and in the first hours of life to minimize hypoxic pulmonary vasoconstriction.

CARE OF THE NEWBORN AFTER DELIVERY ROOM RESUSCITATION

Chest radiographs should be evaluated for endotracheal tube placement, air leaks, and other intrathoracic abnormalities. Generous oxygenation should be maintained as prophylaxis for persistent fetal circulation in mature infants. The infant should be observed for signs of hypoxic-ischemic encephalopathy (HIE); hypoxic-ischemic insult to other organs; gut, liver, and renal injury; metabolic sequelae (e.g., hypoglycemia and hypocalcemia) or postresuscitation trauma of ribs, long bones, or airway.

Table 1–6 Encephalopathy Score (FATES)

	Score		
Factor	**2**	**1**	**0**
Feeding	No problems	Resolved < 8 days	Resolved > 7 days
Apgar (five min)	> 4	3–4	< 3
Tone	No problems	Resolved < 8 days	Unresolved or resolved > 7 days
Extubation	< 7 hours	7–48 hours	> 48 hours
Seizures	None	Onset > 12 hours	Onset < 12 hours

From Becker M, Taeusch W. Unpublished data.

Table 1-7 Encephalopathy Score (FATES) During the First Week of Life and Neurological Outcomes at 5 Years of Life

Encephalopathy Scores	Outcome
5 ± 1	Mild disability
2 ± 1	Moderate to severe disability
1 ± 1	Death

From Becker M, Taeusch W. Unpublished data.

The tests needed at this point usually include gastric aspirate, tracheal aspirate, and amniotic fluid for culture and surfactant measures; placenta for pathological examination; lactate dehydrogenase and creatine phosphokinase from blood and cerebrospinal fluid (CSF); CSF, urine, and blood tests for infection. The syndrome of inappropriate antidiuretic hormone secretion should be anticipated and fluid intake should be minimized. A 2- to 3-day delay in starting feeding should be considered if insult has been severe and the gut may have been injured.

HYPOXIC-ISCHEMIC ENCEPHALOPATHY

HIE is the consequence of central nervous system injury that may be associated with severe perinatal acidosis, hypercarbia, hypoxemia, or hypovolemia. The incidence of HIE is about 0.5/1000 live births. HIE follows hypoxic-ischemic episodes that are usually of sufficient severity to necessitate major resuscitation with intubation. HIE is characterized by abnormal neurological status in the first postnatal week (e.g., feeding problems, abnormalities of motor tone, need for ventilator support, seizures). Magnetic resonance imaging, electroencephalogram, and hearing and ophthalmological examinations are indicated to evaluate the severity of HIE. The degree of encephalopathy in the first week and the neurological status of the patient at discharge bear heavily on the prognosis of an infant with HIE (Tables 1-6 and 1-7).

References

Ambu, Inc, 611 N Hammonds Ferry Rd, Linthicum, MD 21090-1356

American Heart Association and American Academy of Pediatrics. Bloom RS, Cropley C: *Textbook of Neonatal Resuscitation.* American Heart Association 1994.

Anon: Neonatal resuscitation. *JAMA*, 268:2276–2285, 1992.

Barrington KJ, Finer NN, Etches PC: Succinylcholine and atropine for premedication of the newborn infant before nasotracheal intubation: a randomized controlled trial. *Crit Care Med*, 17: 1293–1296, 1989.

Becker M, Taeusch W: Severe perinatal asphyxia. In Taeusch HW, Yogman M (eds): Follow-up Management of the High Risk Infant. Boston, Little Brown, 1987.

Bednarek FJ, Kuhns, LR: Endotracheal tube placement in infants determined by suprasternal palpation: a new technique. *Pediatrics*, 56:224, 1975.

Bent RC, Wiswell TE, Chang A: Removing meconium from infant tracheae. What works best? *Am J Dis Child*, 146(9):1085–1089, 1992.

Black AE, Hatch DJ, Nauth-Misir N: Complications of nasotracheal intubation in neonates, infants, and children: a review of 4 years' experience in a children's hospital. *Br J Anaesth*, 65:461–467, 1990.

Brill J: Cardiopulmonary resuscitation. *Ped Annals*, 15:24, Jan 1986.

Bull DH, Sola A, Wakely A: Meconium and tracheal aspiration [letter]. *Pediatrics*, 90(3):474–476, 1992.

Burchfield DJ, Berkowitz ID, et al: Medications in neonatal resuscitation. *Ann Emerg Med*, 22(Part 2):435–439, 1993.

Cunningham AS, Lawson EE, et al: Tracheal suction and meconium: a proposed standard of care (editorial). *J Pediatr*, 116:153–154, 1990.

Falciglia HS, Henderschott C, et al: Does DeLee suction at the perineum prevent meconium aspiration syndrome? *Am J Obstet Gynecol*, 167(5):1243–1249, 1992.

Freeman J, and Nelson K: Intrapartum asphyxia and cerebral palsy. *Pediatrics*, 82:240, 1988.

Gage J, Taeusch HW Jr, et al: Suctioning of upper airway meconium in newborn infants. *JAMA*, 246:2590–2592, 1981.

Heller RM, Heller TW: Experience with the illuminated endotracheal tube in the prevention of unsafe intubations in the premature and full-term infant. *Pediatrics*, 93(3):389–391, 1994.

Katz L, Bowes WA Jr: Meconium aspiration syndrome: reflections on a murky subject. *Am J Obstet Gynecol*, 166:171–183, 1992.

Keener PA: General pediatrician's role in high risk deliveries. *Pediatr Rev*, 10:119–126, 1988.

Korber TE, Henneman PL: Digital nasotracheal intubation. *J Emerg Med*, 7:275–277, 1989.

Krishel S, Jackimczyk K, Balazs K. Endotracheal tube whistle: an adjunct to blind nasotracheal intubation. *Ann Emerg Med*, 21:33–36, 1992.

Laerdal products (resuscitation models and mannequins), AF Johnson Co., PO Box 10459, Burbank, CA, 91510; (213) 849–7191.

Leviton A, Nelson K: Problems with definitions and classifications of newborn encephalopathy. *Pediatr Neurol*, 8:85, 1992.

Polak MJ, Fazi L: Right sided endotracheal intubation: An alternative method for neonates. *Neonatal Intensive Care*, Jan/Feb 1993, pp 31–33.

Rawlings DJ, Lawrence S, Goldstein JD: Acquired tracheoesophageal fistula in a premature infant. *Am J Perinatol*, 10:164–167, 1993.

Sarnat HB, Sarnat MS: Neonatal encephalopathy following fetal distress. *Arch Neurol*, 33:404, 1970.

Segar JL, Merrill DC, et al: Hemodynamic changes during endotracheal suctioning are mediated by increased autonomic activity. *Pediatr Res*, 33: 649–652, 1993.

Supnet M, Taeusch W: Limits of viability for inner city African American and Latino infants who are extremely premature. *J Natl Med Assoc*, 86:297–302, 1994.

Thiringer K, Hrbek A, et al: Postasphyxial cerebral survival in newborn sheep after treatment with oxygen free radical scavengers and a calcium antagonist. *Pediatr Res*, 22:62–66, 1987.

Vanucci, RC: Current and potentially new management strategies for perinatal HIE. *Pediatrics*, 85:961, 1990.

Verdile VP, Chiang JL, et al: Nasotracheal intubation using a flexible lighted stylet. *Ann Emerg Med*, 19:506–510, 1990.

Yellin PB, Fleischman AR: DNR in the DR? *J Perinat*, 15:232–236, 1995.

Chapter 2

Cardiopulmonary Arrest and Resuscitation: Older Infants and Children

Ronald A. Dieckmann

Pediatric cardiopulmonary arrest is rare. It occurs after a sustained and profound systemic insult (usually hypoxia and ischemia), from respiratory failure, or from hemodynamic collapse. Unlike adults, children almost never suffer pediatric cardiopulmonary arrest as a primary cardiac event. Respiratory failure is by far the most common primary cause, especially during infancy, which is the period of highest risk for childhood cardiopulmonary arrests (Dieckmann, 1991; Dieckmann and Vardis, 1995; Eisenberg, 1983).

Resuscitation from true cardiopulmonary arrest succeeds in fewer than 5% of cases (Dieckmann and Vardis, 1995; O'Rourke, 1986; Zaritsky, 1993a). Several important factors account for poor outcome. First, delayed recognition and response to serious childhood illness and injury in the pre-arrest state sometimes preclude early institution of appropriate therapy that would interrupt and reverse progressive system failure and hypoxia. Technical difficulties in airway management and vascular access, combined with inadequate education and preparation of prehospital and hospital providers for major pediatric emergencies, often limit the quality and timeliness of resuscitative efforts. Second, there is little scientific knowledge about age-related differences in the complex pathophysiology and optimal treatment of pediatric cardiopulmonary arrest. Current pediatric resuscitation guidelines are derived largely from animal models, adult experience, and anecdotal childhood cases. Third, the majority of infant deaths, and hence a substantial proportion of all childhood deaths, are from sudden infant death syndrome (SIDS), a still poorly understood problem that has no known treatment.

ETIOLOGIES

Table 2–1 lists the common causes of cardiopulmonary arrest in children. Table 2–2 indicates the causes and outcomes of 73 consecutive out-of-hospital pediatric cardiopulmonary arrests for which resuscitative efforts were initiated during a 48-month period in San Francisco from 1989 to 1993 (Dieckmann and Vardis, 1995). This population is a representative group of unexpected out-of-hospital cardiopulmonary arrests. The in-hospital pediatric

Table 2-1 Most Common Etiologies of Pediatric Cardiopulmonary Arrest

Sudden Infant Death Syndrome (SIDS)
Respiratory Obstruction
Upper airway obstruction
Croup
Foreign bodies
Bacterial infections
Lower airway obstruction
Bronchospasm
Foreign bodies
Bronchiolitis
Parenchymal lung abnormalities
Drowning
Pneumonia
Hemodynamic Collapse
Hemorrhage
Dehydration
Sepsis
Trauma
Motor vehicle crashes
Fire/smoke inhalation
Falls
Primary Cardiac Problems
Long QT interval
Complete heart block
Congenital heart disease
Cardiomyopathy
Metabolic Disorders
Poisoning
Central Nervous System Abnormalities

Table 2-2 Causes of Prehospital Cardiopulmonary Arrest, San Francisco, 1989-1993*

Medical Conditions	**Total = 65**
SIDS	41
Pneumonia/respiratory failure	2
Asphyxia/drowning	6
Congenital anomalies	5
Upper airway obstruction (infections)	3
Miscellaneous	8
Trauma Conditions	**Total = 8**
Blunt	2
Penetrating	6

*N = 73 children.

Data from Dieckmann RA, Vardis R: High dose epinephrine in pediatric out-of-hospital cardiopulmonary arrest. Pediatrics, June, 1995 (in press).

cardiopulmonary arrest population has slightly different characteristics.

The most frequent etiologies are respiratory failure and SIDS. Less frequently, circulatory failure from exsanguination, dehydration, or sepsis causes cardiopulmonary arrest. Most other acute etiologies are distinctly unusual.

Respiratory Failure

Respiratory insufficiency is the most treatable cause of cardiopulmonary arrest and may develop from upper airway obstruction, lower airway obstruction, or intrinsic lung disease. Croup, foreign bodies, and bacterial infections of the upper airway are the usual causes of upper airway obstruction. Causes of lower airway obstruction include asthma, bronchiolitis, and foreign body aspiration. Bacterial, viral, and mycobacterial pneumonia are the most common conditions contributing to respiratory insufficiency.

Inadequate oxygenation and ventilation from any of these causes can produce progressive hypoxia, hypercarbia, and acidosis, which, if untreated, result in primary respiratory arrest. When effective treatment for respiratory arrest is instituted prior to cardiac arrest, salvage is possible in 75% to 90% of patients (Ludwig et al, 1984). If appropriate interventions (e.g., airway control, oxygenation, artificial ventilation) are not accomplished in a timely manner, secondary hypoxic cardiac arrest, which is exceedingly resistant to therapy, occurs.

SIDS

Of all etiologies for cardiopulmonary arrest, the most frequent is SIDS, which causes up to 40% of all nontraumatic childhood deaths. SIDS usually occurs in infants between 6 weeks and 12 months of age, and it presumably involves sudden loss of autonomic control of breathing. Prevention is the only known approach to SIDS.

Hemodynamic Collapse

Hemodynamic causes of cardiopulmonary arrest include circulatory collapse from hypovolemic, distributive, or cardiogenic shock. Hypovolemic shock is most common and results from acute volume loss associated with hemorrhage from injury, or from water and electrolyte losses caused by conditions such as gastroenteritis or burns. Distributive shock in children is most often caused by sepsis, a condition that is especially prevalent in children under the age of 2 years. Cardiogenic shock is rare, except in children with known congenital heart defects.

Trauma

Trauma deserves special emphasis as a cause of pediatric cardiopulmonary arrest. Injuries are the predominant problem encountered in prehospital pediatric emergency care, and they are the most common cause of death in children over 1 year of age. Critical childhood trauma is usually blunt and multisystem, although penetrating injuries are increasing among urban adolescents. Overall, falls in toddlers, motor vehicle events (with the child as a pedestrian, bicyclist, or vehicle occupant), and fires are the most frequent mechanisms of injury. The magnitude of central nervous system (CNS) insult in critical trauma victims generally determines the overall prognosis for meaningful survival.

Primary Cardiac Arrest

Primary cardiac arrest occurs rarely in children. High-risk patients have long QT intervals, complete heart block, known congenital heart disease, or acquired cardiomyopathy. These patients are susceptible to sudden, lethal dysrhythmias or pump failure, most often in the period following an open-heart operation. Other settings in which children may experience dangerous dysrhythmia include cardiac catheterization, general anesthesia administration, and overdoses of cardiotonic agents (e.g., cyclic antidepressants, potassium, digitalis, calcium channel blockers, theophylline).

PROFILES OF THE CARDIOPULMONARY ARREST VICTIM

There are three distinct clinical profiles of the pediatric cardiopulmonary arrest victim:

1. Infants approximately 3 to 6 months of age who suffer from either respiratory insufficiency or SIDS.
2. Toddlers with severe underlying disease of the cardiopulmonary system or CNS who are admitted to the hospital for treatment of a concurrent infection or for operative therapy and who have an in-hospital arrest.
3. School-age trauma victims who arrest after closed-head and blunt, multisystem injuries sustained in a vehicular crash (Committee on Trauma, 1994).

PROGNOSTIC VARIABLES

For children in true cardiopulmonary arrest, outcome is poor. Positive predictive variables are witnessed collapse, ventricular fibrillation as the presenting rhythm, and early administration of basic life support (BLS) and advanced life support (ALS) (Guidelines for Cardiopulmonary Resuscitation and Emergency Cardiac Care, 1992; Nichols et al, 1986).

Witnessed Collapse

The association of survival with witnessed arrest reflects the much higher rate of survivability when time from collapse to BLS and definitive ALS is short. It may not be an independent variable.

Presenting Rhythm

Of all variables, presenting rhythm may have the highest predictive value for survival. The most common rhythm of childhood arrest is bradyasystole, which is a terminal spectrum of electrical degeneration usually associated with hypoxia-ischemia that probably begins with bradycardia and ends with asystole. Bradyasystole is the first rhythm in approximately 95% of out-of-hospital arrests and in approximately 90% of in-hospital arrests. The survival rate is less than 1%.

Pulseless electrical activity (PEA) is any organized electrical rhythm with no demonstrable perfusion. Some of these patients probably do have minimal pump function, but cardiac output is too low to measure by standard sphygmomanometry or Doppler device. Some authors suggest that PEA patients may represent a heterogeneous arrest category consisting of two groups: Individuals with profound hypoxic-ischemic insult and *no-flow states* (e.g., those with slow rates of $< 20-30$/minute and wide [0.10 second] QRS complexes), whose survival approximates that from bradyasystole; and individuals with *low-flow states* from mechanical problems or hypovolemia, who show narrow complex rates higher than 60/min and possibly have significantly higher rates of survival (Dieckmann and Vardis, 1995).

Ventricular dysrhythmias, primarily ventricular fibrillation and ventricular tachycardia, occur occasionally in pediatric cardiopulmonary arrest victims. Children predisposed to ventricular dysrhythmias are older. When this population receives early electrical countershock, survival ranges from 17% to 50% (Dieckmann and Vardis, 1995; Eisenberg et al, 1983; Friesen et al, 1982).

Advanced Life Support

Another key variable in survival is early management of oxygenation and ventilation. Successful prehospital endotracheal intubation appears to correlate with resuscitation from cardiopulmonary arrest in patients under 18 months of age. Moreover, when respiratory arrest occurs without cardiac arrest, as in airway obstruction or respiratory failure, rapid maneuvers to clear the airway and/or apply mechanical ventilation usually prove successful.

Anticipatory Management

Preparedness is imperative for optimal resuscitation. Preparation includes prior organization of medications and properly sized pediatric equipment, and supplies on a pediatric "crash cart" (Table 2–3), rehearsals, and ongoing personnel training in management of the critically ill or injured child.

A length-based resuscitation tool (e.g., the Broselow tape) helps to avoid common errors in memorization of age-adjusted endotracheal tube sizes, per-kilogram drug formulations, and correctly sized equipment (Luten et al, 1992). A color-coded crash cart that corresponds precisely to the length-based resuscitation tool further facilitates resuscitation organization.

During a resuscitation, one physician (designated the code team captain) must orchestrate all ALS interventions. This physician assigns specific tasks to team members, selects drugs, ensures timely administration of drugs, and orders appropriate procedures. Responsibilities of the code team captain also include limiting the duration of a resuscitation attempt, performing the retrospective critique and debriefing with team members, communicating directly with the patient's family, and contacting the coroner and primary care physician, as needed (Solomon, 1995).

PROCEDURAL CONSIDERATIONS

Securing reliable vascular access is often the rate-limiting step in pediatric resuscitations. Percutaneous and cutdown cannulations of peripheral veins are associated with poor success rates, long delays, and frequent complications. Because of the difficulties associated with conventional techniques, endotracheal and intraosseous drug administration is usually necessary.

Endotracheal Drugs

Epinephrine, atropine, and lidocaine can be given by endotracheal administration. Pharmacokinetic studies of endotracheal drugs in children are poor, although the American Heart Association now suggests that the initial endotracheal epinephrine dose (0.1 mg/kg) be 10 times higher than the standard intravenous epinephrine dose (0.01 mg/kg) to achieve comparable serum levels in first-line drug delivery for cardiopulmonary arrest (Zaritsky, 1993b). For atropine and lidocaine, the endotracheal drug doses are three times the recommended IV doses. When endotracheal drugs are used in resuscitation, the method of administration may be important to pharmacological action. Dilution of the drug to a total volume of no more than 0.5–1 ml/kg may avert interference with gas exchange. The specific sequence for this procedure is as follows:

1. Draw the calculated drug dose into a 3- or 10-ml syringe.
2. Dilute the drug with normal saline to total volume of 0.5 to 1 ml/kg to a maximum of 5 ml.
3. Insert the tip of the umbilical artery catheter or size 5 pediatric feeding tube past the distal tip of the endotracheal tube.
4. Instill solution directly into the trachea.
5. Follow with injected air to clear tubing.
6. Ventilate three times with a bag to disperse the solution into the distal tracheobronchial tree.

Intraosseous Infusions

The intraosseous (IO) or intramedullary infusion technique is now recognized as effective for all resuscitative drugs and fluids, safe to growing bones, and simple to teach and perform (Berg, 1984; Fiser, 1990). This technique is often employed in tandem with the endotracheal route to allow early drug delivery while conventional intravenous access is sought. The procedure is appropriate for both prehospital and in-hospital settings. Although prior studies identified osteomyelitis as the most frequent complication of the IO technique, compart-

Table 2-3 Equipment, Supplies, and Medications for the Care of Pediatric Patients in the Emergency Department

General Equipment Needs	Availability
Pediatric crash cart to store all supplies in an organized manner[1]	
Medication chart, tape, or other system to ensure ready access to proper dosage of medication or proper sizing of resuscitation equipment	CC
Patient warming device	IA
Scales for measuring weights of infants and children	IA
Monitoring Equipment	
Blood pressure cuffs (neonatal, infant, child)	CC
Blood pressure cuffs (adult arm and thigh)	ED
Doppler ultrasound devices	ED
Electrocardiogram (ECG) monitor/defibrillator (0–400 J capacity) with pediatric- and adult-sized paddles	ED
Hypothermia thermometer	ED
Pulse oximeter	ED
End tidal CO_2 detector	IA
Respiratory Equipment and Supplies	
Endotracheal tubes	
uncuffed: 2.5, 3.0, 3.5, 4.0, 4.5, 5.0, 5.5	CC
cuffed: 6.0, 6.5, 7.0, 7.5, 8.0, 9.0	CC
Feeding tubes (5, 8 Fr)	CC
Laryngoscope blades (curved 2.3; straight 0, 1, 2, 3)	CC
Laryngoscope handle	CC
Lubricant (water soluble)	CC
Magill forceps (pediatric and adult)	CC
Nasopharyngeal airways (infant, child, and adult)	CC
Oral airways (sizes 0–5)	CC
Stylets for endotracheal tubes (pediatric and adult)	CC
Suction catheters (infant, child, and adult)	CC and ED
Tracheostomy tubes (Shiley tube sizes (0–6)	CC
Yankauer suction tips	CC and ED
Bag-valve mask (BVM) device, self-inflating, (pediatric size [450 ml] and adult size [1000 ml])	ED
Clear oxygen masks (standard and nonrebreathing) for an infant, child, and adult	ED
Masks to fit BVM adaptor (neonatal, infant, child, and adult sizes)	ED
Nasal cannulae (infant, child, and adult)	ED
Nasogastric tubes (infant, child, and adult)	ED
Vascular Access Supplies and Equipment	
Arm boards (infant, child, and adult sizes)	CC
Butterfly needles (19–25 gauge)	CC
Catheter over the needle (14–24 gauge)	CC
Intraosseous needles	CC
Intravenous (IV) administration sets with calibrated chambers and extension tubing	CC
IV tubing (30 inches)	CC
Stopcocks	CC
Syringes (TB, 3–60 ml)	CC
T-connectors	CC
Umbilical vein catheters[2]	CC
Vascular access supplies utilizing Seldinger technique	CC
Infusion devices with ability to regulate rate and volume of infusate	ED
IV solutions (micro, macro, and blood administration) to include	
Isotonic balanced salt solutions [e.g., normal saline (NS)]	ED
$D_5$0.2 NS	ED
$D_5$0.45 NS	ED
Needles (18–27 gauge)	ED
IV fluid/blood warmer	IA
Fracture Management Devices	
Cervical immobilization equipment or devices suitable for pediatric patients[3]	ED
Spine board (child and adult)	ED

Table continued on next page

Table 2-3 Equipment, Supplies, and Medications for the Care of Pediatric Patients in the Emergency Department (*Continued*)

Specialized Pediatric Trays or Kits	Availability
Lumbar puncture tray	ED
Peritoneal lavage tray	ED
Surgical airway tray	ED
Tube thoracostomy tray	
Chest tubes (infant, child, and adult)	ED
Urinary catheterization kit	
Urinary catheters (infant, child, and adult)	ED
Vascular cutdown tray	ED
Medications[4]	
Atropine	CC
Bretylium	CC
Calcium chloride	CC
Dextrose	CC
Epinephrine (1:1,000 and 1:10,000)	CC
Lidocaine	CC
Naloxone	CC
Sodium bicarbonate	CC
Activated charcoal	ED
Adenosine	ED
Antibiotics	ED
Anticonvulsants	ED
Antipyretics	ED
Benzodiazepines	ED
Beta agonist for inhalation	ED
Dexamethasone	ED
Diphenhydramine	ED
Dopamine	ED
Furosemide	ED
Glucagon	ED
Insulin	ED
Ipecac	ED
Mannitol	ED
Methylprednisolone	ED
Morphine sulfate[5]	ED
Nondepolarizing neuromuscular blocking agents[6]	ED
Phenobarbital	ED
Phenytoin	ED
Potassium chloride	ED
Propranolol	ED
Succinylcholine[6]	ED
Verapamil	ED
Hydralazine	IA
Hydrocortisone	IA
Isoproterenol	IA
Racemic epinephrine for inhalation	IA
3% sodium chloride	IA

CC, on the pediatric crash cart; ED, in the emergency department; IA, immediately available to the emergency department.

[1]In children's hospitals or hospitals with a separate pediatric emergency treatment area, this recommendation may be met by a crash room.

[2]Feeding tubes (size 5 Fr) may be utilized as a UVC catheter.

[3]A cervical immobilization device should be a device that can immobilize the neck of an infant, child, or adult in a neutral position. It may be towel rolls or a commercially available specific neck cradling device.

[4]The following list of medications represents a minimum inventory of medications to be stocked by emergency departments that care for pediatric patients. This list is not meant to be all-inclusive, and it is expected that emergency departments will supplement this inventory based on local resources and needs.

[5]Morphine sulfate or other narcotics (e.g. meperidine) would satisfy this recommendation.

[6]May be available by the Anesthesia Department only. This recommendation may be satisfied if policies exist that ensure the immediate availability of these medications for emergency intubation of the pediatric patient.

From McNeil M, Dieckmann RA, et al: Administration, personnel and policy guidelines for the care of pediatric patients in the emergency department. California EMS Authority, Sacramento, 1994.

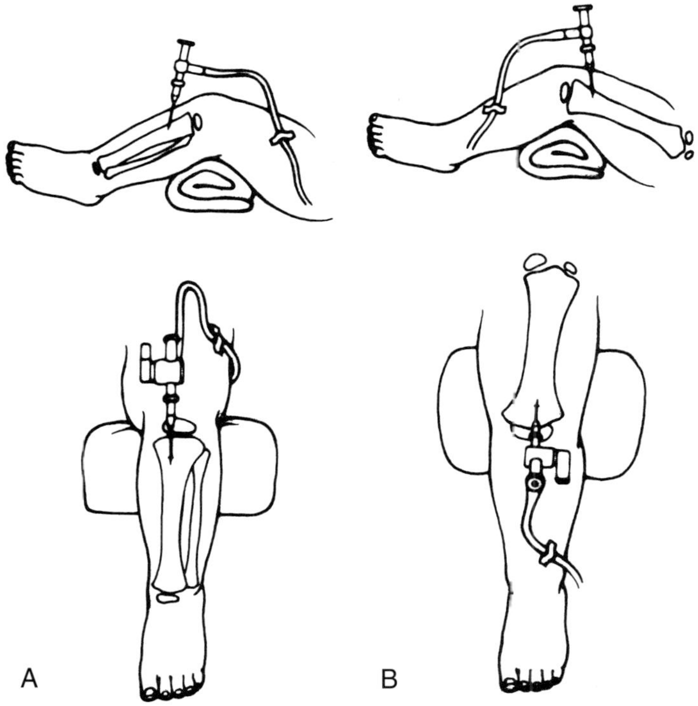

Figure 2–1 Intraosseous infusions. **A.** Proximal tibial insertion site. **B.** Distal femur insertion site. (Redrawn from Grossman M, Dieckmann RA: *Pediatric Emergency Medicine: A Clinician's Reference.* Philadelphia, JB Lippincott, 1991, p 83.)

ment syndrome currently may be the most serious acute complication.

The distal femur or the proximal tibia is a suitable site for needle insertion, although the tibial site is easier. Figure 2–1 illustrates the technical approach. The proper insertion technique is listed below:

1. Prepare the area with antiseptic solution. Use either the midline distal femur (one fingerbreadth above the patella) or the flat surface of the proximal medial tibia.
2. Drape the area.
3. If the child is conscious, infiltrate the insertion site down to the periosteum with lidocaine.
4. Introduce a size 16 bone marrow aspiration or intraosseous needle at a 60° angle directed away from the growth plate.
5. Pierce the bony cortex with a firm, twisting motion.
6. Remove the stylet, and confirm intramedullary placement by instillation (without resistance) of 10 ml of normal saline.
7. Attach stopcock to the hub and infuse fluids, blood products, or drugs directly into intraosseous space.
8. Anchor the needle to overlying skin with tape or sutures.

Electrical Countershock

Electrical countershock is a life-saving procedure in cases of ventricular fibrillation, pulseless ventricular tachycardia, and unstable supraventricular tachycardia. Reperfusion is directly correlated with the timing of electrical current delivery: the sooner after collapse that countershock is administered, the more likely is conversion to sinus rhythm. Electrical dosages and use of the synchronized delivery mode vary with the presenting rhythm (Table 2–4). If the synchronized mode does not work or if the patient is in full cardiopulmonary arrest, the asynchronized or defibrillation mode should be used. The procedure for delivery of electrical countershock is as follows:

1. Ensure that an indication is present: usually shock or full arrest with tachydysrhythmia or ventricular fibrillation. When the patient is conscious, consider a light anesthesia with intravenous diazepam, 0.1 to 0.2 mg/kg.

Table 2–4 Doses for Electrical Countershock

Rhythm	First Electrical Dose	Second Electrical Dose	Third Electrical Dose
Supraventricular tachycardia	0.5 J/kg synch	1 J/kg synch	2 J/kg synch
Ventricular tachycardia	1 J/kg synch	2 J/kg synch	3 J/kg synch
Ventricular fibrillation	2 J/kg asynch	4 J/kg asynch	4 J/kg asynch

Asynch, asynchronized cardioversion (defibrillation); synch, synchronized cardioversion (Note: If synch mode does not work, or if child is in full cardiopulmonary arrest, use asynchronized [defibrillation] mode.)

2. Apply electrode jelly to the lower left sternal border and at the left posterior axillary line at the level of the cardiac apex. When using adult paddles, select locations on the anterior and posterior left chest at the cardiac apex.
3. Use 4.5-cm paddles for infants; use 8-cm paddles for children over 10 kg.
4. Rub jelly into the chest wall to lower skin impedance.
5. Record the ECG.
6. Select the appropriate electrical dose based on the rhythm and the mass of the patient (see Table 2–4).
7. Attempt synchronized cardioversion first if there is tachydysrhythmia. Use asynchronized cardioversion (defibrillation) if the rhythm is ventricular fibrillation or if synchronized cardioversion fails twice to convert tachydysrhythmia.
8. Apply paddles firmly to the chest wall. Ensure that there is no contact between team personnel and the patient or bed.
9. Discharge electrical current.
10. If sinus rhythm does not return, repeat the procedure with double the current.

For infants, 4.5-cm paddles are appropriate; for children weighing over 10 kg, 8-cm paddles are best. Apply pediatric paddles in standard sternoapical locations with conductive jelly, and discharge with firm pressure on the chest wall. When only adult-sized paddles are available, apply them anteroposteriorly on the left chest and left back. Exact paddle size, location, and dose of electricity may be less important than a careful technique that ensures tight contact and timely repeat administrations when indicated. An antidysrhythmic drug, such as lidocaine or bretylium, must be used after electrical countershock for ventricular dysrhythmias.

THE RESUSCITATION SEQUENCE

The code team captain delegates procedures and oversees the following sequence of interventions (Orlowski et al, 1989):

1. *Ascertain unresponsiveness and the quality of cardiopulmonary effort:* Carefully look, listen, and feel to determine that a cardiopulmonary arrest has actually occurred. If the collapse was witnessed, the child may be apneic but not pulseless. Once arrest is diagnosed, help should be called. The second rescuer should be instructed to obtain a pediatric backboard and to initiate chest compressions with proper age-appropriate technique, as illustrated in Figures 2–2 and 2–3. Additional assistance may be required for assembling ALS equipment, medications, and monitoring devices.
2. *Open the airway.* The head-tilt maneuver (Fig. 2–4) should be used, avoiding hyper-

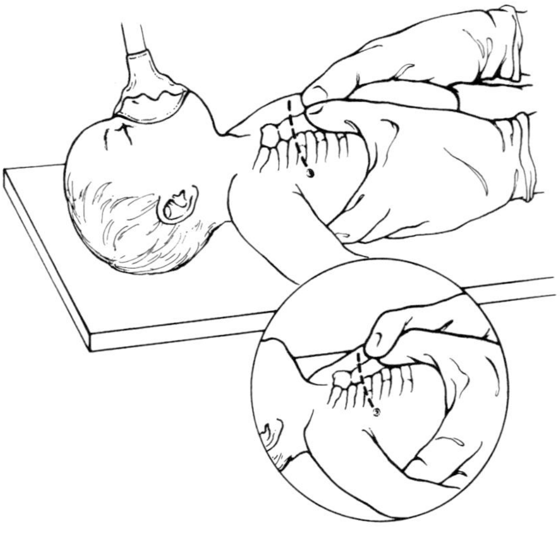

Figure 2–2 Technique of chest compression in an infant.

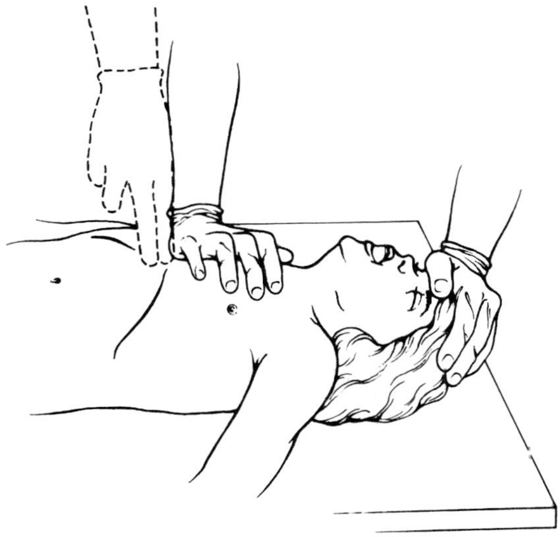

Figure 2–3 Technique of chest compressions in a child. (Redrawn from Emergency Cardiac Care Committee and Subcommittee, American Heart Association: Guidelines for cardiopulmonary resuscitation and emergency cardiac care. *JAMA*, 268:2251–2261. Copyright 1992, American Medical Association.)

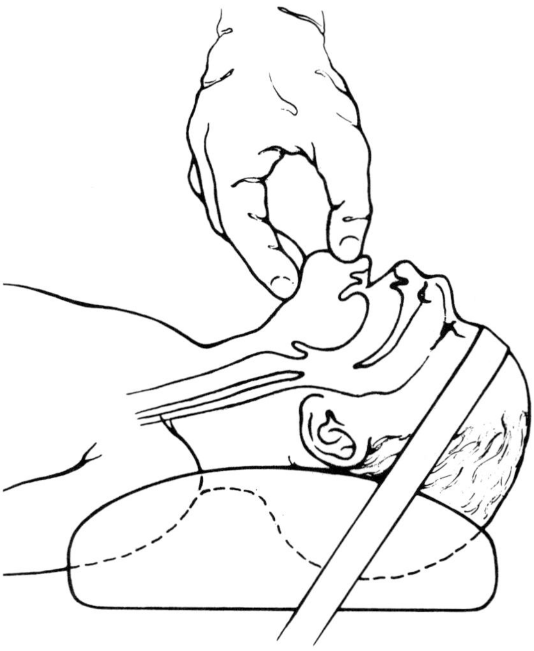

Figure 2–5 Chin-lift maneuver.

extension of the neck. In infants and young children, the larger head size predisposes to cervical flexion, and this age group usually requires a shoulder pad to bring the head and cervical spine into a neutral position. Too-vigorous head-tilt may occlude the trachea or compromise the cervical spine in an injured patient. If spinal injury is suspected, a modified jaw-thrust maneuver (one-person technique) or a chin-lift maneuver (Fig. 2–5) (two-person technique) should be used instead of a head-tilt maneuver. Suction is imperative to clear the airway of secretions, blood, and foreign bodies.

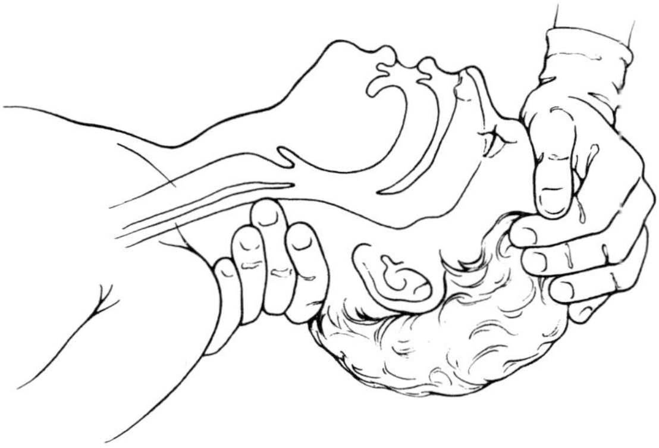

Figure 2–4 Head-tilt maneuver.

If the airway remains obstructed despite initial attempts to establish patency, the following procedures should be implemented to evacuate a possible aspirated foreign body. For children, six to ten rapid subdiaphragmatic abdominal thrusts should be delivered using the heel of the hand (modified Heimlich maneuver) with the patient supine (Fig. 2–6). For infants, four sharp blows to the back should be given with the heel of the hand between securely held shoulder blades. Then, four chest thrusts (instead of abdominal thrusts) should be delivered to the midsternum (Fig. 2–7).

If airway patency still is not established, the sequence should be repeated. If several series of maneuvers fail, an immediate direct laryngoscopy should be performed to visualize the obstructed area. Any obvious foreign body would be removed with Magill forceps. If this procedure does not remove the obstruction, endotracheal intubation should be performed. Very rarely does endotracheal intubation fail to establish an effective airway; however, if this happens, a needle cricothyroidotomy should be performed to bypass the obstruction (Fig. 2–8).

3. *Secure the airway.* When intubation equipment is not immediately available, an ap-

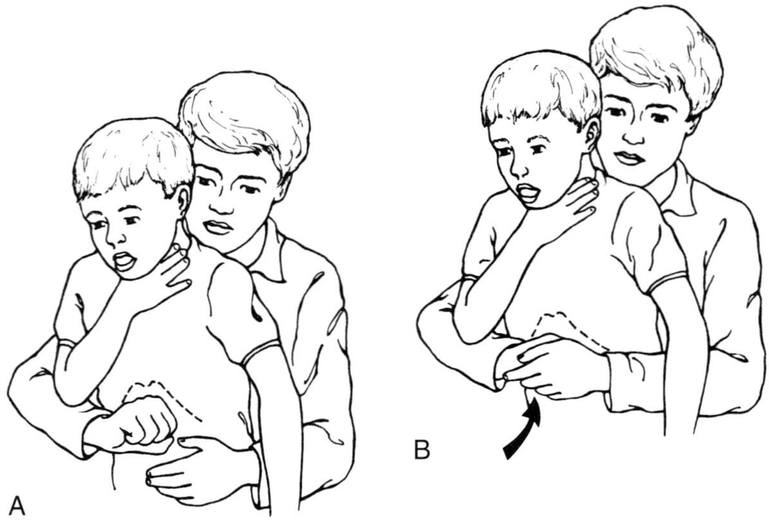

Figure 2–6 Clearing an obstructed airway in a child using a modified Heimlich maneuver.

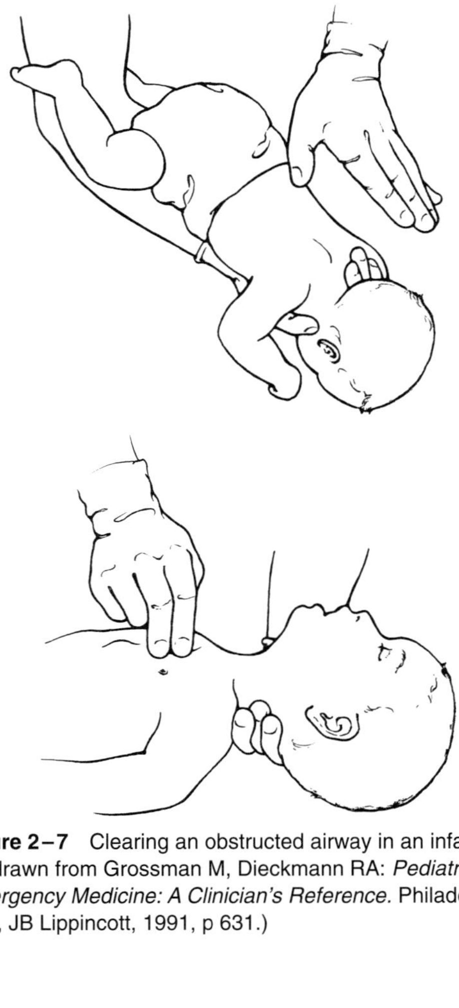

Figure 2–7 Clearing an obstructed airway in an infant. (Redrawn from Grossman M, Dieckmann RA: *Pediatric Emergency Medicine: A Clinician's Reference.* Philadelphia, JB Lippincott, 1991, p 631.)

propriately sized oropharyngeal airway device should be inserted. A conscious child will not tolerate the oropharyngeal device, so a nasopharyngeal device is preferred. When intubation equipment is available, the proper tube should be inserted. Size is estimated from the nail size of the patient's fifth digit or is based on this formula:

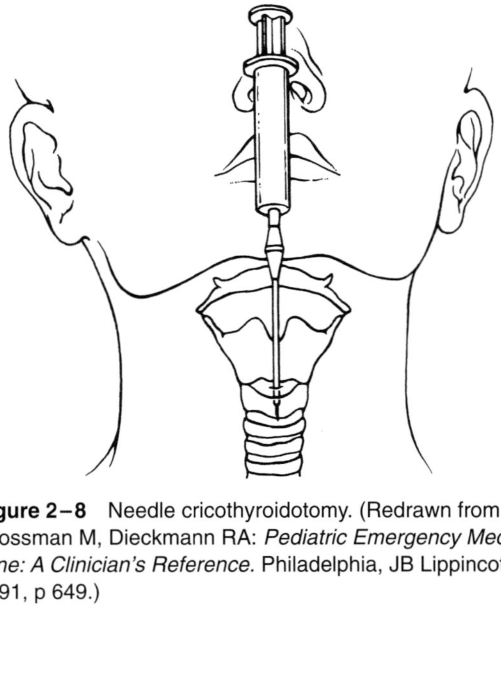

Figure 2–8 Needle cricothyroidotomy. (Redrawn from Grossman M, Dieckmann RA: *Pediatric Emergency Medicine: A Clinician's Reference.* Philadelphia, JB Lippincott, 1991, p 649.)

$$\frac{\text{Age (years)} + 16}{4}$$

4. *Ensure adequate breathing.* After the intubation, attach an end-tidal CO_2 detector to ensure proper tube placement, and apply pulse oximetry. If breathing is absent or ineffective and endotracheal intubation is delayed, the patient's breathing should be assisted with a properly fitted bag-valve-mask apparatus that has an attached inflation bag with a volume of at least 450 ml. This will ensure adequate chest inflation. Bag-valve-mask ventilation is facilitated when one rescuer holds the mask firmly while the second rescuer performs inflations. Slower, controlled chest inflations provide optimal ventilation. (Table 2–5 shows appropriate ventilation rates by ages.) Once the chest rises, insert a nasogastric tube and evacuate stomach contents. An appropriately sized nasogastric tube is usually twice the size of the endotracheal tube. Rarely, equipment for bag-valve-mask ventilation and endotracheal intubation is unavailable, or the intubation maneuver is unsuccessful. In such circumstances, consider either mouth-to-mouth or mouth-to-nose-and-mouth ventilation. Use body substance precautions to prevent disease transmission. When these methods are used, nasal oxygen per cannula applied to the resuscitator may enhance oxygen delivery.
5. *Examine for a pulse.* If a pulse is not palpable, chest compressions (if the second rescuer has not already begun) should be started at an appropriate rate (see Table 2–5) while the patient's back is supported with the opposite hand or with a pediatric backboard. Proper hand placement on the sternum should be used for compressions. Compression effectiveness can be assessed by palpating the brachial or femoral pulse.
6. *Attach "quick look" paddles or a cardiac monitor to assess electrical rhythm.* If ventricular fibrillation, ventricular tachycardia, or supraventricular tachycardia (SVT) is present, electrical countershock should be delivered at appropriate doses (see Table 2–4). Patients with sinus tachycardia, which in infants may be present at rates up to 250 beats/minute, should not be shocked. Countershock should be delivered as soon as proper equipment is available and paddles are charged. This maneuver may precede definitive airway management in patients with unstable ventricular dysrhythmias or SVT. If asystole is present, a second electrocardiographic plane should be obtained to ensure that the rhythm is flatline (as opposed to fine ventricular fibrillation).
7. *Establish vascular access.* IO lines are the preferred conduits for drugs and fluids in children under 2 years of age. An intravenous site in an upper extremity or external jugular vein should also be located if possible. Femoral vein cannulation using a standard percutaneous approach, open venous cutdown technique, or Seldinger guidewire technique is an effective alternative method of rapid access. In patients with difficult access, drug therapy with epinephrine administered through the endotracheal tube should be initiated.
8. *Initiate pharmcological therapy.* The treatment algorithm (Fig. 2–9) indicates the order of interventions and drug administration based on presenting rhythm. Drug doses require careful titration. A validated length-based, drug-dosing resuscitation tool, such as the Broselow tape (Broselow Pediatric Emergency Tape, 1993 ed. Vital Signs, Inc., Totowa, NJ), especially when used in concert with a color-coded pediatric crash cart that matches length and weight categories on the Broselow tape,

Table 2–5 Parameters for Cardiopulmonary Resuscitation in Children

Age	Breathing Rate	Compression Rate/min	Compression Depth	Hand Placement for Compression
< 1 year	20 breaths/min	100–120	1/2–1 inch	Two thumbs at midsternum with hands encircling chest
1–7	15 breaths/min	80–100	1–1 1/2 inches	Two or three fingers above xiphoid; one finger below nipple line
> 7 years	12 breaths/min	80–100	1 1/2–2 inches	Heel of both hands with body pressure two fingers above xiphoid

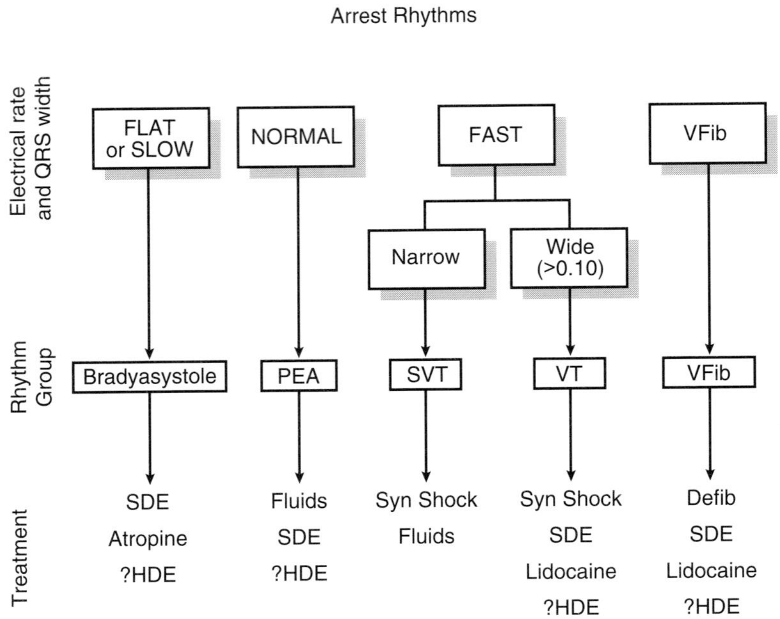

Figure 2–9 Treatment algorithm for pediatric cardiopulmonary arrest. Defib, defibrillation; HDE, high-dose epinephrine; PEA, pulseless electrical activity; SDE, specific dynamic effect; SVT, supraventricular tachycardia; Syn shock, synchronized shock; VFib, ventricular fibrillation; VT, ventricular tachycardia.

Table 2–6 Medications in Pediatric Cardiopulmonary Arrest

Intervention	Dose	Route	Comment
Epinephrine USP 1:10,000 0.1 mg/m 10 ml = 1 mg	0.01–0.2 mg/kg	ET, IV, IO, SL	Repeat every 5 min. Higher doses may be needed, but their effectiveness is unproven
Atropine sulfate 0.1 mg/ml 10 ml = 1 mg	0.02 mg/kg	ET, IV, IO	Repeat every 5 min Minimum dose = 0.1 mg Maximum dose = 1 mg twice
Sodium bicarbonate 8.4% solution 1 mEq/ml 50 ml = 50 mEq	0.5–1 mEq/kg	IV, IO	Use with CAUTION; only with intubated patient
Lidocaine HCl 10 mg/mL 2.5 ml = 25 mg	1 mg/kg	ET, IV, IO	Repeat 1 mg/kg × 3 every 8 min. Follow bolus with infusion at 20–50 μg/kg/min
Bretylium tosylate 50 mg/ml 10 ml = 500 mg	5 mg/kg	IV, IO	Maximum dose = 30 mg/kg. Use after lidocaine fails
D_{25}W and D_{50} Mix D_{50}, 1:1 with water or NS to get D_{25}W or D_{25} NS	< 2 yr: 1–2 ml/kg of D_{25}W > 2 yr: 0.5–1 ml/kg of D_{50}W	IV, IO	Check Chemstix, give for value ≤ 100 mg/dl
Naloxone 0.4 mg/mL 1 ml ampule = 0.4 mg	Children: 0.4–2 mg Neonates: 0.1 mg	ET, IV, IO	Pure opiate antagonist

D_{50}, 50% dextrose; D_{25}NS, 25% dextrose ini normal saline; D_{25}W, 25% dextrose in water. ET, endotracheal; IO, intraosseous; IV, intravenous; SL, sublingual.

helps to minimize errors. Doses can be repeated, if appropriate. If PEA is diagnosed, 20 ml/kg of crystalloid should be infused. Table 2–6 lists drugs by dose, unit form, and route.

9. *Ensure proper chart documentation.* An identified recorder, usually a nurse, must precisely list the time, dose, and exact name and route of every drug and procedure during the resuscitation. Responses to therapy (e.g., rhythm, pulse, blood pressure, neurologic status) are also essential data in the resuscitation record. The code team captain must review and sign the documentation when the resuscitation is complete.
10. *Communicate results of resuscitation to parents immediately.* The parents of a deceased child should be encouraged to view the body following proper clean-up. A private room and a telephone should be provided for the family. Grief support from clergymen, child crisis specialists, friends, and other family members should be facilitated. The primary physician should also be contacted. The need for other health care providers (e.g., child life specialists, social service counselors, psychiatrists) should be considered as well.
11. *Conduct a retrospective critique and stress debriefing involving all resuscitation personnel.* Unclear therapeutic choices and any decision to terminate resuscitation should be explained. Staff questions and concerns should be addressed. Expressions of fear, disappointment, rage, or sadness should be encouraged. Grief reactions should be acknowledged and validated. Critical incident stress debriefings of staff should be arranged when appropriate.

PATHOPHYSIOLOGY AND PHARMACOLOGY

Cardiopulmonary arrest causes hypoxia, as well as respiratory and metabolic acidosis. Actual cell death appears to be mediated by intracellular acidosis and many noxious substances released from cell membranes and anoxic tissues. Even when resuscitation restores spontaneous reperfusion, these agents may cause irreversible cell death. Circulatory arrest for as little as 4 to 5 minutes, in the absence of mitigating factors such as hypothermia, may cause permanent brain injury or death. Circulatory arrest exceeding 8 to 10 minutes is uniformly associated with brain death.

PHARMACOLOGY OF RESUSCITATION

Only a few drugs enhance survival rates. Many drugs that were previously administered routinely during resuscitation (such as sodium bicarbonate, isoproterenol, dextrose, and calcium) are now considered ineffective or dangerous. Furthermore, drugs known to be efficacious in low-flow or shock states (e.g., atropine, naloxone) may be useless in no-flow states.

Drugs Known To Be Effective

The two categories of drugs currently known to benefit cardiopulmonary arrest victims are the alpha agonists and the antidysrhythmics.

Alpha agonists

The alpha agonists are the most effective drugs for cardiopulmonary resuscitation. They work by activating alpha receptors in the aorta to produce vasoconstriction, thereby increasing aortic diastolic pressure and, as a result, coronary artery perfusion. Direct pharmacological action on the myocardium itself does not appear to be a primary mechanism (Paradis et al, 1991).

The most effective alpha agonist is epinephrine, which has both $alpha_1$ and $alpha_2$ properties. The current recommended standard initial dose of epinephrine, 0.01 mg/kg or 10 μ/kg, may be too low, especially in patients with bradyasystolic arrests and slow, wide complex PEA. Increasing 10 to 20 times the current American Heart Association (AHA) initial epinephrine dosing recommendations (i.e., 100–200 μ/kg every 3 to 5 minutes) may be necessary (Brown and Kelen, 1991; Goetting and Paradis, 1991; Paradis et al, 1991). The AHA recommends this higher dose of epinephrine for second and subsequent epinephrine doses.

Several pediatric reports have recommended higher doses in all cardiopulmonary arrest cases, although a recent retrospective study of 65 medical patients showed no benefit from higher initial epinephrine doses (Dieckmann and Vardis, 1995). Larger prospective clinical trials of epinephrine doses are essential to settle the issue of appropriate dose. In children, an important concern is safety, because high epinephrine doses in low-flow states may produce a potentially hazardous sympathomimetic and vasoconstrictive state (Karch, 1991).

Antidysrhythmics

The antidysrhythmics lidocaine and bretylium are secondary agents in cardiopulmonary arrest, used either in postdefibrillation ventricular fibrillation or ventricular tachycardia, or in perfusing ventricular tachycardia. There is no known advantage of one agent over another for these indications. Three boluses of lidocaine (to 3 mg/kg total) should be administered before bretylium is given. *Antidysrhythmics should be administered to patients in arrest only after electrical countershock.* To date, the value of these agents in children is documented only in post–open-heart surgical patients.

Drugs Probably Not Effective in Full Arrest

Two commonly used drugs that actually demonstrate little or no benefit include atropine and naloxone.

Atropine

The anticholinergic drug atropine is useful in the hemodynamically unstable child with rare, primary bradycardia from congenital heart block with secondary hypoperfusion (low-flow state). However, most bradycardia in children results from hypoxia. When used in true cardiac standstill (no-flow state), atropine has no proven benefit. In adults, clinical trials have failed to show any advantage of atropine over normal saline in full arrest, but pediatric studies are not available. Therefore, while atropine is still recommended for bradycardia unresponsive to epinephrine, it is unlikely to improve perfusion, unless the child has a rare congenital heart block.

Naloxone

The opiate antagonist naloxone reliably reverses pulmonary, CNS, and possibly cardiovascular depression in the opiate-overdosed patient in the low-flow state. Naloxone, however, probably has no important action in the no-flow state. In neonates, naloxone administered to an opiate-addicted child may precipitate seizures and therefore should be avoided.

Drugs Possibly Dangerous

Some drugs commonly used during resuscitation may actually be hazardous, including sodium bicarbonate, calcium, and dextrose.

Sodium bicarbonate

Sodium bicarbonate has been used to reverse metabolic acidosis (a condition purported to lower fibrillation threshold) and attenuate pressor response to catecholamines. There are, however, myriad adverse metabolic reactions to bicarbonate administration, including hyperosmolality, hypernatremia, hypokalemia, metabolic alkalosis, and tissue hypoxia from leftward shift of the oxyhemoglobin dissociation curve.

Sodium bicarbonate may also directly depress myocardial and CNS function. The presumed sequence after intravenous administration is an immediate rise in serum CO_2 tension, intracellular diffusion of CO_2, and the resultant increase in intracellular acidosis. Sodium bicarbonate should not be administered unless the child is intubated and well ventilated.

Indications for sodium bicarbonate use are poorly defined. Possible circumstances in which sodium bicarbonate may be helpful include long preintervention times or persistent metabolic acidosis. Sodium bicarbonate may also prove life-saving in unstable patients with cyclic antidepressant overdoses or hyperkalemia.

Calcium

Calcium is indicated only for patients with certain known, specific metabolic disturbances: hypocalcemia, hyperkalemia, hypermagnesemia, and calcium channel–blocker overdose. Except for this extreme minority of arrest patients, calcium will be not only ineffective but also possibly harmful. Calcium is an established endogenous chemical mediator of brain cell injury and death. Calcium administration may cause neuronal and cardiac injury in patients who experience return of spontaneous circulation.

Dextrose

Routine dextrose may injure the brain in no-flow states, because dextrose may increase lactic acidosis in the brain and worsen intracellular acidosis. Rapid bedside glucose determinations identify those few hypoglycemic patients who actually need dextrose. The Chemstrip technique reduces unnecessary administration in the normoglycemic or hyperglycemic patient, in whom the safety of concentrated dextrose solutions is unknown.

TERMINATING THE RESUSCITATION

A patient who experiences an unwitnessed bradyasystolic arrest in unlikely to respond to any therapy. If the child is warm and no extenuating factors are present, resuscitation should be performed with intubation and reversal of hypoxia and respiratory acidosis, electrical countershock when appropriate, and three epinephrine doses. If hypothermia is suspected, more prolonged efforts to revive the child are indicated until the heart is warm.

If the arrest rhythm is ventricular fibrillation (VF), ventricular tachycardia (VT), or supraventricular tachycardia (SVT), resuscitation should usually continue until either reperfusion or asystole occurs. Multiple countershocks may be necessary (O'Marcaigh et al, 1993).

References

Berg R: Emergency infusion of catecholamines into bone marrow. *Amer J Dis Child,* 139:810–811, 1984.

Brown CG, Kelen GD: High dose epinephrine in pediatric cardiac arrest (editorial). *Ann Emerg Med,* 20:104, 1991.

Committee on Trauma, American College of Surgeons: Resources for optimal care of the injured patient. p 57, 1994.

Dieckmann RA: Cardiopulmonary arrest and resuscitation in childhood. In Dieckmann RA, Grossman M (eds): *Pediatric Emergency Medicine: A Clinician's Reference.* Philadelphia, JB Lippincott, 1990, pp 30–37.

Dieckmann RA: Cardiopulmonary arrest and resuscitation. In Rudolph A (ed): *Rudolph's Pediatrics,* 19th ed. Norwalk, CT, Appleton & Lange, pp 1453–1458, 1991.

Dieckmann RA, Vardis R: High dose epinephrine in pediatric out-of-hospital cardiopulmonary arrest. *Pediatrics,* June, 1995 (in press).

Eisenberg M, Bergner L, Hallstrom A: Epidemiology of cardiac arrest and resuscitation in children. *Ann Emerg Med,* 12:672–674, 1983.

Fiser D: Intraosseous infusion. *N Engl J Med,* 322:1579–1581, 1990.

Friesen RM, Duncan P, Tweed WA, et al: Appraisal of pediatric cardiopulmonary resuscitation. *Can Med Assoc J,* 126:1055–1058, 1982.

Goetting MG, Paradis NA: High dose epinephrine improves outcome from pediatric cardiac arrest. *Ann Emerg Med,* 20:22–26, 1991.

Guidelines for Cardiopulmonary Resuscitation and Emergency Cardiac Care. Emergency Cardiac Care Committee and Subcommittees, American Heart Association. Part VI. Pediatric Advanced Life Support. *JAMA,* 268(16):2262–2275, Oct 1992.

Karch SB: Problems with high-dose epinephrine therapy. *Ann Emerg Med,* 20(1):178–179, 1991.

Ludwig S, Kettrick RG, Parker M: Pediatric cardiopulmonary resuscitation. *Clin Pediatr,* 23: 71–75, 1984.

Luten RC, Wears RL, Broselow L, et al: Length-based endotracheal tube sizing for pediatric resuscitation. *Ann Emerg Med,* 21:980–984, 1992.

Nichols DG, Kettrick DG, Kettrick RG, Swedlow DB, et al: Factors influencing outcome of cardiopulmonary resuscitation. *Ped Emerg Care,* 2:1–5, 1986.

O'Marcaigh A, Koenig WJ, Rosenkrans JA, Lynn Berseth C: Cessation of unsuccessful pediatric resuscitation—how long is too long? *Mayo Clinic Proc,* 68:332–336, 1993.

Orlowski JP, Julius CJ, Petras RE, et al: The safety of intraosseous infusions: risks of fat and bone marrow emboli to the lungs. *Ann Emerg Med,* 18:1062–1067, 1989.

O'Rourke PP: Outcome of children who are apneic and pulseless in the emergency room. *Crit Care Med,* 14:466–468, 1986.

Paradis NA, Martin GB, Rosenberg J, Rivers EP, Goetting MG: The effect of standard and high dose epinephrine on coronary perfusion pressure during prolonged cardiopulmonary resuscitation. *JAMA* 165(9):1139–1144, 1991.

Solomon M: Organization of the resuscitation. In Dieckmann RA, Fiser D, Selbst S (eds): *Illustrated Textbook of Pediatric Emergency and Critical Care Procedures.* St. Louis, Mosby, 1995 (in press).

Zaritsky A: Outcome of Pediatric Cardiopulmonary Resuscitation. *Crit Care Med,* 21(Suppl 9): S325–327, 1993a.

Zaritsky A, Members of the Medications in Pediatric Resuscitation Panel: Pediatric resuscitation pharmacology. *Ann Emerg Med,* 22(pt 2):445–455, 1993b.

Section B

Airway/Pulmonary

Chapter 3

Endotracheal Intubation

Katherine I. Schooley

Endotracheal intubation is one of the most commonly performed lifesaving procedures. A systematic approach to a patient needing airway management is essential. At times, the evaluation must be done rapidly, as during an emergency resuscitation. A thorough knowledge of the anatomy of the airway is critical because anatomical considerations are important in diagnosing certain problems (e.g., obstruction of the airway by a foreign body) and in anticipating a problematic intubation, such as may occur with a congenital anomaly. Furthermore, during intubation, anatomical structures may be visible only partially; thus the physician must be able to recognize the structures visually and also be able to recognize their spatial relationships to other structures.

The pediatric airway may pose some very challenging problems. The anatomy of the airway varies with age in size, structure, function, and relative position to other structures. For purposes of describing age-related airway differences, an adult is age 16 or older, a child is between ages 1 and 8 years, and an infant is 1 year of age or younger. By age 8, the airway of the child closely resembles that of the adult, except in size.

ANATOMICAL COMPARISON OF THE ADULT AND INFANT AIRWAYS

In comparison to the adult's, the infant's head is much larger in proportion to the rest of the body. Because of this, when the infant is lying supine, the weight of the infant's head forces the cervical spine to assume a more flexed position. In the absence of muscle tone (e.g., with perinatal asphyxia), this may promote airway obstruction.

The infant's tongue is also proportionately larger than that of the adult. In the absence of muscle tone, the tongue has a tendency to fall posteriorly and occlude the oropharynx. Posterior displacement of the tongue is the most common cause of airway obstruction in both infants and adults, but the displacement is more severe in the infant. Respiratory efforts in the presence of decreased muscle tone tend to pull the tongue in a ballvalve–like fashion into the airway, which further contributes to obstruction.

The infant's larynx is situated at a higher level in relation to the cervical spine, compared to the adult's. At birth, the glottis lies at the level of the C3–C4 vertebral interspace. In adults, it lies at the level of the C4–C5 vertebral interspace. The infant's vocal cords are concave and lie at an anteroinferior angle; in the adult, the vocal cords are less concave and lie more horizontally.

The most narrow area of the airway in the infant is at the level of the cricoid cartilage. In the adult, the airway is most narrow at the level of the glottis. Thus, cuffs are not as important in children under 8 years of age because an uncuffed tube of appropriate size should afford a reasonable seal at the level of the cricoid cartilage.

The epiglottis in an infant is relatively larger and less flexible than in an adult, and it lies in a more horizontal plane. Anterior to the epiglottis, the thyoid bone is attached firmly to the thyroid cartilage, and the tongue and epiglottis consequently are pushed upward toward the pharyngeal cavity.

The trachea and bronchi in infants are significantly shorter and narrower than in adults. The mainstem bronchi branch out at higher angles in infants than in adults. If an endotracheal tube is inserted too far, it will enter the right mainstem bronchus in both infants and adults.

In addition to the above "normal" anatomical differences between pediatric and adult airway anatomies, a variety of congenital malformations and syndromes are more likely to be encountered in infant and pediatric patients, making airway management more challenging. For example, Pierre Robin syndrome and Treacher Collins syndrome are generally first encountered in the delivery room, and intubation is difficult because of the mandibular hypoplasia that is present. Klippel-Feil syndrome is associated with a decreased number of cervical vertebrae, which contributes to difficulty in airway management. Soft tissue may be displaced because of the presence of congenital cysts, hemangiomas, or infection, any of which may distort the anatomy and make airway management very challenging.

Airway management, including endotracheal intubation, requires manipulation of the cervical spine, the atlanto-occipital joint, the mandible, and the soft tissues of the oral cavity and neck. Thus, any disease or congenital abnormality that interferes with mobility of these structures may create difficulties in intubation.

PHYSICAL ASSESSMENT OF THE PATIENT PRIOR TO INTUBATION

Intubations may be elective or performed on an emergency basis. When time is available, a systematic evaluation of the patient helps to anticipate difficulties in airway management.

A global assessment of the patient with particular emphasis on level of consciousness and the ability to breathe spontaneously is pertinent. For nasal intubations, not only is nasal patency important, but evaluation for clotting disturbance is prudent, in view of the higher risk of bleeding from mucosal trauma. The size of the mandible and maxilla and the mobility of the temporomandibular joint all affect how wide the oral cavity can be opened. In addition, the relative size of the tongue should be assessed because the tongue may occlude the oropharynx.

Close examination of the oral cavity may reveal the presence of clefts of the lip and/or palate. The presence of loose teeth in a child may increase the danger of aspiration. Protruding incisors and canines are at risk for fracture during laryngoscopy, so great care must be taken when using the laryngoscope. In an edentulous patient, although visualization of the airway with the laryngoscope is easier, bag-mask ventilation may be more difficult because the normal contour of the face may be distorted and collapsed in the absence of teeth.

The neck and cervical spine should be evaluated for mobility and the patient's vocal quality should be assessed. Patients with diseases of the supraglottic structures have inspiratory stridor, and patients with subglottic diseases have both inspiratory and expiratory stridor.

A cardiorespiratory examination should be done, even in emergency situations. The minimum information needed is vital signs. A thorough cardiorespiratory examination gives some measure of the patient's cardiorespiratory reserve.

Further evaluations including arterial blood gas, chest x-ray, neck films, and pulmonary mechanics testing may be done under elective circumstances, depending on the patient's underlying medical problems.

GENERAL INDICATIONS FOR ENDOTRACHEAL INTUBATION

There are five generally accepted indications for intubation:

1. Ventilatory support

2. Protection of the airway
3. Ensuring airway patency
4. Anesthesia and surgery
5. Suctioning

Respiratory failure with the need for assisted mechanical ventilation is undoubtedly the most common indication for endotracheal intubation in the intensive care unit (ICU). Hypoxemia per se may be treated initially with supplemental oxygen via face mask or nasal prongs; however, intubation and mechanical ventilation should be considered if the patient cannot maintain an oxyhemoglobin saturation of at least 90% or a PaO_2 of at least 60 mm Hg. In addition, if the patient's own minute ventilation is unable to maintain a pH between 7.35 and 7.45, mechanical ventilation should be considered.

Pediatricians commonly encounter the need for emergency endotracheal intubation in the delivery room setting. Perinatal distress may lead to apnea or inadequate respiratory drive, which, if not treated, progresses to postnatal asphyxia.

Other instances in which emergency endotracheal intubation is needed include cardiac arrest, head trauma, facial and neck injuries, and airway burns. Pneumonia and respiratory distress syndrome (RDS) may be progressive and interfere substantially with the patient's ability to maintain normal pH and PO_2 values.

Airway protection in patients with impaired laryngeal reflexes is another important indication for endotracheal intubation. A patient's decreased level of consciousness may lead to emesis and aspiration of gastric contents, which often results in aspiration pneumonitis. Airway burns and diseases causing partial paralysis of the laryngeal musculature also contribute to the instability of the airway.

Patency of the airway is compromised in patients with problems such as epiglottitis, croup, vascular trauma to the neck, and anaphylaxis. In addition, foreign body aspiration contributes to airway obstruction and respiratory failure in many instances.

Occasionally, a patient requires endotracheal intubation in the delivery room because of the presence of tracheobronchial secretions. Endotracheal intubation for suctioning of meconium-stained amniotic fluid is essential to decrease the incidence of meconium pneumonitis in the newborn.

Finally, endotracheal intubation should be performed when neuromuscular blocking agents are used for anesthesia because all protective reflexes are completely obtunded during paralysis. For elective procedures lasting longer than 1 hour, endotracheal intubation is generally indicated to ensure adequate delivery of oxygen and anesthetic gases and to decrease the risk of emesis and aspiration.

SELECTING THE ROUTE OF INTUBATION

Once the decision has been made to intubate a patient, the most appropriate route of intubation must be chosen. There are four main routes of intubation:

1. Orotracheal
2. Nasotracheal
3. Transtracheal
4. Endobronchial

Orotracheal and nasotracheal intubation are by far the most common; however, transtracheal and endobronchial intubation may be considered in special circumstances.

The orotracheal route is used for surgical procedures or for short courses of mechanical ventilation. If the patient requires prolonged ventilation, the nasal route is more comfortable for the patient. In addition, nasal tubes are easier to stabilize than oral tubes. Transtracheal intubation refers to the placement of an endotracheal tube through an already existing tracheostomy stoma. This may be preferred in patients with very complex airway problems. Endobronchial intubation is used when ventilation of only one lung is desired. This occurs in patients with unilateral pulmonary interstitial emphysema, unilateral lung cyst, or bronchopleural or bronchopleuralcutaneous fistulas.

PREPARING THE PATIENT FOR INTUBATION

For all elective intubations, the patient should be adequately sedated; in emergency situations, there might not be time. Inadequate muscle relaxation may interfere with visualization of the vocal cords. In addition, patient anxiety about the procedure may create unnecessary emotional trauma. Sedation is associated with impaired reflex activity, and patients may become apneic or develop laryngeal spasm upon manipulation of the airway. Also, patients who have recently eaten may be at increased risk of aspiration when sedated. Patients undergoing elective surgery should have nothing by mouth for 8 hours prior to surgery to decrease the risk of aspiration. In infants, at least a single feeding should be withheld prior to elective intubation. In newborns, feedings should be withheld approximately 3 to 4 hours prior to intubation.

An "awake" intubation without sedation is the technique of choice in the delivery room setting. It is also the procedure of choice for intubating newborns with intestinal obstruction who are at particularly high risk for aspiration. An "awake" intubation may be the procedure of choice in patients who have significant airway obstruction. If possible, these patients should be allowed to breathe spontaneously.

The use of "anesthetic adjuncts" in the form of muscle relaxants, hypnotics, and opioids to facilitate intubation in emergency and critical care centers is not universally accepted. However, it has gained an increasing acceptance as critical care physicians have witnessed their benefit.

There are several advantages to the use of drug combinations that render patients simultaneously immobile and unconscious. The first is the benefit of creating a nonmoving, nonprotesting "target." The patient in respiratory failure who needs intubation needs it quickly. Immobilizing the patient creates optimal intubating conditions for the physician. The paralyzed tongue does not attempt to dislodge the laryngoscope blade. The pharyngeal muscles and vocal cords do not spasm, and the problem of vomiting is eliminated.

For the patient in respiratory fatiure, the oxygen supply is insufficient relative to oxygen demand, and carbon dioxide elimination is inadequate relative to its production. Physicians have traditionally concentrated on improving the oxygen supply and carbon dioxide elimination to restore physiological balance via artificial ventilation. However, any process that reduces cellular metabolism also exerts a balance-restoring effect, as long as gas exchange by the lung is held constant or is improved.

The patient in respiratory failure is working very hard to breathe, and the respiratory muscles are using abnormally high amounts of oxygen. One of the body's responses to mild-to-moderate hypoxemia is a marked increase in cardiac output. Depending upon the patient's level of consciousness, the brain may or may not have a high metabolic rate.

General anesthesia reduces the body's oxygen consumption by 50% to 60% (to 200–250 ml O_2/min/kg in children, and to 500 ml O_2/min/kg in adults). Although definitive studies of the physiological balance– restoring benefit of muscle paralysis and brain anesthesia are presently lacking for patients in respiratory distress, metabolic reduction combined with rapid intubation and mechanical intervention to improve pulmonary gas exchange should be beneficial. Conversely, it would be very surprising if formal studies demonstrated that awake intubation methods produced, on average, more rapid restoration of physiological balance, as measured by increased arterial and mixed venous Po_2 and pH and decreased Pco_2, blood lactic acid level, and heart rate.

General anesthesia induction carries the risk of passive regurgitation and aspiration. Anesthetic agents abolish the reflexes that close the glottis and expel regurgitated gastric material from the hypopharynx. The risk of passive aspiration can be minimized to an acceptable level, however, by the proper application of external cricoid pressure (the Sellick maneuver).

Succinycholine (1.0–1.5 mg/kg) is the most popular muscle relaxant. It is contraindicated in patients with massive crush injury, electrical injury, spinal cord injury, and burns because these conditions exaggerate the potassium-releasing effect of the depolarizing relaxant, which can lead to massive hyperkalemia and asystole. Vecuronium (0.1–0.25 mg/kg) has a slightly slower onset of action than succinylcholine, and its use requires a modified rapid sequence induction, in which cricoid pressure is applied by the assistant while the operator uses a bag-mask-valve O_2 device to manually ventilate the patient for approximately 90 to 120 seconds prior to laryngoscopy.

Humane care mandates the use of agents that minimize the mental and psychological stress of intubation, particularly when muscle relaxants induce paralysis. Midazolam (0.1–0.3 mg/kg), sodium thiopental (3–7 mg/kg), etomidate (0.2–0.3 mg/kg), and sufentanil (1–2 μg/kg) are among the more popular depressants. The dissociative agent ketamine (1–2 mg/kg) is effective in inducing short-term anesthesia but produces hallucinations and unpleasant dreams in older children and adults. It is not known whether infants and young children experience these side effects. The co-administration of midazolam or other benzodiazepines minimizes the dysphoria-inducing effects of ketamine.

Atropine (0.02 mg/kg) or glycopyrrolate (0.01 mg/kg) can be used prior to intubation to prevent vagotonic bradycardia. They should not be used to treat hypoxemia-induced bradycardia. This is properly treated by ventilation with high-concentration oxygen external chest compression, and, if necessary, epinephrine (which can be delivered via the endotracheal tube if a central venous catheter is not in place). Infants with Down syndrome may be hypersensitive to atropine, and it should be used with caution in such patients.

The use of pharmacological agents to reduce the risk of aspiration pneumonitis is debatable. The patient with respiratory distress who is admitted to the hospital for oxygen therapy and observation and who may be a possible candidate for later intubation should be placed on a histamine H_2-blocker regimen (intravenously if the patient cannot tolerate oral medications) to reduce gastric acid volume and raise gastric pH. The patient requiring emergency intubation may benefit from a single oral or nasogastric dose of sodium citrate solution to reduce gastric acidity.

Occasionally, preintubation topical anesthesia is administered to the mucous membranes of the nose and mouth using a nebulizer, a spray, pledgets, or nose drops. Cocaine solution (4%) has been effective in nasal intubations because of its vasoconstricting properties. A 4% or 10% lidocaine spray may also be administered. Oxymetazoline or phenylephrine nose drops can be administered alone or in combination with lidocaine to reduce the risk of epistaxis, particularly in nasal intubations. Laryngoscopy may be performed to allow more complete application of local anesthesia to the larynx and pharynx.

AIRWAY MANAGEMENT EQUIPMENT

Understanding the design and function of airway management equipment is key to the success of airway management. Perhaps the most common error made by the novice is to waste valuable time attempting, unsuccessfully, to intubate the trachea of a patient in respiratory distress or respiratory arrest instead of simply administering oxygen with a mask and self-inflating bag. The primary goal of airway management is to provide a mechanism for oxygenation of the patient. If oxygenation is inadequate, all other supportive care will fail.

Oxygen Delivery Systems

Commercially available oxygen is obtained from fractional distillation of air and is approximately 99% pure. Oxygen is stored either in liquid form or in large cylinder reservoirs, and it is piped throughout most hospitals to wall outlets. A flow meter is connected to the wall outlet. From the flow meter, oxygen tubing may be directly connected to the oxygen delivery equipment, whether it is a self-inflating bag or a face mask. To ensure adequate oxygen delivery from a wall outlet, it is mandatory to check that the flow meter is properly fitted into the wall outlet and that the liter per minute flow is set at an adequate level. The oxygen tubing must also be connected tightly to the flow meter and must not be obstructed.

Another oxygen delivery system is the portable oxygen cylinder with regulator and flow meter. Oxygen flow from a portable tank (oxygen tanks are green) is initiated by opening the cylinder with a key or wrench. A regulator yoke is attached to the cylinder valve, allowing the clinician to measure the pressure in the tank. A flow meter is likewise attached, and the flow can be set in liters per minute. All connectors must be tight, and the oxygen tubing connecting the flow meter to the resuscitation bag must be unobstructed and tightly fitting.

Supplemental oxygen is needed in patients who do not require immediate mechanical ventilatory assistance. The goal of oxygenation should be to achieve an oxyhemoglobin saturation of at least 90%. In the spontaneously breathing patient, the simplest methods of administering oxygen are via nasal cannula, nasopharyngeal catheter, and mask. The commonly used masks include the simple mask, partial rebreathing mask, nonrebreathing mask, and Venturi mask. The Venturi mask is designed to deliver specified percentages of oxygen, depending on the size of the entrainment ports and/or the jet of oxygen. All of these masks can be used in spontaneously breathing patients who are alert enough to protect the airway from aspiration of secretions or vomitus. If a patient cannot protect the airway (i.e., if the patient is obtunded or does not manifest an adequate gag, cough, or swallow reflex), then an oral or nasal airway should be placed. If the airway is felt to be unstable, then endotracheal intubation should be performed.

Suction Apparatus

Clinicians use either flexible suction catheters or rigid tonsillar tip suction catheters. The tonsillar tip is useful for rapid suctioning of large volumes of fluid from the pharynx, whereas the flexible catheter is useful for decompression of the stomach and suctioning the esophagus, pharynx, and endotracheal tube. Both suction catheters should be available to the clinician for the procedure of endotracheal intubation.

Oral Airways

Oral airways are designed to hold the tongue anteriorly from the pharyngeal wall. Obstruction by the tongue can often be relieved by repositioning the patient's head or by displacing the mandible anteriorly. The oral airway can be applied easily behind the tongue, which is first anteriorly displaced by a wooden tongue blade or a finger. Alternatively, the oral airway may be inserted by placing the tip into the mouth, with the tip initially pointing toward the hard palate, and then advancing the airway and simultaneously twisting it 180° so that the tip slides behind the tongue into the hypopharynx. Loose teeth may become dislodged during this maneuver. Because oral airways can stimulate the gag and vomit reflexes by touching the posterior pharyngeal wall, they should be used only in patients whose protective reflexes are obtunded.

Nasopharyngeal Airway

A nasopharyngeal airway is an alternative to the oral airway. This can be placed via the nasal passage after lubricating with Xylocaine Viscous or K-Y jelly.

Bags and Masks

If the patient's spontaneous ventilation is inadequate, oxygenation can be maintained with bag-and-mask ventilation. The mask should fit over the bridge of the nose, cheeks, and chin to produce an airtight seal. The mask should be pressed against the nasal bridge with the clinician's thumb while the index finger is used simultaneously to exert downward pressure on the base of the mask over the chin. The little finger should engage the angle of the mandible. With the hand held in this position, the mandible can be lifted upward, resulting in the establishment of a patent airway. Bag-and-mask ventilation can be maintained for an extended period of time. A nasogastric tube may need to be placed to adequately vent air trapped in the stomach.

The manual resuscitation bags come in a variety of types. It is preferable to use a self-inflating manual resuscitation bag so that at least room air can be delivered to the patient if an oxygen source is not available. The self-inflating system can deliver enriched oxygen mixtures when it is connected to an oxygen storage tank or oxygen wall outlet. A bag-valve device should be fitted into the self-inflating bag and fitted with a 25 to 30 cm H_2O release valve to avoid the development of excessive airway pressure. An alternative to the self-inflating bag is the anesthesia bag, which can be fitted to deliver positive end-expiratory pressure (PEEP) at a specified level. A manometer can be attached to the anesthesia bag; however, this requires proper connection to oxygen flow for successful mechanical ventilation.

Laryngoscope and Blades

The laryngoscope is a vital instrument in airway management. The laryngoscope consists of a handle, which contains the batteries that power the light, and a blade, which contains a built-in light. The handle is fitted into the blade. In order for the proper electrical contacts to be made, the connection between the laryngoscope handle and blade should be kept clean.

The laryngoscope blades are designed to enter the mouth, displace the soft tissues, elevate the epiglottis either directly (straight blade) or indirectly (curved blade with a tip in the vallecula), and expose the vocal cords. The Miller blade is the straight blade most commonly used, and the MacIntosh blade is the commonly used curved blade. All resuscitation trays should contain at least two laryngoscope handles and a variety of sizes of both straight and curved blades. Thin handles that have AA batteries are generally easier to use for intubating infants and toddlers than are the standard C-battery handles used for older children and adults.

Endotracheal Tubes

In addition to a variety of laryngoscope blades, the resuscitation tray should also contain multiple sizes of endotracheal tubes (Table 3–1). For pediatric intubations, three endotracheal tube sizes should be immediately available: the predicted size, one size larger, and one size smaller. Crucial time can be lost searching for the correct size of endotracheal tube, and tech-

Table 3–1 Approximate Internal Diameter and Length of Pediatric Endotracheal Tubes and Size of Suction Catheter

Age (yr)	Internal Diameter (mm)	Length (cm) Oral	Length (cm) Nasal	Suction Catheter Size
Premature	2.5–3.0	9–11	11–12	5 F
Newborn	3.5	10–12	12–14	6 F
1	4.0	12	14	8 F
2	5.0	13	15	10 F
4	5.5	14	16	10 F
6	6.0	15	17	10 F
8	6.5	16	19	10 F

From Funucane BT, Santora AH: Principles of airway management. In Lowenthal DT (ed): Essentials of Medical Evaluation Series. Philadelphia, FA Davis, 1988, p 233.

nical difficulties often arise from selecting inappropriate tube size. The internal diameter of the endotracheal tube is selected on the basis of the child's age (in years). The following formula is usually accurate in most circumstances:

$$\frac{\text{Age (years)} + 16}{4}$$

This formula applies to uncuffed endotracheal tubes in children up to 8 years of age. The correctly fitting endotracheal tube is one that allows a slight leak with application of 20 cm H_2O pressure to the airway. It has also been suggested that the diameter of the child's little finger is approximately the same as that of the trachea. If one decides to use a cuffed endotracheal tube on a child younger than 8 years of age, a slightly smaller endotracheal tube size may be used to avoid too snug a fit. The child's mucosa in the cricoid area is very prone to edema and pressure trauma.

THE TECHNIQUE OF ENDOTRACHEAL INTUBATION

Proficiency in intubation and ventilatory management requires an understanding of the anatomy of the airway and of the design rationale of the laryngoscope. It is useful to visualize the conducting airway in the form of three separate axes: oral, pharyngoesophageal, and tracheal. The patient should be properly positioned and the laryngoscope should be used to provide a direct line of vision between the mouth and the trachea. There are three steps in providing a direct line of vision:

1. Slight backward rotation of the head (commonly known as the head-tilt)
2. Displacement of the mandible anteriorly (jaw-lift or jaw-thrust)
3. Placement of the laryngoscope blade to the right of the patient's tongue, rather than over it

The first objective can be met by a variety of methods ranging from simple operator hand traction on the head (for premature infants) to placement of various types of padding underneath the shoulders, neck, and head. For example, a rolled towel under a patient's back or shoulders is typically used in infants and toddlers, often without a donut surrounding the occiput to prevent the head from rotating to one side. In older children and adults, a simple 2-inch-thick pillow under the head combined with a manually induced backward head tilt is generally preferred to induce the classic "sniffing" position, in which the lower neck is slightly flexed and the upper neck is slightly extended.

Anatomical differences lead to the laryngoscopic appearance of the glottis as more "anterior" relative to the tip of the laryngoscope blade in infants than in older children. Neonates can generally be intubated without special padding, although some physicians use the same shoulder-neck padding as is used in larger infants.

Anterior displacement of the mandible, the second key to obtaining a straight line of vision to the glottis, is achieved by exerting an anteroposterior traction on the laryngoscope handle. Intubation can generally be achieved without meticulous attention to proper head and neck extension or combined upper extension–lower flexion. Recent work in trauma care has formally established this (see below). Thus, the proper use of the laryngoscope as a mandible-lifting device is probably the most important visualization parameter. Nevertheless, the physician who routinely neglects optimal positioning and relies primarily on the mandible lift may find that a glottis occasionally cannot be visualized; checking if the patient positioning can be improved is wise. Using a shoulder roll for most intubations may occasionally bring an otherwise hidden glottis into full view.

The third key to viewing the glottis, the laryngoscope blade, is used to sweep the tongue leftward and cephalad out of the field of operation. The best method of positioning is to initially place the blade's tip into the potential space underneath the right lateral margin tongue and next to the inner margin of the right jaw. The blade should be advanced in this groove, which displaces the tongue leftward and cephalad. The tip is aimed medially so that it intersects the sagittal plane at the level of the base of the epiglottis.

The correct use of the blade is critical to consistent success. The most common error of the inexperienced physician is to insert the blade in the sagittal plane cephalic to the tongue (as one would use a tongue depressor) or perhaps to the right, but still on top of the tongue so that upon lifting the laryngoscope, the tongue lies underneath (cephalad and anterior to) the blade. This error guarantees frequent failure in fully visualizing the glottis, making intubation a hit-or-miss, semi-blind proposition. This position naturally encourages the operator to lever the tip of the blade anteriorly, using the tongue as an immovable fulcrum. Unfortunately, this results in the proximal portion of the blade's moving posteriorly in a teeter-totter manner, into the patient's upper gingiva or teeth.

Emergency intubations, particularly under anesthesia, require the use of cricoid pressure. This maneuver can also be used to displace the glottis slightly posteriorly, if necessary, to aid visualization.

There are two basic laryngoscope blade designs, curved and straight, with many minor variations of each. The curved blade tip is, by convention, advanced just to the point of resting anterior to the epiglottis in the vallecula. The operator then exerts an anterocaudal force (not a backward levering force) to open the airway and provide a direct line of vision to the glottis. The straight blade tip is advanced to lie just posterior to the epiglottis, and the laryngoscope is lifted anterocaudally, with the epiglottis pinned underneath (i.e., anterior to) the blade. Each blade design has advantages and disadvantages, and the preference for either is based on personal experience and comfort more than anything else. Essentially, the curved blade requires more lifting force than does the straight blade to gain adequate straight-line visualization of the glottis. In the process, the curved blade provides a broader field of view that allows the operator to see more peripheral anatomy, which helps in orientation. However, the curved blade frequently fails to reveal the glottis fully, as the epiglottis hangs down in front of the glottis, obscuring the anterior half or even all of the glottis, so that placement of the endotracheal tube sometimes requires a combination of faith and deductive reasoning (one sees everything but the glottis).

The straight blade, particularly the narrow Miller blade, restricts peripheral vision. Yet, if used correctly, it unfailingly provides a full view of the glottis. The Miller blade has a spoon-shaped tip that encourages the user to insert it and advance it underneath the body of the tongue.

The straight blade has gained wider usage in infants and young children than the curved blade. For infants weighing less than 900 g, the suggested blade is a Miller 00; for larger newborns, Miller 0. Many pediatric physicians use a Miller 1 for older infants, a slightly curved Wis-Hipple 1.5 blade for toddlers, and a Foley curved MacIntosh 2 for children between ages 4 and 12. Other physicians simply use progressively larger Miller blades.

Endotracheal tubes used in respiratory care are made of clear or translucent polyvinylchloride (PVC). Modern endotracheal tubes are constructed with various markers to assist proper distance placement. These include single black-stripe markers located near the tip (on intubation, the stripe should be just at the vocal cords), a set of ruled marks with numbers to allow recording on the medical record of the number located at the lower gingival or dental line (key to diagnosing accidental migrations of the tube), and two longitudinal stripes made of radiopaque material used to judge tube-tip placement radiographically.

Cuffless tubes are used for infants and children to approximately 8 years of age because the addition of a cuff reduces the inner circumference of the tube, which increases airflow resistance.

Air Leaks Around the Endotracheal Tube

The physician should ensure that air leaks past the cricoid ring when a continuous positive airway pressure (CPAP) (approximately 15–20 cm H_2O) is generated. This is to ensure that the pressure imposed by the endotracheal tube on the cricoid submucosa is less than capillary perfusion pressure, while at the same time preventing unnecessary leakage and loss of ventilatory efficiency. If a leak occurs with a CPAP of less than 15 cm H_2O, a larger tube is required. If a CPAP of greater than 25 cm H_2O is required to induce a leak, a smaller tube should be used.

Air leakage at pressures less than 15 cm H_2O is acceptable for neonates, as long as adequate ventilatory pressures and volumes can be generated. If a tube is believed to be correctly sized but the tip resists passage through the cricoid ring, it should not be forced. Rather, a smaller tube should be used, and after it is inserted, the amount of CPAP required to induce a leak should be measured.

Stylets

A malleable stylet is useful for emergency intubations, in which a premium is placed upon inserting the tube as rapidly as possible. A stylet is used to direct the tube just beyond the glottis, at which point the stylet is withdrawn to allow the endotracheal tube to more easily conform to the trachea as the endotracheal tube is advanced. The stylet reduces or eliminates the plastic endotracheal tube's propensity to bend posteriorly at the wrong position. In fact, the stylet not only imparts some helpful rigidity to the tube, but also can be used to bend the endotracheal tube into a desired curve (hockey-stick shape) to facilitate intubation (e.g., in the case of the "anterior larynx"). The stylet should be preplaced within the tube. The stylet tip should rest at $\geq$ 5 mm proximal to the endotracheal tube tip. The proximal end of the stylet should then be bent at a right angle to prevent unintended downward migration of the stylet beyond the endotracheal tube tip. If for some reason a stylet is not available and the pliable endotracheal tube will not go into the intended orifice, the endotracheal tube can be made temporarily rigid by immersing it in ice water for 30 seconds.

Confirming Correct Placement

A common beginner's error is to attempt to hold the endotracheal tube in correct anatomical position throughout the procedure; that is, in the sagittal plane with the concave side upward. This obscures visualization of the glottis because the body of the tube lies between the operator's eye and the glottis. The tube should be held off the sagittal plane to the right with the tip angling in toward the midline as it approaches the glottis. The glottis remains in full view, and the beveled tip of the tube can be manipulated to efficiently separate the cords.

It is imperative to confirm correct placement of the endotracheal tube in the trachea. There are several methods for ascertaining this:

1. Direct observation of the endotracheal tube passing between the patient's vocal cords
2. A rising oxygen saturation within 30 seconds of commencement of artificial ventilation following intubation of the patient
3. A characteristic "feel" learned by experience
4. Bilateral expansion of the chest wall (versus a rising epigastrium)

If the endotracheal tube is not seen to pass through the cords, and the patient shows desaturation despite vigorous ventilatory efforts by the operator, it is safest to assume that the endotracheal tube is improperly placed. The tube should be removed and the patient should be ventilated with the mask.

A universal error of the less-experienced physician who correctly places the tube into the trachea in an emergency condition is overzealous advancement of the tube into the mainstem bronchus (usually the right side). It is imperative to observe the chest rise and fall with ventilation and to listen to the chest and epigastrium. If chest motion and/or breath sounds appear to be unilateral, the patient should be rescoped, and the tube should be withdrawn under direct vision until the black circumferential stripe marker (or cuff) appears. Bilateral chest wall movement and breath sounds should return.

A pulse oximeter should be used in the emergency management of patients with respiratory distress. If the oximeter shows desaturation that is not reversed within 30 seconds of intubation, visible cyanosis substantiates the oximeter read-out, and chest wall motion is absent or indeterminate, the safest course is to remove the endotracheal tube and ventilate the patient by mask while an assistant applies cricoid pressure. Even a correctly placed tube may become kinked or may be obstructed by a mucus plug, blood clot, or foreign body. Nasotracheal tubes can "core out" pieces of adenoidal tissue.

The properly functioning endotracheal tube can be secured by any number of devices, including a piece of tape, a plastic snap-on tube clamp, and tape or stay sutures (for tracheostomy tubes). Tincture of benzoin helps to increase tape adhesion.

After intubation has been performed, a plain radiograph of the chest is routinely obtained to determine the level of the endotracheal tube tip, which should optimally be located equidistant from the larynx and carina to minimize the risks incurred with small amounts of migration, either caudad (occurring mainstem intubation) or cephalad (occurring extubation).

ALTERNATIVES TO STANDARD DIRECT LARYNGOSCOPY

Although classic direct laryngoscopy remains the most useful method of intubating patients, occasionally patients will require other methods.

Nasotracheal Intubation

Nasotracheal intubation is useful in the intraoperative and postoperative care of patients undergoing reconstructive facial surgery. It has traditionally been used for intermediate-length periods of ventilatory management of ICU patients requiring approximately 7 to 14 days of intubation. The nasal tube is less likely to become dislodged than the oral tube, it is more comfortable for the patient, and it cannot be bitten.

The full technique is as follows: Cotton-tipped applicators or pledgets soaked in either cocaine 4% solution (2 mg/kg maximum dose) or lidocaine 4%/phenylephrine 0.025% solution (4 mg/kg maximum lidocaine dose) are inserted into the nose, or the solution is sprayed into the nose with an atomizer. The larger nostril should be chosen. If the patient is awake, lidocaine 10% solution is sprayed into the mouth. The applicators or pledgets are left in place for 10 minutes, then removed. This preparatory sequence serves two functions: to anesthetize the very sensitive nasal passage and to shrink the turbinates, which eases tube passage and reduces the risk of epistaxis. An endotracheal tube is lubricated with lidocaine jelly and is inserted between the middle and inferior turbinates. As body temperature warms the tube, the tube softens and tends to bend easily downward when it reaches the posterior wall of the nasopharynx. A laryngoscope is inserted as it would be for orotracheal intubation. The tube is then advanced into the lower pharynx under direct observation. At this point, the operator may attempt to place the tube into the trachea simply by pushing on the proximal end of the endotracheal tube and perhaps turning the patient's head and/or extending it or flexing it. This method is particularly useful in infants. An alternative is to grasp the distal end of the endotracheal tube with a Magill forceps and then insert the tube into the trachea using forceps.

Nasotracheal intubation poses risk of adenoidectomy, obstruction of a sinus cavity with infection, and epistaxis. Unfortunately, the endotracheal tube must generally be a half-size smaller than one would normally use, and an uncuffed tube cannot be inflated to fill the gap. Packing can be used to minimize an air leak, but this mandates that personnel remember to change it and to remove it prior to extubation. Nasotracheal intubation is useful in patients with acute epiglottitis, when the inflamed glottis requires a smaller-than-normal tube, and when premature extubation can be catastrophic.

In blind nasotracheal intubation, a lubricated endotracheal tube is inserted into the nostril and advanced. As the tip is advanced into the hypopharynx, the operator listens for breath sounds emanating from the tube end. Alternatively, a whistle can be affixed to the proximal end. The tube is advanced until either the breath sounds become very loud (and the patient bucks if local anesthesia has not been performed) or the breath sounds abruptly cease. The former indicates successful placement; the latter indicates esophageal placement. If the attempt is unsuccessful and the patient's head can be moved, it may be helpful to perform rotation and/or extension of the head (or occasionally flexion) and then reattempt to intubate.

Nasotracheal suction is frequently performed by ICU personnel. If intubation is unsuccessful, the endotracheal tube can be withdrawn partially and an attempt made to place a nasotracheal suction catheter through the tube. If this is successfully placed, the endotracheal tube can be guided down the catheter.

For many years, patients with cervical injury were thought to require nasotracheal blind intubation. Recent work has demonstrated that direct laryngoscopy can be performed safely by experienced persons, without causing head extension or damage to the spinal cord, by using manual in-line traction (MIAT) or cervical spine immobilization. This technique places primary emphasis on anterocaudal displacement of the mandible by the intubator, while an assistant uses countertraction to maintain the head and neck in a neutral position. Moreover, the risks of placing a nasal tube in head-injured patients (i.e., epistaxis, sinusitis, the theoretical possibility of placing the tube into the cranial vault if the cribriform plate has been fractured, a higher-than-acceptable failure rate) and the specialized technical expertise required outweigh the benefits.

The nasotracheal tube has a disadvantage in the pediatric patient: The tube is uncuffed, yet it must usually be a half-size smaller (in order to pass through the nose) than is optimal for proper seating in the cricoid ring. As in adults, air leakage can be reduced by packing gauze into the hypopharynx; a piece of gauze should be left hanging out of the mouth to remind personnel to remove the packing when extubation is carried out. Air leakage is not a problem in infants with acute epiglottitis because the glottic opening is reduced severely owing to inflammation.

Fiberoptic Bronchoscope

The fiberoptic bronchoscope is eminently useful for performing both nasotracheal and orotracheal intubations (see also chapter 5). This instrument incorporates two bundles of flexible glass fibers that can be bent up to 90° near the tip by using a control lever operated at the proximal end. This allows the scope to be passed through extremely tortuous channels. The flexible scope can be used as both an instrument to visualize the glottic opening and a flexible stylet for the endotracheal tube. The bronchoscope is particularly useful for intubating infants and children with craniofacial anomalies (e.g., as in Pierre Robin syndrome, Treacher Collins syndrome). New versions of pediatric bronchoscopes, such as the Olympus 6000, are small enough to pass through the lumen of a 3.0 endotracheal tube.

If the bronchoscope is used for orotracheal intubations, a special oropharyngeal airway designed to protect and guide the flexible scope should be used in dentulous patients to prevent damage to the delicate optical fibers of the bronchoscope. This airway also aims the scope tip up toward the glottis. Preparatory methods to anesthetize the upper airway for awake intubations are the same as described for nasal intubation.

The flexible fiberoptic scope allows the operator to turn corners and probe deeply into internal spaces. The eyepiece can be attached to a videocamera, which in turn can be connected to a video monitor. This enables the instrument to be an anatomy-teaching device and allows the senior physician to provide guidance to the trainee. The utility of the flexible fiberoptic scope is limited primarily to elective preoperative intubations, verification of tube placement (e.g., for endobronchial intubation, one-lung ventilation), and endotracheal tube exchanges, uses that allow a leisurely pace. The flexible fiberoptic scope is rarely used in emergency intubation efforts because of the time it takes to set up and operate. It is also prone to image obscurement from blood or mucus.

The primary benefit of the flexible fiberoptic scope—allowing the physician to see structures "around the bend and out of sight"—has been incorporated in a modified conventional laryngoscope known as the Bullard laryngoscope. This instrument has a built-in fiberoptic bundle that runs along a conventional metal blade, and, like the flexible scope, it has an eyepiece that can be used for either direct viewing or videocamera hookup. This instrument is much more durable than the flexible scope, it gives the user most of the advantages of the flexible scope, and it requires no specialized skill beyond that required for conventional direct laryngoscopy. The Bullard scope is available in adult and pediatric sizes.

Tactile Intubation

Recent reports have been published to remind physicians that endotracheal tubes can be placed without instrumentation. Two fingers are placed in the patient's mouth and down to the level of the glottis, followed by insertion of the tube between the fingers. Like all procedures, this method works well in practiced hands. It is inappropriate as a first-line method for the practitioner who is occasionally required to intubate and who is untrained in the method.

Head and neck trauma occasionally creates situations in which conventional methods are useless. In such cases, cricothyrotomy may be called for. The standard emergency procedure, which cannot be used in infants, is to palpate the cricothyroid gap and to make a transverse incision through the cricothyroid membrane with a No. 11 scalpel. A blunt hemostat can be used to enlarge the incision, and a small endotracheal tube can be placed through it.

An alternative method of providing translaryngeal ventilation is to puncture the membrane with an IV needle or catheter attached to an aspirating syringe. When air is obtained, the catheter is slipped off the needle and attached to an oxygen source. In adults, a 14-gauge catheter can be effectively connected to a bag-valve device (Ambu bag). For children, the catheter size (16–18 gauge) mandates the use of a high-pressure device, typically either a manually operated valve or a jet ventilator. The needle cricothyrotomy can be used as a temporary measure until a surgical cricothyrotomy or tracheostomy can be performed. In the rare case of proximal obstruction that does not allow exhalation, a second catheter can be inserted as an exit valve.

The cricothyroid puncture method has also been used successfully to pass a guidewire or epidural catheter in retrograde manner into the oropharynx. The wire is then pulled out of the mouth and an endotracheal tube is passed over the wire or catheter and down into the trachea.

Precautions and Complications

Planning ahead

Achieving a successful outcome requires a well-planned management sequence. Prior to any intubation effort, the caregivers must establish airway patency, using the head-tilt and jaw-lift or jaw-thrust maneuver to lift the tongue off the posterior pharyngeal wall. Oxygen should be delivered via a bag-mask oxygen device. The unconscious patient whose airway might not always be opened by positioning may require placement of an appropriately sized oropharyngeal or nasopharyngeal airway. If this does not yield patency, the airway is likely to be obstructed by a foreign body, and the patient will require laryngoscopic examination and extraction using forceps, a malleable spatula (for hard rounded objects), or a small-bore metal suction tip. Blood (which may have formed clots), gastric fluid, or secretions should be suctioned using a high-vacuum device (80–120 mm Hg negative pressure) and a Yankauer tip.

Intubation is typically performed in the delivery suite without first establishing an intravenous (IV) line. In virtually all other circumstances, an IV should be started while the patient in respiratory distress is given oxygen by mask, open tube, or face tent. The patient in severe failure who is fatigued and unable to struggle should be given assisted ventilation using 100% oxygen by mask while the IV is being placed and intubating materials are being set up.

Maintaining equipment

Integrity of the artificial life support apparatus is vital. Ambu or Laerdal bags should be properly stored and periodically inspected and tested to ensure that parts are not missing, worn, or broken. Black rubber anesthesia bags are particularly susceptible to oxidative disintegration over time, and they should be replaced annually. Oxygen tanks and regulators must be inspected by a licensed service technician. It is mandatory to have two laryngoscopes. The worst time to have to diagnose and repair a malfunctioning laryngoscope is during an intubation attempt. Batteries should be changed every 6 months, and handles and bulbs should be checked after each battery change.

Sites used for intubation must have suction devices capable of generating negative pressure (100 cm H_2O), disposable noncollapsing vacuum tubing, and Yankauer tips. Clear plastic disposable masks with air-filled skirts conform remarkably well to almost all faces and provide very good seals.

The patient's pulse should be assessed frequently (brachial artery for infants, carotid or femoral for older patients). A five-lead electrocardiogram is useful for diagnosing arrhythmias and for providing a continuous indication of heart rate.

The majority of the instruments, drugs, and materials should be kept in a code cart, which can be wheeled to the site. Disconnections or failures to make proper connections can occur at any juncture between the primary oxygen source (tanks or wall outlet) and the endotracheal tube, particularly in the initial resuscitation phase and during and after transport. The routine use of continuous pulse oximetry has been a lifesaver in allowing early detection of such events. Ideal fail-safe monitoring includes end-tidal CO_2 monitoring, minute ventilation monitoring, and circuit pressure monitoring, all with built-in alarm devices.

Intubation, especially under emergency conditions, is not infrequently associated with iatrogenic trauma. Teeth can be chipped; lips and mucosae can be lacerated. Subglottic edema, mucosal ulceration, and subglottic stenosis can occur subsequent to traumatic intubation. The use of too-large endotracheal tubes or overinflated cuffs can cause pressure-induced ischemia.

Barotrauma (i.e., tension pneumothorax) occurs occasionally as a result of overzealous hand-bagging with devices that do not have pressure gauges or pressure relief valves. Barotrauma can also result from improper ventilator settings. It may occur with management of diseases of the pulmonary parenchyma, which require high ventilator pressures. Emergency diagnosis requires a high index of suspicion. Diminished or squeaking lung sounds unilaterally upon auscultation of the lung fields, an appearance of hemidistension, and hyperresonance to percussion are key clinical signs. The differential diagnosis includes endobronchial intubation; however, in patients with hyperresonance to percussion, breath sounds and chest movements will be diminished on the contralateral side. The endotracheal tube distance number at the mouth should have been recorded at intubation. If this shows no change from initial placement, endobronchial intubation is unlikely.

An anteroposterior plain radiograph of the chest determines with certainty which condition applies. If the clinical signs indicate tension pneumothorax, and the patient's condition deteriorates too precipitously to allow x-ray study, a 22-gauge IV catheter can be inserted into the pleural to provide immediate relief. Then, a chest tube should be inserted and connected to a Pleur-Evac.

The key to successful intubations is practice. The physician who is rarely called to intubate should take the opportunity to occasionally refresh his or her skills by visiting the operating room and arranging with the anesthesia team to spend a morning intubating surgical patients. A second key is to use an assistant who is capable of performing the Sellick maneuver properly. On occasion, an inexperienced assistant will apply too much cricoid pressure and distort the airway anatomy to an extent that the glottis is unrecognizable. Moreover, the assistant should help the physician by retracting the right lower lip anteriorly to minimize the risk of the lip's being placed between the patient's teeth and the laryngoscope, which can result in various degrees of laceration.

Chapter 4

Sleep Apnea Testing Using Clinical Polysomnography

Ralph Downey, III, and Ronald M. Perkin

INDICATIONS FOR THE USE OF CLINICAL POLYSOMNOGRAPHY

The Patient History

As William Dean Howells once said, "He who sleeps with continual noise is wakened by silence." This typifies the experience of those who live with patients who suffer from sleep-disordered breathing. The primary indications for polysomnography include snoring, sleepiness, sleep apnea report, and physical findings consistent with upper airway obstruction or hypoxemia. A positive history using the three "S" symptom criteria (i.e., sleepiness, snoring, sleep apnea report) is a good heuristic device to use in the vast majority of appropriate patient evaluations, and these symptoms are likely the most sensitive indications. Other questions include those about the child's school performance, sweatiness, restlessness, enuresis, and triggering of apnea alarms (when the patient is monitored).

Sleepiness

Daytime sleepiness can manifest in extreme ways, such as by the child's falling asleep at school or at the park. More subtly, it is manifest by irritability, school performance below expectations, and an unwillingness to communicate with others or participate in activities.

Snoring

Although snoring in children is usually not as loud as in adults, snoring may reach concert levels (100 dB). The crescendo–decrescendo nature of snoring occurs in children as well as in adults. However, unlike the case in adults with apnea, who snore nearly 99% of the time, children's snoring is likely to be more subtle. Stridor, which is a stellar symptom of laryngotracheomalacia, can be mistaken for snoring by the parent but is unlikely to be missed by sleep technicians who are proficient at analyzing snoring. As children age, parents generally pay less attention to their children's sleep and thus are less likely to report snoring to physicians.

Apnea report

While snoring can be loud and cacophonous, it is the "quiet time" during apnea (without air) that seems endless to the observant caretaker.

The Physical Examination of the Apneic Child

The physical examination is an important component of the overall evaluation of the apneic child. Abnormal facies, such as is typically seen in patients with craniofacial syndromes, is associated with apnea (Dysun et al, 1992). Upper airway evaluation may reveal an elongated soft palate, a narrowed palatal arch, enlarged and erythematous tonsils and adenoids, or other anomalies. Nasal obstruction may also be noted, and the child may present with mouth breathing. A deviated nasal septum can cause sleep apnea. Other causes include neuromuscular diseases, mucopolysaccharide storage disorders, obesity, central hypoventilation syndrome, increased pharyngeal compliance, and gastroesophageal reflux. Cases of systemic and pulmonary hypertension, congestive heart failure, and cardiac arrhythmias are also seen (Guilleminault, 1987).

In essence, anything that during sleep has the potential to cause upper airway collapse may impinge on the airway and may be the cause of sleep apnea. During sleep, upper airway muscles lose tone. The negative intrathoracic pressure may lead to airway collapse during inspiration.

EQUIPMENT AND SUPPLIES REQUIRED TO CONDUCT CLINICAL POLYSOMNOGRAPHY

A commodious room with a comfortable bed and plenty of blankets and pillows to make the environment as home-like as possible is necessary during the recording. Bathrooms near the facility and quiet surroundings with a nearby pediatric emergency intervention team are important (Table 4–1).

An electroencephalogram (EEG) is scored by standard criteria. Before sleep spindles de-

Table 4–1 Functions of Necessary Polysomnogram Equipment

Equipment	Function
Polygraph	Record sleep, EOG, EMG, one-lead ECG using gold- or silver-plated electrodes, Sao_2 printout (cable interface), and CO_2 output (cable interface)
Thermistor probes	Record airflow through the nose and mouth
Co-oximeter	End-tidal CO_2 over nares or mouth replaces one channel for recording respiration with oral-nasal thermistor dual probe
Pulse oximeter	Measure Sao_2
Paper	Display recording
Collodion	Secure electrodes
Hypoallergenic tape	Secure electrode to scalp
Gauze pads	Cut length to fit electrode
Acetone and alcohol	Remove collodion; small amounts are needed
Electrode gel	Improve conductance of electrode; optimal mix in an aqueous solution with enough viscosity to retain consistency throughout recording period
Ink	Produce printable sleep tracing
Computer disks	For computerized polysomnography
O_2 and room air suction	Reduce secretions in tracheostomy-dependent patients when needed per patient evaluation and in treatment of patients with cardiopulmonary needs
Audio-visual recording	Document movements and significant events
	Analyze data from study and generate report
Esophageal balloons	Document upper airway resistance or obstructive sleep apnea
pH recording	Performed by specially trained health specialist when indicated for patients with suspected gastroesophageal reflux

EOG, electro-oculogram; EMG, electromyogram; ECG, electrocardiogram; Sao_2, oxygen saturation in alveolar gas.

velop, the Anders et al criteria are used; after sleep spindles develop, the Rechtschaffen and Kales criteria are used. EEG application can be complicated, and reference to the appropriate texts is mandatory for proper scoring of the EEG (Anders et al, 1971; Rechtschaffen and Kales, 1968).

Respiration, electrocardiogram (ECG), and electromyogram (EMG) measurements are parameters that continue to vary and are qualitative. Recording equipment can be adjusted to give a good signal strength. The EMG spike needs to be approximately 5 mm high at the beginning of the study. The EMG can then be altered, and an absence of EMG tone during rapid eye movement (REM) sleep can be expected.

Sleep technicians can have tremendous difficulty maintaining good-quality respiration signals. Patient movement may distort the signal strength; a secure thermistor is important. Placing electrodes on the patient's belly at the point of maximum stomach excursion (maximum pen scoring to produce sine wave form) is critical. Adjustment of the baseline signal may be required to allow adequate pen scoring to produce a sine wave. Placement of electrodes where there is the least tissue is best in order to obtain the maximum excursion; it is also best to place electrodes while the patient is inhaling and awake. Some laboratories use chest wall bands to secure the patient while observing movement. The lower chest channel placement is typically at the navel level.

The oral-nasal thermistor is essential to assess related breathing; this signal needs to be excellent. Signal strength needs to be of sufficient magnitude for the technician to differentiate among hypopnea (50% amplitude of surrounding airflow [reduction of the amplitude of the sine wave]), obstructive sleep apnea, central sleep apnea, and normal breathing. Vigilant adjustment during the night is recommended, as is making certain that abdominal leads are preserved even at the expense of upper chest leads. Figure 4–1 illustrates a child with appropriately applied electrodes.

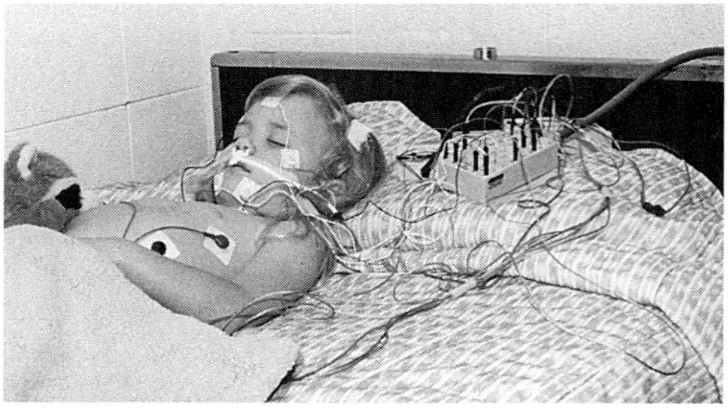

Figure 4–1 Typical placement of electrodes for a child being evaluated for sleep apnea; methods vary.

PREPARATION OF THE PATIENT AND OF THE FAMILY

Polysomnography is intensive, and many parents have waited a good deal of time for the procedure. Having the parents and child arrive early is important so that they feel comfortable with the procedure and the hospital setting. The most successful candidates for polysomnography seem to be children who have not undergone previous hospitalizations. Reassuring young patients that the procedure does not hurt is important, as is letting them know they can stop the test by letting the technician know when they are uncomfortable.

Sedation is rarely used. The caretaker is in the same room with the child throughout the night. Parents are required to stay, and bedding is provided for them. Most parents and children rarely terminate a study. Both parents and children are reassured that if the procedure is not tolerated and insufficient data are gathered to make prudent clinical judgments, they can return another night or under more auspicious circumstances (e.g., during the day when children can see the normal functioning of the center). If observation is consented to by other parents, some children are comforted by watching other children undergoing a polysomnogram.

NECESSARY TRAINING

Ideally, a specialist board certified in sleep disorders by the American Sleep Disorders Association would perform a polysomnogram. Although competent sleep specialists are vital, the backbone of any sleep center is the sleep technician. This individual must stay up all night and endure what, in many cases, is a difficult process of maintaining high-quality recordings when a recalcitrant child may be fighting the study. Patience is the most important virtue of the sleep technician in pediatric sleep medicine. Good communication with the technicians is vital to an excellent sleep center. Respiratory care practitioners, technologists, or ambitious and intelligent medically trained

Table 4–2 Standard Sensitivity and Filter Settings for Polysomnographic Parameters

Parameter	Sensitivity	High-Frequency Filter	Low-Frequency Filter
EEG activity	50 μV/cm	35 Hz	0.3 Hz
EOG activity	50 μV/cm	35 Hz	0.3 Hz
EMG activity	20 μV/cm	75 Hz	10.0 Hz
ECG activity	Varies	15 Hz	1.0 Hz
Respiration	Varies	0.5 Hz	0.15 Hz

From Keenan-Bornstein S: Respiratory monitoring during sleep: Polysomnography. In Guilleminault, C (ed): *Sleeping and Waking Disorders: Indications and Techniques.* Menlo Park, CA, Addison-Wesley Publishing Company, 1982.
EEG, electroencephalogram; EOG, electro-oculogram; EMG, electromyogram; ECG, electrocardiogram.

personnel who are knowledgeable about cardiopulmonary resuscitation and advanced cardiac life support are also critical.

METHODS

The standard settings for recording sleep, respiration (snoring is subjectively recorded or monitored), and heart rate and rhythm are listed in Table 4–2.

Measurement of Vital Functions (Table 4–3)

Sleep

Sleep is critical because during REM sleep, a flurry of physiological changes occur, which leave the apneic sleeper subject to possible pharyngeal collapse. During REM sleep, humans are paralyzed. Obstructed breathing is most likely to occur with anatomical obstruction. Upper airway muscle atonia occurs. The upper airway muscles lose tone, which allows the airway to close under the intense endothoracic pressure changes that occur during sleep. If a child goes through an entire sleep study without REM sleep (which is unlikely the younger the child), then the likelihood of a false-negative finding is increased. Studies are usually repeated when REM sleep comprises less than 10% of the entire night, if obvious apnea is not present. Figure 4–2 illustrates REM sleep. Figure 4–3 illustrates nonREM (NREM) sleep (stage 4) in a child.

EEG arousals have a direct link to excessive daytime sleepiness. Therefore, the number of arousals greater than 10 per hour, which is considered normal (Downey et al, 1989), should be noted during assessment.

Table 4–3 Polysomnogram Sample Table

Function	Values: Abnormal	Values: Normal
Apneic episodes per hour of sleep (obstructive + hypopnea + central apnea index)	5	< 5
Minimum Sao_2	75% (> 100 events below 90%)	90%
Arousals per hour	50	10–20
Pco_2 maximum	55 mm Hg	< 53 mm Hg
Technical report	Appended	

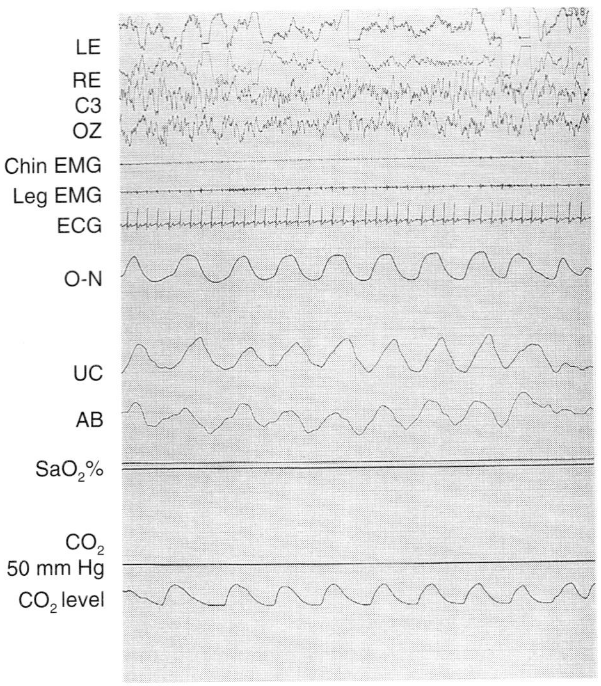

Figure 4–2 REM sleep is apparent from this recording. Notice the wave forms in the presence of muscular atonia (flat EMG) and the conjugate rapid movements of the left eye (LE) and right eye (RE). This figure shows the subtle respiratory variability and heart rate variability in REM sleep. SaO_2 and CO_2 levels are normal. C3 and OZ are EEG channels; O-N is the oral-nasal thermistor; UC is the upper chest lead; AB is the abdominal lead.

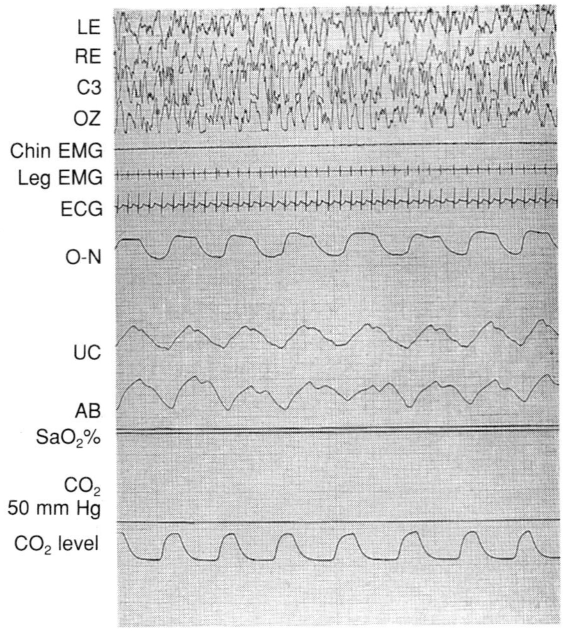

Figure 4–3 NREM sleep (sleep stage 4) is apparent from this recording. Notice that the wave forms are significantly elevated, compared with those in REM sleep in Figure 4–2, and are more sinusoidal. C3 and OZ are EEG channels; O-N is the oral-nasal thermistor; UC is the upper chest lead; AB is the abdominal lead.

Respiration

The second critical vital physiological function is respiration. It is highly unusual for children to desaturate (Sao_2 below 90%) during the course of a sleep study or to have elevations greater than 50 mm Hg in Pco_2 levels (Marcus et al, 1992) (Fig. 4–4). Consistently elevated Pco_2 levels are a harbinger of alveolar hypoventilation (Fig. 4–4).

The amount of hypoxia and desaturation during apnea may depend on three factors: baseline awake Po_2, expiratory reserve volume, and percentage of apnea time during sleep (Singer and Saenger, 1990). The worse the patient's baseline Po_2, the more profound the Po_2 becomes while the patient is asleep.

Snoring

Documentation of snoring is vital, as this symptom is rare among children without sleep apnea. Some sleep centers have found the use of a microphone attached to the side of the neck to be valuable. However, this may be less valuable in children who move frequently during sleep because it leads to artifact. Some of the newer recording machines are able to record snoring. A microphone interface can interdigitate with nearly any recorder.

Time and technique indicate when the snoring measurement is valid in children. Research documenting the predictability of apnea using this technique needs to be completed because quantifying of this variable remains elusive. In general, much like submarine sonar operators who sensitively detect sounds without computer aids, technicians are exquisitely skilled at documenting snoring without a cable snoring interface. However, a reliable snoring technology is desirable.

Oxygen Administration

The use of oxygen during a sleep evaluation may lead to spurious results because oxygen may reduce the drive to breathe, lengthen apneic episodes, and falsify Sao_2. The clinician is then misled to believe the state of apnea is not as profound as in reality. Oxygen administration should be clearly delineated on the patient report. Some patients who are under care need supplemental oxygen; in such cases, oxygen should be provided.

In some circumstances, oxygen will be titrated

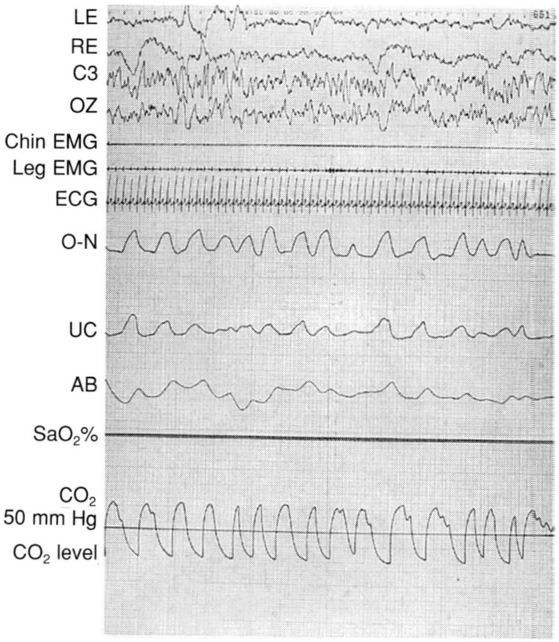

Figure 4–4 Chronic alveolar hypoventilation in REM sleep. Noticeably, the carbon dioxide (CO_2) levels remain above 50 mm Hg during this time period. During NREM sleep, CO_2 levels were normal in this child, emphasizing the importance of obtaining sufficient REM sleep in studies to warrant substantive conclusions. C3 and OZ are EEG channels; O-N is the oral-nasal thermistor; UC is the upper chest lead; AB is the abdominal lead.

in varying increments (0.25–1.0 L/min) to determine the patient's response. However, unless there is an order or a life-threatening requirement for oxygen, oxygen administration is not recommended in a diagnostic study. Oxygen may be used to treat the underlying pulmonary dysfunction.

Heart rate and rhythm

The third vital physiological function is heart rate and rhythm. Patients with sleep apnea often have arrhythmia, which resolves with treatment. The ECG is vital because during the night the technician needs to know when to intervene with cardiac life support and when to let the diagnostic study continue so that the important information can be gathered. The presence of arrhythmias may necessitate the child's being awakened or may require life-support intervention.

POST-PROCEDURE CARE

Removal of electrode paste (collodion) may require acetone, which is generally tolerated well. Tape is removed (nonsticking tape is available for sensitive patients). A typewritten report is sent to and direct contact is usually made with the patient's primary care physician regarding recommendations of care. The physician's availability to discuss options is important because sleep disorder medicine is relatively new, and physicians feel uneasy about treating these patients. Substantial guidance from specialists early in the treatment phase is important, until the responsible pediatricians feel competent to treat the apneic child. Apnea monitors should be ordered by the primary care physician.

Nasal Continuous Positive Airway Pressure (CPAP) Treatment and/or Surgical Follow-up

About half of pediatric patients tolerate nasal continuous positive airway pressure (nasal CPAP), independent of the presenting diagnosis (e.g., Down syndrome, Treacher Collins syndrome); the older the child, the better the tolerance. Half of pediatric patients will not tolerate nasal CPAP despite vigorous efforts to assuage them. Keeping contact with patients and the specialists involved in their care is critical to maintain compliance, because most patients with positive polysomnograms will require intervention.

Most patients require tonsillectomy and adenoidectomy. Perioperative management in these cases can become complicated because of the increased risk produced by anesthetic agents, tissue edema, and airway and pulmonary hemodynamic complications. These factors correlate with a history of prematurity and low birth weight, along with pulmonary hypertension, hypothyroidism, or hypoventilation, as well as continual mouth breathing. On this basis a strong recommendation is made for a follow-up polysomnogram after surgery and once tissue edema resolves (to ensure a normal test). Some patients who are at extreme risk may require tracheostomy or close observation in the hospital with concomitant polysomnograms during the resolution of symptoms.

Nasal CPAP is used when surgery or medical management is contraindicated. Figure 4–5 illustrates a nasal CPAP unit. Nasal CPAP gear is listed below:

1. CPAP unit
2. Humidifier
3. Mask supplies
4. Filters
5. Tubing
6. Head gear
7. Remote (optional)

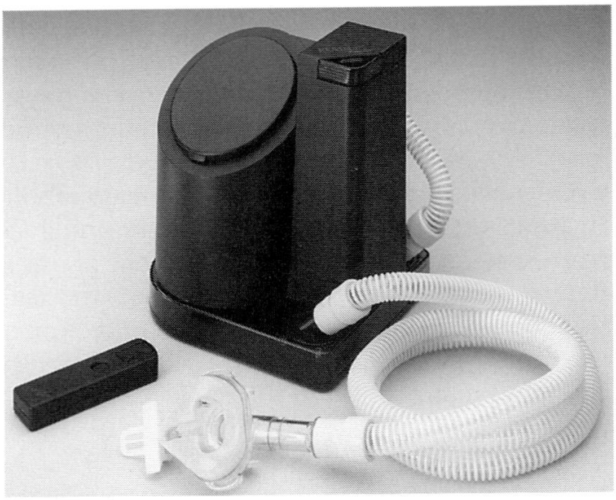

Figure 4–5 A nasal CPAP unit. (Courtesy of C&L Medical and Respironics, Inc., Murraysville, PA.)

Great preparation and care are required for nasal CPAP. Some parents find that the child has taken the CPAP mask off during the night, which is a dangerous situation without monitoring. Various methods have been employed to increase the compliance rate. The best method is to fit the patient for the mask ahead of time in the clinic or in the hospital and let him or her have time to play with it.

Most CPAP supplies come in one package for one patient. Each patient needs to be specially measured for the size of the spacer (a foam rubber or silicone piece between the forehead and mask to secure fit), mask, or nasal pillow. Some patients prefer the nasal pillow instead of the mask to fit directly into the nares for CPAP application. Other specialty masks are also available.

INTERPRETATION OF DATA

Performance and interpretation of polysomnograms require expertise and extensive training. No book chapter can supplant this training. With this rather large caveat, most studies lead to one of four diagnoses:

1. Obstructive sleep apnea
2. Upper airway resistance syndrome
3. Alveolar hypoventilation syndrome
4. Central sleep apnea

Obstructive Sleep Apnea

Figure 4–6 shows a clinical polysomnogram of a patient with obstructive sleep apnea. The patient has vigorous chest wall movement against a blocked airway. Therefore, the upper and/or lower chest may move rapidly, and there is an absence of airflow. In both central apnea and obstructive sleep apnea there is an absence of airflow; however, in obstructive sleep apnea, chest wall movement is present. In typical cases, an EEG arousal, sometimes of brief duration, accompanies the event, with the P_{CO_2} level dropping to zero, which indicates a lack of respiration. The heart rate typically slows during the event (sometimes to clinical bradycardia levels) and then will change to tachycardia when the patient gasps for air, moves, and goes back to sleep. The patient may repeat this sequence hundreds of times each night. Typically, obstructive sleep apnea is accompanied by more profound hypoxia than is central apnea. Negative endothoracic chest wall measurement can be detected, as occurs with snoring (−80 or greater cm H_2O versus −10 cm H_2O for normal sleepers) (Lugaresi et al, 1989).

Upper Airway Resistance Syndrome (UARS)

Patients with upper airway resistance syndrome do not have obvious changes on polysomnograms, unlike patients with obstructive sleep apnea. The negative pressure changes

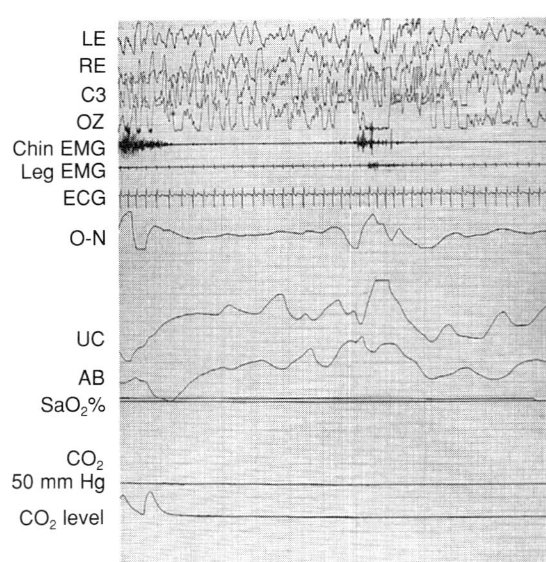

Figure 4–6 This is a recording of obstructive sleep apnea. C3 and OZ are EEG channels; O-N is the oral-nasal thermistor; UC is the upper chest lead; AB is the abdominal lead.

in the chest, as measured by endoesophageal balloons, were first discovered by Guilleminault et al (1982). Upper airway resistance syndrome accounted for approximately 20% of the diagnoses in our pediatric center. The diagnosis is typically made in the presence of a study that shows increased work of breathing as evidenced by tachycardia, chest wall excursions beyond normal, hypoxia without apnea, frequent EEG arousals, or elevations in P_{CO_2} level. Upper airway resistance syndrome patients experience the same hazards as do obstructive sleep apnea patients. A strong positive family history and a sleep study suggestive of increased work of breathing usually help to identify upper airway resistance syndrome. These patients respond well to the same treatments as for obstructive sleep apnea; however, they seem to be highly underdiagnosed in the population of sleep disorder–affected children.

Alveolar Hypoventilation

Sleep studies may be helpful in detecting hypoventilation, because P_{CO_2} levels typically rise during sleep. Without adequate control of P_{CO_2} levels, elevations occur. The norms set by Marcus et al (1992) are helpful in interpreting these data. In their study, it was rare for P_{CO_2} values in sleeping children to exceed 53 mm Hg; the average was approximately 38 mm Hg. End-tidal P_{CO_2} values can be easily measured in sleeping children, and these values are important for diagnosing alveolar hypoventilation (see Fig. 4–4). As Figure 4–4 shows, these children can have elevations of end-tidal P_{CO_2} level during normal sleep that are not associated with the typical clinical sequelae in children with obstructive sleep apnea or upper airway resistance syndrome. Rather, the child sleeps as the P_{CO_2} level remains elevated.

Central Sleep Apnea

Central sleep apnea is most common in infants and young children or in children with neurological disorders. During the first year of life, many children, especially premature infants, will have central sleep apnea. Kahn et al (1992), in a large-scale Belgian study, did not find central sleep apnea to be associated with sudden infant death syndrome (SIDS). Rather, obstructive sleep apnea was found to be a significant predictor of SIDS. Although this does not provide conclusive proof of a causal relationship between obstructive sleep apnea and SIDS, the data are suggestive.

Central sleep apnea can be dangerous, particularly when it is related to gastroesophageal reflux. The clinical polysomnogram shows no oral-nasal airflow and no diaphragmatic movement, indicating an absence of movement of both the upper and lower chest walls. EEG arousals may be present, and snoring may be present before and after the arousals. Oxygen desaturation can be profound, as in obstructive sleep apnea. In one study of 50 apparently normal sleeping children, 30% had episodes of central sleep apnea longer than or equal to 10 seconds. One child had an episode of central sleep apnea associated with an S_{aO_2} less than 90% (Marcus et al, 1992). On this basis, patients who desaturate below 90% may warrant a full diagnostic evaluation.

POSSIBLE COMPLICATIONS

Few complications are associated with polysomnography because it is not an invasive test. Not all possible complications can be foreseen, but these complications are the most common. Most often, the untoward events include allergies to the tape or collodion associated with the tests. The antidote to the sticky collodion is an alcohol/acetone mixture gingerly placed on the scalp when removing electrodes. Technicians need to be careful to avoid getting acetone into the patient's eyes. Eye washing should be immediate and extensive if this should happen, and the injured person should undergo an extensive visual examination by a specialist. Generalizations about which patients will tolerate the procedure are often wrong.

References

Anders T, Emde R, Parmelee AH (eds): *A Manual of Standardized Terminology, Techniques and Criteria for Scoring of Sleep and Wakefulness in Newborn Infants.* Los Angeles, UCLA Brain Information Service/Brain Research Institute, 1971.

Downey R, Bonnet MH, et al.: Comparison of sleep stage and arousal indices in normal young adult sleepers, normal elderly adult sleepers and elderly adult insomniacs. *Sleep Research*, 18:137, 1989.

Downey R, Perkin R: Upper airway resistance syndrome: Sick, symptomatic but underrecognized. *Sleep* (In Press).

Dyson M, Beckerman RC, Brouillette RT: Obstructive sleep apnea syndrome. In Beckerman RC, Brouillette RT, Hunt CE (eds): *Respiratory Control Disorders in Infants and Children.* Baltimore, Williams & Wilkins, 1992, pp 212–230.

Guilleminault C: Obstructive sleep apnea syndrome in children. In Guilleminault C (ed): *Sleep and Its Disorders in Children.* New York, Raven Press, 1987, pp 213–229.

Guilleminault C, Winkle R, Korobkin R, Simmons B: Children and nocturnal snoring—Evaluation of the effects of sleep related respiratory resistive load and daytime functioning. *Eur J Pediatr*, 139:165–171, 1982.

Kahn A, Grosswasser J, Rebuffat E, et al: Sleep and cardiorespiratory characteristics of infant victims of sudden death: A prospective case-control study. *Sleep*, 15:287–292, 1992.

Keenan-Bornstein, S: Respiratory monitoring during sleep: Polysomnography. In Guilleminault C (ed): *Sleeping and Waking Disorders: Indications and Techniques.* Menlo Park, CA, Addison-Wesley Publishing Company, 1982, p 183–212.

Lugaresi E, Cirignotta F, et al: Snoring: Pathogenic, clinical, and therapeutic aspects. In Kryger MH, Roth T, Dement WC (eds): *Principles and Practice of Sleep Medicine*, 2nd ed. Philadelphia, WB Saunders, 1989, pp 621–629.

Marcus CL, Omlin KJ, Basinki DJ, et al: Normal polygraphic values for children and adolescents. *Am Rev Respir Dis*, 146:1235–1239, 1992.

Martin RJ, Block AJ, Cohn MA, et al: Indications and standards for cardiopulmonary sleep studies. *Sleep*, 8(4):371–379, 1985.

Rechtschaffen A, Kales A (eds): *A Manual of Standardized Terminology, Techniques and Scoring System For Sleep Stages of Human Subjects.* Los Angeles, UCLA Brain Information Service/Brain Research Institute, 1968.

Singer LP, Saenger P: Complications of pediatric obstructive sleep apnea. *Otolaryngol Clin North Am*, 23:665–676, 1990.

Chapter 5

Fiberoptic Bronchoscopy

Bruce G. Nickerson

Fiberoptic (or flexible) bronchoscopy is the examination of the airways from the nose to the fourth or fifth generation of bronchi using a flexible fiberoptic bronchoscope. Fiberoptic bronchoscopy is feasible for nearly all pediatric patients; only a few considerations related to size, degree of illness, or underlying medical conditions preclude it. The technique is relatively easy to learn, and in experienced hands it is safe. Fiberoptic bronchoscopy frequently yields important information about the anatomy, degree of obstruction, or dynamics of the airways. It also provides access to specimens from the lower airways. Individual bronchi can be selectively lavaged in order to relieve mucus plugging. Fiberoptic bronchoscopy is most commonly done in sedated, spontaneously breathing patients. A fiberoptic bronchoscope can be threaded through an endotracheal tube or tracheostomy while mechanical ventilation is continued.

INDICATIONS

Fiberoptic bronchoscopy is indicated when the benefits to the patient outweigh the risks involved. It is not indicated when a safer or better course of treatment is available. For example, fiberoptic bronchoscopy is not indicated in an otherwise healthy child with simple pneumonia because the most likely causes include infection with viruses or bacteria, which may be treated with relatively harmless antibiotics. In contrast, fiberoptic bronchoscopy is frequently indicated in an immunocompromised host whose pneumonia is likely to be life-threatening and who requires treatment with potentially toxic antibiotics that could be discontinued based on the results of the bronchoscopy.

UPPER AIRWAY PATHOLOGY

Fiberoptic bronchoscopes may be used for nasal endoscopy to look at the anatomy of the posterior nasal cavity. This is particularly useful in patients who have had a cleft palate repaired. Nasal endoscopy allows the physician to look at the closure of the palate and to evaluate the result of surgery or effectiveness of prostheses or the need for further specific speech therapy.

Fiberoptic bronchoscopes are also useful in

evaluating children with laryngomalacia and other causes of congenital stridor. There are three types of laryngomalacia; the most common type is prolapse of the arytenoids, in which the patient has large and hypotonic arytenoids that prolapse with each breath. With the fiberoptic bronchoscope, the arytenoids can be seen to be vibrating in conjunction with the patient's stridor. Less common and more serious is the stovepipe epiglottis type of laryngomalacia, in which the epiglottis curves on itself and collapses during inspiration. This is often associated with arytenoid prolapse as well. Rarely, children with other congenital anomalies can have an epiglottis that folds on itself in an anteroposterior plane, which creates a trap-door closure of the airway.

Hemangiomas may affect the upper trachea. Rarely, congenital webs may also cause congenital stridor.

Following trauma, intubation, or infection in children, acquired tracheal stenosis may be present and may be evaluated by flexible bronchoscopy.

Vocal Cords

The vocal cords should be carefully evaluated during each fiberoptic bronchoscopic procedure. The bronchoscopist should make sure that both vocal cords abduct and adduct from their neutral position. Patients with meningomyelocele or patients who have recently undergone chest surgery may have unilateral or bilateral vocal cord paralysis. Congenital unilateral or bilateral vocal cord paralysis may also cause congenital stridor.

Trachea and Bronchi

The trachea is well evaluated by the fiberoptic bronchoscope, because during the procedure the patient ventilates spontaneously. Evidence of tracheomalacia with dynamic collapse of areas of the trachea in which the cartilaginous supports are deficient is easily seen. External compression by abnormal blood vessels in patients with cardiac defects (e.g., tetralogy of Fallot) or by lymph nodes (e.g., tuberculosis) may also be seen. Children with glycogen storage diseases may have tracheomalacia demonstrated as short, wide tracheal cartilages. Evidence of bronchial stenosis, malacia, or plugging may also be viewed with the flexible bronchoscope. Using a small scope, four to five generations of bronchi can be visualized and evaluated.

Pneumonia

In patients with suspected infection of the lungs, alveolar washings may be obtained to identify aerobic and anaerobic bacteria, fungi, acid-fast bacteria, viruses, and parasites (e.g., *Pneumocystis carinii*, lung flukes, *Strongyloides*, and *Ascaris*). Also, the macrophages can be evaluated for the presence of fat globules, which suggests recurrent aspiration. In asthmatic patients, the alveolar washings may be filled with eosinophils. There is also interest in cytology of the alveolar washing, although the exact interpretation of cytology results is not yet clear.

Foreign Bodies

Fiberoptic bronchoscopy is usually contraindicated for patients in whom a foreign body is strongly suspected, as these patients are better treated by rigid bronchoscopy. Rigid bronchoscopy allows better control of the airway, and it is done in the operating room with the patient under general anesthesia. Rigid bronchoscopes provide better ventilation and permit the use of instruments for removing large foreign bodies.

CRITICALLY ILL PATIENTS

Fiberoptic bronchoscopy may be done in critically ill patients if the bronchoscopist is experienced and is able to perform bronchoscopy rapidly with minimum compromise of the airway. Critically ill patients also require judicious use of sedation and must be attended by personnel who are skilled in intubation and resuscitation procedures. Monitoring the patient's oxygen saturation, heart rate, blood pressure, and sometimes transcutaneous carbon dioxide level can be helpful.

PREPARATION OF THE PATIENT

Prior to fiberoptic bronchoscopy, there should be a thorough review of the history, physical findings, differential diagnosis, medications, history of adverse reactions to medications, and indications for the bronchoscopy. Radiographic results (and often the actual films) should be available for review. Relevant laboratory tests and reports of previous bronchoscopic or other relevant surgical procedures should be reviewed, as should the patient's allergies and reaction to sedation. The bronchoscopist should discuss the risks and goals of the procedure with the parents and the patient.

The risks of fiberoptic bronchoscopy include sedation, airway compromise due to obstruction by the scope, and post-procedure stridor or bronchospasm. Many patients experience minor nasal bleeding after bronchoscopy, and the patient and parents should be so warned.

Rarely, infection may be introduced by the bronchoscope or spread from one area to another. One or two percent of patients develop fever or increased cough following bronchoscopy. Post-bronchoscopy stridor or wheezing may be easily treated with racemic epinephrine or β-adrenergic aerosols. Rarely, instances of respiratory failure have been reported. There is one report of death following flexible fiberoptic bronchoscopy with extensive alveolar lavage in a critically ill patient with impending respiratory failure.

Prior to the bronchoscopic procedure, the patient should have an empty stomach. Generally, patients should have nothing orally for 3 to 6 hours before. This should be confirmed with the patient's parents and nurses prior to proceeding with the bronchoscopy. In an emergency, the stomach may be emptied using a nasogastric tube, but the bronchoscopist should be aware that this may empty only about half of the stomach contents, and there is consequently an increased risk of aspiration.

Table 5–1 Necessary Equipment and Medication For Fiberoptic Bronchoscopy

Equipment	
Bag and masks of different sizes	
Light source	
Oxygen for the bag and mask	
Oxygen for the mouth	
Phenylephrine	
Specimen labels	
Suction for the bronchoscope	
Suction for the mouth	
Suction traps	
Tube thoracostomy tray	
Various sizes of bronchoscopes	
Various sizes of endotracheal tubes and laryngoscopes	
Lidocaine 1%	
Lidocaine 2% jelly	
Emergency Drugs	
Albuterol	
Atropine	
Calcium gluconate	
Epinephrine 1:10,000	
Furosemide	
Lavage medium (saline, Plasma-Lyte, isotonic bicarbonate)	
Lidocaine (intravenous solution)	
Midazolam	
Naloxone	
Phenobarbital	
Racemic epinephrine	
Sodium bicarbonate 1 mEq/ml	
Sedative Drugs	
Diazepam	Meperidine
Fentanyl	Midazolam
Ketamine	Morphine

EQUIPMENT

The room in which the bronchoscopy will take place should be spacious enough to allow room for the patient, bronchoscopist, and at least two assistants, as well as the equipment for the bronchoscopy and any emergency (Table 5–1). The room should be provided with a variable light source so that the lights can be dimmed to improve viewing through the bronchoscope and to provide a hypnotic atmosphere for the patient. There should be a sink available for washing hands and rinsing the bronchoscope. Monitors should be available for measuring oxygen saturation, blood pressure, transcutaneous oxygen, and carbon dioxide levels, and for the electrocardiogram.

The patient's bed should be able to be raised and lowered. A neck roll is important for adequate positioning of the patient. A papoose board is helpful to securely restrain toddlers.

Suction should be available for attachment to the bronchoscope and for suctioning out the mouth independently. A variety of sizes of suction catheters and tonsil suction should be available. Two sources of oxygen should also be available. During bronchoscopy, most patients wear an oral face mask to receive supplemental oxygen. Oxygen should also be attached to the bag and mask. Occasionally, oxygen may be fed into the bronchoscope to provide additional oxygen during the procedure.

The equipment should be checked to make sure that it is adequately prepared for the bronchoscopic evaluation. The functioning of the bronchoscope, monitors, light source, and video recorder and the availability of suction traps should be checked. Equipment for intravenous medications, including a heparin lock, is helpful. A resuscitation cart should be available with a variety of sizes of endotracheal tubes, chest tubes, and pediatric resuscitation drugs. These should include 0.5% phenylephrine for dilation of the nose and 1% and 2% lidocaine for anesthetizing the nose and posterior airway. Racemic epinephrine should be available to manage postoperative stridor. Albuterol should be available for aerosol treatment of wheezing. A bag and masks in a variety of mask sizes should be available for different-sized pediatric patients. A variety of sizes of endotracheal tubes and laryngoscopes should also be available, in case the patient requires intubation. A chest tube should be available in case of pneumothorax. Naloxone should be available for reversing the effects of narcotics, if there is excessive sedation. Atropine should also be available for reversing vagal spells. Epinephrine, sodium bicarbonate, calcium gluconate, phenobarbital, and lidocaine should be available in the emergency code cart.

A bronchoscopy laboratory can be started with a versatile 3.7-mm bronchoscope with a 1.7-mm suction channel. However, in a busy service, it is helpful to have a variety of sizes of bronchoscopes (Table 5–2). A larger 4.9-mm bronchoscope with a 2.2-mm suction channel can be very helpful for older patients with bronchial plugging who require extensive lavage and suctioning. Smaller bronchoscopes such as the 2.2-mm scopes, which do not have a suction channel, can be helpful for examining the airways of premature infants.

Table 5–2 Flexible Bronchoscopes

External Diameter	Suction Channel Diameter
2.2 mm	0
3.7 mm	1.7
4.9 mm	2.2
6.0 mm	2.2

PERSONNEL

Prior to the bronchoscopy, the bronchoscopist and assistants should discuss the specific goals and anticipated difficulties of the procedure.

It is helpful to have two assistants for a flexible bronchoscopy. One assistant's job is to handle the bronchoscope, suction traps, light source, and video camera and to directly assist the bronchoscopist. The other assistant watches the patient and monitors; he or she must be experienced in recognizing clinical deterioration, malfunction of the monitors, true cyanosis, bradycardia, and arrhythmias. That assistant may also be in charge of administering intravenous drugs.

The bronchoscopist should have extensive experience with children who have lung disease. This experience is best obtained in a residency and a fellowship involving extensive clinical training in a wide variety of pediatric pulmonary problems. The bronchoscopist should first master controlling the scope and smoothly moving it rapidly in the desired direction. This experience can be obtained in a course using mannequins or animal models to obtain technical expertise. The bronchoscopist needs to gain facility in rapidly finding the vocal cords. This requires excellence in moving the scope rapidly, meticulous positioning of the patient, and judicious suctioning of the airways when required.

The bronchoscopist should also be experienced in administering sedation. The bronchoscopist should be comfortable with several different types of sedation, as the patient's previous reactions or allergies may dictate the choice of drug. The bronchoscopist should also have experience recognizing significant pathology of the upper and lower airways. This can be learned by studying some of the excellent atlases of upper airway pathology but is best obtained by attending a large number of bronchoscopies. The bronchoscopist should also be facile in dealing with problems that may be encountered. These include undersedation or oversedation, wheezing, stridor, seizures, apnea, and rashes. Recognition and rapid response to decreases in oxygen saturation or heart rate should also be practiced.

PROCEDURE

When the patient is brought to the bronchoscopy room, the informed consent and confirmation that the patient has had nothing orally for the prescribed period should be checked. The patient should be connected to the pulse oximeter and electrocardiogram monitors. If an intravenous line has not already been started, intravenous access should be established.

It is very important to maintain a calm, hypnotic atmosphere in the bronchoscopy suite. Children who are unafraid and calm require much less sedation than those who are terrified and out of control.

The patient should be positioned near the head or the side of the bed with an adequate neck roll to maintain the chin in the "sniffing" position.

Prior to manipulation of the nose, the patient should be sedated. Administration of midazolam (0.1 to 0.2 mg/kg) repeated every 3 to 5 minutes until an adequate level of sedation is obtained often works well. Midazolam can be alternated with fentanyl at a dosage of 1.5 to 3 µg/kg to provide better analgesia. Alternatives to this regimen include the use of morphine, meperidine, pentobarbital, diazepam, or ketamine. Each of these has its relative advantages and disadvantages. For example, ketamine may cause increased airway secretions; meperidine may cause histamine release; diazepam is longer acting than midazolam.

The patient's nose should be prepared. First, 2 drops of 0.5% phenylephrine are placed in the nostril to be used. Using the left nostril for most flexible bronchoscopic procedures allows the left hand to be used to turn the scope without obstructing the right nostril. After the phenylephrine is administered, the nostril is packed with lidocaine jelly, which may be painted on with a cotton-tipped applicator. After several minutes, the cotton-tipped applicator dipped in 2% lidocaine jelly is positioned in the patient's posterior nostril. The nose can be further anesthetized by dripping liquid 1% lidocaine into the nostrils. This allows for anesthetizing the nose, and as the lidocaine dribbles into the posterior pharynx, it also provides good anesthesia of the posterior pharynx. If adequate anesthesia has been used, the patient should not feel when the cotton-tipped applicator is withdrawn.

When the patient is prepared, the nose is anesthetized, the patient is well sedated, and all the equipment has been checked, the bronchoscopist is ready to proceed. The distance from the nose to the vocal cords should be gauged, and the bronchoscope should be gripped with the left hand at approximately that distance. This allows the bronchoscopist to constantly monitor the position of the end of the bronchoscope relative to the position of the vocal cords, so that time is not wasted searching for the vocal cords in the posterior nares or down the esophagus. The bronchoscope is controlled by turning the scope with the left hand and moving the tip up or down with the thumb of the right hand. The right index finger can be used to apply suction.

The importance of a good neck roll for placing the airway in the proper position so that the vocal cords can be easily visualized cannot be overemphasized. Occasionally, this can be enhanced by having the assistants hold the ends of a piece of gauze to maintain the patient in a jaw-thrust or tongue-pull position. The bronchoscope should be advanced until the larynx is visualized. The motion of the vocal cords in both abduction and adduction should be confirmed.

If the vocal cords are not adequately anesthetized, spraying 1 ml of 1% lidocaine into the larynx via the suction channel usually provides adequate anesthesia so that laryngospasm is not produced by touching the vocal cords with the bronchoscope. Anesthetizing the cords should be done very judiciously. Too much anesthesia may predispose the patient to aspiration of saliva and upper airway secretions, which may contaminate lower airway specimens and may decrease cough. Also, administering anesthetics (e.g., lidocaine) through the bronchoscope may contaminate the scope with bacteriostatic solutions, which may decrease the yield from cultures. On the other hand, the cords should be anesthetized adequately so that the scope can be easily passed without provoking laryngospasm.

Usually, the bronchoscope is advanced using an S-curve motion into the trachea. When entering the larynx, the bronchoscope is advanced anteriorly so that the anterior commissure can be seen. The bronchoscope is turned posteriorly and advanced through the cords near the posterior commissure at their widest opening; it is then turned anteriorly again so that the trachea can be seen.

If keeping the scope sterile for cultures is particularly important, the scope can be kept free of upper airway secretions by blowing oxygen through it at a rate of 2 to 3 L/min or approximately 50 ml/sec. If this is done, the bronchoscopist must be careful at all times not to allow the tip to be occluded.

In patients requiring lavage, aliquots of volumes between 1 ml and 15 ml are usually used, depending on the size of the patient. A total lavage volume of 1/4 of functional residual capacity (or approximately 5 ml/kg) has been suggested. Solutions used to lavage the lungs should be nearly isotonic. Isotonic saline, Plasma-Lyte, or isotonic bicarbonate, which may be prepared by diluting 1 ml of a standard 1-mEq/ml solution of bicarbonate with 6 ml of sterile water, may be used to soften secretions. If hypertonic or hypotonic solutions are used, they may provoke cough or bronchospasm.

The specimen obtained should be viewed for color, consistency, and the presence of casts or chunks, which may suggest a foreign body or the presence of *Aspergillus*. The specimen should be sent for studies appropriate to the differential diagnosis. Studies of specimens obtained by flexible bronchoscopy include

- Bacterial culture and sensitivity
- Gram's stain

- Fungal culture and stain
- Acid-fast bacteria culture and stain
- Viral culture and fluorescent antibody
- Fat-laden macrophages
- Eosinophils
- Direct smear for parasites
- Silver stain for *Pneumocystis carinii*
- Cytology
- Surfactant Constituents

After the bronchoscopic procedure, the patient should be monitored until the sedation has worn off. Because of airway anesthesia, the patient should not have anything orally for at least one hour. The bronchoscopist should discuss the findings of the examination with the parents and reassure them immediately following the bronchoscopy. The parents then may join the child coming out of sedation, if they are cautioned that the child is still under the influence of the medication. The bronchoscopy results should be dictated for the medical record promptly.

If a patient is intubated with an endotracheal tube, bronchoscopy may be performed with a Bodi attachment while the patient is being ventilated. A 3.7-mm fiberoptic scope will fit through a 4.5-mm or larger endotracheal tube. The 2.2-mm bronchoscope will fit through a 3.0-mm endotracheal tube. Precautions should be taken to keep the patient from biting the bronchoscope through the endotracheal tube, which might damage the fibers. Ventilator settings often need to be increased while the bronchoscope is in place, particularly if the bronchoscope is close in size to that of the endotracheal tube. If the patient has a tracheostomy, the bronchoscope may be inserted through the nose and passed posterior to the tracheostomy along the pars membranosa. If this is done gently, the area above the tracheostomy usually can be adequately examined for the presence of granuloma. The scope can then be passed behind the tracheostomy, and bronchoscopy of the lower airways also can be performed while the patient is ventilated through the tracheostomy.

In patients who require intubation, the fiberoptic bronchoscope is inserted nasally. The nose is prepared as described previously. The endotracheal tube of the appropriate size is loaded over the bronchoscope without an adapter. Lubrication with saline or lidocaine may be used to facilitate the sliding of the endotracheal tube over the bronchoscope. The endotracheal tube should be positioned so that it is not sheathing the flexible bronchoscope tip. The bronchoscope can be gripped firmly through the endotracheal tube in order to provide rotation. The scope is passed through the nares, the vocal cords are visualized and anesthetized, the bronchoscope is passed into the trachea, and the endotracheal tube is slid off the bronchoscope. The position of the endotracheal tube can be confirmed by visualizing the carina, and the endotracheal tube then can be precisely positioned. This procedure can be useful in positioning the endotracheal tube below the area of obstruction in patients with conditions such as tracheomalacia or stenosis.

Chapter 6

Aerosols

Paul Lubinsky

The optimum route for administration of many pulmonary therapeutic agents is via inhalation. Drugs are safer, more effective, and better tolerated when inhaled than when administered orally or parenterally. Inhaled therapeutic agents are delivered directly to the site of action, minimizing the vagaries of absorption and metabolism while providing immediate onset of action at lower doses and with minimal systemic side effects. The most commonly inhaled medications are bronchodilators, which affect sympathetic and parasympathetic airway receptors. Anti-inflammatory medications, such as steroids and cromolyn sodium, are also being used more frequently. Other medications delivered via aerosol include mucolytics and anti-infectious agents.

The efficacy of inhaled medications is a function of the amount of drug deposited on the walls of specific airways. The delivery of inhaled medications is dependent on several variables: particle size, particle charge, speed of inhalation, and coordination of inhalation with delivery. These factors are affected by the composition of the delivery solution and addition of substances such as diluents, surfactants, and propellants. The type of delivery system also will affect the delivered dose.

Optimum particle size is 1 to 7 micrometers (μm). Particles $< 1\ \mu m$ behave like a gas and are often exhaled, whereas particles $> 10\ \mu m$ deposit in the mouth, oropharynx, and tubing or spacer device. Deposition in central and peripheral airways is preferred. There is minimal absorption from the proximal airway, and alveolar deposition is associated with rapid absorption and increased systemic effects.

TYPES OF AEROSOL DELIVERY SYSTEMS: NEBULIZERS AND INHALERS

Nebulizers

Nebulizers are used to deliver anti-infectious agents and other drugs that are not available in metered dose inhalers. Because they require only tidal volume breathing, nebulizers are preferred for unconscious, uncooperative, or uncoordinated patients. Nebulizers are also used for continuous administration of aerosolized therapeutic agents, such as albuterol and ribavirin.

Jet nebulizers

Jet nebulizers utilize a jet of air/O_2, in which the Venturi effect draws the medication solution from the nebulizer's reservoir to create the aerosol. The aerosol then strikes a baffle, which further disperses the solution. The baffle and walls of the nebulizer capture the larger droplets, which are then renebulized. The gas stream carries the smaller droplets. The design of a nebulizer, the driving flow of the gas, and the type of solution determine the size of droplets that are delivered. A large proportion of the drug remains on the walls of the nebulizer, and the larger particles deposit in the tubing between the patient and the nebulizer. There is also a considerable amount of wastage when the patient is not inhaling. A jet nebulizer delivers approximately 2% of the drug to the airway. The jet nebulizer should have a reservoir attached that fills with aerosolized medication immediately prior to the next inhalation (Fig. 6–1).

Jet aerosols may also be administered to ventilated patients but require that the respiratory therapist spend more time to achieve the same therapeutic effect. It also requires adjustment of the ventilator settings because the increased flow increases tidal volume and airway-distending pressures. The increase in bias flow also reduces the sensitivity of the system, which makes it more difficult for patients to trigger assisted breaths. Dosing is more accurate with MDIs because a standard dose is delivered with each actuation, solutions are not prepared individually, and there is no judgment involved in deciding when the treatment is completed.

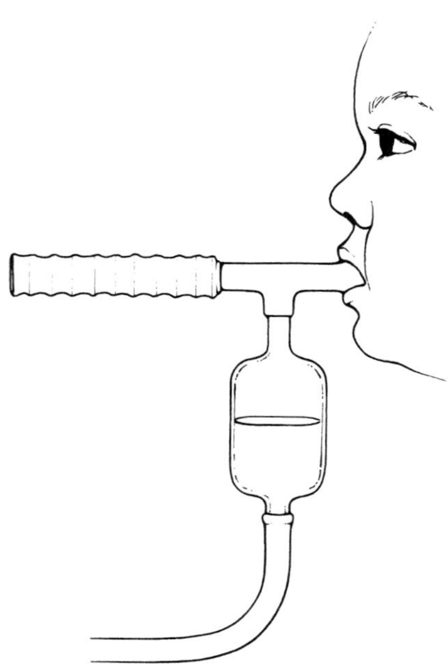

Figure 6–1 Jet nebulizer with reservoir.

Ultrasonic nebulizers

Ultrasonic nebulizers use a piezoelectrical crystal that directs ultrasonic sound waves at an air–fluid interface, which creates a cloud of small particles (Fig. 6–2). The number and size of the particles vary with the frequency and power. For maximum drug delivery, the connecting tubing should be as short and as wide as possible.

Metered dose inhalers

Metered dose inhalers (MDIs) are propellant-driven devices. Chlorofluorocarbons are frequently used as propellants because they are biologically inert and evaporate rapidly on exposure to air, leaving the particles of suspended drug. Some MDIs dispense drug dissolved in the propellant. Other types of MDIs have solid microparticles suspended in a propellant, and these usually contain a surfactant to prevent clumping of the particles. Approximately 10% of the delivered dose reaches the lungs, with the majority of the drug being lost in the mouth and nasopharynx. Delivery of bronchodilators via MDIs is gaining acceptance in patients who are cooperative or in those with whom a spacer device may be utilized (Fig. 6–3). MDIs are also used for ventilated patients. The dose is delivered via an inline adapter attached directly into the ventilator circuit. MDIs have been demonstrated to deliver medications as effectively as nebulizers, while being more cost-effective. The amount of time required to deliver a given therapeutic dose is markedly reduced with MDIs.

Equipment for continuous nebulization

- Ultrasonic or other nebulizers
- Aero mask/trach collar
- Hood
- Blender/flow meter
- Heated humidifier
- Medications prescribed
- One-way valve
- Oximeter
- Oxygen analyzer
- Large-bore tubing

For continuous nebulization with a ventilator, additional necessary equipment includes

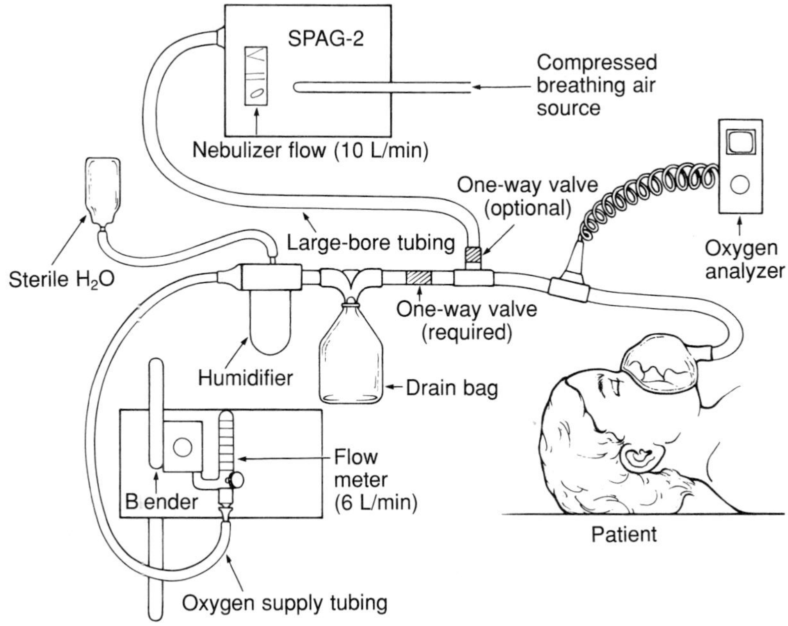

Figure 6–2 Connection of the small particle aerosol generator (SPAG-2) when used for continuous nebulized bronchodilator therapy. (Courtesy of Children's Hospital of Orange County, Orange, CA.)

- A reservoir on the inspiratory limb—for patients < 20 kg, approximately 250 ml (optimal configuration); for patients > 20 kg, approximately 500 ml
- Filter prior to the exhalation valve if necessary

Delivery of medication via an MDI requires an MDI reservoir with a port to accept MDI placed in the inspiratory limb.

MEDICATIONS

Delivery and Dosing

The amount of drug delivered to the lungs is proportional to the size of the endotracheal tube, with the best delivery occurring with larger tubes and inversely proportional to the inspiratory flow rate. Experimental models have been used to study delivery through ventilator circuits, but these cannot compensate for the amount of drug that would settle in the upper airway or be exhaled. In vitro models also cannot mimic flow patterns and distribution within the lung with airways of varying calibers. Aerosol deposition may be determined using radioactive isotopes, but these studies are not performed in children. Dosing is therefore individualized by assessing the severity of the patient's airway dysfunction and titrating the dose to the clinical response and development of side effects, while understanding the unique attributes of the system (e.g., only a small portion of the nebulized drug is delivered). Doses of 5 mg/hr reportedly do not cause side effects in young children; and nebulized doses of 25 mg/hr (even as high as 30–40 mg/hr) in children weighing 1 to 30 kg have been used without causing side effects.

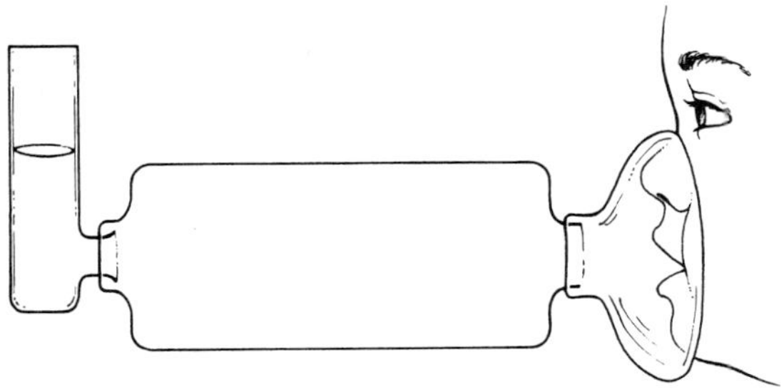

Figure 6–3 Metered dose inhaler (MDI) with spacer.

β-Adrenergic Agonists Agents

β-Adrenergic agonists agents are used commonly in the ICU to reduce bronchospasm by inducing relaxation of the bronchial smooth muscle. β-Adrenergic agonists also inhibit mast cell degranulation, reduce mucous gland secretion, augment mucociliary clearance, and improve respiratory muscle contractility.

These agents are useful for treating many disorders characterized by reversible bronchospasm and difficulty clearing airway secretions. These disorders include acute severe asthma, bronchiolitis, bronchopulmonary dysplasia, cystic fibrosis, and cardiac lesions with left to right shunting. The augmentation of diaphragmatic function is a serendipitous therapeutic effect. Dosage of albuterol (0.5%) is generally 0.02 to 0.04 ml/kg rounded to the nearest 0.05 ml. Peak onset of action is 30 to 60 minutes, and duration of action is 4 to 6 hours. There are increasing data supporting titration of the dose of aerosolized bronchodilator medications delivered by all types of aerosol generators. Because of individual patient variations, the dose should be titrated to the point that therapeutic effects or significant side effects are noted.

Jet nebulizer administration

Medications delivered via a jet nebulizer are usually diluted in 2 to 3 ml 0.9% saline. For patients with severe bronchospasm, pure albuterol without a diluent may be administered via a nebulizer for a total of 12 to 20 breaths or until side effects are evident. This may be repeated as tolerated until a therapeutic response occurs. Alternatively, repeated doses from an MDI with spacer may be administered until a therapeutic response is achieved.

Side effects from these agents are related to β_1 receptor activity and include tachycardia, tremor, and hyperactivity. The development of more selective β_2-adrenergic agents has significantly reduced these side effects. Hypokalemia is associated with β_2-adrenoreceptor stimulation. Serum potassium levels need to be monitored at least daily in patients receiving frequent or continuous aerosol administration.

Continuous aerosol administration

The administration of continuous aerosols of β-adrenergic agonists is supplanting the use of intravenous isoproterenol in the management of acute severe asthma, and it is also superior to frequent intermittent therapy. Continuous aerosol administration is used when the patient is not responding sufficiently to repeated administration of β-adrenergic agonists. (These patients are also receiving oxygen, inhaled parasympathomimetics, steroids, and on occasion intravenous aminophylline.) It is postulated that continuous aerosol administration reduces rebound bronchospasm by providing constant β-sympathomimetic stimulation, which promotes progressive bronchodilation. Continuous aerosol administration decreases the amount of time needed to deliver the bronchodilator; continuous nebulization maximizes the opportunities for the patient to rest.

Continuous aerosols may also be delivered to ventilated patients. Ultrasonic nebulizers are advantageous because they do not introduce a bias flow into the system. Aerosol administration should occur at least halfway up the inspiratory limb of the circuit because the inspiratory limb then acts as a reservoir. Administration immediately prior to the Y adapter or between the Y adapter and the endotracheal tube has been demonstrated to be suboptimal. Delivery of intermittent or continuous aerosols is further enhanced by having a reservoir at least equivalent to the tidal volume on the inspiratory limb of the circuit. Some ventilators may require filters in the expiratory limb to protect their flow transducers when continuous nebulization is employed.

Ultrasonic nebulizer administration

A 1:10 to 1:1 solution of 0.5% albuterol delivered via a small particle aerosol generator (SPAG) ultrasonic nebulizer aerosolizes approximately 10 ml of the solution per hour (see Fig. 6–2). The solution is prepared by the pharmacy in a 250-ml bag of normal saline, which is placed in the reservoir. A 1:10 solution aerosolizes approximately 5 mg/hr, a 1:4 solution aerosolizes 10 mg/hr, and a 1:1 solution aerosolizes 25 mg/hr. This solution may be administered via mask, hood, pup tent, or mist tent or in-line in a ventilator circuit. If possible, the larger tents should be avoided to maximize drug delivery. Another technique uses an infusion pump to drip albuterol into the reservoir of a standard jet nebulizer at a steady rate. The patient must be monitored for side effects. If an aminophylline infusion is being used, the dose needs to be increased and closely monitored because there is increased clearance. The initial solution is usually a 1:2 solution, which is then adjusted depending on the clinical response and the presence of side effects. As the patient improves, the concentration may be decreased or the patient may be switched directly to intermittent therapy.

Specific dose recommendations are not available at present. The volume of drug aerosolized depends on the specific nebulizer used, the fill volume, the type of drug and diluent, the length of connecting tubing, and the mechanism of aerosol delivery to the patient. The dose is also affected by the patient's respiratory rate and tidal volume; therefore, smaller patients with lower minute ventilation receive less drug than larger patients with the same drug concentration and nebulizer setup. Additionally, the narrower the airways, the less aerosol deposition occurs distally. Infants with narrower airways or more severe airway dysfunction receive less of an administered dose than do larger children and adults.

Administration via metered dose inhaler

There are multiple adapters for introducing MDIs into the ventilator circuit. Optimal administration is achieved by having a 250- to 500-ml reservoir just above the Y adaptor on the inspiratory limb of the ventilator circuit. While use of a reservoir optimizes drug delivery, an MDI may be used without one but may require additional actuations to achieve the same therapeutic effect. The MDI is actuated immediately prior to the inspiratory cycle. Alternatively, a spacer can be attached to the endotracheal tube to bag in the treatment. The administration of at least four puffs has been recommended for adults, but in fact the number of puffs should be individualized to the therapeutic response. A study of albuterol administration in neonates by Denjean et al (1992) showed near-maximal benefit with two puffs, but four puffs could be delivered without significant adverse effects.

Parasympathomimetics

Atropine and ipratropium bromide are parasympathomimetic agonists that have a synergistic effect in combination with the β-adrenergic agonists. They are potent bronchodilators and appear to affect the larger airways. Compared to the β-adrenergic agonists they have a delayed onset of action but a longer duration of action. The nebulizer solution of ipratropium was recently approved by the FDA. It is available in a 0.5 mg/2.5 ml vial. Dosing is not yet established in the pediatric patient. A dose of 0.5 mg/10 kg is a reasonable starting point; the dose may then be titrated to the desirable effect.

Racemic Epineprhine

Racemic epinephrine contains equal amounts of dextrorotatory and levorotatory forms of epinephrine. Its activity is mediated by the stimulation of β-sympathomimetic receptors. It induces local vasoconstriction, which reduces mucosal swelling. Racemic epinephrine is utilized in pathophysiological processes characterized by upper airway obstruction and stridor. These conditions include viral croup, postextubation mucosal edema, angioneurotic edema, and acute laryngospasm. Racemic epinephrine is also used to counteract mucosal edema induced by environmental irritants, such as smoke. It is also useful to help ameliorate worsening upper airway obstruction in patients with laryngotracheomalacia. Racemic epinephrine has also been used topically during bronchoscopy to facilitate the removal of impacted foreign bodies. Racemic epinephrine 2.25% is diluted to a volume of 2 to 3 ml and administered via nebulizer in the following doses:

patients $<$ 10 kg: 0.25 ml
patients 20–40 kg: 0.5 ml
patients $>$ 40 kg: 0.75 ml

Racemic epinephrine has an immediate onset of action, and the dose may be repeated as necessary while the patient is monitored for side effects. All children who receive a racemic epinephrine treatment need to be observed for at least 4 hours because it has a short duration of action and does not alter the natural course of the disease.

Racemic epinephrine may also be delivered as a continuous aerosol in a 1:5 solution via an ultrasonic nebulizer or dripped continuously into a jet nebulizer hourly at three times the standard nebulizer dose. A greater proportion of the racemic epinephrine is therapeutically effective because the site of action is the upper airway, and thus the droplets that settle here are active, as opposed to β-adrenegic agonists that are active only when delivered to and absorbed from the distal airways.

Ribavirin

Ribavirin is a virustatic agent with a broad spectrum of activity against RNA and DNA viruses. The indications and clinical efficacy of ribavirin remain controversial, but it is currently recommended by the AAP for patients with respiratory syncytial virus (RSV) infection who fall into a high-risk group. A multi-institutional study was begun in 1993 in pediatric ICUs under the auspices of the Pediatric Critical Care Study Group to evaluate ribavirin use. Provisional reports from this study do not support the use of ribavirin. In some institutions ribavirin is used to treat patients with RSV bronchiolitis and pneumonia who do not fall into the high-risk group.

Aerosolized administration appears to be effective against respiratory pathogens because high concentrations of particles are achieved in respiratory secretions. Systemic absorption is minimal, and no significant patient side effects have been documented. The dose is 6 mg of ribavirin in 300 ml sterile water, which is aerosolized using an ultrasonic SPAG and administered via hood or face mask for 18 hours per day. In another regimen the drug is concentrated and delivered for 2 hours three times per day, but this does appear to be as well tolerated by the patient or the caregivers.

Infants on ventilators as a result of RSV infection are also considered to fall into the high-risk group by many practitioners. Initiation of mechanical ventilation or progressive respiratory failure is also considered an indication for ribavirin therapy. Administration of ribavirin to mechanically ventilated patients can be accomplished safely but has been associated with complications caused by crystallization of the ribavirin at areas of turbulence and at the expiratory valve.

The following recommendations must be followed to administer ribavirin safely:

1. One filter must be placed in front of the expiratory valve, and a second filter must be placed on the inspiratory limb between the humidifier and the one-way valve through which the aerosol enters.
2. The filters must be changed every 2 hours.
3. The one-way valve should enable flow from the nebulizer toward the patient.
4. The circuit should be examined at least every 30 minutes for crystal deposition.
5. The inspiratory and expiratory pressures being delivered to the patient should also be checked every 30 to 60 minutes.

Ribavirin is teratogenic in animals, and it is recommended that pregnant and breastfeeding caregivers avoid exposure. A scavenger hood (Figs. 6–4 and 6–5) is often used for patients who are not intubated and receiving ribavirin. The exhaust gases from mechanically ventilated patients should pass through a filter.

Patients should be in a private room with negative pressure, and the room air should be exchanged six times per hour with outside air or through a high-efficiency particulate air (HEPA) filter. Hospital personnel should also utilize full-barrier protection when caring for these patients (i.e., goggles, mask, gown, gloves).

Equipment used for ribavirin therapy includes

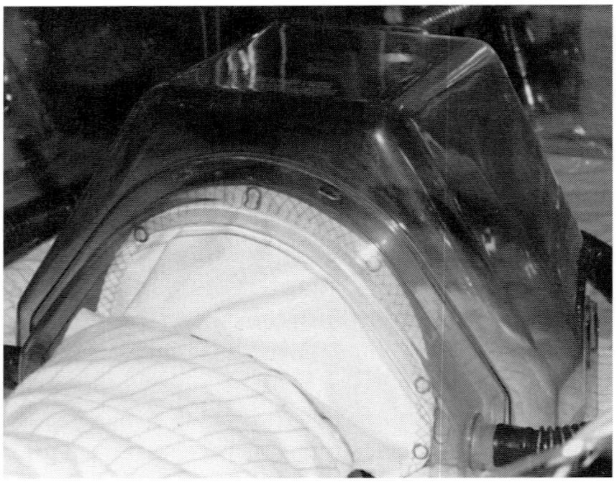

Figure 6–4 Scavenger hood.

- SPAG
- Aero mask, hood, or tent
- Blender/flow meter
- T-connector
- One-way valve
- Vacuum unit
- Hood unit with collar attached
- Disposable filters
- Large-bore tubing
- Oxygen analyzer
- HEPA filter unit

Mucolytics

There are currently two therapeutic agents used to enhance mobilization of secretions. Acetylcysteine (Mucomyst) disrupts the sulfur bonds of the mucoproteins. It is used in patients in whom viscous secretions contribute to airway obstruction. Between 1 and 2 ml of the

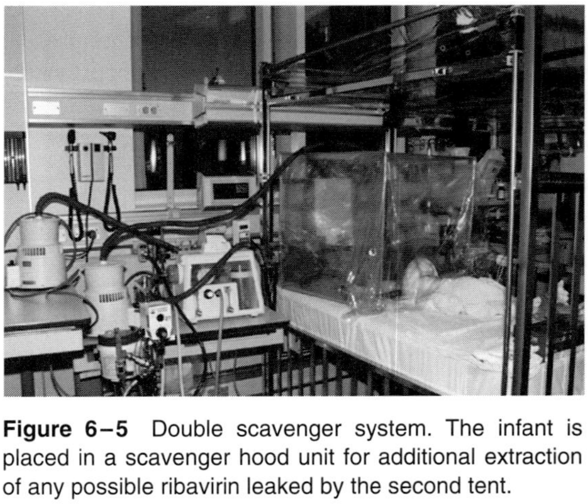

Figure 6–5 Double scavenger system. The infant is placed in a scavenger hood unit for additional extraction of any possible ribavirin leaked by the second tent.

20% solution are administered 3 to 4 times daily with 2.5 ml of 0.9% sodium chloride. It is administered in conjunction with a bronchodilator because it may produce bronchospasm. Administration is followed by percussion and postural drainage.

Pulmozyme (dornase alfa) is a recently approved agent that has undergone extensive study in patients with cystic fibrosis. It is administered as an aerosol with a dose of 1 vial daily and works by breaking down the DNA strands from destroyed white cells in the mucus; this decreases the viscosity of the mucus and thus enhances mucociliary clearance. Further delineation of efficacy in patients with cystic fibrosis and other pathophysiological processes is still necessary.

Antimicrobials

An increasing number of antibacterial agents can be delivered directly to the bronchial tree. Antibiotics such as tobramycin, Coly-Mycin, and gentamicin are used frequently in patients with cystic fibrosis. Pentamidine is used prophylactically in immunocompromised patients.

All aerosolized bronchodilators and mucolytics can be mixed for intermittent therapy. The antimicrobials are also frequently mixed with bronchodilators at the time of administration. Further studies need to be done to see which medications can be mixed for 24-hour periods of continuous administration.

Bibliography

Ackerman AD: Continuous nebulization of inhaled β-agonists for status asthmaticus in children: A cost-effective therapeutic advance? *Crit Care Med*, 21:1442–1444, 1993.

American Academy of Pediatrics, Committee on Infectious Disease, Hall CB (Chairperson): Use of ribavirin in the treatment of respiratory syncytial virus infection. *Pediatrics*, 92:501–504, 1993.

Calacone A, Walkove N, Stern E, et al: Continuous nebulization of albuterol (salbutamol) in acute asthma. *Chest*, 97:693–697, 1990.

Consensus Conference on Aerosol Delivery, sponsored by the American Respiratory Care Foundation and the American Association for Respiratory Care: *Resp Care*, 36:916–921, 1991.

Denjean A, Guimaraes H, Migdal M, et al: Dose related bronchodilator response to aerosolized salbutamol (albuterol) in ventilator-dependent premature infants. *J Pediatr*, 120:974–979, 1992.

Gay PC, Patel HG, Nelson SB, et al: Metered dose inhalers for bronchodilator delivery in intubated, mechanically ventilated patients. *Chest*, 99:66–71, 1991.

Kerem E, Levison H, Schuh S, et al: Efficacy of albuterol administered by nebulizer versus spacer device in children with acute asthma. *J Pediatr*, 123:313–317, 1993.

La Via W, Marks MI, Stutman HR: Respiratory syncytial virus puzzle: Clinical features, pathophysiology, treatment and prevention. *J Pediatr*, 121: 503–509, 1992.

Manthous CA, Hall JB, Schmidt GA, et al: Metered-dose inhaler versus nebulized albuterol in mechanically ventilated patients. *Am Rev Resp Dis*, 103:1567–1570, 1993.

Papo MC, Frank J, Thompson AE: A prospective, randomized study of continuous versus intermittent nebulized albuterol for severe status asthmaticus in children. *Crit Care Med*, 21: 1479–1486, 1993.

Rau JL, Harwood RJ, Groff JL: Evaluation of a reservoir device for metered-dose bronchodilator delivery to intubated adults. *Chest*, 102: 924–930, 1992.

Wilson AF: Aerosol delivery systems. In Weiss EB, Stein M (eds): *Bronchial Asthma, Mechanisms and Therapeutics, 3rd ed.* Boston, Little Brown, 1985, pp 749–755.

Chapter 7

Cystic Fibrosis —Diagnosis

David A. Hicks

Cystic fibrosis (CF) is the most common genetic disease of the Caucasian population. It is also present in African-American and Asian populations. Since the 1930s, when the term fibrocystic disease of the pancreas was first used for CF, advances in the diagnosis and treatment of CF have increased the median age of survival from less than 5 years to 29 years. The pathological changes of malabsorption (leading to weight loss) and recurrent pulmonary infections (leading to destruction and fibrosis of the lungs) are well known. Knowledge of the pathogenesis of these changes has increased rapidly over the last 20 years. The sweat electrolyte abnormality was first recognized in 1953, but it was not until 1983 that the chloride-transport defect was identified. For decades, the genetic basis for transmission of CF was assumed. It was not proven until the CF gene was identified and cloned in 1989.

GENETIC BASIS

The inheritance of CF follows mendelian rules and is autosomal recessive. The incidence in Caucasian populations is between 1:2000 and 1:4500 live births. In the African-American population, it is approximately 1:27,000 live births; and the Oriental population, the incidence of CF is 1:90,000 or more live births. The CF gene is located on chromosome 7. The protein encoded by the gene is called the cystic fibrosis transmembrane conductance regulator (CFTR). There are more than 300 different known mutations of the CF gene. The most common mutation involves the omission of three base pairs, which results in the deletion of phenylalanine at the 508 position on the gene. This mutation is observed in about 70% of individuals of Northern European ancestry. Among patients registered by the Cystic Fibrosis Foundation who were genotyped in 1991, 50% were homozygous for delta 508, 40% were compound delta 508 heterozygous, and 10% had two mutations other than delta 508.

Currently, the phenotypic expression of the CF gene has only one correlation: delta 508 and pancreatic insufficiency. Genotype and a variety of other factors appear to have a role in the progression and severity of pulmonary disease.

DIAGNOSIS

The diagnosis of CF is based upon a combination of patient and family history, physical findings, and laboratory analysis. The family history can often be helpful. The following historical information can increase the suspicion of CF:

A parent with recurrent sinopulmonary disease
A mother who had difficulty in getting pregnant
A family member who died in childhood with lung problems
A family member with CF

Presenting signs and symptoms for CF can be common or uncommon (Table 7–1). Any of these presentations should prompt a suspicion of CF and lead to appropriate laboratory studies. At least 15% of CF patients have a history of meconium ileus. The diagnosis of CF should always be considered in a newborn with meconium ileus or peritonitis because approximately 80% to 85% of these infants have CF. Meconium plugging is a cause for concern and follow-up. One report indicates a 25% chance for CF in infants with meconium plugging. Young children, adolescents, or adults may present with a meconium ileus equivalent or a small bowel obstruction with impacted viscous material. These individuals often have unneeded surgical intervention. The most frequent early presenting problem is failure to thrive, which is caused by pancreatic dysfunction and malabsorption. Families often complain that an infant or child has a voracious appetite with weight loss or failure to gain weight, as well as foul-smelling, large, bulky stools. Malabsorption can lead to hypoproteinemia, loss of fat-soluble vitamin K, hypoprothrombinemia, and rectal prolapse.

Any infant or child with recurrent respiratory disease in the first 1 or 2 years of life should have a sweat test. Repeated attacks of bronchiolitis, wheezing, productive cough, sinusitis, or pneumonia are a cause for concern. A lower respiratory tract infection caused by a *Pseudomonas* organism, specifically the mucoid strain, is also a cause for concern.

Persistent metabolic alkalosis is caused by excessive loss of sodium and chloride in the sweat. Azoospermia results from an absence or atrophy of the vas deferens and seminal vesicles.

The physical signs that may suggest a diagnosis of CF include the following:

- Poor weight gain and growth
- Muscle wasting
- Digital clubbing
- Hyperexpanded chest, bronchiectasis, chronic cough
- Peripheral edema
- Protuberant or distended abdomen
- Wheezing, crackles
- Nasal polyps
- Rectal prolapse
- Cirrhosis of the liver, portal hypertension

Table 7–1 Presenting Signs and Symptoms of Cystic Fibrosis

Common Presentations	Uncommon Presentations
Newborns and Infants	**All Age Groups**
Failure to thrive	Biliary cirrhosis and portal hypertension
Malabsorption	Diabetes mellitus
Meconium ileus	Edema and hypoproteinemia, hypoprothrombinemia
Children	Enlarged submaxillary glands
Failure to thrive	Gallstones, biliary colic
Malabsorption	Hemoptysis
Recurrent nasal polyposis	Meconium ileus equivalent, intestinal obstruction syndrome
Recurrent respiratory disease	Meconium peritonitis
Adolescents and Young Adults	Meconium plug syndrome
Azoospermia	Persistent metabolic alkalosis
Malabsorption	Rectal prolapse
Recurrent sinopulmonary disease	Recurrent hyponatremia/hypochloremia and heat prostration

LABORATORY DIAGNOSIS

The laboratory diagnosis for CF includes prenatal testing and screening examinations in the newborn, sweat analysis, and genetic testing.

Newborn Screening and Prenatal Testing

As newer therapies are developed to treat the underlying pathophysiology of CF, early diagnosis may become more important. Early diagnosis and treatment may help to preserve lung function, reverse abnormal growth, and promote early family–patient education about CF. Data from the Cystic Fibrosis Foundation indicate that there are many months between the onset of symptoms and the final diagnosis.

The use of microvillar intestinal enzyme

analysis by amniocentesis may be helpful for families in whom the affected individual's CF genotype is not known. As treatment and preventive strategies for CF improve, the need for prenatal testing may change.

Newborn screening for CF was introduced several years ago in a number of countries and in a few states in the United States. To date, a highly reliable, cost-effective screening method has yet to gain universal acceptance. Follow-up studies of screened infants have not conclusively demonstrated that diagnosis in newborns results in better survival. Of the two screening tests available, the meconium albumin test and the serum immunoreactive trypsin test, the latter seems to have the most promise.

Normal meconium usually contains little or no albumin.The amniotic albumin, which is swallowed by the fetus, normally is destroyed by pancreatic enzymatic action. Most fetuses with CF produce inadequate amounts of enzymes to catabolize the albumin. High albumin levels can be found in the meconium of newborns with CF. The test does have a high incidence of false negatives and has false positives, as well.

Many newborns with CF have high levels of serum trypsin, which is detectable by radioimmunoassay. The increased levels of trypsin may be caused by a backup of pancreatic trypsin from blocked pancreatic ductules. The test can be performed on a dried blood spit; it is inexpensive, but it may fail to identify the 10% to 15% of newborns with CF who have normal pancreatic function. There appears to be an age-related decline in serum trypsin so that by 6 to 8 weeks of age, the levels may be normal. If the serum immunoreactive trypsin test is done, it must be backed up by careful clinical follow-up, sweat analysis, and possibly genetic analysis.

Sweat Analysis

Since its introduction in 1959, the sweat test has been the single most useful laboratory test for identifying an individual with CF. This test relies upon the stimulation of sweat by pilocarpine iontophoresis (Fig. 7–1). The accurate collection and analysis of the sweat sample is of critical importance. Most errors in the test lie in sample collection and analysis. The Cystic Fibrosis Foundation recognizes only the iontophoretic method. There are two methods for sweat collection: the Gibson-Cooke test by Farrall Instruments and the Marroduct Sweat Collection by Wescor, Inc., which is more simple. The sweat test measures both sodium and chloride. A positive test result is indicated by a sweat chloride value of 60 μg/L or greater. Many physicians who deal with CF believe there is an age distribution for a positive value (i.e., > 60 μg/L before age 20 years, > 80 μg/L after age 20 years). It is important to note the sweat sodium value. There should not be more than a 10-mEq/L difference between the sodium and chloride values. The sweat test is suspect if too great a difference exists. To ensure quality and uniformity, only a few laboratory technologists should be doing the test in each hospital.

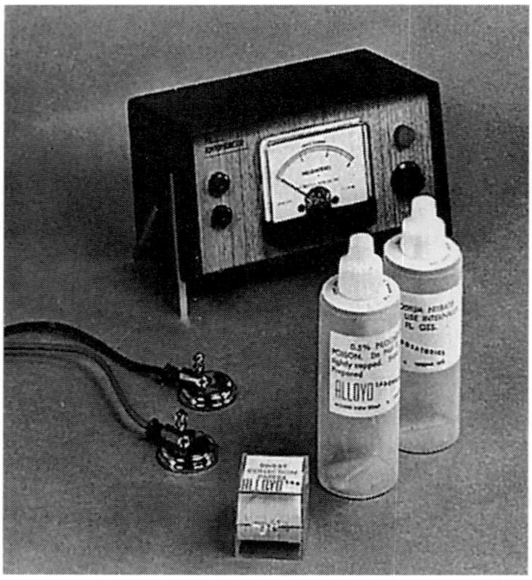

Figure 7–1 Equipment for collection of sweat after pilocarpine iontophoresis. (From Hughes WT, Buescher ES: *Pediatric Procedures.* Philadelphia, WB Saunders, 1980, p 315.)

Diseases that may demonstrate falsely elevated sweat chlorides include the following:

- Untreated adrenal insufficiency
- Ectodermal dysplasia
- Hereditary nephrogenic diabetes insipidus
- Glucose-6 phosphatase deficiency
- Malnutrition
- Hypothyroidism
- Mucopolysaccharidosis
- Fucosidosis

Genetic Testing

Since the discovery of the CF gene in 1989, genetic testing of CF has spread rapidly. The cost of DNA testing has decreased, and ease with which it is done has increased. With the availability of genetic analysis, prenatal testing of fetal tissues can be performed to determine if the CF genotype is present. Most laboratories test for the 10 or 15 most common CF genes. Such genetic testing may be useful to a family with a CF history. What may be particularly useful is to know what CF genotype may exist. Knowing the CF genotype of the pregnant woman, the father, and the person affected with CF can be helpful to the geneticist for determining the possibility of CF in the fetus.

Genetic testing can be very helpful when the clinical examination, history, or sweat test is inconclusive. However, routine screening of the population of individuals with no family history of CF is unwarranted at this time.

Chapter 8

Chest Physical Therapy

Rocky Stone

BACKGROUND AND INDICATIONS

The umbrella term chest physical therapy (CPT) describes a variety of techniques designed to aid in the mobilization of bronchial secretions, the prevention of secretion accumulation, and the improvement of gas exchange in the treatment of acute and chronic lung disease (Burton and Hodgkin, 1984; Committee on Bronchial Hygiene, 1991; Eid et al, 1991; MacKenzie, 1989; Proceedings of the Conference on the Scientific Basis of In-Hospital Respiratory Therapy, 1980; Wade and Badgett, 1990). These techniques include postural drainage and turning; chest percussion and vibration; cough; suction; the forced expiration technique (FET); and newer modalities such as autogenic drainage, positive expiratory pressure (PEP), and high-frequency type devices. Most often, these techniques are used in combination to promote secretion clearance.

CPT has indications for a variety of clinical conditions, including cystic fibrosis, bronchiectasis, and atelectasis (Cole, 1984; Eid et al, 1991; Hammon and Martin, 1981; Lorin and Denning, 1971; Mazzocco et al, 1985; Wong et al, 1977). However, recent studies do not support the efficacy of CPT in patients with uncomplicated pneumonia or uncomplicated exacerbations of asthma, unless those patients produce excessive amounts of sputum. CPT is also not indicated in the treatment of bronchiolitis or in routine care of postoperative patients, unless they have an underlying respiratory disease for which CPT is known to be beneficial (Conners et al, 1980; Kirillof et al, 1985; Murray, 1979; Quittel et al, 1988; Reines et al, 1982; Stapleton, 1985; Sutton et al, 1982; Webb et al, 1985; Wissing et al, 1988).

The effectiveness of CPT has been debated over the years, and more recently its efficacy has been vigorously challenged (Anderson and Falk, 1991; Murray, 1980; Pontoppidan, 1980; Sutton, 1988; Wollmer et al, 1985). Many time-honored therapies have been abandoned following numerous controlled clinical trials, in which the techniques either have shown no demonstrable benefit or have proven to be hazardous to the patients they are intended to help (Campbell et al, 1975; Christensen et al, 1990; Falk et al, 1984; Huseby et al, 1976; McDonnell et al, 1986; Ricksten et al, 1986; Sutton et al, 1983; Wollmer et al, 1985).

CHEST PHYSICAL THERAPY TECHNIQUES

Postural Drainage Techniques

Postural drainage therapy (PDT) is intended to promote mobilization of bronchial secretions and to normalize functional residual capacity (FRC) (Committee on Bronchial Hygiene, 1991; Sutton, 1988). PDT relies on gravitational forces, turning of the patient in various positions to promote drainage, and the external manipulation of the thorax (Burton and Hodgkin, 1984; Committee on Bronchial Hygiene, 1991; Wade and Badgett, 1990). The usefulness of PDT remains controversial. There are studies that support its efficacy (Etches and Scott, 1978; Finner and Boyd, 1978; Reismann et al, 1988) and those that find no appreciable benefit to the patient (Falk et al, 1984; Murray, 1980; Wollmer et al, 1985).

The areas of the lungs to be treated should be determined on the basis of radiographic findings and auscultation of the chest. Prior to initiation of any of these techniques, the procedure should be fully explained in nontechnical language to the patient or the patient's family.

Positioning

Postural drainage begins with placing the child or infant in the proper position, so that the uppermost involved segments receive treatment first (Burton and Hodgkin, 1984; Carlo and Chatburn, 1979). If possible, the child or infant should be placed on a bed, warmer, or table that can be adjusted to the Trendelenburg position or the reverse Trendelenburg position. However, neonates should not be placed in the Trendelenburg position because it may increase the risk for developing intraventricular hemorrhage (Ravel et al, 1985). Studies have also reported incidents of hypoxemia in neonates during PDT (Fox et al, 1978). Additionally, if the patient is receiving enteral feeds or has just eaten, feeding should be stopped and therapy should be delayed at least 1 hour to reduce the risk of emesis or of aspiration of gastric contents.

During postural drainage, pillows should be used for support, as well as comfort. The infant or child should be as comfortable and as relaxed as possible to achieve maximum benefit from therapy. Infants tend to relax when held; therefore, the infant may be held or laid across an adult's knees when practical. The infant should be supported with a firm hand and percussed with the other.

Percussion

Percussion is the rhythmic application of kinetic energy to the external thorax by use of a cupped hand or a mechanical percussor. Percussion is performed directly over the pulmonary segments being drained. During this procedure, the cupped hand should make a "popping" sound as it strikes the chest. The procedure should be continued throughout the inspiratory and expiratory cycle (Burton and Hodgkin, 1984; Carlo and Chatburn, 1979; Committee on Bronchial Hygiene, 1991; Wade and Badgett, 1990).

Electric and pneumatic percussors are frequently used in the home and hospital settings. Many practitioners and patients prefer them to traditional hand percussion; however, there is no convincing evidence that demonstrates the superiority of one method over the other (Committee on Bronchial Hygiene, 1991). Electric percussors or vibrators must never be used on a patient who is in an oxygen-enriched environment (e.g., tent, isolette).

Vibration

Vibration is best described as a fine tremulus or a repetitive isometric contraction of the practitioner's shoulder and forearm, manually performed over the affected area during expiration (Burton and Hodgkin, 1984; Ravel et al, 1985). Currently, there is no conclusive clinical evidence to support the efficacy of vibration therapy or the superiority of the manual method versus the mechanical method (Committee on Bronchial Hygiene, 1991).

There is no standard amount of time that each segment or lobe should undergo percussion, vibration, and postural drainage. The therapy must be tailored to the particular needs of the patient. Generally, if there is no increase in cough or in expectorated secretions after 2 to 10 minutes, the practitioner should proceed to another segment or lobe (Burton and Hodgkin, 1984). The patient should be encouraged to cough forcefully following treatment in each of the various positions.

Cough

The ability to cough effectively is one of the most important factors in the management of bronchial secretions. In infants, gentle cricoid pressure is sometimes effective in stimulating a cough (Burton and Hodgkin, 1984; Wade and Badgett, 1990). However, there may be factors that impair an infant's or a child's ability to cough effectively, including the presence of an artificial airway, tracheal or laryngeal stenosis from prolonged intubation, tracheomalacia, neuromuscular disease, muscular weakness secondary to prolonged mechanical ventilator support, sedation, and pharmacologically induced paralysis (Burton and Hodgkin, 1984; Carlo and Chatburn, 1979; Committee on Bronchial Hygiene, 1991; Wade and Badgett, 1990).

Suction

When the patient is unable to clear secretions, tracheal suction may be indicated. Endotracheal or nasotracheal suctioning, which is an important component of CPT (Committee on Bronchial Hygiene, 1992), involves the insertion of a suction catheter through an endotracheal tube, a tracheostomy tube, or the nasal passages into the trachea of a patient to remove secretions or foreign material.

Tracheal suction is indicated to maintain airway and endotracheal tube patency or to remove accumulated secretions that remain following the patient's best cough efforts (Committee on Bronchial Hygiene, 1992). The practitioner should assess the effectiveness of the child's cough and auscultate the chest for indications for suction. Therapy is judged effective on the basis of improved breath sounds and the removal of secretions.

Because suctioning is considered such a routine part of a patient's respiratory care, there may be the tendency to minimize the potential complications. The procedure, even when performed properly, is a risky and somewhat complicated modality that should be undertaken only by those who understand the potential hazards and complications (Burton and Hodgkin, 1984; Committee on Bronchial Hygiene, 1992; Kerem et al, 1990; Riegel and Forshee, 1985). Whenever this procedure is performed, the following signs should be monitored:

- Skin color
- Oxygenation (with pulse oximeter when available)
- Pulse rate (with electrocardiogram monitor if available)
- Breath sounds
- Respiratory rate
- Cough

In the acute-care setting or for a potentially unstable patient, the following equipment should be utilized or available:

- Oxygen
- Resuscitation bag with manometer
- Mask of appropriate size
- Protective equipment for personnel

Forced Expiratory Technique

FET involves a series of forceful expirations from mid- to low-lung volumes, while maintaining an open glottis ("huff cough"). Huffing consists of one or two forced expirations (i.e., short, sharp, expiratory blasts) from mid-lung volume, followed by relaxed, controlled diaphragmatic breathing. Secretions that are mobilized are then expectorated, and the procedure is repeated until maximal clearance of the bronchi is achieved (Gaskell and Webber, 1980; Pryor et al, 1979). Studies comparing FET to coughing exercises or classic or traditional CPT (i.e., postural drainage, percussion, vibration) have shown FET to be superior in the enhancement of secretion removal (Sutton et al, 1983; Sutton et al, 1985). A study by Pryor and associates documented an increase in sputum production and clearance when FET was combined with cough and CPT (Pryor et al, 1979). In addition to these benefits, FET is a procedure that can easily be taught to age-appropriate patients and employed for home therapy. It does not require any special skills or equipment.

Autogenic Drainage

Autogenic drainage (AD) appears to be an effective technique for aiding the mobilization of accumulated bronchial secretions and excessive secretion production associated with cystic fibrosis and bronchiectasis. AD attempts to mobilize secretions in the peripheral airways first, progressing toward the central airways last, where secretions can be removed by "huff" cough (Chevaillier, 1984).

AD assumes that by using systematic breathing and control of expiratory flows, the airway can be stabilized and secretion removal enhanced. AD begins with low-volume breathing, inspiratory breath holds, and controlled expiration; it progresses toward increased inspiratory volumes and increased expiratory flow rates. This procedure is repeated for 1 to 3 minutes, or until crackles or rales are heard near or at the beginning of exhalation. Crackles heard at the beginning of exhalation indicate that the patient should be advanced to the next lung volume level. Several huff coughs are then performed to expectorate secretions (Chevaillier, 1984; Kraemer et al, 1986).

Advantages of AD include the following:

- Patients can perform the technique without assistance.
- Special equipment is not necessary.
- The technique can be performed anywhere.

However, AD is difficult to teach, and its usefulness in seriously ill patients is somewhat doubtful (Anderson and Falk, 1991).

Positive Expiratory Pressure

Positive expiratory pressure (PEP) is used to assist in removing bronchial secretions from patients with chronic pulmonary disease (Christensen et al, 1990; Mahlmeister et al, 1991; Sutton et al, 1982). PEP therapy enhances secretion mobilization by stabilizing compliant airways, by reducing airway collapse, and by increasing collateral ventilation (Eid et al, 1991; Paul and Downs, 1981). The mobilized secretions are then cleared by the use of FET or cough. PEP has also been effectively used in the treatment of postoperative atelectasis (Paul and Downs, 1981).

PEP, like AD and FET, does not require the assistance of gravity to promote secretion removal. However, PEP does require specialized training and some simple equipment.

The PEP system consists of a face mask or mouthpiece, a T-assembly, and a one-way valve, on which an expiratory resistance device can be placed. A pressure manometer is placed into the assembly between the one-way valve and the resistance device to determine the PEP level. The appropriate level of resistance is determined for the individual patient to produce a steady 20 to 30 cm H_2O of PEP during mid-expiration. With the patient seated, different levels of resistance are tested. The size of the hole in the resistance device is gradually reduced until the correct level of PEP is reached. During this adjustment period, diaphragmatic breathing is utilized, with the patient breathing at a volume slightly larger than tidal volume. The patient is instructed to actively but not forcefully exhale to maintain a PEP of 10–20 cm H_2O (Anderson and Falk, 1991; Mahlmeister et al, 1991). Expiration should be twice as long as inspiration. The patient takes 10 to 20 breaths following the above procedure, then does several huff coughs to raise secretions (Pryor et al, 1979).

PEP therapy is attracting increasing interest, and clinical results are very encouraging. Clinical studies have indicated that PEP therapy is more effective than classical CPT for secretion mobilization (Falk et al, 1984; Tonnesen and Stovring, 1984). Also, one study demonstrated an improvement in measured oxygen tension during and after treatment (Falk et al, 1984).

Contraindications for PEP include active hemoptysis and an unresolved pneumothorax. As always, the practitioner should evaluate the patient carefully before initiating any therapy.

High-Frequency CPT

High-frequency chest wall oscillation (HFCWO) was proposed as a mechanism for improving mobilization of secretions from the peripheral airways (Chang, 1989; King et al, 1983; Selsby and Jones, 1990). Hansen and Warwick (1990) developed the high-frequency chest compression (HFCC) system, which is an updated version of CPT used in the CF population.

The system uses an inflatable vest that fits snugly over the patient's thorax. The vest is linked via flexible hoses to a variable-frequency, air-pulse delivery system. Air pulsates through the entire vest and oscillates the thorax, which produces airflows that are intended to enhance the movement of secretions toward the large airways. The patient then uses huff coughs to clear secretions from the airway.

HFCC has shown promise in initial clinical studies (Hansen and Warwick, 1990; Warwick and Hansen, 1990). In contrast to those studies, McEvoy and associates (1982) found that high-frequency oscillation (HFO), when applied to the airway opening, reduced the rate of secretion clearance in the peripheral airways. Multicenter studies are needed to further evaluate the role and efficacy that these high-frequency devices have in clearance of bronchial secretions.

HAZARDS AND COMPLICATIONS

The caregiver must closely monitor the patient for signs of distress or pain during CPT. Evidence of hypoxemia, increased intracranial pressure, pulmonary hemorrhage, dysrhythmias, acute hypotension, vomiting and aspiration, pain, and bronchospasm is an indication to stop therapy and consult the physician. Therapy may need to be modified in postsurgical patients, as well as those with cardiac disease, fractures, chest tubes, or gastroesophageal reflux. The Trendelenburg position should be avoided in patients with increased intracranial pressure, premature infants, patients with uncontrolled hypertension, and patients at risk for aspiration.

References

Anderson JB, Qvist J, Kann T: Recruiting collapsed lung through collateral channels with positive end expiratory pressure. *Scand J Respir Dis*, 60:260–266, 1979.

Anderson JB, Falk M: Chest physiotherapy in the pediatric age group. *Respir Care*, 36:546–554, 1991.

Burton GG, Hodgkin JE: *Respiratory Care: A Guide to Clinical Practice, 2nd ed.* Philadelphia, JB Lippincott, 1984.

Campbell AH, O'Connell JM, Wilson F: The effect of chest physiotherapy upon the FEV in chronic bronchitis. *Med J Aust*, 1:33–35, 1975.

Carlo WA, Chatburn R: *Neonatal Respiratory Care, 2nd ed.* Chicago, Year Book Medical Publishers, 1979.

Chang HK: Transthoracically-induced high frequency ventilation. *Brit J Anaesth*, 64:24S–31S, 1989.

Chevaillier J: Autogenic Drainage. In *Cystic Fibrosis: Horizons.* New York, John Wiley & Sons, 1984, p 235.

Christensen EF, Nedergard T, Dahl R: Long-term treatment of chronic bronchitis with positive expiratory pressure mask and chest physiotherapy. *Chest*, 97:1645–650, 1990.

Cole PJ (ed): Strategies for the management of chronic bronchial sepsis. Oxford, England, Medical Publishing Services, Ltd., 1984.

Committee on Bronchial Hygiene, American Association for Respiratory Care. Postural drainage therapy. *Respir Care*, 36:1418–1426, 1991.

Committee on Bronchial Hygiene, American Association for Respiratory Care. Nasotracheal Suctioning. *Respir Care* 37:898–901, 1992.

Conners AF, Hammon WE, et al: Chest physical therapy: The immediate effect on oxygenation in acutely-ill patients. *Chest*, 78:559–564, 1980.

Eid N, Buchheit J, et al: Chest physiotherapy in review. *Respir Care*, 36:270–282, 1991.

Etches PC, Scott B: Chest physiotherapy in the newborn: Effect on secretions removed. *Pediatrics*, 62:173–175, 1978.

Falk M, Kelstrup M, et al: Improving the ketchup bottle method with positive expiratory pressure, PEP, in cystic fibrosis. *Eur J Respir Dis*, 65: 423–432, 1984.

Finner NN, Boyd J: Chest physiotherapy in the neonate: A controlled study. *Pediatrics*, 2:285, 1978.

Fox WW, Schwartz J, Shaffer T: Pulmonary physiotherapy in neonates: Physiologic changes and respiratory management. *J Pediatr*, 92:977–981, 1978.

Gaskell DV, Webber BA: *The Brompton Hospital Guide to Chest Physiotherapy, 4th ed.* Oxford, England, Blackwell Scientific Publications, 1980.

Hammon WE, Martin RJ: Chest physical therapy for acute atelectasis. *Phys Ther* 61:217–220, 1981.

Hansen LG, Warwick WJ: High-frequency chest percussion system to aid clearance of mucus from the lung. *Biomed Instrum Technol*, 24: 289–294, 1990.

Huseby J, Hudson L, Stark K, Tyler M: Oxygenation during chest physiotherapy. *Chest*, 70:430, 1976.

Kerem E, Yatsiv I, Gotein KJ: Effect of endotracheal suctioning on arterial blood gases in children. *Intens Care Med*, 16:95–99, 1990.

King M, Phillips DM, Gross et al: Enhanced tracheal mucus clearance with high frequency chest wall compression. *Am Rev of Respir Dis*, 128: 511–515, 1983.

Kirillof LH, Owens GR, et al: Does chest physical therapy work? *Chest*, 88:436–444, 1985.

Kraemer R, Aumbuhl C, et al: Autogenic drainage. *Pediatr Prax*, 33:223–232, 1986.

Lorin ML, Denning CR: Evaluation of postural drainage by measurement of sputum volume and consistency. *Am J Phy Med*, 50:215–219, 1971.

MacKenzie CF (ed): Chest Physiotherapy in the Intensive Care Unit. Baltimore, Williams & Wilkins, 1989, p 31.

Mahlmeister MJ, Fink JB, et al: Positive expiratory pressure mask therapy: Theoretical and practical considerations and a review of the literature. *Resp Care*, 36:1218–1229, 1991.

Mazzocco M, Kirilloff L, et al: Chest percussion and postural drainage in patients with bronchiectasis. *Chest*, 88:360–363, 1985.

McDonnell T, McNicolar WT, FitzGerald MX: Hypoxemia during chest physiotherapy in patients with cystic fibrosis. *Ir J Med Sci*, 155:345–348, 1986.

McEvoy RD, Davies NJH, et al: Lung mucociliary transport during high frequency ventilation. *Am Rev Respir Dis*, 126:452–456, 1982.

Murray JF: The ketchup-bottle method (editorial). *N Engl J Med*, 300:1155–1157, 1979.

Murray JF: Indications for mechanical aids to assist lung inflation in medical patients. *Am Rev Respir Dis*, 122 (Part 2, Suppl):121–125, 1980.

Paul WL, Downs JB: Postoperative atelectasis, intermittent positive pressure breathing, incentive spirometry, and face mask positive end-expiratory pressure. *Arch Surg*, 116:861–863, 1981.

Pontoppidan H: Mechanical aid to lung expansion in nonintubated surgical patients. *Am Rev Respir Dis*, 122 (2, Suppl):109–119, 1980.

Proceedings of the Conference on the Scientific Basis of In-Hospital Respiratory Therapy, Atlanta, Georgia, November 14–16, 1979. *Am Rev Resp Dis*, 122:1–16, 1980.

Pryor JA, Webber BA, et al: Evaluation of the forced expiration techniques as an adjunct to postural drainage in treatment of cystic fibrosis. *Br Med J* 2:417–418, 1979.

Quittel LM, Wolfson MR, Schidlow DV: The effectiveness of chest physical therapy (CPT) in infants with bronchiolitis (abstract). *Am Rev Respir Dis*, 137:406, 1988.

Ravel D, Cuevas D, et al: The efficacy of chest physiotherapy (CPT) on the first postnatal day in infants with RDS (abstract). *Pediatr Res*, 19 (Suppl):359A, 1985.

Reines D, Sade R, et al: Chest physiotherapy fails to prevent postoperative atelectasis in children after cardiac surgery. *Ann Sur*, 195:451–455, 1982.

Reismann JT, Rivington-Law B, Corey M: Role of conventional physiotherapy in cystic fibrosis. *J Pediatr*, 133:632–636, 1988.

Ricksten SE, Bengtson A, et al: Effects of periodic positive airway pressure by mask on postoperative pulmonary function. *Chest*, 89:774–781, 1986.

Riegel B, Forshee T: A review and critiques on preoxygenation for endotracheal suctioning. *Heart Lung*, 14:507–518, 1985.

Selsby D, Jones JG: Some physiological and clinical aspects of chest physiotherapy. *Br J Anaesth*, 64:621–631, 1990.

Stapleton T: Chest physiotherapy in primary pneumonia (letter). *Br Med J*, 291:143, 1985.

Sutton P, Pavia D, et al: Chest physiotherapy: A review. *Eur J Respir Dis*, 63:188–201, 1982.

Sutton PP, Parker RA, Webber BA: Assessment of the forced expiration technique, postural drainage, and directed coughing in chest physiotherapy. *Eur J Respir Dis*, 64:62–68, 1983.

Sutton PP, Lopez-Vidriero MT, et al: Assessment of percussion, vibratory shaking and breathing exercises in chest physiotherapy. *Eur J Respir Dis*, 66:147–152, 1985.

Sutton PP: Chest physiotherapy: Time for reappraisal. *Br J Dis Chest*, 82:127–137, 1988.

Tonnesen P, Stovring S: Positive expiratory pressure (PEP) as lung physiotherapy in cystic fibrosis: A pilot study. *Eur J Respir Dis*, 65:419–422, 1984.

Wade B, Badgett D: *Essentials of Pediatric Intensive Care*, St. Louis, Quality Medical Publishing, 1990, p 930–932.

Warwick W, Hansen L: Vest bronchial drainage therapy two-year follow-up (abstract). *Pediatr Pulmonol*, 5 (Suppl): 251, 1990.

Webb M, Martin J, et al: Chest physiotherapy in acute bronchiolitis. *Arch Dis Child*, 60: 1078–1079, 1985.

Wissing DR, Boggs PB, George RB: Use of respiratory care procedures in the management of hospitalized asthmatics. *Ann Allergy*, 61:407–419, 1988.

Wollmer P, Ursing K, et al: Inefficiency of chest percussion in the physical therapy of chronic bronchitis. *Eur J Respir Dis*, 66:233–239, 1985.

Wong J, Keens T, et al: Effects of gravity in tracheal transport rates in normal subjects and in patients with cystic fibrosis. *Pediatrics*, 60:146–152, 1977.

Chapter 9

Thoracentesis and Thoracostomy Tubes

James Swift

Drainage of the pleural space as a therapeutic technique has been performed for centuries. The first recorded procedure was by Hippocrates, when he described the drainage of empyemas with incision and placement of metal tubes (Adams, 1886). In the middle of the 19th century, the procedure known as thoracentesis was modified by Hunter, who inserted the newly developed hypodermic needle into the pleural space (Castiglion, 1947). Routine use of chest tubes with a water seal was introduced by Playfair in 1872, and in 1876, Hewitt published an account of a closed-tube drainage of an empyema (Hewitt, 1876). Widespread use of thoracentesis and thoracostomy tubes was not established until the influenza outbreak of 1917, when they were used to treat the accompanying effusions (Garrison, 1929). By the 1920s, both procedures had gained acceptance in the medical community. During the last half of the 20th century, both procedures became instrumental in diagnosing and treating pulmonary disease.

THORACENTESIS

Indications

The pleural space normally contains a small amount of fluid between the visceral and parietal pleurae. In patients with abnormal conditions, this fluid may increase and result in a pleural effusion and respiratory compromise (e.g., infection, heart failure, renal failure). Trauma to the chest may cause bleeding into this space (i.e., hemothorax), thus compromising respiratory function. In a pneumothorax, air fills the pleural space and creates a life-threatening condition.

Thoracentesis is indicated in the treatment of each of these problems. A large pleural effusion, hemothorax, or tension pneumothorax may require emergent evacuation. In most cases, however, thoracentesis is performed on an elective basis to evaluate pleural fluid collections. With mild-to-moderate pleural effusions, thoracentesis may be used to eliminate fluid, which results in functional improvement of the patient.

Procedure

There are two approaches to performing a thoracentesis: An anterior approach is used for the emergent treatment of a tension pneumothorax, and a posterior approach is most commonly used for the diagnosis and treatment of pleural effusions.

Thoracentesis for pneumothorax

Pneumothoraces in the pediatric population may be classified into four groups:

1. *Spontaneous* pneumothorax occurs in patients with underlying lung disease (e.g., cystic fibrosis, asthma).
2. *Idiopathic* pneumothorax occurs generally in tall, slender males during adolescence.
3. *Iatrogenic* pneumothorax occurs most commonly in patients who are undergoing invasive procedures (e.g., central line placement) or mechanical ventilation with positive end-expiratory pressure (PEEP).
4. *Traumatic* pneumothorax results from blunt or penetrating trauma to the chest.

A pneumothorax is further categorized by its position and location in the hemothorax (e.g., apical, medial) and also by the degree of lung collapse, usually expressed as a percentage. The most important characterization of a pneumothorax is whether tension is present.

A tension pneumothorax is a medical emergency. Patients with tension pneumothorax present with profound dyspnea and chest pain. There is a progressive collection of air in the pleural space, which results in increased pleural pressure, lung compression, mediastinal shift, and decreased venous return to the heart. The condition may progress to cardiac tamponade, and patients may die if they are untreated. The usual treatment for all patients with significant (> 20%) pneumothorax, including those with tension pneumothorax, is tube thoracostomy. However, the immediate intervention prior to chest tube placement in patients with tension pneumothorax is thoracentesis of the involved hemithorax. This intervention is most easily performed from an anterior approach.

The equipment for performing a thoracentesis for pneumothorax includes the following:

- Povidone-iodine solution
- Sterile drapes
- Lidocaine (1%)
- Needles (18-gauge, 20-gauge, and 25-gauge)
- Syringes (5-ml, 10-ml, and 60-ml)
- Three-way stopcock
- Collection bag and tubes

The site of the pneumothorax may be confirmed by auscultation (decreased or absent breath sounds) and percussion (hyperresonance). Treatment should not be delayed by waiting for a confirming chest radiograph. The patient is placed in a supine position with the head of the bed at 20 to 30 degrees. The site of insertion is the second intercostal space in the midclavicular line. The site should be prepared with povidone-iodine or an equivalent solution. Sterile drapes can be placed if time permits. Lidocaine (1%) is instilled locally for anesthesia, first intradermally then deep to the edge of the third or fourth rib. An 18- to 20-gauge needle is placed on a 5- to 10-ml syringe and inserted at the anesthesia site. The needle is advanced deep toward the superior edge of the third rib and "walked" over the rib to avoid the intercostal vessels, which are located on the inferior surface of the ribs.

Once the pleura is penetrated (noted by a small "pop"), free air should be aspirated easily into the syringe. Alternatively, an 18- to 20-gauge intravenous catheter may be used (without a syringe attached). Upon penetrating the pleura, a rush of air can be heard, and the catheter may be advanced into the pleural space and the needle removed simultaneously. Free air can then be aspirated by attaching a syringe to the catheter. The patient tends to experience significant symptomatic relief with this procedure, and chest radiograph can determine the status of the pneumothorax. Patients almost always require tube thoracostomy for full resolution of the pneumothorax.

Few contraindications to thoracentesis in the patient with tension pneumothorax exist. Sites of infection on the chest wall should be avoided. In the case of a bleeding diathesis, care should be taken to avoid bleeding.

Thoracentesis for pleural effusion

The pleural fluid balance is maintained by Starling (fluid transport) forces, lymphatic drainage, and membrane surface area (Light et al, 1972). Alteration of any of these parameters may result in increased fluid accumulation in the pleural space.

Pleural effusions can be divided into two categories: transudates and exudates. The etiologies of transudates and exudates are listed

Table 9-1 Causes of Pleural Effusions

Transudates	Exudates
Congestive heart failure	Infections
Cirrhosis	Neoplasms
Hypoalbuminemia	Collagen vascular disease
Nephrotic syndrome	Pancreatitis

in Table 9–1. The difference in these two categories is based on the laboratory analysis. Exudates have a specific gravity higher than 1.016; a protein concentration greater than 3 gm/dl, a protein–serum protein ratio greater than 0.5, a lactate dehydrogenase (LDH) level greater than 200 IU/L, and a LDH–serum LDH ratio greater than 0.6 (Light et al, 1972).

Thoracentesis for a pleural effusion has two roles. The primary utility is in the diagnosis of the effusion. In moderate-to-large effusions, however, thoracentesis can serve a therapeutic role by removing fluid that is restricting lung mechanics.

When using thoracentesis for a pleural effusion, the posterior approach is most common. However, there are instances in younger children (or in those who cannot sit) in which a lateral approach is preferable.

The equipment needed for the procedure includes the following:

- Povidone-iodine solution
- Sterile drapes
- Lidocaine (1%)
- Needles (18-gauge, 25-gauge)
- Three-way stopcock
- Scalpel (number 11)
- Large and small hemostats
- 3-0 Silk suture
- Gauze
- Syringes (20-ml to 60-ml)
- Collection bottle or bag
- Chest tubes

The effusion should be confirmed by auscultation (diminished breath sounds), percussion (dullness), and certainly by chest radiograph. The patient is placed in a sitting position and is subsequently leaned forward over a table. The site of entry is determined by percussion, and an area 2 cm below the level of dullness is used. The entry site is then aligned along the midscapular region or the posterior axillary line. This area is prepared with povidone-iodine solution and draped with sterile towels. Anesthesia is accomplished with lidocaine (1%), instilled with a 25-gauge needle first intradermally, then deep to the level of the rib and pleura. An 18-gauge needle is then placed on a 20-ml to 60-ml syringe. Between the needle and the syringe is a three-way stopcock. The needle is inserted at the entry site and is introduced over the superior aspect of the rib. The needle is advanced into the pleural space, which is identified when fluid is obtained. Once fluid is obtained, it can be collected with the three-way stopcock and a collection bag. Care should be taken not to remove more than 1000 ml in a 30-minute period. Following the procedure, a chest radiograph should be performed to evaluate the effusion and rule out a pneumothorax as a complication.

THORACOSTOMY TUBES

Indications

Indications for chest tube placement in the pediatric population include tension pneumothorax, large (> 20%) idiopathic, spontaneous, iatrogenic, or traumatic pneumothorax; hemothorax; parapneumonic effusions (empyemas); and post-thoracic surgery.

Procedure

The equipment needed for tube thorocostomy includes the following:

- Povodine-iodine solution
- Sterile drapes
- Lidocaine (1%)
- Syringe (20-ml)
- Needles (20-gauge, 25-gauge)
- Scalpel (number 11)
- Large and small hemostats
- 3-0 Silk suture
- Gauze
- Collection system
- Chest tubes

The chest tube sizes for children range from 10 French for neonates, 12 to 16 French for children younger than 12 months, 16 to 20 French for children 1 to 5 years, and 20 to 32 French in children older than 5 years. A collection system is necessary and is available commercially. The collection system is composed of three chambers. The chamber attached to the chest tube is the collecting reservoir. The second chamber contains a small amount of saline and acts as a one-way valve with a water seal. The third chamber controls the amount of suction in the system.

The best approach for the pediatric population is from the lateral chest wall in the midaxillary line. Patients tolerate the procedure better with some sedation (ketamine [1 mg/kg] and fentanyl [1 μg/kg] are well tolerated). The fifth intercostal space (third to fourth in newborns) is prepared with povidone-iodine solution and draped in sterile fashion. Lidocaine (1%) is instilled first intradermally, then deep to the level of the rib and pleura. A 1-cm incision is made 1 to 2 cm below the site of insertion through the intercostal space. This creates an oblique tract to prevent infection and facilitate wound healing when the chest tube is removed. Following the incision, a hemostat is used for blunt dissection down to the intercostal muscles. The pleura is penetrated with the hemostat, and the chest tube is either inserted or clamped at the end and inserted with the tip of the hemostat. Once the tube has penetrated the pleura, it is advanced so all the side holes of the chest tube are in the thoracic cavity.

An anterior chest tube can be placed by rotating the hemostat anteriorly and advancing the chest tube after release by the hemostat. Caudal, cephalic, or posterior placement can be facilitated similarly by rotating the curved mosquito hemostat. The most frequent placement errors include not "burying" all the side holes of the chest tube under the chest wall within the pleural space and placing the tube subcutaneously rather than intrapleurally. Palpation around the insertion site can detect subcutaneous placement, and careful inspection of the tube as it enters the chest wall can detect incorrect side hole positioning. "Steaming" of the tube with condensed water vapor is an indication of proper placement of the tube within the pleural space. Also, holding the end of the tube in a bottle of water causes a rush of bubbles as air egresses from the pleural space, indicating entrance of the chest tube into the pleural space and removal of extrapulmonary air under pressure. After placing a purse-string suture around the tube where it penetrates the skin, we wrap the two long suture ends in opposite directions upward around the tube in an "argyle sock" pattern and use two locking knots to crimp the tube. In this way slippage into and out of the chest wall is prevented (Stiles, 1987).

For emergency situations, insertion of a chest tube using a trocar may be done. This is a more risky approach than the method using curved hemostats to push the tube through the chest wall because inadvertent excessive pressure can allow the trocar and tube to penetrate areas other than the pleural space, such as the liver or the heart. Nonetheless, for a dying child with a tension pneumothorax for which needle aspiration is insufficient, rapid trocar insertion of a chest tube is lifesaving. A curved Kelly clamp attached to the tube with trocar 2 cm from its end can be used as a guard to prevent accidental insertion into the chest. The skin can be stretched with the thumb after a splash preparation and the trocar and tube applied perpendicularly to the chest immediately superior to the rib. A sharp downward push is given until the curved Kelly clamp meets the curve of the chest wall. The clamp and then the trocar are removed and the tube sutured after proper placement and function are ascertained, as described above.

The chest tube is placed to suction at −15 to −20 cm H_2O using a Pleur-Evac system. On rare occasions with massive air leaks, more than one chest tube per hemithorax must be placed to prevent recurrence of pneumothorax.

The chest tube is removed following a 24-hour period in which the patient has been stable both on water seal and with the tube clamped. The patient's underlying process (i.e., pneumothorax or pleural effusion) must have improved sufficiently to warrant removal. If the patient has no reaccumulation on chest radiograph, then the tube may be removed, and a dressing may be placed.

References

Adams F: *The Genuine Works of Hippocrates.* New York, William Wood and Co., 1886.

Castiglion A: *A History of Medicine.* New York, Alfred A. Knopf, 1947.

Garrison FH: *Introduction to the History of Medicine, 4th ed.* Philadelphia, WB Saunders, 1929.

Hewitt FC: Thoracentesis: The plan of continuous aspiration. *Br Med J*, 1:317, 1876.

Light RW, MacGregor MI, Luchsinger PC, et al: Pleural effusions: The diagnostic separation of transudates and exudates. *Ann Intern Med*, 77: 507, 1972.

Stiles AD: Air leak. In Cloherty JP, Stork AR (eds): *Manual of Neonatal Care,* 2nd ed. Boston, Little Brown, 1987, pp 185–190.

Chapter 10

Oxygen Saturation Monitoring

Nick G. Anas

CONTINUOUS PULSE OXIMETRY

Continuous pulse oximetry represents one of the most important advances in critical care technology in the last 10 to 15 years. Its use is widespread, and it represents the standard of care in the resuscitation or intensive care of children. Pulse oximetry is a safe procedure that provides a rapid determination of the patient's pulmonary or cardiac status. A thorough knowledge of oxygen physiology (particularly the relationship of SaO_2 to PaO_2) is required before the oximeter can be used safely to monitor patients and to assess the response to therapy.

Continuous pulse oximetry is simple to use, provides reliable data, and is a noninvasive way to quickly assess the severity of disease or the response to therapeutic interventions. Continuous pulse oximetry is valuable in the following situations:

- Cardiorespiratory management of critically ill patients in the emergency department or in the pediatric intensive care unit (PICU)
- Transport of patients (both intra- and interfacility)
- Perioperative monitoring by an anesthesiologist
- Postoperative assessment of systemic oxygenation
- Monitoring during invasive bedside procedures that require sedation or anesthesia
- Assessment of the patient during radiographic procedures that limit access for examination (e.g., magnetic resonance imaging [MRI])
- Sleep studies utilized to determine the occurrence of sleep hypoxemia or the impact of apnea on gas exchange
- Home care of the oxygen-dependent child
- Follow-up monitoring of the child with chronic lung or heart disease

Arterial oxygen saturation (SaO_2) and arterial oxygen tension (PaO_2) are measured in patients with cardiopulmonary dysfunction to assess the adequacy of systemic oxygenation. The product of the patient's cardiac output and arterial oxygen content (CaO_2) determines oxygen delivery (DO_2) to the vital organ system. CaO_2 is primarily determined by the hemoglobin concentration and the SaO_2. The patient's PaO_2 represents the maximal tension that drives oxygen to the mitochondria for use in aerobic metabolism.

A variety of clinical disorders result in hypoxemia (i.e., $PaO_2 < 60$ mm Hg; $SaO_2 <$ 90%) and therefore interfere with systemic oxygen delivery. These problems are almost entirely related to one of the following pulmonary disturbances:

- Reduced alveolar oxygen tension (PAO_2), such as hypoventilation syndromes
- Intrapulmonary shunting (e.g., pulmonary edema)
- Low ventilation-perfusion matching (e.g., focal pneumonias)
- Dead space ventilation (e.g., pulmonary hypertension syndromes)
- Diffusion abnormalities (e.g., interstitial fibrosis)

The relationship of SaO_2 and PAO_2 is not linear but is expressed by the sigmoid oxyhemoglobin dissociation curve (Fig. 10–1). This nonlinear relationship represents a potential limitation of oxygen saturation monitoring as a tool for assessing respiratory function. As the curve demonstrates, at PaO_2 values greater than 60 mm Hg, the SaO_2 approaches its maximum (100%). The physiological benefit is that hemoglobin molecules exposed to the high oxygen tension in the alveolus ($PAO_2 \sim 1250$ mm Hg) are transported to the peripheral vascular beds nearly 100% saturated. At PaO_2 values less than 60 mm Hg, the SaO_2 falls rapidly, demonstrating that oxygen unloading to the mitochondria (where PO_2 values are low) occurs more readily and efficiently.

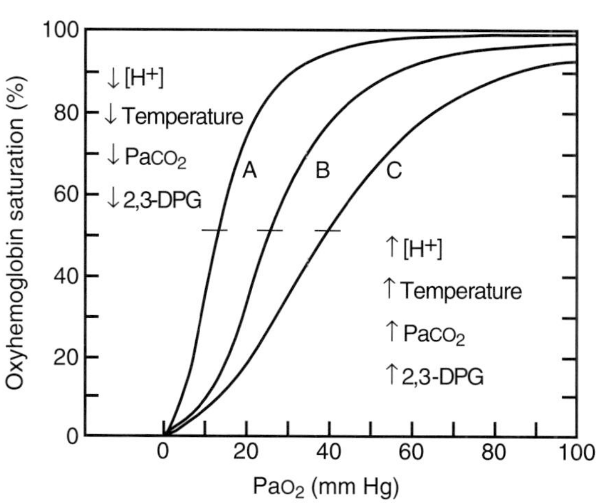

Figure 10–1 Oxyhemoglobin saturation curve. A. Abnormalities that result in an increased affinity of the hemoglobin molecule for oxygen. B. The normal curve. C. Decreased affinity of hemoglobin for oxygen. The P_{50} value for each curve is represented by a horizontal *dash* at the 50% oxygen saturation level. 2,3-DPG is 1,2,3-diphosphoglycerate; $[H^+]$ is hydrogen ion concentration; $PaCO_2$ is partial pressure of carbon dioxide in arterial blood; PaO_2 is partial pressure of oxygen in arterial blood.

The relationship of SaO_2 and PaO_2 is also determined by the position of the oxyhemoglobin dissociation curve relative to normal. That is, the position of the curve may shift to the right or to the left, reflecting changes in the affinity of hemoglobin for oxygen (see Fig. 10–1). The quaternary structure of the hemoglobin molecule regulates its affinity for oxygen and is altered by several factors:

- The arterial carbon dioxide tension ($PaCO_2$)
- The negative log of the hydrogen ion concentration (pH)
- The body temperature
- The hemoglobin concentration of 2,3-diphosphoglyceride (2,3-DPG)
- The type of hemoglobin

The PaO_2 value at which the hemoglobin molecule is 50% saturated (P_{50}) is used as a marker of the position of the oxyhemoglobin dissociation curve. Under normal conditions, the $P_{50} =$ 27 mm Hg. That is, the $SaO_2 = 50\%$ when the $PaO_2 = 27$ mm Hg.

Most pathological conditions result in a shift of the oxyhemoglobin dissociation curve to the right. Acidosis, hypercapnia, and hyperthermia increase the P_{50} value, which indicates a lowered affinity of hemoglobin for oxygen and a more efficient delivery of oxygen to the tissue mitochondria. Alkalosis, hypocapnia, and hypothermia reduce the P_{50} value, which indicates an increased affinity of hemoglobin for oxygen. This situation results in a reduced PaO_2 relative to SaO_2 and inhibits the unloading of oxygen from the hemoglobin molecule. Very few pathological clinical conditions naturally shift the curve to the left. Rather, therapeutic maneuvers, such as inducing alkalosis for the treatment of pulmonary hypertension or purposely hyperventilating ($PaCO_2 < 35$ mm Hg) a patient to treat intracranial hypertension, may result in impaired oxygen delivery and consumption, due to the leftward shift of the oxyhemoglobin dissociation curve.

2,3-DPG also lowers hemoglobin affinity for oxygen by binding to beta chains of hemoglobin A or to gamma chains of hemoglobin F (fetal hemoglobin). For example, anemia leads to increased 2,3-DPG levels (i.e., increases the P_{50}), whereas storage of blood with acid-citrate dextrose (ACD) preservative results in depletion of 2,3-DPG, thereby lowering the P_{50} value.

The type of hemoglobin also determines the avidity of oxygen binding to hemoglobin. For example, fetal and sickle-cell hemoglobin molecules shift the curve to the left (i.e., reduce the P_{50} value). Methemoglobin (HbMet) is a hemoglobin molecule in which iron is oxidized; therefore, it cannot bind oxygen as readily, and inadequate oxygen delivery ensues. Tissue hypoxia and acidosis occur when HbMet levels exceed 30%. Carbon monoxide has a greater affinity for hemoglobin than does oxygen, and therefore, carbon monoxide poisoning is characterized by a reduced Sao_2 and hence Cao_2. Importantly, carbon monoxide also shifts the oxyhemoglobin dissociation curve to the left, which further limits oxygen delivery and consumption.

EQUIPMENT AND CLINICAL UTILITY

Sao_2 monitoring gauges pulmonary function by demonstrating trends that reflect the adequacy of gas exchange. If Sao_2 monitoring is simultaneously performed with mixed venous saturation (Svo_2) monitoring, the determination of oxygen consumption (Vo_2) relative to delivery (Do_2) can be used to direct therapy and perhaps to predict patient outcome (see Chapter 15). During the last decade, noninvasive Sao_2 monitoring has surpassed intermittent intra-arterial sampling of the Pao_2 as the optimal method for continuously detecting the adequacy and degree of systemic oxygenation in critically ill children. Pulse oximetry has proved to be an ideal monitoring system for children for a number of reasons:

1. It instantly provides continuous data. In an emergency or in life-threatening conditions, the patient's Sao_2 can be obtained within seconds to provide medical personnel with valuable information regarding the severity of the patient's cardiopulmonary compromise.
2. It is noninvasive and therefore can be employed painlessly and rapidly. Minimal patient cooperation is necessary, which makes pulse oximetry an ideal system for treating children.
3. It provides information that is invaluable in guiding ventilator and hemodynamic management.

The technique of continuous pulse oximetry is based on the following principles:

- The color of blood is a function of the Sao_2.
- The optical properties of hemoglobin determine the color of blood at various Sao_2 values.
- The total absorption of a system of absorbent agents is the sum of the individual absorbances of each agent (Beer-Lambert law).

The pulse oximeter takes into account the effect of the absorption of light by tissue and venous blood by assuming that only arterial blood pulsates. (This is not true under certain clinical conditions of high venous pressure, such as tricuspid regurgitation.)

In practice, pulse oximeters use only two wavelengths of light: 660 nanometers (nm) (red light) and 940 nm (near-infrared light). The two wavelengths permit calculation of the ratio of deoxygenated hemoglobin to oxyhemoglobin. Specifically, visible red light (660 nm) is absorbed 10 times as much by reduced oxyhemoglobin (deoxyhemoglobin), whereas at the near-infrared wavelength (940 nm), the absorption coefficient of oxyhemoglobin is greater than that of deoxyhemoglobin. Therefore, most commercially available pulse oximeters use two light-emitting diodes (LEDs) and one photodiode as transmitting and sensory transducers, respectively (Fig. 10–2). The two LEDs are activated alternately, and the difference between the ratios of the absorbances of oxyhemoglobin and deoxyhemoglobin provides the Sao_2 value. Although light absorbance technology has existed for 50 years,

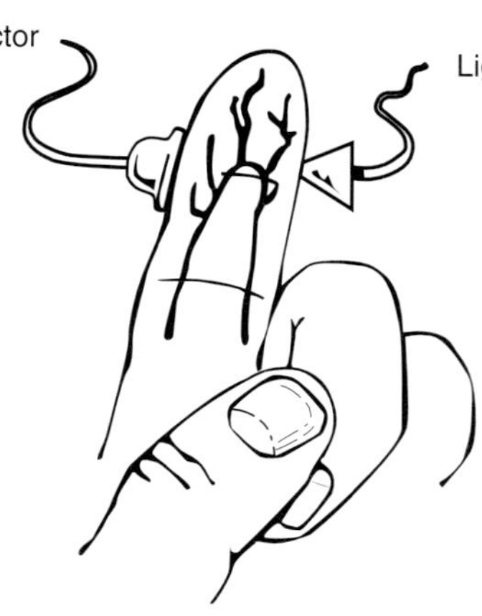

Figure 10–2 Oximeter probe photodetector and light source. (Redrawn from Hicks DA, Anas NG: Oxygen saturation monitoring. In Levin DL, Morriss FC [eds]: *Essentials of Pediatric Intensive Care.* St. Louis, Quality Medical Publishing, Inc., 1990, p 866.)

the use of the pulse principle and the use of LEDs representing a narrow range of the electromagnetic spectrum have resulted in the widespread adoption of this equipment.

Continuous pulse oximetry also provides measurement of heart rate independent from the heart rate obtained from impedance chest wall leads. The pulsating vascular bed in the site chosen for monitoring creates a change in the length of the light path, which modifies the amount of light that is detected. The oximeter determines the pulse rate from the change in the amount of light that is absorbed, comparing systole to diastole. Importantly, the Sao_2 value is accurate only if the heart rate measured by the pulse oximeter correlates with the heart rate determined either by chest wall impedance (heart rate monitor) or by auscultation of the heart rate.

Application of the continuous pulse oximeter is simple and safe. The digits (or the heel in a newborn) provide easy access and multiple sites. Heat pretreatment to "arterialize" the cutaneous vascular supply is not necessary, as it is when using transcutaneous oxygen monitoring systems or when analyzing capillary blood samples. A microprocessor performs the calibration, measurements, and digital display, making it a user-friendly system (Fig. 10–3). The initial reading occurs within 10 to 15 seconds of application of the probe. The digital probes are small, relatively inexpensive, easily transportable, disposable, and durable.

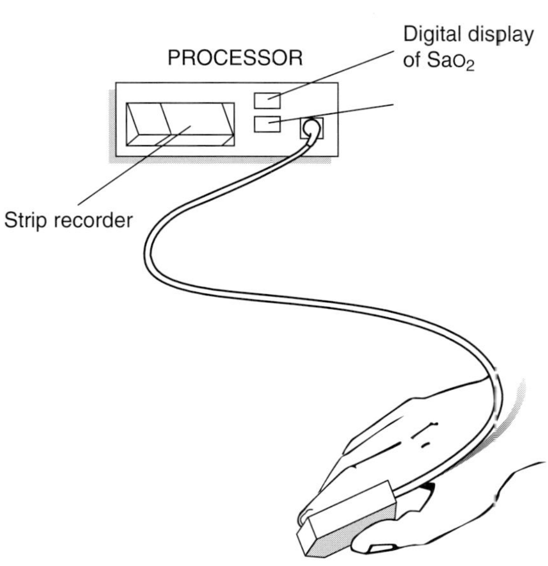

Figure 10–3 Finger pickup and oximeter. The strip chart can be useful for providing a permanent record. (Redrawn from Hicks DA, Anas NG: Oxygen saturation monitoring. In Levin DL, Morriss FC [eds]: *Essentials of Pediatric Intensive Care.* St. Louis, Quality Medical Publishing, Inc., 1990, p 866.)

RISKS AND LIMITATIONS OF TECHNOLOGY

Noninvasive, continuous Sao_2 monitoring utilizing the systems described above provides inaccurate data when there is a reduction in measured vascular pulsation, which is detected by a discrepancy between the oximeter heart rate measurement and the heart rate measurement obtained by chest wall impedance techniques, by palpation of the patient's pulse, or by chest auscultation. Clinical situations in which this inaccuracy is likely to occur include shock states, dysrhythmias, and motion artifact. Motion artifact limits the use of oximetry in circumstances in which the patient either is uncooperative or is not being observed (e.g., home sleep studies). There is great danger in relying on untrained observers (e.g., parents) for determining the validity of the Sao_2 measurements. An additional source of error is introduced by extraneous light sources consisting of wavelengths near the measured frequency (e.g., infrared radiation heaters, ultraviolet phototherapy for treating hyperbilirubinemia). Injection of dyes (see Table 32–3), such as methylene blue (for treatment of methemoglobinemia), results in a falsely low Sao_2 measurement. Finally, the present technology does not provide accurate data when the $Sao_2 < 70\%$, and because of the sigmoid shape of the oxyhemoglobin dissociation curve, the present technology is rather insensitive to large changes in Pao_2 at the high end (plateau) of the curve.

Misleading information can be obtained under a number of circumstances. Because only oxyhemoglobin and deoxyhemoglobin are detected by pulse oximeters, the presence of abnormal hemoglobin molecules can lead to an overestimation by the oximeter of the true Sao_2. For example, carboxyhemoglobin (HbCO) has an absorbance similar to that of oxygenated hemoglobin (Hbo_2), and therefore the pulse oximetry value can be falsely high. Studies have shown that when HbCO is 50%, the Sao_2 measured by the pulse oximeter is 95%. Methemoglobin (HbMet) has a larger absorbance than either of the two major types of hemoglobin at 940 nm but simulates deoxyhemoglobin at 660 nm. Therefore, at high Sao_2 levels ($>85\%$), the reading underestimates the true value; at low Sao_2 levels ($<85\%$), the measured value is falsely high. In the presence of high HbMet ($>50\%$), the measured SaO_2 approaches 85%, independent of the actual SaO_2. In these circumstances, intra-arterial sampling and measurement of SaO_2 by co-oximeter is necessary for accurate determination of the true SaO_2. Finally, in neonates, there is a large amount of hemoglobin F (HbF). Because HbF has almost the same absorption spectrum as HbA, there is no major effect on SaO_2 measurement by oximetry. Additionally, hyperbilirubinemia in the newborn does not adversely affect the SaO_2.

Several problems in interpreting the data are related to the fact that the SaO_2 and PaO_2 are not linearly related throughout the wide range of possible PaO_2 values (particularly in the patient receiving supplemental oxygen). For example, a significant reduction in PaO_2 (e.g., from 200 mm Hg to 95 mm Hg) can occur as a result of ventilation-perfusion ($\dot{V}/\dot{Q}$) mismatching, and yet the oximeter value will remain between 98% and 100%. In this circumstance, a physiologically significant event is not detected by the oximeter. Even a reduction in SaO_2 from 98% to 90% might not be appreciated as significant, although it reflects an important decrease in the PaO_2 (e.g., from 100 mm Hg to 60 mm Hg) and places the patient much closer to the "steep" portion of the oxyhemoglobin dissociation curve. Another clinical situation in which the shape of the oxyhemoglobin dissociation curve may be responsible for providing misleading information is that in which hypoxemia occurs as a result of alveolar hypoventilation. The alveolar gas equation shows that the reduction in PaO_2 that results from hypoventilation (assuming no $\dot{V}/\dot{Q}$ mismatch) is proportional to the increase in $PaCO_2$ in a 1:1 relationship. For example, in a patient breathing room air, an increase in $PaCO_2$ from 40 mm Hg to 60 mm Hg results in a reduction in PaO_2 from 110 mm Hg to 90 mm Hg with little diminution in the SaO_2 value. This phenomenon is further masked (and will be underappreciated) if, for example, the administration of supplemental oxygen increases the PaO_2 to 150 mm Hg. The decrease to 130 mm Hg under the condition of hypoventilation described is even less likely to be appreciated.

Misleading information also occurs because of changes in the position of the oxyhemoglobin dissociation curve. As mentioned earlier, a reduced P_{50} value indicates that oxygen is bound to hemoglobin more avidly. Therefore, for any given PaO_2 value, the SaO_2 will be higher than if the curve were in the "normal" position. A patient in whom alkalosis or hypocapnia has been induced therapeutically will demonstrate a greater SaO_2 value relative to the PaO_2, and the degree of intrapulmonary shunt will not be appreciated (or accurately calculated) using the SaO_2 measurement as a guide.

Bibliography

Barker SJ, Tremper KK: Advances in oxygen monitoring. Pulse oximetry: Applications and limitations. *Int Anesthesiol Clin*, 15:3, 1987.

Benumof J: Respiratory physiology and respiratory function during anesthesia. In Miller RD (ed): *Anesthesia*, 3rd edition. New York, Churchill Livingstone, 1990, p 505.

Boyson PG, Broomer JA: Noninvasive monitoring of lung function during mechanical ventilation. *Crit Care Clin*, 4:527, 1988.

Brown M, Vender JS: Noninvasive oxygen monitoring. *Crit Care Clin*, 4:493, 1988.

Bryan-Brown CW, Baek SM, Makebali G, et al: Consumable oxygen: Availability in relation to oxyhemoglobin dissociation. *Crit Care Med*, 1:17, 1973.

Cohen DE, Downes JJ, Raphaely RC: What difference does pulse oximetry make? *Anesthesiology*, 68:181, 1988.

Fanconi S, Doherty P, Edmonds J, et al: Pulse oximetry in pediatric intensive care: Comparison with measured saturations and transcutaneous oxygen tension. *J Pediatr*, 107:362, 1985.

Helfaer MA, Nicholas DG, Rogers MC: Developmental physiology of the respiratory system. In Rogers MC (ed): *Text of Pediatric Intensive Care*. Baltimore, Williams and Wilkins, 1992, p 104.

Hicks DA, Anas NG: Oxygen saturation monitoring. In Levin DL, Morriss FC (eds): *Essentials of Pediatric Intensive Care*. St. Louis, Quality Medical Publishing, Inc., 1990, p 864.

Marin JJ: Monitoring during mechanical ventilation. *Clin Chest Med*, 9:73, 1988.

Moon RE, Campores EM: Respiratory monitoring. In Miller RD (ed): *Anesthesia*, 3rd ed. New York, Churchill Livingstone, 1990, p 1129.

Tremper KK, Barker SJ: Fundamental principles of monitoring instrumentation. In Miller RD (ed): *Anesthesia*, 3rd edition. New York, Churchill Livingstone, 1990, p 957.

Chapter 11

End-Tidal Carbon Dioxide Monitoring (Capnography)

Nick G. Anas

INDICATIONS FOR CAPNOGRAPHY

End-tidal carbon dioxide monitoring (capnography) is the measurement and display in waveform of carbon dioxide tension or partial pressure in exhaled gases ($PETCO_2$). In the intensive care unit, capnography may provide a continuous assessment of the following:

1. The adequacy of alveolar ventilation
2. The patency or proper placement of an endotracheal tube
3. The relationship of alveolar ventilation and pulmonary perfusion (i.e., the amount of dead space ventilation)
4. The cardiac output during resuscitation
5. The function of the patient's mechanical ventilator.

The utility of capnography is a function of the multiple factors that determine the $PETCO_2$:

1. The arterial carbon dioxide tension or partial pressure ($PaCO_2$)
2. The cardiac output
3. The percent dead space ventilation (dead space volume divided by tidal volume [V_D/V_T])
4. Airway–time constants
5. Carbon dioxide production (i.e., the metabolic rate)
6. The exogenous administration of sodium bicarbonate

Interpretation of the capnogram requires knowledge of these physiological determinants; $PETCO_2$ monitoring in the pediatric intensive care unit (PICU) is useful only if the data are logical and are consistent with the clinical assessment of the patient's problems.

PHYSIOLOGY

Under the circumstances of ideal ventilation-perfusion ($\dot{V}/\dot{Q}$) matching (i.e., $\dot{V}/\dot{Q} = 1$), venous blood entering the pulmonary circulation has a $PETCO_2$ equal to 46 mm Hg ($PvCO_2$ = 46 mm Hg). Carbon dioxide diffuses rapidly across the alveolar–capillary membrane to the alveolus. By the time the blood leaves the alveolus, the PCO_2 in the end-capillary blood and the alveolus are in equilibrium; that is, the $PaCO_2 = PACO_2$ (again, assuming $\dot{V}/\dot{Q} = 1$). Moreover, the $PETCO_2$ approximates the value of the P_ACO_2 of all functional lung units. Based on the relationship of $PaCO_2$ to P_ACO_2 and the relationship of P_ACO_2 to $PETCO_2$, the $PETCO_2$ closely approximates the $PaCO_2$ when $\dot{V}/\dot{Q} = 1$. The difference between the $PaCO_2$ and $PETCO_2$ is known as the arterial to end-tidal CO_2 gradient ($PaCO_2$–$PETCO_2$), which has a normal value of ± 5 mm Hg.

The P_ACO_2–$PETCO_2$ gradient may be significantly altered by changes in $\dot{V}/\dot{Q}$ matching. The $PaCO_2$ value is determined by the PCO_2 of perfused alveoli (whether or not they are ventilated), whereas the $PETCO_2$ value represents the PCO_2 of all ventilated alveoli (whether or not they are perfused). The primary $\dot{V}/\dot{Q}$ disturbance causing a change in the $PaCO_2$–$PETCO_2$ gradient is the creation of increased dead space ventilation i.e., $\dot{V}/\dot{Q} = \infty$ The lung units that lack perfusion but still continue to be ventilated will have $PETCO_2$ concentrations that approximate that of the atmosphere ($PCO_2 = 0$). The resulting dilution of the end-tidal gas causes the $PETCO_2$ value to be lower, and thus the $PaCO_2$–$PETCO_2$ gradient widens.

These relationships are best expressed by the modified Bohr equation, which states the following:

$$\frac{V_D}{V_T} = \frac{PaCO_2}{PaCO_2}$$

or

$$V_D = \frac{(PaCO_2 - PETCO_2)\ V_T}{PaCO_2}$$

V_D represents the dead space volume and V_T the tidal volume. Therefore, the greater the volume of dead space, the more the $PETCO_2$ will be diluted. As dead space increases, the $PETCO_2$ underestimates the $PaCO_2$. That is, to ensure a constant ($PaCO_2$–$PETCO_2$) gradient as dead space volume increases, the tidal volume for a given $PaCO_2$ value must increase.

Capnography provides a marker of alveolar ventilation and pulmonary perfusion. Pathophysiological conditions that increase dead space ventilation, and therefore reduce $PETCO_2$, are all characterized by interfering with pulmonary blood flow:

1. Reduced cardiac output (e.g., hypovolemia, cardiac arrest)
2. Increased pulmonary vascular resistance (e.g., pulmonary hypertension, excessive positive end-expiratory pressure [PEEP])
3. Reduced area of the pulmonary vascular bed (e.g., multiple pulmonary emboli, aggregation of white blood cells in the pulmonary capillary beds)
4. Large pulmonary artery obstruction (e.g., pulmonary embolus, infarction)

In all of these situations, the increasing ($PaCO_2$–$PETCO_2$) gradient makes capnography a marker of pulmonary perfusion. In pathophysiological conditions in which the gradient remains constant (i.e., ideal pulmonary perfusion and alveolar ventilation matching exists), capnography provides a means of following alveolar ventilation. Alveolar ventilation may be altered by changes in respiratory rate, tidal volume, airway resistance, or pulmonary compliance. Changes in $PETCO_2$ also may reflect obstruction or malposition of the patient's endotracheal tube. Table 11–1 provides a comparison or the $PaCO_2$ and $PETCO_2$ values in critically ill PICU patients.

EQUIPMENT AND METHODS

In the intensive care unit or in the operating room, capnography is generally used in patients with either an endotracheal tube or a tracheostomy, which provides easy access to the airway. In the sleep laboratory, detecting the end-tidal CO_2 concentration during spon-

Table 11–1 The $PaCO_2$–$PETCO_2$ Gradient in the PICU Patient

$PaCO_2$	$PETCO_2$	Diagnosis
Reduced	Reduced	Improved alveolar ventilation Reduced CO_2 production
Unchanged or increased	Reduced	Reduced cardiac output Cardiac arrest Increased pulmonary vascular resistance Pulmonary embolus
Increased	Increased	Reduced alveolar ventilation Increased CO_2 production Bicarbonate administration
Unchanged	Increased	Increased airway resistance Excessive alveolar compliance

$PaCO_2$, partial pressure of carbon dioxide in arterial blood; $PETCO_2$, end-tidal pressure of carbon dioxide; PICU, pediatric intensive care unit.

taneous breathing is accomplished by attaching a sampling catheter to the patient's chin (or upper lip). This technique requires patient cooperation and physician flexibility. For example, an intravenous catheter can be threaded into the common lumen of a pair of nasal oxygen cannula so that the tip lies midway between the two nasal prongs. The extension tube that is normally connected to the oxygen source is tied off, and the intravenous catheter is connected to a sidestream capnometer.

The $PETCO_2$ value in an exhaled gas mixture can be determined either by infrared absorption analysis or by mass spectroscopy. Although the use of the mass spectrometer allows the measuring of multiple gas concentrations, its use in the clinical setting is limited because of its high cost, its slow response time, its bulkiness, and the requirement for labor-intensive repair. An infrared absorption spectrophotometer is much more commonly used and consists of an infrared energy source, optical filter, sample chamber, reference chamber, and detector. Light from the infrared source strikes the optical filter, which excludes all wavelengths of light except for those corresponding to the absorption peak of CO_2. This narrow band-width light is passed alternately through the sample and reference chambers. In the sample chamber, CO_2 absorbs the narrow band-width light. No CO_2 absorption takes place in the reference chamber. At the end of the chamber, opposite the infrared source, a solid-state detector converts light to voltage. Because the absorption of infrared light by CO_2 is proportional to the CO_2 concentration, the patient's CO_2 concentration can be determined by comparing its absorbance to that of a standard known concentration. The CO_2 measured by the monitor is usually expressed as a partial pressure in mm Hg or torr. Some capnometers display the percent (%) of CO_2, which is obtained by dividing the CO_2 in mm Hg by the atmospheric pressure. For example, the normal $PETCO_2$ = 38 mm Hg or 5% at an atmospheric pressure of 760 mm Hg.

Sidestream Analyzers

Sidestream analyzers (Fig. 11–1A) draw gas from the patient's airway (by means of a sampling adapter) through fine-bore tubing into the capnometer. Because the gas sample must be transported to a remote measurement site, a delay in response occurs. The response time of sidestream capnography is determined by the

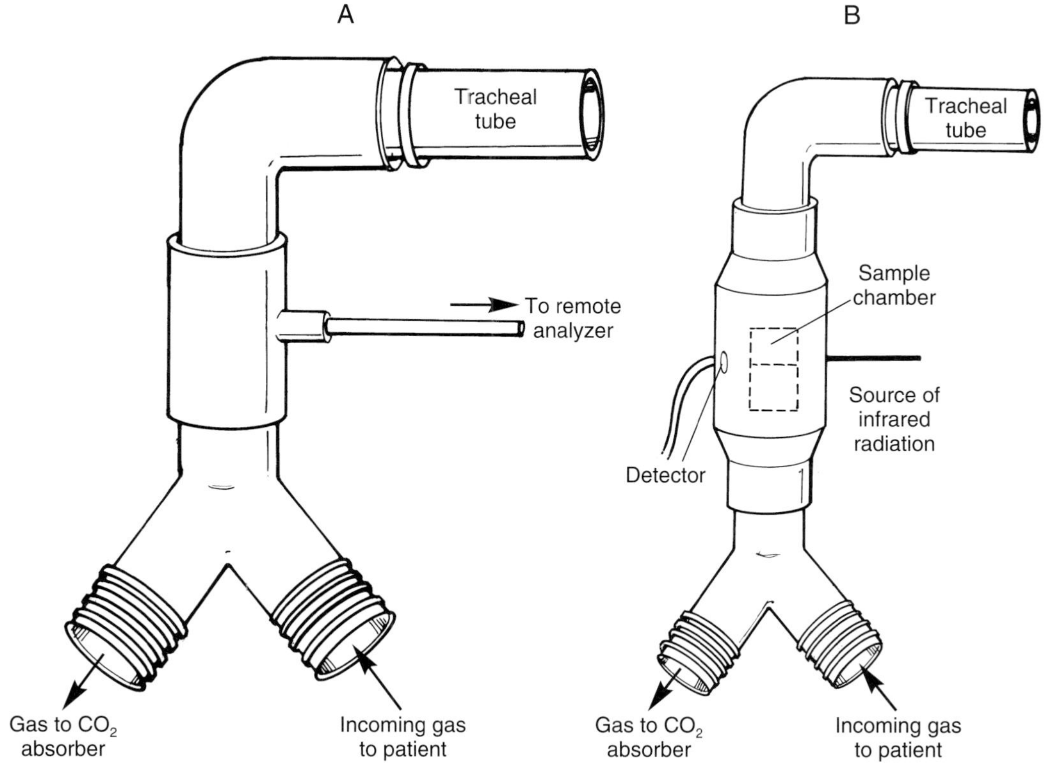

Figure 11–1 Sidestream **(A)** and mainstream **(B)** end-tidal CO_2 analyzers.

flow rate at which the sample gas is aspirated from the airway. Sample gas transport through the fine-bore tubing may be reduced or occluded by condensed water vapor or accumulated airway secretions.

Mainstream Analyzers

Mainstream analyzers (Fig. 11–1B) are in line; that is, the sample measurement chamber is attached directly to the endotracheal tube or tracheostomy. The measurement chamber contains the infrared light source and the photodetector; therefore, the delay in response time is negligible. The measurement chamber is usually heated to 40°C to prevent water condensation; the heated sensing head must be kept away from direct contact with the patient's skin. Additionally, the window of the sensor must be kept clean of mucus and particles to prevent a false reading. Mainstream analyzers are heavy and must be supported to prevent endotracheal tube kinking or dislodgment. Portable, battery-operated CO_2-monitoring devices that are suitable for emergency areas, patient transport, and intensive care units are now available.

INTERPRETATION OF DATA AND CLINICAL USE

To properly interpret the $PETCO_2$ value, the practitioner must understand the essential characteristics of the capnographic waveform (Fig. 11–2). The waveform can be divided into four components: the zero baseline; a rapid, sharp upstroke; an alveolar plateau; and a rapid, sharp downstroke. The $PETCO_2$ is measured at the point of highest CO_2 concentration. The value for $PETCO_2$ represents the average CO_2 concentration ($PACO_2$) for all ventilated lung units. Unless significant maldistribution of perfusion or ventilation is present, the value of $PETCO_2$ is assumed to be the best estimate of $PaCO_2$.

Changes in the $PETCO_2$ must be compared to the $PaCO_2$ value to determine the cause of the gas exchange derangement (see Table 11–1). When $PETCO_2$ and $PaCO_2$ correlate (i.e., the dead space ventilation is unchanging), hypoventilation can be diagnosed by an increase in the height of the capnogram (Fig. 11–3). Hyperventilation can be diagnosed by a reduction in the height of the $PETCO_2$ plateau (Fig. 11–4). If a reduction in the $PETCO_2$ value occurs in the presence of an unchanged or increasing $PaCO_2$, then increased dead space volume is occurring, and clinical correlation (e.g. cardiac arrest) is necessary to determine the most likely cause. Figure 11–5 demonstrates the capnogram typical of cardiac arrest ($\dot{Q}$ =

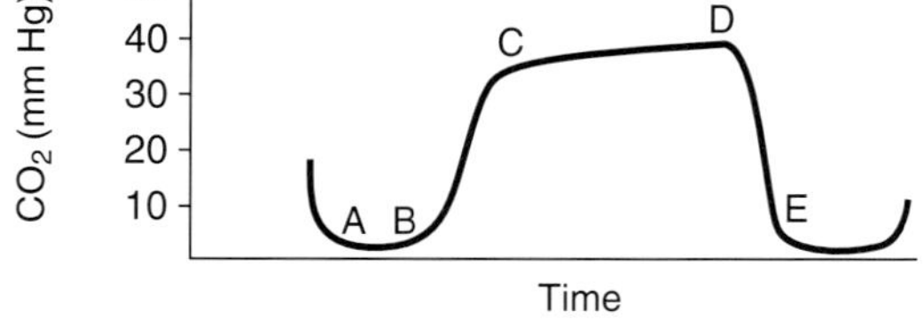

Figure 11–2 Capnographic waveform. Segment AB represents the first gas expired during a normal exhalation and measures gas from the anatomic dead space, which does not contain CO_2. As the exhalation continues, a second phase (BC) occurs as a rapid upstroke, representing the increasing concentration of CO_2 in the expired gas. The third phase (CD) is the alveolar plateau, which reaches a peak (D) during the final phase of exhalation. The PCO_2 value at point D is the $PETCO_2$. Segment DE represents the initiation of the inspiratory phase of the respiratory cycle; this rapid downstroke occurs as the inhaled (ambient) air contains no CO_2.

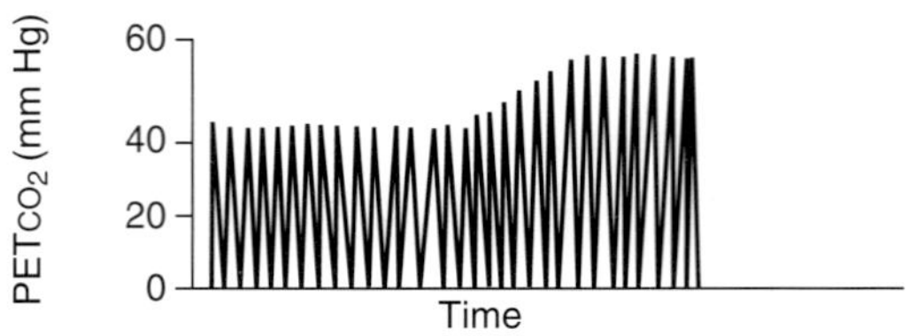

Figure 11–3 Capnogram of a patient with hypoventilation. With a reduced paper speed compared to the waveform demonstrated in Figure 11–2, this pattern provides the $PETCO_2$ values of a number of successive breaths. The left side of the tracing ($PETCO_2$ = 40 mm Hg) is consistent with normal alveolar ventilation. The right side is consistent with hypoventilation, as the $PETCO_2$ values approach 60 mm Hg.

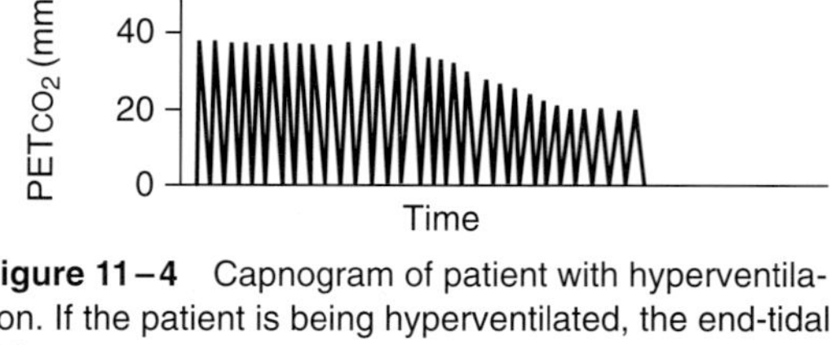

Figure 11–4 Capnogram of patient with hyperventilation. If the patient is being hyperventilated, the end-tidal CO_2 value will decrease to values below 40 mm Hg. Confirmation is achieved by the simultaneous measurement of the $PaCO_2$ value, which will also be less than 40 mm Hg.

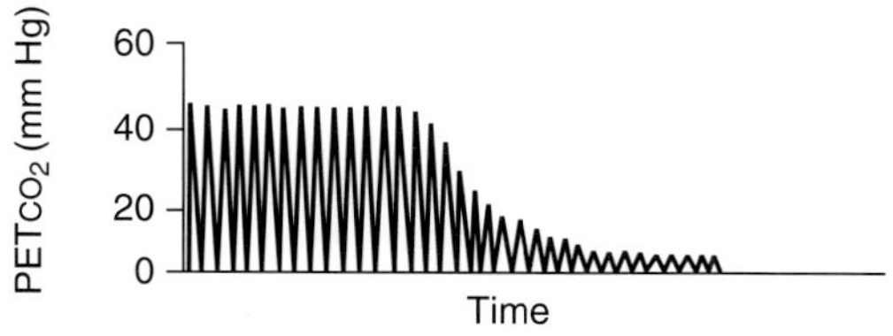

Figure 11–5 Capnogram of patient with cardiac arrest. In the patient with an arrested heart, pulmonary perfusion rapidly approaches 0 (i.e., increased dead space volume), and therefore the PETCO_2 value also approaches 0.

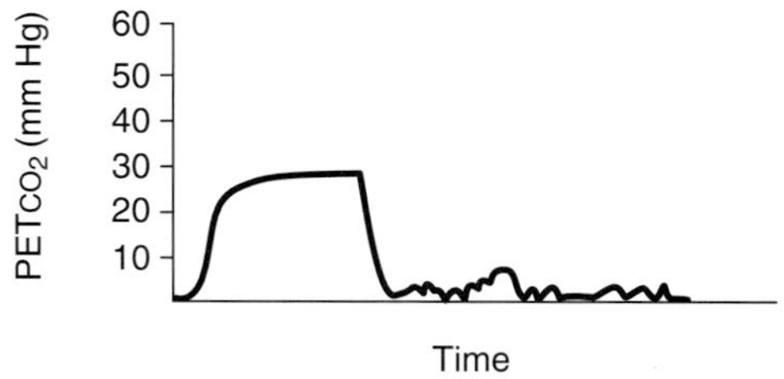

Figure 11–7 Sudden loss of waveform. The rapid reduction of the PETCO_2 value to 0 is consistent with apnea, ventilator malfunction, or esophageal intubation.

0); Fig. 11–6 demonstrates a more gradual reduction in PETCO_2, with reduced pulmonary perfusion due to hypovolemia or excessive positive pressure (e.g., PEEP). A rapid reduction of PETCO_2 from baseline to 0 mm Hg (Fig. 11–7) is consistent with situations in which no alveolar ventilation is occurring (e.g., apnea) or those in which there is ventilator malfunction or an esophageal intubation.

The integrity of the airway and the distribution of ventilation may be assessed by analysis of waveform morphology. In situations of airflow obstruction, such as bronchospasm, the capnographic waveform is characterized by an increased slope of the alveolar plateau or absence of the alveolar plateau (Fig. 11–8). Elevation of the capnographic waveform baseline indicates rebreathing of previously exhaled gas (Fig. 11–9), which can be caused by the addition of excessive mechanical dead space, a malfunctioning expiratory valve, or inadequate gas flow through a T-piece system. The appearance of a downward cleft in the alveolar plateau (Fig. 11–10) may be observed in patients recovering from neuromuscular blockade. The cleft represents a diaphragmatic contraction that does not result in an adequate inspiratory flow. This ineffective diaphragmatic contraction results in brief entrainment of a small amount of CO_2-free gas into the airway, which results in the appearance of the cleft in the expiratory phase of the capnographic waveform.

COMPLICATIONS

Complications of PETCO_2 monitoring include misinterpretation of the displayed data and mechanical dysfunction of either the monitoring or the ventilating apparatus. An example of inadequate understanding is failure to compare the PETCO_2 value to a simultaneously obtained PaCO_2. Pulmonary perfusion or the CO_2 production (i.e., the metabolic rate) cannot be assumed to have remained constant.

A change in the PETCO_2 can result from mechanical malfunction, not patient malfunction. The infrared spectrophotometer measurement of CO_2 can be affected by changes in atmospheric pressure or the presence of halogenated anesthetic vapors and nitrous oxide, which can falsely elevate the PETCO_2 value. A sudden reduction in the PETCO_2 to 0 may indicate one

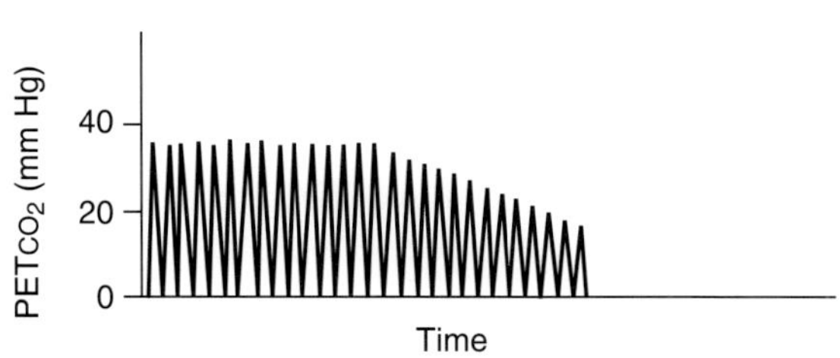

Figure 11–6 Capnogram of patient with compromised pulmonary perfusion. The gradual reduction in the PETCO_2 value over time is consistent with compromised pulmonary perfusion as occurs in a patient with hypovolemia, one with increased pulmonary vascular resistance, or one in whom the positive end-expiratory pressure exceeded the pulmonary capillary pressure.

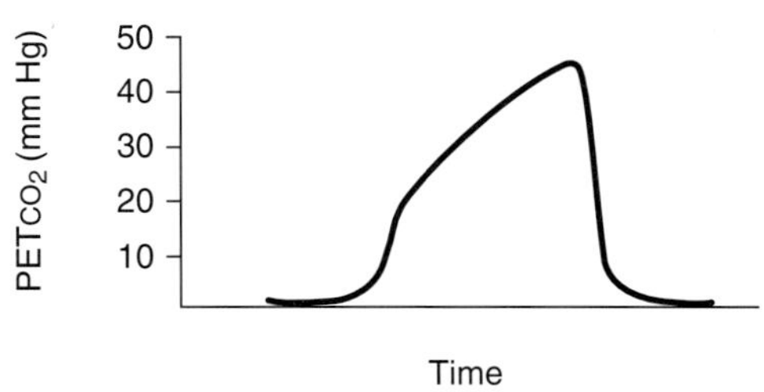

Figure 11–8 Capnogram of a patient with airflow obstruction. An alveolar plateau is never reached, as the slowest-emptying lung units contain increasing concentrations of CO_2.

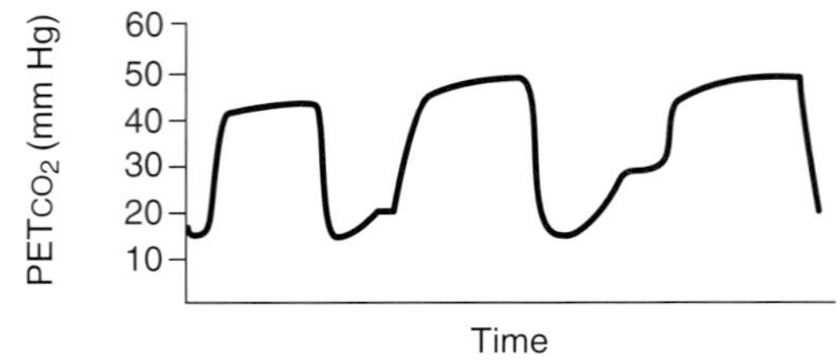

Figure 11–9 Capnogram of a patient rebreathing exhaled gas. The baseline rises above 0, as the inhaled gas contains CO_2. Causes of rebreathing might include the addition of excessive mechanical dead space to the ventilator tubing, a malfunctioning expiratory value, or inadequate gas flow through a T-piece system.

or more of the following mechanical defects: an obstructed endotracheal tube, a defective CO_2 analyzer, a ventilator malfunction, or an endotracheal tube malposition. A sudden increase in the $PETCO_2$ baseline may be caused by a saturated CO_2 absorber, the presence of water in the analyzer, or a calibration error.

CAPNOGRAPHY: PURCHASE CONSIDERATIONS

Before a physician or facility decides to purchase the equipment necessary for performing capnography, the following issues need to be considered.

1. Location of use: operating room, emergency department, intensive care units, transport ambulance, sleep laboratory
2. Availability of power source
3. Types of procedures to be monitored
4. Presence of other monitoring equipment
5. Durability requirements (e.g., if the equipment will be frequently transported to different patient care areas and therefore be exposed to more mechanical shocks)
6. Training level of user
7. Cost
8. Ease of servicing
9. Types of patients

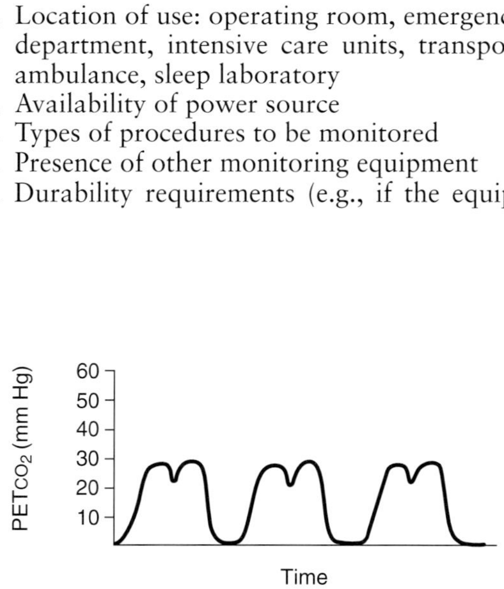

Figure 11–10 Capnogram of a patient recovering from neuromuscular blockade. The cleft in the capnographic waveform represents a diaphragmatic contraction, during which a small amount of CO_2-free gas is entrained into the airway.

Bibliography

Anas NG: End-tidal carbon dioxide monitoring (capnography). In DL Levin, FC Morris (Eds): *Essentials of Pediatric Intensive Care.* St. Louis, Quality Medical Publishing, Inc., 1990, p 869.

Bhende M, Thompson A, Orr R: Utility of an end-tidal carbon dioxide detector during stabilization and transport of critically ill children. *Pediatrics,* 89:1042, 1992.

Burrows FA: Physiologic dead space, venous admixture, and arterial to end-tidal carbon dioxide difference in infants and children undergoing cardiac surgery. *Anesthesiology,* 70:219, 1989.

Callahan M, Barton C, Matthay M: Effect of epinephrine on the ability of end-tidal carbon dioxide readings to predict initial resuscitation from cardiac arrest. *Crit Care Med,* 20:337, 1992.

Callahan M, Barton C, Matthay M: Prediction of outcome of cardiopulmonary resuscitation from end-tidal carbon dioxide concentration. *Crit Care Med,* 18:358, 1990.

Falk JL, Rackow EC, Weil MH: End-tidal carbon dioxide concentration during cardiopulmonary resuscitation. *N Engl J Med,* 318:607, 1988.

Hatle L, Rokseth R: The arterial to end-expiratory carbon dioxide tension gradient in acute pulmonary embolism and other cardiopulmonary diseases. *Chest,* 4:352, 1974.

Hunt GE: Capnography—uses and interpretation. *J Respir Care Practitioners,* July:71, 1993.

Morley TF, Giaimo J, et al: Use of capnography for assessment of the adequacy of alveolar ventilation during weaning from mechanical ventilation. *Am Rev Respir Dis,* 148:339, 1993.

Murray JP, Modell JM: Early detection of endotracheal tube accidents by monitoring carbon dioxide concentration in respiratory gas. *Anesthesiology,* 59:344, 1983.

Murray JP, Modell JM, et al: Titration of PEEP by the arterial minus end-tidal carbon dioxide gradient. *Chest,* 85:100, 1984.

Nobel JJ: Carbon dioxide monitors: Exhaled gas. *Ped Emer Care,* 9:244, 1993.

Nunn FJ, Hill DW: Respiratory dead space and arterial to end-tidal CO_2 tension differences in anesthetized man. *J Appl Physiol,* 15:383, 1960.

Raemer DB, Francis D, et al: Variation in PCO_2 between arterial blood and peak expired gas during anesthesia. *Anesth Analg* 62:1065, 1983.

Schena J, Thompson J, Crone RK: Mechanical influences on the capnogram. *Crit Care Med*, 12:672, 1984.

Sivan Y, Eldadah M, et al: Estimation of arterial carbon dioxide by end-tidal and transcutaneous $P{CO_2}$ measurements in ventilated children. *Pediatr Pulmonol*, 12:153, 1992.

Stock MC: Noninvasive carbon dioxide monitoring. *Crit Care Clin*, 4:511, 1988.

Weil MH, Bitera J, et al: Cardiac output and end-tidal carbon dioxide. *Crit Care Med*, 13:907, 1985.

West J: Ventilation, blood flow, and gas exchange. In Murray J, Nadel J (Eds): *Textbook of Respiratory Physiology.* Philadelphia, WB Saunders, 1988, p 47.

Chapter 12

Ventilatory Support in Infants and Children

David M. Habib, J. Scott Brandeburg, and J. Warren Bradley

Assisted ventilation is a supportive technique; it is not curative. It can do no more than maintain blood gas tension homeostasis within acceptable physiological limits for a time. Its goals are to provide alveolar ventilation (i.e., carbon dioxide removal) and optimal systemic oxygenation, to reduce the work of breathing, and to protect airway patency.

To safely and effectively provide assisted ventilation for infants and children, one must understand the physiological effects of mechanical ventilation. A working knowledge of pulmonary mechanics and the ventilator's design and operation is required, and an appreciation is needed of the disease process for which assisted ventilation is indicated.

INDICATIONS FOR ASSISTED VENTILATION

Children may need assisted ventilation for conditions that may or may not have a primary pulmonary cause. The most common indication for pediatric patients is respiratory failure, defined as either a reduction in arterial oxygen tension (i.e., $PaO_2 < 50$ mm Hg) despite supplemental oxygen or an increase in arterial carbon dioxide tension (i.e., $PaCO_2 > 55$ mm Hg). Hypoxemia (actual or impending), not hypercapnia, is the usual indication for ventilatory support. Progressive hypercapnia and acidosis, however, are important predictors of impending central nervous system depression, additional alveolar hypoventilation, apnea, and hypoxemia.

The clinical indications for assisted ventilation are best stated in terms of categories based on neurological and cardiopulmonary pathophysiological processes (Table 12–1). The decision to begin assisted ventilation should be a clinical judgment based on the potential for respiratory failure. Generally, elective intubation is wise, especially if the underlying disease process is unlikely to improve rapidly.

PULMONARY MECHANICS

Compliance

Transthoracic compliance of the respiratory system (C_{rs}) is defined as the change in volume per unit change in distending airway pressure.

Table 12–1 Indications for Assisted Ventilation

Central Nervous System Dysfunction
Head and spinal cord injuries
Mass lesions
Abnormal breathing pattern
Loss of airway protection or patency
Infection
Status epilepticus
Drug effect
Respiratory Pump Failure
Neuromuscular failure
Diaphragmatic paralysis
Nutritional debilitation
Respiratory muscle fatigue
Respiratory Failure Caused by Intrinsic Pulmonary Disease
Alveolar disorders (i.e., adult respiratory distress syndrome)
Interstitial disorders (i.e., pneumonia)
Airway diseases (i.e., asthma, bronchiolitis)
Circulatory Problems
Cardiac arrest
Shock syndrome
Pulmonary arterial hypertension
Surgical Indications
After cardiac surgery
Intraoperative trauma to lung or airway
Extensive abdominal surgery
Need for high-dose analgesics
Trauma

($\Delta V/\Delta P$). Because a greater negative intrapleural pressure must be generated to inflate a less compliant lung, the patient's work of breathing increases, and gas exchange in general becomes less efficient. Static compliance of the normal pediatric respiratory system ranges between 1 and 1.5 ml/cm H_2O/kg body weight (American Thoracic Society/European Respiratory Society, 1993). Disease states associated with reduced lung or chest wall compliance are listed in Table 12–2.

Functional Residual Capacity

Functional residual capacity (FRC) is the volume of gas retained in the lung at the end of the expiratory phase of the respiratory cycle. The normal FRC is between 18 and 25 ml/kg body weight (Gerhardt et al, 1986). It is decreased in patients with respiratory failure that results from alveolar or interstitial disease. A decrease in FRC reduces lung compliance and increases the work of breathing. A major goal of assisted ventilation is to return FRC toward normal and therefore improve systemic oxygenation.

Airway Resistance

Airway resistance is the pressure difference between the mouth and the alveoli, or the driving pressure needed to move respiratory gases through the airways at a constant flow rate. The most important determinant of airway resistance is the airway radius (i.e., resistance is inversely related to the fourth power of the radius as defined by Poiseuille's law) (Martin, 1992).

Time Constant

The time constant of a patient's respiratory system is a measure of how quickly the lungs can inhale or exhale. More than 95% of the proximal airway pressure is delivered to the distal alveoli after a period of three time constants

Table 12–2 Conditions Associated with Decreased Lung or Chest Wall Compliance

Increased Elastic Recoil Forces
Severe bronchiolar-alveolar pneumonia (bacterial, viral, fungal, aspiration, opportunistic organisms)
Severe diffuse pulmonary edema (cardiogenic, hydrostatic, neurogenic, postobstructive)
Neonatal or adult respiratory distress syndrome (permeability pulmonary edema)
Diffuse atelectasis
Interstitial inflammation; fluid or fibrotic process
Radiation pneumonitis and chronic changes (bronchopulmonary dysplasia)
Reduced Chest Wall, Lung, and Diaphragmatic Excursion
Thoracic trauma and abdominal surgery
Pleural effusions
Pneumothorax
Reduced diaphragmatic excursion caused by abdominal distention (ascites, gastric or intestinal gas, peritoneal dialysis, after gastroschisis repair)
Paralysis of diaphragm
Thoracic bone deformities (severe kyphoscoliosis)
Alveolar Overdistention
Asthma
Bronchiolitis
Severe meconium aspiration
Severe bronchopulmonary dysplasia
Severe laryngotracheobronchomalacia
Excessive positive end-expiratory pressure or continuous positive airway pressure
Inadequate assisted ventilator expiratory time

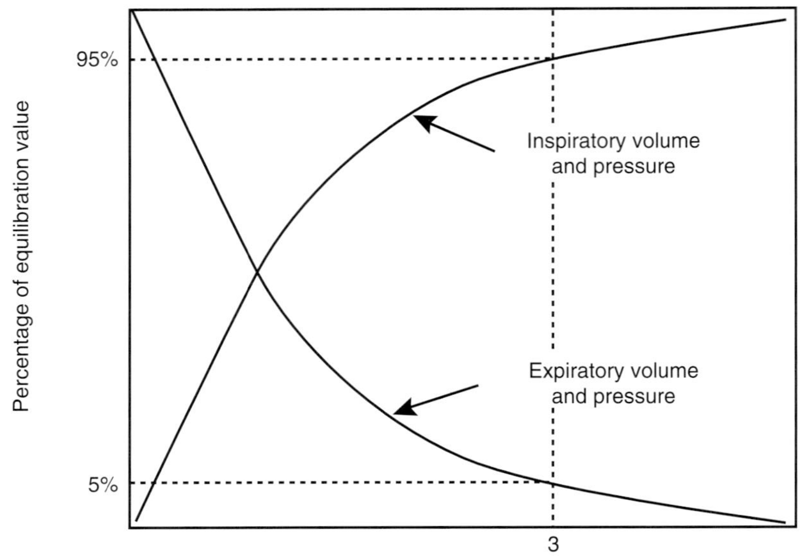

Figure 12–1 The time constant of a patient's respiratory system is a measure of how quickly the lungs can inhale or exhale. More than 95% of the proximal airway pressure is delivered to the distal alveoli after a period of three time constants.

(Fig. 12–1). In a normal infant, one time constant equals approximately 0.15 second, and three time constants equals 0.45 second.

Because the airways tend to collapse during exhalation, expiratory time constants are normally longer than inspiratory time constants. In diseases associated with increased airway resistance, such as asthma, bronchiolitis, or bronchopulmonary dysplasia, the time constants of alveolar units increase, which causes slower filling and emptying of the diseased alveolar units. Inadequate expiratory time can lead to air trapping and inadvertent positive end-expiratory pressure ($PEEP_i$), also called auto-PEEP (Bancalari, 1986). Patterns of ventilation involving prolongation of inspiration should be avoided in these types of mechanically ventilated patients (Martin, 1992). Signs of gas trapping include overexpansion of the chest, decreased chest wall movement, retention of carbon dioxide with decreased end-tidal carbon dioxide, decreased PaO_2 in infants with extrapulmonary right-to-left shunting, and deterioration of cardiovascular function (i.e., reduced cardiac output).

In diseases that result in decreased compliance (e.g., adult respiratory distress syndrome [ARDS]), the time constant decreases, which causes the alveolar unit to have a faster filling and emptying time. This allows longer inspiratory time, which may improve overall alveolar gas distribution with less risk of $PEEP_i$.

HYPOXEMIA

Physiological mechanisms that give rise to inadequate pulmonary capillary oxygen uptake and hypoxemia include ventilation-perfusion ($\dot{V}/\dot{Q}$) mismatching, shunting, hypoventilation, low inspired oxygen concentration, and diffusion abnormalities.

Hypoxemia can be corrected (i.e., PaO_2) by several methods. The appropriate choice is based on the specific pathophysiological process that caused the hypoxemia. Increasing the oxygen concentration of the delivered gas increases the PaO_2, when the cause of the hypoxemia is hypoventilation, a diffusion impairment, or $\dot{V}/\dot{Q}$ mismatching. However, when severe shunt (> 20%) is the cause of hypoxemia, increasing the inspired oxygen concentration is not effective (Chatburn, 1991).

PEEP and continuous positive airway pressure (CPAP) are the cornerstones of treatment for patients with intrapulmonary shunt and refractory hypoxemia associated with reduced FRC (Tyler, 1983). Furthermore, in normal infants and young children the difference between resting FRC and airway closing pressures is larger, thus increasing their risk for hypoxia.

POSITIVE END-EXPIRATORY PRESSURE

PEEP is the residual pressure above atmospheric pressure that is maintained at the airway opening at the end of expiration. CPAP is higher than atmospheric pressure and is maintained at the airway opening throughout the respiratory cycle during spontaneous breathing (Martin, 1992). The mechanisms important for improving arterial oxygenation that occur with PEEP or CPAP include increasing FRC by distention and recruiting collapsed alveolar units.

PEEP or CPAP is most likely to benefit patients with acute or diffuse lung disease associated with reduced FRC. When FRC is increased, gas flow to poorly ventilated or collapsed alveoli improves, lung compliance improves, intrapulmonary shunt decreases, and $Pa{O_2}$ increases. If hypoxemia persists despite supplemental oxygen administration (e.g., > 50%), a trial of PEEP or CPAP is indicated.

Uses of PEEP and CPAP

- Acute lung injury
  - ARDS
  - Hyaline membrane disease
  - Diffuse pneumonia
  - Aspiration syndromes
- Other conditions
  - Apnea
  - Asthma and bronchiolitis
  - Tracheobronchomalacia
  - Chronic lung disease
  - Postoperative care
  - Pulmonary edema
  - Artificial airways
  - Intracardiac left-to-right shunts
  - Weaning from mechanical ventilation

PEEP or CPAP is generally increased in small increments (2–3 cm H_2O); oxygenation and hemodynamic performance must be monitored during these changes. As $Pa{O_2}$ improves, the fraction of inspired oxygen ($F{IO_2}$) can be reduced. A goal of PEEP or CPAP is to achieve a $Pa{O_2}$ greater than 70 mm Hg with use of nontoxic levels of oxygen (i.e., < 50%). The optimal amount of PEEP or CPAP administered must be guided by the ability to reduce $F{IO_2}$ while adequate tissue perfusion (i.e., cardiac outout) and oxygenation are maintained (Suter, 1975). Inappropriately high levels of PEEP can lead to overinflation of alveoli, increased dead space ventilation, decreased pulmonary compliance, and increased intrapulmonary shunt.

Therapy with PEEP and CPAP has long been known to reduce cardiac output. Two separate mechanisms have been identified: an increase in intrapleural pressure that decreases venous return, and an increase in lung volume that causes ventricular dysfunction (Dorinsky and Whitcomb, 1983; Schulman et al, 1992). The reduction in cardiac output can be severe enough to offset the benefits of increased arterial oxygen content and can result in an actual decrease in systemic oxygen transport. It is recommended that cardiac output be monitored when PEEP or CPAP is greater than 15 cm H_2O.

The use of PEEP or CPAP may result in or intensify intracranial hypertension, cerebral ischemia, or both (Cooper et al, 1988; Shapiro and Marshall; 1978). Decreased cerebral perfusion pressure may be related to a decrease in cardiac output and mean systemic arterial blood pressure as well as to an increase in intracranial pressure.

POSITIVE-PRESSURE VENTILATION

Before positive-pressure ventilation can be instituted, a stable airway must be established, usually by placement of an endotracheal tube. The narrowest part of the pediatric airway is at the subglottic region (Miyasaka, 1993). The subglottic region is completely surrounded by cricoid cartilage and is susceptible to edema and inflammation. To minimize laryngeal damage, uncuffed endotracheal tubes must be used, and a small air leak at 20 to 30 cm H_2O positive pressure should be present. The presence of air leaks, however, may cause difficulties in adequately ventilating a child, especially when pulmonary compliance is decreased.

Most clinicians are familiar with the terms volume-cycled ventilator and pressure-cycled ventilator. Regardless of which term is applied, a ventilator can control only two of four parameters during inspiration: pressure, volume, flow, or time (gas flow and time are inversely related and are the regulators of tidal volume) (Table 12–3). When volume flow is controlled, the delivered tidal volume is a function of the preset flow pattern, and time is independently determined by the ventilator. If volume and time are controlled, tidal volume is a function of the preset time, and flow is internally regulated. When pressure is controlled, the tidal volume is a function of time, the amplitude of the pressure waveform (the difference between the peak and end-expiratory pressure), and the compliance (C_{rs}) and resistance (R_{rs})of the respiratory system.

An important mechanical distinction between volume and pressure ventilators is the

Table 12–3 Ventilator Types: Controlled Versus Determined Parameters

	Ventilator Type	
Parameter	**Time-Cycled, Pressure-Limited**	**Volume-Cycled**
Flow	Controlled	Controlled/ Determined*
Volume	Determined	Controlled
Pressure	Controlled	Determined
Inspiratory time	Controlled	Determined/ Controlled*
FIO_2	Controlled	Controlled

*When flow rate is controlled by the clinician, inspiratory time is determined by the ventilator, and vice versa.

type of flow pattern generated by the power drive. The flow pattern for pressure-cycled ventilators is decelerating (i.e., low-pressure generator); a constant proximal airway pressure is generated, but the accumulation of alveolar volume and pressure is nonlinear. When the pressure drive is high (i.e., volume-cycled ventilator), a constant flow is generated and the accumulation of lung volume and airway pressure is linear (Fig. 12–2). This difference results in a higher peak airway pressure but a lower mean airway pressure for volume-cycled ventilation in comparison to time-cycled, pressure-limited ventilation. Also, in pulmonary diseases with high alveolar critical opening pressures (e.g., ARDS), a constant flow pattern may leave less time for the alveolus to fill than does the constant pressure pattern. This could result in a lower level of ventilation and poorer oxygenation with volume cycling.

It is important to distinguish between limit and cycle. A parameter is limited if it reaches a constant value before inspiration ends. Inspiration is cycled off when a variable (pressure, volume, time, or flow) reaches a preset threshold value. For example, during time-cycled, pressure-limited ventilation, pressure is limited to some preset peak value, but inspiration is terminated when the inspiratory time meets the

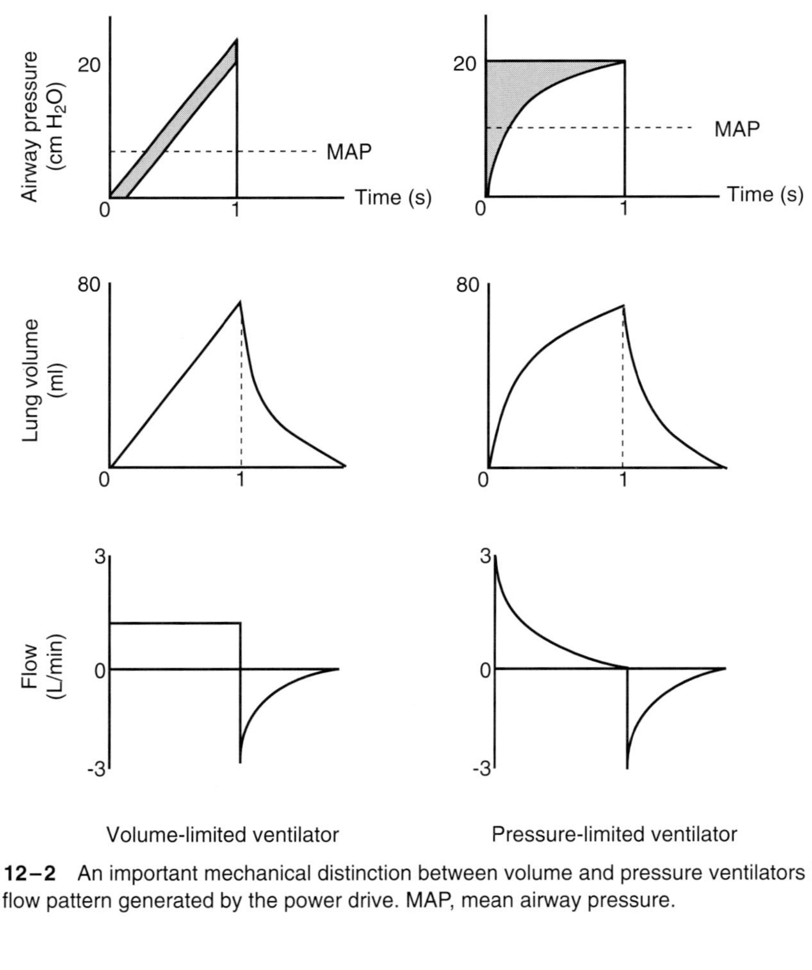

Figure 12–2 An important mechanical distinction between volume and pressure ventilators is the type of flow pattern generated by the power drive. MAP, mean airway pressure.

value set by the clinician. On the other hand, volume-cycled ventilators usually deliver a preset rectangular or constant flow waveform. Inspiration is terminated when the inspiratory time has reached the duration necessary to deliver the preset tidal volume. Most neonatal and infant ventilators are pressure limited and time cycled; those used in children and adults are volume limited and either volume or time cycled. Ventilators may thus be classified according to what parameter ends the ventilator cycle.

A ventilator may use any of the four parameters for triggering, limiting, cycling, and controlling baseline pressure. For example, the pressure support mode is pressure-limited ventilation that is pressure triggered and flow cycled.

Volume-Cycled Ventilation

A ventilator is volume cycled when the inspiratory phase ends at the moment a preset volume has been delivered into the patient circuit. Driving pressure is variable and determined by the patient's respiratory compliance and resistance. The clinician determines the volume to be delivered. Once the desired tidal volume is established, usually 10 to 15 ml/kg body weight, provisions must be made to ensure that the volume is delivered within a reasonable time. With most volume-cycled ventilators, a flow rate control is present and provides the necessary means of regulating the length of the inspiratory phase.

A major advantage of volume-cycled ventilation is the delivery of consistent tidal volume despite any changes in lung compliance or airways resistance. However, not all of the volume selected at the ventilator reaches the patient. Some compressible volume is lost in the ventilator circuit as a consequence of the system's compliance and the driving pressure. For neonates and infants, the use of short, small-diameter, thick-walled ventilator tubing has reduced the compliance factor to less than 1 ml/cm H_2O of applied pressure (Martin, 1992). Volume may also be lost because of a leak (uncuffed tubes) or if the patient is disconnected from the circuit. The usual method of correcting for lost volume is by slowly increasing delivered volume until the desired return volume is achieved. The flow rate may then need further adjustment to maintain inspiratory time. Use of pressure-cycled ventilation can avoid this problem.

Another advantage of volume-cycled ventilation is that a change in driving pressure reflects a change in the mechanics of the patient's respiratory or ventilator system. For example, if the patient's lung compliance decreases, more pressure is needed to deliver the same tidal volume. Conversely, if the patient's compliance improves, less pressure must be developed by the ventilator to deliver the same tidal volume. Ventilator circuit problems that may produce increased pressure readings include kinked ventilator tubing, malpositioned or obstructed endotracheal tube, water condensate in ventilator tubing, increased airway resistance caused by secretions or bronchospasm, and changes in the patient's position. In this case, the ventilator vents excess gases through a relief valve at a preset limited pressure.

Pressure-Cycled Ventilation

Pressure-cycled ventilators terminate the inspiratory phase when a preselected airway pressure is achieved, regardless of the volume delivered or the time elapsed. The major advantage of pressure-cycled ventilation is avoidance of excessive inflating pressures, which decreases the risk of barotrauma (Fig. 12–3). A short inspiratory time can result from a decreased pulmonary compliance, a restriction or obstruction in the endotracheal tube (i.e., accumulation of secretions) or in the ventilator circuit, or an increase in the patient's airway resistance. Regardless of the cause, a smaller tidal volume is delivered because the cycling pressure is reached prematurely. The corrective procedure is with the cycling pressure, which must be increased.

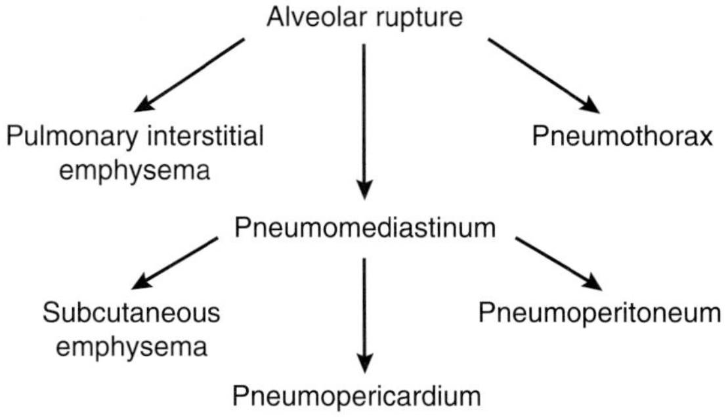

Figure 12–3 Barotrauma complicating mechanical ventilation. (Adapted from Habib D, Perkin R: Continuous distending pressure. In Levin D, Morriss F [eds]: *Essentials of Pediatric Intensive Care.* St Louis, Quality Medical Publishing, 1990, p 908.)

The pressure-cycled mode can provide better compensation for gas leakage when the leak is not great enough to prevent cycling. In the event of a large airway leak or ventilator disconnection, cycling pressure cannot be achieved, and inspiration is prolonged indefinitely. This disadvantage of pressure-cycled ventilation can be avoided by the use of the time-cycled, pressure-limited mode.

Time-Cycled Ventilation

Ventilators that are time cycled change from the inspiratory phase of the breathing cycle to the expiratory phase only after an adjusted time has elapsed. The cycling is independent of the volume delivered to the patient or the pressure required to deliver the volume. The frequency of ventilation is determined by the inspiratory and expiratory controls. If tidal volume is increased by prolonging the inspiratory time, respiratory rate decreases unless expiration time is decreased. Conversely, if the inspiratory time is decreased to reduce the tidal volume, the ventilatory rate increases unless expiratory time is increased. Time-cycled ventilators do not control volume directly but deliver a volume proportional to the product of flow rate and inspiratory time. If one plans to manipulate the tidal volume without changing inspiratory time, the flow rate can be manipulated. In practice, time-cycled ventilation is used in conjunction with pressure-limited or volume-controlled modes.

Time-Cycled, Pressure-Limited Ventilation

Time-cycled, pressure-limited ventilation is the most widely used method of assisted ventilation in neonatal critical care (McWilliams, 1987). In time-cycled, pressure-limited ventilation, mandatory breaths are not cycled even when a preset airway pressure is reached. Rather, the preset airway pressure is sustained during inspiratory time and produces a pressure plateau. This allows improved distribution of inspired gases owing to recruitment of alveoli with prolonged time constants (Chatburn, 1991) (see Fig. 12–2). Pressure-limited ventilation can be applied by two different methods: (1) inspiratory gas flow is constant and excess gas is vented through a separate pressure relief valve; (2) during inspiration, gas flow is gradually decreased by a servoregulated pressure control mechanism.

There is no simple way to predict the initial requirements of the pressure limit because the extent of the patient's pulmonary dysfunction is not established. Clinical judgment is needed to select the pressure limit, which is customarily in the range of 10 to 20 cm H_2O for infants and children. (Higher pressures are commonly necessary for newborns and those with severe lung disease.) The exact setting for flow rate is also impossible to establish but is initially adjusted to provide an adequate inspiratory time (e.g., 0.3–0.6 second), equal to approximately three times the normal inspiratory time constant.

Once the preliminary settings are made, the patient is connected to the ventilator. The optimal tidal volume and minute ventilation of infants and children are then assessed by listening for air entry and exit, observing chest expansion, obtaining arterial blood samples for blood gas tension and pH analysis, and measuring exhaled volume. In pressure-limited ventilation, the delivered tidal volume may vary and is influenced by changes in respiratory compliance and airways resistance.

VENTILATOR MODES

Intermittent mandatory ventilation (IMV) was initially developed as a technique of weaning. It is the most widely used technique in pediatric critical care. IMV allows the patient to breathe spontaneously and yet provides a certain preselected number of mechanically delivered breaths. Mandatory breaths can be synchronized with spontaneous breaths (synchronized IMV), but not all spontaneous breaths are assisted. Some of the advantages of IMV include (1) ventilation with lower mean airway pressures, leading to less cardiovascular depression and less barotrauma; (2) reduced need for sedation or paralysis in patients requiring mechanical ventilation; (3) less tendency for alveolar hyperventilation or hypoventilation; (4) maintenance of spontaneous respiratory activity, which results in the continuous exercise of respiratory muscles; and (5) more even distribution of ventilation and pulmonary blood flow, which improves overall $\dot{V}/\dot{Q}$ matching.

Controlled mechanical ventilation delivers mechanical breaths at a predetermined interval; no gas flow is available for spontaneous ventilation. Therefore, if the patient attempts to breathe, airway pressure is decreased, but no gas will flow into the lungs. Respiration is fully supported by controlled mechanical ventilation, and administration of high-dose sedatives or muscle relaxants is usually necessary.

Assisted mechanical ventilation is a mode in

which preset mandatory breaths are delivered on all spontaneously triggered efforts to breathe by the patient. This is less advantageous in pediatric critical care because triggering is not always obtainable in pediatric patients and may significantly increase the work of breathing. In addition, respiratory rates of infants and children are relatively higher, promoting alveolar hyperventilation and respiratory alkalemia.

COMPLICATIONS AND PROBLEMS

Two important clinical complications associated with high mean or peak airway pressure are impaired cardiac filling and barotrauma. Mean airway pressure is the area under the pressure curve of one ventilatory cycle. Mean airway pressure rises with decreased C_{rs}, increased R_{rs} or PEEP, and ventilator parameters that increase tidal volume. With volume-cycled ventilators, the main parameters affecting mean airway pressure are tidal volume, inspiratory time, and PEEP. For time-cycled, pressure-limited ventilators, they are peak inspiratory pressure, inspiratory time, and PEEP. Mean airway pressure is also increased by $PEEP_i$, where distal airway pressures are positive at end-exhalation even though the machine's proximal airway pressure manometer indicates zero pressure (Fig. 12–4). PEEP is evidenced by air trapping on the chest film and is promoted by airway obstruction, rapid respiratory rates, slow inspiratory flow rates, and nearly equal inspiration to expiration (I/E) ratios (Schuster, 1990).

Elevation of mean airway pressure may cause arterial hypotension by either a decrease in venous return or right ventricular dysfunction, particularly if preset PEEP or $PEEP_i$ is high (Biondi et al, 1988; Potkin et al, 1987). Cardiac output can usually be maintained with fluid therapy and positive inotropes. Other causes of hypotension include tension pneumothorax, intravascular volume depletion, sedatives and paralytic drugs, and reduced catecholamine levels.

Peak airway pressure is determined by the tidal volume and the compliance and resistance of the respiratory system. High peak airway pressure, greater than 45 cm H_2O, is a significant risk factor for barotrauma (Schuster, 1990). Barotrauma and alveolar rupture are the most life threatening complications of assisted ventilation, and sometimes avoiding their sequelae is more important than achieving normal blood gas values (see Fig. 12–3). For example, in severe asthma, excessive peak airway pressure, mean airway pressure, and $PEEP_i$ can occur when the goal is to achieve a normal Pa_{CO_2}. If peak airway pressure exceeds 45 to 50 cm H_2O, permissive hypercapnia should be instituted by decreasing the ventilator rate, lengthening the expiratory phase, and tolerating blood pH as low as 7.25 (Dworkin and Kattan, 1989).

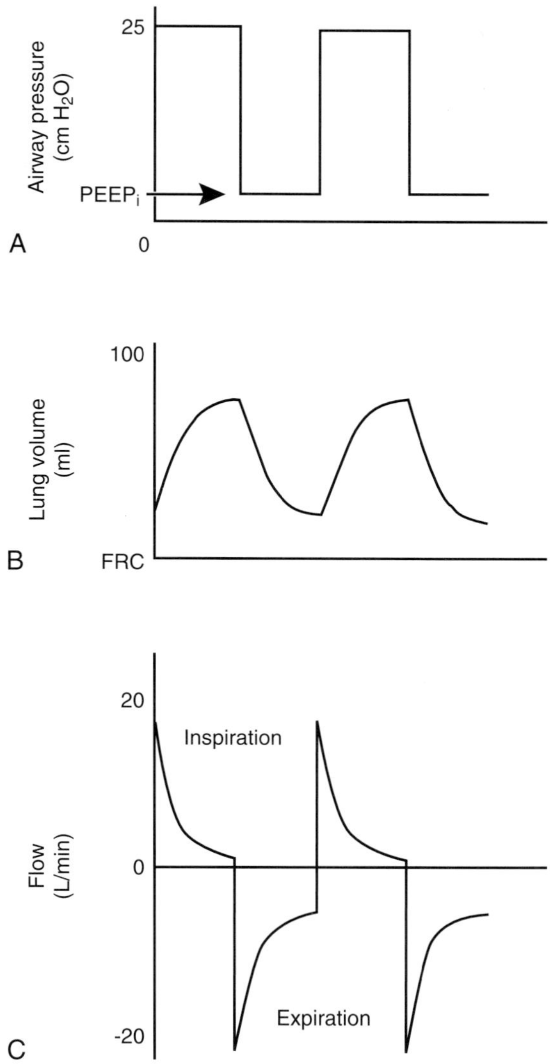

Figure 12–4 Comparison of pressure, volume, and flow curves during pressure control–inverse ratio ventilation. **A**. Development of inadvertent positive end-expiratory pressure ($PEEP_i$); airway pressure never reaches baseline. **B**. Elevation of functional residual capacity (FRC) due to gas trapping. **C**. Representation of flow showing expiratory flow never reaching baseline before initiation of next breath. (Adapted from Chatburn R: Principles and practice of neonatal and pediatric mechanical ventilation. *Respir Care,* 36:580, 1991.)

To prevent unwanted patient-ventilator asynchrony, struggle, or anxiety, administration of respiratory depressant drugs or induction of neuromuscular blockade is indicated (McEvoy, 1993; Taketomo et al, 1993) (Table 12–4). Sedation facilitates the patient's breathing in phase with the ventilator so that peak airway pressure and barotrauma are kept to a minimum. Muscle relaxants increase chest wall compliance, reduce oxygen consumption, and maximize the patient's cooperation. The use of sedation or muscle relaxants is generally limited to the following situations: (1) requirement for high airway pressures, such as in a patient with asthma; (2) critically inadequate oxygenation, such as in ARDS; (3) ventilator intolerance, such as in an anxious infant; and (4) nonpulmonary indications, such as severe head injury.

The use of adequate humidification and the proper regulation of inspired gas temperature during mechanical ventilation are essential for precluding complications. Because medical gases such as oxygen and compressed air are dry, they must always be rehumidified before delivery to the patient. In addition, artificial airways, such as endotracheal or tracheostomy tubes, reduce the normal respiratory surface available for heating and humidification of inspired gases by 25%. Inadequate humidification may result in increased respiratory insensible water loss, inspissated secretions, decreased mucociliary function, and airway obstruction. In pediatric patients, obstruction may be potentiated further by the smaller caliber of their airways, and failure to provide adequate thermal regulation may result in inadvertent hypothermia or pulmonary burns.

Humidity represents molecular water in its gaseous or vapor state; the actual weight of water per volume of gas at normal body temperature (37°C) equals 43.8 mg/L (body humidity). Relative humidity is the percentage of the water vapor content of a gas in comparison to its potential water vapor capacity at any given temperature (relative humidity-content/capacity × 100). Because gas at 100% relative humidity and room temperature (22°C) contains less than 40% body humidity, inspiratory gases must be heated to approximately 32 to 37°C to provide 90% to 100% relative humidity. All humidifiers should be capable of providing servocontrolled gas temperatures of 32 to 37°C and 90% to 100% relative humidity across the full spectrum of clinical gas flow rates. In addition, both the humidifier and ventilator should have circuit temperatures digitally displayed and be equipped with both inspiratory and expiratory heated wire circuits to prevent excessive humidity rainout. To prevent unnecessary compressed volume loss, the humidifier unit should be of a minimum volume and equipped with internal self-test and diagnostic circuitry to continuously monitor the system's function.

Acute respiratory distress occurring in the patient on ventilatory support may be caused by the patient or by the ventilator's malfunction. Common ventilator problems and their possible causes are listed in Table 12–5.

WEANING FROM MECHANICAL VENTILATION

Weaning is the gradual withdrawal of assisted ventilatory support in those patients in whom recovery from respiratory failure is incomplete. The principle of weaning includes high-intensity work for short periods, followed by adequate rest. In general, weaning is not instituted until hemodynamic stabilization is achieved and the patient is alert and responsive.

As ventilatory support is reduced, signs of increased work of breathing and fatigue must be monitored carefully. Signs of fatigue often precede deterioration of blood gas and pH values. Clinical manifestations of distress include anxiety, tachypnea, tachycardia, hypotension, diaphoresis, paradoxical chest wall–abdominal breathing, and alternating use of intercostal muscles and diaphragm. Frequent assessment of arterial blood gas values (i.e., every 4–12 hours) and observation of the child's clinical status are essential throughout the weaning process. Also, loss of body weight is a sign of inappropriately high levels of work of breathing.

Nutritional support and correction of metabolic abnormalities are important for successful weaning. Malnutrition diminishes the diaphragm's muscle fiber cross-sectional area, which enhances fatigability. A balanced intake of carbohydrates, protein, and fat is recommended. Calorie supplementation that is high in carbohydrates should be avoided and has been associated with elevated carbon dioxide production, which increases both minute ventilation and the work of breathing (Taketomo et al, 1993). Metabolic abnormalities such as hypocalcemia, hypokalemia, and hypophosphatemia may prevent successful weaning.

Weaning may be inhibited by other causes of increased carbon dioxide production, including fever (10% increase per 1°C increase), seizures, and shivering. In addition, other con-

Table 12–4 Drugs Commonly Used to Facilitate Mechanical Ventilation

Trade Name	Generic Name	Route	Dose	Side Effects	Comments
Aquachloral Noctec	Chloral hydrate	PO, PR	20–50 mg/kg	CNS depression Vomiting Gastrointestinal irritation	Do not exceed 2 g/24 h Hepatic metabolism
Versed	Midazolam	IM, IV	0.05–0.15 mg/kg 2–8 μg/kg/min as continuous infusion	Respiratory depression	Hepatic metabolism
Ativan	Lorazopam	PO, IV	0.05 mg/kg	Respiratory depression	Hepatic metabolism
Morphine	Morphine	IM, IV	0.05–0.2 mg/kg 0.02–0.1 mg/kg/h as continuous infusion	CNS depression Hypotension Histamine release Constipation and delayed gastric emptying	Hepatic metabolism Half-life; 2–2.5 hr
Sublimaze	Fentanyl	IM, IV	1–3 μg/kg 2–10 μg/kg/h as continuous infusion	Respiratory depression Chest wall muscle rigidity associated with rapid IV administration	Hepatic metabolism
Ketalar	Ketamine	IV	0.5–2 mg/kg	Tachycardia Hypertension Hypersalivation ↑ Intracranial pressure	Analgesic and amnestic agent Emergence reactions (hallucinations)

continued

Table 12–4 Drugs Commonly Used to Facilitate Mechanical Ventilation *(Continued)*

Trade Name	Generic Name	Route	Dose	Side Effects	Comments
Pavulon	Pancuronium	IV	0.1–0.15 mg/kg	Tachycardia Hypertension	Renal excretion (55%–70%) Hepatic metabolism (30%–40%)
Metubine	Metocurine	IV	0.2–0.4 mg/kg	Hypotension Histamine release	Renal excretion
Tracrium	Atracurium	IV	0.3–0.5 mg/kg 0.3–1 mg/kg/h as continuous infusion	Histamine release	Nonenzymatic degradation by Hofmann elimination and ester hydrolysis Metabolite, laudanosine, stimulates CNS
Norcuron	Vecuronium	IV	0.08–0.1 mg/kg 1–3 μg/kg/min as continuous infusion	Minimal histamine release Prolonged paralysis	Biliary elimination Renal excretion (10%–20%)
Romazicon	Flumazenil	IV	0.01 mg/kg (max dose 0.2 mg)	Seizures (with long-term benzodiazepine use) Dysrhythmias	Benzodiazepine antagonist of CNS depression Onset: 1–3 min; duration: < 1 h Potential for sedation
Narcan	Naloxone	IV, IM, SC	0.1 mg/kg	Hypertension Tachycardia	Narcotic antagonist May precipitate withdrawal syndrome Onset: 2–5 min; duration: 20–60 min

CNS, central nervous system; IM, intramuscular; IV, intravenous; PO, oral; PR, rectal; SC, subcutaneous.

Table 12-5 Ventilator Dilemmas

Problem	Possible Causes
High peak airway pressure and normal plateau pressure	High peak inspiratory flow rate High resistance in endotracheal tube or ventilator circuit: small endotracheal tube; malpositioned endotracheal tube; kinking; obstruction; secretions High airway resistance: bronchospasm; edema; foreign body; tracheobronchomalacia or stenosis
High plateau and high peak pressures	Alveolar overdistention Lung edema Consolidation Atelectasis Main stem intubation Pneumothorax Chest wall constriction Abdominal distention Agitation, seizures
Increased respiratory rate	Change in respiratory mechanics Low tidal volume Insufficient flow rate
No spontaneous breaths	Respiratory alkalosis Sedation Central nervous system problems

ditions that cause failure to wean include diaphragm paralysis, increased chest wall compliance, pulmonary hyperinflation with increased alveolar dead space, inadequate sleep, excessive sedation, and incompletely treated heart failure.

Weaning Techniques

The specific weaning technique employed is often less important than the care with which it is applied (Schuster, 1990). The most frequently chosen methods for weaning are IMV, CPAP trials, and pressure support ventilation.

IMV is a weaning technique that facilitates a gradual shift between the amount of ventilation provided by the patient and that provided by the machine. The IMV rate is usually decreased by 2 to 4 breaths/minute at intervals tailored to the capabilities of the patient. Most normal infants and children can be extubated from rates between 4 and 8 breaths/minute. However, protracted periods at low rates require the patient to sustain the work of breathing through a high-resistance endotracheal tube, which creates the potential for respiratory muscle fatigue. To avoid this problem, a combination of moderate IMV rates (8–12 breaths/minute) with alternating periods of CPAP (1–3 hours, three to four times/day) is often used successfully.

Pressure support ventilation is useful when respiratory muscle weakness or severe patient-ventilator asynchrony limits successful weaning. In the pressure support mode, a limited amount of positive pressure is delivered into the ventilator circuit; the peak inspiratory flow rate, tidal volume, and respiratory rate are governed by the patient. Each cycle is terminated when the flow rate decreases to 25% of the peak flow rate. Initial limits of positive pressure vary from 10 to 20 cm H_2O so that each tidal volume is 10 to 15 ml/kg. As the patient improves, the pressure limit is gradually decreased to 5 cm H_2O. Pressure support ventilation can be provided alone or in combination with synchronized IMV or CPAP when either complete ventilatory support or end-expiratory pressure is needed. A pitfall of pressure support ventilation occurs when low lung compliance along with excess initial gas flow leads to premature termination of gas flow and autocycling.

When oxygenation failure is the clinical indication for positive-pressure support and the patient's FIO_2 is less than 50%, PEEP should be gradually withdrawn to physiological levels (3–5 cm H_2O). PEEP or CPAP must be reduced in a carefully controlled fashion (i.e., in increments of 2 to 3 cm H_2O) while a PaO_2 above 70 mm Hg is maintained. Premature withdrawal or sudden discontinuation of PEEP or CPAP may lead to a precipitous fall in PaO_2 and FRC. During this time, the ventilator mode, rate, and tidal volume should be adjusted to maintain a normal pH and minimize the work of breathing. Once the PEEP required to maintain oxygenation is 5 cm H_2O or less, further weaning can usually be rapid.

Criteria for withdrawal of positive-pressure support are nonspecific and insensitive in adults, and few data exist for infants and children. However, useful clinical guides for ensuring adequate oxygenation include a PaO_2 of 60 mm Hg or greater with FIO_2 of 40% or less, or alveolar-arterial oxygen gradient less than 350 mm Hg, or a PaO_2/FIO_2 ratio above 200 (Martin, 1992). A spontaneous minute ventilation less than 10 L/min with a respiratory rate less than 30 breaths/minute implies a relatively low work of breathing to maintain adequate gas exchange. A vital capacity of 10 to 15 ml/kg and a maximal negative inspiratory force of 30 cm H_2O are useful as indices of respiratory muscle strength and for predicting effective cough (Martin, 1992; Schuster, 1990).

MONITORING MECHANICAL VENTILATION

The success of assisted ventilation is directly related to the skill with which it is applied, and complications associated with its use can be limited only through careful monitoring. After ventilation is initiated, attention should be directed to the adequacy of alveolar ventilation and systemic oxygenation. This is established by clinical observation of chest excursion, vital signs, and quality of breath sounds and by assessment of peripheral circulation. Serial monitoring should then be performed a minimum of every 2 to 3 hours to detect changes in the mechanics of the ventilator-patient system. In many modern ventilators, this is facilitated by the use of extended electronic pressure, flow and volume monitoring capabilities, graphic display, and recording options.

NONCONVENTIONAL MODES OF MECHANICAL VENTILATION

New methods of ventilatory support, designed for specific problems and made possible by new mechanical ventilators, have been developed (Hazelzet et al, 1993). These newer methods of mechanical ventilation include pressure support ventilation, high-frequency ventilation, mandatory minute ventilation, differential lung ventilation, inverse ratio ventilation, airway pressure release ventilation, and flow synchronization. Most of these ventilatory modes are currently available, and even though few clinical studies have assessed their value, they are used when conventional modes of ventilation (i.e., volume-cycled or time-cycled; pressure-limited) fail to maintain adequate gas exchange.

Pressure Control–Inverse Ratio Ventilation

Pressure control–inverse ratio ventilation (PC-IRV) is nothing more than a variation of pressure-limited ventilation. The use of inverse ratio ventilation with a pressure-limited device was first popularized in the 1970s in the management of infants suffering from idiopathic respiratory distress syndrome (Boros, 1979). PC-IRV was introduced as an adult mode of ventilation in the early 1980s for the management of the patient suffering from ARDS.

The primary goal of PC-IRV is to improve gas exchange and recruit collapsed or flooded alveoli while decreasing peak airway pressure, thereby reducing lung parenchymal stress and barotrauma (Marcy and Marini, 1991). This is probably related to the fact that PC-IRV uses a decelerating inspiratory waveform, which aids in reducing $\dot{V}/\dot{Q}$ mismatching by ventilating more lung units (Fig. 12–5). Studies have shown that PC-IRV is effective for improving gas exchange in the patient suffering from severe ARDS, compared with conventional volume-controlled ventilation (Abraham and Yoshihara, 1989; Papadakos et al, 1991). PC-IRV has also been shown to significantly reduce peak airway pressure, total respiratory resistance, ratio of dead space to tidal volume (V_D/V_T), and alveolar-arterial oxygen gradient (Al-Saady and Bennett, 1985).

Initiation criteria

Initiation of PC-IRV should be limited to caregivers who are familiar with the pathophysiological processes as they are affected by this mode of ventilation. In general, the indications for the use of PC-IRV are diffuse bilateral infiltrates on chest film with refractory hypoxemia ($PaO_2 <$ 60 mm Hg with an $FIO_2 \geq 0.80$) despite the use of PEEP of 10 cm H_2O or greater and peak airway pressure greater than 65 cm H_2O (Blanch et al, 1993). However, some evidence supports early initiation of PC-IRV in patients diagnosed with ARDS (Papadakos et al, 1991).

Initiation on PC-IRV

Most patients require deep sedation or paralysis during PC-IRV (Abraham and Yoshihara, 1989; Papadakos et al, 1991; Tharratt et al, 1988). However, this needs to be judged on an individual basis.

Before placing the patient on PC-IRV, the clinician will need to determine whether the ventilator in use is capable of pressure control ventilation. The ventilator must be capable of delivering a decelerating inspiratory waveform in the pressure control mode. Inverse ratio is usually begun at 2:1 (Abraham and Yoshihara, 1989; Papadakos et al, 1991; Tharratt et al, 1988), but some clinicians believe a ratio of 1:1 may be a safer starting point (Lanin et al, 1989). To further improve oxygenation, the I/E ratio may be gradually increased in a period of several hours. The preset PEEP level is usually

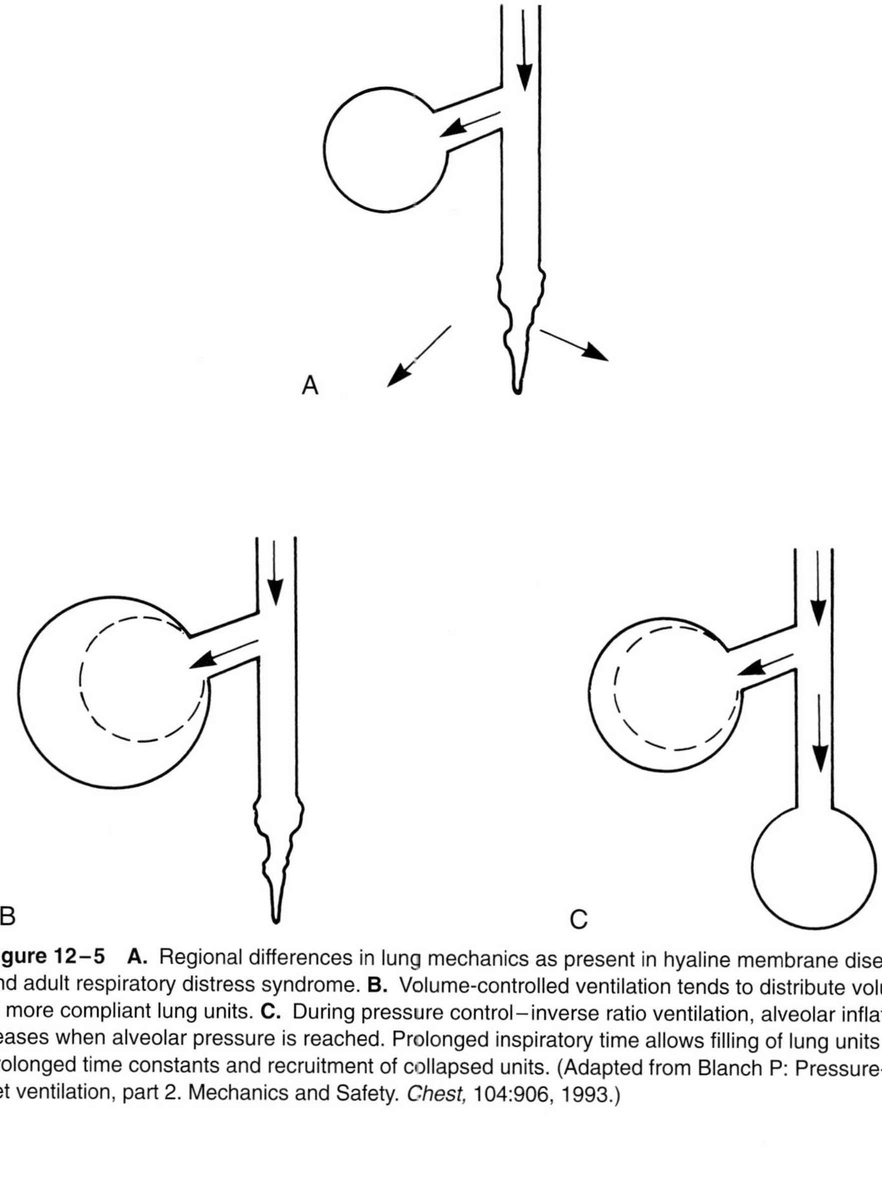

Figure 12–5 **A.** Regional differences in lung mechanics as present in hyaline membrane disease and adult respiratory distress syndrome. **B.** Volume-controlled ventilation tends to distribute volume to more compliant lung units. **C.** During pressure control–inverse ratio ventilation, alveolar inflation ceases when alveolar pressure is reached. Prolonged inspiratory time allows filling of lung units with prolonged time constants and recruitment of collapsed units. (Adapted from Blanch P: Pressure-preset ventilation, part 2. Mechanics and Safety. *Chest,* 104:906, 1993.)

reduced by 50% on initiation of PC-IRV (Lanin et al, 1989; Tharratt et al, 1988), and the respiratory rate should be adjusted so that zero expiratory flow is not reached before the initiation of the next breath (Tharratt et al, 1988) (see Fig. 12–4). Peak inspiratory pressure is reduced as needed to maintain a tidal volume of 10 to 15 ml/kg (Abraham and Yoshihara, 1989; Papadakos et al, 1991) and is usually less than the peak inspiratory pressure required to move the same volume of gas during volume-cycled ventilation.

Ventilation

Unlike in conventional modes of mechanical ventilation, expired volume (V_E) is inversely related to respiratory rate. Increases in respiratory rate often lead to decreases in expired volume V_E and thus an increase in Pa_{CO_2}. Ventilation may also be affected by changes in tidal volume; however, it is strongly recommended not to use volumes greater than 15 ml/kg. The use of a large tidal volume (> 15 ml/kg) is associated with an increased risk of pulmonary barotrauma (Tharratt et al, 1988). Oxygenation is controlled by increasing mean airway pressure. The usual method of increasing mean airway pressure with PC-IRV is to first increase the I/E ratio, up to a maximum of 4:1; however, some authors suggest increasing PEEP levels before increasing I/E ratios above 3:1 (Lanin et al, 1989).

Monitoring

Complete cardiopulmonary monitoring should be in place before the initiation of any change in mechanical ventilation. Ventilator monitoring of peak inspiratory pressure, PEEP, gas flow, tidal volume, mean airway pressure, and expired volume should be closely observed for any sudden changes in pulmonary mechanics. PEEP should be monitored for total PEEP ($PEEP_T$), which consists of preset PEEP plus $PEEP_i$. Many of the new microprocessor-controlled ventilators offer an "expiratory hold" maneuver that can be used to determine $PEEP_i$.

Tidal volume should be continuously monitored during PC-IRV. Tidal volume is a function of compliance (C_{rs} and R_{rs}), and changes in either C_{rs} or R_{rs} may alter the delivered tidal volume, thus affecting $Pa{CO_2}$ (Blanch et al, 1993). Special emphasis should be placed on setting the high and low minute volume alarms tightly to alert the clinician of any sudden changes in C_{rs} or R_{rs}.

Respiratory monitoring should consist of oximetry, arterial blood gas analysis, transcutaneous monitoring, and capnography. This is of great importance during the initiation of PC-IRV when rapid changes in pulmonary mechanics may occur. Cardiac function should be monitored by heart rate, blood pressure, filling pressures, and cardiac output. This is of particular importance because PC-IRV may greatly increase mean airway pressure (Tharratt et al, 1988), leading to hemodynamic compromise.

High-Frequency Ventilation (see also Chapter 13)

High-frequency ventilation was first introduced during the 1960s, and success in the infant and pediatric population has been encouraging (Fields, 1993). The primary goal with any high-frequency device is to maintain gas exchange and oxygenation by use of lower ventilatory pressures (Carlo and Chatburn, 1988). The two major types of high-frequency ventilation currently available are (1) high-frequency jet ventilation (HFJV) and (2) high-frequency oscillatory ventilation (HFOV).

HIGH-FREQUENCY JET VENTILATION: HFJV is accomplished by use of a high-pressure gas source and a small-bore cannula that delivers a tidal volume of 2 to 5 ml/kg and ventilatory rates between 60 and 600 breaths/minute (Bunnell, 1990; Villar et al, 1990). Inspiratory times are small, ranging from 20 to 34 milliseconds with long exhalation times (I/E > 1:6). Expiration during HFJV is passive. A back-up conventional ventilator is usually placed in parallel with the high-frequency device to provide a fresh gas source for entrainment of additional volume and for supplying PEEP and sigh breaths to the patient.

HFJV has been found to be effective in the treatment of neonatal pulmonary interstitial emphysema (Keszler et al, 1991); success has been limited in the treatment of diaphragmatic hernia, meconium aspiration, persistent pulmonary hypertension of the newborn, and pneumonia/sepsis. HFJV has been reported to be effective in the treatment of respiratory failure after surgery for congenital heart disease (Kocis et al, 1992). The beneficial effect is due to the ability of the jet to decrease intrathoracic pressure, thereby improving venous return while at the same time improving ventilation.

HIGH-FREQUENCY OSCILLATORY VENTILATION: HFOV operates by setting a mean airway pressure and superimposing a sinusoidal pressure waveform, generated through the oscillation of a piston within the device. HFOV delivers small tidal volumes at high respiratory frequencies (3–18 Hz) (Gerstmann et al, 1991). The major advantage of HFOV is an active expiratory phase of ventilation (Kinsella and Clark, 1993) which promotes a zero net flow of gas delivered to the patient.

HFOV has been used in infants suffering from hyaline membrane disease, persistent air leak, meconium aspiration, pneumonia, and pulmonary hypoplasia and as a rescue treatment before the application of extracorporeal membrane oxygenation (Frantz, 1993; Null et al, 1990). Reports have described positive results in the use of HFOV in pediatric patients with ARDS (Arnold et al, 1993). However, these are small study groups, and no large studies have been performed that show HFOV is advantageous over conventional ventilation (Fields, 1993).

References

Abraham E, Yoshihara G: Cardiorespiratory effects of pressure controlled inverse ratio ventilation in severe respiratory failure. *Chest,* 96:1356–1359, 1989.

Al-Saady N, Bennett ED: Decelerating inspiratory flow waveform improves lung mechanics and gas exchange in patients on intermittent positive-pressure ventilation. *Intensive Care Med,* 11:68–75, 1985.

American Thoracic Society/European Respiratory

Society: Respiratory mechanics in infants: physiologic evaluation in health and disease. *Am Rev Respir Dis,* 147:474–496, 1993.

Arnold JH, Truog RD, et al: High-frequency oscillatory ventilation in pediatric respiratory failure. *Crit Care Med,* 21:272–278, 1993.

Bancalari E: Inadvertent positive end expiratory pressure during mechanical ventilation. *J Pediatr,* 108:567–569, 1986.

Biondi JW, Schulman DS, Matthay RA: Effects of mechanical ventilation on right and left ventricular function. *Clin Chest Med,* 9:55–70, 1988.

Blanch PB, Jones M, et al: Pressure-preset ventilation, part 2: mechanics and safety. *Chest,* 104:904–911, 1993.

Boros SJ: Variations in inspiratory:expiratory ratio and airway pressure wave form during mechanical ventilation: the significance of mean airway pressure. *J Pediatr,* 94:114–117, 1979.

Bunnell JB: High-frequency ventilation of infants. In Manohar R *Current Perinatology, Vol II.* New York, Springer-Verlag, 1990, pp 172–200.

Carlo WA, Chatburn RL: High frequency ventilation. In Carlo WA, Chatburn RL (eds): *Neonatal Respiratory Care, 2nd ed.* Chicago, Year Book Medical Publishers, 1988, pp 366–393.

Chatburn RL: Principles and practice of neonatal and pediatric mechanical ventilation. *Resp Care,* 36:569–592, 1991.

Cooper KR, Boswell PA, Choi SC: Safe use of PEEP in patients with severe head injury. *J Neurosurg,* 63:552–555, 1988.

Dorinsky PM, Whitcomb ME: The effect of PEEP on cardiac output. *Chest,* 84:210–216, 1983.

Dworkin G, Kattan M: Mechanical ventilation for status asthmaticus in children. *J Pediatr,* 114: 545–549, 1989.

Fields AI: Newer modes of mechanical ventilation for patients with adult respiratory distress syndrome. *Crit Care Med,* 21:S367–S368, 1993.

Frantz ID: High-frequency ventilation. *Crit Care Med,* 21:S370, 1993.

Gerhardt T, Reinfenberg L, et al: Functional residual capacity in normal neonates and children up to 5 years of age determined by an N_2 washout method. *Pediatr Res,* 20:668–671, 1986.

Gerstmann DR, deLemos RA, Clark RH: High-frequency ventilation: issues of strategy. *Clin Perinatol,* 18:563–580, 1991.

Hazelzet JA, Petru R, et al: New modes of mechanical ventilation for severe respiratory failure. *Crit Care Med,* 21:S366–S367, 1993.

Keszler M, Donn SM, et al: Multicenter controlled trial comparing high-frequency jet ventilation and conventional ventilation in newborn infants with pulmonary interstitial emphysema. *J Pediatr,* 119:85–93, 1991.

Kinsella JP, Clark RH: High-frequency oscillatory ventilation in pediatric critical care. *Crit Care Med,* 21:174–175, 1993.

Kocis KC, Meliones JN, et al: High-frequency jet ventilation for respiratory failure after congenital heart surgery. *Circulation,* 86 (suppl II): II-127–II-132, 1992.

Lanin DC, DiBenedetto R, et al: Pressure control inverse ratio ventilation as a method to reduce peak inspiratory pressure and provide adequate ventilation and oxygenation. *Chest,* 95:1081–1088, 1989.

Marcy TW, Marini JJ: Inverse ratio ventilation in ARDS: rationale and implementation. *Chest,* 100:494–504, 1991.

Martin L: Principles of respiratory support and mechanical ventilation. In Rogers MC(ed): *Textbook of Pediatric Intensive Care.* Baltimore, Williams & Wilkins, 1992, pp 134–203.

McEvoy GK: *American Hospital Formulary Service Drug Information.* Bethesda, MD, American Society of Hospital Pharmacists, 1993.

McWilliams BC: Mechanical rentilation in pediatric patients. *Clin Chest Med,* 8:597–609, 1987.

Miyasaka K: Mechanical ventilation. In Holbrook PR (ed): *Textbook of Pediatric Critical Care.* Philadelphia, WB Saunders, 1993, pp 442–464.

Null D, Berman LS, Clark R: Neonatal and pediatric ventilatory support. In Kirby RR, Banner MJ, Downs JB (eds): *Clinical Applications of Ventilatory Support.* New York, Churchill Livingstone, 1990, pp 199–238.

Papadakos PJ, Halloran W, et al: The use of pressure-controlled inverse ratio ventilation in the surgical intensive care unit. *J Trauma,* 31: 1211–1214, 1991.

Potkin RT, Hudson LD, et al: Effect of positive end-expiratory pressure on right and left ventricular function in patients with the adult respiratory distress syndrome. *Am Rev Respir Dis,* 135:307–311, 1987.

Schulman DS, Biondi JW, et al: Left ventricular diastolic function during positive end-expiratory pressure. *Am Rev Respir Dis,* 145:515–521, 1992.

Schuster DP: A physiologic approach to initiating, maintaining, and withdrawing mechanical ventilatory support during acute respiratory failure. *Am J Med,* 88:268–278, 1990.

Shapiro HM, Marshall LF: Intracranial pressure responses to PEEP in head-injured patients. *J Trauma,* 18:254–256, 1978.

Suter P: Optimal end-expiratory airway pressure in patients with acute pulmonary failure. *N Engl J Med,* 292:284–289, 1975.

Taketomo CK, Hodding JH, Kraus DM: *Pediatric Dosage Handbook*, 2nd ed. Hudson, OH Lexi-Comp, 1993.

Tharratt RS, Allen RP, Albertson TE: Pressure controlled inverse ratio ventilation in severe adult respiratory failure. *Chest,* 94:755–762, 1988.

Tyler DC: Positive end-expiratory pressure: a review. *Crit Care Med,* 11:300–307, 1983.

Villar J, Winston B, Slutsky AS: Non-conventional techniques of ventilatory support. *Crit Care Clin,* 6:579–603, 1990.

Chapter 13

High-Frequency Oscillatory Ventilation

James P. Cappon

High-frequency oscillatory ventilation (HFOV) is one of several methods of high-frequency mechanical ventilation currently in clinical use for neonates and older children with respiratory disease. The ability of this technology to provide adequate oxygenation and ventilation has been established in numerous animal and human investigations and has led to licensure by the Food and Drug Administration of several different types of high-frequency ventilators. These include high-frequency flow interrupters, jet ventilators, and oscillating ventilators. Much of the use of high-frequency ventilation to this point has been as a rescue therapy for the most critically ill, although prospective studies with HFOV for less severely ill children are underway.

The ability of ventilatory frequencies in the supraphysiological range (i.e., adults > 60 breaths/minute; children > 100 breaths/minute) to sustain normal blood gas tensions was demonstrated in 1967 by Sjöstrand; animals were ventilated at respiratory rates of 60 to 100 breaths/minute with small tidal volumes, and normal ventilation was sustained. In 1972, Lukenheimer et al first described HFOV, in which airway oscillation with a loudspeaker in paralyzed animals did not produce arterial hypercapnia. Numerous animal and clinical investigations followed, confirming the feasibility of oxygenation and ventilation with respiratory frequencies well above normal ranges.

HFOV produces a biphasic pressure waveform through the to-and-fro oscillation at high frequency of a piston within an enclosed cylinder. This provides active inspiratory and expiratory phases of ventilation, unlike other modes of mechanical ventilation, in which expiration is a passive process dependent on the intrinsic elastic recoil properties of the lung and chest wall. Classical explanations of gas exchange in conventional positive-pressure ventilation, in which minute ventilation is the product of tidal volume (V_T) and respiratory rate, and V_T is the sum of the alveolar volume and the dead space volume (V_D), do not explain ventilation during HFOV, where V_T is less than V_D and, hence, no alveolar ventilation should occur. There is also an inverse relationship between frequency and V_T; moreover, the V_T has more effect on carbon dioxide elimination, compared with conventional mechanical ventilation (CMV).

Oxygenation during HFOV is related to lung volume and the concentration of inspired oxygen and inspiratory time. The maintenance of an adequate alveolar volume for gas exchange is of paramount importance and is controlled by manipulation of the mean airway pressure ($\overline{Paw}$), because peak inspiratory pressure and positive end-expiratory pressure (PEEP) cannot be directly controlled in this ventilatory mode. The rapid fluctuations of small tidal volumes (and, hence, pressure) about the lung volume at a given $\overline{Paw}$ provide the basis for the protective effect from barotrauma; numerous investigations have shown that peak inflation pressures and the amplitude of change between inspiratory and expiratory pressures are associated with lung injury (Fig. 13–1). The incidence of atelectasis and air trapping is also reduced. Finally, in air leak syndromes, high-frequency ventilation of all types minimizes further air leak; HFOV, with its active expiratory limb, may enhance this benefit.

Initial applications of HFOV were directed toward the neonate with air leak syndromes or respiratory distress syndrome, with varying rates of success. Those studies demonstrating successful use of HFOV had in common the attainment and maintenance of adequate lung volumes during therapy; this "high-volume strategy" is now commonly used in both neonatal and pediatric centers using this alternative method of lung support. Prospective series of HFOV use in severe respiratory failure are well-established in the neonatal literature, and early reports in older children are promising.

INDICATIONS

HFOV is one of several alternative therapies available for the support of gas exchange in the infant and child with severe respiratory failure; others include extracorporeal membrane oxygenation (ECMO), surfactant, intravascular oxygen and carbon dioxide exchange, nitric oxide, and liquid ventilation.

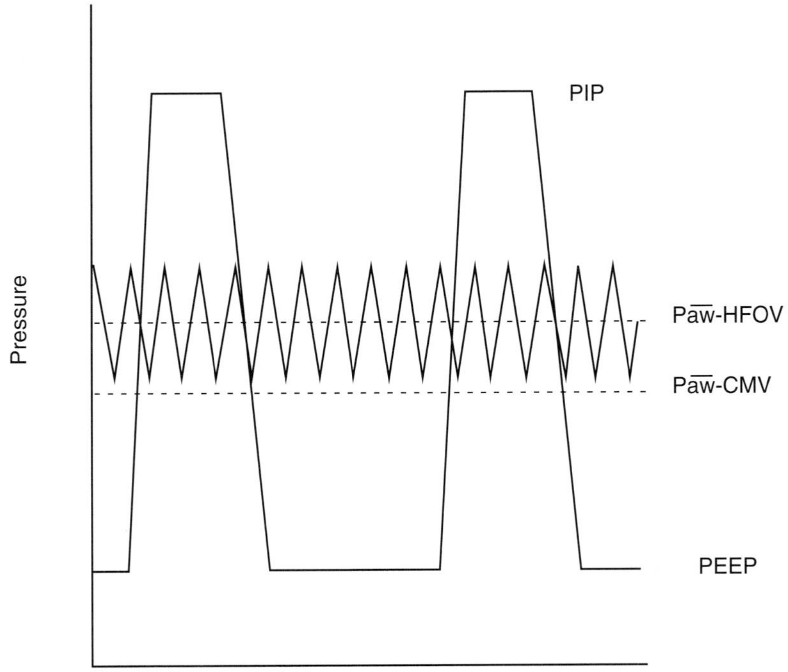

Figure 13–1 Schematic representation of airway pressure and ventilator frequency in conventional mechanical ventilation (CMV) versus high-frequency oscillatory ventilation (HFOV). PIP, peak inspiratory pressure; PEEP, positive end-expiratory pressure; $\overline{Paw}$-HFOV, mean airway pressure during HFOV; $\overline{Paw}$-CMV, mean airway pressure during CMV. Although the $\overline{Paw}$ of HFOV is higher than that of CMV, the magnitude of the respiratory cycle pressure change during HFOV is decreased.

The SensorMedics 3100A (SensorMedics, Inc., Yorba Linda, CA) high-frequency oscillator is currently licensed for use in infants less than 10 kg with primary pulmonary disease or respiratory failure. Non-neonatal HFOV has to date been used as rescue therapy for hypoxemic and hypercapnic respiratory failure refractory to "maximal" conventional ventilation, often with the compounding problem of air leaks.

Much of the HFOV experience has been in infants and children who meet ECMO criteria, that is, those with the most profound deficiencies in oxygenation or the highest conventional ventilator settings. Although these criteria (e.g., the alveolar-arterial oxygen gradient [$AaDo_2$] and the oxygenation index [OI]) are well-established indicators of more than 80% mortality in the neonate, similar predictors for the pediatric population have not yet been fully established, and there is no broad consensus. This is in part due to the differences in the disease processes in the two age groups: the majority of neonatal pulmonary disease is of homogeneous lung injury, particularly respiratory distress syndrome, often complicated by barotrauma and air leak. Meconium aspiration syndrome, in contrast, is an example of heterogeneous pulmonary disease of the newborn, and HFOV has not consistently demonstrated equal efficacy in this syndrome until several days into the disease course, when the lung damage becomes more uniform. Non-neonatal pulmonary disease is of a much broader spectrum, with etiologic factors including bacterial, viral, and other infectious pneumonia as well as aspiration pneumonia, near-drowning, trauma, and chronic fibrotic disease. Reflecting the diverse underlying pathophysiological processes, the natural history and response to therapy are highly variable for each of these entities. The result is that predictors of morbidity and mortality are harder to develop, and meaningful comparisons between groups of patients and treatment modalities are more difficult to substantiate.

With use of currently recommended protocols, HFOV has demonstrated improvement in gas exchange and survival in severely ill neonates with respiratory distress syndrome, pulmonary interstitial emphysema, meconium aspiration syndrome, persistent pulmonary hypertension, and refractory respiratory failure (Table 13–1). There are indications that the incidence of bronchopulmonary dysplasia can also be reduced by early use of HFOV. Older children with severe respiratory failure of diverse causes have also been successfully treated with HFOV. Viral pneumonia (particularly due to respiratory syncytial virus) and air leak syndromes have demonstrated the best response to date. A limiting factor in the use of this type of ventilation in the pediatric intensive care setting is a maximal weight limit of 30 to 35 kg; beyond this, ventilation with current oscillators is inadequate. A prototype for larger patients is now in early clinical trials. In both populations of patients, the need for ECMO can be decreased by early intervention with HFOV.

Table 13–1 Indications for High-Frequency Oscillatory Ventilation

Neonatal
Severe respiratory failure
Respiratory distress syndrome
Pulmonary interstitial emphysema
Meconium aspiration syndrome
Persistent pulmonary hypertension
Pneumonia
Congenital diaphragmatic hernia*
Pediatric
Severe respiratory failure
Pneumonia
Viral
Bacterial
"Adult" respiratory distress syndrome
Aspiration pneumonitis
Extensive/persistent air leak
Bronchopulmonary fistula
Bronchoscopy
Asthma/reactive airway disease*

*Minimal reported experience to date.

EQUIPMENT AND SUPPLIES

Other than the oscillating ventilator itself, special equipment and supply needs for HFOV are few. Back-up tubing circuits are recommended, as are additional exhalation valves. The valves, a balloon-type apparatus on the exhalation limb of the system, have shown an increased tendency to leak and, occasionally, break. A low-volume compressible humidifier is typically used with the HFOV system. Because of the importance of maintaining adequate lung volume during oscillation, efforts are made to reduce circuit interruption. For pediatric patients, a one-way valve adapter that fits onto the end of the endotracheal tube allows suctioning of the airway without compromising circuit integrity. Clinical experience has demonstrated that the approximately 1- to

5-ml dead space of this adapter significantly interferes with ventilation of the neonatal patient, particularly the premature infant; $Paco_2$ increases of 20 mm Hg or greater are commonly seen.

Two major exceptions exist with regard to the routine management of the mechanically ventilated child. First, capnography, the measurement of end-tidal carbon dioxide magnitude and waveform, is not accurate with high-frequency ventilation. Determination of arterial oxygen saturation and transcutaneous determination of Pao_2 and $Paco_2$ are therefore more valuable, particularly given the limitations of the auscultatory examination of the thorax in HFOV (see later). Second, aerosolized medications cannot be effectively delivered with oscillation. Alternatives include bagging the medication into the airways and the use of metered-dose inhalers via a spacer device placed in continuity with the HFOV circuit. An extension of this restriction is that administration of continuously nebulized medications is not possible during HFOV. As with all patients receiving mechanical ventilation, periodic measurements of arterial (and, if feasible, mixed venous) Po_2, Pco_2, and oxygen saturation are also required. Pulmonary function testing can be performed with minor pneumotach circuit modifications. Although bulk flow measurements (i.e., pressure-volume curves) cannot be obtained, lung compliance and airways resistance can be determined. Finally, the 24-hour availability of portable radiographs is mandatory for serial determinations of lung expansion.

PREPARATION OF THE PATIENT AND FAMILY

Although HFOV is currently considered a novel form of mechanical ventilation and can be lifesaving, there is little additional risk to the patient by its use. The majority of patients ventilated with this technology thus far either have demonstrated severe respiratory failure refractory to maximal conventional ventilation or have been thought likely to do so. Many of these infants and children have also met existing ECMO criteria. Given the background and alternatives, most families are comfortable with trials of HFOV, whether under licensed or compassionate use guidelines.

Such patients are commonly transported to a tertiary care facility by referral. It is thus mandatory to stabilize the patient at presentation per usual institutional protocols, while confirming the ongoing refractory nature of the disease process (i.e., hypoxemia, pulmonary hypertension, bronchopleural fistula) as preparations for HFOV are underway. Specific preparations of the patient include maximizing the diameter of the endotracheal tube because ventilation is improved with larger artificial airway sizes. Strong consideration should be given to nasotracheal intubation. The external circuit of existing oscillators is made of rigid, noncompliant tubing, and adequate securing of the endotracheal tube is imperative. This, as well as the patient's comfort, is improved by nasotracheal tube placement.

The hemodynamic status of the patient bears attention as well. Reports of impaired cardiac output and metabolic acidosis with HFOV have focused on impaired stroke volume secondary to the high, essentially constant $\overline{Paw}$ as a cause. When efforts are made to keep the central venous pressure at high-normal or supranormal values, series have not demonstrated this problem. Once intravascular volume is maximized, cardiac output—both right- and left-sided—should be optimized with inotropes and vasoactive drugs to improve gas exchange and oxygen delivery. Arterial and central venous cannulas, if not already present, should be placed to facilitate ventilator, fluid, and blood pressure management.

NECESSARY TRAINING

Mechanical ventilation largely remains a hands-on technique, with success highly correlated with experience; this is even more the case with HFOV. As mentioned, many of the traditional precepts of CMV do not apply to oscillation (Table 13–2). Previous clinical experience, as garnered by trial and error, provides the foundation for many of the techniques of HFOV management.

RESPIRATORY THERAPY: Manufacturers of oscillating ventilators provide multiday, intensive institutional training with purchase of a device. It is then recommended that the respiratory therapy department provide inservice education to all staff members, with annual follow-up of competency. Ongoing clinical training with a therapist experienced in HFOV is provided before independent patient care is initiated. The limitations of various therapeutic and diagnostic interventions (i.e., aerosols, capnography, and pulmonary function testing) must be understood. Indications for periodic changes in the patient's position and for chest physiotherapy are usually unchanged from CMV.

Table 13–2 Conceptual Differences in Ventilator Management between Conventional Mechanical Ventilation and High-Frequency Oscillatory Ventilation

Parameter	CMV	HFOV
Alveolar oxygenation	F_{IO_2}	F_{IO_2}
Rate	IMV (bpm)	Hz (cps)
Breath size*	V_T	Pressure amplitude (ΔP)
Inflation pressure*	PIP	Pressure amplitude, power
Lung volume	PEEP	$\overline{Paw}$

*Note that each of these parameters allows indirect assessment of lung compliance.

CMV, conventional mechanical ventilation; HFOV, high-frequency oscillatory ventilation; F_{IO_2}, fraction of inspired oxygen; IMV intermittent mandatory ventilation; bpm, breaths per minute Hz, hertz; cps, cycles per second; V_T, tidal volume; PIP, peak inspiratory pressure; PEEP, positive end-expiratory pressure; $\overline{Paw}$, mean airway pressure.

NURSING: Inservice education and orientation to the ventilator are recommended for all nursing staff with exposure to the device. Specifically, familiarization with the oscillator "on-off" switch should be mandatory; experience has demonstrated the SensorMedics device to be sensitive to electrical power supply transients (e.g., during periodic hospital back-up generator checks). Because of the rigid circuit tubing and use of one-way valves, airway suctioning is often best coordinated with respiratory therapists. Tension on the endotracheal tube due to the inflexible ventilator circuit predisposes the patient to pressure wounds of the nares and mouth. Similarly, because the head of these critically ill children is often more immobilized than usual, dependent scalp edema is more common. The physical examination of the patient on HFOV is altered, largely in terms of auscultation of the heart and lungs. Although chest expansion (oscillation is a more appropriate description) occurs, there are no appreciable inspiratory and expiratory breath sounds. This is due to the high frequency and small V_T of HFOV as well as loud transmitted sounds of the ventilator itself. The auscultatory examination of the heart is similarly limited, and appreciation of the point of maximal impulse, thrills, and ventricular heaves and lifts is difficult. Central and peripheral pulses and perfusion, however, remain intact.

PHYSICIANS: Previous experience with HFOV physiology and clinical management is a necessary requirement in use of this technology. A premise is that patients requiring HFOV are severely ill to begin with, and that any transition in care (transport, reintubation, initiation of HFOV) may be poorly tolerated. The changeover to HFOV is frequently unnerving, requiring multiple oscillator adjustments, patient care interventions, and diagnostic assessments. The limitations of the chest physical examination are described earlier.

METHODS AND ONGOING CARE

Because oxygenation is usually the critical factor in these patients, the fraction of inspired oxygen (F_{IO_2}) is usually at or near 1.0 during transition to HFOV. An inspiratory time (I-time) of 33% of the respiratory cycle is generally set as default but can be increased. The $\overline{Paw}$ should be set at least 1 to 2 cm H_2O *above* the $\overline{Paw}$ on CMV for premature neonates (3–5 cm H_2O for older children), and lung inflation of approximately nine posterior ribs should be confirmed radiographically.

A traditional beginning ventilator frequency for neonates is 10 to 12 Hz. This rate may not provide adequate V_T for the larger infant or child, however, and these patients may require an initial rate of 5 to 8 Hz. The pressure amplitude (ΔP) setting controls the degree of piston displacement during the oscillatory cycle (and hence the ventilator pressure wave amplitude) and is adjustable across a large pressure range. The initial ΔP should be sufficient to generate oscillatory chest wall movement. A power control that increases the amperage necessary for piston displacement can be varied from 1 to 10 arbitrary units and should be set at or below 3 during changeover from CMV to HFOV.

Improvements in oxygenation are often rapid, occurring within minutes, if adequate lung volume has been established (Fig. 13–2). Carbon dioxide elimination is occasionally more difficult, requiring manipulation of the frequency and pressure amplitude before acceptable levels of carbon dioxide are achieved (Fig. 13–3). The use of transcutaneous oxygen and carbon dioxide monitoring, as well as Sa_{O_2}, gives instantaneous information as to adequacy of gas exchange; after stability of the patient is achieved, invasive sampling of blood gases can be lessened. Frequent chest radiographs are needed to obtain objective data regarding lung volume as well as to observe areas of parenchymal and pleural abnormalities

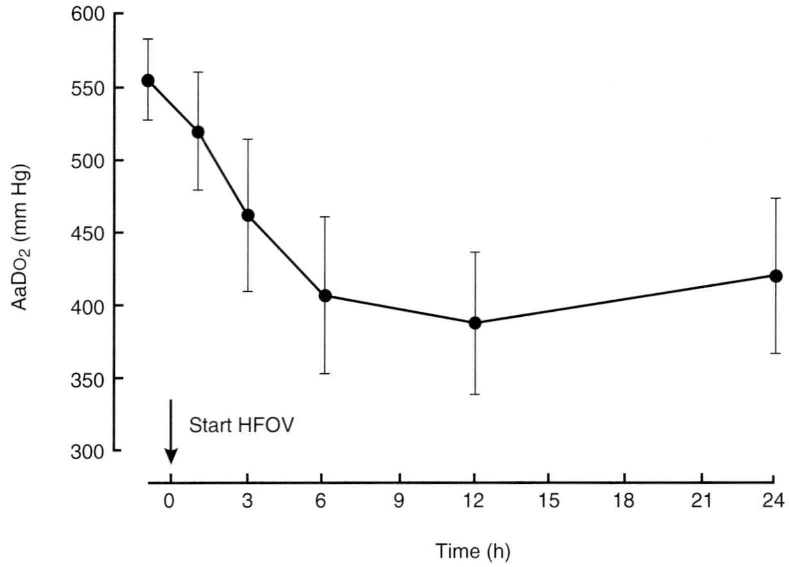

Figure 13–2 Early improvement in oxygenation, as represented by the alveolar-arterial oxygen gradient ($AaDo_2$), after transition from CMV to HFOV in 12 pediatric patients. $AaDo_2$ = [(PB − PH_2O) FIO_2 − $Paco_2$/R] − Pao_2; PB, barometric pressure (760 mm Hg); PH_2O, water vapor pressure (47 mm Hg); FIO_2, fraction of inspired oxygen; $Paco_2$, partial pressure of arterial carbon dioxide; R, respiratory quotient; Pao_2, partial pressure of arterial oxygen. (Redrawn from Cappon JP, Anas NG: High-frequency oscillatory ventilation in ECMO-eligible children with severe respiratory failure. *Am Rev Respir Dis,* 147:A887, 1993. Abstract.)

(i.e., consolidation, edema, or air leak). It is reasonable to obtain these films every 6 to 8 hours early in the course of HFOV and every 12 hours thereafter. Underexpansion of the lung fields is treated with increases of 1 to 2 cm H_2O in the $\overline{Paw}$ until the desired expansion is obtained; overinflation of the lungs (e.g., flattened diaphragms, evidence of gas trapping) is responded to in reciprocal fashion.

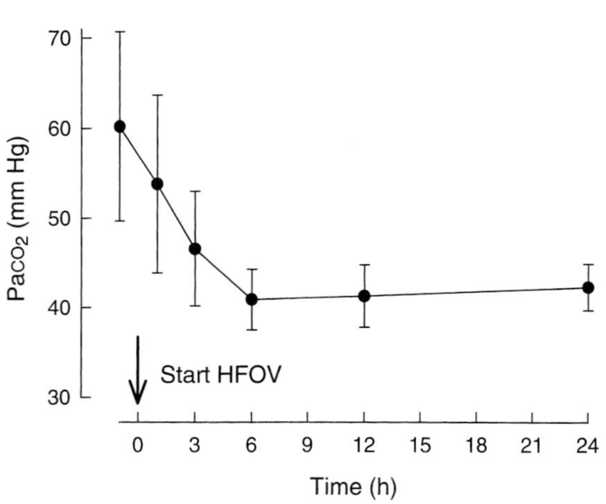

Figure 13–3 Early $Paco_2$ response to HFOV after transition from CMV. (Redrawn from Cappon JP, Anas NG: High-frequency oscillatory ventilation in ECMO-eligible children with severe respiratory failure. *Am Rev Respir Dis,* 147:A887, 1993. Abstract.)

Inadequate oxygenation is improved through adjustment of the FIO_2 and $\overline{Paw}$, with the I-time percentage of lesser importance. It is important to allow adequate time after a ventilator change for results to be seen; this guideline is even more applicable to management of ventilation. To decrease ventilator settings, some degree of hypoventilation may be desirable if normal acid-base status can be maintained. For more severe carbon dioxide retention, efforts should be made to increase the V_T by decreasing the frequency and increasing the pressure amplitude. The liberal use of chest radiographs to determine lung volume should again be reinforced.

The first 24 hours of oscillation frequently require shorter intervals between airway suctioning, compared with CMV. The increased production of secretions is most likely secondary to alveolar recruitment, with elaboration of the contents of previously atelectatic lung units. This increased suctioning regimen usually resolves by HFOV day 2 and is worse with the various pneumonias.

Nonrespiratory care of the patient on HFOV centers on maintenance of intravascular volume and oxygen transport, nutritional support, and adequate sedation. High-normal to supranormal central venous pressure values maintain ventricular filling pressures and cardiac output in the presence of high $\overline{Paw}$; with appropriate intravascular volume status, transition to HFOV does not cause significant hemodynamic alterations (Fig. 13–4). Inotropic agents may also increase cardiac output, improving gas exchange by normalizing ventilation-perfusion relationships and concurrently improving oxygen transport and uptake through increased oxygen delivery. Although there are no contraindications to enteral feedings, many pediatric patients on HFOV initially require parenteral nutrition. Efforts should be made to meet estimated anabolic calorie and protein needs while maintaining a "normal" respiratory quotient of 0.8. All of these children require sedation per usual guidelines, both for comfort and to reduce pulmonary vascular reactivity and optimize gas exchange. Because of the critical and unstable condition of many patients, muscle relaxants are frequently used before as well as after transition to HFOV. Continued neuromus-

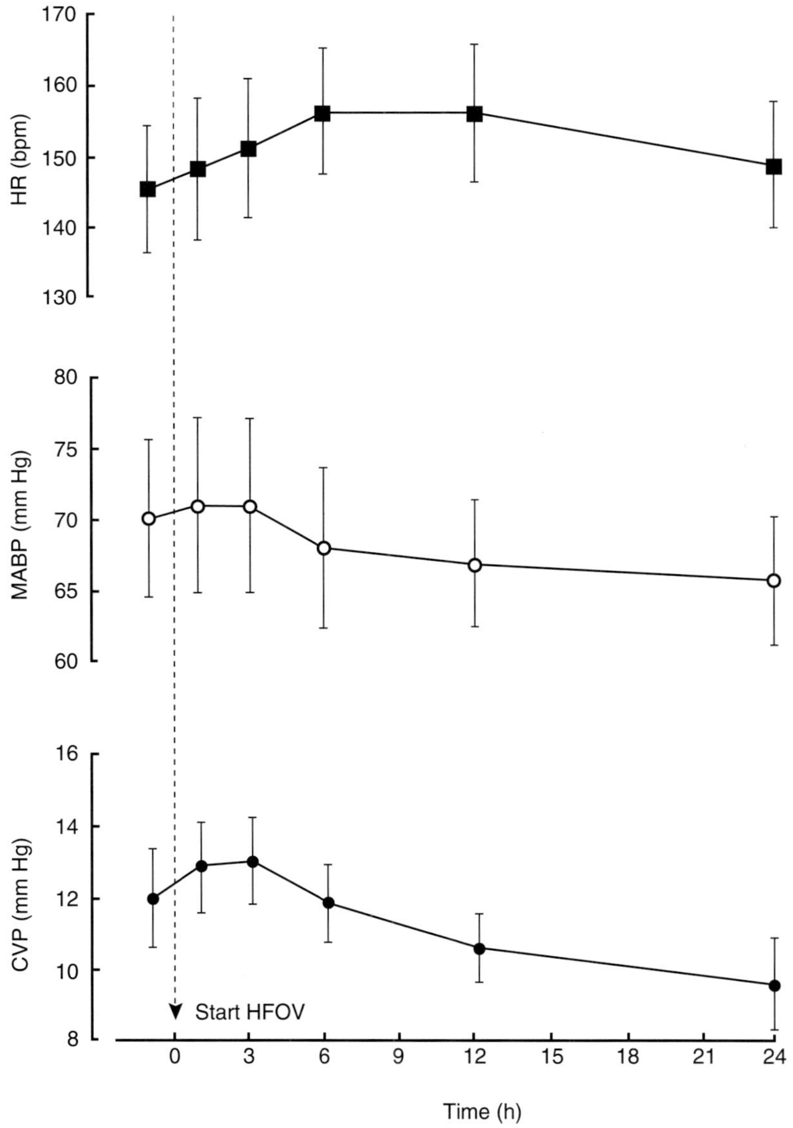

Figure 13–4 The early hemodynamic response to HFOV. Note the stability in all parameters after transition from CMV to HFOV. HR, heart rate; bpm, beats per minute; MABP, mean arterial blood pressure; CVP, central venous pressure. (Redrawn from Cappon JP, Anas NG: High-frequency oscillatory ventilation in ECMO-eligible children with severe respiratory failure. *Am Rev Respir Dis,* 147:A887, 1993. Abstract.)

cular blockade is the norm for older infants and children, but it is less so for neonates undergoing oscillation.

The early improvement in oxygenation seen in HFOV is thought to be due to the recruitment of previously underventilated or nonventilated alveoli and forms the basis of the high-volume strategy of HFOV currently advocated by numerous investigators. Although most clinical series have used changes in the $\overline{Paw}$ to establish adequate lung inflation, animal studies have documented use of periodic prolonged positive-pressure breaths ("sustained inflations") with the same results. These sustained inflations, lasting many seconds at pressures and volumes well above maintenance conventional ventilator settings, increase lung volume and improve both ventilatory status and pulmonary mechanics without lung parenchymal damage because recruited lung units can be subsequently ventilated at much lower pressures and remain open. In situations of potential repeated volume loss and atelectasis, for example, suctioning of the neonatal patient with interruption of the HFOV circuit, sustained inflations may play a crucial role in clinical management.

Weaning oscillator settings during HFOV can usually be begun within hours of transition from CMV. Once oxygenation has improved, the FIO_2 is preferentially decreased rather than the $\overline{Paw}$ for reasons outlined before. The pressure amplitude may also be gradually decreased after acceptable carbon dioxide elimination is established, with careful attention to maintenance of chest wall movement and transcutaneous and blood gas determinations of PCO_2. With an FIO_2 of 0.6 or less, the $\overline{Paw}$—often 5 to 8 cm H_2O greater than that originally on CMV—is weaned in increments of 1 to 2 cm H_2O while SaO_2 is kept at 90% or above.

No absolute indications exist as to when to resume conventional ventilation. Although infants were weaned from HFOV directly to supplemental oxygen in one neonatal series, most studies have included a return to CMV once severe respiratory insufficiency has resolved. Broad guidelines for neonates include an FIO_2 of 0.5 or less and a $\overline{Paw}$ of 10 to 12 cm H_2O; pediatric series have shown an FIO_2 of 0.6 or less and a $\overline{Paw}$ of 18 to 20 cm H_2O to be appropriate. If obtainable, measurements of improved lung compliance may provide further objective evidence for discontinuation of HFOV. Clinically, the patient should be able to tolerate brief (i.e., < 60 seconds) periods off oscillation for suctioning before a return to CMV. The advantages of resuming CMV include facilitation of the patient's spontaneous tidal breaths, retraining of respiratory muscles, and increased comfort of medical personnel with this type of mechanical ventilation before discontinuation of artificial ventilatory support. The average duration of HFOV varies from approximately 7 to 10 days in the neonate and older child, respectively; however, ranges from hours to 28 days are reported.

POSSIBLE COMPLICATIONS

Complications with HFOV are rare. Early concerns with air trapping have not been demonstrated in children with use of recommended $\overline{Paw}$ and oscillator frequencies. Airway damage is minimal and comparable to that seen in CMV, in contrast to other types of high-frequency ventilation. Mechanical failure of the device itself is uncommon.

Continued hypoxemia with HFOV is usually a function of inadequate lung inflation and responds to maneuvers to optimize alveolar recruitment. Conversely, overexpansion of the lung, determined radiographically and confirmed clinically by hypoxemia and hypoventilation, usually results from too high a $\overline{Paw}$, which should be incrementally decreased (Table 13–3). This is not an unusual problem during the later course of HFOV as lung compliance improves. Isolated hypoventilation generally reflects a low V_T and, because of the inverse relationship between V_T and frequency, is best responded to by deceasing the respiratory rate. Inadequate pressure amplitude to allow

Table 13–3 Therapeutic Maneuvers for Specific Clinical Problems During High-Frequency Oscillatory Ventilation

Problem	Therapy
Hypoxemia	↑ $\overline{Paw}$, ↑ FIO_2, ↑ I-time
Hypercapnia	↓ Hz, ↑ ΔP, ↑ power*
Hyperinflation	↓ $\overline{Paw}$, ↓ ΔP
Persistent air leak	↓ $\overline{Paw}$, ↓ ΔP, ↓ I-time
Unexplained hypoxemia, tachycardia, hypotension, acidosis	Rule out pneumothorax, ↑ CVP, ↑ sedation

*Note that all act directly or indirectly to increase tidal volume.
$\overline{Paw}$, mean airway pressure; FIO_2, fraction of inspired oxygen; I-time, inspiratory time of ventilatory cycle; Hz, hertz (ventilator frequency); ΔP, pressure amplitude; CVP, central venous pressure.

carbon dioxide elimination is more commonly seen in the older infant and child. Because of the rigid HFOV circuit, inadvertent changes of endotracheal tube position are a constant possibility and may not be detectable by auscultation of the lung fields.

Barotrauma is lessened in HFOV versus CMV; hence, the frequency and magnitude of air leaks are decreased. Pneumothorax, pneumomediastinum, and other types of leak still occur, however, given the degree of underlying lung damage, particularly if there is large parenchymal heterogeneity. The value of routine chest radiography is supported by experiences in which large tension pneumothoraces did not become clinically significant owing to the efficiency of gas exchange with HFOV. Unexplained tachycardia and hypercapnia, often without concurrent hypoxemia, are useful indicators of this complication. High-frequency ventilation is the treatment of choice for persistent air leak syndromes, with emphasis on keeping the $\overline{Paw}$ at the lowest level that allows acceptable oxygenation. Transthoracostomy tube pleurodesis is feasible while the patient is on HFOV.

Animal studies have demonstrated hypotension and metabolic acidosis during HFOV when either high $\overline{Paw}$ or repeated, prolonged, sustained inflations are used. Clinical investigations in which the intravascular volume is optimal have not shown this effect. In fact, studies have shown no significant changes in heart rate, mean arterial blood pressure, cardiac index, systemic and pulmonary vascular resistance, or oxygen delivery and consumption. Once pneumothorax is ruled out, fluid challenge is a reasonable consideration for the triad of tachycardia, hypotension, and hypoxemia.

An increased occurrence of severe intracranial hemorrhage was seen in one study of premature infants receiving HFOV versus CMV therapy for respiratory failure. This finding, attributed to relatively constant and high $\overline{Paw}$ of HFOV interfering with systemic venous return and thereby elevating intracranial pressure, has not been substantiated in other neonatal or pediatric series. Clinical management protocols of the premature infant at risk for intracranial bleeding should be strictly adhered to during HFOV.

Subtherapeutic levels of sedation and neuromuscular blockade are poorly tolerated by the critically ill patient on HFOV. Furthermore, oscillation itself may mask some of the easily recognized clinical signs of this state (for instance, small movements representing inadequate muscle relaxation). Careful attention to frequent twitch monitoring and detection of unexplained tachycardia or systemic oxygen desaturation help ensure adequate sedations and induced paralysis of the patient.

ILLUSTRATIVE CASE

N.R. was a 9-week-old 3.8-kg boy with a 9-day history of upper and lower respiratory tract infection due to respiratory syncytial virus requiring mechanical ventilation for apnea and respiratory distress. He was transferred for consideration for ECMO from the referring pediatric intensive care unit on day 9 of hospitalization, after 192 hours of conventional ventilation, with progressive hypoxemia and hypercapnia despite maximal conventional ventilator settings and the initiation of inotropic and vasoactive support. The past medical history was significant for a 35-week twin gestation and respiratory distress syndrome requiring 1 week of mechanical ventilation and 10 additional days of oxygen therapy during a 3-week total hospitalization. He was discharged home off of oxygen or diuretics, requiring only metoclopramide for gastroesophageal reflux. Well-child examinations at 4 and 8 weeks of life were unremarkable.

CMV settings before helicopter transport were as follows: FIO_2, 1.0; peak inspiratory pressure, 39 cm H_2O; PEEP, 12 cm H_2O; ventilator rate, 40; I-time, 0.6 second; and $\overline{Paw}$, 18 cm H_2O. Arterial blood gas (ABG) results were pH, 7.54; $PaCO_2$, 30 mm Hg; PaO_2, 35 mm Hg; HCO_3^-, 31 mEq/L; and SaO_2, 75%. The $AaDO_2$ was 641 mm Hg, and OI was 51. The $AaDO_2$ had been greater than 500 mm Hg and the OI greater than 30 for 24 hours. He was receiving continuous infusions of dopamine 5 μg/kg/min and nitroprusside 4 μg/kg/min as well as infusions of fentanyl and vecuronium and intermittent vancomycin and cefotaxime. He had received 3 days of ribavirin therapy earlier in the hospitalization. A tracheal aspirate on hospital day 4 grew *Moraxella (Branhamella) catarrhalis*, without evidence of inflammation. The chest radiograph showed bilateral alveolar and interstitial infiltrates and normal heart size.

After transport, the patient was placed on HFOV, with initial settings of FIO_2, 1.0; $\overline{Paw}$, 22 cm H_2O; ΔP, 41 cm H_2O; rate, 6 Hz; and I-time, 33%. ABG analysis after 1 hour of HFOV revealed pH, 7.61; $PaCO_2$, 29 mm Hg; PaO_2, 93 mm Hg; and SaO_2, 93%. The $AaDO_2$ was 591 mm Hg, and OI 23. To improve oxygenation, he required incremental increases in $\overline{Paw}$, to a maximum of 30 cm H_2O. ABG values at 6 hours were pH, 7.51; $Paco_2$, 36 mm Hg; Pao_2, 87 mm Hg; and Sao_2, 97%. $AaDo_2$ was 590 mm Hg, and OI 34. Clinical improvement continued, and oscillator settings after 12 hours of HFOV were Fio_2, 0.85; $\overline{Paw}$, 24 cm H_2O; ΔP, 33 cm H_2O; rate, 8 Hz; and I-time, 33%. ABG analysis at this time demonstrated a pH of 7.47; $Paco_2$, 47 mm Hg; Pao_2, 68 mm Hg; and Sao_2, 94%. $AaDo_2$ was 479 mm Hg, and OI 30. The patient's preexisting systemic hypertension resolved during transport, which allowed the discontinuation of nitroprusside. Continuous infusions of midazolam, fentanyl, and vecuronium were maintained during oscillation. Dopamine was continued at 5 μg/kg/min for the first 36 hours of HFOV and then weaned. There were no significant changes in heart rate, mean arterial pressure, or central venous pressure during or in the first 24 hours after transition to HFOV.

The patient subsequently showed gradual improvement during a 134-hour HFOV course. There was no evidence of air leak, and culture was negative for respiratory syncytial virus on the second day of HFOV. He tolerated continuous nasoduodenal formula feedings without difficulty. Oscillator settings at the time of return to CMV were Fio_2, 0.56; $\overline{Paw}$, 11 cm H_2O; ΔP, 30 cm H_2O; rate, 5 Hz; and I-time, 33%. ABG results were pH, 7.42; $Paco_2$, 33 mm Hg; Pao_2, 67 mm Hg; and Sao_2, 94%. $AaDo_2$ was 291 mm Hg, and OI 9. He required an additional 8 days of conventional ventilation and 5 days of supplemental oxygen after extubation. Seven days after stopping HFOV, and while still on CMV, the patient had right lung collapse, subsequently proved by rigid bronchoscopy to be due to mucus plugging. The final chest radiograph before hospital discharge revealed slight bilateral hyperinflation and increased interstitial markings. He was discharged home in good condition without need for supplemental oxygen, diuretics, or new medications.

SUMMARY

HFOV is a novel form of mechanical ventilation that can improve gas exchange and outcome of patients in the neonatal and pediatric population. Its use in severe respiratory failure refractory to maximal CMV has become accepted in neonatology and has been extended to older infants and children. HFOV also provides an additional means of managing persistent pulmonary air leaks and, when optimally used, may decrease the sequelae of chronic lung disease. The role of HFOV in less severely ill children awaits the results of ongoing and future investigations.

Bibliography

Arnold JH, Truog RD, et al: High-frequency oscillatory ventilation in pediatric respiratory failure. *Crit Care Med,* 21:272–278, 1993.

Bond DM, Froese AB: Volume recruitment maneuvers are less deleterious than persistent low lung volumes in the atelectasis-prone rabbit lung during high-frequency oscillation. *Crit Care Med,* 21:402–412, 1993.

Boynton BR, Villanueva D, et al: Effect of mean airway pressure on gas exchange during high-frequency oscillatory ventilation. *J Appl Physiol,* 70:701–707, 1991.

Bryan AC, Froese AB: Reflections on the HIFI trial. *Pediatrics,* 87:565–567, 1991. Editorial.

Cappon JP, Anas NG: High-frequency oscillatory ventilation in ECMO-eligible children with severe respiratory failure. *Am Rev Respir Dis,* 147:A887, 1993. Abstract.

Carter JM, Gerstmann DR, et al: High-frequency oscillatory ventilation and extracorporeal membrane oxygenation for the treatment of acute neonatal respiratory failure. *Pediatrics,* 85: 159–164, 1990.

Chan V, Greenough A, Milner AD: The effect of frequency and mean airway pressure on volume delivery during high-frequency oscillation. *Pediatr Pulmonol,* 15:183–186, 1993.

Clark RH, Gerstmann DR, et al: Prospective randomized comparison of high-frequency oscillatory and conventional ventilation in respiratory distress syndrome. *Pediatrics,* 89:5–12, 1992.

Gerstmann DR, deLemos RA, Clark RH: High-frequency ventilation: issues of strategy. *Clin Perinatol,* 18:563–580, 1991.

HIFI Study Group: High-frequency oscillatory ventilation compared with conventional mechanical ventilation in the treatment of respiratory failure in preterm infants. *N Engl J Med,* 320:88–93, 1989.

HIFI Study Group: High-frequency oscillatory ventilation compared with conventional mechanical ventilation in the treatment of respiratory failure in preterm infants: assessment of pulmonary function at 9 months of corrected age. *J Pediatr,* 116:933–941, 1990.

Kinsella JP, Gerstmann DR, et al: High-frequency oscillatory ventilation versus intermittent mandatory ventilation: early hemodynamic effects in the premature baboon with hyaline membrane disease. *Pediatr Res,* 29:190–196, 1991.

Kohelet D, Perlman M, et al: High-frequency oscillation in the rescue of infants with persistent pulmonary hypertension. *Crit Care Med,* 16:510–516, 1988.

McCulloch PR, Forkert PG, Froese AB: Lung volume maintenance prevents lung injury during high-frequency oscillatory ventilation in surfactant-deficient rabbits. *Am Rev Respir Dis,* 137: 1185–1192, 1988.

Tamburro RF, Bugnitz MC, Stidham GL: Alveolar-arterial oxygen gradient as a predictor of outcome in patients with nonneonatal pediatric respiratory failure. *J Pediatr,* 119:935–938, 1991.

Timmons OD, Dean JM, Vernon DD: Mortality rates and prognostic variables in children with adult respiratory distress syndrome. *J Pediatr,* 119:896–899, 1991.

Utah Valley Regional Medical Center: *SensorMedics 3100A High-Frequency Oscillatory Ventilator Training Program.* Provo, UT, March 1993. Manual.

Wetzel RC, Gioia FR: High-frequency ventilation. *Pediatr Clin North Am,* 34:5–38, 1987.

Section C

Critical Care Medicine

Chapter 14

Neonatal Extracorporeal Membrane Oxygenation

Carrie Worcester

Extracorporeal membrane oxygenation (ECMO), a modified heart-lung bypass system, was first used in 1975 in critically ill neonates with potentially reversible lung disease (Bartlett et al, 1976). This was followed by other successful neonatal cases (Bartlett et al, 1977), and by the mid-1980s, 40 newborn infants treated with ECMO had been described (Bartlett et al, 1982). Currently, there are more than 70 ECMO centers that have treated more than 6000 patients with an overall survival rate greater than 80% (Extracorporeal Life Support Organization, 1990, 1993). Two prospective randomized studies have demonstrated the effectiveness of ECMO in neonates (Bartlett et al, 1985; O'Rourke et al, 1989), and further studies have also demonstrated cost-effectiveness (Schumacher et al, 1992; Short and Pearson, 1986). ECMO is a high-tech, labor-intensive, expensive procedure that results in good outcome at less cost, resource use, and morbidity than with conventional modes of treatment. Moribund infants with acute cardiorespiratory failure recover on ECMO because of the "lung rest" from high pressures and high oxygen concentration of conventional ventilatory support.

INCLUSION CRITERIA

ECMO is indicated when conventional, maximal medical management fails. Inclusion criteria for neonatal ECMO are those listed in Table 14–1 plus an 80% mortality risk. Mortality risk is estimated by measuring pulmonary dysfunction and the level of ventilator support. These factors have been combined into measurements to estimate the severity of pulmonary dysfunction in the alveolar-arterial oxygen gradient or the oxygenation index with 80% mortality criteria commonly used (Table 14–2). The usefulness of these criteria depends on the method and type of ventilation management. The alveolar-arterial oxygen gradient ($AaDO_2$) is calculated as follows:

$$AaDO_2 = [FIO_2 \times (760 - 47) - PaCO_2/R] - PaO_2$$

where 760 is barometric pressure (PB) and 47 is water vapor pressure (PH_2O). The oxygenation index (OI) is calculated as follows:

$$OI = \left(FIO_2 \times \frac{P\overline{aw}}{PaO_2}\right) \times 100$$

where $P\overline{aw}$ is the mean airway pressure.

Table 14-1 Inclusion Criteria for ECMO

Gestational age ≥ 34 weeks, or
Birth weight ≥ 2000 g
No significant coagulopathy or bleeding complications
No major intracranial hemorrhage
Mechanical ventilation < 10 to 14 days
Reversible lung injury
No major cardiac lesion
No major nonpulmonary disease
Life-threatening cardiac or respiratory failure unresponsive to conventional treatment

Most centers use the alveolar-arterial oxygen gradient to monitor the severity of ventilation-perfusion mismatch in infants with respiratory distress syndrome. The oxygenation index has an advantage because it reflects the conventional ventilation support being used to achieve any given PaO_2 and is used exclusively in some centers. Criteria for patients with congenital diaphragmatic hernia may differ.

ECMO may be contraindicated if a patient has

- severe underlying nonpulmonary disease (e.g., untreatable congenital heart disease, major malformation syndromes or chromosomal anomalies, untreatable renal dysfunction)
- intracranial hemorrhage recognized before ECMO (grade I intraventricular hemorrhage may be an exception)
- severe coagulopathy
- birth weight less than 2 kg if due to prematurity
- evidence of severe and irreversible brain damage (e.g., history of severe or prolonged ischemia, including cardiac arrest and seizure activity)

Table 14-2 Commonly Used Neonatal ECMO Criteria

$AaDo_2$ (normal, 10–15 mg Hg) Range: 605 to 620 mm Hg × 4 to 12 hours
Oxygenation index Range: > 35 to > 60 × 0.5 to 6 hours
Pao_2 Range: < 35 to < 50 mm Hg × 2 to 12 hours
Barotrauma pH < 7.25 × 2 hours or with hypotension
Acute deterioration Range: Pao_2 < 30 to 40 mm Hg

ECMO may occasionally be used as part of a diagnostic work-up when cardiorespiratory failure precludes further analysis of an unusual congenital anomaly and death is imminent without ECMO stabilization. If this guideline for ECMO is used, and if the diagnosis of an irreversible anomaly is made after the patient is placed on ECMO, it may be necessary to discontinue ECMO therapy even though death may result.

Disease processes amenable to ECMO include meconium aspiration syndrome, persistent pulmonary hypertension of the newborn, sepsis, pneumonia, congenital diaphragmatic hernia, and congenital heart defects that cannot be stabilized with medical management but are surgically treatable.

PRE-PROCEDURE EVALUATION AND CONSENT

Before ECMO, each patient must have a central nervous system ultrasound examination to rule out significant intracranial hemorrhage; coagulation studies, including partial thromboplastin time, prothrombin time, measurement of fibrinogen and fibrin degradation products, and platelet count; electrolyte determinations; complete blood count with differential; and cardiac evaluation. Many ECMO candidates have been paralyzed, which makes the neurological status difficult to assess. The history of Apgar scores, resuscitation, and seizures and a description of neurological status before paralysis are helpful in assessment.

Informed consent must be obtained from the patient's family or legal guardians. All therapeutic options and risks should be discussed.

EQUIPMENT AND CIRCUIT

Equipment used for ECMO is an adaptation of modified cardiopulmonary bypass. There is no one ECMO circuit. Rather, each center devises an ECMO system. Essential components of the system are listed in Table 14-3.

The ECMO circuit is a type of cardiopulmonary bypass through venoarterial bypass or single-cannula venovenous bypass. In venoarterial bypass, blood drains by gravity from the right atrium through a cannula inserted into the internal jugular vein. It then flows through the servoregulator and is pumped through the membrane oxygenator, where gas exchange

Table 14–3 ECMO System Components

Roller occlusion pump
Pump base
Venous return monitor
Heating unit
Coagulation timer
Membrane mounting board
Oxygen blender
Carbon dioxide or carbogen tank
Oxygen and carbon dioxide flow meters
Temperature probes, in-line
Oxygen saturation monitor, in-line

takes place. Finally, the arterialized blood passes through a heat exchanger, where it is rewarmed to body temperature and then returned to the patient through the carotid artery cannulas. Venoarterial bypass provides effective cardiac support as well as gas exchange.

Venovenous bypass is performed with a single venous double-lumen catheter introduced into the right internal jugular vein to the midportion of the right atrium (Anderson et al, 1989). The circuit is otherwise similar to that described for venoarterial bypass.

The usual criteria for ECMO apply to neonates for venoarterial or venovenous bypass. With venovenous bypass, the 14 French catheter may be a physical limitation in patients weighing less than 2.5 kg. Other considerations that may be contraindications to venovenous ECMO include severe right- or left-sided cardiac failure as seen on echocardiographic evaluation, as in "crash on" ECMO cannulation situations. Use of inotropes is not a contraindication to venovenous bypass (Cornish et al, 1993).

On either venoarterial or venovenous bypass, the unoxygenated blood passes through a membrane oxygenerator, which separates the blood and gas. The membrane lung consists of a large silicone rubber envelope wound around a spool and enclosed in a watertight jacket. Ventilating gas flows on the inside of the envelope in one direction, and blood passes on the outside in the opposite direction between the turns of the coil. Gas and blood come into close contact across a large surface area, much as they do in the natural lung. Adjusting the flow of ventilating gas controls $PaCO_2$ of blood after oxygenation. To prevent hypocapnia, 5% carbon dioxide is blended into the gas as necessary. PaO_2 after oxygenation depends on FIO_2 of the ventilating gas and the time the blood spends in the oxygenator. Seventy percent to 80% bypass flow is usually required initially. Drainage is by gravity (passive) and therefore limited by the diameter of the venous cannula and the vertical distance from the baby to the pump. The patient's PaO_2 is determined by the proportion of fully saturated blood returning from the artificial lung to that of desaturated blood shunting through the nonfunctional natural lungs.

TRAINING

ECMO requires a highly trained and skilled team consisting of physicians, perfusionists, neonatal nurses, and ECMO technicians. The ECMO technical specialist may have a background in medicine, nursing, respiratory therapy, or as a perfusionist. All personnel involved in the ECMO team undergo didactic instruction, laboratory and bedside experience, and water drills on the ECMO circuit. One study reported the average length of clinical preceptorship or supervision to be 34.2 hours (Arensman and Cornish, 1993). Careful training is essential in the recognition and management of complications. Both a nurse and an ECMO technician are assigned to a patient on ECMO each shift. The nurse is responsible for ongoing assessment, hemodynamic monitoring, data collection, and pulmonary care. The ECMO technician is responsible for checking and monitoring the circuit, adjusting gas and pump flow, maintaining heparinization, drawing blood specimens, and administering fluids and medications into the circuit. The team approach is of utmost importance in ECMO care, which requires constant, diligent round-the-clock surveillance.

METHODS

Preparing the Circuit

While the infant is cannulated, the ECMO circuit is primed. The circuit is flushed with carbon dioxide to remove all nitrogen and filled with crystalloid-containing solution. This solution is displaced with washed packed red blood cells to which calcium and heparin have been added. The pH of the blood is corrected with tromethamine (THAM). The system has a volume of approximately 350 ml.

Cannulation

Cannulation (either venoarterial or venovenous) and initiation of bypass occur in the neonatal intensive care unit under local anesthesia with the operating room staff in attendance. Before cannulation, the patient is paralyzed with 0.1 mg/kg pancuronium (or vecuronium 0.1 mg/kg); 100 U/kg heparin is given for anticoagulation. The right internal jugular vein is the location of choice for venous access. It has the largest internal diameter and accepts the shortest catheter that usually permits the desired blood flow of approximately 100 to 120 ml/kg/min. For venoarterial bypass, the right common carotid artery is the vessel of choice because it is large enough to accept a large arterial catheter and provides flow directly into the aortic arch. Details of the cannulation technique are available (Arensman and Cornish, 1993). After the cannulas are secured, they are carefully connected to the ECMO circuit to avoid air bubbles. A chest radiograph is obtained to confirm proper catheter placement. Bypass is initiated at low flow and gradually increased in 5 to 10 minutes until maximal bypass is achieved at 70% to 80% of the infant's cardiac output.

MANAGEMENT OF THE PATIENT ON ECMO

Routine

Most patients require 3 to 7 days on ECMO support. Daily parameters are recorded and include hematocrit, platelet count, activated clotting time (ACT), mean blood pressure, the patient's PaO_2 and $PaCO_2$, and the pump's $PaCO_2$. Careful routine care must be done because of the use of routine heparinization. No intravenous line insertions, heel sticks, or nasal suctioning should occur. Vital signs are monitored continuously. Daily laboratory values include complete blood count with differential, serum electrolyte, determinations, serum plasma free hemoglobin concentration, blood culture, fibrinogen level, prothrombin time, and platelet count. Hourly tests include bedside ACT.

Packed red blood cells are used when 10% of blood volume has been removed and to maintain a hematocrit of 45%. Fresh frozen plasma or cryoprecipitate is used for bleeding complications. Platelet counts are maintained above 75,000. Daily chest films are taken to evaluate pulmonary status and any change in catheter placement.

Lung compliance studies can be helpful in determining successful decannulation. Evaluation of lung compliance (Arensman and Cornish, 1993) and functional residual capacity has been advocated. Hand bagging the infant with good chest wall movement at 20 cm H_2O or less is a predictor of success in weaning from ECMO (Arensman and Cornish, 1993).

Because of the systemic heparinization, the patient on ECMO is at risk for intracranial hemorrhage. Daily central nervous system ultrasound examinations are needed, and significant changes may play an important role in the length of the patient's ECMO support.

Evaluation of any bleeding source is mandatory. Bleeding from the neck incision may occur. If it exceeds 5 to 10 ml/h, the surgeon should re-explore the site. Packing with Gelfoam and topical thrombin often stops the bleeding. Bleeding from chest tubes may often be extensive and difficult to control. A plan for replacement of blood loss must be devised. Tracheal bleeding occurs at times and may be managed with the use of higher pressures on the ventilator.

Also of major concern in ECMO bypass is clot formation. The circuit is checked daily, and ACTs are carefully monitored. Clots on the post-membrane side of the circuit require a circuit change. Hematology consultation should be obtained in cases of excessive bleeding or clot formation.

Fluids and Electrolytes

Maintenance fluids are calculated at 80 to 100 ml/kg/d. Many patients are receiving drip infusions and frequent fluid boluses for blood pressure instability, which creates significant edema on ECMO. ECMO patients in the first several days typically have decreased urine output and edema. Furosemide (Lasix) may be used. If a patient is oliguric or anuric, hemofiltration may be indicated.

Hyperalimentation is usually started on day 3, and initiation of intralipid therapy is considered. Fluids are increased to 120 to 140 ml/kg/d after edema improves and urine output increases.

Heparin

Continuous heparin infusion is necessary to prevent the ECMO circuit from clotting. The goal of heparin management is to decrease the risk for fibrin and clot formation in the circuit while minimizing the risk of bleeding complications in the patient. ACTs are measured hourly at the bedside. Normal ACT values are 80 to 120. ACTs are kept at approximately 200 to 220 (1 1/2 times normal). This generally requires 30 to 60 units of heparin per kilogram per hour. Heparin is bound to platelets and excreted in the urine. Larger doses are required during diuresis and platelet transfusion; smaller doses are required in renal failure and thrombocytopenia. If bleeding complications occur, ACTs may need to be kept in a lower range (190–220).

Sedation

Patients are sedated with fentanyl and midazolam continuous infusions at the author's institution. Fentanyl infusion for pain control is maintained at 1 to 10 μg/kg/h in combination with midazolam at 0.1 to 0.5 mg/kg/h. Patients frequently develop tolerance to these drugs and must be weaned slowly to avoid withdrawal responses.

Pulmonary Management

After a few hours of ECMO bypass, a "white-out" of the lung is frequently seen. The etiology is unknown, but contributing factors may include activation of complement because of interactions between blood and the artificial lung surface, transient capillary leak syndrome, alteration in ventilation-perfusion relationships, surfactant deficiency, and left-to-right shunt across a patent ductus arteriosus. Use of higher positive end-expiratory pressure (12–13 cm H_2O) (Kestler et al, 1989) and use of artificial surfactant replacement therapy (Lotze et al, 1990) may improve lung compliance.

Once the patient is stabilized on ECMO, ventilator settings are reduced to allow lung rest. Routine ventilator settings on ECMO based on central registry data (Extracorporeal Life Support Organization, 1990, 1993) include FIO_2, 0.27 ± 0.11; peak inspiratory pressure, 21 ± 6 cm H_2O; rate, 17 ± 7 breaths/minute; positive end-expiratory pressure, 6 ± 4 cm H_2O; and mean airway pressure, 9 ± 3 cm H_2O. Routine chest physiotherapy and careful suctioning through the endotracheal tube can be performed.

During the first several days of ECMO, most patients require 60% to 70% bypass and are primarily dependent on the pump for oxygenation. If a significant left-to-right shunt develops through the patent ductus arteriosus, oxygenation may decrease and fail to respond to increased pump flow. Ways to increase oxygenation during ECMO are to (1) increase pump flow, (2) decrease left-to-right shunt, and (3) increase hemoglobin concentration.

Venous saturation monitoring is used to determine sufficiency of oxygenation. For venous saturations to give a true indication of arterial oxygen content, (1) the cardiac output must remain stable, (2) the hemoglobin concentration must stay stable, and (3) the metabolic rate of the patient cannot change. Any of these factors can cause a change in venous saturation. Arterial blood gas analysis is necessary to determine the PaO_2 and $PaCO_2$. $PaCO_2$ values on ECMO are adjusted by management of gas flow rates rather than blood flow rates, that is, by (1) changing the ventilation to membrane lung or (2) decreasing or increasing the concentration of carbon dioxide in the membrane gas mixture.

Weaning from ECMO

After 3 to 4 days on ECMO, lung compliance usually begins to improve, with improvement in arterial blood gas values allowing a decrease in ECMO blood flow. In the first several days on ECMO, there may actually be a worsening in arterial blood gas values if a left-to-right shunt develops across the patent ductus arteriosus. After closure of the patent ductus arteriosus, the patient is slowly weaned (10- to 20-ml decreases every hour) off ECMO flow, and arterial blood gas values are monitored. When ECMO flow is decreased to 30% of cardiac output (120–150 ml/h), ventilation settings are increased. A "trial off" is indicated at this point. The patient is taken off ECMO by clamping the catheters. This is done for up to 30 minutes. The response to a trial off, as well as compliance studies, determines the patient's ability to come off ECMO. Ventilation settings after decannulation are usually FIO_2, 0.3 to 0.4; peak inspiratory pressure, 15 to 20 cm H_2O, and rate, 40 to 45 breaths/minute.

Decannulation

Detailed decannulation technique has been reviewed (Arensman and Cornish, 1993). After decannulation, routine laboratory studies are obtained at 4 hours. Platelet counts need to be observed closely in the first 24 hours. Care after ECMO is virtually the same as care of ventilator-dependent babies.

Before discharge, the ECMO patient should have cranial computed tomography, basal auditory-evoked responses, and neurological assessment as well as formulation of a neonatal developmental follow-up program.

RESULTS

Complications of ECMO can be short- and long-term. A registry of the outcomes of these patients and their complications is maintained yearly by the Extracorporeal Life Support Organization, a study group to which all ECMO centers send their data. Neonatal cases by year are shown in Table 14–4. The distribution of diagnosis by year is shown in Table 14–5. Complications in descending order of frequency are noted in Table 14–6. Mechanical complications occurring with ECMO are related to each major component of the circuit in Table 14–7.

Neonatal ECMO survivors should be followed closely for possible complications caused by hypoxia and acidosis before ECMO as well those caused by ECMO itself. Survivors are evaluated for their growth and development, respiratory status, and neurological status. Overall outcome is fairly good; the frequency of pulmonary or neurological handicap is approximately 20% (Glass et al, 1989). Detailed reviews have been published regarding these outcome studies (Arensman and Cornish, 1993; Glass et al, 1989; Krummel et al, 1984; Van Meurs et al, 1993.)

SUMMARY

The use of ECMO for certain neonates has been proved to be beneficial. Considering the morbidity of the disease processes amenable to ECMO, the morbidity of ECMO itself with careful selection of patients is acceptable. ECMO is labor intensive and requires an experienced team with standardized techniques. Because of the expertise required and the expense of maintaining a qualified team, ECMO programs should be regionalized in tertiary-level neonatal centers with an appropriate cardiovascular service for backup and consultation. High-risk infants failing maximal therapy should receive consultation with an ECMO physician as soon as possible. The referring physician should consider the need for ECMO when the patient has a PaO_2 of 50 to 60 mm Hg, peak inspiratory pressure is greater than 35 cm H_2O, and the FIO_2 is 1.0. After consultation with an ECMO physician, the time and type of transport should be determined. Diagnostic studies before transfer should include (1) central nervous system ultrasound examination; (2) prothrombin time, partial thromboplastin time, fibrinogen level, and platelet count; (3) calcium and electrolytes determinations; (4) complete blood count with differential; (5) blood type; and (6) cardiac ultrasound. Early consultation with an ECMO center and safe transfer of the ECMO candidate are critical in outcome of the patient.

Table 14–4 Neonatal ECMO Cases by Year

Year	Total	Number Survived (%)
1986	808	644 (80)
1987	647	555 (86)
1988	1006	825 (82)
1989	1114	911 (82)
1990	1333	1078 (81)
1991	1383	1117 (81)
1992	1379	1088 (79)
1993	350	278 (79)

From Extracorporeal Life Support Organization: *ECMO Registry Report.* Ann Arbor, MI, University of Michigan, July 1993.

Table 14–5 Neonatal ECMO Cases by Diagnosis

Primary	Total	Number Survived (%)
Meconium aspiration syndrome	2997	2798 (93)
Respiratory distress syndrome/hyaline membrane disease	982	821 (84)
Congenital diaphragmatic hernia	1543	900 (58)
Pneumonia/sepsis	1197	914 (76)
Air leak	32	21 (66)
Persistent pulmonary hypertension of the newborn/persistent fetal circulation	1008	840 (83)
Other	261	202 (77)

From Extracorporeal Life Support Organization: *ECMO Registry Report.* Ann Arbor, MI, University of Michigan, July 1993.

Table 14-6 Complications of ECMO (%)

Intracranial	16
Seizures	15
Surgical site	13
Cardiac dysfunction	11
Hemofiltration/dialysis	11
Hypertension	9
Abnormal creatinine concentration	9
Electrolyte disturbance	9
Hemolysis	8
Pneumothorax	5
Positive blood culture	5
Gastrointestinal hemorrhage	4
Arrhythmias	3

From Extracorporeal Life Support Organization: *ECMO Registry Report*. Ann Arbor, MI, University of Michigan, July 1993.

Table 14-7 Mechanical Complications of ECMO

	Incidence (%)	Survival (%)
Cannula problem	8	75
Oxygenator failure	5	66
Clots in major vessel	5	77
Tubing rupture	2	83
Pump failure	2	86
Heat exchanger	1	71
Air in circuit	1	73
Mechanical—other	11	81

From Extracorporeal Life Support Organization: *ECMO Registry Report*. Ann Arbor, MI, University of Michigan, July 1990.

References

Anderson HL, Otsu T, et al: Venovenous extracorporeal life support in neonates using a double lumen catheter. *ASAIO Trans*, 35:650–653, 1989.

Arensman RM, Cornish JD: *Extracorporeal Life Support*. Cambridge, MA, Blackwell Scientific Publications, 1993.

Bartlett RH, Andrews AF, et al: ECMO for newborn respiratory failure: 45 cases. *Surgery*, 92: 425–433, 1982.

Bartlett RH, Gazzaniga AB, et al: Extracorporeal membrane oxygenation (ECMO). Cardiorespiratory support in infancy. *Trans Am Soc Artif Intern Organs*, 22:80–88, 1976.

Bartlett RH, Gazzaniga AB, et al: ECMO in neonatal respiratory failure. *J Thorac Cardiovasc Surg*, 74:826–833, 1977.

Bartlett RH, Roloff DW, et al: Extracorporeal circulation in neonatal respiratory failure. A prospective randomized study. *Pediatrics*, 76:479–487, 1985.

Cornish JD, Heiss KF, et al: Efficacy of venovenous extracorporeal membrane oxygenation for neonates with respiratory and circulatory compromise. *J Pediatr*, 122:105–109, 1993.

Extracorporeal Life Support Organization: *ECMO Registry Report*. Ann Arbor, MI, University of Michigan, July 1990 and July 1993.

Glass P, Miller M, Short B: Morbidity for survivors of extracorporeal membrane oxygenation: neurodevelopmental outcome at 1 year of age. *Pediatrics*, 83:72–78, 1989.

Kestler M, Subramanian KN, et al: Pulmonary management during extracorporeal membrane oxygenation. *Crit Care Med*, 17:495–500, 1989.

Krummel TM, Greenfield LJ, et al: The early evaluation of survivors after extracorporeal membrane oxygenation for neonatal pulmonary failure. *J Pediatr Surg*, 19:585–590, 1984.

Lotze A, Whitsett JA, et al: Surfactant protein A concentrations in tracheal aspirate fluid from infants requiring extracorporeal membrane oxygenation. *J Pediatr*, 116:435–440, 1990.

O'Rourke PP, Krone R, et al: ECMO and conventional medical therapy in neonates with persistent pulmonary hypertension of the newborn. A prospective randomized study. *Pediatrics*, 84: 957–963, 1989.

Schumacher R, Roloff DW, et al: Neonatal ECMO. A prospective randomized study of cost effectiveness. *ASAIO Trans*, 1992.

Short BL, Pearson GD: Neonatal extracorporeal membrane oxygenation: a review. *J Intensive Care Med*, 1:47–54, 1986.

Van Meurs KP, Robbins ST, et al: Congenital diaphragmatic hernia: long-term outcome in neonates treated with extracorporeal membrane oxygenation. *J Pediatr*, 122:893–899, 1993.

Bibliography

Bartlett RH, Andrews AF, et al: Extracorporeal membrane oxygenation for neonatal respiratory failure: a report of 50 cases. *J Thorac Cardiovasc Surg*, 97:706–714, 1989.

Bartlett RH, Toomasian JM, et al: Extracorporeal membrane oxygenation in neonatal respiratory failure: 100 cases. *Ann Surg*, 204:236–244, 1986.

Donn SM: ECMO indications and complications. *Hosp Pract*, 25:143–157, 1990.

Short BL, Miller MR, Anderson KP: Extracorporeal membrane oxygenation in the management of respiratory failure in the newborn. *Clin Perinatol*, 14:737–748, 1987.

Chapter 15

Pulmonary Artery Catheters

Adam J. Schwarz

INDICATIONS

The pulmonary artery (PA) catheter was first introduced in 1970 when Swan, Ganz, and colleagues described catheterization of the human heart with the use of a flow-directed balloon-tipped catheter (Swan et al, 1970). Shortly thereafter, Forrester was able to directly measure cardiac output by thermodilution using a triple-lumen catheter with a thermistor at the distal tip (Forrester et al, 1972). Information gathered through the PA cathether is used to directly assess and monitor a wide array of cardiopulmonary physiological parameters, including cardiac output, left and right ventricular filling pressure and vascular resistance, blood oxygen content, oxygen delivery, and tissue oxygen use. This hemodynamic information can be extremely valuable in the management of critical illness involving cardiovascular and respiratory diseases. Some of the common uses for PA catheters are the management and evaluation of therapeutic efficacy in different shock states, such as hypovolemic, cardiogenic, and septic shock; differentiation of adult respiratory distress syndrome from cardiogenic pulmonary edema; monitoring of pulmonary hypertension; and optimizing of cardiac output after cardiac surgery. PA catheterization is therefore a frequent procedure in the intensive care setting, and its use in children is becoming increasingly common (Katz et al, 1984).

The use of a PA catheter is not without risk, and the overall benefit of its placement and use must outweigh the risk. There are only a few absolute contraindications to PA catheter placement. The first is refusal of the patient or the family to give consent (Victor, 1989). In addition, patients with known heparin allergy should not have a heparin-coated PA catheter placed. There are, however, myriad relative contraindications. In terms of the simple financial considerations, the PA catheter is an expensive piece of technology. As of 1990, the PA catheter industry in sales and related costs, including physician fees, laboratory charges, and setup, amounted to 2 billion dollars in the United States alone (Shoemaker, 1990). There is little justification for placement of a PA catheter unless the data obtained will be used both to improve the understanding of the patient's illness and to provide beneficial therapeutic interventions (Robin, 1985). The decision to place a PA catheter should be based on the determination that the information gathered will guide a course of action.

PA catheter placement must be performed by a physician skilled in the procedure. The physician should be able to identify, evaluate, and treat possible complications of PA catheter placement and should possess the understanding to interpret and apply the data obtained in a meaningful therapeutic fashion. Whereas these prerquisites appear self-evident, a large multicenter study evaluating physicians' knowledge of the PA catheter and its application nevertheless revealed that nearly half of all physicians surveyed, in a study sample in which PA catheter use was common and familiarity assumed, could not correctly identify a pulmonary capillary wedge pressure (PCWP) from an obvious tracing, and revealed that misinterpretation of the data occurred frequently (Iberti et al, 1990). Concern regarding misuse of PA catheters and misinterpretation of the data they generate has led some to recommend the establishment of credentialing committees to evaluate and certify competence in their insertion and use. A task force established by the American College of Physicians, American College of Cardiology, and the American Heart Association has suggested not only initial certification but also that a minimum of 12 hemodynamic monitoring procedures be performed each year to maintain accreditation. Swan himself believes a minimum of 50 procedures is required to maintain therapeutic skills (Swan, 1993). The proper indications for PA catheterization therefore are (1) placement in a patient with critical illness, in whom the objective data generated assist in assessing cardiopulmonary dysfunction; (2) use of the data to affect therapy that has an impact on cardiopulmonary management; and (3) insertion and management by a physician well versed in the technical preparation, procedure, risks, and interpretation of the data generated.

EQUIPMENT

There are a number of different PA catheter models, but the basic design is the same. A PA catheter consists of a flexible, radiopaque catheter made of polyvinyl chloride with four or five lumens. Black markings at 10-cm intervals along the outside of the catheter indicate length, and a balloon at the distal tip inflates with 1.0 to 1.5 ml of air. Sizes vary from 4 to 8 French; 5 and 7 French catheters are the most commonly used in pediatrics. The 7 French catheters are generally placed in children who weigh more than 18 kg; the 5 French catheters are used in children less than 18 kg (Katz et al, 1984), including neonates, although the sequelae of long-term catheter placement in small infants remain poorly defined. The lumens include a distal lumen, which is used to monitor PA pressures and the PCWP and is the most common source of mixed venous blood sampling; a proximal lumen, which is used to monitor central venous pressure (CVP) as well as being the injection port for calculating cardiac output by thermodilution; an injection port for inflating the balloon; and, in some larger (7.5 French) catheters, a second proximal lumen for additional intravenous access. A thermistor catheter typically is located within a few centimeters of the distal tip and its connection port at the proximal end of the catheter, which is connected to a cardiac output computer or monitor. There are 2 and 3 French double lumen catheters for small patients that consist only of a thermistor and a distal lumen for pressure monitoring, but these require a separate right atrial catheter for injecting saline when cardiac output is calculated.

In addition to the catheter itself, a pressure-monitoring system must be set up, consisting of three components: the tubing, transducer, and monitor. The tubing should be stiff, short, and liquid filled so that pressure waves are accurately transmitted to the transducer. The transducer has a thin diaphragm that converts the pressure wave transmitted in the tubing to an electrical signal that is displayed on a monitor. A cardiac output computer is also necessary; it may be integrated into the monitor or exist as separate equipment that plugs into the monitor for display purposes.

The PA catheter itself is inserted through a catheter sheath introducer, which consists of a soft catheter with a one-way valve at the proximal end and a side port that can be used for the administration of fluid or medicines. The equipment commonly used to cannulate central veins is used for insertion of the catheter sheath. This equipment includes povidone-iodine; sterile gowns, gloves, and drapes; 1% lidocaine; finder (Cook) needle; J-tipped guidewire; dilator; suture material; saline flush; and the catheter sheath.

A PA catheter should be placed only in a controlled environment with monitoring and resuscitation equipment that includes an electrocardiographic (ECG) monitor, atropine, a defibrillator, appropriate sedation, and preexisting intravenous access.

PREPARATION

The placement of a PA catheter is an invasive procedure that carries a significant risk of complications, so it is essential that informed consent be obtained before insertion. The aforementioned equipment should be gathered and immediately available. The pressure system should be assembled, filled with heparinized 0.9% saline, flushed, and calibrated before catheter insertion. The patient must be made comfortable with appropriate sedation. The site selected for catheter insertion needs to be exposed and unobstructed by blankets, intravenous lines, ventilator tubing, or other obstacles. If the site selected is a subclavian or internal jugular vein, the patient should be placed on the left side in the Trendelenburg position to allow neck vein distention and landmark identification and to prevent the rare but potentially fatal complication of air embolism by facilitating air trapping in the right side of the heart. The patient should be connected to an ECG and oxygen saturation monitor.

PROCEDURE

PA catheters can be inserted in a number of major central veins. Common sites include the internal jugular, external jugular, subclavian, femoral, and median basilic vessels within the antecubital fossa. Each site has its advantages and disadvantages. The internal jugular vein is rapidly accessible and provides easy passage of the catheter to the heart, but it is associated with pneumothorax, carotid artery puncture, and tracheal puncture as well as potential thoracic duct injury when the left side is used. The subclavian vein allows rapid access, free neck and arm movement, and ease of sterile maintenance but is associated with an even greater risk of pneumothorax as well as hemothorax, subclavian artery puncture, and brachial plexus injury. External jugular vein placement is relatively easy and safe, but it may be hindered by valves that prevent catheter or guidewire insertion. Femoral placement avoids the possibility of pneumothorax, but it may increase the risk of sepsis and femoral artery puncture with associated hematoma; the femoral site is more difficult to keep clean, and passage of the PA catheter through to the heart may be more difficult because of the additional length of insertion (Amin et al, 1993). Placement is generally more successful when the patient's right side rather than from the left side is used because a more direct approach to the heart is afforded. The great neck veins, subclavian veins, and femoral veins are usually accessed by use of a percutaneous modified Seldinger approach, and it is this technique that is described in detail. However, a venous cutdown, typically of the median basilic vein in the antecubital fossa, can be used as an alternative technique and may be preferred if the patient has a bleeding disorder necessitating local compression. Access should be obtained by whichever route the operator is most comfortable with and skilled in.

After all equipment has been gathered, the transducer system assembled and calibrated, and the patient positioned and sedated appropriately, the selected site is scrubbed well with a sterile povidone-iodine solution. Sterile technique should be observed at all times to minimize the risk of infection; the physician should wear a hat, mask, and sterile gown as well as sterile gloves. Landmarks are determined and 1% lidocaine is infiltrated into the skin at the insertion site, with aspiration back before injection to ensure that lidocaine is not inadvertently injected into the central vein. If the Seldinger approach is used, the Cook finder needle attached to a syringe is inserted, and negative pressure is applied until venous access is obtained and ensured with good blood return. The J-tipped guidewire is then passed through the finder needle into the vein. Care should be taken not to force the wire if resistance is encountered, which may indicate needle displacement or cannulation of an artery. If resistance is encountered, the wire should be gently withdrawn and the needle repositioned with negative pressure until venous access is regained. Care should be taken not to force wire removal because the sharp end of the needle may catch and shear the wire as it is withdrawn. The ECG should be monitored for the presence of spontaneous arrhythmias, which indicate that the wire has been passed through to the heart to a distance in excess of that necessary to serve simply as a venous guidewire. The finder needle is removed, with care taken not to withdraw the guidewire accidently, and the wire is left in the vein. A small nick in the skin is then made with a No. 11 scalpel at the guidewire insertion site. To dilate the vein, the dilator is passed onto the guidewire and held close to the skin between the thumb and index finger. It is inserted with a small amount of gentle torque, slid over the guidewire into the vein up to the hub, and then withdrawn. Enough wire must protrude from the skin to extend through the proximal end of the dilator or catheter sheath assembly at all times, or else the wire could accidentally be inserted completely into the vein.

At this point, the placement of the PA catheter sheath differs somewhat from the insertion of a simple central venous catheter. The dilator is placed through the catheter sheath via the one-way valve, and the catheter-dilator combination is passed over the guidewire. The dilator and guidewire are withdrawn from the catheter sheath, and sheath placement in a large vessel is confirmed by aspirating blood from the side port. The catheter sheath may then be flushed with saline and sutured into place.

Once the catheter sheath has been inserted, the PA catheter may be removed in sterile fashion from its package. The balloon should be tested before insertion by injecting 1.0 to 1.5 ml of air into the air injection port, and it is allowed to deflate by opening the air port to atmospheric pressure. In patients with intracardiac shunts, the risk of air embolism should balloon rupture occur may be reduced by using carbon dioxide for balloon inflation. The proximal and distal lumens are flushed with sterile heparinized saline and attached to the CVP and PA pressure monitors by means of the pressure tubing, stopcocks, and transducers. A plastic sleeve is slipped over the catheter before insertion through the introducer sheath to preserve a sterile length of catheter after insertion. The catheter is then ready to be placed into the pulmonary artery.

With the balloon deflated, the PA catheter is passed into the central vein through the introducer sheath. The natural curve to the catheter is used to facilitate passage to the right side of the heart. The catheter should pass smoothly through the sheath and central vein. Forcing the catheter against resistance may damage, kink, or bend it and subsequently render it unusable. The catheter is inserted to an intrathoracic location (which varies in distance, depending on the location of insertion and size of the patient, but may be estimated by noting the distance from the catheter insertion site to the sternomanubrial joint), and the balloon is inflated. A continuous pressure tracing from the distal lumen of the catheter is then monitored as the catheter is "floated" through the right atrium, right ventricle, and pulmonary artery until it is wedged in the pulmonary capillary bed.

Characteristic pressure changes recorded from the transducer attached to the distal port are seen as the catheter traverses each cardiac chamber and vessel (Fig. 15–1). A typical sawtooth pattern with rapid systolic rise followed by a diastolic fall nearly to zero indicates passage into the right ventricle. As the catheter passes into the pulmonary artery, the waveform changes to an arterial waveform with a similar ventricular systolic pressure but a diastolic pressure higher than that of the right ventricle, a narrowed pulse pressure, and a dicrotic notch. This waveform becomes dampened when the catheter is advanced into the wedge position. At this point, the balloon occludes the vessel proximal to the distal lumen of the PA catheter. A continuous column of

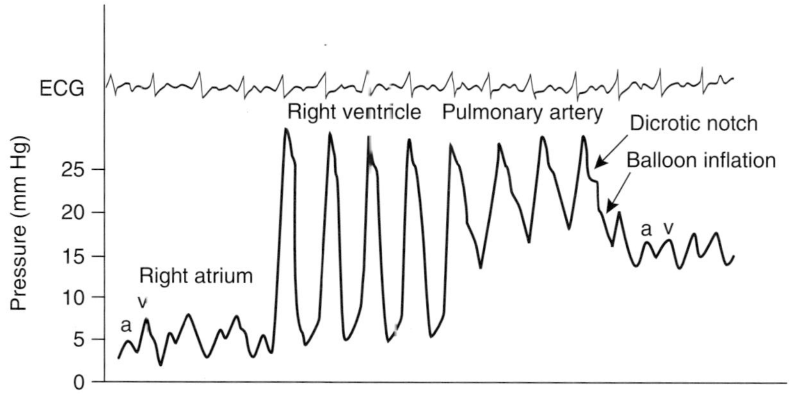

Figure 15–1 Characteristic pressure changes recorded from the transducer attached to the distal port are seen as the catheter traverses each cardiac chamber and vessel. The a wave occurs during atrial systole; the v wave occurs during ventricular systole. ECG, electrocardiogram.

blood, sealed off from the right ventricular pulse, transmits pressure from the pulmonary veins draining into the left atrium to the distal catheter lumen. This PA wedge pressure tracing represents the left atrial pressure under most circumstances and is in turn equivalent to left ventricular end-diastolic pressure, which reflects left ventricular end diastolic volume. The wedge pressure tracing varies with respiration, cough, or Valsalva maneuver and should be measured at end-expiration for greatest accuracy. Once the wedge pressure is read, the balloon should be allowed to deflate, and the waveform should immediately revert to the pulmonary arterial waveform. If the waveform remains wedged, the catheter may have been inserted too far and should be withdrawn until an arterial waveform reappears (Fig. 15–2).

PA catheter placement may be more difficult in patients with tricuspid regurgitation, pulmonary hypertension, or decreased cardiac output. In these situations, PA catheter placement might be facilitated in a conscious and cooperative patient by having the patient take deep inspirations to increase blood flow to the right side of the heart. In refractory situations, placement under fluoroscopy with or without the use of a guidewire might be necessary. Difficult PA insertion may also be guided by echocardiography.

If, during insertion, an excessive length of catheter is passed into the heart without appearance of a wedge tracing, the catheter may curl within the right atrium or ventricle, possibly knotting on itself, which could impede or prevent catheter removal. After the PA catheter is in a satisfactory position that wedges easily with balloon inflation and returns to an arterial waveform immediately when the balloon is deflated, a radiograph should be taken to confirm placement and exclude such complications as pneumothorax. The insertion length where the catheter has wedged should be noted in case manipulation through the sterile plastic sheath is necessary to reobtain a wedge tracing. Once the cardiac monitor is connected to the thermistor outlet, the PA catheter is ready to calculate cardiac output and a wide range of hemodynamic cardiopulmonary data.

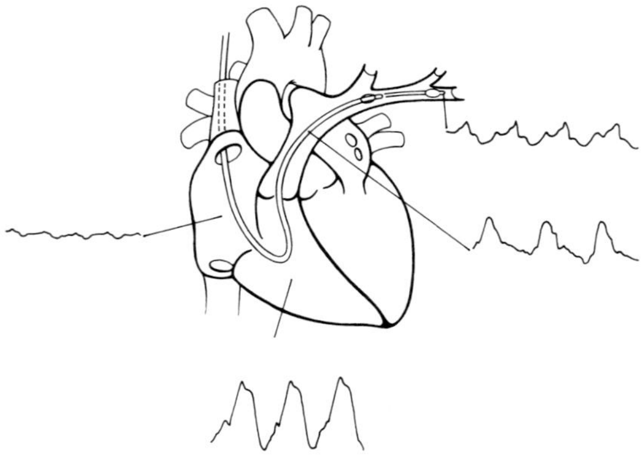

Figure 15–2 As the catheter passes into the pulmonary artery, the waveform changes to that of an arterial waveform with a similar ventricular systolic pressure but a diastolic pressure higher than that of the right ventricular pressure, a narrowed pulse, and a dicrotic notch. (From Amin DK, Shah PK, Swan HJ: The technique of inserting a Swan-Ganz catheter. *J Crit Illness,* 8:1147–1156, 1993.)

INTERPRETATION OF THE DATA

The utility of PA catheter data requires a thorough understanding of cardiac physiology, which can then be applied toward evaluation of the patient and therapy. Values may be directly measured or derived. Those values that are directly measured can be easily remembered from Ohm's law describing the relationship of pressure, flow, and resistance. One needs only to recall the alphabet to remember the relationship of these variables, as P is followed by Q and R; $P = QR$, where P is pressure, Q is flow or cardiac output, and R is resistance. Pressure and cardiac output are directly measured from the PA catheter. Resistance and all other variables are obtained from these two variables with knowledge of arterial and venous oxygen content obtained by drawing mixed venous and arterial blood samples to analyze for hemoglobin content and oxygen saturation.

Cardiac output, Q, is directly measured off the PA catheter. The technique of thermodilution is used, in which 3 to 10 ml of 5% dextrose in water or 0.9% normal saline of a certain temperature (ranging from 0°C to room temperature, depending upon technique and style), measured by an external thermistor fed into the cardiac output computer, is rapidly injected through the proximal PA catheter lumen; the temperature change sensed by the distal catheter thermistor is integrated over time to calculate the cardiac output. The derivation of the calculus is omitted from this discussion (Wetzel et al, 1991). Several cardiac output values (generally between three and five) are generated and averaged for greatest accuracy. Accuracy of measurement depends on a rapid injection rate, accurate measurement of injectant temperature, thorough mixing, and no loss of injectant. Variation between measurements is due to both variations in procedure technique, such as different rates of saline injection, and spontaneous variations in cardiac output. Other sources of error in cardiac output measurement are mechanical ventilation, intracardiac shunts, and tricuspid regurgitation (Armengol et al, 1981; Jansen et al, 1986; Okamoto et al, 1986).

Absolute cardiac output can vary widely, depending on the patient's size, and is therefore indexed to body surface area. The cardiac index is the cardiac output divided by body surface area. Because cardiac output is equal to heart rate multiplied by stroke volume, the stroke volume is cardiac output divided by heart rate, and the stroke volume index is the cardiac index divided by heart rate. These equations demonstrate that cardiac index can be increased by any intervention that raises either the heart rate or stroke volume, such as fluid or inotropic support.

The second directly measured variable described in Ohm's law for fluids is pressure. The PA catheter can measure the pressure of both the right and left sides of the heart. The CVP is the pressure in the great veins leading to the right side of the heart and is measured using a catheter lumen either within the great veins or in the right atrium. It is useful as an indicator of blood volume, venous capacitance, and right atrial pressure. In patients with normal lungs and ventricular function, it is used as a guide to determine adequate intravascular volume status for fluid replacement therapy. CVP ranges from 0 to 5 mm Hg in a normal, healthy, upright patient and 3 to 6 mm Hg in the supine position. Values greater than 10 to 12 mm Hg indicate increased intravascular volume, increased intrathoracic pressure, cardiac tamponade, tricuspid regurgitation, pulmonary hypertension, or right ventricular failure. Values less than 3 mm Hg in the supine position imply relative hypovolemia.

The limitation in using CVP as an indicator for myocardial preload is that the CVP measures right-sided pressures, not left-sided, and therefore not systemic filling pressures. In addition, measurements of pressure are used to infer volume status $\Delta V/\Delta P$ which presumes normal left ventricular function and compliance. When there is altered compliance, such as in congestive heart failure, a stiff noncompliant left ventricle may lead to high CVP readings without increased intravascular volume. Toussaint et al (1974) demonstrated poor correlation between CVP and PCWP in patients without myocardial compromise and even worse correlation in patients with cardiovascular dysfunction. In a controlled trial of parameter-guided therapy of postoperative surgical patients compared with the study cohort using PA catheter data for PCWP, Shoemaker et al (1988) showed that in conjunction, CVP monitoring and standard noninvasive data such as heart rate, ECG, and urine output alone were "neither sensitive nor accurate descriptors of circulatory decompensation."

The PCWP is the most accessible means of evaluating the amount of stretch of the myocardial fibers and is therefore used as an indicator of preload. This assumes that PCWP reflects left ventricular end diastolic pressure and volume. This assumption may not hold true if there exists a disease state that affects end-diastolic pressures without affecting volume status, such as restrictive cardiomyopathies. Moreover, the position of the PA catheter within the lung may affect the accuracy of the wedge pressure. Classically, the PA catheter should be located within zone 3 of the lung as described by West, where the arterial pressure exceeds the venous pressure, which in turn exceeds the alveolar pressure. In zone 1, where alveolar pressure is greater than both arterial and venous pressures, and in zone 2, where alveolar pressure is less than arterial but greater than venous pressures, the wedge reading may reflect a significant contribution from alveolar pressure and render it inaccurate. This is of concern when a patient is on a great deal of positive end-expiratory pressure (PEEP), which can convert zone 3 lung into non–zone 3 conditions and make wedge readings inaccurate. The level at which PEEP begins to affect wedge readings is controversial; different studies claim no false elevation up to 30 cm H_2O, whereas others claim an increasingly significant PEEP effect at pressures above 10 cm H_2O (Berryhill and Benumof, 1979; Goldenheim and Kazemi, 1984; Tooker et al, 1978). A normal PCWP is generally between 8 and 12 mm Hg. Values above 18 mm Hg can imply hypervolemia, increased intrathoracic pressure as with PEEP, or congestive heart failure. A PCWP below 8 mm Hg might imply hypovolemia.

When cardiac output (CO), mean arterial pressure (MAP), and CVP are known, systemic vascular resistance (SVR) can be calculated by use of Ohm's law: SVR is equal to MAP − CVP/CO multiplied by a constant 79.9 to get units of dyne-sec/cm^{-5}. Similarly, knowlege of the PCWP allows calculation of pulmonary vascular resistance (PVR), where PVR is equal to mean pulmonary artery pressure (MPAP) − PCWP/CO multiplied by 79.9 dyne-sec/cm^{-5}. Indexed values are obtained by dividing the SVR and the PVR by body surface area. These values are often thought of as the afterload of the right- and left-sided circulation. Decreased SVR may therefore imply arterio-venous shunting as occurs in septic shock, cirrhosis, and fistulas; increased SVR is most commonly found in patients with cardiogenic shock and occasionally increased systemic blood pressure. Likewise, increased PVR implies pulmonary hypertension. These values are useful indicators of overall resistance, but they may not accurately reflect regional differences in resistance because they consider the vascular bed as a whole in series when in reality it is composed of multiple systems in parallel. Normal SVR index is 800 to 1600 dyne-sec/cm^{-5}; normal PVR index is 80 to 240 dyne-sec/cm^{-5}.

The left and right ventricular stroke work index (LVSWI and RVSWI) can be calculated and used to evaluate cardiac and individual ventricular function. The stroke index (SI) is the cardiac index over heart rate (SI = CI/HR). LVSWI is the product of SI multiplied by MAP and the constant 0.0136 in g = m/m^2:

$$LVSWI = SI \times MAP \times 0.0136 \text{ g} = \text{m/m}^2.$$

Similarly, RVSWI is the product of SI multiplied by MPAP and 0.0136:

$$RVSWI = SI \times MPAP \times 0.0136 \text{ g} = \text{m/m}^2.$$

Normal LVSWI and RVSWI values are listed in Table 15–1.

A sample of blood drawn from the distal lumen of the PA catheter and hence from within the pulmonary artery represents the mixing of blood from the entire venous return of the body. This blood sample can be analyzed for the mixed venous oxygen tension ($P\bar{v}O_2$) and saturation ($S\bar{v}O_2$). Although these values are not diagnostic of any specific physiological function, they are necessary to calculate systemic oxygen delivery and consumption and may themselves contribute useful insight into various clinical situations. A normal $S\bar{v}O_2$ is approximately 75%. Values significantly below this are most commonly due to decreased cardiac output but can also imply hypoxia; poor tissue perfusion, as in shock; or increased oxygen demand due to seizures, shivering, hyper-

Table 15–1 Hemodynamic Values Obtained by Pulmonary Artery Catheterization

Parameter	Formula	Normal	Units
Cardiac output (CO)	CO = HR × SV	Varies	L/min
Cardiac index (CI)	CI = CO/BSA	3.5–5.5	L/min/m^2
Stroke volume index (SVI)	SVI = CI/HR	30–60	ml/beat/M^2
Systemic vascular resistance index (SVRI)	SVRI = 79.9(MAP − CVP)/CI	800–1600	dyne-sec/cm^{-5}/m^2
Pulmonary vascular resistance index (PVRI)	PVRI = 79.9(MPAP − PCWP)/CI	80–240	dyne-sec/cm^{-5}/m^2
Left ventricular stroke work index (LVSWI)	LVSWI = SI × MAP × 0.0136	56 ± 6	g-m/m^2
Right ventricular stroke work index (RVSWI)	RVSWI = SI × MPAP × 0.0136	6.0 ± 0.9	g-m/m^2
Left cardiac work index (LCWI)	LCWI = CI × MAP × 0.0136	4.0 + 0.4	kg-m/m^2
Right cardiac work index (RCWI)	RCWI = CI × MPAP × 0.0136	0.5 + 0.06	kg-m/m^2
Arterial-venous oxygen content difference ($Cavo_2$)	$Cavo_2$ = Hgb × 1.34 × (Sao_2 − Svo_2)	3.0–5.5	ml/dl
Oxygen delivery (Do_2)	Do_2 = Cao_2 × CI × 10	620 ± 50	ml/min/m^2
Oxygen consumption (Vo_2)	Vo_2 = $Cavo_2$ × CI × 10	120–200	ml/min/m^2
Oxygen extraction ratio	Vo_2/Do_2	28%–33%	

BSA, body surface area; CVP, central venous pressure; Hgb, hemoglobin; HR, heart rate; MAP, mean arterial pressure; MPAP, mean pulmonary artery pressure; PCWP, pulmonary capillary wedge pressure, SI, stroke index, SV, stroke volume.

Adapted from Katz RW, Pollack M, Weibley R: Pulmonary artery catheterization in pediatric intensive care. *Adv Pediatr,* 30:169–190, 1984.

thermia, or other hypermetabolic states. Values in excess of an $S\bar{v}O_2$ of 75% may indicate decreased tissue oxygen uptake and use, arteriovenous shunting as in severe septic shock, cirrhosis, arteriovenous fistula, or inappropriately increased cardiac output.

The $S\bar{v}O_2$ allows calculation of tissue oxygen consumption (VO_2). VO_2 is equal to arterial-venous oxygen content difference ($CavO_2$) multiplied by cardiac index (CI) multiplied by a constant 10 to obtain units of ml/min/m²:

$$VO_2 \, CI \times CavO_2 \times 10 \text{ ml/min/m}^2$$

The $CavO_2$ is equal to the oxygen content of hemoglobin (Hgb) multiplied by the arterial-venous oxygen saturation difference:

$$CavO_2 = (Hgb \times 1.34)(SaO_2 - SvO_2) \text{ ml } O_2\text{/dl blood}$$

This value, which in normal patients is generally 120 to 200 ml/min/m_2, describes systemic tissue oxygen consumption.

The amount of oxygen being delivered to the tissues for consumption (DO_2) is equal to the CI multiplied by the arterial oxygen content (CaO_2) multiplied by the constant 10 for units of ml/min/m²:

$$DO_2 = CI \times CaO_2 \times 10 \text{ ml/min/m}^2$$

The CaO_2 is described by the following formula:

$$CaO_2 = (Hgb \text{ x } 1.39)(SaO_2) + (PaO_2 \times 0.00031) \text{ ml } o_2\text{/dl blood}$$

Oxygen extraction, the ratio of VO_2/DO_2, is typically 0.28 to 0.33. The hemodynamic values of VO_2 and DO_2, and the VO_2/DO_2 ratio are clinically useful indicators of tissue perfusion.

The hemodynamic values obtained by a PA catheter are most valuable in states of shock. In shock, where tissue perfusion is inadequate to meet the metabolic demands of the tissues, an oxygen debt exists at the tissue level, and DO_2 is inadequate for that clinical state. A given DO_2 value must be taken in the context of the clinical condition, and a "normal" DO_2 value may thus still be insufficient for a patient who has sustained a cumulative oxygen debt secondary to prolonged shock. This situation can be confirmed by observing the initial DO_2 and VO_2 of a patient at clinical baseline and giving a trial of therapy (such as administering fluid or adding inotropic support) to raise DO_2. If the VO_2 is noted to increase concurrently, this may be interpreted as increased oxygen consumption at the tissue level as more oxygen is delivered, that is, as tissue perfusion is improved. An oxygen debt can then be assumed to have existed because the tissues used the additional oxygen delivered, and consideration of an additional trial of therapy is warranted. If DO_2 is increased without any improvement in VO_2, tissue perfusion may already have been maximized. Maximizing DO_2 and VO_2 is associated with increased survival in some clinical studies (Shoemaker et al, 1988).

PA catheter data have inherent limitations. The mathematical coupling of VO_2 and DO_2, which depend on a single variable, the $S\bar{v}O_2$, may lead to inaccurate calculations of oxygen consumption. Marik and Sibbald (1993) demonstrated that DO_2 and VO_2 as determined from PA catheter data increase after blood transfusion, whereas VO_2 measured with indirect calorimetry did not. In addition, spontaneous variation in oxygen demand coupled with methodological errors may allow enough error in calculated DO_2 and VO_2 to render an inaccurate picture of true peripheral organ perfusion and oxygen consumption (Seear et al, 1993). Nevertheless, in conjunction with other clinical data, the PA catheter provides valuable information that helps direct optimal management of the patient's compromized hemodynamic status. Table 15–1 summarizes the hemodynamic values that may be obtained by PA catheterization.

COMPLICATIONS

Complications can arise at any stage of the PA catheter's introduction, passage, or use. The insertion of the introducer sheath may cause different complications, depending on the site of insertion. Pneumothorax may result from insertion in upper thoracic venous sites, such as the internal jugular or subclavian veins. Bleeding and hematoma formation are common complications observed at all sites. Arteries that lie near central veins, such as the carotid, subclavian, and femoral arteries, may accidently be entered; they may be cannulated in situations in which shock and hypoxia do not allow clear differentiation of arterial from venous blood. Air may enter through a Cook finder needle and cause air embolism. Patients with a suspected air embolism should be placed left side down in the Trendelenburg position to trap air in the right atrium until a catheter can be placed to evacuate it.

Passage of the PA catheter through the introducer may cause dysrhythmias as the catheter passes through the right atrium and ventricle. Sprung et al (1981) report a

48% frequency of dysrhythmia with PA catheter placement. Premature atrial contractions, premature ventricular contractions, ventricular tachycardia, bradycardia, complete heart block, and right bundle branch block may all be seen. These dysrhythmias usually resolve on removal of the catheter. Special attention should be paid to placing a PA catheter in a patient with left bundle branch block because new-onset right bundle branch block may induce complete heart block. Medical intervention with lidocaine or defibrillation may be necessary in refractory arrhythmias. ECG monitoring during PA placement is mandatory, and antiarrhythmics, resuscitation medications, and defibrillation equipment must be readily available.

PA catheter placement may cause direct damage to the heart or blood vessels. Care should be taken not to overinflate the balloon, which could cause its rupture or, more important, rupture of the pulmonary artery in which the balloon is wedged. In addition, only air or carbon dioxide should be used to inflate the balloon because it may not be possible to withdraw liquid once it is injected. The catheter may be passed accidentally into the coronary sinus or through the myocardial wall. Pulmonary infarct may occur if the catheter is wedged despite decompression of the balloon, or overinflation of the balloon can cause pulmonary arterial rupture. The catheter might pass through an intracardiac shunt, such as a patent foramen ovale or ductus arteriosus. Tricuspid valve and pulmonary valve injury and ruptured chordae have been reported (Ducatman et al, 1975; O'Toole et al, 1979; Smith et al, 1976). The catheter may curl on itself within the ventricle, potentially knotting on itself and preventing or hindering withdrawal. The catheter should not continue to be advanced if, once it is in the right atrium, no waveform change is observed to occur despite advancing the catheter 10 cm.

Finally, the risk of sepsis increases the longer the catheter remains in place. Aseptic conditions should be maintained from the time of insertion until the catheter is removed to reduce this risk. The risks of thrombosis, emboli, erosion of pulmonary arteries, or other cardiovascular damage also increases with time. Hence, PA catheters should be removed as soon as they are no longer essential for understanding the patient's cardiovascular status or are no longer directly guiding therapy.

The PA catheter can be a valuable tool in diagnosing and managing critically ill patients with life-threatening hemodynamic and pulmonary conditions. They are used to differentiate among different cardiopulmonary disorders and can be used to guide and evaluate therapy in cases such as adult respiratory distress syndrome, shock, or pulmonary hypertension. Their use is not trivial, and the potential benefits must be weighed heavily against their cost, morbidity, and mortality. However, in skilled hands, the PA catheter remains the most direct and accurate means by which to measure, evaluate, and manipulate cardiopulmonary performance.

References

Amin DK, Shah PK, Swan HJ: The technique of inserting a Swan-Ganz catheter. *J Crit Illness,* 8:1147–1156, 1993.

Armengol J, Godfrey CW, et al: Effects of the respiratory cycle on cardiac output measurements: reproducibility of data enhanced by timing thermodilution injections in dogs. *Crit Care Med,* 9:852–854, 1981.

Berryhill RE, Benumof JL: PEEP-induced discrepancy between pulmonary arterial wedge pressure and left atrial pressure. *Anesthesiology,* 51: 303–308, 1979.

Ducatman BS, McMichan JC, Edwards WD: Catheter-induced lesions of the right side of the heart. *JAMA,* 253:791–795, 1975.

Forrester JS, Ganz W, et al: Thermodilution cardiac output determination with a single flow-directed catheter. *Am Heart J,* 83: 306–311, 1972.

Goldenheim PD, Kazemi H: Cardiopulmonary monitoring in critically ill patients. *N Engl J Med,* 311:717–721, 776–780, 1984.

Iberti TJ, Fischer EP, et al: A multicenter study of physicians' knowledge of the pulmonary artery catheter. *JAMA,* 264: 2928–2932, 1990.

Jansen JR, Scjreider KK, et al: Thermodilution cardiac output—an in vitro model of low flow states. *Crit Care Med,* 14:57–59, 1986.

Katz RW, Pollack M, Weibley R: Pulmonary artery catheterization in pediatric intensive care. *Adv Pediatr,* 30:169–190, 1984.

Marik PE, Sibbald WJ: Effect of stored-blood transfusion on oxygen delivery in patients with sepsis. *JAMA,* 269:3024–3029, 1993.

Okamoto K, Komatsu T, Kumar V: Effects of intermittent positive-pressure ventilation on cardiac output measurements by thermodilution. *Crit Care Med,* 14:977–980, 1986.

O'Toole JD, Wurtzbacher JJ, et al: Pulmonary-valve injury and insufficiency during pulmonary artery catheterization. *N Engl J Med,* 301:1167–1168, 1979.

Robin ED: The cult of the Swan-Ganz catheter: overuse and abuse of pulmonary flow catheters. *Ann Intern Med,* 103:445–449, 1985.

Seear M, Wensley D, et al: Oxygen consumption–oxygen delivery relationship in children. *J Pediatr,* 123:208–214, 1993.

Shoemaker WC, Appel PL, et al: Prospective trial of supranormal values of survivors as therapeutic goals in high-risk surgical patients. *Chest,* 94: 1176–1186, 1988.

Shoemaker WC: Use and abuse of the balloon tip pulmonary artery (Swan-Ganz) catheter: are patients getting their money's worth? *Crit Care Med,* 18:1294, 1990.

Smith WR, Glauser FL, Jemison P: Ruptured chordae of the tricuspid valve: the consequence of flow-directed Swan-Ganz catheterization. *Chest,* 70:790–792, 1976.

Sprung CL, Jacobs LJ, et al: Ventricular arrhythmias during Swan-Ganz catheterization of the critically ill. *Chest,* 79:413–415, 1981.

Swan HJ: What role today for hemodynamic monitoring? *J Crit Illness,* 8:1043–1050, 1993.

Swan HJ, Ganz W, et al: Catheterization of the heart in man with use of a flow-directed balloon-tipped catheter. *N Engl J Med,* 283:447–451, 1970.

Tooker J, Huseby J, Butler J: The effect of Swan-Ganz catheter height on the wedge pressure–left atrial pressure relationship in edema during positive-pressure ventilation. *Am Rev Respir Dis,* 117:721–725, 1978.

Toussaint G, Burgess J, et al: Central venous pressure and pulmonary wedge pressure in critical surgical illness. *Arch Surg,* 109:265–269, 1974.

Victor LD: *Hemodynamic Monitoring, Manual of Critical Care Procedures.* Rockville, MD, Aspen Publishers, 1989, p. 55.

Wetzel RC, Tabata BK, Rogers MC: Hemodynamic monitoring considerations in pediatric critical care. In Rogers M (ed): *Textbook of Pediatric Intensive Care.* Baltimore, Williams & Wilkins, 1991, pp 624–629.

Chapter 16

Left Ventricular Assist Devices

Paul Lubinsky

The ventricular assist device (VAD) is developing a specialized niche in cardiac surgery. The term ventricular assistance implies use of a device designed to provide temporary support for one or both ventricles but does not include total cardiopulmonary bypass (CPB), extracorporeal membrane oxygenation (ECMO), or a total artificial heart. The intra-aortic balloon pump also provides left ventricular assistance and is discussed elsewhere, as are techniques for ECMO. The intra-aortic balloon pump is often limited in pediatric use by the size of the balloon, and its effectiveness in augmenting diastolic pressure is compromised by the compliance of the arterial tree and the high heart rates required. Advantages of ECMO are that it provides biventricular support and improves systemic oxygenation, and cannulas do not need to be placed through a sternotomy incision. However, ECMO is more complex than nonpulsatile ventricular assistance, exposes the blood to a greater surface area of foreign material, and requires higher levels of anticoagulation.

In the pediatric intensive care unit, ventricular assistance is most frequently instituted to allow a period of cardiac rest during which functional recovery may occur. The use of mechanical assistance as a bridge to recovery is predicated on the premise that there exists myocardial stun that will recover with time. The goals are to decrease preload, and thus ventricular wall tension and myocardial oxygen consumption, while coronary perfusion and systemic blood flow are optimized.

To achieve maximal myocardial rest, as much preload as possible should be diverted from the target ventricle, minimizing pressure or volume work and maximizing subendocardial perfusion. The VAD is also used as a bridge to transplantation.

The VAD may support either ventricle. Historically, the VAD has been used mostly for left ventricular failure. However, right ventricular failure is a common cause of mortality in patients requiring left ventricular assistance, and biventricular assistance is being initiated more frequently.

SELECTION OF PATIENTS

Patients requiring implementation of ventricular assistance fall into three broad clinical groups:

1. Patients who cannot be weaned from CPB after a technically successful operation or those who have low cardiac output states within 48 hours of surgery, a syndrome now described as postcardiotomy cardiogenic shock
2. Patients with a potentially reversible cause for cardiac failure, such as digitalis intoxication or myocarditis
3. Patients with acute cardiogenic shock after myocardial infarction (a rare event in pediatrics)

Patients should meet the criteria listed in Tables 16–1 and 16–2. These criteria are guidelines only and need to be established for each institution.

INDICATIONS (see Table 16–1)

The decision to initiate cardiac support is often based on clinical judgment because thermodilution catheters are often not present, and systemic-to-pulmonary shunts will skew the results obtained from these catheters. The decision is based on evidence of left- or right-sided heart failure, pulmonary hypertension, decreased peripheral perfusion, and systemic acidosis. Inability to be weaned from CPB after successful repair and otherwise uncomplicated surgery identifies an obvious candidate for mechanical circulatory assistance. This group of patients has been shown to have a 44% survival rate (combined adult and pediatric data).

The rapidly deteriorating patient will clearly benefit from mechanical circulatory support. Intervention before the development of irreversible multiple system organ failure is necessary for optimal results. It is the patients with marginal hemodynamic function receiving maximal medical therapy who present the most difficult problems in defining who should receive assistance. Patients who have VADs placed after weaning from CPB have much lower survival rates than do those patients who have VADs placed intraoperatively.

Table 16–1 Indications for Ventricular Assist Device

Cardiac index < 1.8 L/min/m^2 with SVRI < 1000 dyne-sec/cm^{-5}/m^2
Left atrial pressure > 20 mm Hg (optimal preload)
Inadequate systolic blood pressure for age
Failure to respond to maximal inotropic, vasodilator, and vasopressor support
Mechanical ventilatory support
Reversible left ventricular dysfunction*
Failure to respond to IABP†

*Unless instituting as a bridge to transplant.
†Not usually attempted in pediatric patients.
IABP, intra-aortic balloon pump; SVRI, systemic vascular resistance index.

CONTRAINDICATIONS (see Table 16–2)

Some contraindications are relative and are also device dependent.

Analysis of the registry data has revealed that significant predictors of an inability to be weaned from bypass are renal failure, biventricular failure, neurological event, coagulopathy, and infection. The presence of multiple complications further reduces the odds of weaning from bypass.

In the adult population, many bridge-to-transplant patients are not undergoing CPB when the decision to initiate prolonged circulatory support is made. This is less true of the pediatric population.

CANNULATION

For left ventricular support, a drainage cannula is placed in the left atrium through the left atrial appendage, in the right superior pulmonary vein, or directly through the roof of the left atrium. The return cannula is placed in the aorta. For biventricular assistance, the right-side drainage cannula is placed in the right atrium, with the return cannula in

Table 16–2 Contraindications to Ventricular Assist Device*

Multiple organ failure
Intracranial hemorrhage
Acute cerebral injury (fixed dilated pupils/flat EEG)
Severe coagulopathy
Unsuccessful surgical procedure

*Some contraindications are relative and are also device dependent.
EEG, electroencephalogram.

the main pulmonary artery. If assistance is initiated as a bridge to transplantation, the drainage cannulas may be placed directly through the ventricular apex; this is the most efficient technique for unloading the ventricle. Cannulas are placed by use of standard technique with purse-string sutures, pledgets, and rubber tourniquets. Particular effort is made to minimize leaks; hemorrhage from surgical sites is a common complication during long-term ventricular assistance.

Once the drainage line is secured, it is allowed to fill with blood and is then connected to the inflow line of the preprimed pump. All air must be excluded from the system at this time. The return cannula is then connected to the outflow line, again with all air excluded.

The small size of the thoracic cavity may not allow closure of the sternum with the cannulas in place because this may produce a tamponade. In these instances, only the skin is closed.

DEVICES

VADs are divided into three basic categories: centrifugal, rotary, and pulsatile. The pulsatile devices are more complex and expensive to operate and have been restricted by investigational requirements of the Food and Drug Administration (FDA); thus, the centrifugal devices have been more widely used and accepted. The choice of device depends on whether recovery is expected or it is a bridge to transplantation. An important factor in choosing the type of device is availability and experience at individual institutions. This chapter concentrates on centrifugal devices and briefly highlights rotary and pulsatile devices.

Centrifugal Devices

The centrifugal pump consists of acrylic rotator cones, sealed in a vortex housing, that impart a centrifugal force to the blood. There is a drive magnet sealed in the housing attached to the cones. A rotational force is imparted to this magnet by a magnet on the external drive console. This design prevents induction of air and environmental contamination. The centrifugal force generated by the spinning cones creates pressure and flow. The flow path of the pump is hydrodynamically designed to virtually eliminate turbulence, cavitation, and associated damage to blood elements. The blood flow is proportional to the revolutions per minute, which is controlled from the drive console; the flow is measured by an in-line electromagnetic flow probe and adjusted to maximize myocardial rest, coronary perfusion, and systemic perfusion.

Centrifugal devices are more frequently used because they are less expensive, less complex, and more readily available than pulsatile VADs. Outcomes for short-term support are not statistically different for the two types of devices. Centrifugal systems have a higher frequency of hemorrhage, however.

The most commonly used centrifugal pump is the Biomedicus Biopump (Eden Prairie, MN). A 50-ml pediatric and an 80-ml adult pump are available (Fig. 16–1).

Additional equipment required

- Appropriate-sized cannulas for the patient
- Biomedicus pump console and disposable pump head
- Biomedicus flow transducer and disposable flow probe
- Battery pack
- Four tubing clamps
- 3 L of priming solution (5% albumin/Plasma-Lyte A)
- 10 feet of 3/8 × 3/16-inch sterile tubing
- Appropriately trained personnel to manage the device and patient
- Spare pump console, pump head, and flow probe

Once the pump is connected, flow is incrementally increased so that total systemic flow (pump and native ventricle) is 2.2 L/min/m^2 or

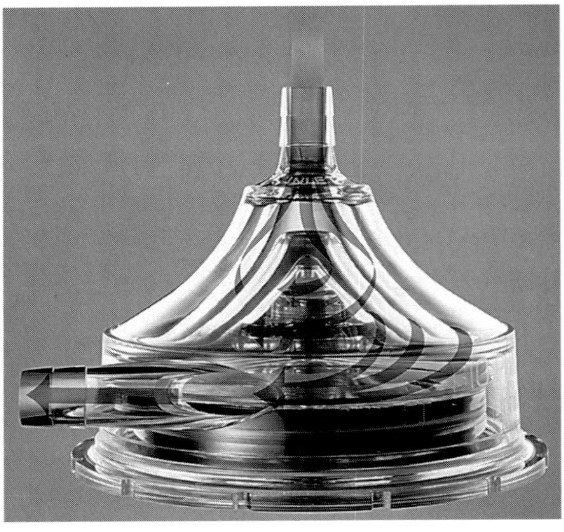

Figure 16–1 Biomedicus cone showing blood flow.

greater and left atrial pressure is maintained in the range of 8 to 15 mm Hg. After initiation of ventricular assistance, inotropic agents may be weaned to reduce some of the deleterious effects associated with large doses of these agents (tachycardia or arrhythmias, increased myocardial oxygen demands, and increased afterload).

Vasoactive medications may still be required to optimize hemodynamic function, augmenting the unassisted ventricle and maximizing systemic and coronary perfusion pressure. These pharmacological agents may provide either a decrease in systemic vascular resistance (sodium nitroprusside, amrinone) or an increase in systemic vascular resistance (epinephrine, norepinephrine).

Pharmacotherapy to reduce the pulmonary vascular resistance may also be required (prostaglandin E_2, amrinone). Amrinone is an ideal agent because it increases ventricular inotropy and decreases pulmonary and systemic vascular resistance. Amrinone is administered with an initial loading dose of 0.75 to 1.5 mg/kg followed by constant infusions of 5 to 30 μg/kg/min. Thrombocytopenia is a common side effect of amrinone administration and may necessitate discontinuation of the drug. Milrinone is a newer phosphodiesterase inhibitor that does not induce thrombocytopenia. The loading dose is 50 μg/kg by bolus over 15 minutes followed by a continuous infusion of 0.35 to 0.75 μg/kg/min.

If the left ventricular assistance is unable to maintain adequate flow despite adequate volume loading, good cannula placement, and maximal pharmacological manipulation, then right ventricular assistance must be initiated. Because the pumps are in series, manipulation of the pumps needs to be coordinated to maintain left atrial pressure and systemic blood flow.

If possible, atrial septal defects should be closed before isolated ventricular assistance is initiated. Shunting at the atrial level will compromise the function of the unassisted side.

In most institutions, a perfusionist manages the pump. Some facilities are now training nurses to manage the patient.

Heparinization

If the patient was on CPB, heparinization is reversed with protamine. Once bleeding from chest tubes has decreased to an acceptable level, heparin therapy is initiated and titrated to achieve activated clotting time (ACT) of approximately 150. Starting dose is 10 U/kg/h. Concentration of the infusion is adjusted so that only 1 to 2 ml/h of fluid is required. If pump flows are less than 2 L/min, ACT should be 180 to 200; at pump flows less than 1 L/min, ACT should be 200 to 225. Some authors recommend routine changing of the pump head every 48 to 72 hours. If a stethoscope is placed over the pump head, a smooth "whirring" sound is heard. If this begins to chatter and there is adequate inflow pressure, thrombus formation must be seriously considered.

Respiratory support

Routine ventilator management is per unit protocols. PaO_2 is maintained above 70 mm Hg. The pH may be maintained in the normal range (7.35–7.45) or may be adjusted upwards (7.45–7.55) in attempt to relax the pulmonary vascular bed. The alkalotic pH is achieved by judicious hyperventilation combined with metabolic alkalinization.

General supportive therapy

Heating or cooling blankets may be required, and VAD lines may need to be insulated against heat loss with silver foil. Nutrition is of paramount importance in these patients, and total parenteral nutrition should be initiated by the second postoperative day. This should be supplemented by enteral nutrition as soon as possible with a view toward total enteral nutrition. Air fluidization therapy beds should be an early consideration because many of these patients may remain immobilized for an extended time. Range-of-motion exercises should also be instituted per unit protocol. The provision of adequate analgesia and sedation is mandatory and is discussed elsewhere.

Routine laboratory tests include white blood cell count every 6 hours initially; hematocrit; platelet count; prothrombin time and partial thromboplastin time; and fibrinogen, sodium, potassium, bicarbonate, blood urea nitrogen, creatinine, and calcium concentrations. Initial laboratory studies also include liver function tests and determination of serum albumin and magnesium and free serum hemoglobin concentrations.

The care of these and other complex patients in the intensive care unit may be streamlined by the development of standard order sheets, which need to reflect the preferences of the cardiac and intensive care unit teams at the individual institutions.

Complications

Device-Related Complications

HEMOLYSIS: The frequency of hemolysis is far less with centrifugal pumps than with roller pumps; for this reason, centrifugal pumps are preferred for providing nonpulsatile flow. Urine and free serum hemoglobin concentrations should be monitored. Immediate postoperative hemolysis may be due to long CPB times or may be a side effect of multiple transfusions. If hemolysis occurs beyond 24 hours, the device is implicated; adjustment of revolutions per minute may reduce this. It is also important to monitor the pressure in the inlet line (i.e., patient to pump). Pressures in excess of −60 mm Hg are associated with increased hemolysis due to pressure effects on the red blood cells.

THROMBOEMBOLISM: Exposure of blood to artificial surfaces predisposes to thrombus formation. High flows and complete emptying of pulsatile devices reduce thrombus formation. Anticoagulation is also used as discussed previously, and heparin-bonded surfaces are now in use but are not yet effective for prolonged support. Newer textured surfaces are being developed that encourage the formation and adherence of a pseudointimal surface. This is a biological lining that is not recognized as foreign and may contain cells that actively create a nonthrombogenic surface.

MECHANICAL FAILURE: Mechanical failure does occur, and a back-up system must be available. All tubing junctions must be secured and monitored for rupture.

Patient-Related Complications

BIVENTRICULAR FAILURE: A left VAD can only pump blood delivered from the right side of the heart. Poor right ventricular function thus diminishes the benefits of a left VAD. Right ventricular function may be enhanced by the addition of an inotropic agent or a pulmonary vasodilator. If pharmacotherapy and volume loading are inadequate, biventricular assistance needs to be initiated.

HEMOSTASIS/BLEEDING: Bleeding is a common and serious complication that may require exploration to achieve control. Serum coagulation studies (prothrombin time, partial thromboplastin time, fibrinogen level, and platelet count) should be monitored at least daily and more frequently while there is bleeding that requires correction. Platelet count should be maintained above 100,000/mm^3. Fresh-frozen plasma is used for prolonged clotting times. Cryoprecipitate is used if the serum fibrinogen concentration is less than 100 mg/dl, although some institutions believe that the use of cryoprecipitate is associated with increased thrombus formation. Topical agents such as fibrin glue or Surgicel are also used, but surgical hemostasis and control of any coagulopathy are the most important ways to control bleeding.

RENAL FAILURE: Renal function is frequently suboptimal because of renovascular hypotension. If this remains inadequate with low-dose dopamine (3–5 μg/kg) and administration of furosemide, then continuous arteriovenous hemofiltration may be instituted and can be modified to provide dialysis. The circuit can easily be adapted to provide this.

INFECTION: Patients are at high risk for infections owing to the premorbid state, which may include malnutrition and nonspecific immunosuppression as well as pre-existing infections. Surgical procedures are associated with immunosuppression, and multiple invasive lines are present after the procedure. In addition, translocation of bacteria from the intestinal tract may occur, particularly after periods of low mesenteric blood flow. Prevention is the key, and strict aseptic technique must be observed. Some institutions recommend reverse isolation. Prophylactic cefazolin is administered at 100 mg/kg/d in four divided doses, until all lines are removed. Some institutions also use regimens to reduce bacterial colony counts in the gastrointestinal tract. In the event that the patient becomes febrile, blood, urine, and tracheal cultures should be obtained and antibiotics changed to nafcillin and cefotaxime. Culture-specific antibiotics are initiated when an organism is identified. *Candida* infections are not uncommon in patients on long-term support.

NEUROLOGICAL COMPLICATIONS: The exact frequency of neurological complications is not known at this time. There is certainly a risk of embolic central nervous system (CNS) injury as well as the possibility of CNS compromise resulting from the inadequate cardiac function that necessitated the initiation of ventricular assistance. In addition, children with cyanotic congenital heart disease may have CNS injuries before surgery.

TRANSFUSION REQUIREMENT: The patient requires multiple transfusions, and this must be discussed with the family and, if appropriate, the patient at the outset. Anemia occurs as a result of losses due to hemorrhage and drawing of laboratory samples, hemolysis, and decreased marrow production.

Weaning

No weaning is attempted during the first 24 hours. After this initial stabilization period, pump flows are decreased and native ventricular activity is assessed by monitoring the arterial pressure waveform, pulmonary artery pressures, left and right atrial pressures, cardiac output by echocardiogram or thermodilution catheter, and peripheral perfusion. If it appears that cardiac function is adequate to support the circulation, pump flows are weaned in approximately 10% increments, allowing gradual volume loading of the ventricle. The risk of thrombosis is much higher at low-flow rates and particularly at flows below 1 L/min. In some pediatric patients, it is necessary to reduce flows to less than 500 ml/h to ensure adequate cardiac function before discontinuing the VAD. The minimal safe flow for the circuit is 200 ml/min for 1 to 2 hours. Heparin administration and ACTs need to be adjusted as described before. If both ventricles are being supported, they may be weaned simultaneously or separately in a stepwise manner. Decannulation may occur in the operating room, although it is frequently accomplished in the postanesthesia recovery area or in the intensive care unit with use of strict aseptic technique; the sternum is closed at that time.

Rotary Devices

The Hemopump (Fig. 16–2) is a percutaneous cable-driven axial blood pump. This device is placed by femoral artery cutdown and is advanced to the left ventricular chamber. The pump is 7 mm in diameter and 16 mm long. It is positioned across the aortic valve, and a rotating Archimedean screw pumps blood from the left ventricle into the ascending aorta. Hemolysis has not been a significant problem with this device. The two major problems are device migration and its 21 French size, which limits its use to adults without atherosclerotic disease of the femoral artery. A smaller version that may be useful in pediatric patients is under development.

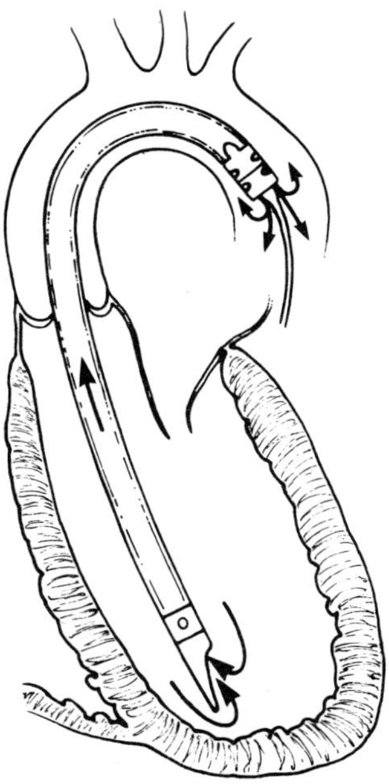

Figure 16–2 The Nimbus Hemopump. (From Locke T, Mcgregor C: Ventricular assist devices. In *Techniques in Extracorporeal Circulation*, 3rd ed. London, Butterworth-Heinemann, 1992, pp 268–281.)

Pulsatile Devices

For short-term use, pulsatile devices have not been demonstrated to be superior to centrifugal systems. They are more expensive and complex than centrifugal devices and are restricted by the FDA. Centrifugal systems have therefore been used more frequently to provide a bridge to recovery. The advantage of the pulsatile devices is that they may be used for more extended periods without the same degree of complications seen with the nonpulsatile systems. Pulsatile devices are thus the optimal system for providing a bridge to transplantation. More recently, increasing data have demonstrated that although the optimal time frame for the use of a centrifugal system is less than 7 days, ventricular assistance may be required for longer periods as a bridge to recovery.

Pulsatile pumps have a lower frequency of bleeding, hemolysis, and thromboembolic events than centrifugal systems do. Another advantage of the pulsatile systems is that should the myocardium not recover as expected, the appropriate long-term support system is already in place.

There has been a proliferation of different devices, internal and external, pneumatic and electromechanical, and it will be some time before we define the optimal indications for each system. A few of the more commonly used systems are profiled here.

Pneumatic pumps

THORATEC VAD: The Pierce-Donachy or Thoratec VAD (Thoratec Laboratories Corporation, Berkeley, CA) is a pneumatic pulsatile device. This device has a seamless 65-ml flexible polyurethane blood pumping chamber in a rigid plastic housing with inflow and outflow connections and a pneumatic drive console.

These pumps are connected to the drive console, which provides alternating negative and positive pressure to the space surrounding the pumping chamber, thus creating pulsatile flow. These pumps may be operated in three modes: (1) asynchronous (fixed rate); (2) synchronous; and (3) volume (fill-to-empty). The volume mode is preferred because it adjusts to venous return. These devices do use negative pressure to assist flow in the drainage line, which may be associated with complications. Bubbles may form by vacuolation, or external air may be sucked in.

These devices require less anticoagulation than nonpulsatile devices do because the chamber is emptied on each beat, which provides less opportunity for stasis to occur. In larger patients with flows above 4 L/min, only low-molecular-weight dextran infusion is required, with addition of heparin at flow rates below 4 L/min. Patients may also be maintained on oral anticoagulants long term. The Symbion AVAD (Ethicon Inc., Somerville, NJ) is a pulsatile univentricular assist device.

ABIOMED BVS 5000: The BVS 5000 (Abiomed Cardiovascular, Inc., Danvers, MA) is a gravity-filled, pneumatically driven external assist device placed at the bedside (Fig. 16–3). This device has three unique characteristics:

1. It is a dual chamber device with a filling and pumping chamber. This design maintains constant flow to the pump with pulsatile flow to the patient. Pulses of compressed air from the control system produce pulsatile flow from the "ventricular" chamber, with passive filling.
2. It has two polyurethane valves to ensure unidirectional flow.
3. It has an automated control system that adapts to the patient's condition but restricts the operator's input. This has the advantage of making this a simple system to operate. The flow can be adjusted in 0.1-L/min increments to a minimum of 0.5 L/min for weaning.

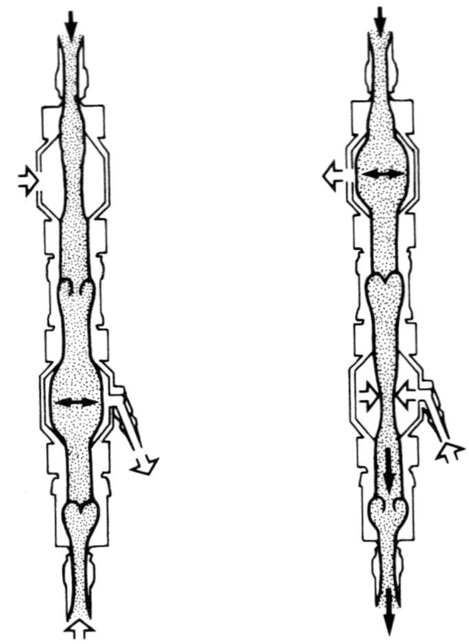

Figure 16–3 Schematic illustration of the BVS 5000 blood pump during pump systole (left) and diastole (right). The ventricular bladder collapses during pump systole and fills during diastole. The atrial bladder fills continuously. (From Guyton AC, Schonberger JP, et al: Clinical evaluation of the BVS 5000. *Ann Thorac Surg,* 56:347, 1993. Reprinted with permission from the Society of Thoracic Surgeons.)

This device has received FDA approval.

IMPLANTABLE DEVICES: Implantable left ventricular assist systems have also been developed, such as the TCI Heartmate LVAD (TCI, Woburn, MA) and the Novacor LVAS (Baxter Healthcare Corporation, Oakland, CA) (Fig. 16–4).

OUTCOME

Combined registry experience showed that in 90% of patients discharged from the hospital, circulatory support was discontinued by 1 week. Patients requiring univentricular support had a better prognosis, and outcome results did not differ between pulsatile and nonpulsatile devices. Overall survival was 24.6% for the period of data analysis (1985 to December 1990). Mortality is highest on the pump, but there is still a 47% mortality in the group weaned off circulatory assistance. Those patients receiving postcardiotomy support have a 29% to 50% survival rate, which is better than

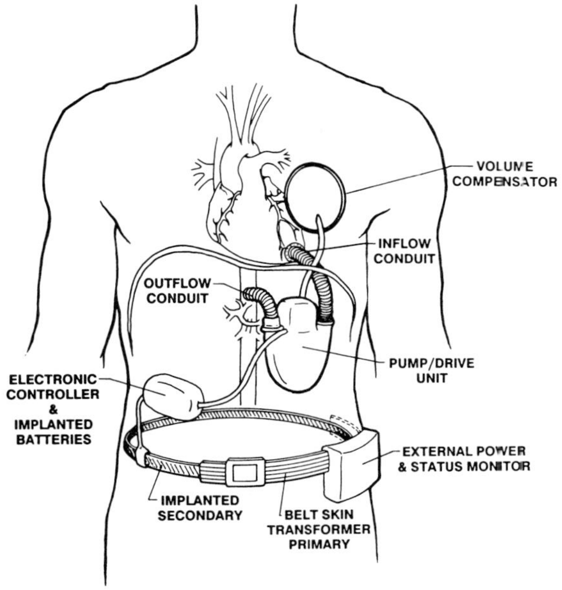

Figure 16–4 Novacor Left Ventricular Assist System (LVAS). The totally implantable LVAS is designed for long-term support as an alternative to transplantation. (Courtesy of Baxter Healthcare Corporation, Oakland, CA.)

the survival rate of the entire population of patients receiving assistance.

REPORT TO REGISTRY

There is a voluntary registry for all cardiac mechanical assist devices. Cases should be reported to facilitate data analysis and a better understanding of the clinical circumstances under which VADs should be used and which type of VAD should be used. The registry is maintained at the Division of Cardiothoracic Surgery, Department of Surgery, The Pennsylvania State University, P.O. Box 850, Hershey, PA 17033.

Bibliography

Chang AC, Hanley FL, et al: Left heart support with a ventricular assist device in an infant with myocarditis. *Crit Care Med,* 20:712–715, 1992.

Joyce LD, Toninato C, Hansen JB: Centrifugal ventricular assist devices. In Quaal SJ (ed): *Cardiac Mechanical Assist Beyond Balloon Pumping.* St, Louis, CV Mosby, 1993.

Karl TR, Sano S, et al: Centrifugal pump left heart assist in pediatric cardiac operations. *J Thorac Cardiovasc Surg,* 102:624–630, 1991.

Locke T, Mcgregor C: Ventricular assist devices: In *Techniques in Extracorporeal Circulation,* 3rd ed. Oxford, Butterworth-Heinemann, 1992, pp 268–281.

Loisance DY: Mechanical circulatory support in the 1990s. *Eur J Cardiothorac Surg,* 6(suppl 1): S107–S112, 1992.

Louis PT, Bricker JT, et al: Nonpulsatile total left ventricular support in pediatric partients. *Crit Care Med,* 20:704–707, 1992.

Ott RA, Gutfinger DE, Gazzaniga AB: Mechanical cardiac assist. *Cardiac Surg,* 7:2, 1993.

Pae WE, Miller CA, et al: Ventricular assist devices for postcardiotomy cardiogenic shock. *J Thorac Cardiovasc Surg,* 104:541–553, 1992.

Scheinin SA, Radovancevic B, et al: Postcardiotomy LVAD support and transesophageal echocardiography in a child. *Ann Thorac Surg,* 55: 529–531, 1993.

Chapter 17

Intra-aortic Balloon Pump

Sana Al-Jundi

The intra-aortic balloon pump (IABP) is a form of mechanical support of the left ventricle in the failing heart and a way to augment cardiac output in patients with cardiogenic shock. Its clinical application was first reported by Kantrowitz et al in 1967, and it gradually became standard therapy for congestive heart failure mainly in the adult population. Its use in children has been limited in the past owing to some technical difficulties, although reports of successful use in children have been published (Al Mofada et al, 1990; Anell et al, 1990; del Nido et al, 1988; Park et al, 1993; Pennington and Swartz, 1993; Pollock et al, 1980; Veasey et al, 1981; Veasey et al, 1983; Webster and Veasey, 1985). Adjustment of the equipment and availability of small catheters for pediatric use in the last few years have made the IABP a valuable addition to conventional medical therapy in the treatment of refractory cardiogenic shock.

MECHANISM OF CARDIAC SUPPORT

A balloon catheter is surgically placed in the descending thoracic aorta (Fig. 17–1). The balloon inflates during ventricular diastole and deflates right before the onset of ventricular systole. Helium and carbon dioxide are the usual gases used to inflate the balloon. Balloon inflation causes forward displacement of blood volume into the peripheral circulation. Meanwhile, the retrograde displacement of blood volume enhances the coronary perfusion. During the rapid deflation of the balloon, the left ventricle ejects against less resistance, which provides an afterload reduction effect. Depending on the cardiac output and the size of the balloon, this mechanism could provide an increase in the cardiac output by 10% to 20% (Smith and Cleavinger, 1991).

INDICATIONS

Indications in children involve the following:

1. Inability to wean off the bypass circuit in patients undergoing cardiac surgery
2. Acute cardiogenic shock (e.g., myocarditis, Kawasaki's disease)
3. Congestive heart failure, end stage
4. Postoperative left ventricular dysfunction with low cardiac output
5. Preoperative use for patients who are un-

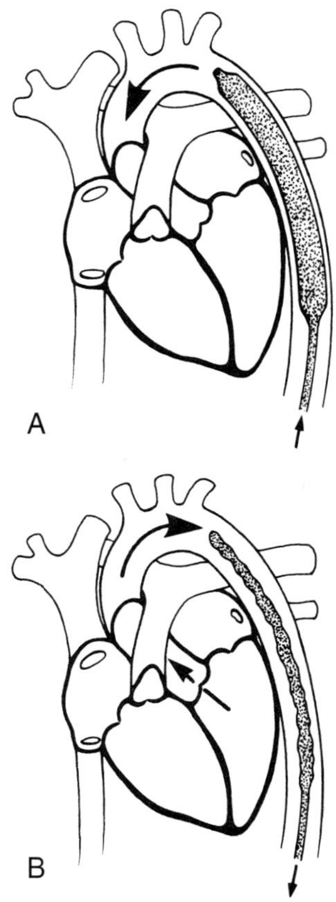

Figure 17–1 Effects of intra-aortic balloon pump (IABP) counterpulsation. **A.** Diastolic augmentation with balloon inflation. **B.** Systolic afterload reduction with rapid balloon deflation. (From Quaal SJ: *Comprehensive Intra-aortic Balloon Pumping.* St. Louis, CV Mosby, 1984 pp 78–86.)

dergoing heart transplantation as a bridge for transport

6. Cardiac support during transportation to referral specialty centers, especially when the referral is for cardiac transplantation

Data on criteria for initiating intra-aortic balloon counterpulsation in pediatric patients are limited. Veasey et al (1981, 1983) recommended considering IABP with a cardiac index less than 2 L/min/m^2, venous partial pressure of oxygen less than 20 mm Hg, and urine output below 1 ml/kg/h.

In adults, all the pediatric indications apply, plus the main indications of acute myocardial ischemia due to coronary occlusion and for patients with unstable angina. Mitral regurgitation with congestive heart failure is another indication in the adult population. Georgeson et al (1992) suggested the use of IABP prophylactically in high-risk cardiac patients undergoing noncardiac surgery.

CONTRAINDICATIONS

1. Aortic regurgitation, which permits backward flow into the left ventricle in diastole
2. Aortic aneurysm or dissection in the area in which the balloon will be placed
3. Presence of a prosthetic graft in the aorta, although some authors (Kantrowitz et al, 1992) suggested that this would be a contraindication only if it is less than 12 months old as long as there are no signs of instability of the graft

EQUIPMENT

Insertion of the IABP can be done in the intensive care unit. Equipment required is the balloon catheter and the drive unit. There are four manufacturers of the balloon pump systems. The most commonly used in pediatrics is the Datascope 90; the pumping console is adjusted for pediatric use by a volume-limiting chamber that regulates the amount of helium used to inflate the balloon (Fig. 17–2). Balloon catheters are now made as small as 4.5 French in diameter and up to 12 French for adults. The standard balloon size for adults is 30 to 40 ml, maxi-

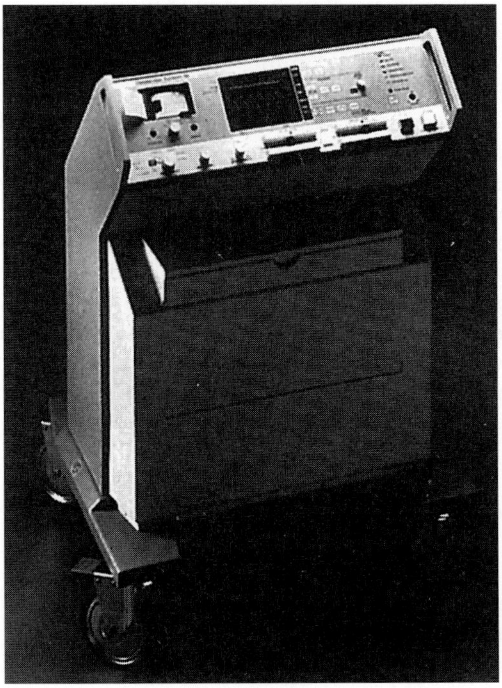

Figure 17–2 Datascope IABP System 90, one of the systems commercially available in the United States. (Courtesy of Datascope Corporation, Montvale, NJ.)

mum 60 ml. In pediatrics and according to Datascope Corporation guidelines (1985), the suggested balloon size is 0.5 ml/kg for children less than 30 kg body weight and 1 ml/kg for children more than 30 kg. In general, pediatric balloon size ranges from 5 to 20 ml. The balloon catheter is a double-lumen catheter. The outside lumen is used to deliver the inflation gas, and the central lumen is used to monitor the central aortic root pressure. An introducer sheath is usually used for percutaneous insertion. Helium is the preferred gas because it is lighter than carbon dioxide and allows rapid inflation that will meet the demand of the high heart rate of children. Anticoagulation is necessary unless contraindicated.

Insertion Technique

The common femoral artery is the preferred site for percutaneous insertion. Cutdown is often necessary in children. Insertion is occasionally done transthoracically or under direct vision in patients undergoing heart surgery. The introducer sheath is inserted in sterile fashion by use of the standard Seldinger technique. The balloon catheter is advanced through the sheath after the helium channel is connected to a one-way valve. The catheter is advanced to approximately 1 cm below the origin of the left subclavian, which is the standard position for the balloon catheter, although Robicsek et al (1990) had recommended that proper position of the balloon catheter be determined by appropriate hemodynamic measurements in different locations. They used three different locations in the aorta: the transverse/ascending aorta, high descending aorta near the left subclavian, or low descending aorta near the diaphragm. A chest film should be obtained unless the procedure is done under fluoroscopic control, and both sheaths and the balloon catheter should be sutured in place. The one-way valve is then disconnected, and the balloon catheter is connected to the IABP console. The pressure monitor is also connected so the waveform can be used for the timing of the pump. Heparin should be given as soon as the IABP starts.

Specific Technical Problems in Pediatric IABP

In small children, the aorta is small; the smallest balloon could extend below the diaphragm, which could impair the renal and the mesenteric circulation. Pediatric patients with severe reduction of cardiac output can have too small of a stroke volume to allow significant balloon augmentation. They also have rapid heart rates that necessitate rapid inflation and deflation; balloon pumping is usually used as every other beat, when necessary.

Operating the IABP

The console programming requires both the waveform from the electrocardiogram and the waveform from the central aortic pressure (the dicrotic notch) to be identified. Timing is set so deflation occurs at R wave on the electrocardiogram before the next systole. Lead II is recommended for the identification of the tall R wave. The arterial line waveform can also be used, and deflation should occur right before systole or at the upstroke of the waveform on the arterial line. Timing is evaluated in 1:2 ratio inflation frequency mode to compare assisted and unassisted pressure waveforms. The aortic pressure waveform during

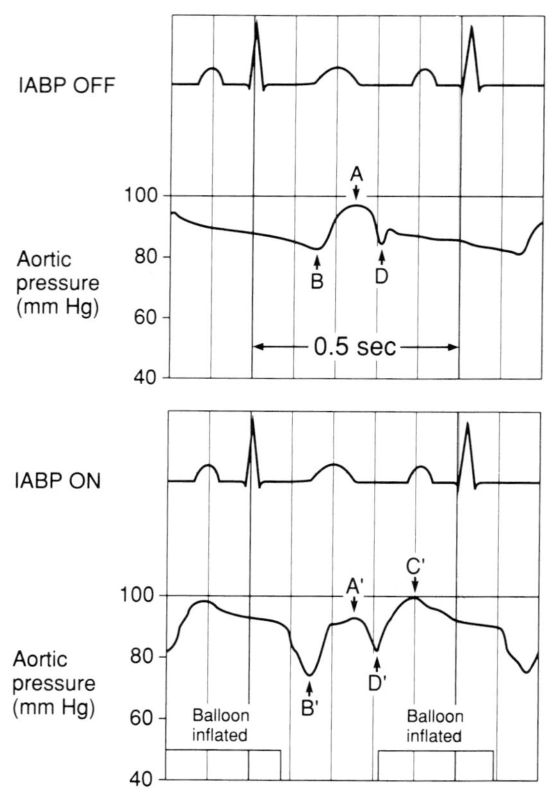

Figure 17–3 Central aortic pressure waveform illustrating optimal IABP timing. A–A′, peak systolic pressure; B–B′, end diastolic pressure; C′, peak assist pressure; D′, dicrotic notch. (From Kantrowitz A, Cardona RR, Au J, et al: Intraaortic balloon pumping in congestive heart failure. In Hosenpud JD, Greenberg BH [eds]: *Congestive Heart Failure: Pathophysiology, Differential Diagnosis, and Comprehensive Approach to Therapy.* New York, © Springer-Verlag, New York, Inc., 1994.)

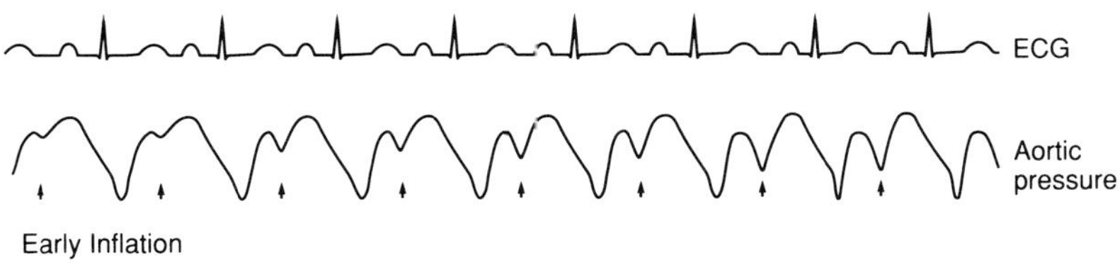

Figure 17–4 Electrocardiographic (ECG) and central aortic pressure waveforms during IABP illustrating early inflation (*left*). Inflation is continuously delayed so that it is correct (*right*). (From Kantrowitz A, Cardona RR, Au J, et al: Intraaortic balloon pumping in congestive heart failure. In Hosenpud JD, Greenberg BH [eds]: *Congestive Heart Failure: Pathophysiology, Differential Diagnosis, and Comprehensive Approach to Therapy.* New York, © Springer-Verlag, New York, Inc., 1994.)

balloon pumping has a certain character (Fig. 17–3).

Incorrect timing can occur in the following situations:

1. Early inflation. The aortic valve is still open, which can cause incomplete emptying of the left ventricle and ultimately decreased cardiac output (Fig. 17–4).
2. Late inflation. The balloon is inflated well after aortic valve closure and the appearance of the dicrotic notch. In this case, the diastolic augmentation is minimal (Fig. 17–5).
3. Early deflation, which causes shorter duration of diastolic augmentation; left ventricular afterload reduction may not occur. The waveform in this case has a wide U-shaped region between the peak systolic and the diastolic pressure (Fig. 17–6).
4. Late deflation. Deflation lasts into systole, which impedes ventricular emptying and causes increased preload and afterload. It is important to become accustomed to the characteristics of the waveform in all four situations (Fig. 17–7). In the event of arrhythmia, IABP may or may not be able to produce an effective waveform. Most clinicians would turn the IABP off until the arrhythmias are treated.

POSTPROCEDURE CARE

The heparin drip should be started after the bolus. The partial thromboplastin time should be measured 6 hours after the bolus administration and once or twice a day thereafter and should be kept about 1 1/2 to 2 times normal value. Patients should have close monitoring of their cardiac output, acid-base balance, urine output, and peripheral perfusion (especially in the leg in which the catheter is inserted). It is important to try to wean the patient from the vasopressors as soon as the aortic pressure is satisfactory. Patients should be kept well sedated; on most occasions, neuromuscular blockade is needed. It is important to give the family adequate support and to explain the mechanics of IABP, especially because the term "pumping" may sound like cardiac compressions to some parents.

WEANING

When the child is clinically stable and not receiving inotropic agents and has adequate cardiac output and pulmonary capillary wedge pressure, weaning from IABP should be considered. This is done either by reducing the ratio of assisted heart beats from 1:1 to 1:2,

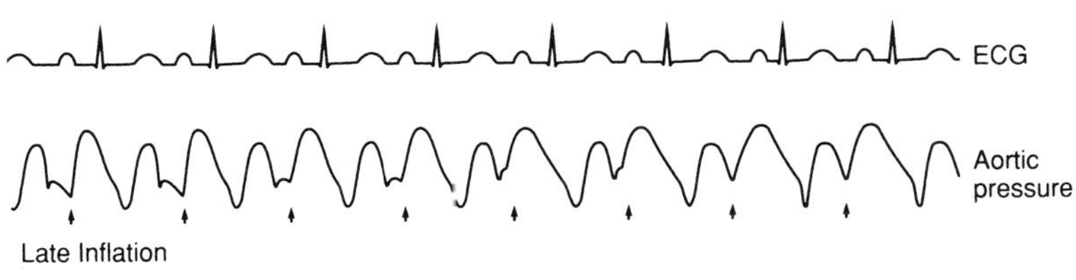

Figure 17–5 ECG and central aortic pressure waveforms during IABP illustrating late inflation. Note the time interval between dicrotic notch and balloon inflation. Inflation delay is gradually reduced; at right, timing is correct. (From Kantrowitz A, Cardona RR, Au J, et al: Intraaortic balloon pumping in congestive heart failure. In Hosenpud JD, Greenberg BH [eds]: *Congestive Heart Failure: Pathophysiology, Differential Diagnosis, and Comprehensive Approach to Therapy.* New York, © Springer-Verlag, New York, Inc., 1994.)

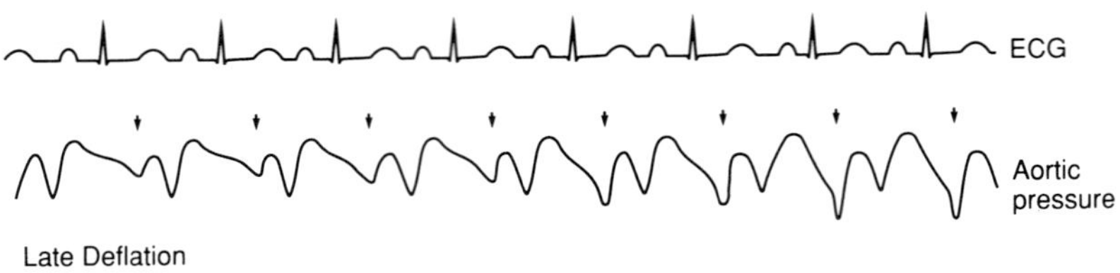

Figure 17–6 ECG and central aortic pressure waveforms during IABP illustrating early deflation (*left*). Note wide valley after deflation. Deflation is gradually delayed so that correct timing is achieved (*extreme right*). (From Kantrowitz A, Cardona RR, Au J, et al: Intraaortic balloon pumping in congestive heart failure. In Hosenpud JD, Greenberg BH [eds]: *Congestive Heart Failure: Pathophysiology, Differential Diagnosis, and Comprehensive Approach to Therapy.* New York, © Springer-Verlag, New York, Inc., 1994.)

1:3, and so on or by reducing the volume of the balloon gradually. Afterload reduction agents as well as vasopressors might be needed for 24 to 48 hours after IABP is stopped.

COMPLICATIONS

1. Bleeding either at the site of the insertion or elsewhere due to heparinization or thrombocytopenia
2. Thrombocytopenia, which could be related to recent bypass during cardiac surgery, although it has been observed in patients who were not on the bypass before they were put on IABP
3. Sepsis, although it is difficult to assess the frequency of sepsis related to IABP because most of these patients have other catheters in place at the same time
4. Ischemia and altered pulses in the lower extremities, especially in the leg in which the catheter is inserted
5. Abdominal distention and renal insufficiency

Published pediatric data include only a small series of children, and it is difficult to assess the frequency of these complications. Adult literature reported vascular complications as a major problem with frequency ranging from 20% to 38% (Miller et al, 1992). It seems that the risk of complications increases with prolonged use. In the pediatric experience, the length of IABP use was mostly 24 to 96 hours (Park et al, 1993), although there are reports of IABP use up to 20 days (Anell et al, 1990). Lazar et al (1992) reported successful prolonged use of IABP (5–46 days) in adult patients with end-stage heart disease.

OUTCOME

Published pediatric experience is limited. In the adult literature, the survival rate to discharge for patients with severe heart failure due to myocardial infarction without shock ranged from 25% to 68% (Kantrowitz et al, 1992). In children in a large study (Al Mofada et al, 1990), 41 patients who could not be weaned from the bypass after cardiac surgery were put on IABP. Nineteen of 41 patients survived; renal failure occurred in more than half of these patients, and limb ischemia occurred in 5 of 41 patients. Webster and Veasey (1985) had 9 of 18 patients survive, and they were mostly

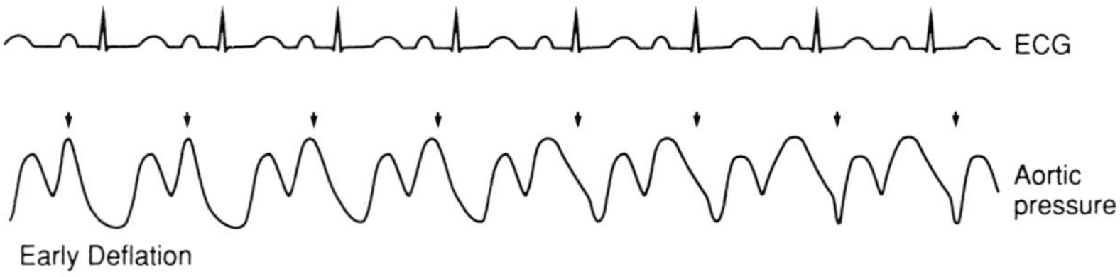

Figure 17–7 ECG and central aortic pressure waveforms during IABP illustrating late deflation (*left*). Note aortic pressure at end diastole is higher than pressure at dicrotic notch. Deflation delay is gradually reduced to result in proper timing (*right*). (From Kantrowitz A, Cardona RR, Au J, et al: Intraaortic balloon pumping in congestive heart failure. In Hosenpud JD, Greenberg BH [eds]: *Congestive Heart Failure: Pathophysiology, Differential Diagnosis, and Comprehensive Approach to Therapy.* New York, © Springer-Verlag, New York, Inc., 1994.)

younger than 5 years. In another study (Anell et al, 1990), 5 of 14 patients survived weaning off the IABP; 1 received a heart transplant and subsequently died, 2 lived to discharge, and the other 2 died within 5 days of stopping the IABP.

References

Al Mofada S, Edmonds J, et al: Intra-aortic balloon pumping (IABP) in children. *Crit Care Med,* 18:S230, 1990.

Anell J, McCloskey A, Vieweg C: Nursing dynamics of pediatric intra-aortic balloon pumping. *Crit Care Nurse,* 4:24–37, 1990.

del Nido PJ, Swan PR, et al: Successful use of intra-aortic balloon pumping in a 2 kilogram infant. *Ann Thorac Surg,* 46:574–576, 1988.

Georgeson S, Coombs AT, Ekman M: Prophylactic use of IABP in high risk cardiac patients undergoing noncardiac surgery: a decision analytic view. *Am J Med,* 92:665–677, 1992.

Kantrowitz A, Cardona RR, Freed PS: Percutaneous intra-aortic balloon counterpulsation. *Crit Care Clin,* 8:819–837, 1992.

Lazar JM, Ziady GM, et al: Outcome and complications of prolonged intra-aortic balloon counterpulsation in cardiac patients. *Am J Cardiol,* 69:955–958, 1992.

Miller JS, Dodson TF, et al: Vascular complications following intra-aortic balloon pump insertion. *Am Surg,* 58:232–238, 1992.

Park JK, Hsu DT, Gersony WM: Intra-aortic balloon pump management of refractory congestive heart failure in children. *Pediatr Cardiol,* 14:19–22, 1993.

Pennington DG, Swartz MT: Circulatory support in infants and children. *Ann Thorac Surg,* 1:233–237, 1993.

Pollock JC, Charlton MC, et al: Intra-aortic balloon pumping in children. *Ann Thorac Surg,* 29:522, 1980.

Robicsek F, Masters TN, et al: Enhancing the applicability and effectiveness of intra-aortic balloon counter pulsation. *J Cardiovasc Surg,* 5:321–327, 1990.

Smith RG, Cleavinger M: Current perspectives on the use of circulatory assist devices. *AACN Clin Issues Crit Care Nurs,* 2:488–499, 1991.

Veasey LG, Blaylock RC, et al: Preclinical evaluation of intra-aortic balloon pumping for pediatric use. *Trans Am Soc Artif Intern Organs,* 27:490, 1981.

Veasey LG, Blaylock RC, et al: Intra-aortic balloon pumping in infants and children. *Circulation,* 68:1095, 1983.

Webster H, Veasey G: Intra-aortic balloon pumping in children. *Heart Lung,* 14:548–555, 1985.

Bibliography

Bolooki H: *Clinical Application of IABP,* 2nd ed. Mt Kisco, NY, Futura Publishing, 1984.

Holbrook PR. *Textbook of Pediatric Critical Care.* WB Saunders, Philadelphia, 1993.

Quaal SJ. *Comprehensive Intra-aortic Balloon Pumping.* St Louis, CV Mosby, 1984.

Chapter 18

Intracranial Pressure Monitoring

Sana Al-Jundi

In cases of severe head trauma, continuous recording of the ventricular fluid pressure provides an important method of evaluating the intracranial dynamics and, subsequently, modes of treatment. This chapter discusses the different intracranial pressure (ICP)–monitoring catheters and the advantages and disadvantages of each, the indications for ICP monitoring, the monitoring procedures, and the potential complications of this procedure. The most common ICP catheters used in pediatric patients are the intraventricular catheter, the epidural bolt or the subarachnoid bolt, and the fiberoptic catheter. The placement and the mechanics of each of these catheters are different (Fig. 18–1).

INTRACRANIAL PRESSURE–MONITORING CATHETERS

Intraventricular Catheter

Technique of insertion

The intraventricular catheter can be placed in the operating room, the emergency department, or the intensive care unit with use of adequate local anesthetics and intravenous sedation. After the head is shaved and the skin prepared with povidone-iodine solution, a hole is made in the skull with a twist drill. Location is just anterior to the coronal suture in line with the pupil. This is usually done on the right side (Fig. 18–2). The intraventricular catheter is then inserted through the hole and advanced until fluid is obtained, that is, approximately 7 cm in adults. This requires a small incision in the dura. The catheter is then tunneled under the scalp and connected to a pressure transducer, which should be kept at the same level as the head. The catheter is then sutured in place.

Advantages

- Use of intraventricular catheters is the "gold standard" and the most accurate way of measuring ICP. It also provides a way to drain the cerebrospinal fluid (CSF) and quickly relieves the increased ICP.

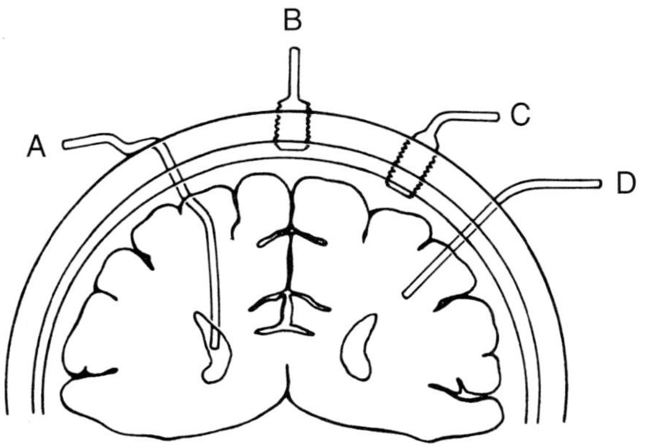

Figure 18–1 Diagram illustrating intraventricular catheter (A), epidural bolt (B), subarachnoid bolt (C), and fiberoptic catheter for intracranial pressure measurement (D). (Redrawn from Doyle DJ, Mark PWS: Analysis of intracranial pressure. *J Clin Monit* 8:81–90, 1992.)

Disadvantages

- There is a high risk for ventriculitis.
- There is a risk of bleeding, especially because the catheter travels through the brain parenchyma, which is rich in blood vessels.
- In severe cerebral edema, placement in the ventricles can be difficult when they are compressed.
- Occlusion is possible when the ventricle collapses around the catheter.
- There is a questionable risk for seizure after removal of the catheter due to the scarring around the catheter site.

Subarachnoid Bolt

The technique for drilling the bur hole is the same as the ventriculostomy for intraventricular catheter insertion. After a small incision is made in the dura to allow the CSF to fill the bolt and the catheter to go through to the transducer device, a bolt that has the same caliber as the hole, filled with normal saline, is screwed in.

Advantages

- It is a simple procedure that does not require invasion of the brain tissue.
- The risk of bleeding is lower than with the ventriculostomy.
- When infection occurs as a complication, it is normally more superficial and not ventriculitis.
- It is useful in severe edema, even when the ventricles are compressed.

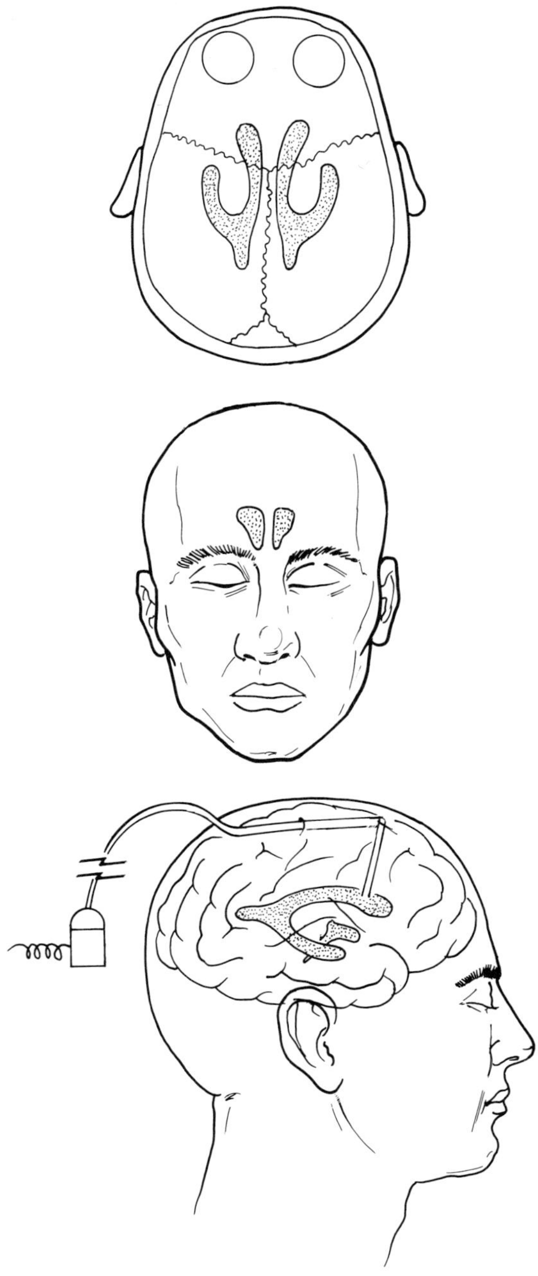

Figure 18–2 Ventriculostomy placement. (Redrawn from Kanter MJ, Narayan RK: Intracranial pressure monitoring. *Neurosurg Clin North Am* 2:257–265, 1991.

Disadvantages

- The reading of the ICP from the subarachnoid space given by the subarachnoid bolt may be lower than the actual ICP near the ventricles (Lehman, 1990; Mendelow et al, 1983; Raftopoulos et al, 1988).
- CSF cannot be withdrawn.

- It is impossible to use in newborns and infants younger than 6 months because of the thin skull, which cannot provide support for the bolt.

Fiberoptic Intracranial Pressure Catheter

In recent years, the fiberoptic intracranial pressure catheter has been used in pediatric populations more commonly than the intraventricular catheter or the subarachnoid bolt. It is a fiberoptic transducer-tipped catheter (made by Camino Laboratories, San Diego, CA). This catheter can be placed in the subdural, intraparenchymal, or intraventricular space. It uses a monitor that senses the variations in the amount of light reflected from a pressure-sensitive diaphragm located at the catheter tip and gives a continuous digital reading of the ICP.

Advantages

- It is a closed system and has less risk for infection.
- There is no need for calibration after the initial insertion.
- It appears to maintain accuracy of the ICP reading for several days. A downdrift of 0.6 mm Hg/d is reported in adult patients by Crutchfield et al (1990), who suggest catheter replacement every 5 days.
- The accuracy and reliability have been challenged by Schickner and Young (1992), who found a difference of 9.2 ± 7.2 mm Hg between the fiberoptic catheter and the intraventricular catheter when ICP values were recorded up to 118 hours in 10 adult patients.
- There is no risk for occlusion because it is not a fluid-filled system.

Disadvantages

- Inability to drain CSF
- Accuracy, as mentioned before

Transcranial Doppler Ultrasonography

This technique is still under investigation, but it is a promising noninvasive method of recording blood flow velocity from the basal intracranial arteries. It is done by placing the ultrasound transducer externally on the skull with use of a low 2-MHz ultrasound frequency, which allows better bone penetration.

In acute head trauma, there is an increased velocity due to the hyperemia and the vasospasm. With increased ICP, ultrasonography may show increased pulsatility, progressive reduction in diastolic velocity, and decreased mean velocity (Hassler et al, 1988). Shigemori et al (1992) studied transcutaneous Doppler ultrasonography in patients with severe head injury and correlated the results with cerebral perfusion pressure in both focal and diffuse brain injury. They found that flow velocity decreased significantly in patients with focal injury when cerebral perfusion pressure decreased to 40 mm Hg or below. They also found that correlation was more complex and less reliable in dealing with diffuse brain injury.

INDICATIONS

In general, ICP monitoring is indicated whenever there is evidence of risk for increased ICP and when controlling ICP will improve outcome.

Head Trauma

Especially when there is a risk for development of brain swelling, ICP monitoring is indicated. Patients at risk may have altered consciousness. A Glasgow Coma Scale score less than 7 was associated with increased ICP in 90% of adults (Eisenberg et al, 1988) and 72% of children (Muizelaar et al, 1989). Other criteria include a computed tomographic (CT) scan of the head showing high-density lesions (hematomas) or low-density lesions (edema). When the lesion on the CT scan is small and is associated with good physical and neurological examination findings (the patient is following commands), ICP monitoring may not be needed. On the other hand, the CT scan could be normal and the patient could still be at risk for the development of increased intracranial hypertension (Narayan et al, 1982). In this case, clinical criteria, such as motor posturing, help identify patients who are at risk.

In head trauma patients who have evidence of mild elevation of ICP when heavy sedation and paralysis are used for other reasons, ICP monitoring becomes the only way of assessing the intracranial dynamics.

ICP monitoring is also recommended in diffuse traumatic brain injury, especially in association with a Glasgow Coma Scale score less than 7, brain swelling on CT scan, and subarachnoid hemorrhage (Sganzerla et al, 1989).

Multiple Trauma Patients

ICP monitoring is indicated for patients who have mild head injury associated with severe trauma when they require prolonged general anesthesia for non-neurosurgical procedures.

Reye's Syndrome

In advanced stages of Reye's syndrome, aggressive ICP control is shown to improve the outcome (LeRoux et al, 1991; Shaywitz et al, 1980).

Meningitis

ICP monitoring is indicated especially when meningitis is associated with abnormal CT scan of the brain and clinical findings of increased ICP. Other criteria include a Glasgow Coma Scale score less than 7 (Goitein et al, 1983; LeRoux et al, 1991).

Note: In hypoxic ischemic injury, as in near-drowning or after cardiopulmonary resuscitation, ICP monitoring is not indicated and is potentially futile. Studies fail to document improvement of the outcome even when ICP was controlled (Bohn et al, 1986; Frewen et al, 1985).

MONITORING PROCEDURES

When the ICP catheter is connected to the transducer, a pressure waveform is obtained; its characteristics are similar to the arterial pressure waveform in the absence of severe cerebral edema. The waveform shows an initial sharp rise and subsequent downward slope. It also shows a change in the excursion with respiration owing to the transmission of the pleural pressure to the intracranial cavity (Fig. 18–3). It is important to recognize the characteristics of the ICP waveform in different stages of cerebral edema because the waveform becomes more rounded as the edema develops or the mass expands. Changes in the waveform are reported to occur before the ICP pressure is actually elevated (Portnoy and Chopp, 1980).

When the waveform has the shape of a plateau, it reflects a poor prognosis, indicating prolonged elevation of the ICP, ischemic changes with compression of the brain stem, and herniation.

Charting of the cerebral perfusion pressure (cerebral perfusion pressure equals mean arterial pressure minus intracranial pressure) is important. A 24-hour trend of the ICP is helpful in evaluating the response to different values in $Pa{CO_2}$.

When CSF is drained from the ventriculostomy as a mode of treatment for increased ICP, the collection bag should be kept at the height, in relation to the patient's head, that maintains the CSF pressure gradient at 5 to 10 cm H_2O. A drainage time should be limited to 1 to 2 minutes. The catheter should then be clamped because it is not possible to monitor ICP when the drain is open; also, there is a

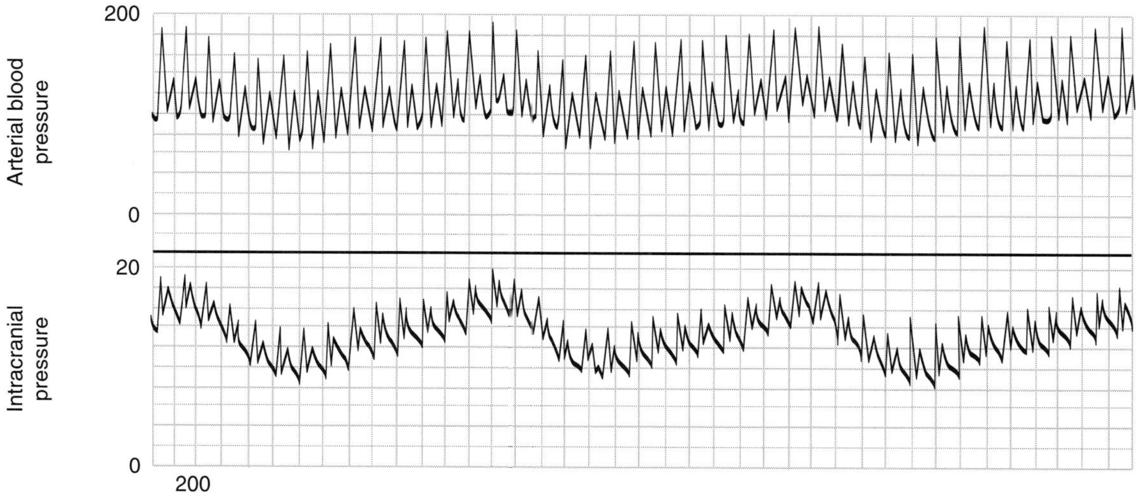

Figure 18–3 Effect of respiratory excursions on intracranial pressure. This effect is mediated both by transmission of intrapleural pressure to the intracranial vault and by effects on cardiac output. This patient was on a positive-pressure ventilator. (From Rogers MC: *Textbook of Pediatric Intensive Care*, 2nd ed. Baltimore, Williams & Wilkins, 1987.)

high risk for clogging when the catheter is left open in a collapsed ventricle (Schultz et al, 1993). The head is normally kept elevated at 30 degrees, and the transducer is kept at the same level as the head. Prophylactic antibiotics are used in most institutions. Routine or surveillance cultures of the CSF are recommended every 2 or 3 days. Analysis of the CSF protein and lactate level is suggested by some authors as an early way of detecting CSF infection (Schultz et al, 1993; Venes, 1989). Patients are kept sedated and occasionally paralyzed. It is important to use restraints in children who are not receiving neuromuscular blockade. Routine change of catheters every 3 to 5 days as suggested in some adult studies is not usually done in children; at this point, there is no proof that this adds extra benefit. ICP monitors should be discontinued as soon as the patient shows signs of clinical recovery or when there is no evidence of increased ICP over the first 3 to 5 days from the time of injury (especially because increased ICP is usually observed in the first 24 to 96 hours after trauma). Unterberg et al (1993) reported a phenomenon of secondary rise of ICP after the initial increase, and this could occur as late as 3 to 10 days from the time of injury. They suggested prolonged use of the ICP monitor. No similar observations have been documented in the pediatric population.

COMPLICATIONS

Infection occurs more frequently in intraventricular catheters compared with the fiberoptic intracranial pressure catheter and the subarachnoid bolt. The frequency of infection ranges from 2% to 11% in ventriculostomy; it was reported to be less than 2% with subarachnoid bolts. One adult study suggested that use of ventriculostomy for longer than 5 days was associated with increased risk of infection and recommended routine replacement of the ICP monitors every 5 days; but other authors (Kanter and Weiner, 1984) observed that ventriculostomy-related infections occur normally in the first week, presumably due to the contamination at the time of insertion. In this case, prophylactic use of antibiotics rather than routine replacement of the ICP catheter is suggested. It is also reported that the frequency of infection is higher in patients who are receiving steroids (Chesnut et al, 1991). Infection is prevented by efforts to avoid invasion of the catheter and to keep the system closed and by antibiotic use prophylactically, although this issue is still controversial (Chesnut et al, 1991; Schultz, 1993).

ICP catheters are associated with a low risk for bleeding, reported to be between 1% and 2% (Narayan et al, 1982). Bleeding is usually in the subdural or subarachnoid space with subarachnoid bolts; intracerebral or ventricular hemorrhage is associated with ventricular catheters.

Edema around the catheter in ventriculostomy was observed to last up to a few days (Raftopoulos et al, 1988). No evidence of morbidity due to this edema has been documented.

There is a potential for scarring and risk for development of seizures. Assessment of this risk is difficult because of the high risk for post-traumatic seizure development with and without ICP monitors.

Plugging of the catheter and potentially inaccurate reading of the ICP could mask the evidence of increased pressure and the need for therapeutic intervention.

References

Bohn DJ, Biggar WD, et al: Influence of hypothermia barbiturate therapy and intracranial pressure monitoring on morbidity and mortality after near-drowning. *Crit Care Med,* 14:529, 1986.

Chesnut RM, Marshall LF: Treatment of abnormal intracranial pressure. *Neurosurg Clin North Am,* 2:267–283, 1991.

Crutchfield JS, Narayah RK, et al: Evaluation of a fiberoptic intracranial pressure monitor. *J Neurosurg,* 72:482–487, 1990.

Eisenberg HM, Frankowski RF, et al: High-dose barbiturate control of elevated intracranial pressure in patients with severe head injury. *J Neurosurg,* 69:15, 1988.

Frewen TC, Sumabat WO, et al: Cerebral resuscitation therapy in pediatric near-drowning. *J Pediatr,* 106:615, 1985.

Goitein KJ, Amit Y, Musaffi H: Intracranial pressure in central nervous system infections and cerebral ischaemia of infancy. *Arch Dis Child,* 58:184, 1983.

Hassler W, Steinmetz H, Gawlowski J: Transcranial Doppler ultrasonography in raised intracranial pressure and in intracranial circulatory arrest. *J Neurosurg,* 68:745–751, 1988.

Kanter MJ, Narayan RK: Intracranial pressure monitoring. *Neurosurg Clin North Am,* 2:257–265, 1991.

Kanter RK, Weiner LB: Ventriculostomy related infections. *N Engl J Med,* 3:987, 1984.

Lehman LB: Intracranial pressure monitoring and treatment: contemporary view. *Ann Emerg Med,* 19:295, 1990.

LeRoux PD, Jardine DS, et al: Pediatric intracranial pressure in hypoxic and nonhypoxic brain injury. *Childs Nerv Syst,* 7:33, 1991.

Mendelow AD, Rowan JO, et al: A clinical comparison of subdural screw pressure measurements with ventricular pressure. *J Neurosurg,* 58:45, 1983.

Muizelaar JP, Marmarou A, DeSalles AA: Cerebral blood flow and metabolism in severely head-injured children. Part 1: Relationship with GCS score, outcome ICP and PVI. *J Neurosurg,* 71:63, 1989.

Narayan RK, Kishore RSP, et al: Intracranial pressure: to monitor or not to monitor? A review of our experience with severe head injury. *J Neurosurg,* 56:650, 1982.

Portnoy HD, Chopp M: Special analysis of intracranial pressure. In Shulman K, et al (eds): *Intracranial Pressure IV,* New York, Springer-Verlag, 1980, pp 167–172.

Raftopoulos C, Baleriaux D, et al: The traumatic aspect of ventricular catheterization demonstrated by magnetic resonance imaging. *Clin Neurol Neurosurg,* 90:47, 1988.

Schickner DJ, Young RF: Intracranial pressure monitoring: fiberoptic monitor compared with the ventricular catheter. *Surg Neurol,* 37:251–254, 1992.

Schultz M, Moore K, Foote AW: Bacterial ventriculitis and duration of ventriculostomy catheter insertion. *J Neurosci Nurs,* 25:158–164, 1993.

Sganzerla EP, Tomei P, et al: Clinicoradiological and therapeutic considerations in severe diffuse traumatic brain injury in children. *Childs Nerv Syst,* 5:168–171, 1989.

Shaywitz BA, Rothstein P, Venes JL: Monitoring and management of increased intracranial pressure in Reye syndrome: results in 29 children. *Pediatrics,* 66:198, 1980.

Shigemori M, Kikuchi N, et al: Monitoring of severe head-injured patients with transcranial Doppler (TCD) ultrasonography. *Acta Neurochir (Wien),* 55:6–7, 1992.

Unterberg A, Kiening K, et al: Long-term observations of intracranial pressure after severe head injury. The phenomenon of secondary rise of intracranial pressure. *Neurosurgery,* 32:17–24, 1993.

Venes JL: Infections of CSF shunt and intracranial pressure monitoring devices. *Infect Dis Clin North Am,* 3:289–299, 1989.

Bibliography

Doyle DJ, Mark PWS: Analysis of intracranial pressure. *J Clin Monit,* 8:81–90, 1992.

Holbrook PR: *Textbook of Pediatric Critical Care.* Philadelphia, WB Saunders, 1993.

Newell DW, Aaslid R: Transcranial Doppler: clinical and experimental uses. *Surg Neurol,* 4:122–143, 1992.

Chapter 19

Arterial Catheterization

Sandra C. Short-Bartlett

INDICATIONS

Arterial catheters are indicated in a wide variety of medical situations. For all types of arterial catheters, there are significant risks that must be weighed against their usefulness. Principal uses are

Beat-to-beat blood pressure monitoring
Frequent blood gas monitoring
Exchange transfusion
Frequent blood sampling
Hemodialysis outflow
Bedside aortogram/access for cardiac catheterization (via umbilical artery catheter [UAC])
Continuous Po_2 monitoring (via UAC)
Indocyanine green cardiac output determination
Infusion of crystalloid, blood products, and medications (via UAC)

EQUIPMENT AND SUPPLIES

Common Equipment

1. Setup

   Intravenous tubing
   Pressure transducer
   Infusion pump
   Monitor with alarm
   Light source

2. Safety equipment

   Mask
   Eye shields
   Sterile gloves

3. Sterile surgical field (umbilical, Seldinger, cutdown)

   Sterile gown
   Sterile drapes
   Surgical cap

4. Flush solutions: usually infused at 1 to 2 ml/h

   Half-normal saline can be used during placement; in UAC, hypertonic glucose–containing solution may be infused.
   Heparin 1/4 U/ml to 5 U/ml reduces clotting and should be added to the infusion unless the patient is systemically heparinized. A higher concentration may prolong patency of peripheral artery

catheters. As little heparin as 1/4 U/ml (< 4 U/kg/h) has been shown to prolong the patency of UACs without any increased risk of intraventricular hemorrhage. Heparin-bonded umbilical catheters are available.

Papaverine 60 mg/500 ml, a smooth muscle vasodilator, reduces the risk of catheter failure. It is not recommended for use in neonates or with atrioventricular complete block, increased intracranial pressure, or hepatic failure.

5. General

   3- to 10-ml syringe with 18- to 23-gauge needle for flush
   Sterile gauze (2 × 2 or 4 × 4)
   Iodine solution with applicators (can use half strength for extremely premature infants)
   Benzoin with applicators (optional)
   Suture with 4–0 silk or nylon with or without needle holder (optional for peripheral artery lines)
   Adhesive tape
   Restraints as needed
   Iodine ointment (optional; not used for UACs)

6. Analgesia (peripheral, Seldinger, cutdown)

   Lidocaine 0.5% to 1%
   1- to 3-ml syringe
   18- to 23-gauge needle
   25-gauge needle
   EMLA (eutectic mixture of local anesthetics) cream (optional)

Peripheral Artery Catheters

1. Percutaneous*

   Catheter-over-needle; 1 to 2 inches long

   Premature infant: 24-gauge
   Term newborn: 22- to 24-gauge
   Infants and toddlers: 22-gauge
   School-age children: 20- to 22-gauge
   Adolescent to adult: 20-gauge

   Kits with guidewire

   Arrow radial artery catheterization set: 22-gauge, 1 3/8-inch/3.49-cm radiopaque polyurethane catheter over 23-gauge needle with spring wire guide tube assembly
   Cook 2.5 French (21-gauge) 2.5-cm (1-inch) polyethelyene catheter; 22-gauge 2-cm needle; 0.015-inch-diameter 15-cm guidewire

2. Seldinger technique (can use a central venous catheter kit)†

   Representative catheter sizes:
   24-gauge, 9-cm/3.5-inch
   22-gauge, 4.45-cm/1.75-inch
   20-gauge, 12.5-cm/5-inch
   18-gauge, 15-cm/6-inch
   Appropriate guidewire, introducer needle, and vessel dilator
   Measuring tape

3. Cutdown technique
4. Other equipment

   T-connector or stopcock
   Armboard or footboard for peripheral sites
   Cotton or gauze padding
   Alcohol
   Needle slightly larger than catheter or No. 11 blade to make skin puncture

Umbilical Artery Catheterization/ Subumbilical Cutdown

UAC trays contain some of the necessary materials.

3.5 French (< 1500 g) or 5 French (> 1500 g) umbilical catheter (2.5 French Argyle available)
Stopcock
Umbilical tape
Scalpel No. 11 or No. 15
Two 5-inch curved or straight hemostats
Small scissors
Small smooth forceps (curved or straight; sometimes microforceps)
Measuring tape

Optional:
Blunt needle for Argyle catheters
Tissue forceps (toothed)
Catheter introducer (Becton-Dickinson)
Gelfoam

PREPARATION OF FAMILY AND PATIENT

Preparation of the Family

Whenever possible, *informed consent* should be obtained from a parent or legal guardian

*Somewhat larger for axillary or femoral lines (2.5 to 4 French; 18- to 22-gauge); dorsalis pedis is the smallest artery and is often absent.

†Steven and Cohen (1990) use a 23-gauge butterfly needle as an introducer with a 15-cm/0.015-inch outer diameter straight angiographic guidewire for infants.

(see "Indications" and "Complications" sections). Parents should also be told that every effort will be taken to minimize discomfort to the child. When catheters are placed urgently without informed consent, I make an effort to discuss the indications and risks as soon as possible with the family and to document this in the chart.

Preparation of the Patient

Peripheral artery catheterization and arterial cutdowns can be painful. The age of the patient must be taken into consideration. Young children and infants often require sedation, whereas older children and adolescents often cooperate. EMLA cream and lidocaine are helpful in the alert patient, but neither of these numbs nerves in the arterial wall. Immobilization of the extremity also increases the likelihood of success. In most cases, I prefer to have the family step out.

UAC causes some discomfort from pinching of the skin by the cord tie, clamps, or forceps and the one skin suture; however, most newborns are disturbed more by the iodine preparation than by the procedure itself. The infant does not usually require sedation for the procedure. Arms and legs should be restrained to prevent the baby from contaminating the field.

NECESSARY TRAINING

The individual learning the procedure should first observe the procedure a few times with an experienced individual explaining all of the steps. For peripheral artery catheters, mastery of arterial puncture before attempting this procedure is helpful. UAC can be taught on placentas. As in all procedures, emphasis should be placed on monitoring vital signs and the patient's tolerance of the procedure. A drop in blood pressure, for example, may make arterial cannulation difficult and generally needs treatment. The student should be observed performing the procedure a few times before attempting it alone.

METHODS

Peripheral Arterial Catheterization

Sites (Fig. 19–1)

Radial
Posterior tibialis
Ulnar

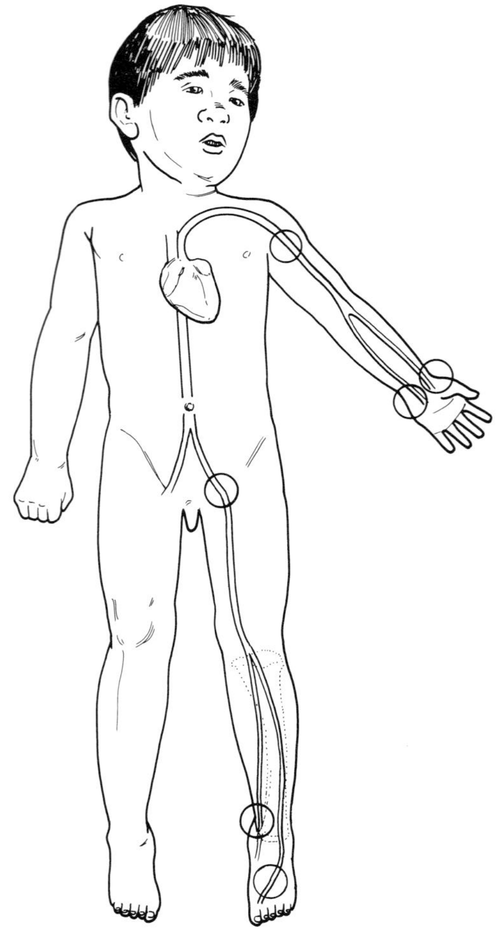

Figure 19–1 Sites for peripheral arterial catheterization.

Dorsalis pedis: Small, can be absent; inadequate in severe peripheral vasoconstriction.

Axillary: The axillary and sometimes the femoral pulses remain strong in shock when peripheral pulses are poor or absent. The axillary artery has excellent collateral blood flow and more accurately reflects central systolic arterial pressure than more peripheral sites do. The patient's mobility is relatively unimpaired.

Femoral: Some risk of fecal or urinary contamination, increased risk of infection, apparently adequate collateral circulation. Transient vascular insufficiency increases in patients younger than 6 months and is especially common in neonates when a 20-gauge catheter is used.

Brachial: Generally not recommended because of poor collateral flow with possible damage to a large area.

Temporal: Not recommended because of proximity to the brain.

Side selection

For catheters in the upper extremity the nondominant side is most appropriate. This facilitates the patient's use of the dominant hand and protects the dominant side from any injury. The left axillary is preferred to the right because of lower risk of carotid artery obstruction or embolization. If the patient is to have subclavian flap repair of coarctation, one should never place a catheter in the corresponding arm. Catheters placed distal to a cross-clamped aorta may cause more complications. Extracorporeal membrane oxygenation (ECMO) criteria for neonates are based on postductal PO_2values; however, preductal PaO_2/saturations are a better indication of brain oxygen delivery. On venoarterial ECMO, there is preferential streaming to the right upper extremity, which makes the PaO_2 unrepresentative in a patient of any age. Transcutaneous PO_2 monitors and pulse oximeters can be used in conjunction with arterial catheters.

Position the patient for best access:*

- Radial, ulnar: Wrist dorsiflexed 30 degrees
- Posterior tibialis: Foot in anatomical position
- Dorsalis pedis: Foot in anatomical position, slight plantar flexion
- Femoral: Frog-leg position
- Axillary: Arm hyperabducted and supinated; rest occiput on ipsilateral hand

Flush T-connector and catheter.
EMLA cream may be applied in advance.
Prepare the area with iodine solution three times followed by an optional alcohol wipe (which makes the area less sticky).
Palpate pulse. Transillumination or Doppler flow may help locate the artery.
Overlying skin and soft tissue may be infiltrated with 0.5% to 1% lidocaine.
Skin may be punctured with large needle or blade to prevent buckling of catheter.

Direct percutaneous technique (all sites) (Fig. 19–2A)

Enter the skin at a 10- to 30-degree angle.
When a flash of blood is observed in the hub, advance the catheter up to 0.5 mm more, then bring the angle down to 10 degrees and advance the catheter over the stylet.
Remove the stylet and attach a T-connector if desired.
Attach intravenous tubing and pressure transducer.

Transfixion technique (all sites) (Fig. 19–2B)

Enter the skin at a 30- to 45-degree angle.
Continue advancing the catheter and stylet together beyond the point of blood return.
Remove stylet.
Pull back the catheter slowly at a 10- to 30-degree angle until blood pulsates back. Rotation of the catheter may be helpful.
Advance the catheter to the hub at a 10-degree angle.
Connect to the catheter a T-connector if desired.
Attach tubing and a pressure transducer.

Seldinger technique (described for axillary; also used for femoral and occasionally other sites) (Fig. 19–2C)

Measure the distance from the axilla to the first portion of the subclavian.
Palpate the artery high in the axilla.
Flush the catheter through with saline or heparinized saline.
Prepare and drape the area.
Infiltrate the skin with lidocaine.
Keep traction on the skin with tape or manually.
Insert an introducer needle into the artery distal to the humeral head.
Place a wire through the introducer needle not more than 3 cm beyond the tip, and remove the needle.
Skin may be nicked at the top of the entry site with No. 11 scalpel blade or large needle.
Vessel dilator tip may be threaded over the wire just through the artery.
Thread the catheter over the wire.
Remove the wire.
Suture the catheter in place so that the tip lies in the axillary artery or in the subclavian artery distal to the innominate artery and to the origin of the common carotid artery.
Apply pressure to prevent hematoma formation and brachial plexus injury.
Document placement radiographically.

ALL PERIPHERAL ARTERY CATHETERS: Secure the catheter with adhesive tape and dressing. Taping methods vary. The most common method is to

*Must be able to assess distal circulation (i.e, see fingers and toes). The Allen test on the hand or foot to assess collateral circulation was originally used in cases of thromboangiitis obliterans; it has not been shown to predict collateral flow or thromboembolic/ischemic damage to tissues. Fortunately, most pediatric patients have good collateral flow. Young children and infants do not cooperate, which makes the test more difficult to perform.

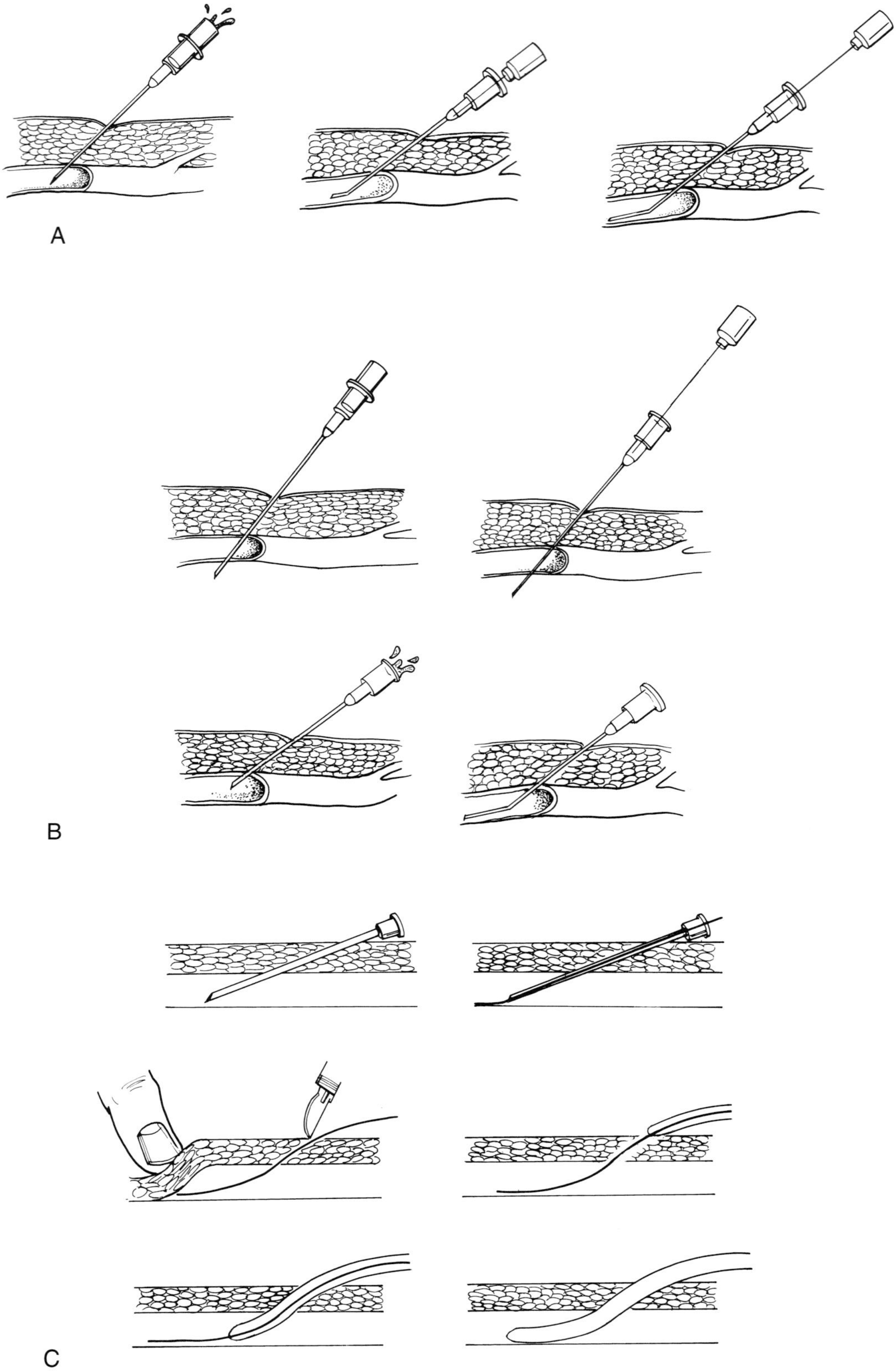

Figure 19–2 Direct **(A)**, transfixion **(B)**, and Seldinger **(C)** techniques for arterial catheterization.

place tape over the tip of the catheter where it enters the skin with or without tincture of benzoin (liquid adhesive). Wings on some catheters can be used as anchors for tape, or they can be sutured to the skin. Suturing the catheter in place is a serious consideration in the vigorous, uncooperative patient. Sometimes the catheter needs to be propped with cotton or gauze to achieve an optimal waveform and blood return. Extra tape needs to go around the T-connector or intravenous tubing to minimize the chance of the line's being accidentally pulled. Recheck all connections; a disconnected arterial catheter can cause massive hemorrhage within minutes.

HELPFUL HINTS AND CAVEATS: The direct technique takes somewhat more skill than the transfixion technique because the entry angle is critical and variable. Even though the tip of the stylet is in the artery, the tip of the catheter is set back from the tip of the stylet and sometimes buckles rather than penetrating the artery. Other reasons for failure include disruption of the intima of the artery as the catheter is advanced and arterial spasm. The needle or catheter can develop clots even after a short period. A guidewire can be any obstruction threaded through the catheter to help bypass any obstruction. Pushing small amounts of flush through the catheter as it is advanced can also facilitate the procedure. Too much flush can cause tissue ischemia and can carry air or thrombi retrograde to the brain.

Excessive bleeding can be controlled with pressure over the artery or by quickly connecting the T-connector. A sterile site can be reused without repreparation if it is dried with sterile gauze. Some recommend placing iodine ointment over the insertion site. Many arteries have nearby veins that can be punctured accidentally. A hematoma from a previous attempt may make the exact location of the arterial pulse difficult to interpret and increases the risk of complications. Transillumination or Doppler techniques may facilitate finding the artery when the pulse is difficult to locate. Multiple punctures of the same artery increase the risk of laceration of the vessel, intimal damage, emboli, thrombosis, spasm, damage to surrounding structures, and infection. Always re-evaluate the distal circulation between attempts.

Cutdown Technique

See Chapter 28.

Umbilical Artery Catheterization

This technique is generally not possible beyond 2 weeks of age.

Most newborns have two umbilical arteries and one umbilical vein. The arteries can be distinguished by their thick muscle wall; the vein is thin walled and bleeds more easily when the cord is cut.

Place the newborn infant supine in an open warmer and restrain all extremities. Measure the distance from the acromioclavicular joint to a line extending laterally from the umbilicus. A low-lying UAC generally needs to be placed about two thirds of this shoulder-to-umbilicus distance plus extra for the length of the umbilical stump.

Select an appropriate-sized catheter.
Attach a stopcock if it is not already a part of the catheter. (Argyle catheters come with blunt needles that can be used to reduce dead space in the catheter. The catheter is trimmed until the needle fits, and the blunt needle is introduced to get a secure fit. The stopcock is then attached to the blunt needle.)
Flush the stopcock and catheter. Leave the syringe on the stopcock. Make sure that all other stopcock ports are off.
Have an assistant hold up the cord while you prepare it and the surrounding skin with iodine solution three times.
Place a cord tie around the skin at the base of the cord.
Cut the cord 1 to 2 cm above the skin. (Excessive bleeding usually responds to tightening the cord tie; however, direct pressure or clamping is occasionally necessary.)
Identify the two umbilical arteries.

Direct technique (Fig. 19–3A)

Grasp the side of the cord with one hand or a hemostat.
Dilate one of the arteries by use of tissue forceps, microforceps, or a catheter introducer. This takes patience.
Thread the catheter into the vessel. The catheter may be threaded through an already dilated vessel, between the two ends of the forceps, or along the side of the introducer.

Side technique (Fig 19–3B)

Identify the approximate course of one of the arteries along the side of the cord.
Cut partway through the cord until the scalpel transects the artery about one third to one half of the way through.
Insert a catheter introducer into the artery.
Thread the catheter along the introducer into the artery.

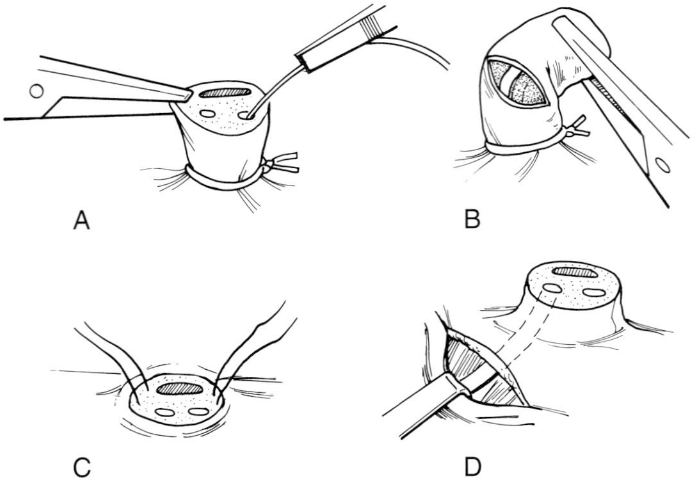

Figure 19–3 Techniques for umbilical artery catheter placement. **A.** Direct technique. **B.** Side technique. **C.** Variation for older umbilical cords. **D.** Subumbilical cutdown.

Variation for older umbilical cords (Fig. 19–3C)

Soften the cord with sterile gauze soaked in saline.
Prepare the cord with iodine solution.
Trim off any excess dried cord.
An umbilical cord tie is not usually necessary.
Attempt to identify the umbilical arteries and veins. They are sometimes impossible to distinguish from each other at this stage.
Dilate the umbilical artery and thread the catheter by the direct technique.
If the cord is sunken, it may be pulled up with a piece of suture placed through either side of what is left of the Wharton's jelly. This often brings the vessels into view.

Document that the catheter draws and flushes well. Make sure that the stopcock is off to the patient while the catheter is sutured to the skin with 3–0 or 4–0 silk.

Suturing techniques vary. The Wharton's jelly will disintegrate, so it is necessary to place one suture through the skin. A second knot higher up on the catheter is also useful.

Remove the cord tie. If there is excessive bleeding, place a purse-string suture through the cord or place pressure followed by Gelfoam on the site.

Taping techniques also vary. The most common is the "goalpost" or "H-type" method. Two pieces of tape that stick up on each side of the umbilicus are placed, then the catheter is taped with a third piece of tape to the two "posts." Another method involves placing tape around the catheter and suturing the tape to the skin. This reduces skin irritation, which can be a potentially serious problem on small premature infants.

Subumbilical cutdown (Fig. 19–3D)

Prepare the umbilicus and the area below.
Inject 0.5% to 1% lidocaine into the site.
Make a 1-cm skin incision 1 to 2 mm below and slightly to the side of the umbilicus (over the projected path of one of the arteries).
Expose the artery with parallel blunt dissection with a hemostat. (The artery can be distinguished from the urachus. The artery sometimes has pulsations. Lidocaine squirted directly into the wound often increases arterial pulsation and helps distinguish the artery from other structures. The urachus widens as it approaches the bladder.)
Elevate the artery with a curved hemostat and place stay sutures as for peripheral cutdown.
While pulling on the distal stay suture, incise the artery one third to one half its circumference as in the side technique. (Remember: distal is closest to the umbilicus.)
Advance the catheter in a similar manner.
Suture the wound with single stitches. Tape the stay sutures to the skin (may be removed when there is less chance of bleeding). Place extra adhesive or suture around the catheter.

ALL TECHNIQUES: Document placement with a chest film or kidney, ureter, and bladder radiograph. Acceptable placement is between T6–T10 or L3–L4. This avoids having the tip of the catheter near the ductus, heart, brain, celiac artery, superior mesenteric artery, renal artery, and femoral artery. Alternatively, the location of the catheter may be documented sonographically. Arguments for high versus low line placement are discussed later. Connect the UAC to tubing with flush or maintenance solution and transducer.

HELPFUL HINTS AND CAVEATS: Several problems can prevent UAC placement. If the vessel has not been dilated long enough, you might not be able to introduce the catheter. If the cord tie is on too tight, it may prevent threading of the catheter. The catheter can get stuck at the peritoneum. It might be in a false passage. The catheter can take a wrong turn and head down a femoral vessel. The artery can be in spasm. This sometimes responds to turning down the FIO_2 until the saturation is around 90%, but the risks of doing this must be weighed against the benefits of the catheter. Alternatively, the catheter can be held at the point of resistance for a few minutes. There can be some resistance when the catheter passes from the hypogastric to the femoral artery, which again usually responds to gentle pressure. Never force a UAC because you can perforate the peritoneum or even rupture the artery, causing a massive hemoperitoneum.

POSTPROCEDURE CARE

Assessment of distal neurological function should be done immediately after placement of a peripheral artery catheter. Frequent assessment of distal circulation is critical for both peripheral artery catheters and UACs. Cannulated arteries can develop spasm and thromboembolic phenomena at any time. For peripheral arterial lines, this involves assessment of skin color and capillary refill. For UACs, circulation to the lower extremities and internal organs must be assessed. Subtle changes, such as hypertension, might indicate early thromboemboli.

The insertion site needs to be monitored every shift for signs of infection or bleeding. Peripheral arterial line dressings should be changed approximately every 1 to 3 days. Bleeding sometimes responds to pressure. The line should be removed if there is severe bleeding or hematoma formation. Some recommend changing axillary or femoral catheters over a guidewire every 4 days to reduce infectious complications. It is prudent to leave the infant supine for the first day after UAC placement; this is when there is the highest risk of bleeding from the umbilicus.

For peripheral artery catheters, transient arterial spasm sometimes responds to repositioning the catheter, warming the oppposite extremity, or injecting 0.3 ml of 0.1% lidocaine into the artery. A dampened waveform sometimes returns spontaneously but often indicates that the catheter is failing. Clots in the catheter are difficult to remove. Changing the catheter over a wire is sometimes successful but is not without risk.

For umbilical catheters, transient ischemia in the toes or even the leg can be relieved by warming the opposite foot, which causes reflex vasodilatation. The affected extremity needs very careful monitoring. Any evidence of ischemia that is recurrent or does not go away easily should prompt removal of the catheter.

Once either type of catheter is removed, pressure should be applied until the site is no longer bleeding. Care should be taken to remove any skin sutures.

Blood Sampling

For peripheral catheters, blood may be withdrawn by use of the drip method or a syringe. In the drip method, the T-connector is clamped, and a straight needle (ususally 23-gauge, 1-inch) is inserted into the hub. Three to five drops of blood are allowed to fall onto sterile gauze. Subsequent drops are collected in a capillary tube or other container of choice. A syringe can also be attached directly to the needle in the hub (after wasting three to five drops of blood).

In another method, the syringe is attached to a stopcock. With the stopcock off to the flush solution, an amount equal to approximately three times the dead space is collected in the first syringe; then the sample needed is collected in a second syringe. This method is also used for umbilical lines. Some return the original blood back through the arterial or a venous catheter, but the risks of introducing clots or air must be considered. Air bubbles may be "tapped" or drawn out of the system. The hub should point upward so that any microbubbles are trapped at the top.

Flushing of Catheters

Catheters should be flushed gently after blood is withdrawn to reduce the risk of clotting. The flushing apparatus can be in-line for older children and teen-agers. For younger children and infants, the syringe/stopcock method is better because it allows better regulation of the amount of flush. The minimal volume of flush solution injected as a bolus into the radial artery that can travel to the central circulation is directly proportional to height:

0 to 18 months: 0.3 to 0.75 ml

18 months to 3 years: 0.75 to 1.0 ml
3 to 8 years: 1 to 2 ml (Edmonds et al, 1980)
Adults: 3 ml

Selldén et al (1987) suggest that use of 0.5-ml volume in a 5-second period minimizes the chance of microbubble embolization. *Bolus flushing of axillary catheters is not recommended* except when it is absolutely necessary because of the proximity to the carotid artery.

Infusion of Blood Products and Medications Through Umbilical Artery Catheters

Good case-control studies on this controversial practice are not available. Infusion of blood products, medications, lipids, and hypertonic glucose solutions varies widely.

Feeding Practices

There are no studies that show whether it is safe to feed a patient with an indwelling UAC. Feeding practices vary widely.

INTERPRETATION OF DATA

Normal Blood Pressure for Infants and Children (Fig. 19–4)

NORMAL TRACING: An arterial tracing has the following features.

There is a dicrotic notch halfway down the downslope corresponding to aortic valve closure and electrocardiographic T waves/ventricular repolarization. This is easily detected at aortic and proximal arterial sites. It moves down in hypovolemia or decreased systemic vascular resistance.

The area under the upstroke corresponds roughly to stroke volume. Slow upstroke with narrow pulse pressure can be due to decreased contractility or high impedance to flow (such as aortic stenosis; venoarterial ECMO, which also has a component of nonpulsatile flow). A narrow, spiked tracing corresponds to low stroke volume due to hypovolemia. The rate of diastolic decay (and usually pulse pressure) correlates with systemic vascular resistance—rapid in thyrotoxicosis, fever, anemia, and run-

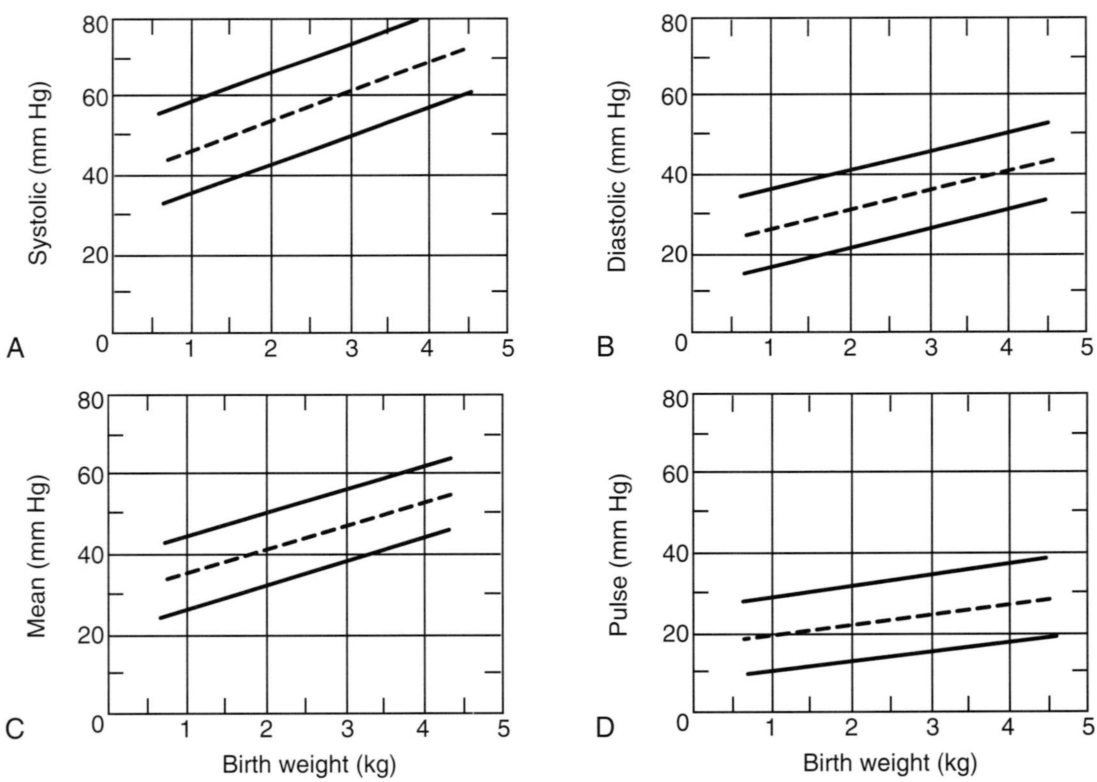

Figure 19–4 Normal blood pressures for newborns during the first 12 hours. **A.** Systolic. **B.** Diastolic. **C.** Mean. **D.** Pulse. (Redrawn from Versmold HT, Kitterman JA, et al: Aortic blood pressure during the first 12 hours of life in infants with birth weight 610 to 4220 grams. *Pediatrics,* 67[5]:607–613, 1981. Reproduced by permission of Pediatrics.)

off lesions (such as patent ductus arteriosus, aortic insufficiency, or arteriovenous malformations).

There is normally no variation in peak pressures in relation to pleural pressures. Variation above 10 mm Hg (pulsus paradoxus) occurs in conditions causing decreased filling of the heart, such as hypovolemia, pericardial effusion, and high intrapleural pressure. With spontaneous breaths, pressure decreases with inspiration; with positive-pressure ventilation, pressure increases during inspiration.

The waveform becomes more pointed as it travels to the periphery, with some increase in systolic pressure, a decrease in diastolic pressure, and a relatively stable mean (Fig. 19–5).

Direct measurements of blood pressure usually give values 5 to 20 mm Hg higher than indirect measurements for a variety of reasons. Invasive monitoring measures both kinetic and static elements of the presssure wave; noninvasive monitoring measures only static components. Hydrostatic differences can also exist if pressure is measured at different levels. Differences are more marked in obesity and edema; and in cases of shock or hypothermia, the indirect measurement is falsely low by 20 to 30 mm Hg. If the indirect measurement is higher, there is a technical problem with one of the systems or there is peripheral vascular disease.

Overshoot can be caused by anything that causes reflection of waves, such as small bubbles; long tubing; small, noncompliant vessels, such as the dorsalis pedis; or resonance phenomena in the catheter-manometer system.

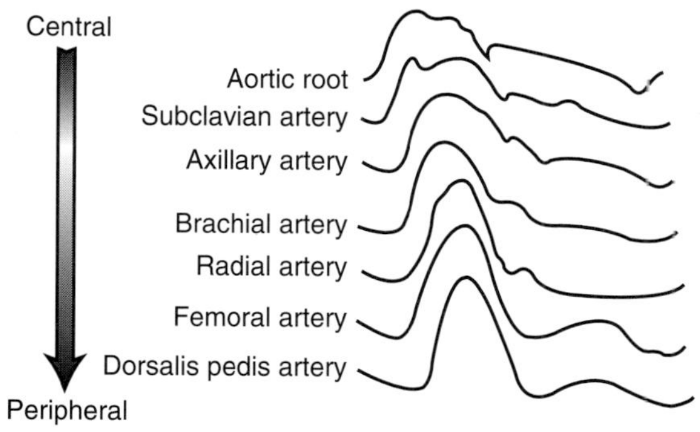

Figure 19–5 The waveform in an arterial tracing becomes more pointed as it travels to the periphery, with some increase in systolic pressure, a decrease in diastolic pressure, and a relatively stable mean. (From Bedford RF. Invasive blood pressure monitoring. In Casey D, Blitt ED [eds]: *Monitoring in Anesthesia and Critical Care Medicine*, 2nd ed. New York, Churchill Livingstone, 1990 p 102. Modified by Morgan GE, Mikhail MS: Patient Monitors, In *Clinical Anesthesiology*. Norwalk, CT, Appleton & Lange, 1992, p 70.)

Dampening of the waveform can be caused by long tubing, large air bubbles, narrowing of an already small catheter with fibrin deposition, vasoconstriction in shock (especially pedal vessels), or compliant tubing.

The waveform can be useful in determining how a dysrhythmia affects stroke volume and in assessing the effectiveness of cardiopulmonary resuscitation.

COMPLICATIONS

All Arterial Catheters

Ischemia/necrosis: Risk increases with shock, large catheter/small vessel, multiple attempts, prolonged use; permanent clinical damage less than 1%.

Thrombosis: Some degree is universal; risk factors are similar to those for ischemia. Peripheral Teflon catheters are less thrombogenic than polypropylene and polyethylene. Polyurethane may be less traumatic. Although 71% of radial arteries can be occluded after catheter removal, most recanalize within 14 days. Radial artery thrombosis is more likely to persist after a cutdown procedure. Polyvinyl chloride UACs are somewhat thrombogenic but easy to use. Seibert et al (1991) found that 26% of UACs had sonographically detectable aortic clots, and half of these resulted in moderate to severe symptoms. Smith et al (1991) have shown a risk of clinically important thrombosis of 1%.

Emboli (air, clot): By arteriography, 23% of radial lines had thromboemboli. Emboli can travel retrogradely to the brain if the catheter is flushed too fast or if too much volume is used. A multicenter trial (Umbilical Artery Trial Study Group, 1992) failed to show any correlation between UAC position and intracranial hemorrhage.

Vessel damage: Laceration, arterial-intimal flaps/aneurysm, arteritis; associated with infection.

Infection (local, systemic): The frequency of sepsis is 5%.

Bleeding/hematoma formation

Disconnection with hemorrhage

Severed catheter

Electrocution (system must be grounded)

Leg length discrepancy: Femoral, umbilical; more common in younger patients, but rare overall.
Arteriovenous fistula formation

Peripheral Artery Catheters

Peripheral nerve damage due to trauma, hematoma
Vascular compromise to distal extremity

Umbilical Artery Catheters

Vascular compromise in lower extremities (especially low-lying UAC)
Vascular compromise in kidneys (hypertension, renal insufficiency)
Vascular compromise in spine (paralysis—especially if in shock)
Vascular compromise in intestines—abdominal symptoms, possible necrotizing enterocolitis (high-lying UAC, prolonged use)
Hemoperitoneum
Bladder rupture due to dissection through the umbilical artery to the urachus with possible avulsion of the urachus from the bladder (more common in subumbilical cutdown)
Hypoglycemia due to malposition with glucose infusing near pancreatic blood supply
Aortic thrombi (more common with high-lying UAC; have been successfully treated with urokinase)

Failure of the catheter is the most common complication and occurs earliest with peripheral arterial lines, then low-lying UACs, then high-lying UACs. Frequency of blood draws influences peripheral artery catheter patency more than UAC patency. Peripheral catheters fail sooner if heparinized 5% dextrose in water is infused rather than heparinized normal saline. It is the author's opinion that because of the more severe complications with high-lying UACs, low-lying UACs are preferred in all but the most immature or critically ill newborns, in whom the longer patency and ease of placement of the high-lying catheter outweigh the risk of complications. A high-lying UAC can also be used for a bedside aortogram to rule out interrupted or hypoplastic arch or coarctation. Some prefer attempting placement of peripheral artery catheters in more stable neonates.

References

Edmonds JF, Barker GA, Conn AW: Current concepts in cardiovascular monitoring in children. *Crit Care Med,* 8:548, 1980.

Seibert JJ, Northington FJ, et al: Aortic thrombosis after umbilical artery catheterization in neonates: prevalence of complications on long-term follow-up. *AJR,* 156:567, 1991.

Selldén H, Nilsson K, et al: Radial arterial catheters in children and neonates: a prospective study. *Crit Care Med,* 15:1106, 1987.

Smith PK, Miller DA, et al: Urokinase treatment of neonatal aortoiliac thrombosis caused by umbilical artery catheterization: a case report. *J Vasc Surg,* 14:684, 1991.

Steven JM, Cohen DE: Anesthesia equipment and monitoring: In Motoyama EK (ed): *Smith's Anesthesia for Infants and Children,* 5th ed. St Louis, CV Mosby, 1990, pp 217–253.

Umbilical Artery Catheter Trial Study Group: Relationship of intraventricular hemorrhage or death with the level of umbilical artery catheter placement: a multicenter randomized clinical trial. *Pediatrics,* 90:881, 1992.

Bibliography

Abrahamson EL, Scott RC, et al: Catheterization of posterior tibial artery leading to limb amputation. *Acta Paediatr,* 82:618, 1993.

Allen EV: Thromboangiitis obliterans: methods of diagnosis of chronic obstructive lesions distal to the wrist with illustrative cases. *Am J Med Sci,* 178:237, 1929.

Ankola PA, Atakent YS: Effect of adding heparin in very low concentration to the infusate to prolong the patency of umbilical artery catheters. *Am J Perinatol,* 10(3):229, 1993.

Barr PA, Summers J, et al: Percutaneous peripheral arterial cannulation in the neonate. *Pediatrics,* 59:1058, 1979.

Bedford RF: Percutaneous radial-artery canulation—increased safety using Teflon catheters. *Anesthesiology,* 42:219, 1975.

Bedford RF: Radial artery function following percutaneous cannulation with 18–20 gauge catheters. *Anesthesiology,* 47:37, 1977.

Bedford RF, Wollman H: Complications of percutaneous radial-artery cannulation: an objective prospective study in man. *Anesthesiology,* 38: 228, 1973.

Boros SJ, Thompson TR, et al: Reduced thrombus formation with silicone elastomere (Silastic) umbilical artery catheters. *Pediatrics,* 56:981, 1975.

Bosque E, Weaver L: Continuous versus intermittent heparin infusion of umbilical artery catheters in the newborn infant. *J Pediatr,* 108:141, 1986.

Brown M, Gordon LH, et al: Intravascular monitoring via the axillary artery. *Anaesth Intensive Care,* 13:38, 1984.

Brown MS, Phibbs RH: Spinal cord injury in newborns from use of umbilical artery catheters: report of two cases and a review of the literature. *J Perinatol,* 8:105, 1988.

Bryan-Brown CW, Kwun KB, et al: The axillary artery catheter. *Heart Lung,* 12:492, 1983.

Bryant BG: Drug, fluid, and blood products administered through the umbilical artery catheter: complication experiences from one NICU. *Neonatal Network,* 9:27, 1990.

Bull MJ, Schriner RL, et al: Neurologic complications following temporal artery catheterization. *J Pediatr,* 93:1071, 1980.

Butt WW, Whyte HW: Blood pressure monitoring in neonates: comparison of umbilical and peripheral artery catheter measurements. *J Pediatr,* 105:630, 1984.

Butt WW, Gow R, et al: Complications resulting from use of arterial catheters: retrograde flow and rapid elevation in blood pressure. *Pediatrics,* 76:250, 1985.

Butt W, Shann F, et al: Effect of heparin concentration and infusion rate on the patency of arterial catheters. *Crit Care Med,* 15:230, 1987.

Cantwell GP, Holzman BH, Caceres MJ: Percutaneous catheterization of the axillary artery in the pediatric patient. *Crit Care Med,* 18:880, 1990.

Carey BE, Zeilinger TC: Hypoglycemia due to high positioning of umbilical artery catheters. *J Perinatol,* 9:407, 1989.

Dalton B, Laver MB: Vasospasm with an indwelling radial artery cannula. *Anesthesiology,* 34:194, 1971.

Damen J, van der Tweel I: Positive tip cultures and related risk factors associated with intravascular catheterization in pediatric cardiac patients. *Crit Care Med,* 16:221, 1988.

Davis FM: Radial artery cannulation: influence of catheter size and material on arterial occlusion. *Anaesth Intensive Care,* 6:49, 1978.

Diamond DA, Ford C: Neonatal bladder rupture: a complication of umbilical artery catheterization. *J Urol,* 142:1543, 1989.

Dmochowski RR, Crandell SS, Lowiere JN: Bladder injury and uroascites from umbilical artery catheterization. *Pediatrics,* 77:421, 1986.

Downs JB, Rackstein AD, Klein EF Jr: Hazards of radial artery catheterization. *Anesthesiology,* 38: 283, 1973.

Downs JB, Chapman RL Jr, Hawkins IF: Prolonged radial-artery catheterization. An evaluation of heparinized catheters and continuous irrigation. *Arch Surg,* 108:671, 1974.

DuCharme FM, Gauthier M, et al: Incidence of infection related to arterial catheterization in children: a prospective study. *Crit Care Med,* 16:272, 1988.

Evans DH, Lark GM, et al: The continuous measurement of intra-arterial pressure in the neonate—method and accuracy. *Clin Phys Physiol Meas,* 7:179, 1986.

Fok TF, Ha MH, et al: Sciatic nerve palsy after umbilical artery catheterization. *Eur J Pediatr,* 145:308, 1986.

Fukutome T, Kojiro M: Doppler-guided "percutaneous" radial artery cannulation in small children. *Anesthesiology,* 69:434, 1988.

Gilhooly J, Lindenberg J, Reynolds J: Survey of umbilical artery catheter practices. *Crit Care Med,* 18:247, 1990.

Glenski JA, Beynen FM, Gracy J: A prospective analysis of femoral artery monitoring in pediatric patients. *Anesthesiology,* 66:227, 1987.

Goetzman BW: Arterial access in the newborn. *Am J Dis Child,* 141:841, 1987.

Graves PW, Davis AL, et al: Femoral artery cannulation for monitoring in critically ill children: prospective study. *Crit Care Med,* 18:1363, 1990.

Greenough A: Where should the umbilical catheter go? *Lancet,* 341:1186, 1993.

Greenwald BM, Notterman DA, et al: Percutaneous axillary artery catheterization in critically ill infants and children. *J Pediatr,* 117:442, 1990.

Gupta JM, Robertson, NR, Wigglesworth JS: Umbilical artery catheterization in the newborn. *Arch Dis Child,* 43:382, 1968.

Gurman GM, Kriemerman S: Cannulation of big arteries in critically ill patients. *Crit Care Med,* 13:217, 1985.

Harris MS, Little GA: Umbilical artery catheters: high, low or no. *J Perinat Med,* 6:15, 1978.

Hecker JF: Thrombogenicity of tips of umbilical catheters. *Pediatrics,* 67:467, 1981.

Henry M, Harrison D, et al: Umbilical artery catheter position and aortic thrombus: a randomized trial. *Pediatr Res,* 29:257A, 1991.

Heulitt MJ, Farrington EA, et al: Double-blind, randomized, controlled trial of papaverine-containing infusions to prevent failure of arterial catheters in pediatric patients. *Crit Care Med,* 21:825, 1993.

Horgan MJ, Bartoletti A, et al: Effect of heparin infusates in umbilical arterial catheters on frequency of thrombotic complications. *J Pediatr,* 111:774, 1987.

Hustead VA, Wicklund BM: Treatment of neonatal aortic thrombosis with urokinase. *Am J Pediatr Hematol/Oncol,* 12:336, 1990.

Jackson JC, Truog WE, et al: Efficacy of thromboresistant umbilical catheters in reducing aortic thrombosis and related complications. *J Pediatr,* 110:102, 1987.

Kaye W: Invasive monitoring techniques: arterial cannulation, bedside pulmonary artery catheterization, and arterial puncture. *Heart Lung,* 12:395, 1983.

Kempley ST, Gamso HR: Randomized trial of umbilical arterial catheter position: Doppler ultrasound findings. *Arch Dis Child,* 67(special issue):885, 1992.

Kirpekar M, Augenstein H, Abiri M: Sequential development of multiple aortic aneurysms in a neonate post umbilical arterial catheter insertion. *Pediatr Radiol,* 19:452, 1989.

Lally KP, Sherman NJ: Iliac artery pseudoaneurysm following umbilical artery catheterization. *Surgery,* 101:636, 1986.

Landers S, Moise AA, et al: Factors associated with umbilical catheter–related sepsis in neonates. *Am J Dis Child,* 145:675, 1991.

Lawless S, Orr R: Axillary arterial monitoring of pediatric patients. *Pediatrics,* 84:273, 1989.

Lowenstein E, Little JW, Lo HH: Prevention of

cerebral embolization from flushing radial-artery catheters. *N Engl J Med,* 285:1414, 1971.

Malik M, Wilson DP: Umbilical artery catheterization: a potential cause of refractory hypoglycemia. *Clin Pediatr,* 26:181, 1987.

Mandel MA, Dauchot PJ: Radial artery cannulation in 1000 patients: Precautions and complications. *J Hand Surg,* 2:482, 1977.

Mata JA, Livne PM, Gibbons MD: Urinary ascites: complication of umbilical artery catheterization. *Urology,* 30:375, 1987.

McGregor AD: The Allen test—an investigation of its accuracy by fluorescein dye. *J Hand Surg,* 12:82, 1987.

Miyasaka K, Edmonds JF, Conn AW: Complications of radial artery lines in the paediatric patient. *Can Anaesth Soc J,* 23:9, 1976.

Mokrohisky ST, Levine RL, Blumhagen JD: Low positioning of umbilical artery catheters increases associated complications in newborn infants. *N Engl J Med,* 299:561, 1978.

Mortensen JD: Clinical sequelae from arterial needle puncture, cannulation, and incision. *Circulation,* 35:1118, 1967.

Neal WA, Reynolds JW, et al: Umbilical artery catheterization: demonstration of arterial thrombosis by aortography. *Pediatrics,* 50:6, 1972.

Park MK, Robothan JL, German VF: Systolic pressure amplification in pedal arteries in children. *Crit Care Med,* 11:286, 1983.

Parker MM: Prevention of arterial catheter failure in children—new use for an old drug? *Crit Care Med,* 21:815, 1993.

Prian GW, Wright GB, et al: Apparent cerebral embolization after temporal artery catheterization. *J Pediatr,* 93:115, 1978.

Rais-Bahrami K, Karna P, Dolanski EA: Effect of fluids on life span of peripheral arterial lines. *Am J Perinatol,* 7:122, 1990.

Rajani K, Goetzman BW, et al: Effect of heparinization of fluids infused through an umbilical artery catheter on catheter patency and frequency of complications. *Pediatrics,* 64:552, 1979.

Randel MD, Tsang HL, et al: Experience with percutaneous indwelling peripheral arterial catheterization in neonates. *Am J Dis Child,* 141:848, 1987.

Rodriguez M, Sosenko I: Catheter-induced aortic thrombus masquerading as coarctation of the aorta. *Clin Pediatr,* 28:581, 1989.

Ruderman JW, Morgan MA, Klein AH: Quantitative blood cultures in the diagnosis of sepsis in infants with umbilical and Broviac catheters. *J Pediatr,* 112:798, 1988.

Schick JB, Beck AL, DeSiva M: Umbilical artery catheter position and intraventricular hemorrhage. *J Perinatol,* 9:382, 1989.

Schwartz N, Eisenkraft JB: Transillumination aids the percutaneous cannulation of peripheral vessels. *J Cardiothorac Anesth,* 3:675, 1989.

Seldinger SI: Catheter replacement of needle in percutaneous arteriography: new technique. *Acta Radiol Diagn (Scand),* 39:368, 1953.

Singh S, Nelson N, et al: Catheter colonization and bacteremia with pulmonary and arterial catheters. *Crit Care Med,* 10:736, 1982.

Soderstrom CA, Wasserman DH, et al: Infected false femoral artery aneurysms secondary to monitoring catheters. *J Cardiovasc Surg,* 24:63, 1983.

Squire SJ, Hornung TL, Kirchhoff KT: Comparing two methods of umbilical arterial catheter placement. *Am J Perinatol,* 7:8, 1990.

Stewart DL, Wilkerson S, Fortunato SJ: New technique for stabilizing umbilical artery catheters in very low birthweight infants. *J Perinatol,* 9:458, 1989.

Stringel G, Mercer S, et al: Catheterization of the umbilical artery in neonates: surgical complications. *Can J Surg,* 28:143, 1985.

Stromquist C, Perez J: Neonatal radiology casebook. *J Perinatol,* 12:1992, 1992.

Taylor LM, Troutman R, et al: Late complications after femoral artery catheterization in children less than five years of age. *J Vasc Surg,* 11:297, 1990.

Urbach J, Kaplan M, et al: Neonatal hypoglycemia related to umbilical artery catheter malposition. *J Pediatr,* 106:825, 1985.

Vohra K, Shah P, et al: Broken umbilical artery catheter: a rare occurrence. *J Perinatol,* 9:347, 1989.

Wagner CW, Vinocur CD, Weintraub WH: Retrieval of an umbilical artery catheter: a potential for misadventure. *South Med J,* 80:1434, 1987.

Wetzel RC, Tabata BK, Rogers MC: Hemodynamic monitoring considerations in pediatric critical care. In Rogers MC (ed): *Textbook of Pediatric Intensive Care,* 2nd ed. Baltimore, Williams & Wilkins, 1992, pp 620–624.

Wilkins RG: Radial artery cannulation and ischaemic damage: a review. *Anaesthesia,* 40:896, 1985.

Chapter 20

Therapeutic Plasma Exchange

David Moromisato

PLASMAPHERESIS

Apheresis, or bloodletting, comes from the Greek term *aphairesis*, which means to remove. It is one of the oldest of medical therapies and has been practiced for thousands of years. Plasmapheresis, the withdrawal of plasma, is a term coined by Abel in 1914 (Abel et al, 1914). His initial intention was to collect animal antiserum by removing whole blood, separating the plasma, and returning the cell portion back to the body. The practical benefit of plasmapheresis was first appreciated during World War II, when the technique was used to obtain plasma for the treatment of wounded soldiers. However, because the technique was performed manually and the equipment was cumbersome, its only clinical use for many years was to alleviate the hyperviscosity complications in Waldenström's macroglobulinemia. In the 1970s, reports of its possible benefit in patients with systemic lupus erythematosus and myasthenia gravis emerged. Moreover, the development of highly automated machines broadened the scope of conditions that might benefit from plasmapheresis. Since then, plasmapheresis, or plasma exchange, has been used for a variety of diseases that might possibly benefit from plasma removal.

INDICATIONS

In the past 20 years, plasmapheresis has been used for a wide variety of immunological and nonimmunological diseases that might possibly benefit from plasma removal. However, the range of disorders that have proved to benefit from the procedure has narrowed in the past decade. The rationale for the use of plasmapheresis is the removal of a constituent (e.g., plasma proteins or toxins) in the plasma phase that is contributing to the disease process. The diseases treated with plasmapheresis can be broadly categorized into neurological, hematological, renal, and collagen-vascular in origin (Table 20–1). Extensive reviews discussing the use of plasmapheresis in specific disease states have been published (Rossi et al, 1991).

Neurological disorders are the most common category of diseases for which plasmapheresis is used, and approximately half of the plasma exchanges performed today are for neurological disorders (Consensus Confer-

Table 20-1 Diseases for Which Plasmapheresis Is Commonly Used

Neurological
Acute Guillain-Barré syndrome
Chronic Guillain-Barré syndrome
Myasthenia gravis
Multiple sclerosis
Hematological
Hemolytic-uremic syndrome
Thrombotic thrombocytopenic purpura
Leukemia
Hyperviscosity syndromes (dysproteinemias)
Collagen-Vascular
Systemic lupus erythematosus
Vasculitis
Renal
Rapidly progressive glomerulonephritis
Goodpasture's syndrome

ence, 1986). The majority of patients in this category have Guillain-Barré syndrome, which is a demyelinating disorder of the peripheral nervous system. The disease is believed to be immune mediated, and plasma exchange apparently removes or dilutes circulating factors associated with its pathogenesis. Its beneficial effects have been demonstrated in three large clinical studies (French Cooperative Group, 1987; Guillain-Barré Study Group, 1985; Osterman et al, 1984). In all three studies, plasma exchange shortened the duration of illness. Duration of mechanical ventilation and time to unassisted ambulation were decreased by approximately 50%; and in two studies, the long-term outcome appeared to be improved with the use of plasma exchange. In the North American study, a better outcome was associated with the use of continuous flow plasma exchange, compared with the discontinuous method (Guillain-Barré Study Group, 1985). The French study demonstrated a higher frequency of adverse effects associated with the use of fresh-frozen plasma as replacement fluid compared with albumin (Bouget et al, 1993). Despite the evidence favoring the use of plasmapheresis in the three studies, all have been criticized for not employing sham-controlled treatments.

Plasma exchange should be performed in Guillain-Barré patients with rapidly progressive disease, an inability to ambulate, or deteriorating respiratory function. The typical volume for exchange in the treatment of Guillain-Barré syndrome is 50 ml/kg body weight on alternate days for a total of five treatments in a 10-day period. More recently, it has been suggested that therapy be extended to at least 14 days (Bleck, 1993). Although the efficacy of intravenous immunoglobulin therapy has been shown to be comparable to plasmapheresis in a Dutch multicenter study, evidence suggests that relapse rates are high in patients treated with immunoglobulins (Castro and Ropper, 1993; Irani et al, 1993). Therefore, plasma exchange, for the present, is still the treatment of choice in severe Guillain-Barré syndrome.

Several types of clinical situations are encountered in the critical care setting in which plasmapheresis can be used as a unique tool with advantages over more conventional modes of therapy (Wayne and Fosburg, 1993). With the use of plasma exchange, it is possible to rapidly and relatively safely alter hematocrit to a desired level. Plasma is removed while blood with a higher hematocrit is returned to the patient. This maneuver would be used with profound anemia (e.g., hemolytic-uremic syndrome, severe hemolytic anemia, and newly diagnosed acute leukemia) in a 1- to 4-hour period in patients who would otherwise receive slow transfusion for 24 to 48 hours. In the patient with a coagulopathy and renal failure, plasma exchange allows the delivery of large volumes of blood products for correction of the coagulopathy and, at the same time, control of the blood volume. Thus, plasmapheresis, when used selectively by an experienced hematology service, can serve an important role in the management of the critically ill child.

TECHNIQUE

Plasma exchange involves separation of the blood into its component parts by filtration or centrifugation and return of some components to the patient. In the filtration method, blood is passed through hollow fibers or between flat-plate membranes with pore sizes that prevent platelets and cellular constituents from passing through. The efficiency of the separation depends on pore size, transmembrane pressure, and other factors in the apparatus used. In the centrifugal method of separation, blood is passed into a spinning bowl, in which the components are separated by their density. This yields red blood cell, buffy coat, and plasma layers in the chamber. In this manner, plasma exchange by centrifugation can be used to remove specific types of cells as well as to separate plasma. In contrast, the use of filtration separation does not provide the option of cytapheresis.

The process of plasma exchange may be carried out in a continuous or discontinuous manner. In the continuous system, separation of the components is carried out as blood is removed from the patient through one port, and the separated components are simultaneously returned through another port. With the discontinuous system, sequential aliquots (50 to 200 ml) of whole blood are removed and processed. The processed components are then returned through the same intravenous catheter. The only advantage of the discontinuous system over the continuous method is the need for only one intravenous lumen. However, the duration of the procedure is markedly longer, and the patient can at times be alternately hypovolemic and hypervolemic with use of the discontinuous system.

Anticoagulation

Anticoagulation is required during plasma exchange to prevent clotting in the machinery. This can be accomplished by use of heparin, acid-citrate-dextrose (ACD), or both. More than 50% of the heparin or ACD, when infused into the proximal limb of the machinery, is removed along with the discarded plasma. Therefore, less than half of the anticoagulant infused reaches the patient. When heparin is used, activated clotting times are measured at the bedside every 20 to 40 minutes, with maintenance of a value 1.5 to 2.5 times control. Even in patients at high risk for hemorrhage, bleeding is rare (Sutton et al, 1989).

ACD is the anticoagulant used more often in plasma exchange. The mechanism for the anticoagulant effect of ACD is reduction of ionized calcium levels. Standard infusion rates of 0.5 to 1 mg/k/min lower ionized calcium levels by 20% to 30%, and the side effects that arise from the use of ACD are associated with this reduction in the ionized calcium level (Morse et al, 1980). The most common side effects are paresthesias in the extremities, agitation, and diaphoresis. However, tetany, hypotension, and shock have been reported, and any of these may be the presenting signs of citrate intoxication. Risk factors associated with a higher frequency of citrate toxic effects include renal failure, receipt of large volumes of citrated blood products, and age younger than 6 years (Collins, 1974; Dzik and Kirkley, 1988; Fosburg et al, 1983).

Replacement Solutions

Several types of solutions are currently used to replace the plasma that is discarded during plasma exchange. All of them fulfill the basic requirements that they contain roughly the same volume, electrolyte composition, and oncotic pressure as the plasma removed. The fluids used are fresh-frozen plasma, 5% albumin, synthetic plasma expanders, and saline. Five percent albumin is currently the most widely used replacement solution because of its low frequency of side effects. Its only drawback is its high cost.

Fresh-frozen plasma was commonly used when the plasma exchange technique was in its infancy. Today, because of its potentially severe side effects, plasma replacement is reserved for situations in which its use is absolutely necessary. These include thrombotic thrombocytopenic purpura and other states in which clotting factors or other plasma proteins need replacement. Patients with otherwise normal pretreatment clotting status do not usually need replacement of clotting factors. Other types of replacement solutions have been used as well. Packed red blood cells or intravenous gamma globulin has been used in states of anemia or hypogammaglobulinemia, respectively.

Vascular Access

The ability to obtain adequate vascular access in the pediatric patient is often a major consideration in the decision to use (or not use) plasma exchange. In general, peripheral veins are not large enough to accommodate catheters for plasma exchange to be performed. Pediatric patients as small as 4 to 5 kg require a 7 French double-lumen catheter that is sufficiently stiff so as not to collapse when blood is removed. A 9 French hemodialysis catheter is ideal for the larger child or teen-ager. The most common sites for catheter insertion are the femoral, subclavian, or internal jugular veins. The catheter should draw blood easily and rapidly without "catching." If any catching occurs during aspiration, no matter how easily it otherwise draws, the catheter will not function for the procedure (Wayne and Fosburg, 1993).

COMPLICATIONS

Adverse reactions and complications occur in 2% to 30% of patients undergoing plasma exchange procedures. The Canadian Apheresis Study Group (CASG) reported an adverse reaction in 12% of 5235 procedures (Sutton et al, 1989). Of these reactions, 96% were classified as mild to moderate and not requiring termination of the procedure. Reactions in this group included fever, paresthesias, muscle cramps, hypotension, nausea, and headache. The remaining 4%, 0.5% of procedures in the entire study, were severe enough to require termination of the procedure. The reactions in this group included hypotension, arrhythmias, seizures, respiratory arrest, and one patient with an intracranial hemorrhage. Although only 12% of the procedures in the CASG study were associated with an adverse event, 40% of the patients in the report experienced a side effect at least once in their treatment course. Patients with Guillain-Barré syndrome or hemolytic-uremic syndrome appeared to experience a higher rate of side effects during the course of therapy at 55% and 70%, respectively. The mortality from complications due to plasmapheresis is estimated to be 3 per 10,000 procedures (Consensus Conference, 1986). More than 50 deaths had been associated with plasma exchange in the literature by 1985, and most of the deaths were associated with the use of plasma as fluid replacement (Council on Scientific Affairs, 1985). Many of the reactions reported in the CASG study were also related to the use of plasma as the replacement fluid. Reactions have also been related to the effects of the anticoagulant. ACD decreases ionized calcium levels and results in mild symptoms in 25% of patients (Wayne and Fosburg, 1993). Manifestations of hypocalcemia include paresthesias, twitching, muscle cramps, tetany, or hypotension. Hypotension may be the first sign of hypocalcemia and should be treated as such until calcium levels are obtained. Complications associated with plasmapheresis may occur during or after the procedure and, for this reason, necessitate adequate monitoring as well as the presence of experienced personnel to anticipate any adverse event.

Technical Complications

As with the placement of any large catheter, obtaining vascular access for plasma exchange carries the usual risks of vessel thrombosis or perforation, catheter-related infection, and sepsis. In the CASG study, continuous flow plasmapheresis was associated with a lower frequency of hypotension compared with discontinuous flow plasma exchange (Sutton et al, 1989). There is also some evidence that continuous flow plasma exchange results in a better outcome in patients with Guillain-Barré syndrome (Guillain-Barré Study Group, 1985). Hemolysis caused by a poorly functioning apparatus, tube kinking, or clotting within the machine can occur rarely.

Cardiovascular Complications

Hypotension is one of the most common hemodynamic side effects, and the cause of this occurrence is often unknown. However, volume and protein depletion has been implicated as a common cause of hypotension, and with careful monitoring of fluid balance its occurrence has been minimized (Rodnitzky and Goeken, 1982). Hypocalcemia secondary to ACD, as stated earlier, has also been suggested as a cause of hypotension (Fosburg et al, 1983). Administration of supplemental calcium or slowing the rate of citrate infusion may decrease the frequency of citrate toxic effects (Buskard et al, 1976; Olson et al, 1977). If hypotension occurs in a patient receiving citrate, the procedure should be temporarily discontinued, an ionized calcium level obtained, and volume and calcium administered. Citrate intoxication has also been implicated as the cause of arrhythmias (Olson et al, 1977). Although they are usually brief and self-resolving, they are occasionally severe and can result in sudden cardiac arrest (Sutton et al, 1989).

Complications Associated with Replacement Fluids

The use of plasma as replacement fluid is associated with a high frequency of complications in a number of studies (French Cooperative Group, 1987; O'Conner et al, 1981; Sutton et al, 1989). In the CASG study, plasma replacement was associated with a higher frequency of fever, chills, and urticaria (Sutton et al, 1989). In fact, all of the patients who experienced severe urticaria, dyspnea, or bronchospasm and both patients who had respiratory arrest received plasma. Bouget et al (1993), in a large prospective multicenter trial, evaluated the morbidity associated with plasma replacement compared with albumin replacement in patients with Guillain-Barré syndrome. A higher rate of reactions was observed in the plasma replacement group (46% versus 32%), leading the authors to conclude that fresh-frozen plasma should be abandoned as replacement fluid in Guillain-Barré syndrome. Given the risks associated with transfusion, plasma replacement should be restricted to situations in which bleeding or coagulopathy exists.

Hematological Complications

Clotting factors are decreased by 60% after a single 1.5-volume plasma exchange procedure and, except for fibrinogen level, return to normal in 12 to 24 hours (Urbaniak, 1990). Wood and Jacobs (1986) observed return of normal fibrinogen levels by 48 hours. They also observed platelet counts to decrease by 30% with plasma exchange but return to baseline levels in 48 hours. Despite these decreases in clotting factors, bleeding complications due to platelet or factor depletion are rare. Because of this, replacement of clotting factors is rarely indicated. However, in situations in which plasma exchange is performed on a daily or prolonged basis, progressive declines in factors may occur. Therefore, it is still important to monitor the patient's clotting status during a course of plasma exchange. Paradoxically, a hypercoagulable state may occur, and several cases of spontaneous clotting have been reported (Rubenstein et al, 1983). The mechanism for this occurrence, although not completely understood, may be due to antithrombin III depletion or depressed antithrombin III activity, or both (Chirnside et al, 1981; Sultan et al, 1979).

SUMMARY

Plasmapheresis is one of the oldest modalities in medicine in use today. Absolute indications are rare in the pediatric population; however, it is the treatment of choice in severe Guillain-Barré syndrome. Although immunoglobulin has been studied as a less invasive alternative, its long-term efficacy has yet to be determined. The potential use and safety of plasmapheresis as an alternative mode of therapy in profound anemia and renal failure have not been fully recognized. To avoid complications associated with its use, studies suggest using heparin alone or in combination with ACD, continuous flow devices, frequent monitoring of calcium levels and activated clotting times, careful monitoring of fluid balance, and avoidance of plasma as replacement fluid. Plasma exchange, when used in select patients by an experienced staff, can serve as a valuable tool in the management of the critically ill pediatric patient.

References

Abel JJ, Rowntree LG, Turner BB: Plasma removal with return of corpuscles. *J Pharmacol Exp Ther,* 5:625, 1914.

Bleck TP: Treatment strategies for patients with the Guillain-Barré syndrome. *Crit Care Med,* 21: 641, 1993.

Bouget J, Chevret S, et al, The French Cooperative Group: Plasma exchange morbidity in Guillain-Barré syndrome: results from the French prospective, double-blind, randomized, multicenter study. *Crit Care Med,* 21:651, 1993.

Buskard NA, Varghese Z, Willis MR: Correction of hypocalcemic symptoms during plasma exchange. *Lancet,* 2:344, 1976.

Castro LHM, Ropper AH: Human immune globulin infusion in Guillain-Barré syndrome: worsening during and after treatment. *Neurology,* 43:1034, 1993.

Chirnside A, Urbaniak SJ, et al: Coagulation abnormalities following intensive plasma exchange on the cell separator. *Br J Haematol,* 48:627, 1981.

Collins JA: Problems associated with the massive transfusion of stored blood. *Surgery,* 75:274, 1974.

Consensus Conference: The utility of therapeutic plasmapheresis for neurological disorders statement. *JAMA,* 256:1333, 1986.

Council on Scientific Affairs: Current status of therapeutic plasmapheresis and related technique. *JAMA,* 253:819, 1985

Dzik WH, Kirkley SA: Citrate toxicity during massive blood transfusion. *Trans Med Rev,* 2:76, 1988.

Fosburg M, Dolan M, et al: Intensive plasma exchange in small and critically ill pediatric patients: techniques and clinical outcome. *J Clin Apheresis,* 1:215, 1983.

French Cooperative Group on Plasma Exchange in Guillain-Barré syndrome: Role of replacement fluids. *Ann Neurol,* 22:753, 1987.

Guillain-Barré Study Group: Plasmapheresis and acute Guillain-Barré syndrome. *Neurology,* 35: 1096, 1985.

Irani DN, Cornblath DR, et al: Relapse in Guillain-Barré syndrome after treatment with human immune globulin. *Neurology,* 43:872, 1993.

Morse EE, Hohnadel DC, et al: Decreased ionized calcium during therapeutic plasma exchange pheresis and platelet pheresis. *Johns Hopkins Med J,* 146:260, 1980.

O'Conner PC, Erskine JG, Pringle TH: Pulmonary oedema after transfusion with fresh frozen plasma. *Br Med J,* 282:379, 1981.

Olson PR, Cox C, McCullough J: Laboratory and clinical effects of the infusion of ACD solution during platelet pheresis. *Vox Sang,* 33:79, 1977.

Osterman PG, Lundemo G, et al: Beneficial effects of plasma exchange in acute inflammatory polyradiculoneuropathy. *Lancet,* 2:1296, 1984.

Rodnitzky RL, Goeken JA: Complications of plasma exchange in neurological patients. *Arch Neurol,* 39:350, 1982.

Rossi EC, Simon TL, Moss GS (eds): *Principles of Transfusion Medicine.* Baltimore, Williams & Wilkins, 1991.

Rubenstein MD, Wall RT, et al: Complications of therapeutic apheresis including a fatal case with pulmonary vascular occlusion. *Am J Med,* 75:171, 1983.

Sultan Y, Bussel A, et al: Potential danger of thrombosis after plasma exchange in the treatment of patients with immune disease. *Transfusion,* 19:588, 1979.

Sutton DMC, Nair RC, Rock G, Canadian Apheresis Study Group: Complications of plasma exchange. *Transfusion,* 29:124, 1989.

Urbaniak SJ, Robinson FA: Therapeutic apheresis. *Br Med J,* 300:662, 1990.

Wayne AS, Fosburg MT: Therapeutic plasma exchange and cytapheresis. In Nathan DG, Oski FA (eds): *Hematology of Infancy and Childhood,* 4th ed. Philadelphia, WB Saunders, 1993, p 1819.

Wood L, Jacobs P: The effect of serial therapeutic plasmapheresis on platelet count, coagulation factors, plasma immunoglobulin, and complement levels. *J Clin Apheresis,* 3:124, 1986.

Chapter 21

Management of Pain and Sedation

Robert H. Levin, Sylvia Fernandez Villarreal, Ivy Luong, and Teresa Allard

ANALGESIA AND SEDATION FOR PEDIATRIC PROCEDURES

Guidelines for Monitoring

The guidelines that follow list the usual pediatric procedures that require analgesia or sedation and the usual medications for those procedures (Tables 21–1 to 21–5). Whenever drugs are used to produce conscious sedation or anesthesia, appropriate medical specialty guidelines for conscious sedation and anesthesia should be used to ensure the proper monitoring of patients. These guidelines categorize drugs into four levels of monitoring: minimal (usual), mild (extended precautions), moderate (conscious sedation), and maximal (deep sedation). There is considerable variability in a patient's response to these medications. The doses listed in the tables are meant as starting doses and may have to be titrated upward to achieve the desired effect for individual patients. The use of medications for conscious sedation is covered in more detail to ensure proper use.

Minimal (usual monitoring)

The use of medications in pediatric procedures to produce analgesia and sedation is well established. Many of these medications used to produce analgesia are also used by pediatricians, family practitioners, and internists during routine clinic visits to induce conscious sedation by employing larger doses. Usual clinic procedures should be employed to monitor children who have been given therapeutic doses of analgesics and sedatives.

Mild (extended precautions)

Additional monitoring of the patient is required for medications that have the tendency to cause severe respiratory depression when they are administered in larger doses (e.g., oral midazolam, oral ketamine, and rectal thiopental). Patients given these medications (which are marked with a dagger in the tables) should be put on a pulse oximeter, monitored continuously with use of prepared monitoring guidelines in the examination room by a reliable parent or caretaker, and monitored by a health care practitioner every 15 minutes.

Table 21-1 Analgesia and Sedation for Pediatric Surgical Procedures

Surgical Procedures	Analgesia[1]	Sedation[1]
Burn care (tubbing)	Morphine PO (preferred), IV	Lorazepam SL or midazolam PO†
Burn dressings	Morphine PO (preferred), IV; or acetaminophen with codeine PO	Lorazepam SL or midazolam PO† or ketamine IV*
Central line (placement or removal, e.g., Broviac)	EMLA and morphine PO (preferred), IV	Lorazepam SL or midazolam PO†
Chest tube or drain (removal)	Morphine PO (preferred), IV	Lorazepam SL or midazolam PO†
Circumcision	Lidocaine penile block, EMLA, or morphine PO (preferred), IV	—
Incision and drainage	Morphine PO (preferred), IV; or fentanyl IV*	Lorazepam SL, midazolam PO†, or nitrous oxide*; or ketamine IV*
Lacerations (suturing)		
Anesthesia	TAC, lidocaine block	—
Sedation	Morphine PO	Midazolam PO†, IN†, PR†; or lorazepam SL
Laceration (complex repair usually done by surgeons)	Fentanyl IV*, lidocaine block	Midazolam IV* (for facial) or ketamine IV*
Digital nail removal (toe/fungi)	Lidocaine digital block	Lorazepam SL or midazolam PO†
Suture/staple removal	EMLA	Lorazepam SL or midazolam PO†
Wound care (packing)	Morphine PO (preferred), IV; or acetaminophen with codeine PO	Lorazepam SL or midazolam PO† (if large or deep wound)

[1]Whenever possible, the oral route should be used when indicated. The oral route is the preferred route in children because it is safer and usually equally effective.

*All intravenously administered medications marked with an asterisk (also inhaled nitrous oxide) should be used only by physicians familiar with their use within established guidelines for conscious sedation. These medications are intrinsically dangerous; physicians using them should be trained in airway management, including endotracheal intubation, or they should be administered under the direct supervision of an anesthesiologist.

†Medications marked with a dagger are less dangerous than those marked with an asterisk, but more dangerous to use than those not marked. Children given these agents (midazolam PO, IN, PR; ketamine PO; and thiopental PR) should be monitored at all times by a pulse oximeter and a knowledgeable parent and every 15 minutes by a health care practitioner.

IN, intranasal; IV, intravenous; PO, oral; PR, rectal; SL, sublingual; TAC, tetracaine, epinephrine (Adrenalin), and cocaine.

Table 21-2 Analgesia and Sedation for Pediatric Orthopedic Procedures

Orthopedic Procedure	Analgesia[1]	Sedation[1]
Aspiration of joints	EMLA and injected lidocaine	Lorazepam SL or midazolam PO†
Fracture or dislocation realignment, casting	Morphine PO (preferred), IV; or fentanyl IV*	Midazolam IV*, PO†; or lorazepam SL; ketamine IV*
Pin insertion/removal	EMLA and morphine PO (preferred), IV	Lorazepam SL or midazolam PO†
Traction realignment	Morphine PO (preferred),IV; or acetaminophen with codeine PO	Diazepam PO (preferred), IV*

[1]Whenever possible, the oral route should be used when indicated. The oral route is the preferred route in children because it is safer and usually equally effective.

*All intravenously administered medications marked with an asterisk (also inhaled nitrous oxide) should be used only by physicians familiar with their use within established guidelines for conscious sedation. These medications are intrinsically dangerous; physicians using them should be trained in airway management, including endotracheal intubation, or they should be administered under the direct supervision of an anesthesiologist.

†Medications marked with a dagger are less dangerous than those marked with an asterisk, but more dangerous to use than those not marked. Children given these agents (midazolam PO, IN, PR; ketamine PO; and thiopental PR) should be monitored at all times by a pulse oximeter and a knowledgeable parent and every 15 minutes by a health care practitioner.

IV, intravenous; PO, oral; SL, sublingual.

Table 21–3 Analgesia and Sedation for Pediatric Diagnostic Procedures[1]

Diagnostic Procedure	Analgesia[2]	Sedation[2]
Electroencephalography, brain stem auditory evoked response	Usually none	Usually nothing; but if needed, use chloral hydrate PO
Magnetic resonance imaging or computed tomography (uncooperative patient)	Usually none	Pentobarbital IV*; or thiopental PR†; or midazolam IV*, PO† with morphine PO (preferred), IV
Voiding cystourethrography (uncooperative patient)	Usually none	Pentobarbital IV* or midazolam PO† with morphine PO

[1]Use sedation only in patients who are uncooperative and to perform the procedure or insert a catheter. Anagesia is seldom needed.

[2]Whenever possible, the oral route should be used when indicated. The oral route is the preferred route in children because it is safer and usually equally effective.

*All intravenously administered medications marked with an asterisk (also inhaled nitrous oxide) should be used only by physicians familiar with their use within established guidelines for conscious sedation. These medications are intrinsically dangerous; physicians using them should be trained in airway management, including endotracheal intubation, or they should be administered under the direct supervision of an anesthesiologist.

†Medications marked with a dagger are less dangerous than those marked with an asterisk, but more dangerous to use than those not marked. Children given these agents (midazolam PO, IN, PR; ketamine PO; and thiopental PR) should be monitored at all times by a pulse oximeter and a knowledgeable parent and every 15 minutes by a health care practitioner.

IV, intravenous; PO, oral; PR, rectal.

Moderate (conscious sedation)

Patients receiving medications for conscious sedation (Tables 21–6 to 21–8) have an altered level of consciousness but should be able to protect their airway and respond appropriately to verbal commands. A health care provider and all emergency equipment and antidotes must be immediately available when these medications are used. The patients must be monitored by a pulse oximeter, sphygmomanometer, and cuff. Intravenous access should be secured.

Maximal (deep sedation)

A number of medications are intrinsically dangerous because they produce loss of protective reflexes and anesthesia in large doses. They should be used (in a properly prepared and monitored clinical setting) only by practitioners familiar with their effects. These medications (e.g., fentanyl, propofol, thiopental, ketamine, midazolam, and methohexital), when administered by the intravenous route (and inhaled general anesthetics like nitrous oxide), are marked with an asterisk in the tables to indicate their dangerous tendency to produce severe respiratory depression. These medications should be administered only under the supervision of a physician trained in airway management, including endotracheal intubation, or under the direct supervision of an anesthesiologist.

MEDICATIONS FOR CONSCIOUS SEDATION

Most frequently, drugs in the following classes are used for conscious sedation: benzodiazepines, opiate agonists, neuroleptics (droperidol), and propofol (a sedative-hypnotic). Most medications used to produce a state of conscious sedation are administered intravenously. However, these medications can also produce a state of conscious sedation when administered by other routes, and patients should be monitored appropriately as outlined before. Midazolam may also be administered by the oral and

Table 21–4 Analgesia and Sedation for Pediatric Sickle Cell Pain Crisis

Sickle Cell Management	Analgesia[1]	Sedation[1]
Bone pain (chronic)	NSAIDs PO and either morphine PO or acetaminophen with codeine PO	Usually none
Vaso-occlusive pain	Morphine IV by continuous infusion, then morphine PO for tapering, then acetaminophen with codeine PO or hydromorphone PO	Usually none

[1]Whenever possible, the oral route should be used when indicated. The oral route is the preferred route in children because it is safer and usually equally effective. Sedation is usually not needed.

IV, intravenous; NSAIDs, nonsteroidal anti-inflammatory drugs; PO, oral.

Table 21–5 Analgesia and Sedation for Other Pediatric Procedures

Other Procedures	Analgesia[1]	Sedation[1]
Bone marrow	EMLA or morphine PO (preferred), IV	Lorazepam SL or midazolam PO†
Nasogastric tube placement	Viscous lidocaine	—
Fine-needle biopsy	Lidocaine or morphine PO	Lorazepam SL or midazolam PO†
Foreign body extraction	Morphine PO (preferred) IV	Lorazepam SL or midazolam PO† or ketamine IV*; or nitrous oxide*; or thiopental† PR
Intubation, rapid sequence	—	Thiopental IV*, ketamine IV*
IV line placement	EMLA	—
Lumbar punctures	EMLA and lidocaine	Lorazepam SL; midazolam IV*, IN†, PO†
Physical therapy	Morphine PO, acetaminophen with codeine PO, or NSAIDs PO	—
Sexual abuse examination	Fentanyl IV*	Midazolam PO† or ketamine IV*
Urinary bladder catheter (uncooperative patient)	—	Midazolam PO† with morphine PO, pentobarbital IV*, or ketamine IV

[1]Whenever possible, the oral route should be used when indicated. The oral route is the preferred route in children because it is safer and usually equally effective.

*All intravenously administered medications marked with an asterisk (also inhaled nitrous oxide) should be used only by physicians familiar with their use within established guidelines for conscious sedation. These medications are intrinsically dangerous; physicians using them should be trained in airway management, including endotracheal intubation, or they should be administered under the direct supervision of an anesthesiologist.

†Medications marked with a dagger are less dangerous than those marked with an asterisk, but more dangerous to use than those not marked. Children given these agents (midazolam PO, IN, PR; ketamine PO; and thiopental PR) should be monitored at all times by a pulse oximeter and a knowledgeable parent and every 15 minutes by a health care practitioner.

IV, intravenous; IN, intranasal; NSAIDs, nonsteroidal anti-inflammatory drugs; PO, oral; PR, rectal; SL, sublingual.

intranasal routes. Diazepam may also be administered per rectum. Morphine may also be given orally and subcutaneously; however, its use by the intramuscular route should be discouraged because it causes severe discomfort in children. Although individual policies and procedures for conscious sedation may differ, deviations from the "standard of practice" for conscious sedation are not advisable. All health care personnel involved with conscious sedation should be aware of dosage ranges, side effects, and available reversal drugs. In addition, when these agents are used in children, the following materials should be readily available: a full pediatric crash cart including all drugs for advanced life support, reversal agents, pediatric dosing guidelines, and pediatric monitoring procedures.

Metabolism of Conscious Sedation Drugs

Benzodiazepines

Table 21–6 lists the agents in this class. All benzodiazepines are metabolized by the liver. There is little clinical evidence to suggest that one benzodiazepine is more effective than another.

Opiate agonists

Like benzodiazepines, opiate agonists (see Table 21–7) are metabolized by the liver and excreted by the kidneys. Metabolism and excretion can be decreased in neonates, infants, or patients with compromised liver or kidney function. Patients in these categories may need decreased dosages of medications or longer time intervals between doses. Meperidine (Demerol) is metabolized in the liver to the active metabolite normeperidine, which may accumulate in patients and cause irritability and seizures.

Other medications

A number of other sedatives (see Table 21–8) are used in children. Droperidol is a more potent, faster onset sedative similar to haloperidol. Propofol is usually used as an anesthetic agent but can be used as a sedative-hypnotic drug in conscious sedation. Propofol is metabolized by hepatic conjugation and is eliminated by the kidneys. Plasma levels of propofol de-

(Text continues on page 195.)

Table 21-6 Conscious Sedation Drugs: Benzodiazepines[1]

Conscious Sedation Drug	Initial Adult Dosage	Initial Pediatric Dosage	Onset of Action (min)	Duration of Action (h)	Half-Life (h)	Contraindications	Comments
Midazolam (Versed)	0.5–1 mg slow IV*	0.05–0.1 mg/kg slow IV	1–3 IV	1–4 IV	2 (1–4) IV	Hypersensitivity to benzodiazepines; acute narrow-angle glaucoma; comatose patients, patients with pre-existing CNS depression, respiratory depression, or severe uncontrolled pain	Shortest acting benzodiazepine Give IV 3 min before procedure and repeat q 3–4 min to desired effect
	Not used PO in adults	0.2–0.4 mg/kg (or 0.5 mg/kg with a repeated dose of 0.25 mg/kg prn) PO	20–30 PO	1–2 PO	Caution: $t_{1/2}$ may be prolonged with repeated dosing		Give PO 30–45 min before procedure; dose can be repeated in 30 min if needed; can be mixed with a calculated 50% dose of acetaminophen elixir; decrease dose by 1/2 if given along with morphine (see Table 21–12) Max: 2.5 mg (0.15 mg/kg) IV or 15 mg (0.75 mg/kg) PO
		< 1 y old: 0.3–0.5 mg/kg IN	10–20 IN				
Diazepam (Valium)	1–2.5 mg IV	0.1–0.2 mg/kg slow IV	3–10	4–8	30–60 (50–100 for metabolites)	Hypersensitivity to benzodiazepines; acute narrow-angle glaucoma; comatose patients, patients with pre-existing CNS depression, respiratory depression, or severe uncontrolled pain	Elimination $t_{1/2}$ may be up to 48–72 h (longer in neonates) Give IV 10–15 min or PR 45–60 min before procedure and may repeat q 10 min IV or 30 min PR prn Decrease dose by1/2 if given along with morphine (see Table 21–12) Max: 10 mg IV or 30 mg PR
	5–10 mg PR	0.5 mg/kg PR	5–10				

Table continued on following page

Table 21-6 Conscious Sedation Drugs: Benzodiazepines[1] *Continued*

Conscious Sedation Drug	Initial Adult Dosage	Initial Pediatric Dosage	Onset of Action (min)	Duration of Action (h)	Half-Life (h)	Contraindications	Comments
Lorazepam (Ativan)	0.5–2 mg IV 1–2 mg PO, SL	0.02–0.09 mg/kg IV 0.02–0.09 mg/kg PO, SL	2–3 15–30	6–8 6–8	Adults: 14 Children: 10 Neonates: 40	Hypersensitivity to benzodiazepines; acute narrow-angle glaucoma; comatose patients, patients with pre-existing CNS depression, respiratory depression, or severe uncontrolled pain	Has no active metabolites Give 1 h before procedure Do not use IM Decrease dose by 1/2 if given along with morphine (see Table 21–12) Max: 0.09 mg/kg IV

*All intravenously administered medications marked with an asterisk (also inhaled nitrous oxide) should be used only by physicians familiar with their use within established guidelines for conscious sedation. These medications are intrinsically dangerous; physicians using them should be trained in airway management, including endotracheal intubation, or they should be administered under the direct supervision of an anesthesiologist.

[1]Benzodiazepines, used for sedation, have no intrinsic analgesic effects; but when used in conjunction with narcotics, they may have a synergistic effect. Benzodiazepines may also produce disinhibition in children. Do not mix any drugs in the same syringe with diazepam.

CNS, central nervous system; IN, intranasal; IV, intravenous; PO, oral; PR, rectal; SL, sublingual.

Table 21–7 Conscious Sedation Drugs: Opiate Agonists

Conscious Sedation Drug	Initial Adult Dosage	Initial Pediatric Dosage	Onset of Action (min)	Duration of Action (h)	Half-Life (h)	Contraindications	Comments
Morphine (various)	1–4 mg slow IV 5–15 mg SC	Neonates: 0.03 mg/kg IV < 6 mo: 0.05–0.1 mg/kg IV > 6 mo: 0.1–0.2 mg/kg IV 0.1–0.2 mg/kg SQ	2–5 IV 20–40 SC	1–3 IV 3–5 SC	Adults: 1–4 IV Neonates: 4–13 IV	Hypersensitivity to morphine; acute bronchial asthma; upper airway obstruction; increased intracranial pressure; severe respiratory depression; shock; occult hemorrhage; relative contraindication: severe hepatic or renal insufficiency	May repeat IV dose q 5–15 min to desired effect; give IV dose 5 min before procedure Because of pain, the IM route should not be used in children Adjust dosage for renal impairment; Decrease dose by 1/2 if given with pentobarbital, hydroxyzine, diazepam, or other benzodiazepines (see Table 21–12).
Fentanyl (Sublimaze)	10–50 μg slow IV*	0.5–1 μg/kg/dose IV	1–2	0.5–2	2–4	Hypersensitivity to fentanyl; acute bronchial asthma; upper airway obstruction; increased intracranial pressure; severe respiratory depression; severe bradycardia; shock; occult hemorrhage; relative contraindication: severe hepatic or renal insufficiency	May repeat dose q 5–10 min prn Respiratory depressant effects may last longer than analgesic effects

Table continued on following page

Table 21-7 Conscious Sedation Drugs: Opiate Agonists *Continued*

Conscious Sedation Drug	Initial Adult Dosage	Initial Pediatric Dosage	Onset of Action (min)	Duration of Action (h)	Half-Life (h)	Contraindications	Comments
Meperidine (Demerol)	12.5–25 mg slow IV	0.5–1 mg/kg IV	1–5	1–3	Adults: 1–2 Infants: 8–10 Neonates: 12–39	Hypersensitivity to meperidine; patients receiving MAO inhibitors within last 14 days; acute respiratory depression or disorders; increased intracranial pressure; severe tachycardias; biliary colic; seizure disorders; shock; occult hemorrhage; relative contraindication: severe hepatic or renal insufficiency	May repeat IV dose every 5 min to desired effect Because of pain, the IM route should not be used in children Adjust dose in renal impairment Max: 2 mg/kg/dose or 100 mg/dose
Hydromorphone (Dilaudid)	1–3 mg slow IV	0.015 mg/kg IV	2–5	3–5	1–3	Hypersensitivity to hydromorphone; acute bronchial asthma; upper airway obstruction; increased intracranial pressure; severe respiratory depression; shock; occult hemorrhage; relative contraindication: severe hepatic or renal insufficiency	This injection contains benzyl alcohol Because of pain, the IM route should not be used in children

*All intravenously administered medications marked with an asterisk (also inhaled nitrous oxide) should be used only by physicians familiar with their use within established guidelines for conscious sedation. These medications are intrinsically dangerous; physicians using them should be trained in airway management, including endotracheal intubation, or they should be administered under the direct supervision of an anesthesiologist.

IM, intramuscular; IV, intravenous; MAO, monoamine oxidase; SC, subcutaneous.

Table 21-8 Conscious Sedation Drugs: Other Sedatives

Conscious Sedation Drug	Initial Adult Dosage	Initial Pediatric Dosage	Onset of Action (min)	Duration of Action (h)	Half-Life (h)	Contraindications	Comments
Droperidol (Inapsine)	0.625–1.25 mg IV	0.088–0.165 mg/kg IV	3–10	2–4, may last 12 h	2.2	Hypersensitivity to droperidol	Not usually used in children Recommended in conjunction with opiates or BDZs for better effect; administration alone may cause a dysphoric or dystonic response, so pretreatment with diphenhydramine 1 mg/kg/dose is recommended; produces a dissociative effect (allays apprehension and provides a state of mental detachment); has no analgesic or amnestic properties Full effect may take 30 min
Propofol (Diprivan)	50 μg/kg/min IV* (individualize dosing)	25–100 μg/kg/min IV (individualize dosing)	1–3	1.5	24–72 Mean effective $t_{1/2}$ is 6–10 min	Hypersensitivity to propofol or components of product	Use only in intubated patients; titrate carefully to sedation; monitor for respiratory depression (larger doses produce anesthesia) Supplied as a 1% emulsion About 3 to 5 min must be allowed between clinical dosage adjustments

Table continued on following page

Table 21-8 Conscious Sedation Drugs: Other Sedatives *Continued*

Conscious Sedation Drug	Initial Adult Dosage	Initial Pediatric Dosage	Onset of Action (min)	Duration of Action (h)	Half-Life (h)	Contraindications	Comments
Pentobarbital (Nembutal)	100–200 mg slow IV 120–200 mg PR	6 mo–5 y = 1–2 mg/kg slow IV 5–12 y = 2 mg/kg slow IV 2–6 mg/kg PR, PO	IV = 1 PO, PR = 15–60	IV = 15 min PO, PR = 1–4	Adults: 35–50 Children: 25	Hypersensitivity to barbiturates; latent porphyria; severe respiratory dysfunction; severe liver impairment; hypovolemic shock; severe CHF	May cause paradoxical excitement (small doses of morphine can ameliorate this) If therapeutic doses of morphine are given, decrease the dose of pentobarbital by 1/2 Give 5–10 min before procedure and may repeat dose once Do not inject > 50 mg/min Do not add any other drug in same syringe Max: 6 mg/kg or 100 mg/dose in children
Thiopental (Pentothal)	3–4 g PR[†]	5–10 mg/kg PR	IV = 0.5–1	IV = 5–30 min	Adults: 3–11.5 Shorter $t_{1/2}$ in children	Hypersensitivity to barbiturates; latent porphyria; severe respiratory dysfunction; severe liver impairment; hypovolemic shock; severe CHF	Should not be used for long procedures; can cause laryngospasm or bronchospasm

Chloral hydrate (Noctec)	0.5–1 g PO	35–50 mg/kg PO	30–60	4–8	Adults: 8–11 Neonates: 8.5–66	Hypersensitivity to chloral hydrate or its derivatives; marked hepatic or renal impairment; severe cardiac disease	Give 30–60 min before BSER or CT procedure MR once after initial dose prn to a max dose of 120 mg/kg or 2 g total Not an analgesic
Ketamine (Ketalar)	0.25–0.75 mg/kg IV* IM not used in adults PO not used in adults	0.25–0.5 mg/kg IV IM not used in children 6–10 mg/kg PO†	3–4 min IV	10–15 min IV unconscious 30–40 min analgesia 1–2 h amnesia	IV for 10–15 min	Hypersensitivity to ketamine; patients in whom a significant elevation of blood pressure would be a serious hazard; psychiatric disorders	Premedicate children with a BDZ (to decrease CNS effects, see doses Table 21–6) before IV use and with atropine 0.01 mg/kg (to decrease oral secretions) before oral use IM dose produces 12–25 min of anesthesia Do not exceed 0.5 mg/kg/min or give dose in less than 1 min Do not mix in same syringe with barbiturates or diazepam

*All intravenously administered medications marked with an asterisk (also inhaled nitrous oxide) should be used only by physicians familiar with their use within established guidelines for conscious sedation. These medications are intrinsically dangerous; physicians using them should be trained in airway management, including endotracheal intubation, or they should be administered under the direct supervision of an anesthesiologist.

†Medications marked with a dagger are less dangerous than those marked with an asterisk, but more dangerous to use than those not marked. Children given these agents (midazolam PO, IV, PR; ketamine PO; and thiopental PR) should be monitored at all times by a pulse oximeter, and a knowledgeable parent and every 15 minutes by a health care practitioner.

BDZs, benzodiazepines; BSER, brain stem auditory evoked response; CHF, congestive heart failure; CNS, central nervous system; CT, computed tomography; IM, intramuscular; IV, intravenous; MR, may repeat; PO, oral; PR, per rectum.

Table 21–9 Reversal Agents

Reversal Agent	Indication	Adult Dosage	Pediatric Dosage	Onset of Action	Duration of Action	Contraindications	Comments
Flumazenil (Romazicon, formerly Mazicon)	Benzodiazepine reversal only	0.2 mg (2 ml) IV in 15-sec period	3–12 y: 0.01 mg/kg IV (max = 0.2 mg), then 0.005 mg/kg	1–2 min	15 min–2.5 h (average, 53 min)	Seizures; head injury; patients given BDZs for life-threatening conditions, such as status epilepticus or increased intracranial pressure; patients taking BDZs for a seizure indication or patients physically dependent on BDZs; concomitant tricyclic antidepressant overdose	Use only in patients with depressed mental status with or without respiratory depression May repeat as much as 0.2 mg q1 min up to total of 1 mg
Naloxone (Narcan)	Opiate reversal only	0.2–2 mg IV	Birth to 5 y or < 20 kg = 0.1 mg/kg IV > 5 y or ≥ 20 kg = 2 mg/dose IV	0.5–2 min	1–4 h (dose- and route-dependent) 20–60 min	Hypersensitivity to naloxone	Initial dosage administration of 0.4 mg in adults may cause complete opiate antagonism, so use with caution in habituated patients Use with extreme caution in neonates to avoid seizures Titrate dosage for opiate reversal (partial or complete reversal) Half-life: neonates, 1.2–3h; adults, 1–1.5h

BDZs, benzodiazepines; IV, intravenous.

Table 21–10 Pain Management

Other Pain Medications	Initial Adult Dosage	Initial Pediatric Dosage	Onset of Action (min)	Duration of Action (h)	Half-Life (h)	Contraindications	Comments
Antipyretic/ analgesics							
Ketorolac (Toradol) IM, IV		3–15 y: 0.2–0.9 mg/kg IM	10	6–8	Children < 7 y = 5.6 Children > 7 y and adults: 4–6 With renal impairment, 9–10	Hypersensitivity to NSAIDs; use with extreme caution in patients with CHF, hypertension, decreased renal or hepatic function, history of bleeding, or currently receiving anticoagulants	Use only for analgesia in patients unable to tolerate opiates or oral/rectal NSAIDs. Give usually only as a single dose in the emergency department (can be used up to 5 days) followed by another analgesic agent Not usually recommended in children because of the painful IM route and lack of data on its use Max = 120 mg IM or IV/d for adults < 65 y 60 mg IM or IV/d for adults > 65 y or < 50 kg
Single adult dose							
< 65 y	60 mg IM						
> 65 y or < 50 kg	30 mg IM						
< 65 y	30 mg IV						
> 65 y or < 50 kg	15 mg IV						
Multiple adult dose							
< 65 y	30 mg IM, IV q 6 h						
> 65 y or < 50 kg	15 mg IM, IV q 6 h						
Ibuprofen (Motrin, Advil) PO	200–400 mg PO	4–10 mg/kg PO	30	4–6	2–4	Hypersensitivity to NSAIDs; use with extreme caution in patients with CHF, hypertension, decreased renal or hepatic function, history of bleeding, currently receiving or anticoagulants	Max = 3.2 g/d for adults

Table continued on following page

Table 21-10 Pain Management *Continued*

Other Pain Medications	Initial Adult Dosage	Initial Pediatric Dosage	Onset of Action (min)	Duration of Action (h)	Half-Life (h)	Contraindications	Comments
Acetaminophen (Tylenol) PO	325–650 mg PO	10–15 mg/kg PO	30–60	3–4	Neonates: 2–5 Adults: 1–3	Hypersensitivity to acetaminophen; severe G6PD deficiency	Max = 4 g/d for adults
Opiate agonists							
Codeine (various) PO	15–60 mg PO	0.5–1 mg/kg PO	20–60	4–6	2.5–3.5	Hypersensitivity to opiates; acute bronchial asthma; upper airway obstruction; increased intracranial pressure; severe respiratory depression; relative contraindication: severe hepatic or renal insufficiency	Adjust dosage in renal impairment More effective when used with acetaminophen
Fentanyl (Sublimaze)	10–50 μg slow IV*	0.5–1 μg/kg/dose IV	1–2	0.5–2	2–4	Hypersensitivity to fentanyl; acute bronchial asthma; upper airway obstruction; increased intracranial pressure; severe respiratory depression; severe bradycardia; shock; occult hemorrhage; relative contraindication: severe hepatic or renal insufficiency	May repeat dose q 5–10 min prn Respiratory depressant effects may last longer than analgesic effects

Hydromorphone (Dilaudid)	1–3 mg slow IV 6 mg PO	0.015 mg/kg IV 0.03–0.08 mg/kg PO	2–5 IV	3–5 IV	1–3 IV	Hypersensitivity to hydromorphone; acute bronchial asthma; upper airway obstruction; increased intracranial pressure; severe respiratory depression; shock; occult hemorrhage; relative contraindication: severe hepatic or renal insufficiency	This injection contains benzyl alcohol Because of pain, the IM route should not be used in children
Morphine (various)	30 mg q 3–4 h PO 5–15 mg SC 1–4 mg slow IV	0.3 mg/kg q 3–4 h PO 0.1–0.2 mg/kg SC Neonates: 0.03 mg/kg IV < 6 mo: 0.05–0.1 mg/kg IV > 6 mo: 0.1–0.2 mg/kg IV	15–30 PO 20–40 SC 2–5 IV	3–4 PO 3–5 SC 1–3 IV	1–4 PO Adults: 1–4 IV Neonates: 4–13 IV	Hypersensitivity to morphine; acute bronchial asthma; upper airway obstruction; increased intracranial pressure; severe respiratory depression; relative contraindication: severe hepatic or renal insufficiency	Give 30–60 min before procedure or for pain control Because of pain, the IM route should not be used in children Adjust dosage for renal impairment Decrease dose by 1/2 if given with pentobarbital, hydroxyzine, diazepam, or other benzodiazepines (see Table 21–12)

*All intravenously administered medications marked with an asterisk (also inhaled nitrous oxide) should be used only by physicians familiar with their use within established guidelines for conscious sedation. These medications are intrinsically dangerous; physicians using them should be trained in airway management, including endotracheal intubation, or they should be administered under the direct supervision of an anesthesiologist.

CHF, congestive heart failure; G6PD, glucose-6-phosphate dehydrogenase; IM, intramuscular; IV, intravenous; NSAIDs, nonsteroidal anti-inflammatory drugs; PO, oral; SC, subcutaneous; SD, single dose.

Table 21-11 Topical Pain Management

Topical Analgesic Agents	Initial Adult Dosage	Initial Pediatric Dosage	Onset of Action (min)	Duration of Action (h)	Half-Life (h)	Contraindications	Comments
TAC, TEC (Most preparations are tetracaine 2%, epinephrine 1:15,000, cocaine 11.8%)	Apply to area for desired effect (about 0.5–1 ml)	Apply to area for desired effect (about 0.5–1 ml)	10–15	1–2, depending on dosage and concentration	Serum $t_{1/2}$ is 75 min	Hypersensitivity to cocaine, epinephrine, or tetracaine Avoid contact with mucous membranes; do not use on fingertips, toes, nose, or penis	Apply to facial laceration with dropper or gauze Use as little as possible in children to avoid cocaine intoxication
EMLA (eutectic mixture of local anesthetics, available as lidocaine 2.5% and prilocaine 2.5% cream)	Minor dermal procedure: 2.5 g/20–25 cm^2 of skin Major dermal procedure: 1.5–2 g/10 cm^2 of skin	Dosage based on weight; maximal application area to intact skin: up to 10 kg = 100 cm^2 10–20 kg = 600 cm^2 > 20 kg = 2000 cm^2	60	Persists 1–2 h after removal	Lidocaine: 1–2.5 (IV)[1] Prilocaine: 0.1–2.5 (IV)	Hypersensitivity to lidocaine or prilocaine Avoid use in infants younger than 3 mo (except for circumcision) and in those aged up to 12 mo who are also receiving methemoglobin-inducing agents	Apply 60 min before procedure In infants aged younger than 12 mo, EMLA should not be applied for more than 4 h Do not apply to mucous membranes
Lidocaine (Xylocaine)	Dosage varies and depends on the area to be anesthetized, vascularity of tissues, individual tolerance, and technique of anesthesia Administer the lowest dose possible	Dosage varies and depends on the area to be anesthetized, vascularity of tissues, individual tolerance, and technique of anesthesia Administer the lowest dose possible	Rapid	0.5–1	1–2.5 (IV) up to 10% of an absorbed dose May be excreted unchanged	Hypersensitivity to lidocaine Use with extreme precaution in patients with severe shock, severe heart block, or severely traumatized mucosa or sepsis in the region of application	Buffer lidocaine injection as a 1:10 mixture of 1 part of sodium bicarbonate solution in 9 parts of lidocaine to reduce pain of injection For topical use, available as 7.5% and 5% ointment, 0.5% cream

IV, intravenous; TAC, TEC, tetracaine, epinephrine (Adrenalin), and cocaine.

Table 21–12 Combination Therapy

Combination Analgesics and Sedative Medications	Recommendation for Dosing	Comments
Morphine and lorazepam	↓ lorazepam dose by 1/2	—
Morphine and midazolam	↓ midazolam dose by 1/2	—
Morphine and diazepam	↓ the dose of each by 1/2	—
Morphine and hydroxyzine	↓ the dose of morphine by 1/2, and use about 50 mg (0.5 mg/kg) of hydroxyzine	Hydroxyzine is not recommended for patients with history of seizures Hydroxyzine is painful when given intramuscularly
Morphine and pentobarbital	↓ the dose of each by 1/2	—

crease to approximately 50% 80 minutes after administration of a 1-hour intravenous infusion. The pharmacokinetics (rate of metabolism and elimination) of propofol are not affected by hepatic dysfunction or chronic renal failure. Pentobarbital and thiopental are both rapid-onset barbiturates. Chloral hydrate is a sedative in small doses (25–50 mg/kg) and a hypnotic in large doses (50–100 mg/kg). Ketamine is a dissociative anesthetic in large doses (1–2 mg/kg) and a sedative in smaller doses (0.25–0.5 mg/kg).

ANTAGONIST DRUGS OR REVERSAL AGENTS

Two agents are available for the reversal of certain drugs used to produce conscious sedation (Table 21–9). Flumazenil (Romazicon, formerly Mazicon) can be used to reverse benzodiazepines. Flumazenil does not reverse opioids or any class of medications except benzodiazepines. Naloxone (Narcan) can be given to reverse opioids.

MEDICATIONS FOR ANALGESIA

Additional systemic analgesic medications may be used to relieve pain associated with procedures (Table 21–10). For mild pain, inflammation, or fever, a nonsteroidal anti-inflammatory drug like ibuprofen can be used orally. Although not approved by the Food and Drug Administration for use in children, ketorolac has been used in 3- to 15-year-olds if the oral route cannot be used and can be given intramuscularly. There are rectal preparations available for indomethacin, aspirin, and acetaminophen, but these are less desirable and therefore rarely used for pain control. For mild to moderate pain or fever, acetaminophen with or without codeine can be employed. For severe pain, morphine can be given intravenously, orally, or subcutaneously.

Local analgesia and anesthesia are also needed for some procedures. A list of agents used for topical analgesia is included in Table 21–11. A combination of tetracaine, epinephrine (Adrenalin), and cocaine (TEC, TAC) has been used for topical application to anesthetize the skin before lacerations are closed. A eutectic mixture of local anesthetics (EMLA) has been developed with lidocaine and prilocaine. This mixture is applied to intact skin before venipuncture or lumbar puncture, for example, to anesthetize the skin. Finally, lidocaine alone is used by instillation for local anesthetic blocks.

MEDICATIONS USED IN COMBINATION

In a number of circumstances, two agents may be used together to produce both analgesia and sedation. There are no well-studied guidelines for adjusting the doses of these agents when they are used together. The recommendations listed in Table 21–12 are initial suggestions for adjusting doses of one or both of the agents employed. In most circumstances, one or the other of the medications is reduced in dose; the other medication may or may not need a reduced dose.

Acknowledgment

Special acknowledgment for helping with the writing of this article to Yvonne Brouard, M.D., Kevin Coulter, M.D., Ron Dieckmann, M.D., Rhonda Nichols, R.N., Colin Partridge, M.D., Nela Ponferrada, R.N., Donna Ferriero, M.D., and J. Renee Navarro, M.D.

Bibliography

Anderson AB, Colecchi C, et al: Local anesthesia in pediatric patients: topical TAC versus lidocaine. *Ann Emerg Med,* 19:519–522, 1990.

Armand JL, Vredevoe LA, et al: Lorazepam and morphine for IV surgical premedication. *Br J Anaesth,* 52:1259–1263, 1980.

Bahal-O'Mara N, Nahata MC, et al: Efficacy of diazepam and meperidine in ambulatory pediatric patients undergoing endoscopy: a randomized, double-blind trial. *J Pediatr Gastroenterol Nutr,* 16:387–392, 1993.

Beyer JE, Levin CR: Issues and advances in pain control in children. *Nurs Clin North Am,* 22: 661–742, 1987.

Bhatt-Mehta V, Rosen DA: Management of acute pain in children. *Clin Pharm* 10:667–684, 1991.

Bonadio W: TAC: a review. *Pediatr Emerg Care,* 5:128–130, 1989.

Cook BA, Bass JW, et al: Sedation of children for technical procedures: current standard of practice. *Clin Pediatr,* March:137–142, 1992.

Dieckmann RA: Rectal diazepam for prehospital pediatric status epilepticus. *Ann Emerg Med,* 23: 216–223, 1994.

Hubbard AM, Markowitz RI, et al: Sedation for pediatric patients undergoing CT and MRI. *J Comput Assist Tomogr,* 16:3–5, 1992.

Joyce TH: Topical anesthesia and pain management before venipuncture. *J Pediatr,* 122:S24, 1993.

Koren G: Use of the eutectic mixture of local anesthetics in young children for procedure-related pain. *J Pediatr,* 122:S305, 1993.

Koren G, Maurice L: Pediatric uses of opioids. *Pediatr Clin North Am,* 36:1141–1155, 1989.

Lefever EB, Potter PS, Seeley NR: Propofol sedation for pediatric MRI. *Anesth Analg,* 76:919–920, 1993.

Lugo RA, Fishbein M, et al: Complication of intranasal midazolam. *Pediatrics,* 92:638, 1993.

Lyons SM, Clarke RSJ, Vulgaraki K: Proceedings of the anaesthetic research society London meeting at the Research Department of Anaesthetics, Royal College of Surgeons, November 30, 1974. *Br J Anaesth,* 47: 630–631, 1975.

Maunuksela EL, Kokki H, Bullingham RES: Comparison of intravenous ketorolac with morphine for postoperative pain in children. *Clin Pharmacol Ther,* 52:436–443, 1992.

McDonald CF, Thomson SA, et al: Benzodiazepine-opiate antagonism—a problem in intensive-care therapy. *Intensive Care Med,* 12:39–42, 1986.

McEvoy GK (ed): *AHFS 94: Drug Information*, Bethesda, MD, American Society of Hospital Pharmacists, 1994.

McQueen KD: Midazolam routes of administration. *Ann Pharmacother,* 25:476–477, 1991.

Moss ML, Buongiorno PA, Clancy VA: Intranasal midazolam for claustrophobia in MRI. *J Comput Assist Tomogr,* 17:991–992, 1993.

Nahata MC: Sedation in pediatric patients undergoing diagnostic procedures. *Drug Intell Clin Pharm,* 22:711–715, 1988.

Rey E, Delaunay L, Pons G: Pharmacokinetics of midazolam in children: comparative study of intranasal and intravenous administration. *Eur J Clin Pharmacol,* 41:355–357, 1991.

Sacchetti A, Schafermeyer R, et al: Pediatric analgesia and sedation. *Ann Emerg Med,* 237–250, 1994.

Schuman AJ: A protocol for pediatric sedation. *Contemp Pediatr,* 11:74–89, 1994.

Selbst SM: Managing pain in the pediatric emergency department. *Pediatr Emerg Care,* 5: 56–63, 1989.

Sherwood KA: The use of topical anesthesia in removal of port-wine stains in children. *J Pediatr,* 122:S36–S40, 1993.

Singh PN, Sharma P, et al: Clinical evaluation of diazepam for relief of postoperative pain. *Br J Anaesth,* 53:831–835, 1981.

Snodgrass WR, Dodge WF: Lytic/"DPT" cocktail: time for rational and safe alternatives. *Pediatr Clin North Am,* 36:1285–1291, 1989.

Steward D: Eutectic mixture of local anesthetics (EMLA): What is it? What does it do? *J Pediatr,* 122:S21–S23, 1993.

Theroux MC, West DW, et al: Efficacy of intranasal midazolam in facilitating suturing of lacerations in preschool children in the emergency department. *Pediatrics,* 91:624–627, 1993.

Tipton GA, DeWitt GW, Eisenstein SJ: Topical TAC (tetracaine, adrenaline, cocaine) solution for local anesthesia in children: prescribing inconsistency and acute toxicity. *South Med J,* 82: 1344–1346, 1989.

Tverskoy M, Fleyshman G, et al: Midazolam-morphine sedative interaction in patients. *Anesth Analg,* 68:282–285, 1989.

US Department of Health and Human Services, Acute Pain Management, Clinical Practice Guideline: *Acute Pain Management in Infants, Children, and Adolescents: Operative and Medical Procedures.* AHCPR 92–0020.

US Department of Health and Human Services, Acute Pain Management, Clinical Practice Guideline: *Acute Pain Management: Operative or Medical Procedures and Trauma.* AHCPR 92–0032.

Watona M, Jones B, et al: Comparison of ketorolac and morphine as adjuvants during pediatric surgery. *Anesthesiology,* 76:368–372, 1992.

Yaster M: Analgesia and anesthesia in neonates. *J Pediatr,* 111:394–395, 1987.

Yealy D, Ellis JH, et al: Intranasal midazolam as a sedative for children during laceration repair. *Am J Emerg Med,* 10:585–587, 1992.

Zeltzer LK (co-ordinator), Altman A, et al: Report of the subcommittee on the management of pain associated with procedures in children with cancer. *Pediatrics,* 86(suppl):826–831, 1990.

Chapter 22

Withholding or Withdrawing Active Medical Treatment in Critically Ill Infants and Children

Neil T. Campbell, Peter M. Loughnan, and Peter N. McDougall

One third or more of deaths in pediatric intensive care units (ICUs) and one half to three quarters of deaths in neonatal ICUs follow withdrawal of life-sustaining treatments (Campbell, 1994; Carse and Yu, 1988; Mink and Pollack, 1992; President's Commission, 1983; Ryan et al, 1993). This chapter assumes that it is sound medical practice to withhold or withdraw (forgo) life-sustaining treatment from babies and young children when death is almost certain or when survival will result in serious permanent handicaps. It does not attempt to define "almost" or "serious." The aim is to describe processes rather than to debate ethical and legal matters.

BACKGROUND

Physicians and nurses working in critical care environments need to gain insight, early in their careers, into their own abilities and limitations and also into the limitations of high-technology medicine. They need to sort out attitudes concerning "quality" of life, "allowing" patients to die, and death itself because up to 15% of infants and children admitted to ICUs die. Unless professionals are able to discuss such matters comfortably with colleagues and patients' families, they should question their own aptitude for practicing critical care medicine. From time to time, they will be involved in patient care with which they feel uncomfortable or with which they actually disagree. This is inevitable; in life and death matters, no two people think exactly alike, and critical care medicine requires a team process.

Physicians and nurses in leadership roles in critical care environments should nurture an ethos in which the usual hierarchies and power relationships do not impede frank communication among all those involved with cases in which forgoing treatment may be an issue. No single professional group has a monopoly on truth in ethical matters. Valid insights vary from one professional to another and from one situation to another. All staff members in ICUs have ethical views that should be respected, and all are implicated ethically, legally, and emotionally in the decisions that are made. Inevitably, some decisions may be contrary to some staff members' individual views, and such differences should be acknowledged.

The ultimate decision to forgo treatment should belong to a child's parents. They must be adequately informed, counseled, and supported by health care workers and others whom the parents choose to involve, such as extended family, religious advisers, and friends. Unless their views are extreme, it is the values and judgments of parents rather than those of health care workers that should prevail.

PROCESS

Parents and health care workers make and implement the best decisions regarding forgoing treatments if they have time to think and adjust. Parents are better able to make decisions if they have established relationships of trust beforehand with physicians and nurses. They can have more difficulty if they are unexpectedly confronted with the need for a decision late in the course of their child's illness by a physician who is a stranger. To avoid this, a senior physician should be involved from the outset with families of children with a high risk of death or permanent handicap. This physician should introduce at the first interview, as one small part of the information given, the concept that forgoing treatment might at some stage need to be considered.

Fortunately, most children admitted to ICUs have a good prognosis for intact survival, so these considerations are irrelevant. Most children whose risks of death or severe handicap are high can be identified at or soon after admission.

In the past, professionals were taught that physicians should not "burden" families with pessimistic prognoses, because to do so indicated they could not handle their own anxieties and so had to unload them onto the parents. This is no longer true (if it ever was) in modern ICUs, where high technology can keep almost any child "alive" for a time, however hopeless the prognosis. Parents are therefore now more often in the position of having to consider forgoing treatment (Stinson and Stinson, 1983).

When hope of intact survival is fading, the need to consider forgoing treatment in a particular patient can be raised by physicians, nurses, other health care workers, or parents. If parents or the nurses are frequently the first to raise this question, it suggests that the physicians are not communicating effectively. In an optimally functioning ICU, the need will most often be raised first by medical staff.

When critical illness in a patient reaches the stage at which the physicians in charge believe that forgoing treatment must be considered, they should begin specific counseling of the parents, who have previously been prepared for such an eventuality. They should also facilitate the development of a consensus among the ICU staff members. How this staff consensus is achieved varies from place to place and time to time. Some units schedule meetings involving staff members of all levels; others have less formal processes. The important point is that all relevant staff members participate and that each member has the opportunity for input. The physician in charge should keep staff members informed of the progress of ongoing discussions with the family and include members of nursing staff in the discussions whenever possible. The unit social worker should be centrally involved both by accompanying the physician and also by meeting with parents at other times. Consensus does not mean that everyone in the team agrees; it means that everyone is committed to supporting and not undermining or obstructing the decisions of the family and the team as a whole. Staff members unable to do this should willingly withdraw from further involvement.

Discussions should occur on multiple occasions, when the clinical situation permits, to repeat and expand information and to answer new questions. In counseling the family, the physician must provide them with all the information needed to participate in the decision, in a language they understand and at a level appropriate to their intelligence and educational background. If they usually speak a language other than English, a professional interpreter experienced in these sorts of discussions, must be used. Family members or friends are often suitable interpreters for routine discussions, but they should not be used in canvassing treatment withdrawal.

Parents' misunderstanding of what seem to be straightforward words and phrases is a major problem. When physicians say a disease is progressing, they usually mean it is getting worse. Many parents think progressing means getting better. Parents can be puzzled by the physician's saying that he or she is "worried we might lose the child." They have no idea this means that the patient might die.

Although every patient is different, most critical care situations that a physician needs to explain to parents can be categorized into a relatively small number of scenarios. It is most useful for physicians involved in critical care to write out verbatim a number of the standard explanations they will use from time to time with parents and then go through each explanation, striking out all medical and technical words and replacing them as far as possible with everyday-English equivalents. Physicians can then rehearse the resulting documents, using this language as the basis for future counseling.

Knowledge about the body's need for oxygen, the circulation of blood, or the function of lungs should not be presupposed even in highly educated parents. The possibilities for misunderstandings never cease to surprise experienced clinicians. In particular, clinicians need to overcome any reluctance to use words such as "death" and "brain damage." "Severe intellectual handicap" has little meaning for many ordinary people, but "your child may never know who he is or who you are" conveys what is meant. "Severe cerebral palsy" or "spastic quadriplegia" may be unhelpful, but "he will not creep, crawl, roll, sit, or walk" has more meaning.

Although all of this information should be given as objectively as possible, the physician should not remain neutral. In most cases, physicians should indicate clearly what they believe should be done for the child. In addition to supplying factual information about the child's current grave situation and prognosis, they should explain what will happen if treatment is withdrawn, including what measures will be taken to ensure that the child does not suffer. They should outline options for the parents' involvement in the withdrawal process and discuss the legal status of what is proposed. Physicians should advise the parents of the availability of other expert opinions and advice. Physicians should counsel parents to include other family members, loved ones, and religious advisers, if any, in their own discussions. In particular, the parents should be advised that they have nothing to hide or be ashamed of in discussing their child's possible death from treatment withdrawal. In general, it is best for parental counseling to be performed by one physician, speaking for all subspecialists involved in the child's care. However, this physician should not conduct the process alone. A second physician should evaluate the clinical situation, including any other subspecialists' views, and meet with the parents at least once to offer an independent opinion and to ascertain that the parents are adequately informed, that they appear to understand, and what their views are. The second physician should summarize this consultation in the medical record. If a subspecialist apart from the physician in charge is centrally involved in the child's management, it is appropriate for that person to also speak with the parents, but care is required to prevent parents' confusion from inadvertent differences of emphasis and interpretation.

Others have proposed that parents not be the principal decision makers; they are in extreme emotional turmoil and may be unable to absorb complex information, and their own long-term interests may conflict with those of their child. Further, it is argued that it is inappropriate to burden them with the guilt of deciding their own child's death—physicians should protect them from this burden by shouldering it themselves. In our experience, almost all parents, given time, are able to absorb information and think rationally despite grief and anxiety. Attempts to relieve parents of possible guilt feelings, by trying to make it appear that decisions are really made not by them but by the professionals, do not succeed and in any case are inappropriate. Most parents wish to be involved in decision making and see it as natural and appropriate that the decision is theirs. A few do not, but with empathy and encouragement, they are able to indicate clearly that they want the intensive care staff to recommend an appropriate choice.

Occasionally, but rarely in our experience, parents insist on continuation of life-sustaining treatments despite all advice, when unit staff members believe and other informed opinion holds that treatment should be stopped. We think this is more likely to occur if no relationship between the parents and a single senior physician was established when the child was first admitted and if the need to consider forgoing treatment was raised with the parents for the first time at a late stage in the child's illness, rather than being a part of the counseling from the outset; it is especially likely when the staff members raising the issue at this late stage are virtual strangers.

There is no satisfactory solution to this dilemma because the caregivers' responsibilities to the child are in conflict with their responsibilities to the parents. The main considerations in our view are, on the one hand, that continuing treatment imposes senseless burdens on the child and on the staff members who have to provide care; on the other hand, a unilateral decision by staff members to withdraw treatment against parents' wishes can set the parents up for a lifetime of bitter anger and unresolvable grief and loss. This risk is especially so if staff members seek formal legal support for their actions.

One compromise is to continue all treatment in good faith while continuing, with sensitivity and avoidance of confrontation, to advocate withdrawal to the parents. If the reason for advocating withdrawal is that staff members believe death is almost inevitable despite all treatment, and the parents' views remain unchanged, then death may occur "naturally." This may mean withdrawal of some aspect of life-supporting treatment without the parents' knowledge. Thus, the interests of the child are protected, and the parents' chances of satisfactory grief resolution are maximized. We recommend this course as a last resort, and only when all informed opinion is that death is virtually inevitable regardless of treatment and parents are adamant that all treatment must be continued. If the medical reasons for advocating withdrawal are based on judgments about the child's future quality of life, then informed parents' views should be respected and treatment should be continued in good faith. However, professionals should continue with care and sensitivity to present their views to the parents.

Continuing treatment in good faith does not necessarily conflict with staff members' responsibilities to the child; the child may still die, or the parents may still change their minds. However, there is no place for half-measures in this situation, because this may bring about a worse outcome in the surviving child.

When the decision to forgo life-sustaining treatment is reached, all treatment modalities likely to prolong life should be withdrawn. Stated plainly, the decision means that caregivers believe the child is going to die soon regardless of treatment, or that quality of life with survival (as judged by the parents) is likely to be so poor that it is better the child not survive. There is no logic to partial withdrawal (for example, inotropic agents or antibiotics), and no interests of the child are served by such an approach because partial withdrawal is likely to prolong the process of dying. Partial withdrawal suggests that caregivers are incompletely convinced of the need to forgo treatment or else are unable emotionally to accept the reality. Decisions for partial withdrawal are thus usually made in the interest of ambivalent professionals rather than that of the child. Intravenous fluids and artificial nutritional techniques such as orogastric, nasogastric, and gastrostomy feeding are life-prolonging treatments and so should be withdrawn along with other measures. Not only does continuation lack logic, but it can also make the dying process symptomatically worse; withdrawal of fluids can be sound palliative care. In some patients, tube feeding may be the only life-prolonging modality to be withdrawn, for example, in babies with severe birth asphyxia who have managed to be weaned off mechanical ventilation but are subsequently found to be profoundly damaged (Frader, 1986; Paris and Fletcher, 1987). There is legal precedent for such decisions in adults in the British courts (Airedale NHS Trust v Bland, 1993).

When treatment withdrawal has been decided, parents should be given options for their involvement in the process. If the child is likely to die quickly (for example, coming off mechanical ventilation or essential oxygen therapy), would the parents like to hold the child in their arms before withdrawal and then through the dying process? Would they like to be given the child only after withdrawal? Or would they prefer no involvement? If the dying process is likely to extend through many hours or days, would they like to live in the hospital, or visit regularly, or take the child home, or have no involvement? Some parents immediately opt for close involvement, but many initially feel they will "not be able to cope" and so choose to distance themselves. Gentle, tactful persuasion, pointing out the naturalness of "not being able to cope," is fully justified and usually changes their minds. We believe that physicians, fearing paternalism, may in these situations abrogate their professional obligations to provide clear advice. In a study of our own experience in the forgoing of treatment,

96% of parents opted for the closest involvement in their child's death, many deciding only after persuasion (unpublished data). At follow-up, they were unanimous and positive in believing their involvement was the right decision—none regretted it.

When life-sustaining treatments are withdrawn, it is essential to ensure that the child is free from pain, fear, and other distress. Hypoxia from withdrawal of oxygen or ventilation is frightening until unconsciousness occurs. Other distress can include dyspnea from heart failure or lung disease; pain from unrelieved bowel obstruction, for example; aspiration or choking episodes from reflux or inability to cough or swallow; and hunger or thirst in children unable to suck or drink. Although many children will be unaware at the time of withdrawal, this is seldom certain. Whether extremely premature infants or children with gross malformations or destructive lesions of the brain are ever aware is a question for neurophysiologists and philosophers. Staff members in ICUs should err on the side of assuming the possibility of awareness. Parents often cannot believe their children are certainly and completely unaware, even when they are reassured repeatedly. In other children, awareness is evident. The only way of guaranteeing freedom from pain and distress is the administration of adequate analgesia and sedation. Concerns that these may cause or accelerate death should not influence staff members in their use. As well as ensuring the child's freedom from distress, analgesic administration serves a second valid function—it reassures parents and caregivers that the child is not distressed. This is especially important because agonal behaviors in moribund children—gasping, stridor, or convulsions, for example—can appear to parents and inexperienced caregivers as signs of severe distress. Adequate analgesia or sedation not only needs to be given, but needs to be *seen* to be given.

When infants in whom awareness is possible are being taken off mechanical ventilation or essential oxygen therapy, we use intravenous opiates, usually morphine, with or without a sedative such as midazolam, diazepam, or phenobarbital. For infants likely to live hours or days, we offer oral feeding and other fluids if possible. For those with evident or probable severe pain, we use intravenous or oral opiates. When pain is less severe, we use paracetamol together with sedatives such as phenobarbital or chloral hydrate.

Most infants for whom forgoing care is considered cannot take oral fluids. They may have craniofacial malformations or esophageal or bowel obstruction for which surgery has been withheld; brain malformation or injury resulting in poor airway reflexes, inability to suck and swallow, reflux, and aspiration; dyspnea from heart failure or chronic lung disease; and central nervous system depression from previously administered analgesics, sedatives, or anticonvulsants. When intravenous fluids and tube feedings are withheld, dyspnea from heart failure or lung disease improves, often remarkably, as dehydration develops. As oropharyngeal and gastric secretions diminish, choking and aspiration from depression of airway reflexes and reflux usually cease. Normal healthy infants are distressed from time to time by hunger and other discomforts, and often without apparent cause. In babies living many hours or days after treatment withdrawal, it is impossible to distinguish "normal" infant distress from distress arising from their medical condition. For the parents' as well as the infant's sake, it is best to err on the side of relieving all distress.

Around the time of withdrawal, parents should be given descriptions of how their child may behave and what physical changes will occur when treatment is withdrawn. They will manage better and have a less frightening experience if they know in advance of the possibility of gasping, stridor, crying, or seizures, especially when the advice is accompanied by strong reassurances about the use of analgesics and the effects these will have on any awareness the child may have. Color changes and the signs of dehydration and wasting also require discussion.

When death is likely to occur quickly, for example, from withdrawal of mechanical ventilation or essential oxygen therapy, there are numerous ways of managing the process. One approach that works well is as follows:

1. The patient, together with life-support systems, can be moved to a private area if this is available.
2. Junior medical and nursing staff members who are to be involved should be counseled and prepared in the same ways as the parents are.
3. Delays in withdrawal, once the decision has been made, impose additional burdens on the child. However, most experienced caregivers believe delays of even days are justi-

fied if they allow time for parents to adjust, arrange religious or cultural rituals, and ensure the presence of all family members and friends whom the parents wish to be involved. Parents should be encouraged to consider the presence of the child's siblings, other relatives, and friends at the withdrawal.

4. Staff members should ensure, by asking the parents, that all required religious and cultural rites have been carried out. Although this seems obvious, some parents are too overawed or distressed to assert these needs themselves.
5. Staff members should encourage and facilitate the gathering of mementos and keepsakes before death, such as photographs, video records, locks of hair, and foot- or handprints.
6. Staff members should cease or reverse muscle relaxants before treatment withdrawal, because movements in the child, especially eye opening, can be meaningful, treasured experiences for the parents.
7. When all is in readiness, the living child can be given to the parents to hold, with life-support systems continuing. Some parents can bear this only for minutes; others prefer to remain longer. Then, with the child in the parents' arms, intravenous morphine can be given if necessary, the parents' attention being drawn to its administration; the endotracheal tube and all other tubes, catheters, skin leads, and probes are removed, except for one intravenous line for further analgesia, if needed. The parents and attendants can then remain in the general ward or move to a private area.

   Alternatively, morphine can be given, and all the technologic devices can be removed, with the child still in the bed, radiant heater, or incubator. The child can then be given free of impediments to the parents. We prefer the former approach, however.

   During the dying process, reassurance and explanation of any distressing behaviors in the child need to be given to parents and junior staff members in attendance. Further intravenous analgesia may be appropriate as part of this assurance. It is important that parents be helped to understand that everything possible is being done to free the child of pain and fear.

   During the dying process and afterward, parents should be attended part of the time by staff members, but they should also be given periods alone with their child. They should be encouraged in rituals such as bathing the dead child, dressing the child in clothing of their choice, and any relevant religious or cultural rites. This is particularly important if tubes and wires have prevented normal cuddling from birth. Some parents will want to leave minutes after death; others will stay for many hours. They should also be given advice about funeral arrangements. As well, a decision about the previously discussed need for autopsy should be sought.
8. Arrangements for aftercare in the ensuing days and weeks by the social worker, or nursing and medical staff, should be made. Follow-up may include phone calls, review of autopsy findings, and counseling or referral if the grief process is atypical or destructive. If questions about brain death and organ donation have occurred, these complex issues should be discussed at a later date by a person knowledgeable in these areas.
9. Senior medical and nursing staff members should debrief junior staff members, encouraging them to discuss the episode and their feelings in relation to the death.

When the dying process is likely to proceed for many hours or days, there are again several valid ways of conducting the process. One that works well is as follows:

1. When death is likely within hours, life-sustaining treatments are continued to give parents time to adjust and to arrange for other family members and friends to be involved, for religious and cultural rites, and for the collection of all mementos as desired.
2. The physician and senior nursing staff should counsel junior staff members who will be involved to answer questions and offer support.
3. When the family is ready, the physician in charge, with attending nursing staff members and the parents, should withdraw current therapy such as oxygen, intravenous lines (except the catheter maintained for analgesia and sedation), and all other tubes, skin leads, and probes. The palliative care treatment orders should be written up in the presence of the parents and attending nurses, with explanation and discussion to ensure that all parties understand. The palliative care orders include what has been discussed and agreed with respect to oral

feedings, analgesics and sedatives, and such matters as airway suction for comfort, dressing of any wounds, and so on.

4. The child should continue to be nursed in the general ward except when taken elsewhere by the parents for privacy. Parents and junior staff members should know that the process is open and that nothing is concealed.
5. The parents should be encouraged to spend as much time with the child as possible. This may be in the ward, around the hospital for "walks," in-parent accommodation, or, if practicable, outside the hospital. Options for taking the child home include periods of a few hours, overnight, 1 or 2 days at a time, or until death.
6. If the dying process occurs for many days, the physician needs to see the parents frequently to repeat information, to answer new questions, and to reassure.

Maintenance of Adequate Medical Records

All senior physicians involved in the child's care should document in the child's hospital record their opinions about diagnosis and prognosis and their reasons for advocating forgoing treatment. They should describe the outcome of their discussions with parents, including remarks about the parents' comprehension and opinions. They should also include their views about the palliative care required, in particular providing supporting statements if drugs and dosages used could be controversial.

If the withdrawal and dying process extends for many days or weeks, the senior physician in charge and the physician giving a "second opinion" should make progress notes from time to time, including descriptions of the condition of the child—in particular noting that no changes have occurred requiring revision of the withdrawal decision, and noting the ongoing understanding of the parents, including that they remain well informed and in continuing agreement with the withdrawal decision. If pallative care includes drugs likely to shorten the child's life, the physicians should document the justification for their use, including the symptoms for which the drugs are being given, their effectiveness or otherwise, and observed side effects. The documentation should indicate that the drugs and symptoms are regularly reviewed for determining whether the drugs are still required; if dosages are increased, the reasons should be stated. Intensive care staff members other than the physicians should also regularly document the progress of the child and parents from their own perspective. This includes nursing staff, social workers, and hospital chaplains, if involved.

When caregivers from differing professional backgrounds are separately documenting progress, different emphasis and perspectives can lead to apparent conflicts. The physician in charge should ensure that information written in the hospital record by various caregivers does not inadvertently conflict, for example, that nursing notes on the child's condition or the parents' understanding of the situation does not inadvertently conflict with the medical documentation.

Inadvertent conflicts of documentation can readily occur and can be serious. For example, junior staff members may report that a baby is "awake and looking around" when the baby has extensive brain damage, or that a parent is "confused and angry" when the parent may be only expressing normal anxiety, grief, and frustrations. Such inadequacies in documentation can on occasion compound and prolong legal proceedings when issues involving the forgoing of active treatment reach the courts. In one case, treated in our department, protracted legal debate occurred as to whether there was documented evidence of distress in an infant receiving palliative care, before analgesia was commenced (Kuhse, 1992). Both medical and nursing staff members were cross-examined at length.

On occasion, true conflict may occur between staff members, or between parents and staff members. It is our opinion that such conflicts are best resolved by discussion between individuals. In rare cases, we have arranged for parents to meet with dissenting staff members so that they can express opposing views directly. In our opinion, institutional ethics committees rarely have a role in individual cases. Law courts are a last resort in the resolution of such conflicts.

For these reasons, ICUs should have written protocols documenting withdrawal processes, including the nature of any written documentation required. Such protocols may require input from informed lawyers.

In conclusion, we strongly support the concept of parental autonomy in these matters. The parents must be fully and adequately informed. Parental counseling and the withdrawal process itself require a considerable input of time from caregivers. On occasion, in some ICUs, high-technology treatment modalities are continued in children with a hopeless prognosis. Good palliative care is more appropriate. Optimal care of the patient in these situations requires a consensus supported not only by all staff members but also by parents.

References

Airedale NHS Trust v Bland. *All England Law Reports,* March 12, 1993, pp 821–896.

Campbell N: When care cannot cure: medical problems in seriously ill babies. In Beller FK, Weir RF (eds): *The Beginning of Human Life.* Dordrecht, Kluwer Academic, 1994.

Carse EA, Yu VYH: Deaths following withdrawal of treatment in a neonatal intensive care unit. *Proceedings 5th Asia-Oceania Congress of Perinatology,* Denpasar, 1988, p 55.

Frader J: Forgoing life-sustaining food and fluid. In Lynne J (ed): *By No Extraordinary Means.* Bloomington, Indiana University Press, 1986, pp 180–185.

Kuhse H: Quality of life and the death of Baby "M." *Bioethics,* 6:233–250, 1992.

Mink RB, Pollack MM: Resuscitation and withdrawal of therapy in paediatric intensive care. *Pediatrics,* 89:961–963, 1992.

Paris JJ, Fletcher AB: Withholding of nutrition and fluids in the hopelessly ill patient. *Clin Perinatol,* 14:367–377, 1987.

President's Commission for the Study of Ethical Problems in Medicine and Biomedical and Behavioral Research: Deciding to Forego Life-Sustaining Treatment. Washington, DC, US Government Printing Office, 1983.

Ryan CA, Byrne P, et al: No resuscitation and withdrawal of therapy in a neonatal and pediatric intensive care unit in Canada. *J Pediatr,* 123: 534–538, 1993.

Stinson R, Stinson P: *The Long Dying of Baby Andrew.* Boston, Little, Brown, 1983.

Section D

Cardiac

Chapter 23

Electrocardiogram

Daniel Stromberg

The electrocardiogram (ECG) is a recording of body surface electrical potentials generated by the heart. It is easily and non-invasively obtained and has therefore been used for many years to provide important information about cardiac anatomy and pathology. More specifically, ECGs are indicated in the evaluation of arrhythmias, atrial or ventricular hypertrophy, electrolyte changes, myocardial or pericardial infections/inflammation, myocardial ischemia/infarction, and congenital heart disease. The technology offers little aid, however, in assessment of myocardial function or measurement of cardiac chamber size.

Optimal use of the pediatric ECG depends on correct interpretation of the electrical recordings, which is in turn predicated on knowledge of normal cardiac electrophysiology and the differences between pediatric and adult ECGs. This chapter attempts to briefly familiarize the reader with those principles essential for understanding and evaluating pediatric ECGs.

EXPLANATION OF BASIC ELECTROPHYSIOLOGY AND WAVEFORMS

In the normal situation, electrical depolarization begins in the sinoatrial (SA) node, located near the junction of the right atrium and superior vena cava (Fig. 23–1). This SA nodal impulse, which usually sets the electrical pace for the entire heart, passes anteriorly, leftward, and inferiorly, depolarizing the right and left atria by contiguous spread and producing the P wave. Thereafter, the wave of depolarization arrives at the atrioventricular (AV) node, through which it passes at a slower velocity. This delay corresponds to the P-R interval on surface recording and functionally allows complete ventricular filling before ventricular contraction. The electrical impulse next moves rapidly through the bundle of His and traverses the right and left bundle branches in the ventricular septum. Septal activation occurs predominantly from left to right, in an anterior, superior direction, inscribing the Q wave on the ECG. The impulse then proceeds

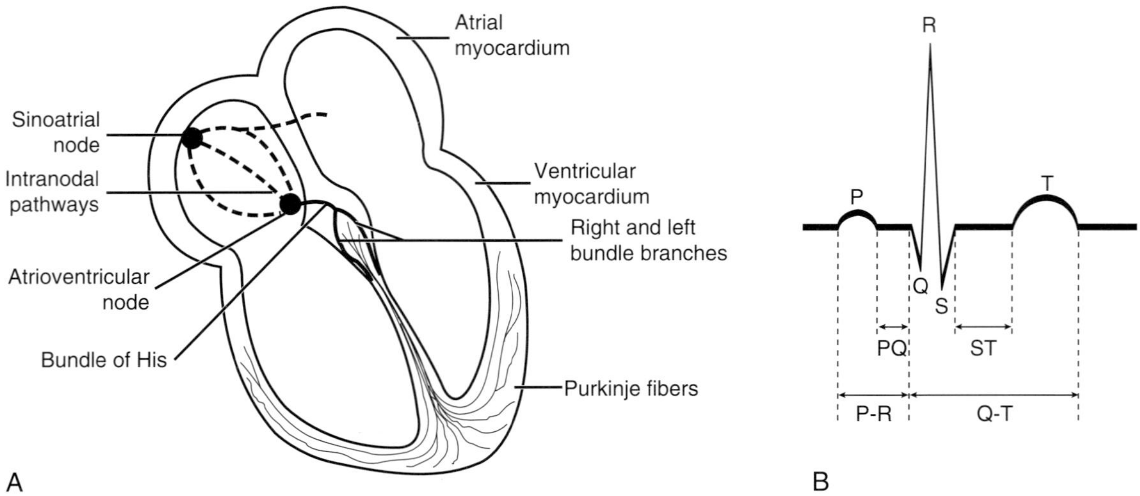

Figure 23–1 A. Diagram of the conduction system of the heart. **B.** Definition of electrocardiographic waveforms and intervals. (**B** redrawn from Park MK, Guntheroth WG: *How to Read Pediatric ECGs.* St Louis, CV Mosby, 1992.)

down the Purkinje fibers to the ventricular free walls, where the myocardium is depolarized from apex to base and from endocardium to epicardium, giving rise to the R and S waves of the QRS complex, which normally correspond to functional ventricular contraction. After a delay, repolarization of the ventricular myocardium ensues, albeit at a slower rate than depolarization, producing the ST segment and T wave of the ECG. Atrial repolarization is not commonly seen on ECG tracings because it is a low-voltage event that usually occurs at the time of higher voltage QRS complex inscription.

EXPLANATION OF RECORDING AXES

Surface tracings in a typical ECG are made in two body planes at right angles to each other—the frontal plane and the horizontal plane. This allows three-dimensional representation of the electrical vectors in the heart. Limb leads I, II, III, aVR, aVL, and aVF record electrical impulses in the frontal plane; precordial leads V_{3R}, V_{4R}, and V_1 through V_6 record voltages in the horizontal plane (Fig. 23–2). Lead I records the potential difference between the left arm and the right arm; lead II, the

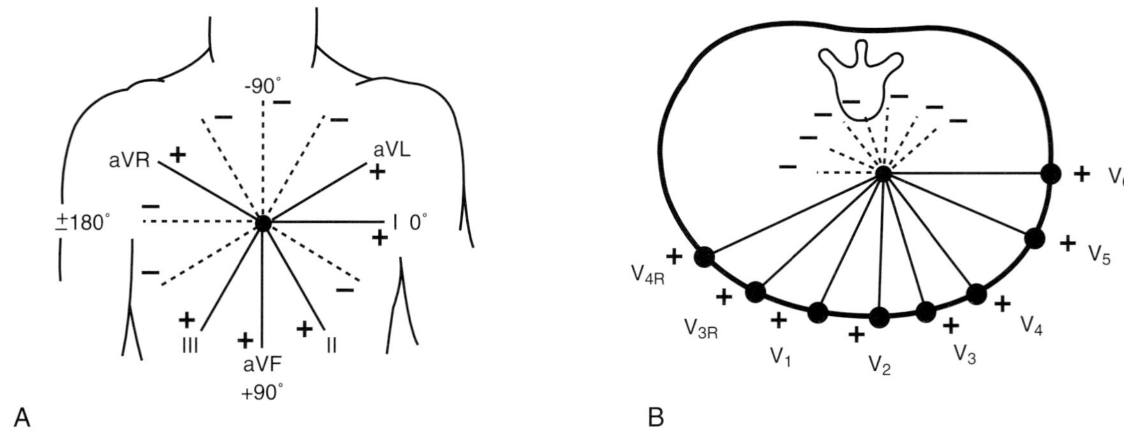

Figure 23–2 A. Hexaxial reference system (as it relates to frontal view of patient). **B.** Horizontal reference system (as it relates to transverse thoracic section). Leads are labeled, and positive poles are indicated by a plus sign. (Redrawn from Park MK, Guntheroth WG: *How to Read Pediatric ECGs.* St Louis, CV Mosby, 1992.)

difference between the left leg and the right arm; and lead III, the difference between the left arm and the left leg. Augmented leads, designated aVR, aVL, and aVF, are so named because the amplitude of voltage deflections is increased by 50% over those of the standard limb leads. Lead aVR inscribes vectors along an imaginary line between the left arm and left leg; aVL extends along an imaginary line between the right arm and left leg; and aVF measures voltages along a theoretical line between the right arm and left arm electrodes.

The leads of each individual plane are superimposed on each other and intersect at a central point of theoretical electroneutrality within the heart. Positivity or negativity of deflections occurring along a lead is determined by convention, as shown in Figure 23–2. Thus, for example, in lead I, impulses passing toward the left are inscribed as positive voltages, and those passing toward the right are inscribed as negative potentials. Similarly, in precordial lead V_1, located at the fourth intercostal space just to the right of the sternal border, impulses passing toward the electrode (i.e., toward the anterior chest) produce positive ECG deflections, whereas those passing posteriorly generate negative waves on the ECG.

By recording the heart's electrical impulses in a number of different locations simultaneously, the direction of the mean electrical vector, or *axis*, for any given part of the cardiac cycle may be determined. The axis is then evaluated relative to the heart's three-dimensional anatomy (i.e., relative to the vector's location in the aforementioned frontal and horizontal planes) to provide data useful in the diagnosis of disorders such as ventricular hypertrophy, bundle branch block, and congenital heart disease, to name a few.

METHODS AND PITFALLS

Given the need to record the heart's electrical activity from both the frontal and horizontal planes, the standard ECG is obtained with use of the previously mentioned limb (I, II, III, aVR, aVL, and aVF) and precordial (V_{3R}, V_{4R}, and V_1 through V_6) leads. Practically speaking, this entails placement of immobile electrodes on the left arm, right arm, left leg, and right leg (the last functioning as an electrical ground) and either eight stationary electrodes on the chest or one "floating" electrode that is moved to the various precordial positions between chest lead recordings (Fig. 23–3). Care must be taken to ensure good electrode contact with the skin. This can be accomplished by removal of hair at the connection site, mild skin irritation with a gauze pad, and removal of skin oil with an alcohol pad. Thereafter, one must either apply conductive gel to the electrode or use only those electrodes with adequate, nondried gel already in place.

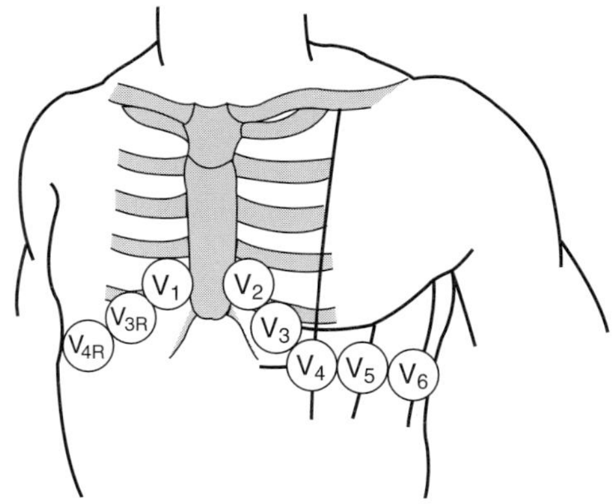

Figure 23–3 Precordial lead placement. V_1: right sternal border, fourth intercostal space (ICS); V_2: left sternal border, fourth ICS; V_3: equidistant between leads V_2 and V_4; V_4: left midclavicular line, fifth ICS; V_5: left anterior axillary line, horizontal to V_4; V_6: left midaxillary line, horizontal to V_4; V_{3R}: (on right chest) mirror image of V_3; V_{4R}: (on right chest) mirror image of V_4; V_{5R}: (on right chest) mirror image of V_5; V_{6R}: (on right chest) mirror image of V_6. (Redrawn from Park MK, Guntheroth WG: *How to Read Pediatric ECGs*. St Louis, CV Mosby, 1992.)

Once the electrodes are properly positioned and good electrical skin contacts are made, the ECG tracing may be recorded. The typical ECG records voltage per unit time at a paper speed of 25 mm/sec. Therefore, each millimeter, or small division on standard ECG paper, equals 0.04 second, and each larger division equals 0.20 second. The electrical sensitivity of the standard ECG is calibrated such that 1 mV of signal produces 10 mm of deflection above baseline (Fig. 23–4). When voltage deflections exceed the ability to properly record them, the voltage sensitivity may be decreased to half the standard setting. This adjustment should be marked prominently on the ECG tracing.

ECG recording quality may be greatly influenced by a number of technical difficulties, leading to significant artifact. Often this artifact is difficult to distinguish from pathological processes and can result in faulty ECG interpretation. One problem commonly encountered is interference from nearby alternating current sources, which produces a widened, fuzzy baseline. This may be avoided by making

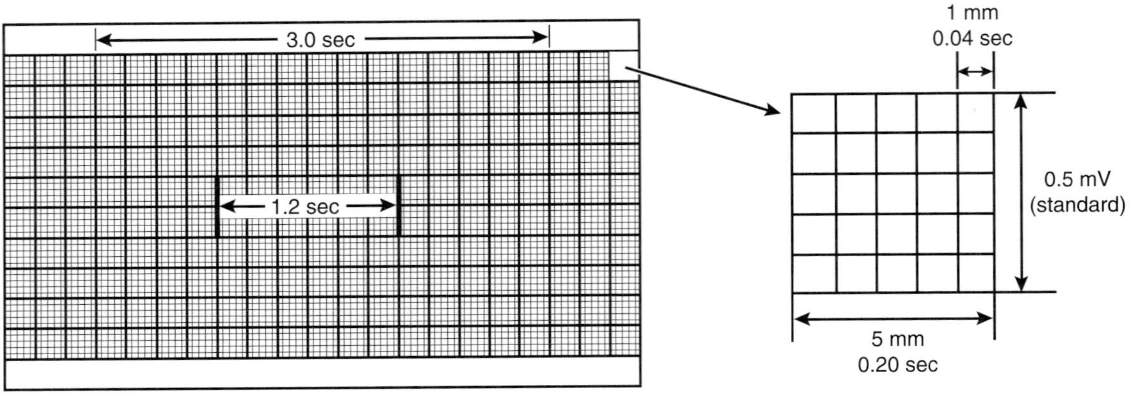

Figure 23–4 Standard ECG paper. Time is measured along the horizontal axis, with each 1 mm equal to 0.04 second and each 5 mm equal to 0.20 second. Three-second intervals are delineated by marks at the top of the ECG strip. The vertical axis measures electrical potential in millivolts. Standard calibration indicates that 1 mV is represented by 10 mm on the ECG record. (Redrawn from Park MK, Guntheroth WG: *How to Read Pediatric ECGs*. St Louis, CV Mosby, 1992.)

sure that the ECG cables are not draped across or parallel to other electrical cables. For the same reason, ECG cables should not touch metal parts of electrical equipment in contact with the patient.

Another common source of ECG artifact comes from the patient's movements. These may be as simple as turning over, shaking due to marked tremulousness, or tapping on an electrode. However, they can lead to marked baseline shifts and irregular deflections. Even normal respiration can produce some degree of cyclic tracing disturbances. Motion artifact can be minimized by obtaining the ECG with the patient in a relaxed posture (usually supine) and by connecting electrodes to areas where there is little skin movement (over bony areas rather than over large muscle masses, skin folds, and joints).

ECG errors may also be avoided by careful attachment of extremity leads to their proper limbs. Improper limb lead connection, such as switching of the right and left upper extremity leads, results in abnormal axes for the P, QRS, and T waves.

Attention should similarly be paid to precordial electrode placement. When precordial leads are applied on infants and small children, pediatric-sized electrodes should be used to guarantee recording from the desired chest position. Moreover, electrode paste from one precordial site should be removed before recording from the next location. Failure to do so may result in large, diphasic precordial ECG deflections resembling biventricular hypertrophy. Care should also be given to accurate placement of the electrode for V_1 in the fourth intercostal space. ECG tracings from the third intercostal space and above may demonstrate smaller precordial voltages.

SYSTEMATIC INTERPRETATION

Accurate reading of pediatric ECGs is accomplished by use of a systematic approach to interpretation, coupled with knowledge of the heart's electrophysiological adaptation to aging and illness. Although a complete discussion of ECG interpretation is beyond the scope of this chapter, information is presented to familiarize the general practitioner with the basic skills needed to examine a pediatric ECG. The following ECG elements must be considered:

- Rhythm (regular or irregular, sinus or nonsinus)
- Heart rate (atrial and ventricular)
- Axes (QRS, T, and QRS-T angle)
- Intervals (P-R, Q-R-S, and Q-T)
- P wave amplitude and duration
- QRS morphology and amplitude
- ST segment and T wave amplitude and morphology

After review of the ECG tracing itself, relevant factors of both the past and present clinical scenario must be examined. Such information should include the patient's age, current medications, and clinical diagnoses and the indication for the ECG study. In addition, prior ECG tracings should be obtained for comparison, if they are available.

Rhythm

The first task commonly associated with ECG interpretation is determination of the heart rhythm. A regular rhythm is described by a tracing in which all distances between consecutive R waves (the R-R interval) are the same. Irregular heart rhythms demonstrate variable R-R intervals. These can be further described as "regularly" irregular or "irregularly" irregular on the basis of the consistency of the abnormal rhythm pattern.

The second task involves differentiating sinus from nonsinus heart rhythms. Sinus rhythm, so named for the SA node initiation of the depolarization impulse, is found normally and meets the following three criteria: (1) there is one (and only one) P wave preceding each QRS complex, (2) the P wave axis must be between 0 and +90 degrees in the frontal plane, and (3) P waves must be uniform in appearance. Nonsinus rhythm is therefore suggested by an abnormal number of P waves before the QRS complex (either absence or more than one) or P waves with an abnormal axis or morphological appearance. This may be seen in a wide variety of conditions, such as third-degree AV block, AV nodal rhythm, and wandering atrial pacemaker.

Heart Rate

Heart rate varies with age (Table 23–1), level of consciousness and anxiety, and disease process. It can be rapidly determined from an ECG tracing by one of the following methods.

Table 23–1 Heart Rate (beats/minute) Variation with Age

Age	5%	Mean	95%
0–24 hours	94	119	145
1–7 days	100	133	175
8–30 days	115	163	190
1–3 months	124	154	190
3–6 months	111	140	179
6–12 months	112	140	177
1–3 years	98	126	163
3–5 years	65	98	132
5–8 years	70	96	115
8–12 years	55	79	107
12–16 years	55	75	102

1. For estimating regular rhythms only, find an R wave whose peak falls on a heavy vertical line on the ECG paper. Then count, in either direction, the number of *heavy* vertical lines until the next R wave peak. One line away corresponds to a rate of 300; two lines away to a rate of 150; three lines away to a rate of 100; four lines away to a rate of 75; and five lines away to a rate of 60. This is based on the fact that 1500 1-mm squares represent 1 minute on the ECG tracing. If one were to count the number of small squares between R wave peaks and divide that number into 1500, this would give the exact heart rate.
2. For irregular rhythms, count the number of cardiac cycles in a 6-second time period, as indicated by the 3-second interval marks at the top of the ECG strip. Multiply this number by 10 to determine the number of cycles, or heart rate, per minute.

In conditions such as complete (or third-degree) AV block and AV dissociation, the atrial and ventricular depolarization rates are different. The individual rates may be determined by the methods delineated before by use of P-P intervals for the atria and R-R intervals for the ventricles.

Axes

The axis of an ECG waveform corresponds to the direction of the mean electrical vector during a depolarization or repolarization impulse. Axis determinations can usually be made separately for each type of wave on the ECG tracing and routinely refer to vectors in the frontal plane.

Knowledge of a waveform's axis may provide information relevant to the diagnosis of a variety of cardiac conditions. The P wave axis is used to help distinguish between sinus and nonsinus rhythm and is normally 0 to +90 degrees in the frontal plane. The QRS axis is used to diagnose conditions such as ventricular hypertrophy and bundle branch block; its value changes with age (Table 23–2; see also later discussion). The T wave axis is evaluated in conjunction with the QRS axis to provide the QRS-T angle.

Because the waveform axes of clinical interest are usually those of the frontal plane, one need only review information from the six limb leads to calculate their values. This may be accomplished by use of the hexaxial reference frame (see Fig. 23–2) and the following evaluative process:

Table 23–2 Changes in QRS Mean Vector (Frontal Plane) with Age

Age	5%	Prevalent Direction	95%
0–24 hours	60	135	180
1–7 days	80	125	160
8–30 days	60	110	160
1–3 months	40	80	120
3–6 months	20	65	80
6–12 months	0	65	100
1–3 years	20	55	100
3–5 years	40	60	80
5–8 years	40	65	100
8–12 years	20	65	80
12–16 years	20	65	80

1. First decide whether the waveform in question is predominantly positive or negative in lead I by estimating the sum of all voltage deflections above (positive) and below (negative) the baseline. If the result is positive, the net vector is in the right hemicircle; if it is negative, the net vector is in the left hemicircle; and if it is zero, the net vector is at a 90-degree angle to the lead.
2. Second, determine the net positivity or negativity of the waveform in lead aVF. If positive, the vector points upward; if negative, it points downward; and if zero, it passes at 90 degrees to the right or left. This information from leads I and aVF should next be integrated to assign the vector to a quadrant consistent with the polarity of both leads.
3. Third, find a lead with an equiphasic form of the complex in question. The axis is perpendicular to this lead in the predetermined quadrant. In the alternative, one may find the lead demonstrating the greatest deflection of the wave in question. The axis is then known to be close to the direction of this lead in the predetermined quadrant.

Intervals

There are two intervals and two waveform durations that are routinely measured from the ECG. These are the P-R and Q-T intervals (see Fig. 23–1B) and the P and QRS durations. They are measured from the left margin of the baseline to the left margin of the baseline (or from right to right) to avoid artificially shortened or prolonged intervals and should be recorded in seconds (Fig. 23–5A).

The P-R interval represents the time required for atrial depolarization and physiological impulse delay in the AV node. Normal values for this time period are influenced by age and heart rate (Table 23–3). Abnormal prolongation may be seen in any process that delays AV nodal conduction, such as myocarditis, rheumatic carditis, digitalis intoxication, and hyperkalemia. Abnormally short P-R intervals can be seen in diseases that use accessory conduction pathways to excite the ventricles. Examples of these illnesses include

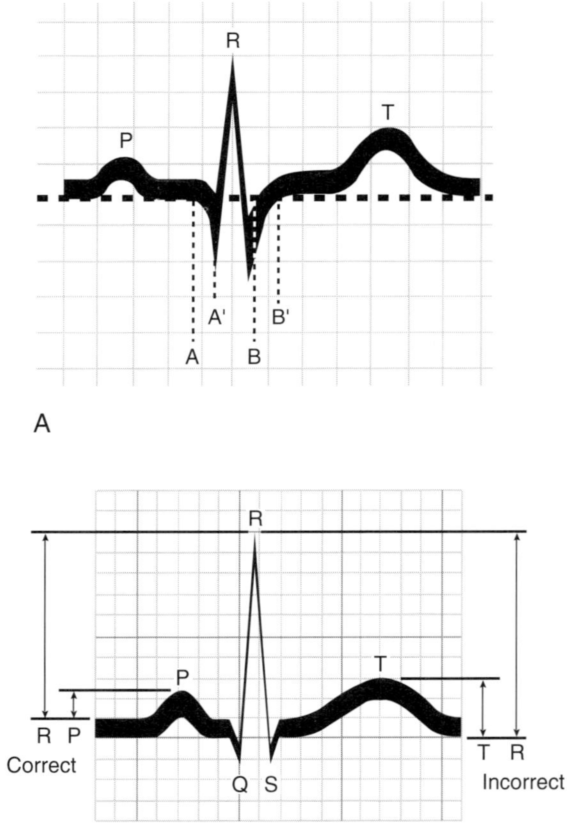

Figure 23–5 **A.** Measurement of waveform duration. Complexes should be measured from either the left to the left (*A–B*) or the right to the right (*A′–B′*) margin of the baseline. **B.** Measurement of waveform amplitude. Correct *(left)* and incorrect *(right)* methods of amplitude determination are demonstrated. (Redrawn from Park MK, Guntheroth WG: *How to Read Pediatric ECGs.* St Louis, CV Mosby, 1992.)

Table 23–3 P-R Interval Variation (and Upper Limit of Normal) with Age and Heart Rate

Rate	0–1 mo	1–6 mo	6 mo–1 y	1–3 y	3–8 y	8–12 y	12–16 y	Adult
< 60						0.16 (0.18)	0.16 (0.19)	0.17 (0.21)
60–80					0.15 (0.17)	0.15 (0.17)	0.15 (0.18)	0.16 (0.21)
80–100	0.10 (0.12)				0.14 (0.16)	0.15 (0.16)	0.15 (0.17)	0.15 (0.20)
100–120	0.10 (0.12)			0.12 (0.15)	0.13 (0.16)	0.14 (0.15)	0.15 (0.16)	0.15 (0.19)
120–140	0.10 (0.11)	0.11 (0.14)	0.11 (0.14)	0.12 (0.14)	0.13 (0.15)	0.14 (0.15)		0.15 (0.18)
140–160	0.09 (0.11)	0.10 (0.13)	0.11 (0.13)	0.11 (0.14)	0.12 (0.14)			(0.17)
160–180	0.10 (0.11)	0.10 (0.12)	0.10 (0.12)	0.10 (0.12)				
> 180	0.09	0.09 (0.11)	0.10 (0.11)					

Wolff-Parkinson-White syndrome and Lown-Ganong-Levine syndrome. Patients with glycogen storage disease type IIA may also demonstrate shortened P-R intervals on the ECG. Variable P-R intervals occur with wandering atrial pacemakers and with Mobitz type I second-degree AV block (Wenckebach phenomenon).

The Q-T interval, measured from the beginning of the Q wave to the end of the T wave, represents the time required for ventricular depolarization and repolarization. It varies with heart rate and is therefore interpreted in relation to it by calculating a "corrected" Q-T interval value (QT_c). The QT_c is determined by the following formula:

$$QT_c = \frac{\text{measured QT}}{\sqrt{\text{R-R interval}}}$$

The QT_c normally does not exceed 0.425 sec, except in infants younger than 6 months, in whom it may nonpathologically reach 0.49 sec. Prolonged QT_c intervals may be found in conditions such as hypocalcemia, myocarditis, and prolonged QT syndrome and with use of the antiarrhythmics quinidine and procainamide. Shortened QT_c intervals are observed with hypercalcemia and digitalis effect.

P Wave Morphology

The P wave represents atrial depolarization. Its axis is normally between 0 and +90 degrees and does not vary with age. An axis greater than +90 degrees is indicative of mirror-image dextrocardia or a complex congenital lesion with the right atrium abnormally located on the left (as in asplenia or polysplenia syndrome). An axis less than 0 degrees may be seen in nodal rhythms with retrograde atrial activation or in the presence of an ectopic low atrial pacemaker.

The normal P wave amplitude is less than 3 mm. Greater amplitudes are seen with right atrial hypertrophy. Left atrial hypertrophy produces a notched, prolonged P wave of duration greater than the 0.10 second upper limit of normal.

QRS Complex Morphology

The QRS complex represents the electrical waveform of ventricular depolarization. Its axis changes with age from a mean of +125 degrees in the neonatal period to +65 degrees by young adulthood (see Table 23–2). Abnormalities of the QRS axis are found with ventricular conduction disturbances, myocardial hypertrophy, and specific forms of congenital heart disease.

The duration of the QRS complex indicates the time required for ventricular depolarization. This period increases with age (Table 23–4), thereby establishing age-specific criteria for the determination of true QRS complex prolongation. Accurate assessment of the QRS

Table 23–4 Changes in QRS Duration with Age: Average (and Upper Limit)

	0–1 mo	1–6 mo	6 mo–1 y	1–3 y	3–8 y	8–12 y	12–16 y	Adult
Seconds	0.05 (0.065)	0.05 (0.07)	0.05 (0.06)	0.06 (0.07)	0.07 (0.08)	0.07 (0.09)	0.07 (0.10)	0.08 (0.10)

duration is important (Fig. 23–5A) because abnormal increases are due to either a delay or an abnormal spread of the depolarization impulse through the ventricular myocardium. This irregularity may be seen in conditions such as bundle branch block, pre-excitation syndromes (e.g., Wolff-Parkinson-White syndrome), ventricular ectopy, ventricular tachycardia, hyperkalemia, or group 1a (e.g., quinidine, procainamide) antiarrhythmic intoxication.

The QRS amplitude is also critical to pediatric ECG interpretation (see Fig. 23–5B for method of accurate amplitude determination). Abnormally large voltage measurements, when positive or negative, may be used to establish the diagnosis of ventricular hypertrophy or ventricular conduction disturbances. Low-voltage QRS complexes may be observed in normal newborn infants, hypothyroidism, or pericarditis. Tables 23–5 and 23–6 show mean and upper limit of normal R and S voltages according to lead and age.

In addition to carefully analyzing the QRS complex for axis, duration, and amplitude, one must look closely for the presence of Q waves, which represent the depolarization of the ventricular septum. These waveforms, defined as the initial downward deflections of QRS complexes, are commonly present in leads I, II, III, aVF, V_5, and V_6. The average Q wave duration should not exceed 0.03 second, and the amplitude should not exceed 6 mm. Unusually deep Q waves may be seen in ventricular hypertrophy. Abnormally deep *and* wide Q waves, or notched Q waves, may be found in the setting of myocardial ischemia, myocardial infarction, and myocardial fibrosis.

ST and T Wave Morphology

The ST segment is that portion of the ECG tracing inscribed after ventricular depolarization (QRS complex) and before ventricular repolarization (T wave). It is usually horizontal and isoelectric, although it may vary normally by 1 to 2 mm, either up or down, in the left precordial leads. ST segment elevation beyond this amount may be associated with acute pericarditis or myocardial ischemia/infarction. ST segment depression may similarly be observed in myocardial ischemia/infarction but is also seen with hypokalemia and digitalis effect. Severe ventricular hypertrophy may produce a

Table 23–5 R Voltage* (and Upper Limit of Normal) According to Lead and Age

Lead	0–1 mo	1–6 mo	6 mo–1 y	1–3 y	3–8 y	8–12 y	12–16 y	Young Adults
I	4 (8)	7 (13)	8 (16)	8 (16)	7 (15)	7 (15)	6 (13)	6 (13)
II	6 (14)	13 (24)	13 (27)	13 (23)	13 (22)	14 (24)	14 (24)	9 (25)
III	8 (16)	9 (20)	9 (20)	9 (20)	9 (20)	9 (24)	9 (24)	6 (22)
aVR	3 (7)	3 (6)	3 (6)	2 (6)	2 (5)	2 (4)	2 (4)	1 (4)
aVL	2 (7)	4 (8)	5 (10)	5 (10)	3 (10)	3 (10)	3 (12)	3 (9)
aVF	7 (14)	10 (20)	10 (16)	8 (20)	10 (19)	10 (20)	11 (21)	5 (23)
V_{4R}	6 (12)	5 (10)	4 (8)	4 (8)	3 (8)	3 (7)	3 (7)	
V_1	15 (25)	11 (20)	10 (20)	9 (18)	7 (18)	6 (16)	5 (16)	3 (14)
V_2	21 (30)	21 (30)	19 (28)	16 (25)	13 (28)	10 (22)	9 (19)	6 (21)
V_5	12 (30)	17 (30)	18 (30)	19 (36)	21 (36)	22 (36)	18 (33)	12 (33)
V_6	6 (21)	10 (20)	13 (20)	12 (24)	14 (24)	14 (24)	14 (22)	10 (21)

* In millimeters; 10 mm = 1 mV.

Table 23-6 S Voltage* (and Upper Limit of Normal) According to Lead and Age

Lead	0–1 mo	1–6 mo	6 mo–1 y	1–3 y	3–8 y	8–12 y	12–16 y	Young Adults
I	5 (10)	4 (9)	4 (9)	3 (8)	2 (8)	2 (8)	2 (8)	1 (6)
V_{4R}	4 (9)	4 (12)	5 (12)	5 (12)	5 (14)	6 (20)	6 (20)	
V_1	10 (20)	7 (18)	8 (16)	13 (27)	14 (30)	16 (26)	15 (24)	10 (23)
V_2	20 (35)	16 (30)	17 (30)	21 (34)	23 (38)	23 (38)	23 (48)	14 (36)
V_5	9 (30)	9 (26)	8 (20)	6 (16)	5 (14)	5 (17)	5 (16)	
V_6	4 (12)	2 (4)	2 (4)	2 (4)	1 (4)	1 (4)	1 (5)	1 (13)

* In millimeters; 10 mm = 1 mV.

"strain" pattern on the ECG with either elevated or depressed ST segments.

The T wave inscribes the electrical events associated with ventricular repolarization. Its amplitude in V_6 should be less than 7 mm when the patient is younger than 1 year and less than 9 mm when the patient is older than 1 year. Tall, peaked T waves are associated with hyperkalemia and cerebrovascular accidents. Low T waves may be seen in a variety of conditions, including hypokalemia, hypothyroidism, pericarditis, myocarditis, myocardial ischemia, and digitalis effect. Low-voltage T waves may also be seen in normal newborn infants. The T wave axis changes with age as described later.

PHYSIOLOGICAL AND NONPHYSIOLOGICAL ALTERATIONS

Changes with Age

ECG findings vary with age as a reflection of the heart's age-related maturation. The predominant changes are due to alteration of the right ventricular to left ventricular weight ratio. At birth, the right ventricle is heavier and thicker than the left ventricle. During the first month of life, the left ventricle's weight increases rapidly, surpassing that of the right ventricle and reaching the doubling point by 6 months (Table 23–7). Although there is a wide range of normality, the ECG demonstrates this by gradual transformation from right ventricular dominant forces to left ventricular dominance. Over time, the right, anterior QRS axis of infancy is directed leftward and posteriorly; R wave amplitude in the right precordial leads decreases, whereas that of the left precordial leads increases; S wave voltages in the right precordial leads increase, whereas those of the left precordial leads decrease. The T wave of ventricular repolarization is upright in V_1 (anterior) in the immediate postnatal period. This becomes posterior by the fourth day of life (failure to do so is suggestive of right ventricular hypertrophy), where it may remain until approximately age 10 years, when it then shifts to an anterior bearing. However, the T wave axis in the frontal plane remains oriented to the left at all ages.

Because the T and QRS vectors do not follow the same progression in childhood, the angle between them (the QRS-T angle) changes over time. In early infancy, the angle may normally be wide (mean of approximately +130 degrees). Thereafter, it falls to less than 60 degrees by the age of 3 months, where it remains. This value is noteworthy because the QRS-T angle is a sensitive indicator of abnormalities in the ventricular repolarization process; widening is seen in conditions such as ventricular hypertrophy with strain, ventricular conduction disturbance, or metabolic or ischemic myocardial dysfunction.

Table 23-7 Changes in Left Ventricle/Right Ventricle Weight Ratio with Age

Age	Left Ventricle/Right Ventricle Weight Ratio
30 weeks' gestation	1.2 : 1
33 weeks' gestation	1.0 : 1
36 weeks' gestation	0.8 : 1
At birth	0.8 : 1
1 month	1.5 : 1
6 months	2.0 : 1
Adult	2.5 : 1

Another notable age-related variation in the ECG is the decrease in heart rate with time (Table 23–1). Normal ranges change from 100 to 175 in the immediate newborn period to 55 to 102 for adolescents and adults. Accompanying the change in heart rate over time is a simultaneous increase in P-R, Q-R-S, and Q-T intervals.

In comparison to full-term newborns, premature neonates manifest several differences in their ECGs. First, because they generally have left ventricles that are heavier than right ventricles (less so with advancing gestational age; see Table 23–7), they demonstrate less right ventricular dominance and greater leftward forces. QRS axes are oriented farther to the left, and T waves in V_1 are commonly negative. Second, the voltages of the QRS complexes and T waves are diminished in the standard limb leads. Furthermore, it has been shown that premature infants have shorter P-R, Q-R-S, and Q-T intervals than do full-term counterparts.

Physiological Changes

The ECG tracing is subject to alteration by physiological benign processes that may produce changes mimicking heart disease. Besides the previously mentioned motion artifact that can be created by normal respiration or purposeful movement, nonpurposeful movements common in the pediatric population may confuse tracing interpretation. Two such examples are the tremors of the "jittery" newborn and hiccoughs. Tremors may give rise to deflections simulating tachyarrhythmias; hiccoughs may produce monophasic or biphasic spiked waves similar in appearance to interpolated beats.

Ingestion of food or cold liquids may also influence the ECG. In both children and adults, iced drinks may cool the esophagus and anatomically related left ventricular inferior wall, causing T wave inversion in the left precordial leads. Likewise, T wave inversion can be observed after a large meal is eaten (an effect thought to be secondary to transient hyperglycemia). These abnormalities are transient and disappear on repeated ECG performed in the fasting state.

Other physiological ECG variants worthy of note include the following:

1. Evidence of early ventricular repolarization before depolarization of all the ventricular myocardium is complete. In this situation, large, upright T waves and elevated ST segments are found in the chest leads, which are suggestive of pericarditis; however, unlike in pericarditis, T waves remain large, and they do not become sharply inverted 2 to 4 weeks later.
2. Isolated inversion of the T waves in leads over the left ventricular apex. This condition, the cause of which is uncertain, may be present intermittently and is found most often in young males.
3. Increased waveform voltages (to the point of ventricular hypertrophy diagnosis) with T wave inversion. These may be normal findings in athletes in peak training condition.

Electrolyte Abnormalities

The ECG may be profoundly altered by abnormalities of both serum potassium and calcium. Hypokalemia, usually at serum potassium concentrations less than 2.5 mEq/L, is associated with depressed ST segments, flat or diphasic T waves, and prolonged Q-T intervals. It is also associated with the appearance of U waves, which are postulated to arise from prolonged repolarization of the Purkinje fibers (Fig. 23–6A). Because electrical instability is increased in this condition, the following dysrhythmias may be observed: premature ventricular complexes (PVCs), atrial tachycardias, junctional tachycardias, ventricular tachycardias, and ventricular fibrillation.

ECG evidence of hyperkalemia moves through a sequence of abnormalities as the serum potassium concentration progressively increases (Fig. 23–6B). Initially tall, symmetrically peaked T waves are seen, followed by QRS widening, P-R interval prolongation, and P wave flattening. With further increments, broad, diphasic sinusoidal waves emerge that may ultimately lead to asystole.

Abnormalities of the serum calcium concentration may result in changes in the ST segment of the ECG tracing. In hypocalcemia, the ST segment is prolonged, lengthening the Q-T interval, without effect on the morphological appearance of the QRS or T waves. Concurrent hypomagnesemia may aggravate these effects, such that clinical improvement may not occur despite calcium repletion, until adequate magnesium has been provided. In hypercalcemia, the ST segment is shortened, with resultant shortening of the QT_c (Fig. 23–7).

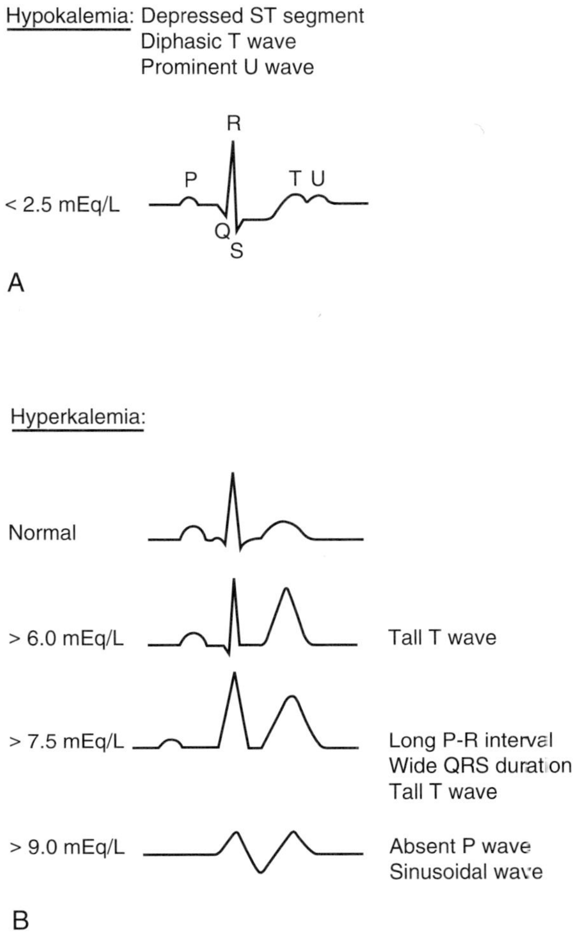

Figure 23–6 **A.** ECG appearance of hypokalemia. **B.** ECG progression with increasing hyperkalemia.

Atrial Hypertrophy

Hypertrophy of one or both of the atria is seen in a variety of clinical circumstances. Identification of this condition by ECG is accomplished by recognition of increased P wave amplitude or duration; P wave axis remains unaltered. Because the right atrium is depolarized first owing to its proximity to the SA node, the initial part of the P wave deflection represents right atrial impulses. The terminal portion of the waveform is contributed by left atrial depolarization. As a result, right atrial hypertrophy is suggested by tall P waves (greater than 3 mm in any lead, but most often seen in lead II), usually of normal duration. Left atrial hypertrophy, however, is associated with P wave prolongation, a "notched" P wave appearance in the limb leads, and a diphasic appearance in V_1. Combined atrial hypertrophy is diagnosed by fulfilling criteria for both right and left atrial hypertrophy, that is, P wave amplitudes in excess of 3 mm *and* durations greater than 0.10 second (Figs. 23–8 and 23–9).

Ventricular Hypertrophy

Making the diagnosis of ventricular hypertrophy in childhood is difficult because (1) variations in the normal position of the heart and the shape of the chest may interfere with accurate surface recording of the cardiac potentials and (2) there is a wide range of normal values for the ECG criteria used in diagnosis. As a result, the ECG should be evaluated fully for a preponderance of evidence supportive of the

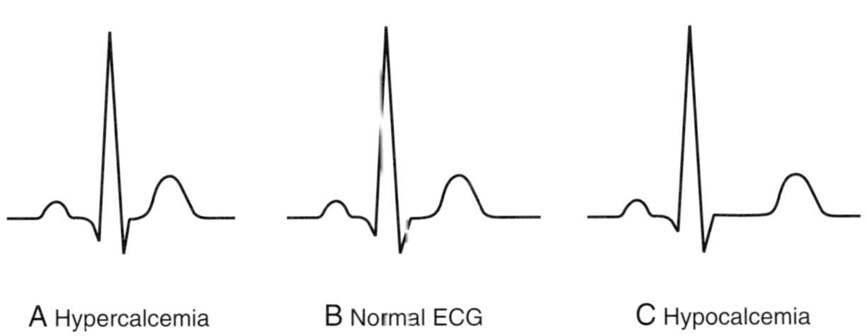

Figure 23–7 **A.** ECG in hypercalcemia. ST segment is shortened, which results in a decreased QT_c. The T wave is unaffected. **B.** Normal ECG. **C.** ECG in hypocalcemia. ST segment is prolonged, with resultant lengthening of the QT_c.

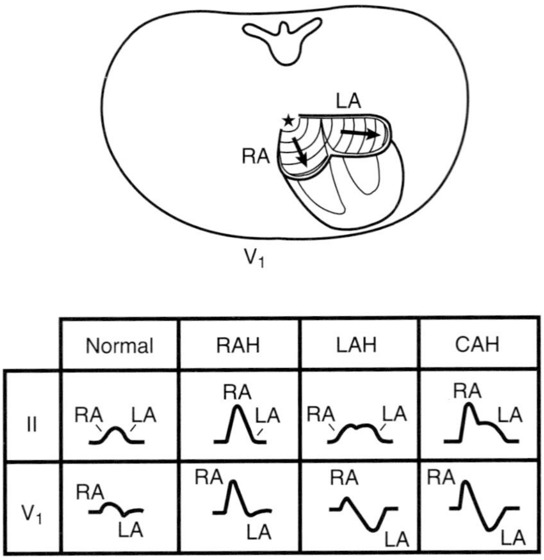

Figure 23–8 Cross-sectional diagram of the heart depicting the direction of the atrial depolarization vector, and expected lead II and V_1 ECG changes in the P wave with right atrial hypertrophy (RAH), left atrial hypertrophy (LAH), and combined atrial hypertrophy (CAH). LA, left atrium, RA, right atrium. (Redrawn from Park MK, Guntheroth WG: *How to Read Pediatric ECGs.* St Louis, CV Mosby, 1992.)

diagnosis of ventricular hypertrophy; no single sign should be relied on, in isolation, for final determination of this condition. ECG abnormalities commonly produced by ventricular hypertrophy include alteration of the QRS axis and QRS voltage, alteration of ventricular repolarization (bringing about a strain pattern), and miscellaneous changes in QRS or T wave appearance. Widening of the QRS complex, as may be seen in interventricular conduction delays or Wolff-Parkinson-White syndrome, precludes the ECG diagnosis of ventricular hypertrophy.

In right ventricular hypertrophy, there is right axis deviation, with an increased rightward and anterior QRS vector. This gives rise to taller R waves and smaller S waves in the right chest leads, and smaller R waves and augmented S waves in the left chest leads. In frontal projection, the bulk of right ventricular mass lies rightward and inferior to the heart's center of gravity, thereby producing increased R voltages in leads aVR and III and increased S voltages in leads I and aVL. Abnormal QRS voltage amplitudes must be interpreted in light of normative values for age because these change in infants and children as they grow. The more abnormal the observed QRS voltages, the more likely the diagnosis of ventricular hypertrophy. Other findings consistent with the diagnosis of right ventricular hypertrophy include a pure R wave or qR pattern in the right chest leads or an upright T wave in V_{4R} and V_1 between 4 days and 8 years of age.

Right ventricular hypertrophy with strain, implying abnormal ventricular repolarization secondary to relative ischemia of the hypertrophied myocardium, is described by presence of a widened QRS-T angle with the T axis outside the normal range of 0 to +90 degrees (usually in the 0 to −90 degree quadrant). ST

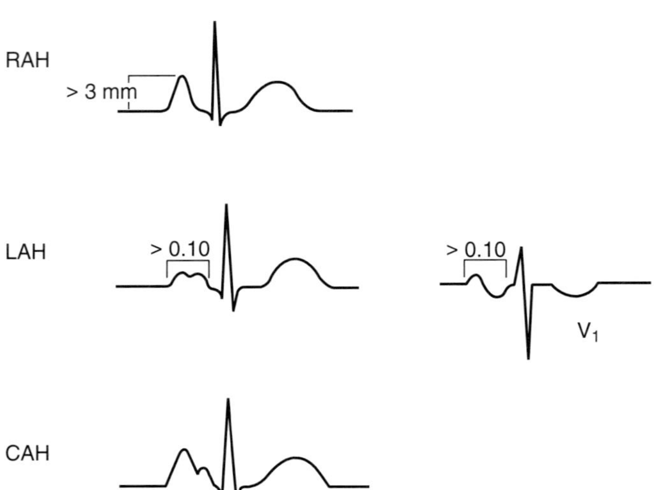

Figure 23–9 ECG appearance of right atrial hypertrophy (RAH), left atrial hypertrophy (LAH), and combined atrial hypertrophy (CAH). Criteria for ECG diagnosis are depicted. (Redrawn from Park MK, Guntheroth WG: *How to Read Pediatric ECGs.* St Louis, CV Mosby, 1992.)

segment depression or elevation may also be observed.

The physiological right ventricular hypertrophy of the newborn resulting from normal right ventricular dominance in utero makes postnatal diagnosis particularly difficult. Upright T waves in V_1 (with an upright T wave in V_6) after 3 days of age are strongly suggestive, as is right axis deviation greater than 190 degrees in infants younger than 1 week, or 105 degrees in infants older than 1 month.

The left ventricular mass lies leftward and inferior in frontal projection and leftward and posterior in horizontal projection. Therefore, left ventricular hypertrophy generates large R waves in leads I, II, aVL, and aVF and tall R waves and small S waves in V_5 and V_6. The QRS axis is similarly influenced by the left ventricle's anatomical position, with left ventricular hypertrophy producing a frontal plane axis between 0 and +90 degrees; values less than 30 degrees in infancy are particularly indicative of left ventricular hypertrophy. In the horizontal plane, the QRS axis is posteriorly directed, thereby giving rise to decreased R waves and increased S waves in V_1. Although axis deviation may be helpful for diagnosis of left ventricular hypertrophy in infants, it is less reliable in older children, who may normally have an axis that is leftward, posterior, and inferior in direction. Therefore, voltage criteria for the diagnosis are used more reliably.

Left ventricular hypertrophy with strain, as with right ventricular hypertrophy, is manifested by a wide QRS-T angle with the T vector in an abnormal quadrant. Furthermore, T waves may appear flat or inverted in aVF or the left precordial leads.

Many forms of congenital heart disease produce biventricular hypertrophy from pressure or volume stresses on both ventricles. This situation may result in ECG waveforms that simultaneously satisfy criteria for right ventricular hypertrophy and left ventricular hypertrophy. However, cancellation of opposing forces from the right ventricle and the left ventricle can occasionally produce normalization of the deflection amplitudes, obscuring this diagnosis.

Ventricular Conduction Disturbances

Ventricular conduction abnormalities are relatively common in pediatrics, the most common disturbance being right bundle branch block (RBBB) or a variant of this condition stemming from right ventricular volume overload. Mechanistically, RBBB arises from actual blockage of the right ventricular depolarization impulse as it travels down the right bundle branch of the Purkinje system, leading to propagation of the normally conducted left ventricular depolarization impulse through the right ventricular myocardium. Because myocardial conduction velocity is much slower than that of the Purkinje fibers themselves, depolarization is delayed, and left ventricular and right ventricular forces, which once opposed each other, are now offset and do not counter one another. This produces (1) prolongation of the terminal portion of the QRS complex, (2) increased leftward and rightward ventricular forces, (3) wide R′ waves in the right precordial leads and aVR (the initial r wave of the QRS complex comes from the unopposed leftward force of normal septal depolarization), and (4) slurred S waves in the left precordial leads and lead I.

The aforementioned variant of RBBB appears as a result of right ventricular volume overload or after open heart surgery involving right ventriculotomy. In these situations, the right bundle branch itself is not blocked, but rather the path of the depolarization impulse is lengthened or disturbed. This increases the duration of right ventricular depolarization compared with that of the left ventricle, although the degree of resultant QRS complex prolongation is usually mild. On the ECG, one may again see an rSR′ pattern in V_1 as well as the other stigmata of RBBB.

True blockage of the left bundle branch impulse (a rare occurrence in pediatrics) proceeds by the same mechanism as true RBBB, in the opposite direction. Septal depolarization occurs from right to left, as does the delayed left ventricular myocardial depolarization. The ECG demonstrates left axis deviation with a terminally slurred QRS complex. There are wide R waves in leads I, aVL, and V_5 and V_6; wide S waves can be found in leads V_1 and V_2. Asynchrony of ventricular depolarization may again produce enhanced QRS complex voltages.

Fascicular blocks, or conduction disturbances in one of the three divisions of the left bundle branch (anterior, septal, or superior), are also exceedingly rare in pediatrics. When such a condition exists in a child, it usually involves blockage of the anterior fascicle, as seen in endocardial cushion defects. The corresponding ECG is characterized by left superior axis deviation, usually without QRS complex prolongation.

Basic Dysrhythmias

Rhythms originating from the sinoatrial node (Fig. 23–10)

SINUS ARRHYTHMIA: This nonpathologic dysrhythmia is characterized by slight variation in the normal sinus heart rate with respiration. Increases are noted on inspiration, and decreases are observed with expiration. The phenomenon is rare in newborns and is more pronounced in adolescence.

SINUS BRADYCARDIA: This entity is defined by comparison of the patient's heart rate to age-adjusted norms. It is rare in healthy children; but in sick children, it is commonly caused by increased intracranial pressure, hypothyroidism, hypothermia, profound hypoxia, hyperkalemia, and drugs such as digitalis and β-adrenergic blockers. Benign sinus bradycardia is observed in well-conditioned athletes. The finding merits treatment when end-organ evidence of compromised cardiac output develops. Atropine is the drug of choice for pharmacotherapy, followed by isoproterenol.

SINUS TACHYCARDIA: Sinus tachycardia is arbitrarily defined as a sinus rhythm with a rate greater than 140 in children and 160 in infants. Common causes of this condition include (but are not limited to) anxiety, pain, fever, infection, anemia, congestive heart failure, myocarditis, thyrotoxicosis, shock, and sympathomimetic medications. Treatment is directed toward alleviation of the inciting disorder.

SINUS PAUSE: The momentary inability of the SA node to initiate an impulse is referred to as a sinus pause. This rhythm interruption is usually of short duration and is often caused by increased vagal tone, hypoxia, or digitalis effect. Treatment is once again aimed at rectification of the underlying, predisposing condition.

On occasion, the quiescent periods during sinus pauses are punctuated by AV nodal or ventricular *escape beats*. These are electrical depolarization impulses that originate from pacemakers in the locations so named as a result of failure of the faster pacemaker.

Ectopic atrial rhythms (Fig. 23–11)

Ectopic rhythms refer to those rhythms generated by parts of the heart other than the SA node. They may originate from the atria, AV node, or ventricles. Ectopic atrial dysrhythmias produce P waves of abnormal axis or contour.

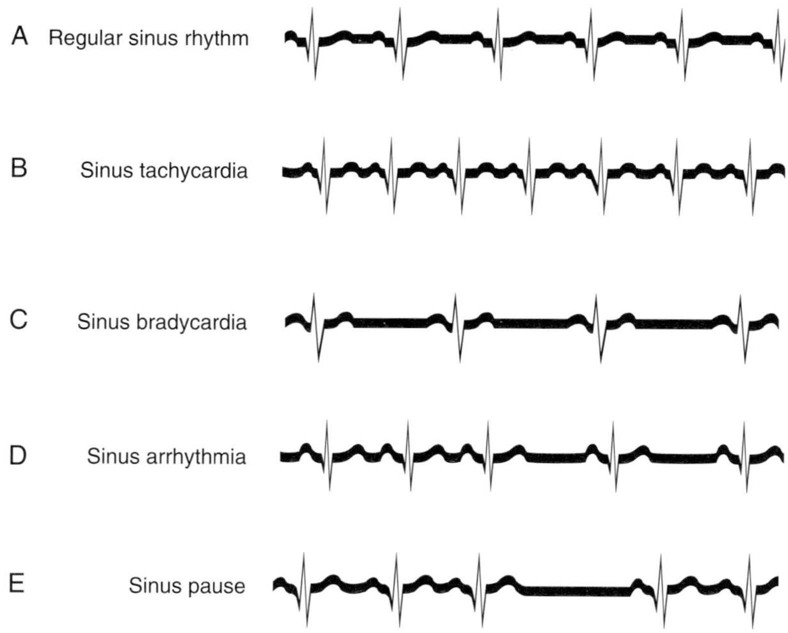

Figure 23–10 Dysrhythmias originating from the sinoatrial node. Each has a normal P-R interval, a P wave preceding every QRS complex, and a P wave axis in the normal range (0 to 90 degrees). **A.** Regular sinus rhythm. **B.** Sinus tachycardia. **C.** Sinus bradycardia. **D.** Sinus arrhythmia. **E.** Sinus pause. (Redrawn from Park MK, Guntheroth WG: *How to Read Pediatric ECGs.* St Louis, CV Mosby, 1992.)

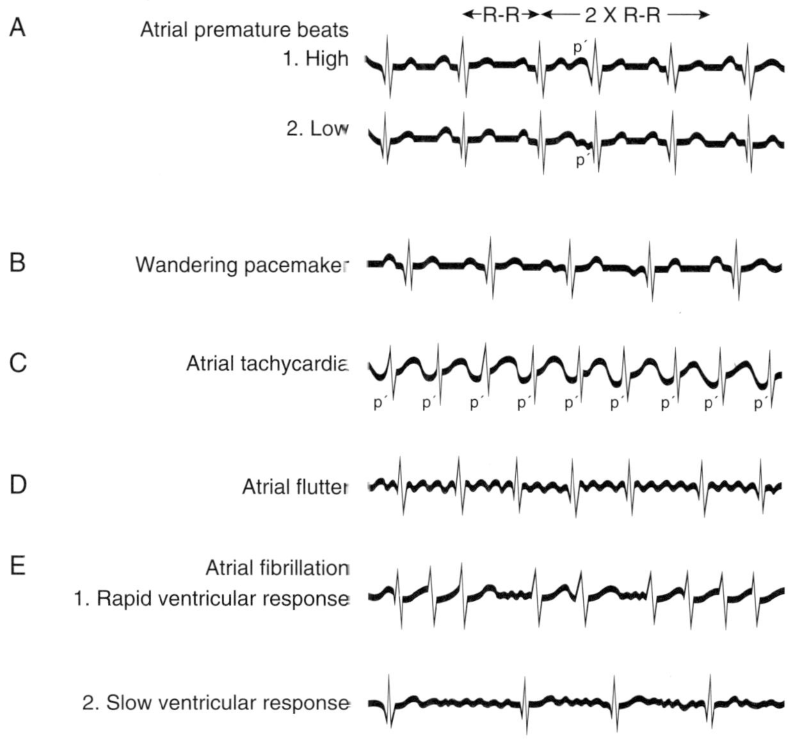

Figure 23–11 Dysrhythmias originating in the atrium. **A.** Atrial premature beats: **1.** Atrial ectopic focus high in atrium; note that the P axis and P-R interval of the premature beat (p′) are normal. The sinoatrial node is reset, leading to an incomplete compensatory pause. **2.** Atrial ectopic focus low in atrium; note the superiorly directed P axis and shortened P-R interval of the premature beat (p′). The sinoatrial node is usually reset, producing a normal R-R interval after the premature QRS complex with an incomplete compensatory pause. **B.** Wandering pacemaker. **C.** Atrial tachycardia; p′ denotes location of P waves. **D.** Atrial flutter. **E.** Atrial fibrillation: **1.** rapid ventricular response; **2.** slow ventricular response. (Redrawn from Park MK, Guntheroth WG: *How to Read Pediatric ECGs.* St Louis, CV Mosby, 1992.)

Furthermore, they may give rise to abnormally conducted P waves, leading to aberrant ventricular response rates and unusually widened QRS complexes.

PREMATURE ATRIAL CONTRACTIONS: These beats occur commonly in healthy children and newborns, although they may also be found in the setting of structural heart disease. They are nonsinus, atrial impulses that fire in advance of the impending normal beat, usually causing ventricular contraction and "resetting" of the SA node. The subsequent QRS complex then appears after a normal interval, which produces an incomplete compensatory pause (i.e., the time elapsed from the normal beat preceding the premature atrial contraction to the following normal beat is less than the length of two regular cycles).

The origin of the atrial ectopic beat can often be deduced by examination of the P wave axis and P-R interval. Premature atrial contractions produced high in the atrium usually have a normal axis (upright in lead II) and P-R interval. Those low in the atrium demonstrate a superiorly directed axis (upright in aVR, negative in leads II and aVF), with a shortened P-R interval. At times, the premature P wave may be buried in the preceding T wave, obscuring localization of the ectopic focus.

ATRIAL TACHYCARDIA: This dysrhythmia, which represents a type of supraventricular tachycardia, is seen in both children with structurally normal hearts (approximately 50%) and those with congenital heart disease. It is characterized by a heart rate in excess of 180 beats/minute and a rhythm that is regular. There is usually a P wave before each QRS complex (although it may occasionally be buried in the preceding T wave), but the P axis is often abnormal. The P-R interval may be prolonged in this dysrhythmia secondary to AV nodal refractoriness that is, insufficient time for nodal recovery of electrical conductivity. QRS complexes are usually of normal appearance. However, atrial impulses conducted to the ventricles by alternative pathways outside the AV node–His–Purkinje system may produce QRS complexes that appear abnormally widened. These waveforms are often difficult to distinguish from ventricular tachycardias.

Rather than rapid firing of a single atrial focus, many atrial tachycardias (such as that found in the Wolff-Parkinson-White syndrome) begin by a "re-entrant" phenomenon, using an accessory conduction pathway. In this situation, an anomalous fiber that can conduct impulses between the atria and ventricles exists in the heart. If a premature atrial contraction occurs in the presence of this abnormal AV connection, the electrical depolarization wave may initially be blocked at the accessory pathway, but not at the AV node. The impulse may then proceed normally through the ventricles, only to re-enter the accessory pathway in retrograde fashion to depolarize the atria. If the AV node is then capable of conducting the newly fired atrial depolarization impulse, a stable circular process is established, the repetition of which may result in tachycardia. The direction of the circular impulses may oppose that described earlier in situations in which both AV node and accessory pathways are able to conduct impulses bidirectionally.

Onset and termination of atrial tachycardias are usually abrupt. The duration of the dysrhythmia may vary from minutes to hours or days. The clinical manifestations vary greatly from those who are asymptomatic to those who are hemodynamically compromised. Deleterious cardiovascular effects result from rapid ventricular rates that shorten diastole and thereby impair ventricular filling. This may in turn decrease coronary blood flow and cause myocardial ischemia (as evidenced by ST segment depression and T wave inversion) and congestive heart failure. Children who experience longer runs of tachycardia are more likely to present with severe congestive heart failure, which may mimic pneumonia or sepsis.

Treatment is determined by the patient's degree of circulatory embarrassment during the acute episode. If the child does not demonstrate congestive heart failure, or has only mild symptoms, then maneuvers designed to increase vagal tone may be attempted, such as rectal stimulation, *unilateral* carotid massage, sudden application of ice water–soaked cloths to the face and nose (diving reflex), and the Valsalva maneuver. These measures are seldom successful in terminating a run of tachycardia in sick infants but may prove effective in older children whose period of tachycardia has been brief. Application of eyeball pressure for vagal stimulation should be completely avoided in young children in favor of safer therapies. The ECG should be recorded before and during the initiation of vagal stimulation both to document the dysrhythmia and to preserve a record of vagally medicated effects on it.

Other therapeutic modalities employed for hemodynamically stable patients with atrial tachycardias include the following:

1. Administration of intravenous adenosine. Begin with 50 to 100 μg/kg as a rapid intravenous push followed by saline push, and increase by 100 μg/kg if no effect to a maximum of 12 mg total dose; the medication should produce transient heart block with dysrhythmia termination.
2. Administration of propranolol, 0.02 mg/kg intravenously every 5 minutes, as needed, to 0.1 mg/kg total, or esmolol, 0.1 to 0.5 mg/kg over 1 minute, followed by an infusion at a rate of 0.2 to 1 mg/kg/minute.
3. Use of procainamide, 2 to 3 mg/kg/dose IV over 5 minutes to a maximum dose of 100 mg, followed by maintenance infusion at a rate of 20 to 80 mg/kg/minute to a maximum of 2 g/24 hours.
4. Administration of medications that increase blood pressure, thereby producing baroreceptor reflex–mediated vagal stimulation (e.g, methoxamine 0.25 mg/kg intramuscularly or 0.1 mg/kg intravenously, or phenylephrine 0.02 mg/kg intravenously slowly).
5. Administration of edrophonium, an anticholinesterase, 2 mg intravenously for infants, 5 mg for ages 1 to 5 years, and 10 mg for older children.
6. Use of verapamil, 0.1–0.2 mg/kg/dose intravenously—only for children older than 1 year.
7. Use of digoxin. This drug often successfully disrupts atrial tachycardias, especially when it is used in conjunction with vagal maneuvers (digoxin sensitizes the heart to vagal stimulation). Avoid digoxin use in patients with Wolff-Parkinson-White syndrome.
8. Atrial overdrive pacing using an esophageal pacing lead.

Children who present with shock or severe

congestive heart failure secondary to atrial tachycardia warrant a rapid trial of vagal maneuvers and intravenous adenosine, followed, if necessary, by synchronized cardioversion (0.5–1.0 joules/kg). Cardioversion may also be indicated when wide QRS complex, supraventricular tachycardias are present that are difficult to distinguish from ventricular tachycardia.

Long-term prevention of atrial tachycardia recurrence is best accomplished with digoxin in infants, who remain at risk for approximately 6 months after an attack. Older children, who are at risk of recurrences for many years, may begin with digoxin but may later require addition of propranolol, sotalol, or quinidine to their medical regimen.

ATRIAL FLUTTER: Atrial flutter is a dysrhythmia characterized by rapid atrial activity (usually between 250 and 350 beats/minute) that is productive of "sawtooth" atrial waves best seen in leads II, III, and V_1. It is thought to occur through a re-entrant mechanism with variable conduction of atrial impulses to the ventricles. Regular or irregular ventricular rates may therefore result. Often the regular ventricular rates demonstrate a ratio of atrial to ventricular activity ranging from 2:1 to 8:1, consistent with impulse blockage in the AV node. If this blockage yields a reasonable heart rate, adequate diastolic filling time, and sufficient cardiac output, then the dysrhythmia may be well tolerated. If, however, the ventricular response rate is too rapid for maintenance of cardiac output, then severe hemodynamic deterioration may ensue.

Atrial flutter is a rare condition in children but may be associated with structural heart disease, such as dilated atria, hypoxia, hypoglycemia, or chronic and severe rheumatic fever. Treatment is directed toward reduction of the rapid ventricular rate and restoration of normal sinus rhythm. Medical management may be attempted initially with use of digoxin; if this does not increase the AV nodal block and slow the ventricular rate, propranolol, sotalol, or quinidine may be added. Cardioversion may be used as a first-line therapy in those patients who are cardiovascularly unstable.

ATRIAL FIBRILLATION: Atrial fibrillation is characterized by disordered atrial activity that inscribes coarse, irregular, rapid deflections along the ECG baseline. The dysrhythmia is usually productive of an irregularly irregular, rapid ventricular response rate that often leads to compromised cardiac output. The condition is found in association with atrial enlargement, hyperthyroidism, hypoglycemia, and intra-atrial surgery. As with atrial flutter, treatment is aimed at reduction of the rapid ventricular rate and restoration of sinus rhythm. This is achieved medically through use of digoxin and, if necessary, quinidine. Cardioversion may also be used to treat this dysrhythmia.

SICK SINUS SYNDROME: This syndrome encompasses a variety of dysrhythmias that arise secondarily from SA node failure. These include sinus bradycardia, SA block, sinus arrest with junctional escape, paroxysmal atrial tachycardia, and variable rate ectopic atrial or junctional rhythms. Sick sinus syndrome is seen most commonly in pediatrics after extensive cardiac surgery, particularly that involving the atria and atrial septum. Treatment is directed toward control of tachydysrhythmias and bradydysrhythmias. Tachycardiac episodes tend to improve with time, although propranolol therapy is often employed. Bradycardia may warrant pacemaker placement.

Rhythms originating from the atrioventricular node (Fig. 23–12)

Rhythms that originate from the AV junctional tissues are generally characterized by (1) P waves that may either be buried within the QRS complex (i.e., inapparent) or appear before or after it in inverted fashion and (2) QRS complexes of normal duration and morphological appearance. In rare instances, junctional rhythms may demonstrate aberrant conduction to the ventricles, thereby inscribing widened QRS complexes on the ECG.

NODAL ESCAPE RHYTHM: This rhythm may appear after a faster intracardiac pacemaker, such as the SA node, persistently delays firing for a period of time sufficient to allow emergence and dominance of AV nodal pacemaker function. This so-called escape rhythm is most often found in patients with sick sinus syndrome (see earlier discussion), with increased vagal tone, or after atrial/open heart surgery. The rhythm is regular, and it usually produces a ventricular heart rate of 50 to 90 or above, corresponding to the nascent depolarization rate of the AV nodal tissues. It also results in the loss of the atrial contribution to ventricular filling (i.e., the "atrial kick") because atrial contraction is no longer appropriately coordinated with ventricular relaxation. If the resultant cardiac output at this nodally determined heart rate is adequate for the patient's meta-

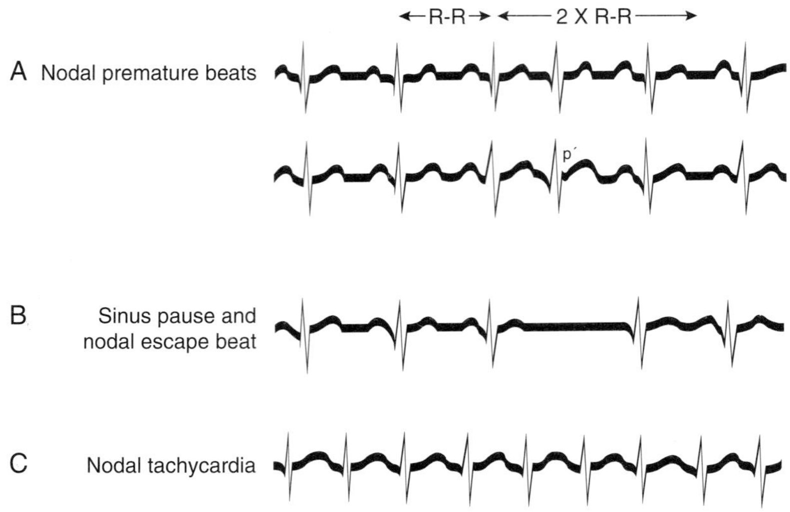

Figure 23–12 Dysrhythmias originating in the atrioventricular node. **A.** Nodal premature beats; note the incomplete compensatory pause (implying that the sinoatrial node *was* reset by the premature beat) and the retrogradely conducted P wave (p′) apparent after the QRS complex. **B.** Sinus pause with nodal escape; note that the escape beat comes later than the anticipated normal beat. **C.** Nodal tachycardia due to persistent slowing or failure of sinoatrial node function. (Redrawn from Park MK, Guntheroth WG: *How to Read Pediatric ECGs*. St Louis, CV Mosby, 1992.)

bolic needs, no treatment for this dysrhythmia is necessary. If, however, the patient has symptoms of cardiovascular compromise, then atropine therapy or artificial pacing may be required.

NODAL ESCAPE BEAT: This impulse arises from a brief interruption in the function of the dominant cardiac pacemaker (as opposed to sustained dysfunction, which may produce the AV nodal rhythm described before). The escape beat arrives later than the anticipated normal beat, and as with all normally conducted nodal impulses, the QRS complex is morphologically normal. P waves, if present, may appear before or after the QRS complex and may be inverted in leads II, III, and aVF. Single, infrequent nodal escape beats have no clinically deleterious effect.

NODAL PREMATURE BEATS: Nodal premature beats originate from an excitable focus in the AV junction and interrupt the underlying heart rhythm. In so doing, they may produce an incomplete or complete compensatory pause on the ECG, depending on whether the SA node is discharged by retrograde activation of the atria. If the SA node is discharged, or "reset," the pause will be incomplete because the next sinus P wave will fire after one normal PP interval has elapsed. If the SA node is not discharged, it continues to depolarize at the original rate, giving rise to a normal beat exactly two P-P intervals from the last sinus beat (i.e., as if the intervening premature junctional beat had not disrupted the sinus rhythm). This is known as a complete compensatory pause.

Nodal premature beats are marked morphologically by the same P wave and QRS complex properties as the aforementioned rhythms of nodal origin. They are observed in the setting of hypoxia or hypoglycemia and after surgery near the AV junction. Treatment of nodal premature beats is warranted only in association with embarrassment of cardiac output. Most nodal premature beats are without clinical consequence. If therapy is indicated, propranolol may be used for this dysrhythmia.

NODAL TACHYCARDIA: This rhythm is generated by a hyperirritable focus within the AV junction that assumes the pacemaker role owing to its rapid rate of discharge (ordinarily 120–180 beats/minute). It is observed with myocarditis, digitalis intoxication, and surgery near the AV node. The QRS complex is usually normal in appearance, although aberrantly conducted impulses from the AV node can occur. This may produce widened QRS waveforms that are difficult to distinguish from tachydysrhythmias of ventricular origin.

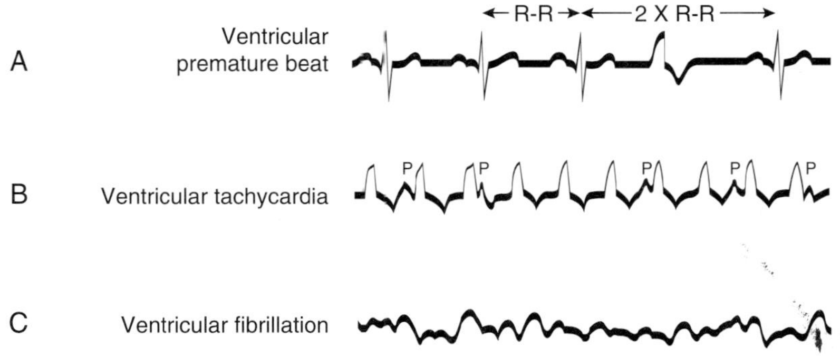

Figure 23–13 Dysrhythmias of ventricular origin. **A.** Ventricular premature beat. Because the sinoatrial node is not usually reset, sinoatrial firing continues uninterrupted, producing a *complete* compensatory pause. **B.** Ventricular tachycardia; note presence of P waves unrelated to QRS complexes. **C.** Ventricular fibrillation. (Redrawn from Park MK, Guntheroth WG: *How to Read Pediatric ECGs*. St Louis, CV Mosby, 1992.)

Patients with nodal tachycardias may experience a reduction in cardiac output from (1) inadequate time for diastolic ventricular filling due to the rapid ventricular rate and (2) loss of the synchronized atrial contribution to ventricular output. Therefore, when treatment is indicated by onset of cardiovascular embarrassment, it is directed toward reducing the rapid ventricular depolarization rate and restoring the dominance of the sinus pacemaker. Patients whose heart rates remain less than 150 are usually able to maintain adequate cardiac output without therapy. However, those children with higher heart rates and evidence of hemodynamic compromise require treatment with either synchronized cardioversion or quinidine.

Patients with poorly tolerated junctional ectopic tachycardia, seen commonly in the early postoperative period, may be treated with induced hypothermia to 34°C, followed by administration of either digoxin or procainamide.

Ventricular dysrhythmias (Fig. 23–13)

Dysrhythmias of ventricular origin are generally productive of bizarre QRS complexes that are long in duration, are randomly related to P waves, and often point in the opposite direction from their associated T waves. These observations are explained by the following: (1) the ventricular impulses originate and travel outside the normal conducting system, and are therefore conducted slowly and abnormally through the myocardium during both depolarization and repolarization, and (2) atrial activation may proceed by retrograde conduction or may be completely unrelated to ventricular depolarization.

PREMATURE VENTRICULAR COMPLEXES: PVCs are extra beats arising from an excitable focus in one of the ventricles. These impulses, which usually interrupt an underlying normal rhythm, may originate from a single focus or from multiple foci. If they are from a single focus, they will inscribe the same waveform in the same lead on each occurrence. If they are from different foci, they will display different configurations. When PVCs occur in alternation with normal QRS complexes in regular fashion, the rhythm pattern is referred to as *ventricular bigeminy*. When one PVC appears regularly after two normal complexes, the rhythm is called *ventricular trigeminy*. *Couplets* describe the repetitive inscription of one normal QRS followed by two PVCs.

Premature ventricular beats may be observed in normal children or those with congenital heart disease, drug intoxication (e.g., digitalis, caffeine, sympathomimetics), electrolyte disturbances (e.g., hyperkalemia and hypokalemia), hyperthyroidism, hypoxia, or hypoglycemia. In healthy children, occasional, unifocal PVCs that disappear with exercise are benign. PVCs that are multifocal, coupled, precipitated by activity, or associated with underlying heart disease usually indicate ventricular irritability. Such irritability may forebode deterioration into more dangerous ventricular dysrhythmias like ventricular tachycardia or ventricular fibrillation, depending on the cause of the PVC. Therefore, further investigation of the underlying cause of the dysrhythmic beats and appropriate treatment of such predisposing conditions may be warranted. Medical therapy may be initiated with either propranolol or lidocaine.

VENTRICULAR TACHYCARDIA: Ventricular tachycardia involves discharge of a ventricular pacemaker at a rate of 120 to 180 beats/minute, producing the aforementioned widened, bizarre QRS complexes with their oppositely directed T waves and temporally unrelated P waves. This dysrhythmia is relatively rare in children and is often difficult to distinguish from supraventricular tachycardia with aberrant interventricular conduction. When truly present, it is indicative of myocardial damage or dysfunction as could be found with severe digitalis intoxication, frank myocarditis, and extreme electrolyte imbalance, or after anesthesia or cardiac surgery. Though it may be well tolerated by some infants, ventricular tachycardia must be treated promptly because there is a significant risk of clinical decompensation with hypotension/hypoperfusion from this rhythm alone or from deterioration to ventricular fibrillation (see later discussion). Therapeutic options include use of synchronized cardioversion and intravenous administration of antiarrhythmic drugs (lidocaine, procainamide, bretylium). If ventricular tachycardia is caused by digitalis intoxication, phenytoin can be employed as a second-line agent.

VENTRICULAR FIBRILLATION: Ventricular fibrillation is a dysrhythmia characterized by chaotic, uncoordinated ventricular depolarization that is inscribed on the ECG as an irregular, fluctuating baseline tracing without discernible P, QRS, or T waves. Clinically, it is often a terminal condition because no effective pulse or cardiac output is produced during the dysrhythmia. This, in turn, results in rapid and severe myocardial and end-organ ischemia and, ultimately, death. Although generally rare in childhood, ventricular fibrillation may be associated with hypoxia, digitalis intoxication, chest trauma, hypothermia, or drug overdose (cocaine, caffeine/theophylline, cyclic antidepressants). It is frequently heralded by some evidence of ventricular irritability (for example, PVCs).

Presence of ventricular fibrillation constitutes a medical emergency and should provoke immediate resuscitation with unsynchronized electrical defibrillation using 2 joules/kg. This maneuver should be repeated three times in a row, if necessary, doubling the electrical energy with each successive attempt at cardioversion. Thereafter, cardiopulmonary resuscitation should be instituted, and epinephrine, lidocaine, and bretylium administration should be interposed between shocks as needed until normal sinus rhythm is restored. If normal sinus rhythm does resume, a prophylactic lidocaine infusion should be initiated, and all conditions predisposing the patient to ventricular fibrillation should be promptly corrected.

Disturbances of atrioventricular conduction (Fig. 23–14)

Atrioventricular Block

A delay or failure of impulse conduction through the AV junction to the ventricles is referred to as an AV block or heart block. There are three classes of this disturbance.

FIRST-DEGREE AV BLOCK: This form of heart block is manifested by prolongation of the PR interval beyond the upper limit of normal, as determined by the patient's age and heart rate (see Table 23–3). The rhythm is regular, is sinus in origin, and produces QRS complexes of normal appearance. The condition may be associated with digitalis intoxication, rheumatic fever, cardiomyopathy, maladies in which there is increased vagal tone (such as increased intracranial pressure, hypertension, gastric dilatation), and structural heart disease (such as atrial septal defect, Ebstein's anomaly). Alternatively, it may occur after myocardial surgery.

There are no clinically deleterious symptoms produced by this conduction disturbance. Therefore, treatment is not usually indicated. However, in the case of suspected digitalis intoxication, intervention to halt the administration of the drug should be undertaken if first-degree AV block is observed on a predose rhythm strip.

SECOND-DEGREE AV BLOCK: This disturbance of AV conduction is characterized by the intermittent failure of some P waves, but not all, to stimulate the ventricles. There are two types of second-degree block, Mobitz type I (referred to as Wenckebach) and Mobitz type II.

Wenckebach block involves progressive lengthening of the P-R interval until a P wave is nonconducted and a ventricular beat is dropped. A pause follows, and the cycle then resumes. This phenomenon is thought to be secondary to successively increased, then normalized, refractoriness of the AV node. Consequently, the duration of the QRS complex is normal, whereas the duration of the R-R interval varies. This gives rise to an irregular rhythm. Of note is that the Wenckebach cycle may begin with a junctional escape beat if the sinus pause is sufficiently prolonged.

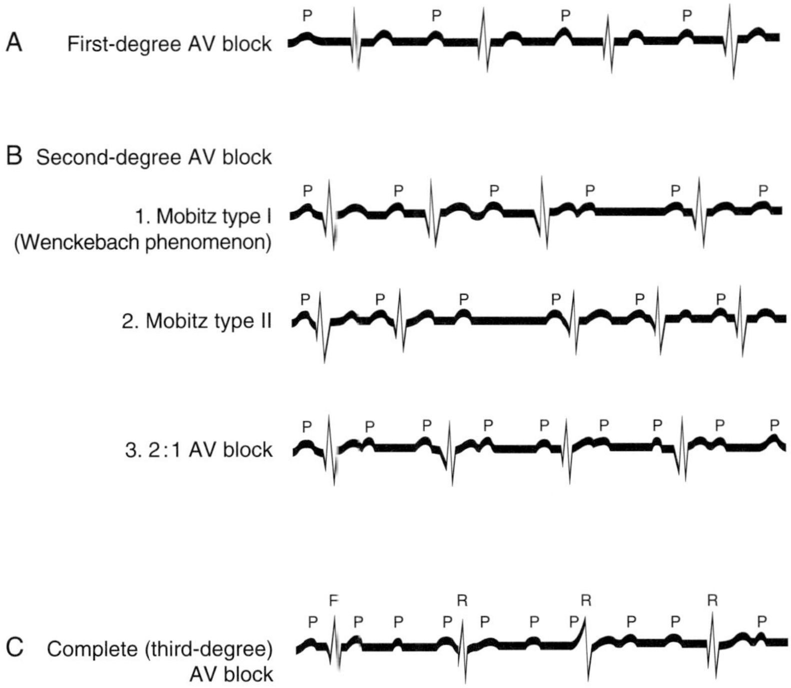

Figure 23–14 Atrioventricular (AV) conduction disturbances. **A.** First-degree AV block. **B.** Second-degree AV block. **C.** Complete (third-degree) AV block. (Redrawn from Park MK, Guntheroth WG: *How to Read Pediatric ECGs*. St Louis, CV Mosby, 1992.)

Wenckebach AV block may be observed in normally functioning hearts, or it may be seen in association with increased vagal tone, myocarditis, digitalis intoxication, structural congenital heart disease, or cardiac surgery near the AV junction. In addition, this form of AV block is seen in acute inferior wall myocardial infarctions (extremely rare in the pediatric population) because both the AV node and this area of the myocardium experience ischemic damage from blockage of the right coronary artery.

No treatment is required for Mobitz type I block. Rather, therapeutic efforts should be directed toward alleviation of the underlying, predisposing condition.

Mobitz type II second-degree AV block originates from failure of impulse transmission at the level of the bundle of His or bilaterally at the level of the bundle branches. On the ECG, it is characterized by P waves that are either normally conducted or completely blocked. P waves that are conducted do so in the usual fashion with a P-R interval that remains constant. P waves that fail to conduct are neither premature nor late—they occur in rhythmic sequence, producing a constant P-R interval. Whereas the atrial rate may be normal and regular, the ventricular response rate may be considerably slower (depending entirely on the ratio of conducted to nonconducted atrial impulses) and irregular (owing to the nontransmitted P waves). Furthermore, the damaged His bundle and bundle branches that give rise to Mobitz type II block may also produce delays in ventricular activation. Such delays in turn inscribe the widened QRS complexes routinely found in this condition.

Type II block is rarely encountered in the pediatric age group because it is usually indicative of extensive myocardial damage, such as that which may be seen with acute anterior wall myocardial infarction. When present in children, it is most commonly associated with surgical damage to the bundle of His or bundle branches. It is a dangerous entity from a clinical perspective because patients are at risk for development of complete heart block and ventricular standstill. Therefore, prophylactic pacemaker therapy may be indicated. Atropine may also be used to augment the ventricular response rate by stimulating the healthy sinus mechanism, thereby increasing the overall rate of conducted beats.

Differentiation between Mobitz type I and type II AV blocks is important for purposes of clinical prognostication and treatment. It is fairly easily accomplished when there are two or more conducted P waves in succession before each dropped ventricular beat because one can look for lengthening or constancy of the PR interval in types I or II, respectively. If there are two P waves for every QRS (i.e., 2:1 conduction), the task of discrimination becomes more difficult. In this situation, one may peruse the ECG strip for a point at which two atrial impulses are consecutively conducted and then compare the corresponding P-R intervals as mentioned before. In addition, one can examine the duration of the QRS complexes. A conduction pattern of 2:1 with a narrow QRS complex usually represents Wenckebach conduction, whereas 2:1 conduction with a widened QRS complex usually indicates a Mobitz type II block.

THIRD-DEGREE AV BLOCK: In this conduction abnormality, also termed complete heart block, all atrial impulses are blocked from initiation of ventricular depolarization. Although the SA node fires normally and produces normal atrial activation (with a regular P-P interval), none of this electrical energy reaches the ventricular conduction system. As a result, the atria and ventricles beat entirely independently from one another, and the P-R interval is inconstant. Ventricular depolarization proceeds at a regular (constant R-R interval) but slower rate compared with atrial activation. This occurs through escape ectopic pacemaker activity. If the pacemaker is in the AV node or at a level higher than the His bundle bifurcation, the QRS complexes will be narrow. If the escape pacemaker is in either ventricle, productive of the so-called idioventricular rhythm, then the QRS complexes will appear widened like those of PVCs.

Third-degree AV block is seen in patients with myocarditis, digitalis intoxication, or congenital heart disease, and after cardiac surgery. Those with congenital complete heart block either as an isolated anomaly or related to structural heart disease (especially transposition of the great vessels) or maternal systemic lupus erythematosus usually have narrow complex QRS waveforms. Patients with acquired or surgically induced complete heart block usually demonstrate QRS complex prolongation.

Treatment of third-degree AV block is unnecessary in asymptomatic children, although there is some controversy about the need for pacemaker placement in these patients during young adulthood. Childhood adaptation to a slow ventricular rate is not uncommon, and it is often accomplished through compensatory mechanisms such as chamber hypertrophy and increased stroke volume. For those in whom congestive heart failure develops from their conduction abnormality, therapy is directed toward augmentation of the ventricular rate to restore adequate circulation. If ventricular activation proceeds from a junctional escape pacemaker, atropine may be used to increase the junctional firing rate. If ventricular activation is initiated by a ventricular pacemaker, isoproterenol administration or ventricular pacing may be attempted.

Atrioventricular Dissociation

Atrioventricular dissociation is a condition brought about by one of the following two conduction disturbances: (1) slowing of atrial impulses with emergence of an "escape" pacemaker, or (2) acceleration of the rate of a subsidiary pacemaker above that of the dominant atrial pacemaker. It appears similar to complete heart block in that one pacemaker usually activates the atria and a second, independent pacemaker usually activates the ventricles. However, AV dissociation is *not* a form of third-degree AV block. It differs from complete heart block in several important ways. First, in complete AV block, atrial impulses cannot be transmitted to the ventricles. In contrast, in AV dissociation, atrial impulses are intermittently conducted to the ventricles if temporal opportunity (i.e., conducting system refractoriness) permits. These "capture beats" occur prematurely relative to the firing of the subsidiary pacemaker, and their morphological appearance is a melding of atrial focus and ectopic focus impulse inscription. Second, in complete AV block, the ventricular rate is usually slower than the atrial rate. However, in AV dissociation, it is usually the atrial rate that lags behind that of the ventricle. Treatment is acutely directed toward maintenance of a ventricular rate adequate for tissue perfusion and oxygenation. This may entail either pharmacological intervention or use of pacemakers, depending on the underlying cause of the dissociative condition. Clinically, AV dissociation usually carries a less ominous prognosis than third-degree AV block.

CHAMBER LOCALIZATION

The anatomical positions of the cardiac chambers relative to one another greatly influence heart physiology and proper function. In many types of congenital heart disease, the normal relationships between right- and left-sided cardiac structures are not preserved. The ECG may simply and noninvasively provide some initial clues to help determine the actual anatomy of the heart until more definitive imaging studies, such as radiography, echocardiography, and angiocardiography, can be performed.

Locating the Atria

Two methods are used for determination of the position of the right atrium (and, by inference, except in cases of situs ambiguus, the position of the left atrium). The first involves examination of the P wave axis. It is based on the fact that the SA node is located in the anatomical right atrium. When depolarization impulses emanate from the SA node, they are directed inferiorly and to the opposite side of the atrium. Therefore, if the SA node, and thus the right atrium, are on the right, then the P wave axis will be between 0 and +90 degrees. If the SA node and right atrium are on the left, as in mirror-image dextrocardia, then the P wave axis will be between +90 and +180 degrees (Fig. 23–15A).

The second method for determining right atrial position has nothing to do with electrocardiography and hinges on the fact that the right atrium and the liver are almost always on the same side. Consequently, one can obtain x-ray films of the chest and upper abdomen to infer the location of the right atrium.

Locating the Ventricles

Discerning the position of the ventricular chambers depends on ECG examination of ventricular septal depolarization. This electromechanical process normally proceeds from embryonic left to right ventricle at the outset of ventricular myocardial activation. When the left ventricle is located to the left of the right ventricle (i.e., normal anatomical position), septal impulse progression advances rightward, thereby inscribing a Q wave in leads I, V_5, and V_6. When the anatomical left ventricle is located to the *right* of the anatomical right ventricle (i.e., ventricular inversion), the direction of septal depolarization points leftward. As a result, Q waves will no longer be seen in leads I, V_5, and V_6 but will instead be found in leads V_1, V_{4R}, and V_{6R}, the last two leads being right precordial leads in mirror-image position from leads V_4 and V_6, respectively (Fig. 23–15B).

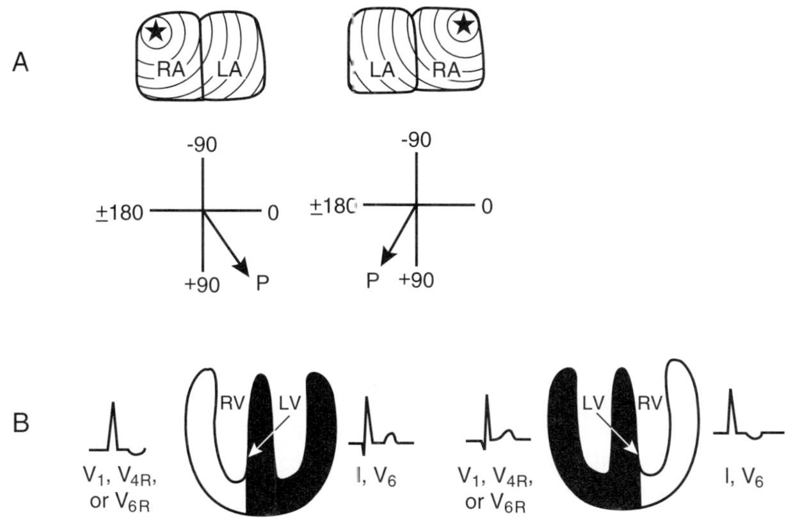

Figure 23–15 ECG clues to abnormal heart chamber localization. **A.** Locating the atria by use of the P axis. Because the sinoatrial node is located in the right atrium, a P axis in the *left* lower quadrant implies that the right atrium is on the right. When the P axis is in the *right* lower quadrant, the right atrium is most likely on the left. **B.** Locating the ventricles. When septal depolarization proceeds from embryonic left to right ventricle, Q waves are inscribed in leads I and V_6. If the anatomical left ventricle is to the right of the anatomical right ventricle, then Q waves are seen in leads V_1, V_{4R}, and V_{6R}. LA, left atrium; LV, left ventricle; RA, right atrium; RV, right ventricle. (Redrawn from Park MK, Guntheroth WG: *How to Read Pediatric ECGs*. St Louis, CV Mosby, 1992.)

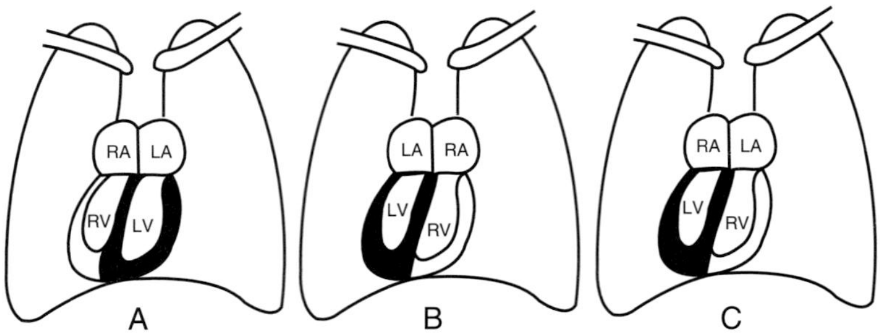

Figure 23–16 Examples of dextrocardia. **A.** Dextroversion. **B.** Mirror-image dextrocardia. **C.** Ventricular inversion (e.g., L-transposition of the great arteries). LA, left atrium; LV, left ventricle; RA, right atrium; RV, right ventricle. (Redrawn from Park MK, Guntheroth WG: *How to Read Pediatric ECGs*. St Louis, CV Mosby, 1992.)

Locating Abnormal Chambers

HEART IN THE RIGHT SIDE OF THE CHEST: It is not infrequent that the heart appears to be located in the right side of the chest on the chest radiograph. This may be due to one of the following conditions: (1) dextroversion, (2) mirror-image dextrocardia, (3) ventricular inversion, or (4) situs ambiguus. Application of the ECG principles of chamber localization described before can aid in the differentiation of these diagnoses.

Dextroversion, or isolated dextrocardia, implies rightward displacement of the cardiac apex with preservation of the normal atrial and ventricular relationships (Fig. 23–16A). It is often secondary to a significant extrinsic abnormality, such as hypoplasia of the right lung, congenital diaphragmatic hernia, or pneumothorax. Because the atria and ventricles are correctly positioned relative to one another, the P wave axis remains between 0 and +90 degrees; Q waves are present in leads I, V_5, and V_6 but not in the right chest leads. Furthermore, there is a progressive decrease from V_1 through V_6 in the amplitude of the QRS complexes as ventricular depolarization is physically distanced from the left precordial leads.

Mirror-image dextrocardia (Fig. 23–16B) is characterized by complete reversal of the laterality of all cardiac structures, with preservation of anterior-posterior anatomical relationships. This may be seen in otherwise normal people with situs inversus totalis or those with Kartagener's syndrome (triad of situs inversus totalis, paranasal sinusitis, and bronchiectasis). Because the anatomical right atrium is to the left of the anatomical left atrium, and the morphological left ventricle is to the right of the right ventricle, the P wave axis is in the right lower quadrant (+90 to +180 degrees) and Q waves are present in the right chest leads V_{5R} and V_{6R}.

Ventricular inversion refers to an abnormality in which the right-to-left relationship of the ventricles is reversed (Fig. 23–16C). In this condition, the ECG demonstrates normal atrial relationships with a normal P wave axis but abnormal laterality of septal activation, leading to Q waves in leads V_{4R} through V_{6R}.

Situs ambiguus exists when persistence of bilaterality of fetal cardiac structures confuses assignment of atrial situs. It is typically associated with asplenia and polysplenia syndromes, in which the cardiac apex is dextroposed in approximately one third of the cases. In the asplenia syndrome, the P wave axis is commonly found in the right lower quadrant, indicating atrial inversion. In the polysplenia syndrome, P wave axis is unreliable for determining atrial situs because of the high frequency of ectopic atrial rhythms. Ventricular morphology is variable in both conditions, ranging from single ventricle to presence of normal biventricular formation. Ventricular inversion is present in approximately one third of cases as well.

HEART IN THE LEFT SIDE OF THE CHEST: Although the cardiac apex lies in the left chest when atrial and ventricular structures are normally positioned, there are conditions in which atrial or ventricular malposition may be coexistent with levocardia. One such example is congenitally corrected transposition, or L-transposition, of the great arteries. In this abnormality, the atria are normally located; however, the ventricles are inverted (along with their atrioventricular valves), and the great vessels are transposed. Thus, deoxygenated blood returns to the right atrium, passes through the mitral valve to the left ventricle, and then moves into the pulmonary artery to the lungs. Correspondingly, oxygenated blood returns to the left atrium, passes through the tricuspid valve into the right ventricle, and out the aorta. Because movement of oxygenated and deoxygenated blood mimics the normal physiological state, this cardiac ailment is termed corrected transposition. Diagnosis of this condition is important because these patients have a high frequency of progressive AV block and Wolff-Parkinson-White syndrome. Analysis of the ECG in corrected transposition can aid diagnosis by revealing a normal P wave axis (i.e., normal atrial position) in the face of right precordial lead Q waves (indicating a reversed direction of ventricular septal activation consistent with ventricular inversion).

SINGLE VENTRICLE: A variety of ECG abnormalities are seen with presence of a single ventricle. First, Q waves are often abnormal—absent in all precordial leads, present in all precordial leads, or present in the right precordial leads only—because of malformations or absence of the ventricular septum. Second, QRS morphological features are abnormal owing to the presence of only one functioning ventricle. One may observe rS, RS, or QR waveforms, along with abnormal R wave progression. Third, abnormalities of the ventricular conduction system commonly give rise to first- and second-degree AV blocks and supraventricular tachycardias.

Bibliography

Ehrat KS: *The Art of Adult and Pediatric EKG Interpretation.* Dubuque, IA, Kendall/Hunt, 1985.

Gillette P, Garson A Jr: *Pediatric Arrhythmias: Electrophysiology and Pacing.* Philadelphia, WB Saunders, 1990.

Hoffman, JIE: Electrocardiogram. In Rudolph AM, Hoffman JIE (eds): *Pediatrics.* Norwalk, CT, Appleton & Lange, 1991.

Liebman J, Plonsey R: Electrocardiography. In Adams FH, Emmanouildes GC (eds): *Heart Disease in Infants, Children, and Adolescents.* Baltimore, Williams & Wilkins, 1983.

Liebman J, Plonsey R, Gillette P: *Pediatric Electrocardiography.* Baltimore, Williams & Wilkins, 1982.

Park MK, Guntheroth WG: *How to Read Pediatric ECGs.* Chicago, Year Book Medical Publishers, 1981.

Van Praagh S, Santini F, Sanders, SP: Cardiac malpositions with special emphasis on visceral heterotaxy. In Fyler DC (ed): *Nadas' Pediatric Cardiology.* Philadelphia, Hanley & Belfus, 1992.

Chapter 24

Cardiac Ultrasonography (Echocardiography)

Daniel Stromberg

Echocardiography refers to the cardiac imaging modality that makes use of sound energy to visualize the heart and its structures. Commonly known as cardiac ultrasonography because it uses sound frequencies above the audible range (i.e., 2–10 MHz), this diagnostic technology noninvasively provides accurate, safe, and easily obtainable information in real time about cardiac anatomy, physiology, and function. Furthermore, it does so without the production of ionizing radiation. Ultrasonography is now widely available in most clinical settings and can readily be taken to the bedside for examination of sick patients without risking transport-related deterioration of their condition.

Although these advantages make echocardiography useful in all age groups, it is particularly well suited for diagnostic evaluation of infants and small children. First, diagnosis of pediatric heart disease often requires delineation of gross anatomical details, for which ultrasound examination is uniquely qualified. In many situations, this imaging modality provides all the information needed to undertake therapeutic intervention. Second, more and better echocardiographic views of the heart are available in the pediatric population because the heart is commonly closer to the ultrasound transducer, and the mass of intervening structures is decreased. The great usefulness of subxiphoid views of the heart in the pediatric population, compared with their relative lack of usefulness in older children and adults, attests to this observation. Third, in keeping with the aforementioned proximity of the pediatric heart to the transducer, the path traversed by emitted sound energy is short. Therefore, high-frequency sound energy may be used to visualize the heart, producing a higher quality cardiac image.

PHYSICAL PRINCIPLES

The physical principles underlying echocardiography are relatively simple and elegant: (1) sound energy propagates through a physical medium with a speed and efficiency dependent on the stiffness and density of the medium, and (2) sound energy is reflected at the interface between media of different sound transmission properties—the greater the difference, the more sound energy is reflected, and the less sound energy passes through to the second medium. Most naturally occurring tissue interfaces, such as that between blood and endocardium, have differential acoustic transmission properties that allow excellent image production. However, interfaces between soft tissues and tissues such as gas-filled bowel, air-filled lung, or bone characteristically reflect all incident sound energy. As a result, those structures beneath the interface cannot be viewed because sound energy does not reach them.

The instruments used to generate an echocardiographic image do so by conversion of electrical energy to mechanical energy and then reconversion of mechanical energy back to electrical energy. Initially, electrical pulses are sent from a pulse generator to a transducer that contains piezoelectric crystals. In response to the electrical stimulation, these crystals emit a short burst of sound energy at a frequency particular to the crystal. The sound waves enter the tissue and are reflected back from tissue interfaces as described before. The transducer then acts as a receiver, converting the reflected echo into an electrical signal. The distance from the transducer to the reflecting target is calculated by use of the known speed of sound energy in soft tissue (1530 m/sec), and a dot representing the signal, the brightness of which is proportional to the intensity of the reflected echo, is placed in its appropriate position on the screen. This process is repeated at a rate of approximately 1000 times/second to build an echocardiographic image.

M-mode, or *motion*, echocardiography directs a thin beam of sound energy into the heart, thereby gleaning specific information about those structures that lie along the beam's path. In this type of study, reflected echoes produce the aforementioned image signals, the movements of which, due to corresponding movements of the cardiac structures, are plotted at successive time intervals. This provides a limited but high-resolution view of the heart that is particularly useful for measuring linear dimensions (such as heart chamber wall thickness) and rate of change of cardiac dimensions.

If one could record simultaneously, or in rapid succession, several adjacent scan lines in a plane, then a two-dimensional cardiac image would be created. *Two-dimensional* echocardiography takes advantage of this possibility to provide cross-sectional views of the heart (Fig. 24–1). This is commonly accomplished through use of a *sector scanner*, which produces triangular images either by rotating

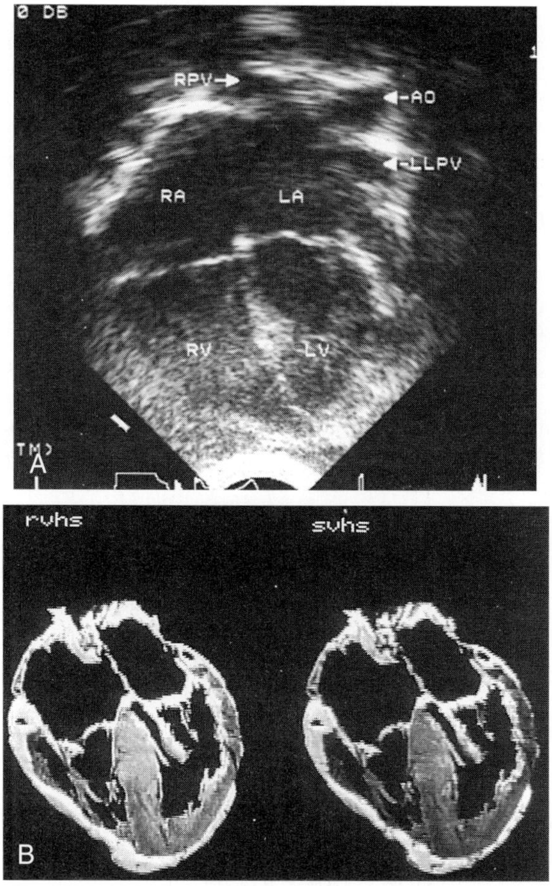

Figure 24–1 A. Apical four-chamber echocardiogram. RA, right atrium; LA, left atrium; RV, right ventricle; LV, left ventricle; AO, aorta; RPV, right pulmonary vein; LLPV, left lower pulmonary vein. **B.** Analogous cross-sectional autopsy photograph.

piezoelectric crystals through an arc with an electrical motor (mechanical sector scanner) or by steering the sound beam through electrical phasing (phased array sector scanner). Higher-frequency scanners provide better axial resolution (ability to discriminate between two closely spaced objects along the axis of the sound beam) and lateral resolution (ability to discriminate between two closely spaced objects perpendicular to the axis of the sound beam), but the ability to penetrate tissue is decreased. Hence, high-frequency transducers (7.5 MHz) give superb images in the near field (i.e., 0–5 cm) and are preferred for use with small infants. Lower-frequency (3.5 MHz), longer-focus transducers are necessary to penetrate the tissues of larger children and adults.

Doppler ultrasonography provides an additional method of sound information processing. This modality makes use of the shift in sound frequency reflected from the surface of an object (e.g., a red blood cell) moving with respect to a sound source (e.g., a transducer). Because this frequency change is proportional to the velocity of the reflector according to the Doppler equation, the frequency increase or decrease can be used to determine the direction of motion of the reflector. The Doppler equation is

$$f_d = (v \times f_o \times \cos \theta) / 2c$$

where f_d is the Doppler frequency shift, v is reflector velocity, f_o is the frequency of the incident sound energy, θ is the angle between the direction of motion of the reflector and the direction of propagation of the sound waves, and c is the speed of sound propagation in tissue. By use of this analysis, Doppler ultrasonography can provide direct measurements of blood flow direction and velocity. Color designations can be added to directional flow, as is done with color Doppler imaging, such that red blood cell movement toward the transducer is depicted in red and movement away from the transducer is depicted in blue. These color images are then superimposed on two-dimensional echocardiograms, allowing the viewer to see blood flow through moving cardiac structures in real time.

METHODS OF EXAMINATION

Echocardiographic examination begins by creating the best possible circumstances for successful evaluation of the patient. This usually entails conducting the study in an area where the room temperature is warm enough for the patient to be comfortable, the surroundings are relatively quiet, and the lighting may be dimmed both to relax the patient and to optimize viewing of the ultrasonic images. The examination area should also be large enough to accommodate at least one parent or caretaker, who may stand at the bedside to provide comfort for the apprehensive child.

Attention should next be focused on proper preparation of the patient for the study. Older children and adolescents usually require no more than a brief explanation of the investigation and the assurance that the test is painless and involves no hazardous radiation. Children between the ages of 12 months and 3 years typically respond to parental soothing combined with the perhaps more mesmerizing distraction of a colorful cartoon video or movie. Patients between 3 months and 1 year of age are often unable to cooperate adequately, despite valiant parental calming efforts, and therefore require sedation for the examination. At the author's institution, pentobarbital (Nembutal) has been used safely and effectively at doses ranging from 3 to 9 mg/kg.* This medication provides excellent sedation by the oral route and can be given in small volumes if the intravenous preparation is provided by mouth. However, care must be taken to adequately monitor patients who have received the drug because significant respiratory depression may result from its use. If a child remains uncooperative despite sedation with pentobarbital, then one should seriously consider temporarily abandoning further outpatient sedation and echocardiographic examination in favor of a more controlled environment for the test. In the inpatient setting, where better monitoring of the sedated patient is available, additional sedative-hypnotic drugs may be administered to achieve compliance with the examination.

After the patient is well prepared for study, the actual echocardiogram is obtained. The examination should be performed by a pediatric cardiologist or an experienced technologist who is thoroughly familiar with the myriad variations in pediatric cardiac anatomy and their physiological implications. The typical study includes identification and evaluation of the four valves, the ventricles, the ventricular septum, the two atria, the atrial septum, the vena cava, the pulmonary veins, the great vessels, and the pericardium. It should also determine the anatomical relationships of these structures to one another. Most examinations proceed through, but are not limited to, several standard two-dimensional echocardiographic views of the heart obtained by placing the transducer at defined anatomical locations. Doppler and M-mode investigations are integrated where indicated. This basic technical approach may, of necessity, be varied considerably to see particular cardiac structures or ab-

*Until recently, chloral hydrate was considered the drug of choice for sedation during outpatient, nonpainful procedures. Its safety and efficacy were seemingly well established, and harmful side effects were rare. The only adverse responses seen after single-dose administration involved a small percentage of patients who exhibited brief periods (15 to 20 minutes) of paradoxical agitation before onset of drug-induced sleep. More recently, however, questions about chloral hydrate's long-term carcinogenic potential have been raised, rendering its use somewhat controversial. Some continue to contend that the benefits of its pharmacological properties (i.e., its short-term safety, efficacy, and lack of side effects that interfere with study interpretation at recommended doses) outweigh the putative carcinogenic risks, thus justifying its limited use for echocardiographic sedation.

normalities. However, the four conventional two-dimensional echocardiographic views, which should be obtained in virtually every patient, offer a standardized frame of reference for sonographic investigation from which the experienced examiner can mentally create three-dimensional cardiac images.

The first echocardiographic view obtained in infants and small children is the subxiphoid view. (For discussion of echocardiography screening of congenital heart disease, see Chapter 41.) This approach provides an excellent window for obtaining an overview of cardiac anatomy by simultaneously imaging the heart and proximal great arteries (Figs. 24–2 and 24–3). The transducer is initially placed in the subxiphoid space, pointing posteriorly, with the scan plane oriented from left to right. This demonstrates visceroatrial situs by pointing out the relationship among the inferior vena cava, the descending aorta, and the spine. The transducer is then slowly angled superiorly and anteriorly to display the atria and the interatrial septum, the left ventricular inflow and outflow tracts, and the right ventricle. Rotation of the transducer clockwise by 90 degrees permits visualization of the junction of both cavae with the right atrium.

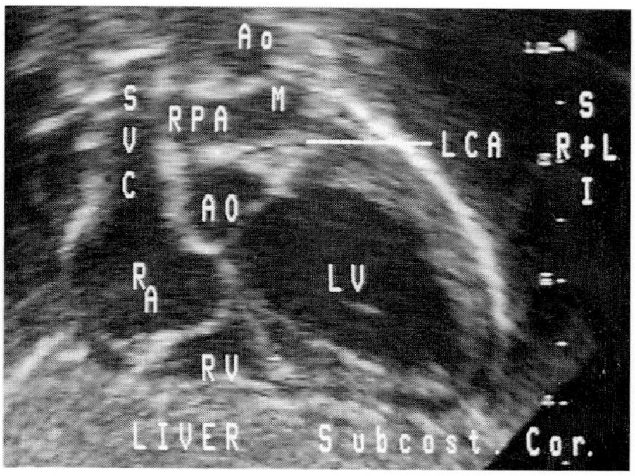

Figure 24–3 Two-dimensional echocardiogram, subxiphoid long-axis view. Ao, aorta; RPA, right pulmonary artery; M, main pulmonary artery; SVC, superior vena cava; RA, right atrium, LCA, left coronary artery; LV, left ventricle; RV, right ventricle.

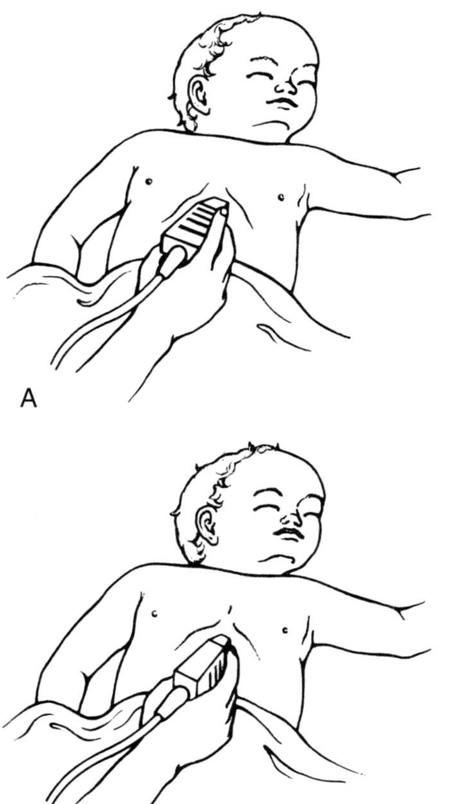

Figure 24–2 **A.** Transducer position for the subxiphoid transverse or long-axis view. **B.** Transducer position for the subxiphoid short-axis scan. (Redrawn from Sanders SP: Echocardiography. In Fyler DC [ed]: *Nadas' Pediatric Cardiology.* Philadelphia, Hanley & Belfus, 1992, p 167.)

Apical views are obtained next by moving the patient into the left lateral decubitus position (to lean the heart toward the chest wall, thereby displacing intervening lung) and then placing the transducer at the tip of the apex impulse of the heart, with the scan plane running from the left shoulder to the right hip (Fig. 24–4). This creates a four-chamber projection of the heart and atrioventricular valves (see Fig. 24–1) from which pulmonary veins may also be observed. If the transducer is angled posteriorly, the coronary sinus may be seen. From there, 90-degree clockwise rotation produces the apical long-axis view of the left ventricle, which is often a good view for examining the left ventricular outflow tract.

Parasternal views are achieved with the transducer in the third or fourth intercostal space, oriented parallel to the plane formed by the right shoulder and left hip. With the patient again in the left lateral decubitus position, images of the left ventricular inflow and outflow tracts, the aortic valve, and the proximal ascending aorta are seen (Figs. 24–5 and 24–6). Clockwise rotation of the transducer yields the parasternal short-axis or transverse view in which the ventricular myocardium is well demonstrated. If this scanning plane is maintained while the transducer is moved superiorly by one or two interspaces, the pul-

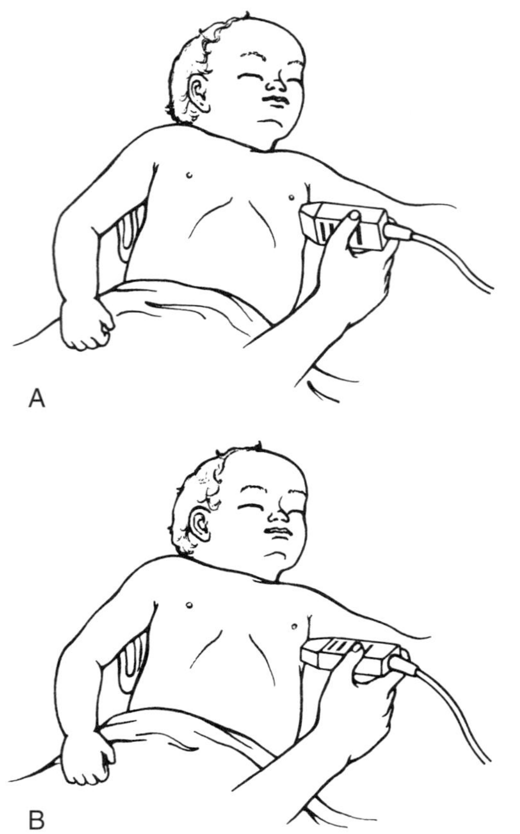

Figure 24–4 **A.** Transducer position for the apical long-axis view. **B.** Transducer position for the apical four-chamber view. (Redrawn from Sanders SP: Echocardiography In Fyler DC [ed]: *Nadas' Pediatric Cardiology.* Philadelphia, Hanley & Belfus, 1992, p 169.)

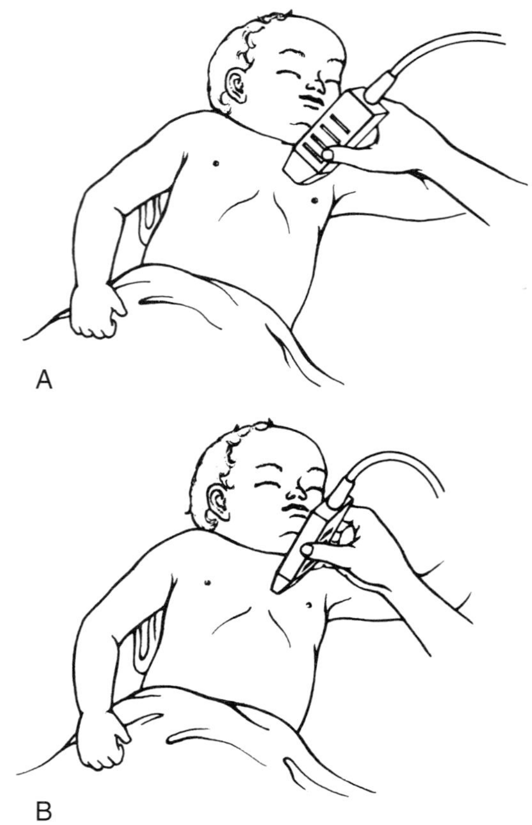

Figure 24–5 **A.** Transducer orientation producing the parasternal long-axis view. **B.** Transducer position for the parasternal short-axis view. (Redrawn from Sanders SP: Echocardiography. In Fyler DC [ed]: *Nadas' Pediatric Cardiology.* Philadelphia, Hanley & Belfus, 1992, p 169.)

monary artery and its proximal branches come into view.

The final standard view that should be obtained during a diagnostic examination is the suprasternal notch view (Figs. 24–7 and 24–8). For useful images to be produced from this perspective, the patient must be positioned to maintain the proper amount of neck extension (that is, moving the chin out of the way of the transducer while not overextending the neck and tightening the skin over the notch, thus limiting transducer access). This may be accomplished by placing a sheet or towel rolled into a flattened cylinder under the patient's shoulders. Because repositioning for imaging from the suprasternal notch may frighten the apprehensive child, this view is usually obtained at the end of the examination. The initial part of the study is begun with the transducer aimed posteriorly and inferiorly, at 45 degrees to the frontal plane, with the scanning plane from left to right. This demonstrates the ascending aorta and the posteriorly situated right pulmonary artery. Thirty-degree counterclockwise rotation, with angulation to the left, reveals the left pulmonary artery. Continued counterclockwise rotation, followed by rightward angulation, brings the aortic arch with the origins of the brachiocephalic vessels into view.

INDICATIONS AND CLINICAL APPLICATIONS

Echocardiographic studies are indicated for situations in which further information is needed regarding structural heart defects, pericardial disease, valvar heart disease, or ventricular function. One of the most common instances in which this technology is applied is in the evaluation of potentially pathological murmurs. Although it is neither necessary nor cost effective to screen every child with a not-clearly-innocent murmur with this imaging

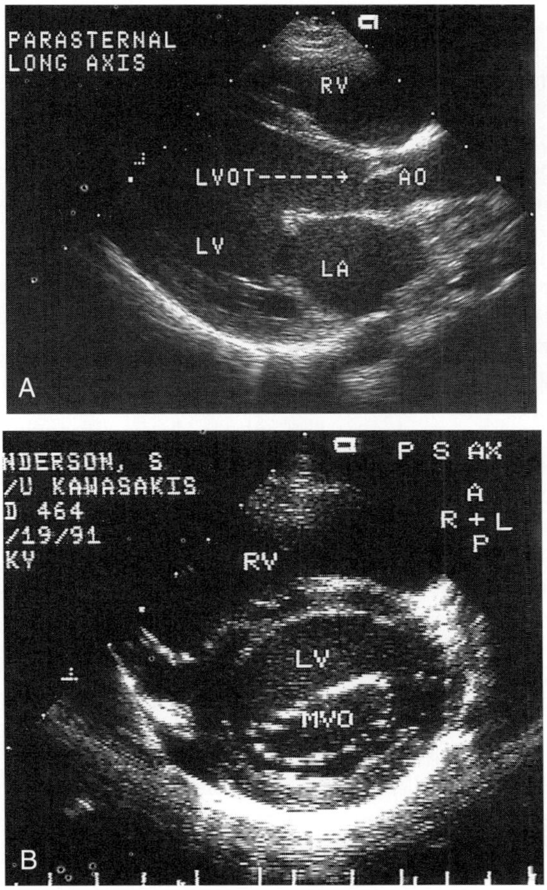

Figure 24–6 A. Echocardiogram, parasternal long-axis view. B. Echocardiogram, parasternal short-axis view. RV, right ventricle; LVOT, left ventricular outflow tract; AO, aorta; LV, left ventricle; LA, left atrium; MVO, mitral valve orifice.

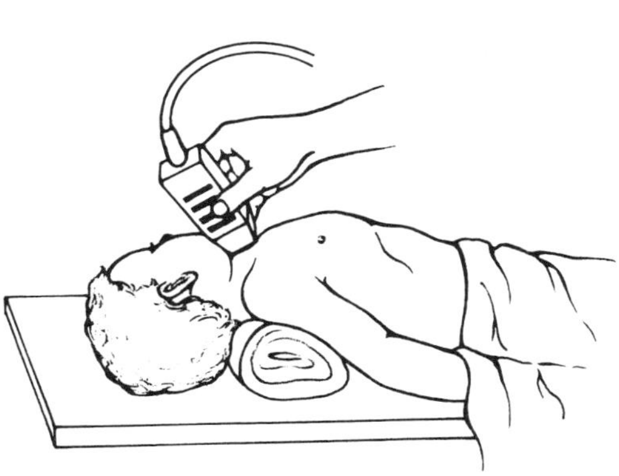

Figure 24–7 Transducer position for the suprasternal notch view. (Redrawn from Sanders SP: Echocardiography. In Fyler DC [ed]: *Nadas' Pediatric Cardiology.* Philadelphia, Hanley & Belfus, 1992, p 170.)

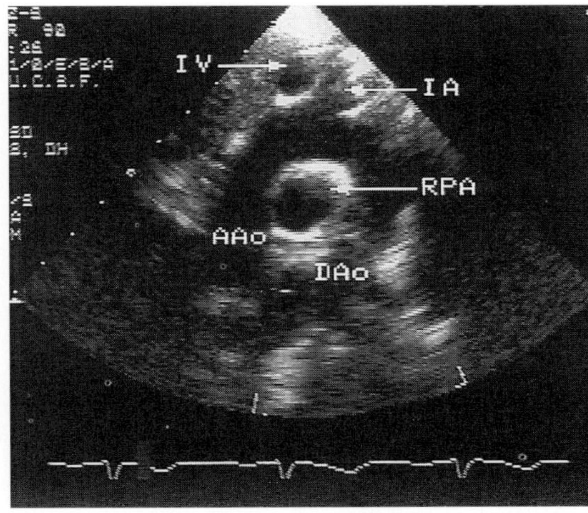

Figure 24–8 Echocardiogram from the suprasternal notch. AAo, ascending aorta; DAo, descending aorta; RPA, right pulmonary artery; IV, innominate vein; IA, innominate artery.

modality (many times, the study can be avoided altogether by referral to a pediatric cardiologist, whose auscultatory skills and expertise may obviate the need for echocardiography), there are those who require cardiac ultrasound examination to reliably exclude significant heart defects or to provide a precise anatomical or physiological diagnosis. Cardiac ultrasonography also frequently suffices as the primary diagnostic imaging study obtained preoperatively for many types of patients (Table 24–1). It is warranted intraoperatively to assess adequacy of congenital heart defect repair, intravascular line tip location, and location of interventional devices. Prenatal use of echocardiography has come into favor for evaluation of fetal cardiac malformations, dysrhythmias, and abnormal cardiac function.

Structural heart defects are accurately screened by echocardiographic study involving assessment of size and position of the cardiac chambers, valves, and great arteries. Further evaluation for intracardiac (e.g., atrial septal defect, ventricular septal defect) and extracardiac (e.g., patent ductus arteriosus) shunts is also essential. This is aided by (1) Doppler color flow mapping, which provides information about the direction and velocity of blood flow in color, on the background gray scale two-dimensional image, and (2) contrast echocardiography. In this latter technique, which is used for detection of intracardiac shunts as well as for confirming the presence of certain

Table 24-1 Surgery on Echo Evaluation Without Catheterization*

Cardiac Lesion	Number of Patients
Secundum ASD	20
Coarctation of the aorta	19
Transposition of the great arteries	18
Patent ductus arteriosus (not neonates)	14
Tetralogy of Fallot	10
Total anomalous pulmonary venous return	9
Perimembranous VSD	9
Taussig-Bing anomaly	7
Atrioventricular canal	7
Interrupted aortic arch	7
Hypoplastic left heart	3
Double-inlet ventricle	3
Subaortic stenosis (fixed)	2
Double-outlet right ventricle	2
Ostium primum ASD	2
Supracristal VSD	2
Miscellaneous	13

*University of California, San Francisco, experience 1993–1994. ASD, atrial septal defect; VSD, ventricular septal defect.

cardiac structures, a small quantity of the patient's blood (0.5–1 ml) is mixed with 20 ml of normal saline and then agitated to produce microcavitations, or microbubbles. Three to 5 ml of the solution is then injected into a peripheral vessel. The injected microcavitations follow blood flow back to the right side of the heart, where they appear as a cloud of reflective structures on echocardiography. Because the contrast microbubbles cannot enter the systemic circulation unless a right-to-left shunt is present, their detection in the left side of the heart provides definitive evidence of such a lesion. By a similar method, injection of microcavitations into the left side of the heart can be used to detect left-to-right shunts.

Valvar heart disease can also be reliably evaluated by cardiac ultrasonography. Doppler and two-dimensional echocardiography, in combination, can demonstrate both the morphological features and function of the heart valves. Atrioventricular valve regurgitation and stenosis, as well as semilunar valve regurgitation and stenosis, are commonly assessed by this technology, which provides information about the anatomical origins of valvar flow velocities and pressure gradients. By use of a modified version of the Bernoulli equation ($\Delta p = 4 \times v^2$), the peak flow velocity (v) across an orifice is measured by the Doppler recording and employed to calculate the peak instantaneous pressure drop (Δp) across that orifice. Prosthetic valves may be similarly studied for evidence of mechanical and circulatory dysfunction caused by wound dehiscence, abnormal leaflet motion, or interfering masses.

Numerous parameters of ventricular size and function, such as ventricular volume, ventricular mass, and ejection fraction, are amenable to echocardiographic evaluation. Because the loading conditions of the left ventricle may be determined by this modality, inference can be made about the contractile state of the ventricles as well. Recent technological advances in automated image-border detection systems hold promise for an even greater role for echocardiographic estimation of ventricular size and function.

Pericardial disease is often assessed by use of echocardiography, especially in the postoperative period when there is great suspicion of pericardial effusion. The thickness of the pericardium may be determined, along with presence of adhesions between the pericardium and the heart wall. If a significant effusion is identified, a safe route for drainage may be chosen by use of this technology.

Cardiac masses, including intracavitary thrombi, vegetations, and tumors, may be visualized using ultrasonographic examination techniques. Thrombi often occur in association with ventricular dysfunction, atrial dysrhythmias, or presence of prosthetic valves or indwelling catheters. They are typically attached to the heart or intracardiac device, and they appear echogenic (compared with myocardium), irregular in outline, and uneven in density. Vegetations are not easily distinguished from thrombi except by their predominant location on valve leaflets and sites of turbulence and their association with clinical signs and symptoms of endocarditis. Intra-cardiac solid tumors such as rhabdomyomas, teratomas, myxomas, and fibromas are easily detected but cannot be differentiated histologically by ultrasonic imaging.

Pacemaker leads and intravascular catheters can be conveniently localized by echocardiographic imaging in several planes. This ability is used to advantage both for catheter guidance during balloon atrial septostomies and for electrode tip localization during electrophysiological procedures.

Since the advent of high-resolution ultrasound scanners that make use of two-dimensional, M-mode, Doppler, and color Doppler imaging, fetal echocardiography has developed into an important discipline within pediatric cardiology. Currently this technology reliably screens for cardiac defects and abnormalities in function in the previable fetus. Such information may help determine the optimal site and route of delivery of the fetus, or it may influence the parents to avail themselves of the opportunity to terminate the pregnancy. Prenatal evaluation is recommended between 18 and 22 weeks of gestation when one of the following historical or clinical criteria is met: (1) there is a family history of congenital heart disease, (2) there is maternal disease that may affect the fetus, (3) there is a history of maternal drug use (including alcohol, lithium carbonate, antitumor drugs, anticonvulsants, and warfarin sodium), (4) there is evidence of other fetal abnormalities, or (5) there is evidence of hydrops fetalis. A wide variety of structural anomalies can be visualized, including atrioventricular septal defects, ventricular septal defects, cardiomyopathies, ventricular outlet obstructions, and complex cardiac defects (e.g., hypoplastic left heart with aortic or mitral atresia, pulmonary valve stenosis or atresia, transposition of the great vessels). In addition, fetal cardiac dysrhythmias may be detected. This is accomplished through timing analysis of mechanical events represented on M-mode or Doppler ultrasonography. The most common dysrhythmias encountered are premature atrial and ventricular contractions; these are usually benign and require no treatment. However, fetal tachydysrhythmias (most often supraventricular tachycardia) and bradydysrhythmias (e.g., complete heart block) are occasionally discovered. These may indicate the need for either early delivery of the infant or intrauterine treatment by administration of medication to the mother to prevent fetal hydrops.

Intraoperative echocardiography represents another technological advance that has found wide applicability. This imaging technique is used to delineate complex cardiac anatomy at the operating table as well as to detect residual structural problems in the immediate postoperative period (e.g., assessment of atrioventricular valve regurgitation after valvuloplasty, localization of residual ventricular septal defects). Ventricular function may also be evaluated, particularly in the period immediately after cardiopulmonary bypass.

Although it is apparent that the uses of cardiac ultrasonography have broadened considerably in recent years, there remain definite limitations to the technology. First, adequate echocardiographic windows must be available to image the heart and great vessels. Fetal ultrasonography poses a particular challenge in this regard, because the examiner has little control over the position of the fetus and thus the views obtained. In the postnatal patient, presence of bandages and chest tubes, chest deformities, and midline abdominal defects may limit transducer access to cardiac structures. In addition, patients with chronic lung disease and pulmonary hyperexpansion or those with pneumothoraces have poor windows for echocardiographic imaging because of ultrasonic energy reflection at air-tissue interfaces. Second, certain cardiovascular structures are practically inaccessible for imaging because of their anatomical proximity to air-containing structures. Examples of these structures include the distal branches of the pulmonary arteries near the lung hila and portions of the pulmonary veins.

Bibliography

Brook MM, Silverman NH, Villegas M: Cardiac ultrasonography in structural abnormalities and arrhythmias: recognition and treatment. *West J Med*, 159:286–300, 1993.

Danford DA, Nasir A, Gumbiner C: Cost assessment of the evaluation of heart murmurs in children. *Pediatrics*, 91:365–368, 1993.

Laird WP: Echocardiography. In Levin DL, Morriss FC, Moore GC (eds): *A Practical Guide to Pediatric Intensive Care*. St. Louis, CV Mosby, 1979.

Sanders SP: Echocardiography. In Fyler DC (ed): *Nadas' Pediatric Cardiology*. Philadelphia, Hanley & Belfus, 1992.

Silverman NH: Ultrasound for pediatric cardiac examination. In Rudolph AM, Hoffman JIE (eds): *Pediatrics*. Norwalk, CT, Appleton & Lange, 1991.

Chapter 25

Cardiac Catheterization

Daniel Stromberg

Cardiac catheterization is an invasive procedure useful for the evaluation and treatment of patients with congenital heart disease. Although the advent of excellent noninvasive imaging techniques in recent years has decreased the demand for cardiac catheterization, it provides accurate data for precise measurement of physiological cardiopulmonary parameters, and it produces high-quality images (especially when it is used in conjunction with angiocardiography) of cardiac anatomical features, some of which are poorly visualized by echocardiography. Cardiac catheterization can also be useful for electrophysiological evaluation and treatment. In certain instances it may be employed to alter intracardiac structures and blood vessels, thereby obviating the need for surgery.

Indications for cardiac catheterization vary enormously from medical center to medical center and from patient to patient, but they generally fall into four broad classes: (1) for delineation of cardiac anatomy, (2) for evaluation of physiological hemodynamics, (3) for purposes of therapeutic intervention, and (4) for purposes of diagnostic intervention. Table 25–1 lists the conditions for which cardiac catheterization is used at the University of California, San Francisco, and the reasons for such investigation.

Parental consent must be obtained for cardiac catheterization. Parents should be apprised in detail of the risks and benefits, especially in situations in which patients are at increased risk for adverse outcomes. Such situations include (1) total anomalous pulmonary venous return, (2) severe pulmonary vascular disease with an intact ventricular septum and no aortopulmonary communication, (3) frequent-onset spontaneous dysrhythmia, (4) severe hypoxemia, (5) severe cardiac failure, particularly due to obstructive lesions, and (6) pulmonic stenosis and ventricular septal defect in those who are prone to hypercyanotic spells. Patients with these maladies may still safely undergo cardiac catheterization if appropriate precautions are taken.

Older children undergoing cardiac catheterization must also be prepared for the procedure. Preparation usually entails explaining the premedication and anesthetic procedures, reassuring the child that pain during the procedure will be minimal, and telling the child that a

Table 25-1 Conditions Warranting Cardiac Catheterization and Their General Indications

Condition	Indication
Tetralogy of Fallot Truncus arteriosus Pulmonary atresia	Delineation of anatomy
Single ventricle Ventricular septal defect Ostium primum atrial septal defect Atrioventricular canal	Measurement of physiological parameters
Pulmonary stenosis Aortic stenosis Ostium secundum atrial septal defect Patent ductus arteriosus Coarctation of the aorta Transposition of great vessels Dysrhythmias	Therapeutic intervention
Myocarditis Dysrhythmias	Diagnostic intervention

number of x-ray pictures of the heart will be obtained.

Premedication of children undergoing cardiac catheterization has, in the past, included meperidine, chlorpromazine, and promethazine. At the author's institution, this regimen has been replaced by a staged approach to premedication. In advance of the patient's arrival at the catheterization suite, sedation is initiated with oral diphenhydramine. A topical anesthetic cream, EMLA (2.5% prilocaine and 2.5% lidocaine), which must remain on the skin for 45 minutes to 1 hour for maximal effect, is placed over the site of anticipated percutaneous catheterization. The child is then transported to the catheterization room, where further sedative is administered in the form of oral pentobarbital. Systemic analgesia is provided by administration of oral methadone. Patients requiring additional sedation are given either more pentobarbital or midazolam. The success of this incremental medication protocol has been remarkable.

Adequate attention should always be paid to aspiration precautions, such that the appropriate amount of time elapses without ingestion of liquids and solids before medications are given. Furthermore, the sedated patient must be properly monitored, and all potentially necessary emergency equipment, medications, and personnel must be available.

Cardiac catheterization involves the placement of a catheter in a peripheral blood vessel, either percutaneously or by cutdown and isolation of the relevant vessel. Percutaneous catheterization poses a lower risk of infectious and arterial complications and allows repeated use of the same vessel. The femoral approach is most commonly used because the vasculature there is readily accessible and is of large enough diameter to permit passage of a venous catheter into the left side of the heart through a patent foramen ovale, an atrial septal defect, or a ventricular septal defect. This avoids the need for retrograde arterial catheterization and its attendant complications.

The type of catheter employed in a given situation depends on the indication for the study. Special catheters with unique properties and abilities are used for interventional procedures, intracardiac electrocardiography, and intracardiac phonocardiography. Despite their differences, however, most catheters are semirigid, and their position is controlled by twisting the catheter or manipulating associated tip-deflecting wires.

Once the proper catheter has been guided into a large vessel, its movements are observed fluoroscopically and by continuous intravascular pressure monitoring during catheter advancement. Both methods reveal catheter position within the heart and great vessels—the former by direct visualization, and the latter by inference from pressure tracings. Differences in pressure from location to location may also facilitate discovery of obstructions to blood flow and permit determination of their severity. Blood oxygen saturation in each of the major vessels and cardiac chambers can be determined by successive sampling to assess the presence of a shunt. Caution must be used in interpreting these data because streaming from different vessels may create significant sampling errors. Normal pediatric pressure and oxygen saturation values within the heart are shown in Figure 25–1.

Blood flow through normal structures and shunts may be determined according to the Fick equation:

$$\text{Pulmonary flow } (Q_p) = \frac{VO_2}{C_{PV} - C_{PA}}$$

$$\text{Systemic flow } (Q_s) = \frac{VO_2}{C_{AO} - C_{MV}}$$

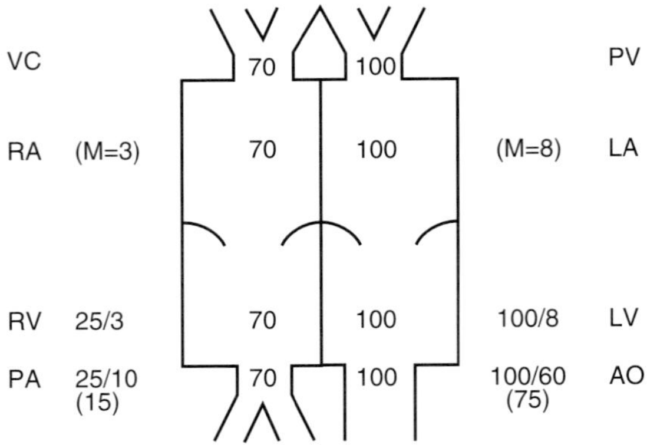

Figure 25–1 Normal pressure and oxygen saturation values in children. AO, aorta; LA, left atrium; LV, left ventricle; PA, pulmonary artery; PV, pulmonary veins; RA, right atrium; RV, right ventricle; VC, vena cava. (Redrawn from Park MK: *Pediatric Cardiology Handbook.* St Louis, CV Mosby, 1991, p 65.)

where flow is given in liters/minute, V_{O_2} is oxygen consumption (ml/min), C is oxygen content at various positions, PV is pulmonary vein, PA is pulmonary artery, AO is aorta, and MV is mixed systemic venous blood. Oxygen consumption is either measured directly during the procedure or estimated on the basis of age, sex, and heart rate. Oxygen content is derived from the multiplication of oxygen capacity (total amount of oxygen that hemoglobin contains when it is 100% saturated) by percentage saturation, plus dissolved oxygen. The Fick equation results may then be used to calculate the magnitude of left-to-right and right-to-left shunts:

$$\text{Left-to-right shunt} = Q_p - Q_s$$

$$\text{Right-to-left shunt} = Q_s - Q_p$$

Catheterization data can also be used to calculate the resistance to blood flow in the pulmonary and systemic circulations according to the following equations derived from Ohm's law:

$$\text{PVR (pulmonary vascular resistance)} = (\text{mean pulmonary artery pressure} - \text{mean left atrial pressure})/Q_p$$

$$\text{SVR (systemic vascular resistance)} = (\text{mean aortic pressure} - \text{mean right atrial pressure})/Q_s$$

The normal SVR varies between 15 and 30 units/m^2 body surface area, such that when pressures are measured in millimeters of mercury, resistance units are equivalent to millimeters of mercury per liter per minute. Normal PVR values vary with age. They are high at birth but diminish to almost adult values (1–3 units/m^2) after 2 to 4 months.

In addition to hemodynamic analysis, cardiac catheterization may be used for angiographic evaluation. In this procedure, a radiopaque dye (usually 1–2 ml/kg) is rapidly injected through a catheter into a particular cardiac chamber, and angiograms are recorded on motion picture film at 60 to 90 frames/second. An image intensifier is used to decrease the patient's exposure to radiation, which, extrapolated from adult cardiac catheterization studies, is in the range of 20 to 47 roentgen (R) (a pediatric barium enema examination involves doses of approximately 4 to 10 R). Several views, and multiple dye injection sites, are usually necessary for complete and accurate delineation of cardiovascular structures. Images obtained in this manner can be examined immediately on a video replay system, facilitating prompt diagnosis.

Interventional cardiac catheterization techniques have been employed effectively in treatment of a number of ailments, many of which formerly required surgical remedies, with their attendant risks, scars, and lengthy postoperative recovery periods. Perhaps the oldest pediatric interventional catheterization procedure involves the creation or enlargement of atrial communications. Many individuals with complicated cardiac abnormalities depend on bidirectional shunting through an atrial septal defect for survival; examples include neonates with D-transposition and a constricted ductus arteriosus, neonates with a single ventricle and a small mitral valve, neonates with mitral atresia, and children with total anomalous pulmonary venous return. Therefore, in an attempt to improve mixing at the atrial level in patients with these lesions, balloon atrial septostomy (Rashkind's procedure) is performed. Rashkind's procedure involves the passage of a balloon-tipped catheter through the foramen ovale under echocardiographic or fluorosopic guidance into the left atrium, followed by balloon inflation, and then rapid and forceful retraction across the septum. This tears the septum and establishes the atrial shunt. If an atrial communication is required in an older infant (> 1 month), who is likely to have a thicker septum less easily torn by an inflated balloon, blade atrial septostomy can be accomplished by use of a special catheter with a retractable knife that cuts open the atrial septum (Park's procedure). Park's procedure may be followed by balloon septostomy to ensure existence of an adequate atrial communication.

Catheterization techniques may also be employed to close intracardiac shunts. Atrial septal defects may be occluded by expandable umbrella devices. This technique is still under development, but 70 patients had been successfully treated with these instruments by 1990. Occlusion techniques for the patent ductus arteriosus that employ a double umbrella wrapped in thrombolytic-soaked cloth have also proved effective. Closure is achieved in more than 95% of cases, and late problems from device migration, embolic phenomena, or endocarditis have not been encountered. Nonsurgical closure of arteriovenous fistulas and bronchial collateral vessels (which often develop in children with tetralogy of Fallot) may be attained by use of catheters with detachable balloons that have valves to prevent subsequent deflation. Alternatively, embolization with metallic coils (10% to 30% larger than the diameter of the vessel to be occluded) may be attempted. Both coil embolization and balloon occlusion have been used successfully to block aortopulmonary shunts. Transcatheter closure of ventricular septal defects remains experimental.

Interventional catheterization has been successfully applied to angioplasty of obstructed vessels. The original impetus for use of this technology was the high mortality rate associated with surgical repair of obstructed lesions in infancy and the high frequency of persistent or recurrent pressure gradients after surgery for coarctation of the aorta. Balloon dilation of native (i.e., not previously repaired) aortic coarctation in neonates and children has shown mixed results. Although immediate findings in all pediatric age groups revealed encouraging pressure gradient reduction, complications from the procedure (particularly the tendency to cause aortic aneurysms from the tearing of the intima and media) have necessarily limited its use. By contrast, balloon angioplasty of coarctations that persist or recur at a site previously repaired by surgery offers a satisfactory alternative to operative therapy. Results and complications compare favorably, because scarring from prior surgery appears to protect against the destructive effects of the dilating balloon. Additional structures that have proved amenable to angioplasty include the various aortopulmonary shunts and stenosed branch pulmonary arteries.

Like balloon angioplasty, balloon dilation valvuloplasty has found utility within pediatric cardiology. Balloon dilation valvuloplasty involves inflation of a balloon that has been positioned across a stenotic valve orifice. The force applied to fill the balloon is transmitted to the surrounding tissues, safely reducing the valvar obstruction. Balloon pulmonary valvuloplasty has proved to be highly successful; postprocedure pressure gradients are typically reduced to 5 to 15 mm Hg, with little or no creation of valvar insufficiency. Balloon aortic valvuloplasty has also met with considerable success. It provides good relief of aortic obstruction while producing variable but usually mild aortic insufficiency. Similar results have been obtained with balloon mitral valvuloplasty performed in patients with either rheumatic or congenital mitral stenosis. For patients who have undergone prior valvar surgery and have reobstruction, balloon valvuloplasty has been used successfully as a means of deferring surgical valve replacement.

Finally, interventional catheterization has been used effectively for retrieval of intravascular foreign bodies and for endomyocardial biopsy. Intravascular foreign bodies, including embolized fragments of venous lines or coils, can be removed by special intravascular instruments that have at their tip either a retractable wire loop or a wire cage. These can be used to grab the misplaced material for eventual disposal. Endomyocardial biopsy may be safely performed with a bioptome advanced through a sheath to the cardiac structure to be sampled.

Despite the technological advances in instrumentation that make cardiac catheterization safer and more precise (e.g., smaller catheters, more flexible shafts, flow-directed balloons, less toxic contrast agents), cardiac catheterization and angiocardiography can lead to serious, albeit uncommon, complications. These complications include serious dysrhythmias, arterial obstruction, hemorrhage, reaction to contrast medium, cardiac perforation, hypoxemic episodes, infection, and death. The risk of encountering such complications generally varies according to the age and severity of illness of the patient, the type of lesion, and the level of experience of those performing the procedure. However, the overall nonfatal complication rate is about 8%, the majority of those being minor complications (6.8%). Less than 1% of patients are left with residual deficits from the procedure. The mortality rate for all ages after catheterization is approximately 0.4%; if only deaths considered directly attributable to catheterization are counted, the mortality rate decreases to 0.2%.

Among the most common problems noted after cardiac catheterization are arterial occlusion and bleeding. Heparinization of catheters along with intermittent monitoring of activated clotting times during procedures has markedly decreased the frequency of arterial occlusion. Nonetheless, although it is extremely rare beyond infancy, arterial occlusion leading to temporary or permanent pulse loss does occur in approximately 2.4% of children undergoing retrograde arterial procedures. Treatment with urokinase has proved effective in restoring pulses in most of these patients. Bleeding complications are observed in approximately 2% of catheterized patients and usually involve local hematomas at the percutaneous wound site; however, significant blood loss requiring transfusion does occur in rare cases.

Bibliography

Bass JL, Tadavarthy SM, et al: Interventional procedures in congenital heart disease. In Tonkin IL (ed): *Pediatric Cardiovascular Imaging.* Philadelphia, WB Saunders, 1992.

Cassidy SC, Schmidt KG, et al: Complications of pediatric cardiac catheterization: a 3-year study. *J Am Coll Cardiol,* 19:1285–1293, 1992.

Hellenbrand WE, Allen HD, et al: Balloon angioplasty for aortic recoarctation: results of valvuloplasty and angioplasty of congenital anomalies registry. *Am J Cardiol,* 65:793–797, 1990.

Lock JE, Keane JF, et al: Cardiac catheterization. In Fyler DC (ed): *Nadas' Pediatric Cardiology.* Philadelphia, Hanley & Belfus, 1992.

Park MK: *Pediatric Cardiology Handbook.* St Louis, Mosby–Year Book, 1991.

Stanger P: Cardiac catheterization. In Rudolph AM, Hoffman JIE (eds): *Pediatrics.* Norwalk, CT, Appleton & Lange, 1991.

Tynan M, Finley JP, et al: Balloon angioplasty for the treatment of native coarctation: results of valvuloplasty and angioplasty of congenital anomalies registry. *Am J Cardiol,* 65:790–792, 1990.

Chapter 26

Patent Ductus Arteriosus

Daniel Stromberg

The ductus arteriosus, a vascular structure derived from the left sixth aortic arch, connects the pulmonary artery to the aorta at a point just distal to the takeoff of the left subclavian artery. During fetal life, the ductus arteriosus (which is often as large as the ascending aorta) carries fetal blood passing through the right ventricle to the descending aorta, effectively routing blood flow from the high-resistance pulmonary arteriolar bed into the low-resistance aortoplacental bed. After birth, the vessel closes rapidly. In so doing, it directs right-sided cardiac output to the pulmonary vasculature and establishes series circulation between the right and left sides of the heart.

If the ductus arteriosus does not close shortly after birth, this abnormality is referred to as a patent ductus arteriosus (PDA). It is commonly encountered as an isolated defect (i.e., a genetically determined deficiency in the amount of ductal smooth muscle) or associated with congenital heart disease. PDAs may also be detected, either persistently or intermittently, in premature infants, in those patients with circulatory or ventilatory problems, and in those patients born of mothers who had rubella infection around the time of conception.

The natural history of a PDA in the normal, full-term newborn involves functional closure within several hours after birth. Patency beyond the first day or two of life is usually permanent unless therapy is provided. In the premature newborn, spontaneous ductal closure is delayed, at times for weeks. In addition, a larger percentage of preterm children have PDA persistence past infancy, compared with their term counterparts in the general population. PDAs are found with increased frequency as birth weight decreases. In one study, 40% of infants weighing less than 1000 g at birth were found to have symptoms attributable to a PDA.

Ductal patency is further prolonged by birth asphyxia and the presence of respiratory distress syndrome (RDS). Those patients without RDS have been found to exhibit ductal closure on the same time scale as term infants; that is, approximately 97% of preterm infants have evidence of spontaneous ductal closure by the fourth day of life, irrespective of gestational age. Those premature infants with RDS have a slightly higher prevalence of delayed closure (11%, compared with 3%) by day four of life, for reasons that are not clearly understood. Exogenous surfactant does not appear to have an adverse impact on ductal patency.

Understanding of functional ductal abnormalities is facilitated by knowledge of the structure's normal anatomical and physiological features. On histological examination, the ductus differs greatly from aortic or pulmonary arterial tissue. Unlike these vessels, the normal ductus arteriosus contains little elastic tissue; it has instead large amounts of mucoid material. It also has copious ground substance containing smooth muscle cells in a spiral arrangement that contract with increasing oxygen exposure. In the fetal environment, the patency of the ductus is maintained by the combined relaxant effects of low oxygen tension and locally synthesized vasodilatory E-type prostaglandins. Near term, ductal responsiveness to prostaglandins decreases, whereas oxygen sensitivity increases. This brings about enhanced ductal closure at birth, with smooth muscle contraction, coalescence of the vessel's mucoid material, and protrusion of the intima into the ductal lumen. Thereafter, intimal proliferation ensues, promoting thrombosis and sealing the ductus completely. This is followed by deposition of fibrous tissue, which transforms the occluded, constricted vessel remnant into the ligamentum arteriosum.

The ductus is influenced physiologically by an infant's first respiratory efforts. With the onset of gasping at birth, the child's arterial Po_2 increases, leading to (1) an abrupt fall in pulmonary arteriolar resistance, and a resultant change in the direction of ductal shunting from right-to-left to predominantly left-to-right, and (2) contraction of the ductal smooth muscle, which brings about the ductal closure cascade. If the ductus does not close, excessive blood flow from the aorta to the pulmonary arteries results in increased circulation through the lungs, left atrium, left ventricle, and ascending aorta. These structures may enlarge in proportion to the size of the left-to-right shunt, and congestive heart failure may supervene. If the ductus remains widely patent, there may be equilibration of the aortic and pulmonary artery pressures, which over time can bring about irreversible pulmonary vascular disease, although this condition is rare before 1 year of age. The patient with a PDA is also at higher risk for endocarditis because high-velocity ductal blood flow can damage vessel endothelium to create a vascular microenvironment predisposed to thrombus formation and subsequent infection.

Clinical manifestations of a PDA vary with the amount of blood passed into the pulmonary circulation. In the neonate, a small shunt may produce nothing more than a systolic murmur. A large shunt may give rise to a widened pulse pressure (greater than approximately 30–40 mm Hg), bounding peripheral pulses, and signs and symptoms of congestive heart failure (feeding difficulty, sweating, tachypnea, dyspnea, intercostal and subcostal retractions, hepatomegaly, and growth failure). Classic auscultatory findings include a crescendo systolic murmur, which peaks in intensity at aortic closure and continues into diastole as a high-frequency decrescendo murmur. These sounds are often accompanied by coarse systolic clicking noises, which produce the "machinery-like" sounds heard best at the second left intercostal space. Although many patients have the characteristic continuous murmur of a PDA, the diastolic component is rarely appreciated in small infants, even if the ductus is large. If pulmonary hypertension develops, auscultatory findings may not be typical. Cyanosis is not evident in PDA patients unless pulmonary edema or irreversible pulmonary vascular disease with right-to-left shunting evolves.

PDA manifestations in the preterm infant being ventilated for RDS may include, in addition to the above-mentioned physical findings, failure to show anticipated improvement after several days of RDS therapy or frank respiratory deterioration with increasing ventilator dependency. Moreover, a PDA must also be considered a possibly negative influence on the development of necrotizing enterocolitis and recurrent apnea.

The diagnosis of a PDA can be established on clinical grounds alone. However, several studies can provide confirmatory evidence of its presence. The electrocardiogram may be normal in the case of a small ductus, or it may show signs of left ventricular hypertrophy with existence of a somewhat larger PDA. If pulmonary vascular disease has developed, evidence of right ventricular hypertrophy may predominate. Enlargement of the aorta, left ventricle, left atrium, pulmonary vessels, and main pulmonary artery occurs in proportion to the magnitude of the left-to-right shunt. The plain chest film may show a cardiac silhouette appropriately altered by these anatomical changes.

Echocardiographic evaluation of a PDA provides a wealth of important information. In addition to screening for concurrent congenital heart disease, this modality permits direct visualization of the PDA. If Doppler analysis is employed, the left-to-right shunt may be quantified, as may the gradient of pressure extant between the aorta and the pulmonary artery (absence of such a gradient is interpreted as a sign of pulmonary hypertension at the systemic level). Cardiac ultrasonography also has the ability to accurately demonstrate the enlargement or hypertrophy of the cardiac chambers and great vessels. Catheterization is reserved for the rare instance in which echocardiographic findings are confusing or nondiagnostic or when complex congenital heart disease is present.

The ductus arteriosus may be closed by either medical or surgical means when left-to-right shunting is clinically detrimental, or its patency may be prolonged to maintain pulmonary or systemic blood flow. Preservation of ductal blood flow has been found advantageous in neonates with heart disease characterized by (1) severe restriction of pulmonary blood flow, (2) poor arterial-venous admixture, or (3) severe systemic hypoperfusion. Manipulation of ductal patency for palliation of symptoms in these conditions is achieved through use of E-type prostaglandins or through endovascular ductal stent placement in the cardiac catheterization laboratory.

As previously mentioned, the fetal ductus remains patent because of the combined relaxant effects of low oxygen tension and locally synthesized prostaglandin E (PGE). After birth, blood oxygen tension obligately increases; however, some ductal sensitivity to prostaglandins is maintained. This provides the rationale for use of PGE_1, another E-type prostaglandin, in forms of congenital heart disease in which temporary ductal patency is required. PGE_1 may be used to keep the ductus open or reopen a ductus that has functionally closed. The medication's efficacy is improved when it is employed early in the neonatal period; infants older than 96 hours are significantly less responsive to it than are younger infants. Once ductal patency is achieved, it may be maintained for as long as 2 months by use of PGE_1.

E-type prostaglandin should be administered continuously (although, in emergency situations, it can be given intravenously or orally every hour), for it is rapidly metabolized in a single pass through the lungs. The initial infusion rate commonly used to obtain a therapeutic response is 0.05 μ/kg/min. This may be increased gradually to a maximum of 0.2 μ/kg/min, although such augmentation is rarely necessary. The onset of action is usually rapid (i.e., within several minutes).

Adverse effects of PGE_1 include cutaneous vasodilation, jitteriness, seizures, diarrhea, apnea/hypoventilation, and hyperpyrexia. The last two side effects occur in 10% to 15% of cases in a dose-independent fashion. Thus, their common appearance and potential for severe complication justify special observation and management of the child receiving PGE_1 therapy. Primarily, the infant must be watched and monitored closely for respiratory compromise in a setting where proper resuscitation equipment and expertise is available. Because the child under treatment is at risk for sudden-onset apnea requiring emergent intubation and ventilation, airway protection should usually be accomplished before interhospital transfer, when such procedures may prove more difficult. Hyperpyrexia in the infant receiving PGE_1 suggests sepsis until the diagnosis is ruled out definitively. Therefore, neonates are often screened with a complete blood count and blood culture, started on broad antibiotic coverage (most frequently ampicillin and gentamycin), and observed closely.

In the setting of severe restriction of pulmonary blood flow (e.g., tricuspid atresia, pulmonary atresia, tetralogy of Fallot), PGE_1 may be used to avoid the overwhelming hypoxemia and metabolic acidosis that would result from natural postnatal ductal closure. By dilating the ductus, prostaglandin frequently augments pulmonary blood flow sufficiently to bring about a 20- to 30-mm Hg increase in arterial Po_2. Most patients respond favorably to an increase in systemic oxygenation of this magnitude, which in turn improves survival during the critical hours required for transfer to a pediatric cardiology center, for diagnostic study, or for mobilization of a surgical team.

Infants with congenital heart disease resulting in poor venous admixture, as might be found in those with transposition of the great vessels and intact ventricular septum, may also benefit from PGE_1 therapy. Ductal dilation in this situation improves mixing of the parallel systemic and pulmonary circulations until such time as an atrial level shunt can be created, usually by balloon atrial septostomy.

In various forms of hypoplastic left heart syndrome, including aortic atresia, critical aortic stenosis, interrupted aortic arch, and severe juxtaductal coarctation of the aorta, ductal patency may again be critical to early neonatal survival. These conditions are marked by extreme left ventricular outflow obstruction and resultant systemic hypoperfusion; virtually all systemic blood flow is supplied by the right heart output, which travels through the ductus. Without such ductal blood flow, shock, acidosis, and death would ensue. Therefore, PGE_1 is used temporarily to maintain ductal patency, and thus viability, in anticipation of surgical correction of the cardiac lesions.

The presence of elevated pulmonary vascular resistance, either as a primary lesion or secondary to cardiopulmonary disease, in combination with a PDA raises the question of whether the ductus should be left open to allow shunting or closed to "force" blood into the pulmonary circuit. The answer to this is not definitively known. Infants have rarely been observed to improve after ductal ligation in the setting of persistent fetal circulation syndrome (i.e., pulmonary vascular constriction unassociated with parenchymal pulmonary disease). Nevertheless, ductal manipulation is currently not recommended because the ductus closes spontaneously in the majority of term infants once the abnormal pulmonary vascular condition is resolved. Therapy is instead directed toward both treatment of the illness predisposing to elevated pulmonary vascular resistance and improved oxygenation. Oxygenation may be improved by dilation of the pulmonary vasculature through hyperventilation (alkalosis gives rise to pulmonary vasodilation) or vasodilating medications (nitric oxide, tolazoline). Extracorporeal membrane oxygenation, a form of cardiopulmonary bypass, may also be required for adequate oxygenation.

Closure of the ductus arteriosus may be warranted to eliminate congestive heart failure and promote growth in an infant, to prevent infective endocarditis, and to preclude development of pulmonary vascular disease. This may be accomplished safely by a transcatheter, surgical, or medical approach. The transcatheter method involves extrusion of an umbrella-like device that occludes the ductus from a cardiac catheter. This procedure is limited by device size to children older than 18 months. Surgical intervention involves ligation or division of the ductus. This proven form of therapy has minimal risks and few recurrences but suffers from the complications attendant to thoracic surgical intervention.

Medical management (beyond therapy for congestive heart failure, which lies outside the scope of this chapter) has centered around the neonatal use of indomethacin for ductal closure. The rationale for this approach is that indomethacin acts as a potent prostaglandin synthetase inhibitor, which promotes ductal closure by inhibition of prostaglandin production and activity; it is thought to be most efficacious if given in the first 14 days of life. Multicenter study of the relative merits of indomethacin treatment versus surgery for PDA closure in premature infants has not demonstrated a difference in the complication rate between the two management methods. Therefore, at the author's institution, PDA treatment commences with medical management based on the infant's birth weight, followed by surgery when medical treatment is unsuccessful.

Contraindications to indomethacin therapy include active bleeding from any source, presence of necrotizing enterocolitis, and renal insufficiency marked by a serum creatinine level above 2.0 mg/dl (levels above 1.7 mg/dl should prompt reconsideration of the risks and benefits posed by medical versus surgical intervention). Presence of intracranial hemorrhage is not a contraindication to initiation of antiprostaglandin therapy.

In keeping with these principles, evaluation of the patient before administration of indomethacin should include a thorough physical examination looking for evidence of a PDA, bleeding, and necrotizing enterocolitis; a platelet count and serum creatinine level should be obtained, and the patient's baseline urinary output should be accurately measured. If the platelet count is less than 50,000, platelet transfusion is recommended before initiation of therapy. Fluid status should be monitored closely because indomethacin may transiently decrease urine output. This, in turn, could cause fluid overload, which promotes ductal patency and worsens pulmonary function. If parenteral diuretics are to be used, furosemide should be used sparingly or in combination with another agent because this medication is known to promote ductal patency by stimulating renal PGE production. An echocardiogram should also be obtained before indomethacin therapy for purposes of definitive diagnosis and to rule out other structural heart disease. The only group that may be exempted from the requirement for a pretreatment echocardiogram is the group of extremely low birth weight infants (< 850 g); 80% of these neonates who have a heart murmur demonstrate a PDA on cardiac ultrasound examination.

Specific medical treatment recommendations are also based on the infant's birth weight. Neonates weighing more than 1000 g at birth should be treated when two or more of the following signs of a PDA are present: (1) heart murmur, (2) increased pulse volume marked by bounding peripheral pulses or palmar pulses, (3) increased pulse pressure (systolic blood pressure − diastolic blood pressure), or (4) increased precordial activity. Infants in the weight category above 1000 g with a majority of these findings have a high likelihood of having a moderate-sized PDA that, if left untreated, would probably prolong the need for oxygen therapy and delay the institution of enteral feedings.

For neonates weighing less than 1000 g at birth, it is known that 70% to 85% of those who have a murmur, even without other signs of a PDA, will eventually have a PDA requiring treatment. Furthermore, 80% of those who have an echocardiographically significant left-to-right ductal shunt on the third day of life, also without clinical signs of a PDA go on to have a symptomatic ductus necessitating therapy. Therefore, infants with birth weight less than 1000 g should receive indomethacin either when either a heart murmur is discovered with other clinical signs of a PDA or when a day 3 echocardiogram reveals a PDA with a significant left-to-right shunt (without regard to the presence of other clinical PDA signs). The earlier infants are treated with indomethacin, the greater the efficacy in producing permanent ductal closure.

Dosage recommendations for antiprostaglandin therapy are also based on the patient's birth weight. Neonates weighing more than 1250 g should receive 0.2 mg/kg of indomethacin intravenously, followed 12 hours later by the same dose, and then a third dose of 0.2 mg/kg at 36 hours from the initial drug administration. If the infant is older than 4 days, the total dose may be given in a 24-hour period (i.e., at times 0, 12 hours, and 24 hours) because children past that age metabolize the medication more quickly. Neonates weighing less than 1250 g should be given 0.2 mg/kg of indomethacin intravenously at time 0, then 0.1 mg/kg at hour 12, followed by 0.1 mg/kg at hour 36. Newer recommendations include the prolonged use of indomethacin at a dose of 0.1 mg/kg for 6 days. This method demonstrated less elevation of the serum creatinine concentration along with a slightly lower PDA recurrence rate. The recurrence rate of ductal patency after one of the standard three-dose regimens ranges from 26% to 40%.

If the success of one of these drug schedules is only temporary and the PDA recurs, the course of medication can be repeated. However, failure of the second round of medical therapy or the occurrence of significant side effects should prompt surgical intervention. Infants weighing less than 850 g are less likely to respond to a second course of indomethacin and, therefore, may require surgical ligation as a second-line treatment.

Studies of prophylactic indomethacin administered to premature infants for prevention of intracranial hemorrhage have also demonstrated significant benefits in ductal closure rates. This work may provide the foundation for future recommendations regarding preventive ductal management strategies.

Bibliography

Archer N: Patent ductus arteriosus in the newborn. *Arch Dis Child,* 69:529–532, 1993.

Clyman R, Sola A: Clinical Consensus Group: indomethacin and the patent ductus arteriosus (unpublished), November 1991.

Fyler DC: Patent ductus arteriosus. In Fyler DC (ed): *Nadas' Pediatric Cardiology.* Philadelphia, Hanley & Belfus, 1992.

Gersony WM: Patent ductus arteriosus in the neonate. *Pediat Clin North Am,* 33:545–559, 1986.

Reller MD, Rice MJ, McDonald RW: Review of studies evaluating ductal patency in the premature infant. *J Pediatr,* 122:S59–S62, 1993.

Section E

Emergencies

Chapter 27

Fluid and Metabolic Therapy

Walter T. Hughes

Parenteral fluid therapy has become a hallmark of pediatrics. A relatively new therapeutic tool in medicine, intravascular infusion of fluids has developed too slowly since Sir Christopher Wren, in 1656, successfully administered opium from a bladder and quill into the veins of a dog. In 1667, Lower and King transfused 9 or 10 ounces of sheep's blood into an arm vein of a human. It was not until the early part of the present century, however, that blood transfusions and intravenous administration of glucose and electrolyte solutions could be safely used therapeutically.

Several routes are available for the administration of fluids:

1. Alimentary

   Oral
   Gastric drip and gavage
   Rectal

2. Intravascular

   Intravenous

3. Hypodermoclysis
4. Intraosseous
5. Intraperitoneal

Only the methods of parenteral administration of fluids are considered in this chapter.

AXIOM: Never administer a solution or drug parenterally that can be equally effective administered orally.

The basic apparatus required for any type of parenteral infusion is made up of a flask or bag to contain the solution or blood, a needle or catheter to enter the subject's blood vessel or other tissue, and a tubing system to connect the flask to the needle or catheter.

PHYSICAL PRINCIPLES RELATED TO INFUSION OF FLUIDS

Hagen-Poiseuille Law

The rate of flow of a solution moving smoothly through a tube in a laminar manner

Supported in part by National Cancer Institute Cancer Center Support (CORE) Grant P30CA21765 and American Lebanese Syrian Associated Charities.

is proportional to the pressure gradient (expressed as *total pressure drop*), the *length of the tube*, and the *fourth power of the diameter of the tube* and is inversely proportional to the viscosity of the fluid. These factors may be expressed as the Hagen-Poiseuille equation (Macintosh et al, 1958):

Volume flow rate =

$$\frac{\text{Pressure}}{\text{Tubing length}} \times \text{Diameter} \times \frac{1}{\text{Viscosity}}$$

EXAMPLE: An infusion flask or bag and tubing are set up with the level of fluid in the flask 0.6 m above the needle. The needle has an inner bore of 0.36 mm and is 3 cm in length. During each minute, 4.5 ml of fluid passes through the needle.

If the flask is elevated so that the level of fluid is 1.2 m above the needle, the flow of fluid is approximately doubled. If the flask is lowered so that the level of fluid is at the original height of 0.6 m and a larger needle with an inner bore of 0.93 mm and the same 3-cm length is used, the flow is about *17 times greater* than with the smaller needle and the same pressure. Thus, use of a large needle to increase flow of an infusion is preferable to increasing the pressure in the small-bore needle.

EXAMPLE: Identical syringes are attached to needles that have different bore sizes. One needle has half the internal diameter of the other.

Identical force is applied to the plungers of the syringes. The volume of fluid expelled in a unit of time is 16 (2^4) times greater from the needle with the large bore. Thus, the same volume of fluid can be ejected from the syringe with the large needle in one-sixteenth the time required for the small needle under the same thumb pressure.

Farman and Powell (1969) compared various different-gauged intravenous needles and catheters and recorded flow rates through them (using both water and blood) under fixed conditions. They showed, for a given gauge, that needles generally outperform plastic catheters with regard to flow rates. There are at least two reasons: (1) intravenous needles are shorter than most plastic cannulas, and (2) their intraluminal diameter is usually greater than that of plastic cannulas of similar gauge because the steel walls can be thinner and still be as strong. Approximate rates of flow through various devices are shown in Table 27–1.

Table 27–1 Expected Flow Rates of Water and Blood Through Needles and Cannulas

Device	Water (ml/min)	Blood (ml/min)
Scalp Vein Needles		
25-gauge	2	0.4
23-gauge	5–6	1–2
21-gauge	20–25	6–8
19-gauge	approx. 60	approx. 20
16-gauge	approx. 250	approx. 8
Plastic Cannulas (4 cm)		
19-gauge	20–40	8–20
18-gauge	90–100	approx. 50
16-gauge	approx. 150	approx. 70
Plastic Cannulas (6 cm)		
18-gauge	45–50	10–15
16-gauge	100–150	50–70
14-gauge	approx. 200	90–100

From Hughes WT, Buescher ES: *Pediatric Procedures.* Philadelphia, WB Saunders, 1980.

Laminar Flow

Laminar flow occurs when a liquid flows smoothly through a tube with the particles composing the liquid moving in lines parallel to the walls of the tube.

Turbulent Flow

Turbulent flow occurs when the lines of flow are not parallel to the walls of the tube but are irregular and disorderly. Points of angulation and constriction produce turbulence. If fluid flowing through a tube ceases to be laminar and becomes turbulent, additional resistance is created, and the flow rate is decreased. If the tubing of the infusion set is angular or constricted, the flow may be impaired by affixing it with tape to the patient, restraint board, or bed.

Viscosity

The property of a liquid that presents a resistance to flow is called viscosity. Because the viscosity of a liquid decreases with a rise in temperature and fluid flow is inversely proportional to viscosity, blood flows proportional to viscosity, blood flows more slowly than water, and cold solutions flow more slowly than warm.

Intravenous Infusion

In most instances, the parenteral administration of fluid is best carried out by infusing directly into the venous system. Many sites are readily adaptable to venocylsis (the injection of fluid into a vein). Figure 27–1 illustrates superficial veins used most frequently. The human peripheral vascular system is symmetrical.

The largest visible vein is not necessarily the preferred one. Also, one must consider the comfort of the patient, position and extent of restraint, ability to maintain a needle in the vessel, solution to be injected, and possible hazards and complications from the selected site.

ACCESSIBLE VEINS FOR VENOCLYSIS

1. Back of Hand

   Dorsal metacarpal
   Dorsal venous network

2. Arm

   Cephalic
   Basilic

3. Antecubital Fossa

   Median cephalic
   Median basilic

4. Forearm

   Accessory cephalic
   Median antebrachial

5. Thigh

   Great saphenous
   Femoral

6. Ankle

   Great saphenous
   Small saphenous

7. Foot

   Venous plexus of dorsum
   Dorsal venous arch
   Median marginal
   Lateral marginal

8. Neck

   External jugular

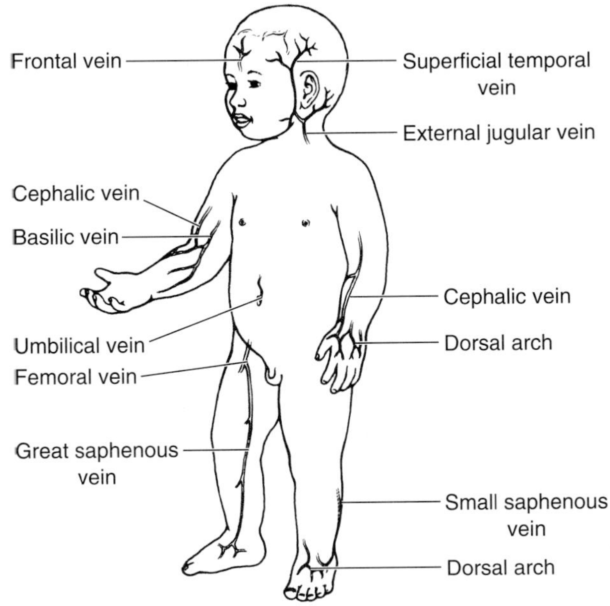

Figure 27–1 Superficial veins accessible for intravascular access. (From Hughes WT, Buescher ES: *Pediatric Procedures*. Philadelphia, WB Saunders, 1980.)

9. Scalp

   In the infant, especially the newborn, the veins of the scalp are the preferred sites for most infusions. Veins of the scalp commonly used are frontal, superficial temporal, supraorbital, and posterior auricular.

10. Umbilicus

   The umbilical vein may be used during the first few days of life for direct infusion if the scalp veins or superficial veins of the extremities are not readily accessible.

Table 27–2 Approximate pH Values for Commonly Used Infusion Solutions

Solution	Approximate pH
D_5W	4.0
D_5W 0.2 NS	4.0
D_5W NS	4.0
$D_{10}W$	4.0
1/2 NS	5.5
NS	5.5
Lactated Ringer's solution	6.5
5% $NaHCO_3$	8.0

From Hughes WT, Buescher ES: *Pediatric Procedures*. Philadelphia, WB Saunders, 1980.

GENERAL COMMENTS

Some general comments about intravenous therapy:

1. The insertion of a needle (or foreign substance) into a vein presents a blood condition that releases the Hageman factor from an inhibitor with which it is combined. Venipuncture results in prompt deposition of clumps of platelets on the endothelium. This clumping is followed by fibrin deposition around the puncture site and sometimes the needle orifice.
2. A right-handed child is more satisfied with an infusion in the left arm.
3. Red goggles used by radiologists for dark adaptation may be helpful in locating small superficial veins. Transillumination of the extremity, even in older children, can be useful in patients with few obvious superficial veins.
4. Try to avoid use of a vein over a joint. If a needle is inserted in these areas, movement at the joint may dislodge the needle from the vessel.
5. When a vein is selected, ensure that the needle and an adjacent length of tubing can be taped snugly against the skin without kinks or constriction.
6. The solution to be infused should be warmed to room temperature. The approximate pH values of commonly used intravenous fluids are listed in Table 27–2. The pH of the solution in use is a major factor in the development of phlebitis and suggests the use of buffering solutions (when possible) for infusion.
7. Methods of distending a vein:

   - A tourniquet may be applied to an extremity sufficiently proximal to the chosen site. The tourniquet is tightened until peripheral pulsation ceases. The tourniquet is then partially released until the arterial pulse is fully palpable. The closer the tourniquet is placed to the venipuncture site, the more pronounced is the venous distention.
   - Exercise plus gravity can be used. The patient should open and close the dependent, hanging hand and keep this hand closed tightly until the vein is punctured. The muscle activity forces blood out of the deeper venous plexus into the superficial veins, where it is held by the venous valve system.
   - Warm, wet compresses are applied over the area for 15 minutes.
   - Place the hand or foot in warm water.
   - Use a warm sponge and antiseptic solution.
   - Probably the most common reason for discontinuing an infusion is infiltration of the solution into subcutaneous tissues. In young children, a relatively small infiltration into a hand vein can cause edema of the entire hand. If this occurs, the infusion should be restarted at another site. If for some reason this is not possible and the infusion must be placed in the same extremity, a useful maneuver is to apply pressure to the dorsum of the hand for 1 to 2 minutes. This squeezes the infiltrated fluid out and displaces it laterally, often revealing a previously hidden vein in the area where pressure was applied. Such a vein is visible for 1 to 2 minutes before the infiltrated fluid redistributes back into the area where pressure was applied. Therefore, the new infusion must be started promptly (Fig. 27–2).

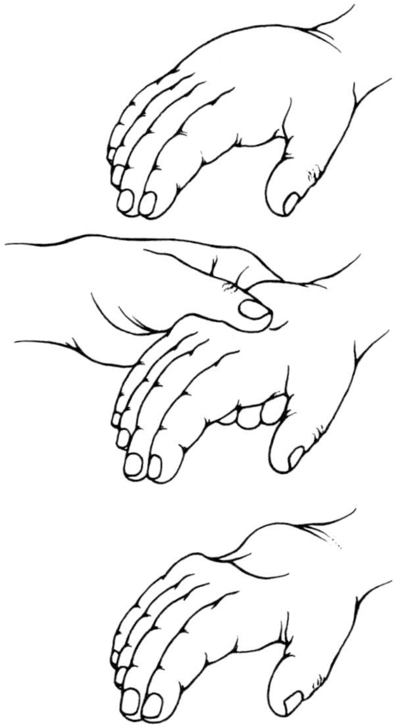

Figure 27–2 Exposure of veins in an edematous hand. (From Hughes WT, Buescher ES: *Pediatric Procedures.* Philadelphia, WB Saunders, 1980.)

VENIPUNCTURE

The method of venipuncture for infusion is the same for all the sites described in this chapter regardless of the site or the patient's age. The scalp needle is preferred for all intravenous infusions to which it can be adapted. Rapid infusion of blood or intravenous fluids may require placement of an intravenous catheter, either percutaneously or by cutdown, but these devices are considered less satisfactory than steel needles because of the increased frequency of complications with catheters.

General Technique for Needle Placement

1. Apply a tourniquet proximal to the venipuncture site if the anatomical site permits.
2. Prepare the skin over the area with an antiseptic solution and allow to dry.
3. Prepare the needle:
    - A few milliliters of normal saline is withdrawn into a 5-ml syringe.
    - Attach the syringe to the needle tubing and determine the patency of the needle by forcing out a few drops of saline. This can also be done by attaching the needle directly to the infusion tubing and running a small amount of fluid through it. A segment of vein that is fairly straight and slightly longer than the needle should be selected; alternatively, one that is fairly straight, is longer than the needle, and originates at the confluence of two venous tributaries may be selected. A site where venous tributaries join is particularly good. The tributaries tend to fix the vein and keep it from sliding under the skin (Fig. 27–3). The needle should be placed in the direction of blood flow. The

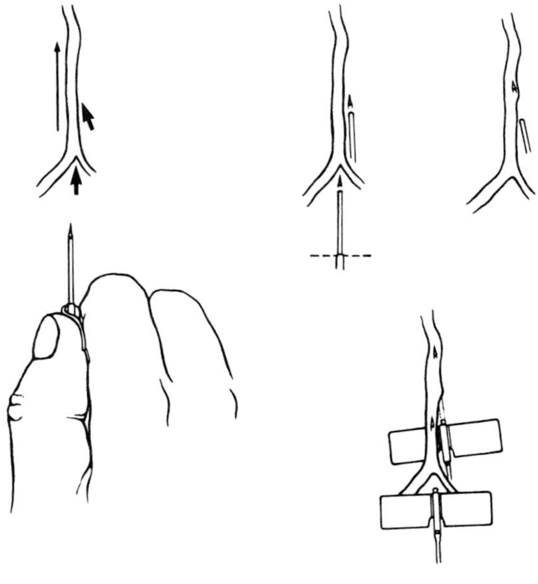

Figure 27–3 Two-stage entry of the needle into veins. (From Hughes WT, Buescher ES: *Pediatric Procedures.* Philadelphia, WB Saunders, 1980.)

gauge of the selected needle should be dictated by the purpose of the infusion. When caustic or irritating agents are to be infused (chemotherapy, certain drugs, and antibiotics), a small-gauge needle in a large vein should be used to maximize dilution of the infused solution. When intravascular volume must be replaced quickly, large-gauge needles in large vessels should be used. When prolonged intravenous therapy is anticipated, smaller needles in peripheral veins should be used, working toward the larger, more central veins after the peripheral sites have been employed.

4. Grasp the needle by the winged tabs. The needle bevel can be either up or down, depending on the size of the vein being used.
5. Anchor the vein with the thumb or index finger of the free hand by stretching the skin overlying it.
6. Hold the needle parallel to the long axis of the vein.
7. Introduce the needle point, bevel up, into and through the skin about 0.5 cm distal to the anticipated site of vessel puncture.
8. Exert suction when using a syringe. The needle is then gently but forcibly introduced into the vessel until blood appears in the tubing. If the needle is being used without an attached syringe, the hub cap must be loosened before the vein is pierced so that blood flows easily into the tubing when the vein is punctured. If the needle being used is already attached to the intravenous setup, then after the skin is pierced, but *before* the vein is pierced, a slight pinch of the tubing will expel a small amount of solution into the subcutaneous tissue. This creates a slight negative pressure in the tubing, so that when the vein is entered, a small amount of blood appears in the clear plastic tubing, signaling venipuncture.
9. Advance the needle as far along the lumen as vein size permits. The more needle under the skin, the more stable the needle will be in situ. In infants and small children, the needle often cannot be advanced without piercing the distal wall of the vein. In these children, most of the needle barrel is left exposed above the skin, and a specific taping method is used (Fig. 27–4) to increase the stability of the needle tip in the vein.

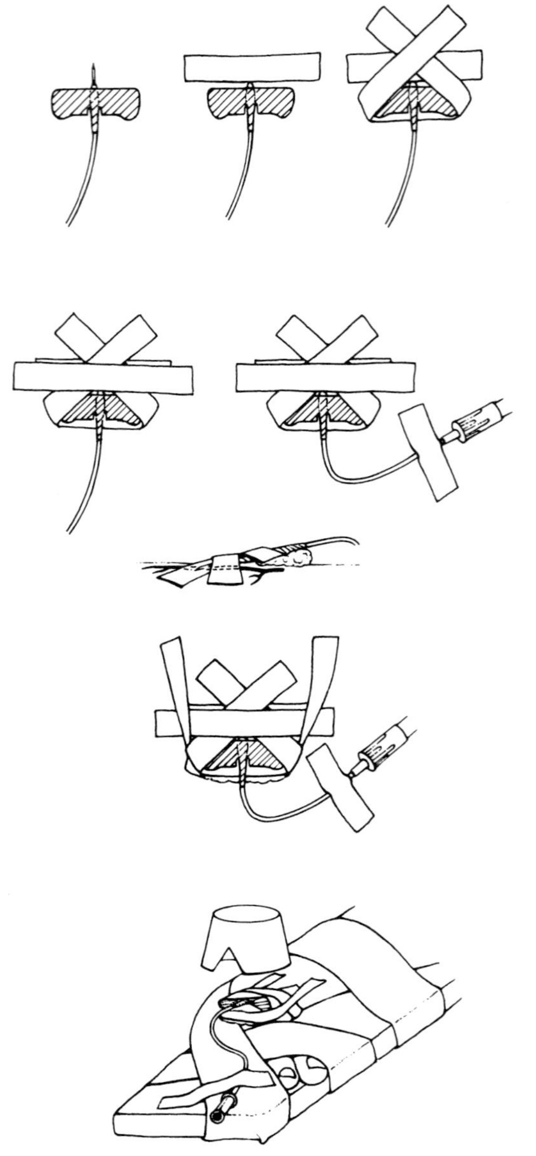

Figure 27–4 Method for securing the needle in a peripheral vein. A disposable cup is cut to fit as a protective cover. (From Hughes WT, Buescher ES: *Pediatric Procedures.* Philadelphia, WB Saunders, 1980.)

10. Release the tourniquet.
11. Apply the needle restraint.

Heparin Lock Needle Placement

One development in intravenous therapy is the use of heparin lock needles or interrupted intravenous infusions. These are standard infusion devices modified so that after the infusion is completed, the intravenous solution can be discontinued. The heparin lock needle is then filled with a heparin solution to avoid clotting.

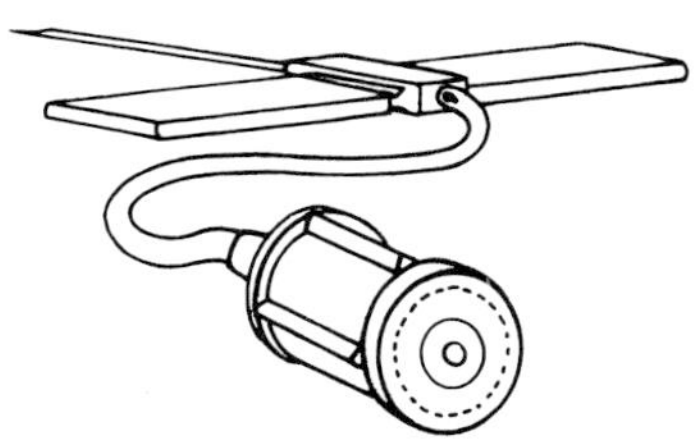

Figure 27–5 Heparin lock device. (From Hughes WT, Buescher ES: *Pediatric Procedures.* Philadelphia, WB Saunders, 1980.)

The standard device is modified by sealing the needle hub with a rubber flange that can be punctured several times (Fig. 27–5). There is an obvious advantage to this type of intravenous device: the patient does not have to be attached to an intravenous fluid line, except when infusions are being given, and therefore has increased mobility.

Equipment

21- or 23-gauge heparin lock needle
Iodine tincture and 70% alcohol
Sodium heparin diluted in bacteriostatic saline to a concentration of 10 U/ml.
Tuberculin syringe with a 25-gauge, 1 1/2-cm needle
25-gauge, 1 1/2-cm needle
Tourniquet
Adhesive tape
4 × 4-cm sterile gauze pads

Site and restraint

With the appropriate restraint, any site amenable to scalp vein needle placement can be used.

1. Prepare the chosen site with iodine tincture; when dry, remove with 70% alcohol.
2. Clean the rubber flange of the heparin lock needle with iodine tincture; when dry, pierce it with the 25-gauge needle.
3. Follow the steps described herein for steel needle placement.
4. Secure the needle in place with the appropriate restraint.
5. Remove the 25-gauge needle from the rubber flange (the attached tubing is usually filled with blood) and inject the heparin solution through the flange into the tubing with use of the tuberculin syringe and 25-gauge needle, flushing out the blood (volume required is approximately 0.4 to 0.8 ml).
6. When it is time to infuse a solution, prepare the rubber flange with the antiseptic solution and pierce the flange with a 23- or 25-gauge needle attached to the intravenous solution tubing, and infuse the solution as usual.
7. After the infusion is finished, remove the needle with the tubing attached and refill the tube of the heparin lock needle with preparing solutions as noted in item 5.

Sites for Intravenous Infusion

Whenever possible, percutaneous intravenous placement is preferable to venotomy and central venous catheter placement.

Veins of the Scalp

Anatomy

The major superficial veins of the scalp that may be used for venoclysis are illustrated in Figure 27–6. In order of preference, they are frontal, superficial temporal, posterior auricular, supraorbital, occipital, and posterior facial.

Arteries closely follow the course of superficial veins of the scalp. Arterial and venous vessels may be differentiated by the following means:

1. Pulsations can be palpated in an artery.
2. A vein is palpated as a furrow beneath the skin. An artery is a more firm and distended vessel. A vein is more clearly visible to inspection than an artery is.

"Stripping" blood from a portion of a vessel with two fingers spread along its course from a midpoint permits determination of the direction of blood flow. Release of the fingers obstructing the vessel allows it to fill. Arterial blood flows away from the heart. Venous blood flows toward the heart.

Equipment

Infusion set, solution, flask, drip chamber, and tubing
23- or 25-gauge scalp infusion needle
3- or 5-ml syringe half-filled with sterile normal saline (if desired)
Material for restraints
Razor, soap, and sponges
Antiseptic solution
Intense light
Rubber band tourniquet

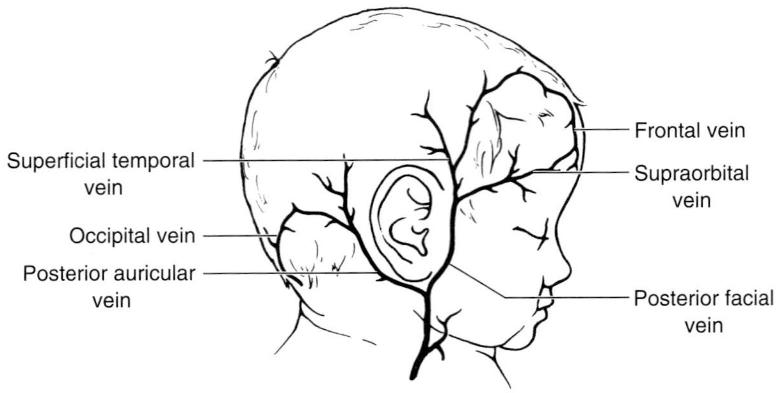

Figure 27–6 Major superficial veins of the scalp. (From Hughes WT, Buescher ES: *Pediatric Procedures.* Philadelphia, WB Saunders, 1980.)

Restraints

With body and needle restraints, an attendant should aid the operator by manually positioning and restraining the patient's head.

Method

1. Shave the selected site clean of hair. This area should be large enough to permit adequate taping of the needle. The frontal vein of the forehead has the advantage of stability; only minimal removal of hair is required, and the needle is easily taped to the forehead.
2. Cleanse the area with antiseptic.
3. Apply a rubber band tourniquet (Fig. 27–7).
4. Perform a two-stage venipuncture as described previously.
5. Apply the needle restraint (Fig. 27–8; see also Fig. 27–4).
6. Check the patency of the system by infusing 2 or 3 ml of saline from the syringe into the vein.
7. Remove the syringe.
8. Attach the hub of the needle tubing to the adapter of the infusion set tubing.
9. Regulate the drip.
10. Remove the body restraint and apply the upper extremity restraints, thus limiting the patient's movement.

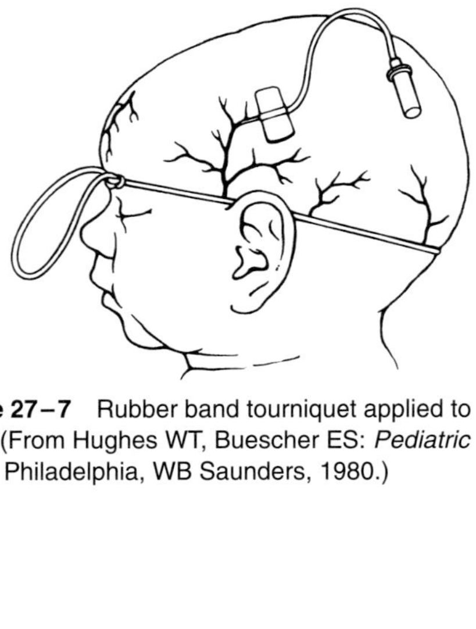

Figure 27–7 Rubber band tourniquet applied to the scalp. (From Hughes WT, Buescher ES: *Pediatric Procedures.* Philadelphia, WB Saunders, 1980.)

Advantages

1. Only the upper extremities need restraining after the infusion is started.
2. Scalp veins are usually the most accessible veins in the infant.
3. Infiltration is easily visible.
4. The needle can be firmly restrained.
5. There are several vessels in the same general area.

Disadvantages

1. Scalp veins can rarely be used after the patient is 2 years old.
2. Scalp vein procedures on children are frequently disturbing to the parents.
3. Veins of the scalp communicate with the intracranial venous sinuses. Pyogenic infection may extend from the scalp and pericranium through the bone to the dura mater and venous sinuses and from these sinuses to the cerebral veins, the pia arachnoid, and the substance of the brain.

Veins of Forearm and Antecubital Fossa

Anatomy

The major superficial veins that may be used for venoclysis in this area are illustrated in Fig. 27–9. In the antecubital space, there is a proximity of veins and arteries. About 10%

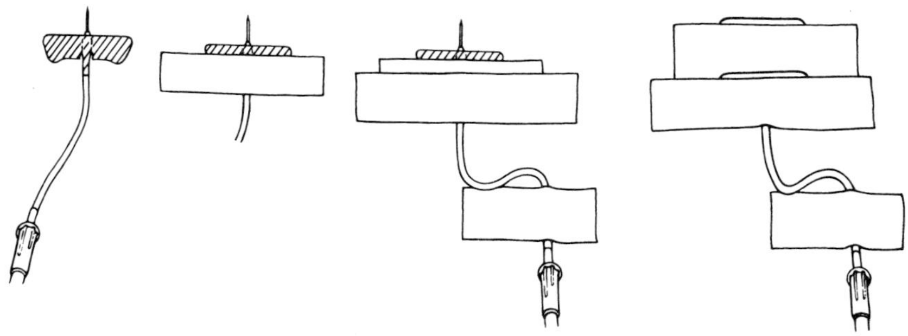

Figure 27–8 Needle restraint for a scalp vein needle in a large peripheral vein. (From Hughes WT, Buescher ES: *Pediatric Procedures*. Philadelphia, WB Saunders, 1980.)

of individuals have an aberrant artery in the antecubital space that may easily be mistaken for a vein. Therefore, care should be taken here to differentiate arterial and venous vessels.

1. An artery pulsates on careful palpation.
2. An artery usually lies more deeply beneath the skin than a vein does.
3. Arterial puncture produces bright red blood in the aspirating syringe. Venous blood is dark red.
4. Intra-arterial injection usually produces pain in the arm and hand. This may be the first indication that an artery has been entered inadvertently.
5. The pressure under which blood enters the syringe in arterial puncture is greater than in venipuncture.

The most frequently used veins are the cephalic, the basilic, and the median basilic.

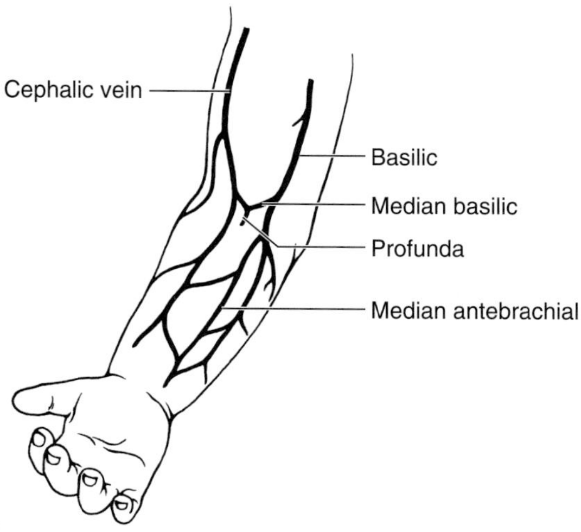

Figure 27–9 Major superficial veins of the forearm and antecubital fossa. (From Hughes WT, Buescher ES: *Pediatric Procedures*. Philadelphia, WB Saunders, 1980.)

Equipment

Infusion set, solution, flask or bag, drip chamber, and tubing
Scalp vein needle in most instances. If an infusion must be given rapidly, a large intravenous device (16- or 18-guage needle) or plastic cannula may be necessary.
A 5- to 10-ml syringe half-filled with sterile normal saline (if desired)
Material for restraints
Intense light
Tourniquet
Antiseptic solution and sponges
Dry, sterile gauze

Restraints

Use an upper extremity restraint, needle restraint, and board-to-bed restraint.

Selection of vein

A vein in the upper third of the forearm is preferable. If possible, avoid the central antecubital area because it is likely to be disturbed by slight flexion of the extremity at the joint, and joint stiffness or pain can be caused by immobilization. The specific vein selected will vary in individual patients. A vein of adequate size, adequately supported by surrounding tissue, and near which needle and tubing can be firmly secured is preferable.

Method

1. Restrain the extremity and prepare the site with antiseptic. Sponge the skin dry with sterile gauze.
2. Apply a tourniquet. If the vein is not readily distended, the other distention methods (described previously) may be used.
3. The tourniquet can be applied to distend the veins.

Advantages

1. Veins are large, easily visible, and palpable (especially in children older than 1 year).
2. The needle and tubing can be firmly secured on the forearm.
3. The tourniquet can be applied to distend the veins.

Disadvantages

1. Vessels are sometimes difficult to locate in infants.
2. The needle, inserted in the antecubital fossa, may be dislodged easily by slightly flexing the patient's forearm.
3. It is difficult to firmly restrain the elbow joint to avoid twisting motions.
4. Proximity of arteries and veins of the antecubital fossa is troublesome.

Veins on Dorsum of Hand

Anatomy

Tributaries of the cephalic and basilic veins (along with the dorsal venous arch) illustrated in Figure 27–10 are potential sites for infusion in infants and children. The fifth interdigital vein is suggested in infants because of its fairly constant position.

Equipment

Infusion set, solution, flask, drip chamber, and tubing
Antiseptic solution and sponges
21-, 22-, 23-gauge scalp infusion needle
5- or 10-ml syringe half-filled with sterile normal saline (if desired)
Material for restraints
Intense light
Tourniquet

Restraints

Use a hand restraint, needle restraint, and board-to-bed restraint.

Method

1. Apply the hand restraint and cleanse the hand with antiseptic. Allow the antiseptic to dry.
2. Apply the tourniquet to the forearm. (If veins are not visible, rub surface briskly with alcohol sponge to distend the vessels.)
3. Select a vein in the metacarpal area, as far distal as the vessel can be clearly identified.
4. With the free hand, stretch the skin taut over the dorsum of the patient's hand and pull distally, in the opposite direction of the needle insertion.
5. Perform a two-stage venipuncture as described previously.
6. Check the patency of the system by infusing 2 or 3 ml of saline from the syringe.
7. Apply the needle restraint.
8. Connect the infusion set and regulate the drip.
9. Apply the board-to-bed restraint.

Advantages

1. Vessel size is adequate in infants and children.
2. A tourniquet can be applied.
3. Several vessels are available in the same general site.

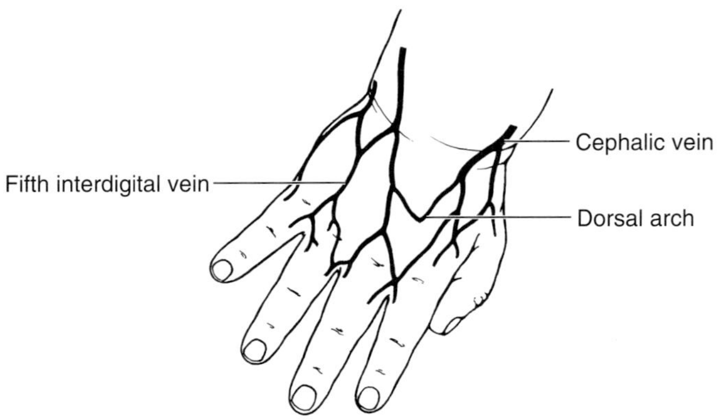

Figure 27–10 Veins of the dorsum of the hand. (From Hughes WT, Buescher ES: *Pediatric Procedures.* Philadelphia, WB Saunders, 1980.)

4. Only one extremity needs to be firmly restrained.

Disadvantages

1. Veins are somewhat mobile and not well supported by surrounding subcutaneous tissue.
2. Space is limited for tape restraint of the needle.
3. Maintaining the proper angle of the needle in the vessel may be difficult.

Veins on Dorsum of Foot

Anatomy
The median and lateral margin veins of the foot are suitable sites for infusions in both infants and children.

Equipment
Same as for dorsum of hand.

Restraints
Use a foot restraint, needle restraint, and board-to-bed restraint.

Method
Same as for dorsum of hand.

Advantages

1. A tourniquet can be applied.
2. It can be used in infants as well as in children.
3. Restraint is effective.
4. The veins are well supported by subcutaneous tissue.

Disadvantages

1. The veins are relatively small.
2. The foot is restrained in an uncomfortable position.
3. An infant's foot may be fat. This can make veins difficult to see or to palpate.

Great Saphenous Vein at the Ankle

Anatomy
The great saphenous vein at the ankle lies between the medial malleolus and the anterior tibial tendon.

Equipment
Same as for dorsum of hand.

Restraints
Use a lower extremity restraint, needle restraint, and board-to-bed restraint.

Method

1. Cleanse the skin with tincture of iodine, which is allowed to dry and is then removed with 70% alcohol or povidone-iodine (Betadine) swabs.
2. Apply a tourniquet just below the knee joint.
3. Select a site for venipuncture at the ankle that is adequate to permit a stable fixation of the needle without interference from flexion of the foot. The skin in this area is tough, and the vein is more deeply situated than those in the scalp, hand, and foot.
4. Perform a two-step venipuncture with a scalp infusion needle (as with infusions in the dorsum of the hand). When use of a needle with a large bore (18- or 19-gauge) is desirable in an older child, a conventional hypodermic needle may be attached directly to the infusion tubing.
5. Release the tourniquet.
6. Use a needle restraint with either a scalp infusion needle or a hypodermic needle.
7. Apply a board-to-bed restraint that is comfortable.

Advantages

1. The vein is large and constant in its anatomical position.
2. A bony landmark (medial malleolus) aids in locating the vessel.
3. The restraint is fairly comfortable and substantial.
4. A large needle can be used.
5. The vessel is rigidly supported by surrounding tissue.
6. A tourniquet can be applied.

Disadvantages

1. Unless it is inserted sufficiently high on the ankle, the needle may be dislodged by flexion of the foot.
2. If attempts at percutaneous venipuncture at this site are unsuccessful, resultant trauma may interfere with a venostomy (cutdown) at this site.

Umbilical Vein Catheterization

A catheter may be inserted into the newborn infant's umbilical vein at the umbilical cord stump. This vein is usually accessible during the infant's first week of life. The greatest advantage of this route, aside from the ease of operation, is its suitability for rapid infusions. The greatest danger of umbilical vein infusion is the ease of circulation overload. Necrotizing enterocolitis, sepsis, cirrhosis, intrahepatic abscess, and the risk of embolization are other hazards. The methods for catheterization of the umbilical vein and the umbilical artery are described in Chapter 19.

Percutaneous Catheterization

A variety of instruments have been devised to catheterize a vein or artery percutaneously without surgical exposure of the vessel. In some instances, venipuncture is performed with a large-gauge needle and a plastic capillary catheter inserted through the lumen of the needle into the vein. When the tubing is in the vein, the outer needle is removed, leaving the catheter in place. This method has the disadvantage of requiring a large needle to insert a small tube. Leakage around the catheter is frequently a problem, as is the risk of severing the tubing in the vein through use of a sharp-pointed outer needle. These cannulas are usually reserved for central venous pressure monitoring or long-term parenteral alimentation.

Another method using an intravenous catheter—over a stylet needle—has become popular. The venipuncture is performed with the catheter-stylet unit. For intravenous placement, the catheter is slipped over and off the needle stylet. The stylet is then totally withdrawn from the catheter, and the infusion solution tubing is attached. This method does not have the disadvantage of requiring a large vein for a large needle. Leakage is not usually a problem because the stylet is totally removed from the catheter, and the catheter is not easily severed from the introducing needle after insertion. Plastic catheters of either type should be used only when large volumes of fluid must be administered rapidly; maintenance of a dependable infusion is an absolute necessity (not just a convenience), or measurement of the central venous pressure is needed.

Equipment (Catheter-Needle-Stylet Device)

16- to 22-gauge catheter-needle-stylet device, with the gauge determined by the size of the vessel to be used; short 3- to 4-cm devices are preferable to 6- to 8-cm devices
1% lidocaine; 1-ml syringe with a 25-gauge, 1 1/2-cm needle
Tincture of iodine and 70% alcohol or povidone-iodine
Straight 16-gauge needle
Tourniquet
Infusion equipment (solution and tubing)
Restraint material
4 × 4-cm gauze sponges
Adhesive tape
Neosporin ointment

Site and restraint

Any adequately sized vein can be used. Restraints employed should be appropriate for the site.

An advantage of using short, plastic catheters instead of steel needles is that they can bend in the vessel lumen without perforating the vessel wall. Therefore, veins not useful for scalp vein needle placement (because of tortuosity or awkward position) can sometimes be used with these plastic catheters. On the negative side, there is a much higher frequency of both infective and chemical phlebitis associated with these devices after 48 to 72 hours than with the steel infusion needles. Phlebitis from plastic intravenous catheters is primarily the result of mechanical trauma to the vein wall; to-and-fro movements of the catheter cause endothelial damage, predisposing to thrombus formation. Placement of plastic catheters in tortuous vessels invites the development of phlebitis.

Method

1. Select an adequate length of vein.
2. Apply the appropriate restraint.
3. Apply the tourniquet.
4. Cleanse the site with iodine tincture; when dry, remove it with 70% alcohol.
5. Anesthetize the selected skin entry site by injecting it with an intradermal bleb of 1% lidocaine. Wait 1 to 3 minutes for the agent to take effect.
6. Use a 16-gauge needle as a trochar and pierce the skin through the anesthetic bleb. Do not enter the vein with the trochar. When small-gauge catheter-needle-stylet devices are used, this step is critical. The skin is tough, and the fine-needle stylets usually bend if they are used to penetrate the skin. This makes it difficult to direct the catheter at a flat angle into a small vein. The trochar needle makes a mini-incision in the skin, larger than the gauge of the catheter. Therefore, no resistance is encountered as the catheter-needle-stylet passes through the skin (Fig. 27–11). This

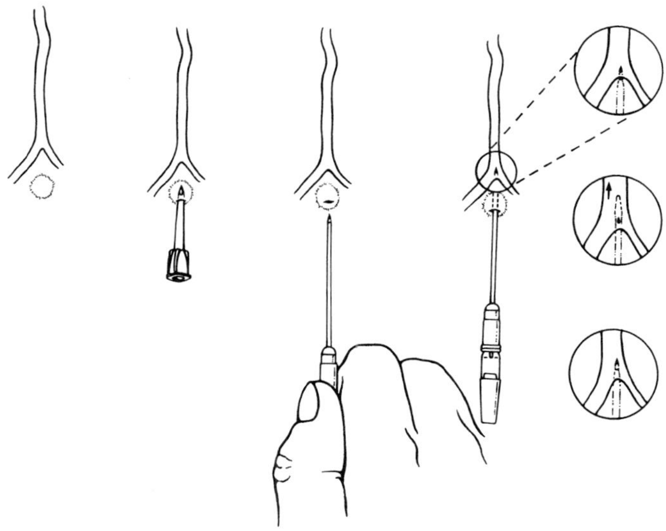

Figure 27–11 Percutaneous catheterization. (From Hughes WT, Buescher ES: *Pediatric Procedures*. Philadelphia, WB Saunders, 1980.)

increases the operator's sensitivity and aids in being able to "feel" when the vein has been entered.

7. Examine the catheter-needle-stylet closely to ensure that the catheter tip is smooth and bur-free. See that the needle-stylet slides easily out of the catheter. Be certain the needle-stylet tip protrudes beyond the catheter tip.
8. Remove the trochar needle and insert the catheter-needle-stylet through the same site. Whether the device is inserted with the bevel up or down is determined by the size of the vessel (Fig. 27–11). Advance the catheter-needle-stylet under the skin until the vein is entered. This is signaled by a recognizable lessening of resistance or by the appearance of blood in the transparent needle-stylet hub.
9. Observe the appearance of blood in the needle-stylet hub. This confirms entry of the needle-stylet point into the vascular lumen (Fig. 27–12). Because the tip of the catheter lies 1 to 2 mm *behind* the needle-stylet point, it is possible for the catheter tip to be extravascular when blood appears in the needle-stylet hub. Removal of the needle-stylet at this point would leave the catheter tip outside the vein, and the cannulation attempt would fail. The catheter can be advanced into the vein lumen (see Fig. 27–11) in one of two ways.

   - The needle-stylet is held carefully in place (tip in lumen), and the catheter is slipped down, along, and over the tip of the needle-stylet into the vein. This is usually the method of choice, although it is more difficult when small veins are used.
   - After blood first appears in the needle-stylet hub, the operator advances the catheter-needle-stylet 2 to 3 mm farther into the vein lumen. The needle-stylet is then pulled back 4 to 5 mm into the catheter (but not removed), and the catheter is advanced into position in the vein lumen. The stylet is removed, and the catheter hub is attached to the infusion tubing.
   - There is one caution in both methods: after the catheter-needle-stylet has been inserted under the skin, if the needle-stylet is pulled back so that the point is within the catheter for any reason, the needle-stylet should never be pushed back into the catheter without the catheter tip's being directly visible. This precaution must be taken because the needle-stylet point can easily clip the catheter if alignment is not exact. This can create either a subcutaneous foreign body or, worse, a free intravascular embolus.
10. Secure the catheter in position by use of the catheter restraint. Observe aseptic technique during insertion of catheters and maintain a careful watch on catheters after insertion.
11. Because there is strong evidence that phle-

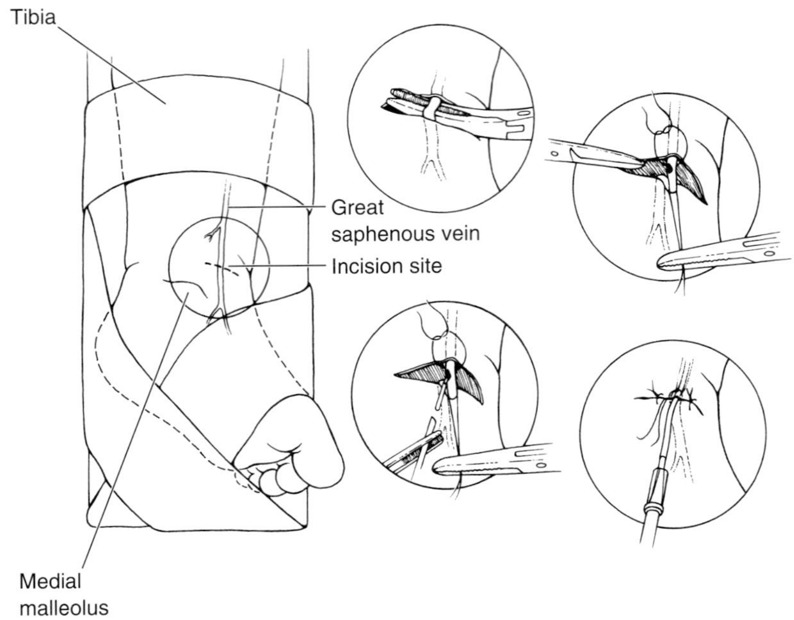

Figure 27–12 Method for great saphenous vein cutdown at the ankle. (From Hughes WT, Buescher ES: *Pediatric Procedures*. Philadelphia, WB Saunders, 1980.)

bitis, bacterial contamination, and septicemia can be related to the use of plastic intravenous catheters, these catheters should be inspected several times daily and be discontinued immediately at any sign of local inflammation, catheter malfunction, or local pain.

VENOSTOMY

When it is not possible to gain suitable intravenous access by percutaneous venipuncture, the physician can expose the vessel to direct incision for venostomy. The great saphenous vein in the ankle area is the vessel most frequently chosen in infants and children. It is the primary choice. If it is not accessible, the small saphenous vein (in the ankle) or the basilic or cephalic veins (in the antecubital fossa) may be used. Under certain circumstances, a venostomy of the great saphenous vein within the femoral triangle may be indicated.

Ankle Cutdown of the Great Saphenous Vein

Anatomy

The great saphenous vein is formed by the union of the medial extremity of the dorsal venous arch with the median, dorsal digital vein of the great toe. The great saphenous vein courses anterior to the medial malleolus, crosses the medial surface of the distal third of the tibia, and ascends to the knee. In the foot and leg, it is accompanied by the saphenous nerve (see Fig. 27–12).

Equipment

Material for restraint
Antiseptic solutions: tincture of iodine and 70% alcohol
Scalpel handle and No. 15 scalpel blade
Curved mosquito hemostat
Straight suture scissors
Disposable measuring tape
Ampule of 1% lidocaine
20-gauge hypodermic needle
25-gauge hypodermic needle
2-ml syringe
10-ml syringe
Needle holder
Small, curved cutting needle
Sterile hand towels (four)
Towel clips (four)
Sterile gauze squares, 6 × 6 cm
Small, sharp-pointed scissors
Tissue forceps
Plastic catheter with attached needle hub. Several sizes of tubing should be available.

Table 27–3 Plastic Tubing and Appropriate Needle Connection

French Scale	Diameter (mM) Inside	Diameter (mM) Outside	Needle Gauge That Fits into Tubing
3.3	0.38	1.09	27 or 26
2.9	0.58	0.965	23
3.6	0.76	1.22	2[illegible]
3.8	0.86	1.27	20
4.5	0.86	1.52	20
4.7	1.14	1.57	18
5.1	1.19	1.70	18
5.7	1.40	1.90	17
6.2	1.57	2.08	16

From Hughes WT, Buescher ES: *Pediatric Procedures*. Philadelphia, WB Saunders, 1980.

Table 27–3 gives information on tubing sizes and appropriate needle connection. In general, tubing with French scale sizes 3.3, 3.6, 4.5, and 5.1 serves most needs.

Sterile rubber gloves
No. 5–0 silk suture
Role of 3-cm adhesive tape
Tourniquet
Sterile normal saline for injection (10 ml)

Restraint

Use a lower extremity restraint.

Method

1. After the extremity is properly restrained, cleanse the site with tincture of iodine and then with alcohol. Don sterile gloves.
2. The operator can easily locate the incision site by placing the thumb over the medial malleolus and the index finger over the anterior tibial tendon. The great saphenous vein lies midway between these points (see Fig. 27–12). With a hypodermic needle, mark the incision site by scratching a line in the skin. The line is transverse and follows the skin creases. It is about 0.5 to 1 cm long. Identify the incision site carefully in this manner, because infiltration with anesthetic may distort the anatomical relationships.
3. Drape the area with four sterile hand towels secured at the inner corners with towel clips. Leave an operative site (about 6 to 9 cm^2) exposed.
4. Use a 25-gauge needle and a 2-ml syringe filled with 1% lidocaine, infiltrate intradermally along the incision site, and then extend the infiltration into the subcutaneous tissue. Attempt aspiration before injection of lidocaine. This is to obviate intravascular administration.
5. Apply a tourniquet just below the knee.
6. Make a transverse skin incision in the previously outlined mark slightly above and anterior to the medial malleolus. The incision should extend in depth through all layers of skin and seldom needs to exceed 1 cm in length.
7. Sponge the incision with gauze to maintain adequate visualization.
8. Dissect bluntly with a curved mosquito hemostat in a direction parallel to the course of the great saphenous vein and down to the surface of the tibia. The vein is identified by its bluish color. Dissection with the hemostat around the vessel will free it in its entire circumference from surrounding tissue and the saphenous nerve (see Fig. 27–12).
9. With a hemostat underneath the vessel positioned with tips up, place a 5–0 silk suture in the clamp tip and pull it through for a guide suture. This suture is not tied. A second suture is placed underneath the vessel in a similar manner at the proximal edge of the wound.
10. Select the proper-sized catheter. A slight bevel is cut onto the catheter tip. Flush a few milliliters of saline through the catheter to check patency. The catheter tip is tailored to a short, blunt bevel.
11. Incise the vein with small, sharp-pointed scissors. The vein is held taut with the distal guide suture, and a V niche is made. This incision should extend about one-third the circumference of the vein and should not exceed half the distance around the vessel (see Fig. 27–12). A free backflow of venous blood should occur to ensure adequate entrance into the lumen. An incomplete incision results in threading of the catheter into the adventitia of the vein. Care should be taken not to sever the vessel completely. Blood flows from the incision when the opening is adequate.
12. Sponge the exposed structures free of blood. The selected catheter is grasped at about 1 cm from its tip with fine forceps. With the opposite hand, the operator exerts gentle traction on the distal guide suture to stabilize the vessel. The catheter tip is inserted, bevel down, into the V inci-

sion. The catheter is threaded into the vein, bevel down, to a distance of 5 to 8 cm (see Fig. 27–12). Venous valves may impede the advancement of the catheter. A slight rotation of the catheter usually overcomes this. Reflux of blood should become visible in the lumen of the catheter.

13. Remove the tourniquet.
14. Tie the suture around the vein proximal to the incision, securing the catheter in place. The ends of this ligature are left long so that when the catheter is eventually removed, they can be pulled up and cut to remove the suture and allow recanalization of the vein. The distal guide suture is not tied. It is gently removed. A small amount of bleeding may occur from the unligated distal portion of the vessel; however, constant pressure with a gauze sponge stops the oozing.
15. Check the patency of the system by injecting a few milliliters of normal saline from a syringe attached to the catheter hub. With gentle pressure on the plunger, the infusion should flow freely. Check for escape of saline around the venostomy site and infiltration around the proximal course of the vein. Attach the catheter to the infusion tubing and regulate the drip.
16. Anchor the catheter firmly to the skin by applying a 6-cm strip of adhesive tape over the catheter.
17. Close the skin incision around the catheter and vessel ligature by placing a single 5–0 silk suture along each side of the tubing. Then apply a folded 6 × 6-cm sterile gauze bandage over the incision. Avoid excessive bandage. A strip of 1 1/2-cm adhesive tape may be applied in a linear fashion over the external length of tubing from the base of the hub to the skin incision. Fold the tape around the tubing, apposing the adhesive sides. This reinforces the tubing and prevents kinking and breaking.

Common sources of error

1. Improper skin incision. If the skin incision is improperly placed, localization of the vein may be difficult or impossible. Mistakes sometimes responsible are
    - Distortion of anatomical landmarks by infiltration of the site with anesthetic before the line of incision is marked.
    - Placing the incision inferior to the medial malleolus.
    - Incision too deep, with severance of the vein.
    - Incision too superficial, making blunt dissection difficult.
    - Incision too short or failure of the operator to subcutaneously extend the full length of a superficial incision.
2. Failure to apply the tourniquet. The distended vessel is more easily located with the use of a tourniquet. Be aware of effects of prolonged tourniquet application.
3. Failure to clearly dissect an adequate segment of the saphenous vein.
4. Inadvertent severance of the vein by dissection.
5. Failure to completely incise into the vessel lumen. Slight bleeding may become apparent after merely cutting the muscular portion of the venous wall. If this is interpreted as retrograde flow from the lumen, the catheter might be guided into the adventitia rather than the lumen.
6. Too extensive a vessel incision. If the vein is completely severed, it retracts immediately, frequently out of the operative field. If this occurs and the vein cannot be retrieved, another skin incision can be made about 2 cm proximal to the initial site and the vessel relocated.
7. Improper bevel of catheter. If the bevel is too long and the point too sharp, the catheter will not pass smoothly into the lumen. If such a catheter is forced past a point of obstruction, perforation of the vessel wall may occur.
8. Catheter too large or too small for the vein. If the tubing diameter is too large, it cannot be inserted a sufficient distance into the vein. If the catheter is too small, leakage may occur between the tubing and the vascular wall.
9. Inadequately secured vessel ligature. This is evidenced by leakage of the infusion fluid from the incision site or by infiltration of surrounding subcutaneous tissue.
10. Failure to firmly secure the catheter to the ankle with adhesive tape. Anchoring the catheter tubing to only the restraint board or bandage allows movement of the ankle to dislodge the catheter. By placing a piece of tape over the tubing and directly onto the skin immediately distal to the skin incision, this can be avoided.

Cutdown of the Small Saphenous Vein

If the great saphenous vein is not accessible at the ankle, the small saphenous vein may be used as an alternative. The vessel is not as constant in its anatomical course as is the great saphenous.

Anatomy

The small saphenous vein is formed by the lateral extremity of the dorsal digital vein of the little toe. It passes posterior to the lateral malleolus lying on the peroneal retinacula, alongside the sural nerve, and along the lateral border of the tendo calcaneus.

Equipment

Same as for great saphenous venostomy.

Restraint

Use a foot restraint.

Method

1. Cleanse the skin with tincture of iodine and then with alcohol. Don sterile gloves.
2. Mark the incision site transversely from the lateral border of the tendo calcaneus (Achilles tendon), extending anteriorly toward the lateral malleolus for a distance of 1 to 2 cm. The mark should be slightly proximal to the level of the lateral malleolus.
3. Drape the operative site with four towels and secure the inner corners with towel clips.
4. Infiltrate the site with 1% lidocaine.
5. Apply a tourniquet just below the knee.
6. Make the cutaneous incision with a scalpel and locate the vessel by blunt dissection. The vessel must be separated carefully from the sural nerve.
7. Release the tourniquet.
8. Follow the technique given previously for great saphenous venotomy.

Common sources of error

1. Failure to locate the vessel. This may result from anatomical variation, inadequate length of the incision, or placement of an incision too far anteriorly.
2. Difficulty in differentiating the vein from the sural nerve. The bluish color of the vessel and blanching on compression identify the vein.

Cutdown at the Antecubital Fossa

A venotomy at the antecubital fossa may be necessary for therapeutic infusions when the routes mentioned previously are inaccessible.

Anatomy

Either the basilic vein on the ulnar side or the cephalic vein on the radial side of the antecubital fossa may be used. The basilic vein is superficial to the deep fascia in the distal third of the arm. It is visible in the medial epicondylar triangle and the distal part of the medial bicipital groove. It is prominent in the medial margin of the antecubital fossa (see Fig. 27–9).

The cephalic vein is identifiable superficially in the lateral margin of the antecubital fossa. It ascends slightly anterior and medial to the lateral edge of the biceps (see Fig. 27–9).

Equipment

Same as for great saphenous cutdown.

Restraint

Use an upper extremity restraint.

Method

1. Cleanse the skin with tincture of iodine and then with alcohol.
2. Apply a tourniquet on the arm above the belly of the biceps muscle.
3. Don sterile rubber gloves.
4. Drape the site with sterile towels and secure the inner corners with towel clips.
5. Palpate the distended vein and outline an incision parallel to the skin creases. Do this by scratching the skin with a hypodermic needle. If the vein is not visible or palpable, estimate the location by its expected anatomical course.
6. Infiltrate the site with 1 or 2 ml of 1% lidocaine.
7. Make the incision (barely) through the skin, and locate the vessel by gentle blunt dissection with a curved mosquito hemostat.
8. Locate the vein. Then strip it clean of surrounding tissue. Release the tourniquet and carry out the remaining procedure as described previously for great saphenous venotomy.

Common sources of error

1. Failure to locate the vessel. This may be due to anatomical variation or an improperly placed incision. During palpation, the bi-

ceps tendon is sometimes confused with the basilic vein.
2. Improper restraint. It is difficult to completely restrain the elbow area against rotation. Unexpected movement may interrupt the procedure or distort the anatomy.
3. Difficulty in inserting the catheter. If the forearm is slightly flexed, curvature in the vessel may inhibit introduction of the catheter. By placement of padding underneath the olecranon, the forearm is hyperextended when restrained, and catheterization is facilitated. Venospasm, too small an incision into the vein, too large a catheter, too sharp a bevel, and insufficient distal retraction are other factors that may prevent catheterization.

Cutdown at the Femoral Triangle

If infusion of an extremely irritating or hypertonic solution is required, a catheter may be inserted into the inferior vena cava from the great saphenous vein at the femoral triangle. Catheterization at this site may also serve as an alternative to umbilical vein catheterization for exchange transfusion if the umbilical vein is inaccessible.

Anatomy

The femoral triangle is a space in the proximal third of the front of the thigh containing the femoral vessels and nerve in the proximal part of their course. It is bounded superiorly by the inguinal ligament, laterally by the sartorius muscle, and medially by the adductor longus muscle.

The great saphenous vein terminates in the femoral vein at the femoral triangle. The femoral vein lies medial and parallel to the femoral artery. The venous course of the femoral vein is to the external iliac vein, to the common iliac vein, and into the inferior vena cava.

Equipment

Same as for great saphenous venotomy.

Restraint

Use a bilateral lower extremity restraint.

Method

1. Cleanse the skin over the groin, the proximal portion of the anterior thigh, and the lower abdomen first with tincture of iodine and then with alcohol.
2. Locate the incision site. An incision high in the groin is a proper approach to the great saphenous vein (Fig. 27–13). A line is drawn between the anterior superior iliac spine and the pubic tubercle. This line is bisected. At 1 to 1.5 cm below this point, which is in the center of the upper thigh, a 1- to 2-cm transverse superficial incision is marked medial and parallel to the inguinal ligament. This incision mark is about 0.5 cm below the inguinal skin crease where the thigh joins the body.
3. Infiltrate the incision site with 1 to 2 ml of 1% lidocaine.
4. Make an incision through the skin along the line described.
5. Separate the skin and subcutaneous fat down to the superficial fascia. Then separate the fascia.
6. Isolate the great saphenous vein. Place two sutures around it, one proximal to the site for incision of the vein and one distal to the site. Tie the distal suture and leave the proximal suture untied.

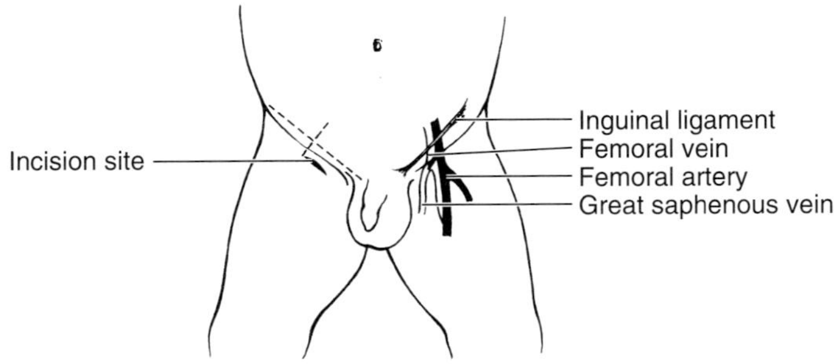

Figure 27–13 Site for venostomy (cutdown) at the femoral triangle. (From Hughes WT, Buescher ES: *Pediatric Procedures.* Philadelphia, WB Saunders, 1980.)

7. Incise the vein transversely with a small, sharp scissors. The incision should be large enough to permit introduction of a catheter that will fit snugly into the vessel.
8. Insert the catheter with a short, blunt bevel through the incision into the great saphenous vein and gently pass it a distance of 4 to 8 cm through the femoral, external iliac, and common iliac veins. Then proceed into the inferi or vena cava. If an adequate pool of blood is encountered in any of these areas, further insertion is not necessary. Careful readjusting of the catheter by slight rotation, advance, or withdrawal may be necessary at times to re-establish a free flow of blood.
9. Tie the proximal suture around the vessel to secure the catheter in the vein. Leave the ends of the sutures long so that when the catheter is eventually removed, the sutures may be retracted and clipped. Recanalization of the vessel is then facilitated.
10. Close the skin incision around the tubing and deep ligature ends with 5–0 silk interrupted sutures.

There is a caution in this method: avoid femoral venipuncture before and after this procedure on the ipsilateral side.

HAZARDS AND COMPLICATIONS OF INTRAVENOUS THERAPY

Although intravenous therapy is undeniably indispensable in the management of illnesses, it should never be undertaken lightly or used indiscriminately. The true perspective of parenteral fluid therapy, that of a substitute for normal alimentation, should always be kept in mind. Although hazards are few and complications are usually trivial, occasional disasters occur. It is important to carefully assess the risks of an intravenous infusion.

1. The needle may be introduced through the vessel wall opposite to the site of introduction and produce a hematoma or infiltrate the surrounding tissue with the infusion solution.
2. Debris or a clot obstructing the needle lumen, if it is dislodged by force into a vein from an attached syringe, can create a hazardous embolus.
3. Venospasm can occur from the trauma of penetration by the needle.

Catheter

1. Irritation of the vessel wall and venospasm may result from frayed edges of a catheter tip.
2. Breakage of a friable catheter is possible.
3. Obstruction of the lumen by debris, clot, or bend in the tubing can result.
4. Infection is one of the leading causes of serious complications from central venous catheters. Septicemia and endocarditis are the most serious types of infections in this regard. Risk factors include prolonged catheterization, frequent manipulations, transparent plastic dressings, improper aseptic techniques, number of lumens, contaminated skin solutions, and location of the catheter (Raad and Bodey, 1992).

THROMBOPHLEBITIS: Thrombi may form on the tip of the catheter and on the adjacent vessel wall. Inflammation of the vein wall often ensues. The phlebitis may subside rapidly or may persist for weeks or months. Veins may not recanalize for a year or more and some perhaps never. Duration of the infusion is perhaps the most common etiological factor.

Dextrose in any concentration is more liable to produce thrombophlebitis than most other solutions are. Heat sterilization of dextrose solutions produces a decrease in pH of approximately 3.5 to 4.0; however, cold-sterilized dextrose solutions are also likely to produce phlebitis. Buffering solution will not entirely prevent an inflammatory response, but it has been shown to decrease the occurrence of postinfusion phlebitis in children.

Thrombophlebitis is more likely to occur with infusions in the leg than with those in the more superior parts of the body. Phlebitis of the lower extremity delays ambulation.

ACCIDENTAL INJECTION INTO AN ARTERY: When the veins in the antecubital fossa are invisible and not palpable, an injection may be given mistakenly into an adjacent artery. An aberrant artery in the antecubital area may be found in 1 person in 10. The proximity of this vessel to nearby veins is a potential hazard. The veins and arteries on the ulnar side of the elbow are separated only by the thin lacertus fibrosus.

Serious complications may arise from intra-arterial injections. In most cases, immediate and intense pain radiates into the hand. The contracture of one or more fingers or necrosis of the fingers or of the arm may occur. When pain is experienced on injection of a drug or solution, stop injecting immediately and evaluate before taking further action.

ISCHEMIA AND GANGRENE OF THE LOWER EXTREMITY: This complication of infusion into the saphenous vein is a hazard that may be fatal. The cause remains obscure. Reflex spasm of the vein with spread into the arterial tree is a possible explanation. Other possible contributory factors are cardiovascular failure, dehydration, prematurity, cachexia, fever, sepsis, local infection, occluding thrombosis or emboli, or any disturbance that interrupts the arterial blood supply to the extremities.

Tubing System

Fatal air embolism may occur when approximately 10 ml of air is introduced into the circulation. If the tubing system becomes empty of fluid, air may be sucked into the venous system. A defect in the tubing or a crack in the fluid container may also permit bubbles of air to enter the blood stream.

Before starting an infusion, the operator must displace all air from the tubing system, leaving only enough to allow observation of the drip mechanism.

Solutions for Infusion

BACTERIAL CONTAMINATION: Contamination with infective material is likely in parenteral solutions left open for several hours. Many solutions are ideal culture media. An open flask covered with a sterile gauze top should never be used. Disposable containers and tubing are far superior to equipment that must be cleaned, sterilized, and reused.

An infusion set of flask and tubing should not be used for a period exceeding 24 hours. It is preferable to change sets every 12 hours when prolonged intravenous infusion is required. Fluids left open for 30 minutes or longer before use should be discarded.

PYROGENIC SUBSTANCES: Pyrogenic substances are noninfectious. They do, however, produce febrile and allergic reactions. These substances are unlikely to be present in commercially prepared solutions in disposable containers.

IRRITATION TO THE VESSEL TISSUE: Several solutions are particularly irritating to the vessel tissue.

1. Hypertonic solutions: Glucose solutions in concentrations greater than 10% should not be given in small, superficial veins. Highly concentrated glucose solutions must be administered into large, deep veins, notably the superior or inferior vena cava.

   Hypertonic saline solutions, although less irritating than glucose, may cause tissue damage if infiltration occurs.
2. Calcium chloride: A brief infusion of 2% calcium chloride may be given in superficial veins without serious complication. Rapid injection may produce flushing, bradycardia, and cardiac arrhythmias. Solutions of greater concentration may cause necrosis in adjacent tissue. The solutions mentioned in items 1 and 2 frequently produce large sloughs when extravasation occurs.
3. Norepinephrine: dye contrast materials used for intravenous radiography; certain cytotoxic agents, such as nitrogen mustard, vincristine, daunorubicin, doxorubicin, and actinomycin D.
4. Alkaline solutions of short-acting barbiturates in 5% or greater concentration are likely to cause pain and frequently thrombosis.

Overloading the Extracellular Fluid Compartment

The most common technical cause of this complication is failure to observe frequently and to regulate the drip flow rate. This hazard can be avoided by placing only small volumes of solutions in the infusion flask or by regulating the intravenous drip rate with an infusion pump. One should never provide more than a total of 100 ml to the infusion container for an infant or 250 ml for an older child.

Administration of hypertonic electrolyte solutions produces rapid, transient increases in intravascular blood volume.

Administration of the Wrong Solution

The solution to be administered must be in a container properly identified by a label that is simple and easy to read. It is preferable to have as much contrast as possible in the size, shape, color, and lettering of the labels on the various solutions.

Cessation of the Drip

No physician has escaped being told that "the IV has stopped dripping." Disturbing as these words may be, such a mishap can be remedied frequently without an adverse display of temperament.

1. Be sure the drip has actually stopped. The regulator may be closed and may need regulation only.
2. Check for a kink in the tubing or for obstruction of the air filter.
3. Examine the tissue around the needle. If it is swollen, the vein wall is damaged, and fluid has infiltrated. In this case, the needle must be removed and inserted into another vein.
4. Look for edema around the needle point. If there is none, blood has probably clotted in the needle. The urge to attach a syringe to the needle and force the clot into the circulation should be suppressed. This maneuver should not be attempted. Compressing or "stripping" the tubing creates the same hazard of releasing a clot that may lodge in a lung capillary and cause a pulmonary infarct. It is safest to remove the clot as follows:

   - Place a tourniquet around the extremity above the needle.
   - Separate the nozzle of the infusion tubing from the needle or catheter hub.
   - Attach a syringe half-filled with saline to the hub of the needle or catheter.
   - By aspiration, try to suck the blood and the clot back into the syringe.

5. Watch for irregular infusion dripping—starting, stopping, or running slowly first and then rapidly. This may occur if the bevel of the needle is pressing against the vessel wall and may be corrected by removing the adhesive tape and retaping the needle while closely observing the drip rate.
6. Spasm of the vein may cause the fluid to drip slowly. This may be caused by mechanical irritation from the needle, local cold, an irritating solution, or a general state of shock. Local irritation may be relieved by injecting 1% lidocaine into the tissue surrounding the vessel or by placing a warm pack over the area to alleviate the cold.
7. The level of fluid in the drip chamber may rise and cover the inner nozzle so that it is impossible to determine whether the drip is running. This situation can be corrected by disconnecting the tubing and turning the bottle upside-down. When the level is sufficiently reduced, the infusion set can be reassembled.
8. See section on use of urokinase in obstructed central venous catheters.

Central Venous Access

In the past two decades, the use of large-bore plastic catheters for central venous access has increased dramatically. They have significantly advanced diagnostic capabilities, methods for monitoring critically ill patients, and intravenous administration of fluid and drugs. Generally, central venous access can be established for short-term or long-term use.

General Uses of Central Venous Catheters

1. Intravenous water and electrolyte administration
2. Drug therapy
3. Measurement of central venous pressure
4. Total parenteral nutrition
5. Collection of blood samples
6. Blood transfusion

Sites for Placement

These large central venous catheters can be peripherally inserted either by cutdown or by percutaneous puncture and advanced into the large central veins (superior or inferior vena cava). The routes of approach to the superior vena cava are the facial vein, the internal and external jugular veins, the innominate vein, the cephalic vein, the basilic vein, and the subclavian vein (Fig. 27–14). The external jugular and the basilic veins are probably the safest for percutaneous puncture because they are visible

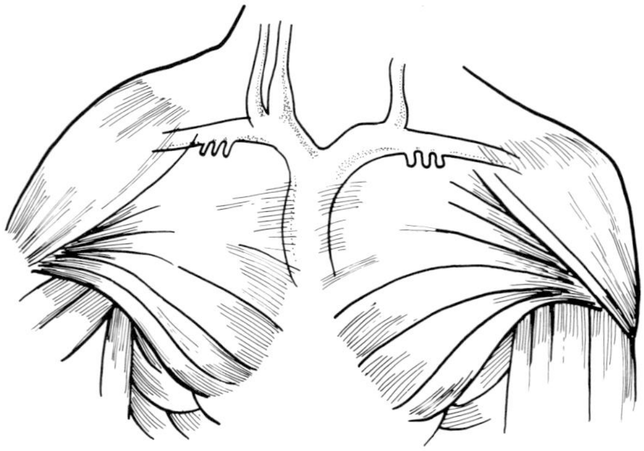

Figure 27–14 Anatomical relationship of major veins used for a central venous catheter. (From Grundfest S, Steiger E: Experience with the Broviac catheter for prolonged parenteral alimentation. *JPEN,* 3:45, 1979.)

and because bleeding can be easily recognized and controlled. Use of the basilic vein at the antecubital fossa or cephalic vein of the arm requires a long catheter. Approaches to the inferior vena cava are the saphenous and femoral veins. However, the inferior vena cava is not usually used for central venous pressure monitoring, because the femoral vein entry site is easily contaminated by excreta. Also, the saphenous vein is susceptible to thrombosis when it is traversed by a catheter that runs the entire length of the vein.

In small children and infants, central venous catheter placement requires great skill. At most sites, it is probably best done by a physician experienced in cutdown and vascular cannulation techniques.

SHORT-TERM CENTRAL VENOUS CATHETERS

Temporary central venous catheters are used when venous access is needed for several days to a few weeks. These catheters should not be used when intravenous lines with steel needles can serve the same purpose without undue stress on the patient.

These commonly used temporary central venous catheters are

- Cook catheter, ranging in size from 2.5 French to 6.3 French single-lumen or 5.0 French and 7.0 French double-lumen or triple-lumen catheters
- Intracaths
- Hohn catheter, sizes 4 French and 5 French

The procedure for percutaneous placement of a temporary catheter in the external jugular vein follows.

Equipment

For infants: 6 cm over-the-needle catheter-needle-stylet device
For children 1 year or older: 10- to 14-cm through-the-needle catheter
Tincture of iodine and 70% alcohol
Intravenous solution and administration set
Adhesive tape
4 × 4-cm gauze pads
Tincture of benzoin
Razor and scissors
Sterile gloves
1% lidocaine and tuberculin syringe (with 25-gauge, 1 1/2-cm needle)
16-gauge straight needle

Position and Restraint

The patient should be placed in a 15- to 30-degree Trendelenburg position, if possible. This causes distention of the external jugular vein. In small children, this distention can be accomplished by making them cry. The patient's head should be turned away from the side of puncture (the right side is the preferred site for placement). The patient should be placed in a body restraint with an assistant holding the patient's head to the side.

Method

1. Shave all hair at the site and any on the neck behind the site.
2. Identify the vein to be used and prepare the skin with tincture of iodine. When dry, remove it with 70% alcohol.
3. Use over-the-needle type catheters in small infants. The skin entry site can be anesthetized with lidocaine and a mini–skin incision made with a 16-gauge needle (as with intravenous catheter placement).
4. Don sterile gloves.
5. Make the infant cry. Each cry causes the external jugular vein to distend and then collapse on inspiration. Place the catheter-needle-stylet in the mini skin incision. With each cry, move it toward the ballooning vein. While the vein is collapsing with each new inspiration, hold the catheter-needle-stylet in position. In this stepwise, determined fashion, the vein is punctured, and blood is seen in the stylet hub. With the next cry, the catheter-needle-stylet is moved slightly into the distended vein, and the stylet tip is pulled back to just inside the catheter tip. The catheter is advanced to slightly above the level of the clavicle. Then the stylet is pulled back almost to the catheter hub but is not

removed. The catheter is then advanced to its full length. During this progression, the catheter may tend to snag at the clavicle as it passes under it. This can be minimized by placing traction on the shoulder, pulling it caudally and posteriorly, and advancing the catheter as before. Remove the stylet and quickly cover the catheter hub with the thumb to prevent a deep inspiration from pulling in a large bolus of air. The intravenous tubing is applied.

6. Loop the intravenous tubing up and over the ear and tape the tubing to the neck behind the intravenous site (Fig. 27–15)
7. For older children, use the through-the-needle catheter, either in a conventional fashion, as described later, or by dismantling the needle-catheter apparatus and using the parts individually. These units have a large-gauge needle (14 to 18) with a small- gauge catheter (16 to 20) 20 to 30 cm long that advances through the needle. Before insertion, the catheter tip is housed inside the needle barrel, and the length of catheter that extends behind the needle hub is enclosed in a sterile, clear plastic envelope (Fig. 27–16). After the vessel has been punctured, the catheter is advanced into the lumen by pushing the catheter hub through the plastic envelope until it locks into the hub of the large-gauge needle. Remove both the clear plastic envelope and the stylet within the catheter. To prevent air from being pulled into the catheter, cover the catheter hub with your gloved thumb and quickly attach the intravenous solution tubing. Then pull out the large-gauge needle from the puncture site and apply the needle guard (a device that splints the catheter as it exits the needle to keep the needle point from shearing the catheter). A satisfactory needle guard can be constructed by taping the needle shaft and proximal catheter to a tongue depressor cut to length; this keeps the catheter from flexing over the needle point and becoming severed.

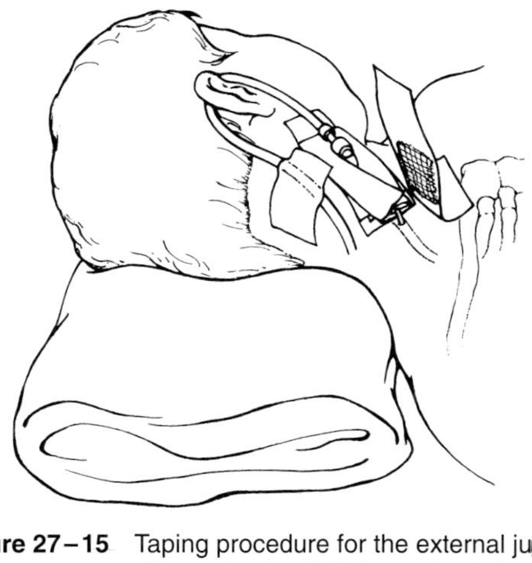

Figure 27–15 Taping procedure for the external jugular venous catheter. (From Hughes WT, Buescher ES: *Pediatric Procedures*. Philadelphia, WB Saunders, 1980.)

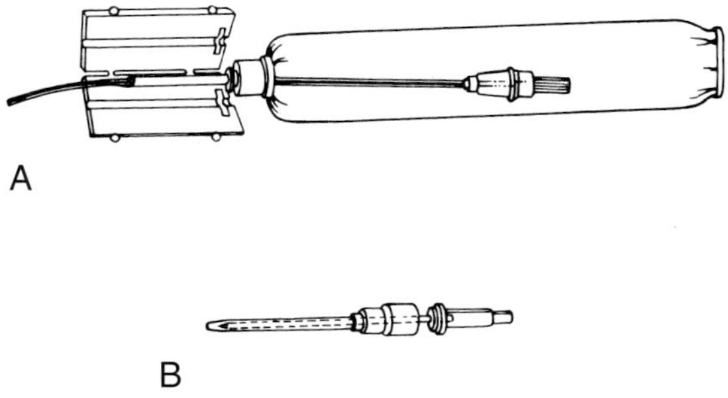

Figure 27–16 Intravenous catheters. **A.** Through-the-needle, **B.** Over-the-needle. (From Hughes WT, Buescher ES: *Pediatric Procedures*. Philadelphia, WB Saunders, 1980.)

An alternative method, using the same equipment, is to dismantle the needle-catheter and attach the large-gauge needle to a 10-ml syringe. Puncture the needle through the skin and apply negative pressure as the needle progresses under the skin. Blood appears in the syringe when the vein is punctured. Then hold the needle in place, detach the syringe, advance the catheter syringe, and advance the catheter through the needle into the vessel lumen. Thereafter, the procedure is as described previously.

8. With the through-the-needle type catheters, there is no need to perform a skin puncture with a trocar needle. If a large-gauge needle is used to puncture the vessel, the bevel should be held downward. This decreases the probability of puncturing the far wall of the vessel when the needle point enters the lumen.
9. Apply the proper catheter restraint, then loop the intravenous tubing behind the ear and tape it to the neck behind the skin puncture site (see Fig. 27–15).
10. After the catheter has been placed, a radiograph to localize the catheter tip is *mandatory*. The catheter should be in the superior vena cava or right atrium above the tricuspid valve. If it is not, it should be

repositioned appropriately. If the catheter is pulled back, it should never be readvanced through the skin site to reposition it. It should be removed completely and a new catheterization attempt made.

11. Examine the skin puncture site daily for signs of inflammation when the separate skin site dressing is replaced. Mark the date and time of change on the separate skin site dressing. The entire dressing should be replaced every 3 days.
12. Care should be exercised with the use of central venous catheters. They are double-edged swords. Although they provide critically useful information in some situations, they are also well-recognized sources of nosocomial infection. When central venous pressure readings are no longer necessary, the central venous catheter should be removed. As with other types of plastic intravenous catheters, their rate of infection rises rapidly after 48 to 72 hours in situ. Other hazards include hematoma formation, catheter embolization, pericardial tamponade, myocardial perforation, large-vessel thrombosis (superior vena cava syndrome), septic thrombophlebitis, and catheter-induced sepsis.

Dressing Change and Site Care for Temporary Central Line

Efforts must be exerted to prevent infection and obstruction related to the catheter. Meticulous care of the site involves changes of the covering bandage and flushing of the lumen. The bandage is usually changed every other day, possibly sparing weekends. Identifying days of the week for this purpose is advisable, such as Monday, Wednesday, and Friday. However, if the bandage becomes soiled or damaged at other times, it should be changed. A ritualistic approach ensures greater compliance from the patient, parents, and nurses.

Equipment

Povidone-iodine
Sterile saline wipes
Alcohol wipes
Sterile cotton-tipped applicators
Neosporin ointment
Splint gauze, 2 × 2
Stopcocks
Normal saline flush syringes
Silk tape
Sterile gloves

Procedure

1. Wash hands thoroughly with an antibacterial agent. Dry thoroughly.
2. Have patient turn head away from the dressing.
3. Carefully remove the old dressing. If the bandage gauze contains blood or exudate, put on sterile gloves to remove the dressing. Put the bandage in an appropriate trash container. An adhesive remover (Uni-Solv wipes) may be needed to clean the skin.
4. Examine the site for evidence of infection (erythema, induration, drainage). If present, take swabs with culturettes for cultures for bacteria and fungi. Drainage should be smeared onto microscope slides for Gram's stain and stain for acid-fast organisms. The findings should be reported to the physician-in-charge and noted in the patient's chart. In some centers, policies require the nurse to describe the site in the chart at the time of dressing change so that the physician and other health care workers will not remove dressings unnecessarily.
5. Don sterile gloves. Prepare stopcocks by flushing with sterile saline using a syringe. Leave syringe on stopcock. Use an alcohol wipe to cleanse the hub of the central venous catheter and the old stopcock. Place the old stopcock in the closed position, stopping the infusion. Quickly change the stopcock, replacing the old with the new unit. Check the blood return from the catheter while flushing with normal saline. Reconnect the infusion tubing to the stopcock of a two-lumen catheter; repeat the procedure.
6. Cleanse the insertion site with a povidone-iodine swab. Swab in circles beginning at the insertion site and moving peripherally.
7. Reswab the area with two sterile saline swabs.
8. Clean the length of the central venous catheter from the proximal area approximate to the insertion site to the distal end of the junction and the intravenous tubing.
9. Apply the Neosporin ointment to the catheter insertion site and suture sites with a sterile cotton-tipped applicator.
10. Apply a split, sterile 2 × 2 gauze sponge to straddle the catheter at the site.
11. Place an occlusive dressing over the gauze.
12. Apply silk tape to secure the catheter to the skin and the dressing to the skin.
13. Document in the chart when the dressing was changed and the appearance of the site.

Collecting Blood Samples from a Temporary Central Venous Catheter

Blood should be drawn from the stopcock nearest the catheter insertion site.

Equipment

Sterile gloves
Syringes
Tubes appropriate for desired tests
10-ml syringe filled with 10 ml heparinized saline (10 U/ml)
10-ml syringe with 1 ml heparinized saline (10 U/ml
Syringe with 5 ml injectable normal saline
Sterile capping devices
Alcohol wipes

Procedure

1. Don sterile gloves.
2. Stop the intravenous infusion. With double-lumen catheter, stop infusions to both lines.
3. Turn stopcock to off position.
4. Clean and swab the stopcock with an alcohol wipe.
5. Disconnect the intravenous infusion tubing and protect the end with a sterile cap.
6. Attach the 5-ml syringe filled with saline to the open stopcock port. Turn the stopcock to the open position and flush the catheter with normal saline.
7. Turn the stopcock to the closed position.
8. Connect the 10-ml syringe containing 1 ml heparinized saline.
9. Turn the stopcock to open position.
10. Aspirate blood gently to the 10-ml volume. (This will later be reinfused.)
11. Close stopcock and remove the blood-filled syringe.
12. Put sterile cap back on syringe.
13. Attach the syringe to contain the sample to the stopcock.
14. Turn stopcock to the open position.
15. Aspirate volume needed.
16. Close stopcock and remove the syringe with blood specimen.
17. Attach the syringe with 10 ml heparinized blood. Check for clots; if clots are seen, do not use.
18. Open stopcock and slowly infuse the 10 ml of heparinized blood, then close the stopcock.
19. Attach the syringe with 10 ml heparinized saline, open the stopcock, and flush the catheter with heparinized saline solution, closing the stopcock as the last 1 ml of the fluid is injected.
20. Disconnect the syringe and clean the stopcock with an alcohol wipe; then flush with 5 ml saline after the infusion of the 10 ml heparinized blood.
21. Reconnect the intravenous infusion line and reopen the stopcock.
22. Label and deliver the blood samples.

Removal of Temporary Central Venous Catheter

Equipment

Sterile gloves
Suture removal kit
Sterile scissors (two)
Culturettes (two)
Povidone-iodine swabs
Neosporin ointment
Dressing (coverlet, adhesive bandage)
Sterile 2 × 2 gauze (three to four packages)
Sterile clamp (hemostat)
Labels

Procedure

1. Wash hands thoroughly with antimicrobial soap.
2. Remove dressing and discard appropriate bag.
3. Clean insertion site with povidone-iodine swabs.
4. Don sterile gloves.
5. Clamp the catheter near where the catheter enters the skin and stop the intravenous infusion.
6. Remove sutures, if present.
7. Apply pressure with sterile gauze pads at the insertion site, then aseptically remove the catheter. After the catheter is out, continue to add pressure. Culture the site if infection is suspected.
8. Culture the tip. Cut the catheter's tip with sterile scissors about 2 cm from the end of the catheter. Place in sterile container and send to the laboratory for cultures.
9. Use the second pair of sterile scissors to cut a second 2-cm segment of the catheter beginning about 0.5 cm below the skin site and place the segment in a sterile container for culture.
10. Hold pressure on the site for at least *1 minute*. Then clean the site with Betadine swabs.
11. Apply Neosporin ointment to the insertion site.

12. Cover the site with two sterile 2 × 2 gauze pads and secure with tape.
13. Document catheter removal in chart.

LONG-TERM CENTRAL VENOUS CATHETERS

The long-term use of indwelling central venous catheters has become a mainstay in the management of infants and children with critical and chronic illnesses. Central venous lines have been developed to infuse fluids and drugs, to provide total parenteral nutrition, and to obtain samples of blood for study. Implantation of catheters for periods of months and years has been a significant advance in the management of patients with cancer and other diseases that require prolonged and intensive intravenous chemotherapy. Management of these indwelling lines demands meticulous attention to rote guidelines and procedures to ensure a functioning system free of complications.

Three general types of catheters for long-term placement are

1. Broviac-Hickman catheters
2. Groshong catheter
3. Implantable subcutaneous ports, such as Port-A-Cath, Infuse-A-Port, MediPort, and P.A.S. Port.

These are described in some detail.

Broviac-Hickman Catheter

In 1973, Broviac, Cole, and Scribner described a silicone rubber (Silastic) catheter for use in long-term intravenous alimentation (Broviac et al, 1973). This catheter initiated a revolution in intravenous therapy, eventually allowing administration of drugs and fluid parenterally at home as well as avoiding the pain and discomfort of multiple venipunctures. The original Broviac catheter was 90 cm long with a thin and flexible intravascular portion allowing it to float within the superior vena cava. This part of the catheter is attached to a thicker extravascular portion with a Dacron cuff in its midportion. The extravascular portion is placed in a subcutaneous tunnel and exits about 35 cm from the venous entry. After placement, the Dacron cuff becomes fixed by fibrous tissue, which in turn serves as a barrier to the migration of microbes from the skin along the catheter tract. A Broviac catheter for children is 62 cm long with the cuff 45 cm from the hub. The Broviac catheter was modified by Hickman to provide a larger bore. The Hickman catheter is available in one size only and may be used in older children and adults. The Broviac catheter is made in different sizes for infants, children, and adults.

In general, the methods for insertion, postoperative care, and long-term maintenance are similar for Broviac and Hickman catheters, so they are discussed as one.

Insertion of the catheter

The insertion is usually done surgically in the operating room under general anesthesia. However, in some older children, the insertion may be done under local anesthesia. Methods are also available for percutaneous insertion of these central venous catheters. The surgical placement of Broviac-Hickman catheters is usually done by a surgeon but can also be done by other physicians who have mastered the technique. Preferably, each medical center will designate the most appropriate individuals for this purpose (Grundfest and Steiger, 1979). Basically, the tip of the catheter is inserted through the cephalic, external jugular, or internal jugular vein into the superior vena cava or the right atrium of the heart (Fig. 27–17). With the patient in the Trendelenburg position and the head turned away from the operative site, the area is prepared with povidone-iodine and draped for sterile surgical incisions. The deltopectoral groove is identified and a cutaneous incision made over the area of the cephalic vein. If the cephalic vein is not accessible, muscular branches of the subclavian vein may be used. It may be necessary to extend the incision medially to below the middle third of the clavicle (Grundfest and Steiger, 1979). The fibers of the pectoralis major muscle are divided; deep to the muscle, one to three muscular tributaries to the subclavian vein are identified. Alternatively, the external or internal jugular veins may be used as access to the subclavian vein. When the selected vein is exposed and identified, it is freed; two silk sutures are placed around the vessel when one suture will be used to ligate the vessel and the other will secure the catheter in place once it is in final position.

From the incision site over the vein, a clamp or probe is used to tunnel through subcutaneous tissue interiorly to a point between the nipple and the sternum. A second small incision is made at this site, and the end of the instrument is visualized. The catheter is then inserted through this tunnel and pulled through as the Dacron cuff is 2 to 5 cm from the skin incision site. The appropriate length of the

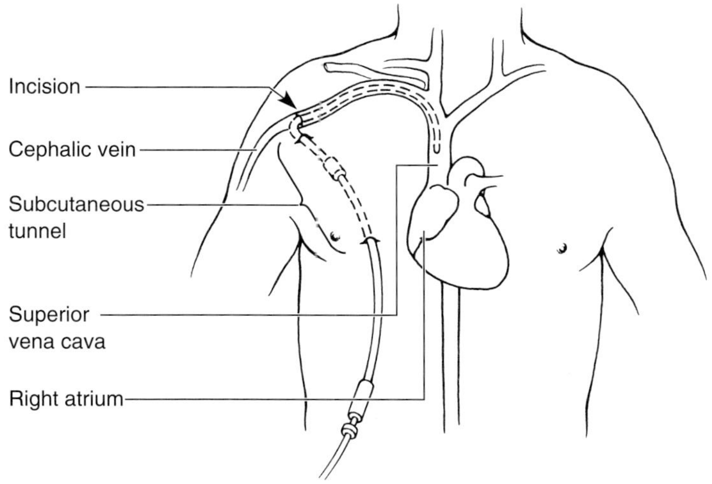

Figure 27–17 Placement of the Broviac-Hickman catheter. (From Nonkin R: The Broviac catheter: OR technique. *AORN J,* 35:216, 1982.)

catheter is estimated by overlaying the catheter from the incision site to the midpoint of the superior vena cava or right atrium. The catheter is cut to the proper length and inserted through an incision into the cephalic or other selected veins. Fluoroscopy or radiography is used to determine the position of the catheter tip. The catheter hub is attached to the tubing of the infusion fluid after the catheter is flushed with 10 ml of normal saline; or the catheter can be flushed with saline and the dead space volume filled with the saline plus 0.5 ml of 1000 U/ml of heparin and capped.

Care of the catheter

Once it is in place, meticulous care and attention must be given to the catheter. Because of the long-term use, spanning months or years, involvement of the patient, parents, or other family members is often required. The most successful approaches to management come through specific, ritualistic, and even obsessive attention to details of dressing changes, drug and fluid administration, and maintenance of catheter patency. Manufacturers of the catheters provide guidelines for care, and medical centers where these catheters are in frequent use establish a team and guidelines to meet their specific needs. The following instructions are in use at St. Jude Children's Research Hospital and are reasonably representative of those from other centers. Prepared as a printed brochure by the departments of nursing and surgery, these are written in terms understandable to parents but are also observed by responsible health care workers. The following instructions are for a single-lumen catheter, but slight modification makes them applicable to double-lumen catheters. Throughout the guidelines, the word "line" means the same as catheter.

Catheter Care at Home (Instructions for Parents)

Some important general principles:

- The dressing must be changed three times a week.
- Keep the dressing dry and clean.
- The catheter must stay clamped at all times when fluid is not moving through it; clamping prevents blood loss when the injection clamp is removed.
- Clamp the catheter only on the reinforced area.

The parent must be taught four procedures: (1) insertion site care, (2) catheter flushing, (3) exit site care and dressing change, and (4) injection cap changes.

INSERTION SITE CARE: As stated before, the insertion site is the small incision near the collarbone or on the side of the neck where the catheter was inserted into a vein. Dissolvable stitches are usually placed beneath the skin to close the incision. They will not have to be removed. The insertion site is strengthened with sterile tape called Steri-Strips. Caring for the insertion site is simple. The only supplies needed for this procedure are soap for handwashing and a package of povidone-iodine swabs, commonly called Betadine swabs. No gauze or other supplies are needed after the first dressing is removed. Just follow these simple steps.

1. Wash your hands for 1 full minute using the antibacterial soap in the catheter care kit.
2. Look at the insertion site for redness, swelling, drainage, or change in appearance. These are signs of possible infection and should be called to the physician or nurse at once.
3. Open the Betadine swabs as shown on the package.
4. Use a Betadine swab to clean the insertion site along the center of the Steri-Strips from one end of the incision to the other.
5. Repeat this cleaning procedure with the two remaining swabs.
6. Allow the Betadine solution to dry on the skin. Do not wipe it off.
7. Wash your hands again.

When your child is discharged from the hospital, the insertion site probably will not be completely healed. You need to paint or cleanse the insertion site with Betadine two times a day for 7 days after insertion of the catheter. For the first 7 days after surgery, your child will not be allowed to fully bathe. After that first week, your child may take a bath or shower and use soap and water to keep the insertion site clean. At the end of the second week, you may gently remove the Steri-Strips if they have not fallen off.

CATHETER FLUSHING: When your child is not receiving intravenous fluids or medications, the catheter must be flushed regularly. The lumen (or opening) of the catheter must be flushed to prevent these hollow tubes from becoming clogged with blood while the catheter is not in use. The catheters are made to stay in place for long periods and to be clamped and unclamped as needed. To prevent damage to the rubber tubing, the catheter clamp should be placed only on the reinforced areas shown for the clamp.

The catheter must be flushed at least one time a day (24 hours apart) with sterile heparin lock flush. Heparin helps prevent the catheter from becoming blocked by a blood clot. If a clot formed and could not be removed, it might be necessary to remove the catheter. Choose the same time each day that best suits your family's routine.

Supplies

10-ml heparin lock flush bottle. The bottle should read **10 USP units/ml.** Check the expiration date to make sure the bottle is not too old.
10-ml Luer-Lok syringe with needle attached
2 alcohol pads
2-inch silk tape
1 Band-Aid (1-inch wide)
Antibacterial soap

Be careful to open all supplies as shown on the packages so that they remain germ free.

If, at any step, anything touches the uncovered needle, you need to get a new syringe and needle and start the whole procedure again from the first step.

Procedure

1. Gather all supplies onto a clean work area.
2. Wash your hands with the antibacterial soap for 1 full minute. Use paper towels to dry your hands and then to turn off the water faucet before throwing it away.
3. Pop off the plastic top from the heparin lock flush bottle by pressing up with your thumb at the edge of the top.
4. Open the alcohol pads. Starting with one alcohol pad, take a corner of the pad and remove it from the package. Clean the bottle's rubber top with an untouched part of the alcohol pad. Allow the top to dry. **Do not blow on the rubber top to dry it. You may fan it with your hand.**
5. Peel open the syringe package and take out the syringe with the attached needle. Keep the clear part of the package to put the syringe and needle covers on. Turn the needle clockwise to twist it on tight.
6. Pull the syringe plunger back to the 5-ml mark. The top edge of the black rubber stopper is on the number 5.
7. Take the cover off the needle by pulling it straight off. Put the cover in the clear syringe package. Do not discard it.
8. Look to see that the bottle's rubber top is dry and push the needle into it. Turn the bottle upside down and push 5 ml of air into it. The added air creates pressure in the bottle and makes it easier for you to take out the solution.
9. Pull the plunger until the solution comes to the 5-ml mark. Keep the tip of the needle below the fluid level.

Before removing the needle from the bottle, look for big "air pockets" in the syringe. Push any air pockets back into the bottle and finish pulling the solution to the 5-ml mark. Pull out the needle from the bottle.

Put the cover back on the needle. Push the cover on until you feel it snap.

10. If air bubbles are in the syringe, do the following:
    - Hold the syringe straight up with the needle pointing to the ceiling.
    - Tap the syringe with your finger to release air bubbles from the bottom or the sides or tap the syringe on a hard surface.
    - All the air bubbles will be at the top.
    - Continue to tap all the bubbles until they are in the center of the needle at the top.
    - Push the plunger until a drop of fluid starts out of the needle.
    - It may be necessary to pull back the plunger to make one big air bubble at the top to remove the smaller air bubbles near the needle end of the syringe.
    - Holding the syringe with the needle pointed straight up, push the plunger until a drop of fluid starts out the needle.
11. Put the syringe down in the clear part of the syringe package while you get the catheter ready to flush.
12. Take off the tape holding the looped catheter on top of the Coverlet-O.R. dressing. You need to uncover only the injection cap and clamp.
13. Remove the Band-Aid over the injection cap and catheter end. You will change this Band-Aid each time you flush.
14. Remove another alcohol pad from the package. Clean the rubber port end of the injection cap with an untouched part of the alcohol pad. Make sure the alcohol completely cleans the rubber port. **After the cap is cleaned, you cannot put it down.**
15. Hold both the syringe and the catheter in the same hand, then pull the needle cover off with your other hand. Do not jerk on the catheter as you remove the needle cover.
16. Push the needle into the rubber port of the injection cap. Stop when you feel resistance. The needle may show. Either way is all right.
17. Unclamp the catheter.
18. Push the 5 ml of heparin lock flush solution into the catheter using a steady and moderately firm pressure to "flush" the catheter. It should flush easily. Do not force the solution. If the catheter will not flush, check to make sure the clamp is opened and the catheter is not kinked anywhere. If you still cannot flush the catheter, please call your physician.
19. When the plunger reaches the 1-ml mark on the syringe, reclamp the catheter. Close the clamp while you are still pushing in the solution. This leaves a positive pressure inside the catheter.
20. After the catheter is clamped, remove the needle from the injection cap. You may now lay the catheter down.
21. Replace the cap on the needle and remove the needle from the syringe by turning it in a counterclockwise direction. The needle should now be thrown away into a hard-sided container.

    Suggestion: Keep a covered hard container to dispose of used needles (a coffee can or jar is fine). When it is full, tape it closed and throw it away.
22. Open the Band-Aid package. Peel paper from back of Band-Aid. Fold over about 1/8 inch on each end of the Band-Aid. Place gauze part of Band-Aid over end of injection cap and press Band-Aid together to cover injection cap and hub of catheter.

    This Band-Aid keeps the injection cap from coming loose and protects the catheter end from germs.
23. Loop the catheter and fasten it in place with the silk tape.
24. Throw away used supplies including the used heparin lock flush bottle. Wash your hands.

EXIT SITE CARE AND DRESSING CHANGE: Care of the exit site (where the catheter comes out of the body) is done at least three times a week. After the first week, your child can get the old dressing wet during short baths and showers (less than 15 minutes), but the dressing must be changed just after the bath.

Supplies

2-inch-wide clear tape and 2-inch-wide silk tape
Sterile cotton-tipped applicators (Q-tips)
Sterile 2 × 2-inch Sof-Wick gauze
Coverlet-O.R. dressing, 4 × 4-inch
Antibacterial soap

Package of Betadine swabs
Two packages of sterile saline wipes
Alcohol pad
Packet of antibacterial ointment (Neosporin)

Procedure

1. Gather all supplies on a clean work area.
2. Wash your hands for 1 full minute using the antibacterial soap provided. Dry your hands with paper towels, then turn the faucets off with the same paper towel before throwing it away.

Open all the supplies as shown on the packages so that they remain germ free. Open the Neosporin packet when you are ready to use it.

3. Remove the old tape and dressing, being careful not to pull the catheter. It is easy to accidentally pull the catheter during this step. Be careful to separate the Sof-Wick gauze underneath the gauze attached to the Coverlet-O.R. dressing as you remove the Coverlet-O.R. dressing. Look at the Sof-Wick for any unusual drainage. Look at the exit site for **redness, swelling, drainage, or any change.** These are signs of possible infection and should be reported to your child's physician or nurse. Also check the location of the marker. Normally, it will be about 2 cm or 1 inch from the exit site. If the marker is not in its normal location, notify your physician or Line Nurse.
4. Wash your hands with antibacterial soap again for 1 full minute as in step 2. (If you are not able to leave your child alone, clean your hands well with an alcohol pad.)
5. Start with the package of Betadine swabs.
    - Hold the catheter up **loosely** to clean completely around the exit site. Cleanse your child's exit site with a Betadine swab starting at the area nearest the catheter. Work outward in a circular motion covering an area about 3 inches across. If you miss an inner spot, do not go back in to clean that spot. Wait and cleanse that area with the next swab.
    - Again starting at the area nearest the catheter, work outward with each of the two remaining Betadine swabs. **Put the catheter down between each step while reaching for new supplies so that you will not pull the catheter.**
    - The Betadine solution on the swabs will not damage the catheter, but it can cause skin irritation with prolonged use. To prevent this, wipe away the Betadine as described in step 6.
6. Take one package of the sterile saline wipes.
    - Before your touch the wipe, fold the entire package in half and squeeze some saline out of the package so the wipes won't get too wet.
    - Take the corner of the wipe with your thumb and one finger, touching only one side of the wipe.
    - Clean the exit site with this saline wipe, starting at the area nearest the catheter, and continue as you did with the Betadine swabs.
    - **The corner of the wipe that starts in the center must stay pointed toward the center as you make your circles, cleaning outward.**
    - Repeat with another saline wipe.
7. Pick up an alcohol pad, fold the package in half, and squeeze out some of the alcohol to prevent it from running down into the exit site.
    - Remove the alcohol pad from the package by grasping a corner.
    - Unfold the alcohol pad by holding two corners.
    - Wrap the alcohol pad around the catheter as close to the exit site as possible without touching the skin. The catheter lies in the fold of the pad.
    - Clean the catheter by using your other hand to push the catheter into the alcohol pad, working the pad from the exit site to the capped end of the catheter.

    Be **gentle** to prevent any pulling of the catheter. If you miss a spot, do not go back and clean it with the same alcohol pad. Get another alcohol pad and do this step again.
8. Pick up both the Neosporin ointment package and the Q-tips, being careful not to touch the cotton ends once they are removed from their package. Tear open the Neosporin packet. **Do not allow the edge of the Neosporin package to touch the Q-tips.**
    - Squeeze all the Neosporin ointment onto the two sterile Q-tips.
    - Use one of the Q-tips to apply part of the Neosporin ointment to the exit site.

- With the other Q-tip, apply the rest of the Neosporin ointment to the exit site.

9. Lift out the sterile gauze (Sof-Wick) from the package. Be careful to **touch only the outer edge.**

   Position the gauze so the catheter passes through the split. Lay the catheter downward on your child's abdomen. (The split of the gauze should be directed toward the top.

   - The bottom of the marker should be almost even with the bottom of the Sof-Wick. The catheter marker helps you see whether the catheter has been pulled out any.

10. Peel open the Coverlet-O.R. dressing, being careful to **touch only the tape edges and not the sterile gauze.**

    Properly place the dressing over the split gauze. Press the tape down firmly on your child's skin. It is okay if there are wrinkles in the Coverlet-O.R. dressing. Make sure the dressing is securely taped to the skin on four sides.
11. This is a special way to tape that keeps the catheter from being pulled at the exit site. You need three pieces of tape as wide as the Coverlet-O.R. dressing.

    - Loop part of the catheter on top of the Coverlet-O.R. dressing. Fasten the catheter with one piece of tape. Tear a small slit in the middle of this tape. Pull the catheter through the slit. You will see the catheter looped into a circle.
    - From the second piece of tape, tear off a skinny piece from the edge. Lay it just underneath the catheter, sticky-side-up. Cross the tape over and make a V to turn the tape sticky-side-down. Place the remainder of this piece of tape over the V to keep the V from coming loose.
    - Place the third piece of tape over the middle of the dressing.

12. Finish fastening remaining catheter on top of the Coverlet-O.R. dressing with the tape, keeping the clamps flat.
13. Throw away used supplies and wash your hands.

Now and then, look at the dressing to be certain the tape is secured. Retape as needed.

INJECTION CAP CHANGES: **Injection caps must be changed once each week** (example: every Monday or when blood specimens are drawn by your local clinic or physician). Do this during a routine catheter flush if possible, either before or after you flush. Do not ever reuse an injection cap. **Once the cap has been removed, a new one should be used.**

Supplies

Injection cap
Alcohol pad
Antibacterial soap
Band-Aid

Procedure

1. Gather supplies on a clean work area.
2. Wash your hands with the antibacterial soap for 1 full minute. Use paper towels to dry your hands and then use these paper towels to turn off the faucet.
3. Open the alcohol pad as shown on the package. Open the injection cap.
4. Remove the Band-Aid from the injection cap.
5. Make sure the catheter is clamped, then unscrew the injection cap and throw it away. Do not put the catheter down or touch the end of the catheter to anything after removing the cap.
6. Remove the alcohol pad from the package by holding only a corner of the pad.
7. Clean the end of the catheter with the alcohol pad thoroughly with the part of the pad that you have not touched.
8. After you clean the end of the catheter, take the injection cap out of the package, being careful not to touch the end of the cap that screws onto the catheter.
9. Screw the cap on securely.
10. Place the new Band-Aid over the connection of the injection cap and the catheter end.
11. Loop and secure the catheter with the silk tape.
12. Throw away all used supplies properly and wash your hands.

ADDITIONAL INFORMATION

1. Remember—the catheter **must** be flushed every 24 hours.
2. Be sure to clamp the catheter as you are flushing the last 1 ml of solution. This prevents a backflow of blood into the catheter and greatly reduces the chance of blood clotting inside the catheter.
3. Tape the connection of the catheter hub and injection cap securely with the Band-Aid.

Your child may wear a tube top as underwear to protect the catheter.
4. Young children, toddlers, and infants should wear a stretch T-shirt dressing. The Line Nurse will show you how this protects the catheter.
5. Your child (if old enough) should always carry a medical I.D. card. You should complete it and carry it with you at all times.
6. Always open supplies as shown on the package so that they remain germ free.
7. If the dressing ever gets a little wet, is soiled, or is not sticking to your child's skin, change it at once regardless of when it was last changed.
8. Never use scissors, hemostats, or any sharp-edged instrument near the catheter.

SOME COMPLICATIONS

Dislodgement: Dislodgement or accidental removal of the catheter can happen easily during the first 4 to 6 weeks after placement of the catheter. The catheter is held in the body by a small Dacron cuff that is on the catheter under the skin about halfway between the insertion and exit sites. The 4- to 6-week period is needed for the tissue of the body to actually grow into this cuff and hold the catheter in place. During this time, it will be necessary to be careful when picking up your child under the arms. You should not swing your child by the arms. The older child should not swing from any type of bar or pick up any heavy packages or objects. Activities that require arm swings, such as baseball, need to be limited for the first 4 to 6 weeks after placement of the catheter.

A marker is placed onto most catheter during surgery that can be used to see whether the catheter has moved out any. This marker is placed one-thumbwidth (1 inch) from the exit site on the catheter. If the marker comes out any farther from the exit site, let your physician know so that the placement of the catheter may be checked by a blood return, a chest x-ray, or a dye flushed through the catheter while x-rays are made (venogram).

One way to help keep the catheter from coming out during the first 4 to 6 weeks is to raise your child's arm (the one on the side on which the catheter was placed) about halfway up just before you place the Coverlet-O.R. on the skin. By doing this, you prevent any possible tension on the catheter.

Many times, especially during the first 6 weeks, you can see the marker move in and out with movement of the arm. If the arm is lifted up, the marker will move in closer to the body. This small movement of the marker is normal.

Infection: One of the most important things to do while changing the dressing is to always look for signs of possible infection. Signs of infection may be redness, swelling, drainage, or other changes in the skin at the exit site or fever. These signs should be reported to your physician at once.

Clotting/Obstruction: If the heparin lock flush cannot be pushed easily from the syringe into the catheter with a moderate amount of pressure, do not use excessive force. This could break the catheter or dislodge a blood clot. If you have problems flushing the catheter:

- Make sure the clamp is open and that the catheter is not kinked or twisted under the tape.

If you are still unable to flush the catheter, do not force it. Remove the needle and the catheter.

Skin Irritation: If the skin under the dressing and tape becomes reddened or irritated, let the Line Nurse know. It might be necessary to change the type of dressing or the tape that is being used. Many times, the use of Skin Prep will decrease the amount of skin irritation caused by the dressing. Before the Coverlet-O.R. dressing is put on, gently apply the Skin Prep to the skin wherever tape or the Coverlet-O.R. outer dressings will be. Let the Skin Prep dry completely. If the skin feels sticky, the Skin Prep is not dry. Then apply the Coverlet-O.R. dressing.

Emergency: If you notice that the catheter is damaged, clamp the catheter at once between your child and the breakage. You may fold the line over on itself and wrap a rubber band around the line to clamp it. Call your physician because the catheter must soon be repaired or replaced.

Reminder: Never use scissors, hemostats, or any sharp-edged instrument near the catheter.

Drawing blood from the Broviac-Hickman catheter

The indwelling central venous catheter provides easy access to blood for diagnostic samples. However, the sampling procedure demands careful attention to details in maintaining sterility to avoid infection. The following procedure applies to the single-lumen Broviac-Hickman catheter.

1. After handwashing with antibacterial soap, don sterile gloves.
2. Stop the intravenous infusion and clamp the catheter at the reinforced site.
3. Wipe the connection site thoroughly with alcohol wipes.
4. Disconnect the intravenous tubing and cap the hub with a sterile cover.
5. Attach a syringe with 5 ml of normal saline to the catheter opening, remove the clamp and flush the catheter, then reclamp the catheter.
6. Disconnect the empty saline syringe and replace with a 10-ml syringe with 1 ml heparinized saline solution. Then aspirate gently to fill the syringe to the 10-ml mark. Clamp catheter at reinforcement site. Remove this blood-filled syringe; do not discard (this is *not* the specimen for tests); keep sterile.
7. Connect a new syringe for collection of the blood sample for testing and aspirate the desired volume.
8. Reclamp the catheter and disconnect the syringe.
9. Attach the syringe with 10 ml of heparinized blood. Open the clamp and infuse back into the patient. If clots are seen, do not infuse but discard the blood.
10. Reclamp the catheter and attach a syringe with 10 ml of heparinized saline; release the clamp and flush the catheter, leaving 1 ml of saline in the syringe. If an intravenous infusion is to be started, flush the catheter further with 5 ml of saline before reconnection.
11. Wipe the catheter hub thoroughly with an alcohol wipe, removing any residual blood.
12. Aseptically reconnect the intravenous infusion or attach a sterile injection cap if no infusion is to be given.

Management of special situations

The following methods have been used with success (Butler et al, 1989).

Emergency Care of a Damaged Catheter: Temporary Splice

When catheters become damaged, whenever possible the permanent repair should be done initially. However, the circumstances may be such that a permanent repair cannot be made. The following procedure is used until permanent repair is done.

1. Clamp the catheter with a guarded hemostat between the damaged part of the catheter and the exit site.
2. Put on sterile gloves.
3. Clean the damaged part of the catheter with an alcohol wipe. Then, clean the entire external catheter with povidone-iodine solution soaked on sterile gauze.
4. Wipe the catheter again with an alcohol wipe.
5. Cut off the damaged end of the catheter with sterile scissors at a right angle. Take an angiocatheter (Jelco) and pull back the stylet slightly to prevent puncture of the catheter while inserting (a blunt needle may be substituted for the angiocatheter).
6. Insert the angiocatheter and remove the stylet. Tape the catheter to the angiocatheter.
7. Attach a sterile syringe to the hub of the angiocatheter.
8. Release the clamp.
9. Aspirate until 2 to 3 ml of blood returns. Send this blood sample for bacterial and fungal cultures.
10. Irrigate the catheter (refer to flushing procedure).
11. Clamp the catheter again and remove the syringe.
12. Attach the intravenous tubing to the spliced catheter and resume infusion or attach a sterile injection cap to the end of the angiocatheter.
13. Tape the angiocatheter to the tongue blade and secure the repaired catheter to the chest.

Permanent Repair

Repair kits are used for permanent repair of damaged catheter. The kit should be for the specific type of catheter (Broviac or Hickman), because these come in different sizes. The kit will usually contain step-by-step instructions. These are generally as follows:

1. Wash hands with antibacterial soap.
2. Prepare the following supplies on the sterile field: 4 × 4-inch gauzes with povidone-iodine solution applied on top of them; alcohol prep pads; scissors and guarded hemostats; fenestrated drape; 3-ml Luer-Lok syringe; and appropriate size repair kit.
3. Prepare 10-ml syringes for normal saline and heparinized saline solutions.
4. Remove the tape holding looped catheter (you may be able to leave the exit site dressing intact).
5. Determine where the catheter will be repaired to make proper preparations.

6. Apply rubber-guarded hemostats on catheter between the exit site and the area to be repaired.
7. Clean the area on the catheter where the repair is to be made with an alcohol prep pad. Have an assistant hold the catheter up for you and do not let it fall back on the patient.
8. Put on sterile gloves and place a sterile fenestrated drape over the catheter. Close the opening of the fenestrated drape with sterile hemostats.
9. Clean the area on the catheter where the repair is to be made with another alcohol prep pad followed by vigorous rubbing of this area with the povidone-iodine–soaked gauzes. Repeat this vigorous cleansing of the catheter with another povidone-iodine–soaked gauze while the assistant is still holding the catheter up for you. Again, clear the catheter with an alcohol prep pad to remove the povidone-iodine solution.
10. Cut off the damaged part of the catheter with straight, sterile scissors and have the assistant who was holding the catheter discard the part cut off.
11. Prepare the Silastic adhesive glue found in the repair kit into a 3-ml Luer-Lok syringe with a blunt, large-gauge needle attached. To best insert the adhesive into the syringe, remove the plunger from the syringe and squirt at least 1 ml of adhesive into the barrel of the syringe. Then reinsert the plunger into the syringe.
12. Prime the repair segment with a heparinized saline (10 U/ml) solution and insert the end of the repair segment into the lumen of the exposed externalized Hickman or Broviac catheter.
13. Inject a small amount of Silastic adhesive onto the repair segment and the end of the exposed Hickman or Broviac catheter after they are joined. Push the end of the catheter and the repair segment together as closely as possible.
14. Slide the large splicing sleeve over the area of the repair. The sleeve will slide much easier if a small amount of Silastic adhesive is used as a lubricant.
15. Once the repair sleeve is in place, inject a moderate amount of Silastic adhesive underneath each end of the sleeve. Roll evenly between your gloved fingers to properly disperse the Silastic adhesive.
16. Attach a sterile syringe to the hub of the catheter.
17. Release the rubber-guarded hemostats from the catheter.
18. Aspirate 1.5 ml of blood and send this blood sample for bacterial and fungal cultures. Observe the splice segment to make sure that no leakage has occurred.
19. Clamp the catheter and remove the syringe with culture specimen. Flush the catheter with normal saline and then with heparinized saline solution (see flushing methods).
20. Clamp the catheter and remove the flush syringe. Attach the intravenous tubing back to the catheter and resume infusion or attach a sterile injection cap to the end of the Hickman or Broviac catheter's hub.
21. Using heavy scissors, trim a tongue blade to use as a splint over the area of the catheter repair. Use of benzoin compound may help attach Steri-Strips to the splint. The splint is to be left in place a minimum of 24 hours.

Removal of the catheter

Removal of the catheter should be done by a physician trained in this procedure and capable of dealing with complications. The procedure is as follows:

1. Explain the procedure to the patient and parents.
2. Wash hands with an antibacterial soap and dry thoroughly.
3. Remove the dressing, place it in a plastic bag, seal it, and discard it in a trash container.
4. Wash hands again.
5. If redness, edema, or drainage is present at the exit site, use culturettes to culture the site for bacteria and fungi.
6. Stop infusion of fluids if necessary.
7. Close the clamp if it is not already closed.
8. Clean the line with an alcohol prep pad from the exit site to the end of the catheter.
9. Clean the exit site with three povidone-iodine swabs.
10. Put on sterile gloves.
11. Wrap the catheter around the hand and pull firmly and steadily, stretching the line with constant pressure. Jerking may break the line. Maintain constant pressure on the line for several minutes so that fibrous tissue that has formed around the cuff loosens and the line breaks free. Continue constant pressure on the line until the entire catheter is brought through the exit site. The Dacron cuff often detaches from the catheter and re-

mains in the patient's subcutaneous tissue. If this occurs, a decision may be made to leave it in place if the tissue around it does not appear to be infected.

12. Once the line is removed, apply immediate pressure over the old insertion site for several minutes.
13. Cut the tip of the catheter 2 cm from the tip with sterile scissors; place it in a sterile container and label "catheter tip."
14. With a separate pair of sterile scissors, cut a second 2-cm segment beginning 0.5 cm below the skin exit site. Place this specimen in a separate sterile container and label "catheter-skin site."
15. If drainage is present, milk the catheter's old subcutaneous tunnel toward the exit site.
16. Clean the exit site with povidone-iodine swabs.
17. Apply one packet of Neosporin ointment.
18. Place a sterile Coverlet-O.R. dressing over the exit site.
19. Remove gloves and wash hands.
20. Send specimens immediately to the laboratory.
21. *Instruct the patient or parents to remove the dressing the next day to keep the old exit site clean with soap and water. Reinforce the need for them to notify their attending physician if signs or symptoms of infection occur.*

Groshong Catheter

The Groshong catheter (Catheter Technology Corporation, Salt Lake City) is a silicone, clear catheter with a closed tip and a two-way valve at the proximal end. It is radiopaque and has a Dacron cuff. The following procedure as suggested by the manufacturer is used for *percutaneous placement* of the Groshong catheter.

1. Wash hands with antibacterial soap and put on sterile gloves.
2. Prepare the venipuncture, tunnel, and tunnel exit sites with povidone-iodine swabs.
3. Infiltrate the venipuncture site with local anesthetic.
4. Place the patient in the Trendelenburg position with the head turned away from the intended venipuncture site.
5. Use a 22-gauge, 1 1/2-inch needle attached to a 3-ml syringe to locate the desired vessel. (See section on venous access procedures.)
6. Attach an 18-gauge, 2 1/2-inch needle to a 5-ml syringe and insert it into the vessel alongside the 22-gauge needle.
7. Remove the 5-ml syringe from the 18-gauge needle after verifying its location in the vessel.
8. Insert the desired tip of the spring wire guide through the 18-gauge needle into the vessel. If a J tip is used, prepare for insertion by sliding the plastic tube over the J to straighten it. Advance the spring wire guide to the desired depth. Advancement of the J tip may require a gentle rotating motion. Do *not* pull the wire back through the needle because it is possible to shear off the wire with the needle bevel.
9. Holding the spring wire guide in place, withdraw the 18-gauge needle.
10. If desired, enlarge the cutaneous puncture site with a mini-scalpel.
11. Advance the tapered tip of the sheath-dilator assembly over the spring wire guide into the vessel using a slight twisting motion. Do not allow the spring wire guide to advance completely into the vessel.
12. Irrigate the catheter-style assembly with any isotonic intravenous fluid through the Luer-Lok lock adapter of the stylet.
13. Holding the peel-away sheath in place, remove the spring wire guide and dilator. Insert the catheter-stylet assembly into the lumen of the sheath and advance to desired position in the vessel by using the graduations on the catheter, which are in 2.5-cm or 5-cm intervals from the distal tip.
14. Verification of catheter and tip location should be accomplished radiographically or fluoroscopically.
15. Grasp the two handles of the peel-away sheath and pull outward and upward at the same time. Peel the sheath away from the catheter completely. Make sure that the catheter is not dislodged from the vessel as the sheath is removed.
16. Slide catheter off stainless steel shaft of stylet adapter. Gently withdraw the stylet from the catheter with a straight, even motion. Do not permit the catheter to be withdrawn from the vessel while the stylet is being removed.
17. Measure the catheter against the chest wall of the patient to determine desired location of the Dacron felt cuff and exit site. Perform local anesthetic infiltration along the tunnel and at the exit site.
18. With the trocar, create a subcutaneous tunnel through to the exit site. The sharp point of the trocar should be used to cre-

ate the exit site. Pass the trocar point through the exit site, then attach the catheter to the trocar extension. Secure the catheter to the trocar with a suture. Continue passing the trocar through the exit site. Because the trocar creates a tight, small tunnel, initial resistance may be encountered where the Dacron cuff meets the tissue. The catheter should not be forced. Holding the catheter segment above the cuff while gently pulling on the trocar should result in a smooth passage of the cuff into the subcutaneous tunnel.

19. Care should be taken not to kink the catheter subcutaneously at the curvature point from venipuncture site to tunnel.
20. Cut the catheter from the trocar extension and trim the external segment of the catheter to desired length.
21. Secure the connector to the catheter per enclosed instructions.
22. After placement is complete but before the venipuncture site is sutured, draw blood through the catheter to ensure patency. If necessary, adjust the catheter at the curvature point to relieve restriction. Irrigate the catheter with 20 ml of isotonic solution.
23. Twist on and securely tighten the latex injection cap or connect it to an intravenous fluid source.
24. Suture the venipuncture site, as necessary.
25. Secure the catheter at the exit site with a dressing. The external segment of the catheter should be coiled and taped. Many institutions have recommended the use of an extension set. Straight pulling tension on the external segment should be avoided. It may result in dislodgement of the catheter.

Implantable Ports

Implantable ports ("ports of entry") may be preferred for some older children and adolescents. The implantable device consists of a self-sealing injection port with a preconnected or attachable silicone catheter that is inserted into a large vein. These units, such as Port-A-Cath, Infuse-A-Port, and MediPort, are placed entirely under the skin for each entry into the system. The Port-A-Cath is described here in some detail.

The Port-A-Cath has two major parts: (1) the subcutaneous port, used for entry into the system, is a silicone-covered metallic chamber with a self-sealing silicone septum; and (2) the plastic catheter. The installment of the Port-A-Cath is similar to that of the Broviac-Hickman catheters. The catheter is inserted into the large central vein, such as the superior vena cava, and the port is placed under the skin and sutured to the chest wall. The target surface of the port is easy to locate and access. The skin covering the port must be in a healthy condition. The self-sealing septum can withstand at least 2000 punctures with a 22-gauge noncoring needle or 1000 punctures with a 19-gauge noncoring needle.

Only special noncoring needles are used for accessing the port. The needles are available in several shapes and sizes. The 90-degree noncoring needle is angulated and may be secured into the port with a dressing for infusions. The maximum time that the needle can be left in place is approximately 7 days.

The unit should always be filled with heparinized saline after each use. The heparin lock helps prevent thrombotic occlusion of the catheter.

The system is flushed the first 3 days postoperatively once per day with 5 ml heparinized saline using 100 units of heparin per milliliter or by continuous infusion of fluids. When there are extended periods between injections, infusions, or blood sampling, the system must be flushed with heparinized saline once every 2 weeks.

Access to the system

1. Wash hands with antibacterial soap.
2. Palpate the location of the port with two fingers, placing them on both sides of the port.
3. Take the cap off a bottle of normal saline and wipe the rubber top with an alcohol pad. Set it aside and allow to dry.
4. If necessary, apply topical anesthetic to the skin directly over the port.
5. Take the 10-ml syringe and needle out of the package.
6. Draw the syringe's plunger back to the 10-ml mark and remove the needle cover (do not discard it).
7. Make sure the rubber top on the normal saline vial is completely dry and insert the needle into it.
8. Turn the vial upside-down and push 10 ml of air from the syringe into the vial; draw 10 ml of fluid into the syringe and the pull the needle from the vial.
9. Replace the cover on the needle.
10. Put on sterile gloves. Open the package containing the 90-degree noncoring needle

and extension set (Gripper) and remove it from the package, leaving the needle covered and the tubing capped.

11. Twist off the needle that is attached to the syringe and remove the cap from the extension set tubing. You must avoid touching either the tip of the syringe or the hub of the uncapped tubing.
12. Twist the syringe tightly onto the hub of the extension set tubing.
13. Flush the set with normal saline; close the clamp.
14. Using an alcohol prep pad, begin cleaning the skin directly over the port in a circular motion away from the port. Clean an area 3 to 5 inches in diameter. If the pad appears dirty after cleaning one time, use another pad until dirt is not visible on the pad.

    Open the package of povidone-iodine swabs. Beginning with a swab at the center of the port, clean the skin in a circular motion away from the port. Cover a 3- to 5-inch area. Use three swabs in the same fashion, beginning in the center of the port and moving outward.
15. Remove the needle guard.
16. With the other hand, locate the port again by placing a finger on either side of it (be careful not to touch the center of the port, because this will contaminate the injection site). Grasp the Gripper tab and insert the needle perpendicularly (straight up and down, or 90 degrees) into the port; push the needle firmly through the skin and port until the needle hits the bottom of the chamber.
17. Open the clamp and aspirate blood into the extension set only to verify correct placement of the noncoring needle. If you are unable to aspirate any blood at this point, flush the system with 2 to 3 ml of saline and attempt to aspirate blood again. If you are still unable to aspirate any blood and the system flushes easily, complete flushing the system with normal saline. If fluid cannot be pushed into the port, the needle may not be properly in place. If the needle is on the bottom of the chamber and fluid still cannot be pushed, STOP. Ascertain that the needle is correctly placed in the center of the port by feeling the location of the port again. It might be necessary to get another noncoring needle and reaccess the port.
18. Flush the port with steady pressure. While flushing in the last 1 ml, close the clamp on the tubing. It is important that you are flushing at the same moment that you close the clamp. This helps prevent blood from backing into the catheter tip.

Procedures for continuous infusion

1. Access the system.
2. Remove the syringe from the extension set tubing.
3. Connect a primed intravenous set to the extension tubing. Release the clamp and begin infusion. When using a pump or controller, turn it on before opening the clamp to keep positive pressure in the port.
4. Clean the needle insertion site with a sterile saline wipe with an outward spiral motion to remove the povidone-iodine. Repeat this step with one more sterile saline wipe.
5. Apply Neosporin ointment to the needle insertion site using a sterile cotton-tipped applicator. Be careful not to touch the edge of the Neosporin packet to the cotton-tipped applicator. Place a sterile Sof-Wick split sponge around the needle insertion site and under the 90-degree angle of the needle (use as many of these as you need to provide support and stabilization).
6. Place an occlusive dressing over the needle. Loop and tape the extension tube on top of the dressing to provide a "safety loop" if the tubing and needle are pulled.

Injections into the Port-A-Cath

1. Access the system.
2. Wash hands and put on gloves.
3. Make sure the clamp is closed and wipe the connection on the extension tube with alcohol before disconnecting whatever tubing, syringe, or injection cap that is present.
4. Attach the 5-ml syringe of normal saline, open the clamp, a flush the line with normal saline to confirm that fluid flows through the port.

Note: If chemotherapy is to be given, the nurse or physician must check for a blood return at this point by gently aspirating blood into the extension tubing and flushing the blood back in with the saline.

5. Clamp the extension tube and remove the syringe.
6. Attach a 5-ml or larger syringe containing the medication to be injected to the extension tube.

7. Open the clamp and inject the medication.
8. When the injection is finished, clamp the extension tube and remove the syringe. If more than one drug is administered, check for blood return before each drug and follow each injection with a normal saline flush. If chemotherapy was given, check for a final blood return during the last saline flush. Close the clamp.
9. Remove the syringe and wipe the end of the extension tube with an alcohol prep pad.
10. At this point, you will either restart the continuous infusion intravenous fluids or you will use the appropriate heparinized saline flushing procedure.

Flushing with heparinized saline

The Port-A-Cath system should always be left filled with heparinized saline after each use. The system is flushed the first 3 days postoperatively once per day with 5 ml heparinized saline using 100 U/ml. If the child weighs less than 25 kg, the dose of heparin recommended for flushing should be calculated on 15 U/kg. When there are prolonged periods between injections, infusions, or blood sampling, the system should be flushed with heparinized saline at least once every 2 weeks.

If the system is already accessed:

1. Attach the correct-size syringe with appropriate heparinized saline solution. Flush the system with heparinized saline, clamping as the last 1 ml is infused (to maintain positive pressure or to leave a "heparin lock").
2. After the system is flushed with heparinized saline, a sterile injection cap may be attached if the unit will be used again that day. If the port is no longer needed for use, the needle may be removed. Press down on each side of the port with two fingers while simultaneously withdrawing the needle.

If the system is not accessed:

1. Wash hands well with an antibacterial soap.
2. Take the cap off a bottle of heparin lock flush and wipe the rubber top with an alcohol pad. Set aside and allow to dry.
3. Apply topical anesthetic (e.g., ethyl chloride spray or 5% lidocaine) to the skin directly over the port. *Note*: The topical anesthetics are not sterile and need to be applied before the skin is cleaned.
4. Draw the 10-ml syringe's plunger back to the 5-ml mark and remove the needle cover (do not discard it). Make sure the heparin lock flush vial's rubber top is completely dry and insert the needle into it.
5. Draw 5 ml of fluid into the syringe and pull the needle from the bottle. Replace the cover over the needle. Remove the air bubbles from the syringe.
6. Open the package containing the Gripper extension set and remove it from the package, leaving the needle covered and the tubing capped.
7. Twist off the needle that is attached to the syringe and remove the cap from the extension set tubing. You must avoid touching either the tip of the syringe or the hub of the uncapped tubing.
8. Twist the syringe tightly onto the hub of the extension set tubing.
9. Flush the set with the heparin (until you see a drop of fluid in the needle guard); close the clamp.
10. Using an alcohol prep pad, begin cleaning the skin directly over the port; clean in an outward circular motion. Clean 3 to 5 inches in diameter. If the pad appears dirty after cleaning, reclean with another alcohol pad.
11. Open the package of povidone-iodine swabs. Beginning with a swab at the center of the port, clean the skin in a circular motion. Cover a 3- to 5-inch area. Use all swabs in the same fashion, beginning in the center of the port and moving outward.
12. Remove the needle guard.
13. With the other hand, locate the port again by placing a finger on either side of the port (be careful not to touch the center of the port). Grasp the Gripper tab and insert the needle perpendicularly (straight up and down, or 90 degrees) into the port; push the needle firmly through the skin and port until the needle hits the bottom of the portal chamber.

Note: If fluid cannot be injected into the port, the needle may not be on the bottom of the chamber. If the needle is on the bottom and fluid still cannot be pushed, stop and call the perioperative nurse.

14. Open the clamp and flush the port with a steady pressure. While flushing in the last 1 ml, close the clamp. It is important that you are flushing at the same moment you slide the clamp closed. This helps prevent blood from backing into the tip of the catheter.

15. With your fingers placed on either side of the port, use the other hand to grasp the Gripper tab and pull the needle out of the port.

Obtaining blood samples from the Port-A-Cath

The following procedure is for the sampling of blood from ports that are already accessed. If the port is not accessed, see the preceding section on access to the system.

1. Wash hands with an antibacterial soap and put on sterile gloves.
2. Make sure the clamp is closed and wipe the connection on the extension tube with alcohol before disconnecting whatever tubing, syringe, or injection cap is present. Attach the 5-ml syringe of normal saline. Open the clamp and flush the catheter with normal saline before drawing the blood sample to clear the catheter of any possible contaminants.
3. Withdraw at least 3 ml of blood, close the clamp, and discard the blood.
4. Connect the sterile syringe for a blood sample. Open the clamp and withdraw the desired amount of blood without pulling aggressively on the plunger so as not to collapse the catheter or damage blood cells. Close the clamp.
5. Attach a syringe with 10 ml normal saline, open the clamp, and flush the system with 10 ml of normal saline with a pulsating action (push, stop, push, stop). Close the clamp. Remove the syringe and wipe the end of the extension tube with an alcohol prep pad.
6. At this point, you will either restart the continuous infusion or intravenous fluids or use the appropriate heparinized saline flushing procedure.
7. Inject blood into lab tubes. The port should not be accessed for blood specimens if adequate samples can be obtained by finger sticks.

Dressing the needle site of the Port-A-Cath

1. Wash hands thoroughly.
2. Remove the old dressing carefully, place in a plastic bag, seal, and discard in a trash container.
3. Inspect the site for redness, swelling, or drainage. If any of these signs of infection is present, culture the site for bacteria and fungi by use of culturettes. Document the appearance of the site in the patient's chart.
4. Wash hands again.
5. Cleanse the needle insertion site with a povidone-iodine swab using an outward spiral motion to prevent contamination of the site by adjacent skin flora. Repeat with all three swabs. The area cleaned should be approximately 3 to 5 inches around the needle site.
6. Wipe off the povidone-iodine with a sterile saline wipe. Repeat this step with one more sterile saline wipe.
7. Apply Neosporin ointment to the needle insertion site with a sterile cotton-tipped aplicator.
8. Apply Sof-Wick sponges around the needle site (apply enough to support 90-degree-angle needle).
9. Apply a transparent dressing or an appropriate occlusive covering over the entire needle and secure to the skin. If a transparent dressing is used, place a small 2 × 2 gauze over the needle before applying the transparent dressing. The small gauze makes it easier to remove the dressing without dislodging the needle.
10. Loop and tape the tubing on top of the occlusive dressing to provide a "safety loop" if the line is accidentally pulled. *Note:* The extension tubing is easy to kink; therefore, be careful when taping tubing to avoid kinking.

Port Implantable System (P.A.S. Port)

The P.A.S. Port (Pharmacia Deltec, Inc., St. Paul, Minnesota) is a recently introduced implantable port and catheter similar to the Port-A-Cath but smaller. The unit may be inserted by a surgical cutdown or a percutaneous method. The percutaneous method uses a sheath introducer for the location of the vein, after which the small catheter is passed into the vein and the introducer is peeled away. This port can be placed in the arm with the catheter inserted peripherally into the cephalic or basilic vein and passed into the superior vena cava. Management of the system is similar to that of the Port-A-Cath.

Infusion Pumps

Accessory equipment for intravenous infusions is often used to monitor and to regulate the delivery of drugs and fluids. These units vary in complexity. Calibrated volume control chambers such as Buretol or Solu-Set regulate the amount of fluid to be infused. A special dropper unit aids in calculation of the flow rate because a prescribed number of millimeters per hour equals the number of drops per minute. If the order is to infuse 30 ml/h, the infusion is regulated to deliver 30 drops/minute (Whaley and Wong, 1991). These control chambers are applied to gravity drainage bags and flasks. Pumps are available to regulate the volume of fluid infused. The infusion pumps may be used for small infusions or may be used as continuous infusion. The manufacturer's instructions must be followed closely.

Advances in biotechnology have provided several devices to allow continuous or intermittent infusions on an outpatient basis for patients with indwelling central catheters. The Intelleject system is a programmable four-channel syringe pump able to administer multiple drugs on different schedules for up to 31 days at a time. The CADD-1 is an electronic pump with battery-powered operation. The battery supplies power that lasts approximately 5 days under continuous operation. These infusion pumps, preprogrammed for specific infusion volumes at specified times, provide a remarkable accurate delivery system.

Filters

In-line filters provide a useful mechanism for preventing bacterial contamination of the proximal delivery system and also remove particulate material from the infusion solution. Filters are important for central venous infusion, especially when parenteral nutrition admixtures are used. Although attention must be given to the specific content of the infusion, generally a 1.2 μmi air-eliminating filter is used for lipid-containing infusion and a 0.22 μm air-eliminating filter for non–lipid-containing solutions. The type and position of the filter may affect drug delivery, depending on the flow rate and the drug's specific gravity. Dye studies have shown that when slow infusion rates are used and when drugs with specific gravities less than that of the intravenous fluid are used, back-effusion may occur, retarding drug delivery. The reverse is true with drugs that have specific gravities greater than that of the infusion fluid (Holbrok, 1993).

Use of Urokinase for Occluded Central Venous Catheter

If the central venous catheter becomes internally occluded, or partially occluded, the use of urokinase may be tried. When doing so, it is essential to ensure that the tip of the catheter is properly placed in the superior vena cava.

Procedure

1. Urokinase is available in 1-ml vials and is kept in the stock concentration in a refrigerator. The final concentration is 5000 U/ml.
2. The dose to be administered is based on the internal volume of the catheter. Some appropriate volumes are listed in Table 27–4.
3. Wash hands with antimicrobial soap.
4. Draw up amount of urokinase needed in a tuberculin syringe, unless instilling into a subcutaneous port. You must *use a 5-ml syringe with the port*. Urokinase should be reconstituted immediately before instillation. (It loses its efficacy if it sets too long after reconstitution.)
5. Turn off intravenous fluids if infusing; clamp line.
6. Clean the connection with an alcohol wipe and disconnect the tubing, placing a

Table 27–4 Internal Volume of Central Venous Catheters

Type	Volume Capacity
Long-Term Vascular Access Devices	
Single-lumen	
Hickman 9.6 Fr	1.8 ml
Broviac 6.6 Fr	0.7 ml
Broviac 4.2 Fr	0.3 ml
Subcutaneous port (e.g., Port-A-Cath) 9.6 Fr	2.1 ml
Subcutaneous port (e.g., Port-A-Cath) 6.6 Fr	1.2 ml
Dual-lumen	
Hickman 12 Fr #1	1.8 ml
Hickman 12 Fr #2	1.8 ml
Hickman 9 Fr #1	1.3 ml
Hickman 9 Fr #2	0.6 ml
Short-Term Vascular Access Devices	
Single-lumen	
Cook catheter, regular, 4 Fr/12 cm	0.1 ml
Cook catheter, hard and soft, 5 Fr/15 cm	0.2 ml
Cook catheter, soft, 6 Fr/15 cm	0.3 ml
Cook catheter, hard, 6.3 Fr/15 cm	0.4 ml
Hohn catheters, 4 Fr/34 cm (before cut)	0.2 ml
Hohn catheters, 5 Fr/34 cm (before cut)	0.3 ml
Double-lumen	
Cook catheter, 5 Fr (overall) #1 or #2	0.2 ml

sterile cap on the intravenous tubing. Always instill urokinase at the hub of the catheter.

7. If possible, flush the line with normal saline. If no fluids will infuse through the line, do not flush. *Never* force fluids through an occluded line because you could either rupture the line or break off the clot.
8. Administer the urokinase slowly into the catheter. It may take a gentle "push, pull" method to instill. Push in urokinase and aspirate back, and continue this until you are able to instill the urokinase. It may take several minutes to instill. Be patient and never force urokinase in.
9. Clamp the catheter and apply the injection cap.
10. Leave urokinase in the line for 1 hour.
11. When urokinase is to be withdrawn, follow these steps:

    - Remove the cap, attach an empty syringe and *gently* aspirate from the line.
    - Aspirate 2 to 3 ml of blood from the line. If you are unable to aspirate blood, try to flush the line.
    - Flush the line with 10 ml of saline—whether or not blood return is present. If you are unable to flush, do not force.
    - If urokinase was not successful, a second dose may be ordered and repeated. No more than two doses should be tried without success.
    - If the line is functional, reconnect intravenous fluids or flush and clamp the line.

Hypodermoclysis

Isotonic solutions can be administered subcutaneously under certain circumstances. This method, although technically simple to perform, is not a suitable substitute for the oral or intravenous route. It should not be used as the sole means of administering fluids to patients who are in shock or who are severely dehydrated. However, hypodermoclysis is sometimes advocated as a complement to intravenous infusion of fluid to avoid the hazard of rapid infusion of potent substances. This procedure is rarely indicated in developed countries.

EQUIPMENT

Material for restraints
Ampule of hyaluronidase (Hyazyme, 150 USP units)
21- or 22-gauge needle, 6 cm long
Tincture of iodine and 70% alcohol
Sponges and tape
Dry, sterile cotton balls
2-ml syringe
Infusion set and flask of isotonic solution

SITES

1. Thighs: Inner aspect of the midthigh region.

2. Scapulae: Inferior aspect of the scapular region of the back. This site should not be used if the infant is dyspneic, because infiltration of the fluid about the chest will impair respiration.

3. Abdomen: Lower abdominal wall. Care should be taken not to introduce the needle through the thin abdominal wall into the peritoneal cavity. A long needle, the shaft of which has only been partially inserted beneath the skin of the lower abdomen, may subsequently be pushed into the cavity by unexpected movements of the infant, such as flexion of the thigh on the abdomen.

Method

1. Restrain the infant properly with extremity restraints, then cleanse the site with tincture of iodine followed by alcohol.

2. Attach a 21- or 22-gauge, 6-cm needle to the 2-ml syringe. The contents of the ampule of hyaluronidase are then withdrawn.
3. Pick up a fold of skin between thumb and forefinger in the selected site. Insert the needle into the fold and advance it the full length of the shaft.
4. Attempt aspiration with the syringe to ensure that the needle is not in a blood vessel. Then inject 0.5 to 1 ml of hyaluronidase.
5. Remove the syringe and attach the nozzle of the infusion flask tubing to the needle hub. The tubing must be filled with solution and be free of air before this is done.
6. Fasten a piece of adhesive tape across the hub of the needle to secure it firmly to the skin. Although a single tube infusion set is usually adequate, some physicians prefer a Y tube assembly for hypodermoclysis in the thighs so that both thighs may be infused simultaneously.
7. Allow the desired amount of fluid to drip into the subcutaneous tissues. Then withdraw the needle and apply pressure over the puncture site with a dry, sterile cotton ball. A needle should not be kept in one site for longer than 12 hours. The fluid administered should not exceed 40 ml per kilogram of the infant's weight for each hypodermoclysis, and the solution must be iso-osmotic.

Hazards and Complications

1. All hypertonic solutions are given subcutaneously to a patient with a diminished circulating volume, as in dehydration from diarrhea; the plasma volume will be further compromised by fluid's leaving the vascular-space and entering the site of clysis. If hypotonic solutions are used in hypodermoclysis, shock may result when electrolytes leave the vascular compartment and come into equilibrium with the subcutaneous pool.
2. Cellulitis may occur if the needle is not properly sterilized or is left in the skin too long.
3. Impairment of respiration could result from excessive infiltration of hypotonic solutions into the thoracic area.
4. Perforation of the peritoneal or pleural cavity may occur.

Intraperitoneal Infusions

Although isotonic solutions can be absorbed from the peritoneal cavity, advice strongly contraindicates this route. Several risks are involved. Introduction of bacteria into the peritoneal cavity, perforation of the intestine, and chemical peritonitis are all real dangers. Under certain circumstances, such as with liver disease, cardiac decompensation, and hypoproteinemia, an even absorption of isotonic fluid will not occur. There is perhaps no indication for this route in the parenteral administration of fluids.

References

Broviac JW, Cole JJ, Scribner BH: A silicone rubber atrial catheter for prolonged parenteral alimentation. *Surg Gynecol Obstet,* 136:602, 1973.

Butler C, Hawkins D, et al: *Blood Aspiration/Line Care Module.* Memphis, TN, St Jude Children's Research Hospital, 1989.

Farman JV, Powell D: The performance of disposable venous catheters, needles, and cannulas. *Br J Hosp Med,* 2:(suppl 2):37, 1969.

Grundfest S, Steiger E: Experience with Broviac catheter for prolonged parenteral alimentation. *JPEN,* 3:45–47, 1979.

Holbrook PR: *Textbook of Pediatric Critical Care.* Philadelphia, WB Saunders, 1993.

Macintosh R, Mushin WW, Epstein HG: *Physics for the Anaesthetist,* 2nd ed. Springfield, IL, Charles C Thomas, 1958.

Raad II, Bodey G: Infectious complication of indwelling catheter. *Clin Infect Dis,* 15:197–210, 1992.

Whaley LF, Wong DL: *Nursing Care of Infants and Children,* 4th ed. St Louis, Mosby–Year Book, 1991.

Chapter 28

Central Venous Access

John German

Gauderer (1992) reported that modern vascular access catheters and techniques have made the traditional cutdown largely obsolete. Seldinger (1953) introduced percutaneous cannulation techniques, in which a needle is used to enter a large vein, a wire guide is passed through the needle, and then the catheter is placed over the wire guide. Kerri-Szantu (1956) first described percutaneous subclavian cannulation. Dudrick and later Filler et al (1969) reported long-term parenteral nutritional support techniques made possible by placement of long-term central venous access catheters in neonates and infants (Coran and Filler, 1979; Wilmore and Dudrick, 1969). Broviac and later Hickman and their colleagues reported the use of cuffed, silicone rubber long-term central venous catheters for management of patients with malignant neoplasms and for blood sampling (Broviac et al, 1973; Hickman et al, 1979).

Most institutions practice percutaneous catheter placement almost exclusively, which has had an impact on the training of critical care physicians. Fewer cutdowns are done, and chances to learn appropriate cutdown techniques are reduced. This can lead to an increased risk of complications when it is necessary for an inexperienced physician to perform a cutdown. The purpose of this chapter is to familiarize the reader with the technical aspects of cutdowns and to encourage the early use of cutdown techniques rather than wasting time with repeated attempts at venipuncture, especially in those severely ill infants who require early intervention.

INDICATIONS

In general, venous cutdown is justified for the placement of intermediate or long-term central catheters, although it should also be considered in any emergency setting. The selection of a vascular access site and catheter material is strongly influenced by the purpose for which the catheter is being placed and the expected duration of its use (Gauderer, 1992). For short-term use (i.e., hours to days), short plastic cannulas have been the mainstay for venous access. They are the first choice in any patient in whom intermediate or long-term use or venous monitoring or sampling will not be necessary.

Intermediate duration of use is defined as central catheter placement for periods of up to 1 month or for shorter periods when monitoring or blood sampling is required.

There are problems involving vascular access in peripheral veins. Use of a dominant upper extremity should be avoided because many children may suck their fingers or thumbs or require their dominant upper extremity for feeding. Access in the foot is best used for infants who are not walking.

Cannulation of a central vein allows month-long antibiotic therapy for orthopedic infections or systemic yeast infections or in severely injured or infected patients. These catheters may have single or multiple lumens. They are used extensively in the operating room or critical care setting because they allow access for sampling, monitoring, and administration of fluids and medications. Most of these catheters are now available in a kit form that has all of the necessary materials for percutaneous technique, such as a needle, a flexible wire, a vein dilator, and a tear-apart sheath that allows placement of catheters made of flexible materials. Most such catheters are somewhat rigid and can irritate the vascular endothelium as well as the exit site. Their insertion requires greater skill, and they are associated with a higher rate of complications. Because they are semirigid, they cannot be tunneled far under the skin, and the risk of catheter infection is increased. The typical catheter is a polyurethane catheter that can be placed by percutaneous or cutdown techniques. Uncuffed silicone rubber catheters are commonly used as a single-lumen device in small children or neonates. Because they are soft they produce less vascular irritation, but placement of the soft, pliable catheter can be time-consuming. With use of local anesthesia, placement may be difficult because of the patient's mobility. Blood sampling is almost impossible, and these catheters tend to occlude early.

Catheter placement for longer than 1 month's duration is considered long term. The usual catheters employed are cuffed silicone rubber catheters, known as Broviac or Hickman catheters. These have become the mainstay for vascular access in long-term parenteral nutrition or for management of malignant neoplasms. They are especially useful in those children with poor vascular access who require long-term blood sampling and administration of medication and blood products. The clinical needs of the individual patient indicate whether a single- or double-lumen catheter is necessary.

Implantable vascular devices, such as ports, are also used long-term. A port consists of a small, implantable metal or plastic reservoir with a silicone rubber diaphragm placed under the skin. This device is connected to a catheter and tunneled to the vein. This system provides immediate access in the operating room; once the wound is closed, a noncoring needle can be used to pierce the chamber of the reservoir, and infusion of heparin or intravenous fluids can be initiated.

The subclavian vein is the preferred site for central venous access in adults and children. Use of the jugular system is an alternative to subclavian cannulation. However, puncture of the internal jugular vein has a higher complication rate and the catheter is more difficult to secure, and puncture of the external jugular vein is no easier and is associated with a higher frequency of catheter malposition outside the thorax than occurs with use of the subclavian vein (Nicolson et al, 1985).

Transfemoral catheterization of the vein or artery is increasingly being employed in the acute care setting, particularly in the immobile child in the intensive care unit, by either percutaneous technique or cutdown. Use of the femoral vein poses more difficulties outside the intensive care unit or operating room and may not be suitable for long-term vascular access in the ambulatory patient. Venous cutdowns are typically required when peripheral sites have been used repeatedly for short-term vascular access or when more central access is necessary for intermediate or long-term use.

PROCEDURE

Details of cutdown technique are described in Chapter 27. The step-by-step technical aspects of all cutdowns vary from program to program and are personalized by the operator. Some of the techniques that come with experience are listed here. One point is not to rely on introducers because they are not always available. The venotomy can be done with whatever is available on the tray. The vein should be isolated with both proximal and distal suture loops. The distal suture loop is used as a traction suture to pull the vein up into the wound and allow better visualization of the anterior surface of the vessel. The proximal cut end of the vein should be elevated and the venotomy site dilated. This can be done with whatever is on the tray, such as fine forceps, the blade of fine scissors as described by Kosloske and

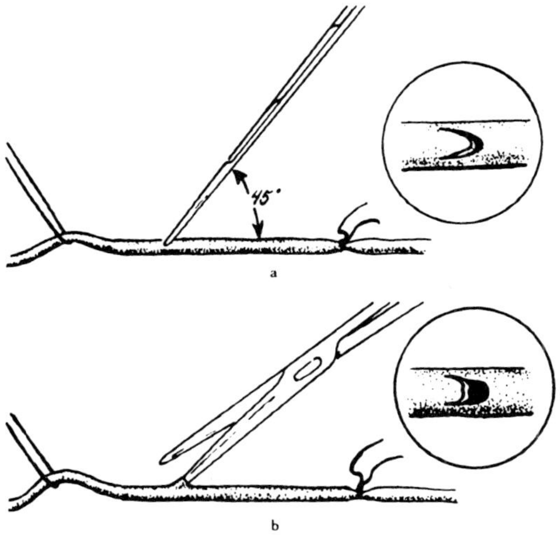

Figure 28–1 Incision is placed obliquely on the surface of the vein, and the blade of the scissors is used to dilate the opening. (From Kosloske AM, Klein MD: Techniques of central venous access for long term parenteral nutrition in infants. *Surg Gynecol Obstet,* 154:394–399, 1982. By permission of Surgery, Gynecology and Obstetrics, now known as the Journal of the American College of Surgeons.)

Klein (1982) (Fig. 28–1), or even the bevel of a needle tip or a fine suture used as a traction suture. Two sutures may be placed on the anterior edge of the venotomy site, which permits opening of the vein by traction on the sutures for direct cannulation. The final step is to flush the catheter and ensure that one is able to aspirate blood. The catheter should be secured with the proximal suture loop tied tightly around the vein. The catheter should again be flushed before closing to be sure that the catheter tie is not too tight. The distal suture may or may not be tied, depending on the tightness of the fit of the cannula through the venotomy site. It should be tied when venotomy has been done by incision, which is usually larger than the catheter. It is seldom necessary when the Seldinger technique has been used.

Except in rare emergency situations, cutdowns should be performed like any other operation in the appropriate setting. Delicate instruments, direct lighting, and assistance are necessary to reduce operative time and trauma to the patient. Improved sedatives and local anesthesia minimize movement in the patient and distraction of the operating team. Oximeter monitoring should be available. The use of a fiberoptic headlight, loupes with a short focal length, portable imaging equipment, and an open intensive care isolette has improved conditions to the point that operative time and trauma are minimized for even the most critically ill patient. Multiple previous catheterizations and thrombopenia or cytopenia are not considered contraindications to the selection or duration of catheterization.

SITES

Use of the greater saphenous vein at the ankle as a peripheral cutdown site is seldom justified in modern pediatric practice, although in the acute situation, this is the safest and fastest venous access procedure for any health care professional to perform. The American Heart Association publication *Pediatric Advanced Life Support* has an excellent discussion regarding cannulation of the greater saphenous vein at the ankle. This site should not be used for catheter placement in chronically ill patients because it is usually occluded or has the potential for producing significant venous complications later (Fig. 28–2).

The most traditional site for short-term venous cutdown cannulation is the basilic vein in the antecubital fossa (see Fig. 28–2). Indications for the use of this upper extremity site are short-term cannulation and cases in which advancement of the catheter will provide blood sampling and allow infusion of intermediate concentrations of hyperalimentation solution.

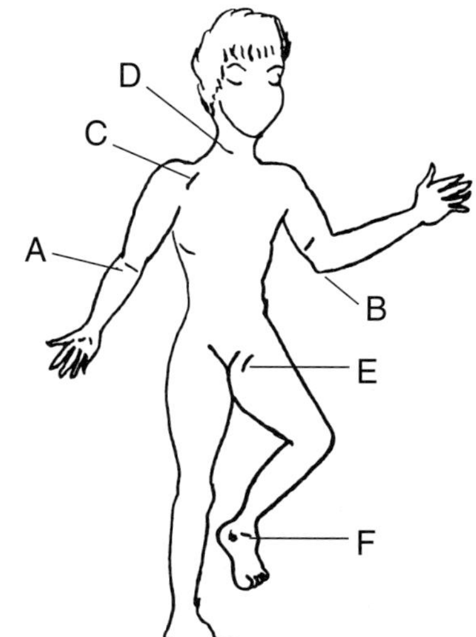

Figure 28–2 Common cutdown sites demonstrated on this figure are the right antecubital (A), the left supracondylar (B), the right deltopectoral (C), the jugular (D), and the greater saphenous at the left fossa ovalis (E) and the left ankle (F).

Deep dissection of the brachial vein is thought to have a higher chance of complications in inexperienced hands. In my experience, these two sites may be useful for intermediate catheter placement in neonates with chronic conditions when central venous sites have been used and when the remaining central venous sites must be spared for expected later long-term catheterization or for preservation of central venous circulation sites. Conservation of central venous circulation sites is important in the premature neonate with intracranial or intra-cerebral hemorrhage who may require a cerebrospinal fluid shunt at some later date.

The basilic vein is superficially located in the subcutaneous tissues of the antecubital fossa. In those patients who have not frequently undergone distal intravenous administration, it should be patent. The routine techniques described previously are then employed to isolate the vessel and cannulate it. The catheter may exit through the wound or tunnel for a few centimeters and exit distal to the wound through a separate stab incision. This allows better immobilization and fixation of the catheter on the volar surface of the forearm.

However, in a patient who has had multiple distally placed peripheral intravenous lines so that intravenous access presents a problem, the basilic vein is usually scarred and nonpatent. When the basilic vein is not patent, a deeper dissection for the brachial vein may be necessary; this poses a higher potential risk of injury to the median nerve or the brachial artery. The anatomical relationship of the nerve, artery, and vein is maintained from lateral to medial and is the same for the femoral region. The overlying lacertus fibrosus is pierced bluntly to find the intramuscular groove where the neurovascular structures are located. The operator can appreciate this by palpating the pulse of the brachial artery. Once the neurovascular bundle is opened, dissection of the neurovascular structures is carried out in a longitudinal direction with a mosquito clamp. The artery should be visualized first. In infants the brachial artery is much larger than the vein. In situations in which an inexperienced surgeon encounters this structure and the patient is hypotensive, it is difficult to determine whether arterial pulsations are present. The operator may inadvertently isolate this structure as the venous structure, perform a "venotomy," and discover that blood spurts from this vessel. The artery is an important landmark because the nerve is located lateral to it, and dissection should proceed medially. The rule of thumb is that a large vessel in the neurovascular sheath in small children is usually the artery; dissect the vein that lies deeper and medial to this artery. The brachial vein may be occluded in patients who have undergone multiple peripheral venous access procedures. In this case, the venae comitantes should be enlarged, or veins overlying the artery may be suitable for cannulation. The venae comitantes, basilic vein, and brachial vein merge into the brachial vein in the mid to upper arm and continue on as the axillary and subclavian veins. The cephalic vein is not for catheterization except in extreme desperation; it seems to become easily inflamed, and advancing the catheter into the subclavian is rarely possible.

If all of these veins are occluded or too small for cannulation, or if a prior cutdown site exists in the arm in the supracondylar area, it is not reasonable to dissect further in the neurovascular sheath. The last vein in the antecubital fossa that is suitable for cannulation is the vein accompanying the ulnar nerve. This dissection should be performed only by experienced surgeons. Repeated cutdowns at this area may be required to find the vein that accompanies the ulnar nerve. The dissection is carried onto the epicondylar area, where the vein and nerve are visualized. One can often appreciate the difference between the two. However, the ulnar nerve and the vein have similar characteristics: they can branch; they appear pink; and the vein is flatter than normal, resembling the nerve. The apparent venous structure is isolated between loops of sutures that are not tied. The approach to this structure should be not a transverse incision but a small longitudinal incision to ensure that this structure has a lumen and contains blood. If the surgeon has made a longitudinal incision on the ulnar nerve, much less damage to the nerve occurs, and the identification of the nerve with a small superficial incision is made easily. Cannulation of the accompanying vein of the ulnar nerve requires a little more mobilization to allow the catheter or cannula to exit distal to the cutdown site. This allows normal mobility of the elbow. This vein is fairly large in younger children and may accommodate a multiple-lumen catheter. Again, only experienced surgeons should attempt this cannulation.

The next site for consideration is the greater saphenous vein at the fossa ovalis in the thigh (Fig. 28–2). The incision and dissection in this particular case are not as clear because there are essentially no landmarks. The incision should be located half a fingerbreadth distal to the inguinal ligament and the same distance medial to the femoral arterial pulsation. An oblique incision is made, extending from lateral to medial and following the fullness of the thigh at that point. The greater saphenous vein is deep in the fatty tissue in a healthy child and is situated obliquely in the thigh, nearly paralleling the inguinal ligament as it courses to the fossa ovalis. This is a reliable site for dissection in an infant or child; the greater saphenous vein pierces the fossa ovalis to join the femoral vein. The angle at the point of merging of these two vessels is often 90 degrees. The operator needs to be aware of this point because when cannulation of the greater saphenous vein is performed, the tip of the catheter may tend to be advanced distally. Retracting the distal suture loop laterally places the junction of the vessels obliquely to allow easier cannulation of the common femoral vein. If the greater saphenous vein has been occluded by long-term use of venous sites below the groin, cannulation of the common femoral vein should be considered. The common femoral vein should not be tied distally; this will produce a swollen, blue leg with a high potential for venous insufficiency. The most suitable way to cannulate this vessel is to place a small purse-string suture of fine monofilament; perform a small venotomy centrally in the purse-string suture, usually with the tip of a No. 11 blade; and insert the catheter through the venotomy site, advancing the catheter for a premeasured distance, extending to the xyphoid process for central venous cannulation. The purse-string suture is tied around the cannula at this point. The cannula should be tunneled and brought out through a separate stab wound, after tunneling back underneath the skin either to the anterior abdominal wall or for a few centimeters distally on the thigh in an immobilized patient, such as a neonate or a small infant.

A final word concerning the anatomy of the common femoral vein and iliac vein: either direct cannulation using the Seldinger technique or cutdown of the femoral vein can result in malpositioning of the catheter in a lumbar vein. The femoral vein joins the iliac vein in its course over the brim of the pelvis at such an angle that there may exist a straighter course into the lumbar system than into the common iliac vein. Radiographic verification of the position of the catheter before closure of the wound is particularly important to prevent this complication. If this is not recognized, high concentrations of sugar and protein solutions can be infused into this area, which will lead to infiltration into the retroperitoneal space. Such an infiltration can lead to severe inflammation and sepsis.

Before the widespread use of percutaneous subclavian cannulation in children and infants, the cephalic vein at the deltopectoral groove was the preferred site for placement of central venous catheters for long-term use (see Fig. 28–2). It remains a useful alternative site when the subclavian site has been used or cannot be cannulated after several attempts. It is small in infants and is not as anatomically consistent as the subclavian or greater saphenous veins. This dissection requires the expertise of a surgeon skilled in vascular access. As a primary approach or after multiple percutaneous attempts through a small incision in the apex of the deltopectoral triangle have been unsuccessful, the incision is extended obliquely to follow the pectoral lines of the deltopectoral groove. Blunt dissection is deepened through the subcutaneous tissues to pierce the deltopectoral fascia bluntly with a mosquito clamp and may include a few fibers of the pectoral muscle. The vein enters the deltopectoral groove, away from the operator toward the subclavian vein. It can easily be missed if one is not expecting this course to be directed away from the visual axis. The vein may be enlarged or may be almost sclerotic if the extremities have been used extensively for intravenous access. If a small venous tributary that is not suitable for cannulation and central vascular access is found, perhaps a smaller single-lumen catheter can be used, permitting central venous access but not sampling because of the small size of the catheter. However, if there is a tributary of significant size, this can be cannulated for venous use for both long-term or intermediate use and sampling. The problem at this area, in about 10% of the cases, is that the cephalic vein does not enter the subclavian vein but rather communicates with the external jugular vein and some other deep plexus. Cases in which the catheter is seen to advance upward into the external jugular vein may indicate a tortuous communication of this system, and cannulation may be virtually impossible. Also, the catheter may be advanced across into the opposite subclavian vein. Use of a wire guide may help direct cannulation into the central venous position, or the catheter tip can be placed within the confluence of the innominate vein.

The jugular system and its tributaries are reliable sites for direct central venous access (see Fig. 28–2). The selection of the external vein, internal vein, or internal branches, such as the common facial vein or the inferior thyroid vein, obviously depends on the anatomy encountered in each patient (Toufanian and Knight, 1983; Zumbro et al, 1971). With the introduction of long-term parenteral nutritional support, considerable experience was gained in premature and other small infants who had central venous lines placed before the development of long-term vascular access as described initially by Filler et al (1969). This experience with the vascular system and the use of smaller, cuffed catheters led to the development of subcutaneous tunneling to the anterior chest walls as described by Andrassy and Mahour (Pereya et al, 1980) (Fig. 28–3). It is expected that jugular system cutdown for the critical care patient would be preferentially performed by a surgeon familiar with such procedures, such as a pediatric surgeon experienced in central venous cannulation in premature neonates for total support and venous sampling.

Percutaneous techniques at the bedside in critically ill neonates are comparable in risk and complications to the traditional cutdown techniques for cannulation of vascular sites for long-term support. The placement of a soft silicone rubber catheter into the right atrium of the small premature infant to allow for growth of the child in the next few months is improper (Durand et al, 1986) (Fig. 28–4). To expect that the patient will grow so dramatically that the catheter's length will become inadequate and the catheter will become peripherally located is conjecture. The proper placement of a catheter in the superior vena cava where it joins the right atrium is the goal for all such procedures.

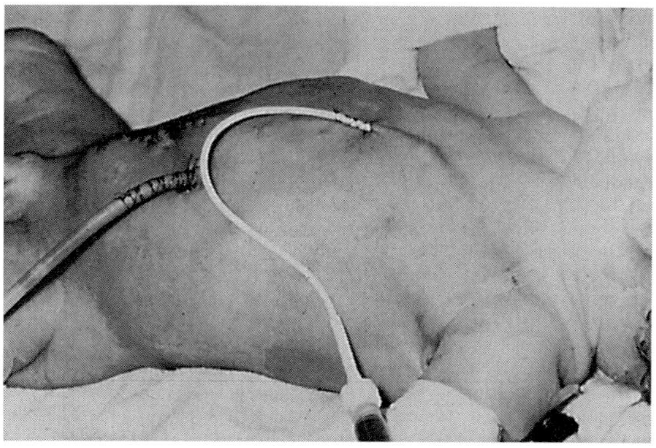

Figure 28–3 Broviac catheter placed at the time of surgery in the neonate. (From Gauderer MWL: Vascular access techniques and devices in the pediatric patient. *Surg Clin North Am,* 72:1267–1285, 1992.)

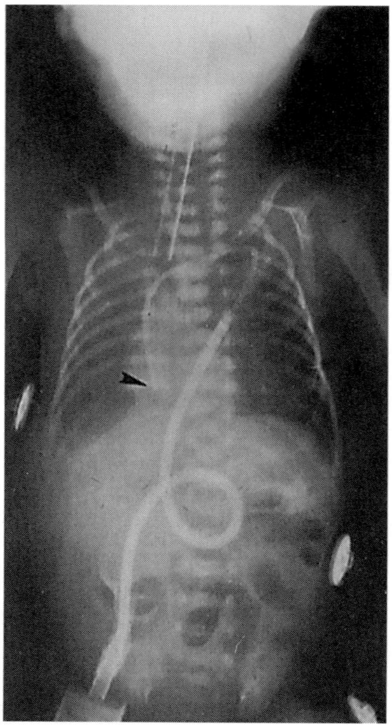

Figure 28–4 Placement of a catheter within the right side of the heart to allow growth of the patient, as shown here, is improper. The goal is to place one catheter tip in the superior vena cava at the tip of the right atrium. (From Durand M, Rangasamy R, et al: Prospective evaluation of percutaneous central venous Silastic catheter in newborn infants with birth weights of 510 to 3920 grams. Reproduced by permission of *Pediatrics,* 78:245–250, 1986. Copyright 1986.)

Another site that has been used when the usual access sites have been thrombosed is the inferior vena cava as reported by Fonkalsrud and others (Donahoe and Kim, 1980; Fonkalsrud et al, 1982). Their experience is comparable to the placement of a superior vena cava line. The inferior vena cava can be used initially or preferentially when other central venous sites have been used or are expected to be used for other problems, such as the conversion of a cerebrospinal fluid drain to a ventriculovascular shunt. The preservation of these central venous vessels is important for these patients.

CONTRAINDICATIONS AND COMPLICATIONS

Contraindications to the use of specific venous cutdown sites reflect the area of injury or the site of the disease process. For example, catheterization of the inferior vena cava may be a problem in patients with burns and infections in the groin, peritonitis, blockage or injury to the inferior vena cava, increased intra-abdominal pressure, paralysis of the lower extremities, confinement to bed, nonpalpable femoral pulses, and history of pulmonary embolisms. Problems restricting the use of a superior vena cava catheter include severe chest trauma, respiratory insufficiency or failure, apical lung disease, emphysema, arterial pressure greater than 180 mm Hg systolic, coagulopathy, aneurysms at the base of the neck, blockage or injury of the superior vena cava, presence of pneumothorax, infections or burns close to the neck, and inability or unwillingness of the patient to cooperate (Parsa and Tabora, 1985).

Formal, closely supervised training in these techniques is essential because of the necessity of intravenous access in most severe disease processes. The most experienced individuals are usually those involved with critical care patients, such as general surgeons, vascular surgeons, thoracic surgeons, and critical care specialists, who form the pool from which individuals are chosen to perform these procedures. An experienced team can provide and supervise long-term care for these catheters so that most complications can be anticipated or prevented. Parsa and Tabora (1985) have stated that the greater the individual and institutional experience, the lower the rate of complications with central venous lines. Therefore, well-trained, concerned, experienced personnel should be available 24 hours a day, 7 days a week, to provide this important surgical service. Gauderer (1992) indicates that vascular access in children requires skill, time, patience, and the appropriate equipment. Fortunately, with attention to detail, most complications can be avoided.

References

Broviac JW, Cole JJ, Scribner BH: A silicone atrial catheter for prolonged parenteral nutrition. *Surg Gynecol Obstet,* 136:602–606, 1973.

Coran AG, Filler RM: Total parenteral nutrition in pediatric surgery. In Ravitch MM, Welch KJ, et al (eds): *Pediatric Surgery,* 3rd ed. Chicago, Year Book Medical Publishers, 1979, pp 53–62.

Donahoe PK, Kim SH: The inferior epigastric vein as an alternative site for central venous hyperalimentation. *J Pediatr Surg,* 15:737–738, 1980.

Durand M, Rangasamy R, et al: Prospective evaluation of percutaneous central venous Silastic catheter in newborn infants with birth weights of 510 to 3920 grams. *Pediatrics,* 78:245–250, 1986.

Filler RM, Eraklis AJ, et al: Long-term total parenteral nutrition in infants. *N Engl J Med,* 281:589–594, 1969.

Fonkalsrud EW, Berquist W, et al: Long-term hyperalimentation in children through saphenous central venous catheterization. *Am J Surg,* 143: 209–211, 1982.

Gauderer MWL: Vascular access techniques and devices in the pediatric patient. *Surg Clin North Am,* 72:1267–1285, 1992.

Hickman RO, Buckner CD, Clift RA: A modified right atrial catheter for access to the venous system in marrow transplant recipients. *Surg Gynecol Obstet,* 148:871–875, 1979.

Kerri-Szantu M: The subclavian vein: a constant and convenient intravenous injection site. *Arch Surg,* 72:179–181, 1956.

Kosloske AM, Klein MD: Techniques of central venous access for long term parenteral nutrition in infants. *Surg Gynecol Obstet,* 154:394–399, 1982.

Nicolson SG, Sweeney MF, et al: Comparison of internal and external jugular cannulation of the central circulation in the pediatric patient. *Crit Care Med,* 13:747–749, 1985.

Parsa MH, Tabora F: Establishment of intravenous lines for long-term intravenous therapy and monitoring. *Surg Clin North Am,* 65:835–865, 1985.

Pereya R, Andrassy RJ, Mahour GH: Central venous cannulation in neonates. *Surg Gynecol Obstet,* 151:253–254, 1980.

Seldinger SI: Catheter replacement of the needle in percutaneous angiography. *Arch Radiol,* 38: 368–387, 1953.

Toufanian A, Knight P: The middle thyroid vein: an alternate route for central venous catheter insertion. *J Pediatr Surg,* 18:156–157, 1983.

Wilmore DW, Dudrick ST: Safe long-term catheterization. *Arch Surg,* 98:256–258, 1969.

Zumbro GL, Mullin MJ, Nelson TG: Catheter placement in infants needing total parenteral nutrition utilizing common facial vein. *Arch Surg,* 102:71–73, 1971.

Chapter 29

Intraosseous Access and Infusion

Ronald M. Perkin and Daved van Stralen

Intravenous access is vital for drug and fluid administration but may be difficult, time-consuming, or impossible to achieve in pediatric patients. In one pediatric emergency department, establishing intravenous access took more than 10 minutes in 24% of pediatric cardiopulmonary arrest victims. In 6% of these patients, intravenous access was never obtained. In another study, venous cutdowns, even when performed by experienced pediatric surgeons, required 11 minutes, 8 minutes, and 6 minutes in neonates, 1- to 5-year-olds, and 6- to 16-year-olds, respectively. Such experiences have led to a resurgence in the use of the intraosseous route to obtain vascular access for pediatric resuscitation efforts.

Intraosseous infusion offers a "safe, rapid, and reliable alternative to intravenous infusion when resuscitation must proceed rapidly," according to a policy statement issued by the American Academy of Pediatrics Committee on Pediatric Emergency Medicine (see Appendix). Both the Academy and the American Heart Association have endorsed intraosseous infusion in their pediatric advanced life-support course as a key step in resuscitating children younger than 6 years.

The latest American Heart Association guidelines (developed from The Fifth National Conference on Cardiopulmonary Resuscitation in 1992) advocate a simple protocol for rapidly securing an intravascular line:

In a child 6 years of age or younger, attempt to place an intraosseous line if reliable venous access cannot be achieved in 90 seconds or three attempts, whichever comes first. The effectiveness of the intraosseous route is limited in children older than 6 years because of replacement of red marrow by fat in the long bones.

If an intraosseous or intravenous line cannot be established in 3 to 5 minutes, give medications by the endotracheal route.

Keep in mind that any method of administering resuscitation medication into the vascular system is preferred to endotracheal administration. In the majority of cases, an intraosseous line can be established in less than 1 minute, even by unskilled personnel. Resuscitation fluids and medications can be effectively administered by this route, and complications are rare. Also, other studies have shown that successful intraosseous line placement can be achieved in older children and that age should not be a limitation for placement.

HISTORY

The technique of intraosseous infusion is not a new one. Drinker and Drinker published their first work on circulation in mammalian bone marrow in 1916 in the *American Journal of Physiology*.

In 1934, Josefson described the first use of the intraosseous route in humans when he infused liver concentrate into the sternum for treatment of pernicious anemia. Intraosseous infusion gained wide acceptance in Europe in the 1930s but was not extensively used in the United States. Tocantins, however, reported successful intraosseous infusions of blood products, dextrose, and saline in 1940.

After extensive use in the 1940s and 1950s, intraosseous infusion fell into obscurity with improvements in the types and quality of intravascular catheters available. A resurgence of interest has primarily focused on its use in the management of emergencies in children, both in the emergency department and before admission to the hospital.

Within the last decade, studies have shown that the proportion of successful cannulation attempts is higher for intraosseous infusions than for all other forms of intravenous access, including percutaneous peripheral, central venous, and surgical cutdown. Other investigations have demonstrated that the intraosseous catheter can be quickly placed even when the operator is inexperienced in the technique.

Emergency medical technicians–paramedics (EMT-Ps) may be trained and authorized to perform intraosseous infusion, but in practice, the opportunities to attempt the technique are infrequent. However, a Milwaukee study (Glaeser, 1993) is reassuring. In a 5-year period, Glaeser monitored the ability of their EMT-Ps to remain proficient. In all, there were 165 attempts on 152 patients (14 were 10 years or older), with a success rate of 76% per patient and 70% per attempt; the rate dropped the older the patient, so that success was significantly higher in patients younger than 3 years (85% in 1- to 2-year-olds). As an indication of infrequency of need, five EMT-P units performed five or fewer intraosseous infusions during the study period, but their success rate was still 65%. Although additional training was limited to an update after 1 year, the individual units may have maintained their proficiency by continuing informal self-education.

ANATOMY

In the long bones, the marrow sinusoids drain into medullary venous channels, and nutrient and emissary veins drain into the systemic venous system. An anatomical advantage of the marrow cavity is that it functions as a rigid vein that does not collapse in the presence of hypovolemia or profound peripheral circulatory shock. Investigators have demonstrated that substances injected into the bone marrow are absorbed almost immediately into the general circulation in animals and humans. Blood from the bone marrow of the tibia passes from intramedullary veins into the general circulation through the popliteal vein. The popliteal vein joins the femoral vein, whose branches drain the distal femur.

INDICATIONS AND CONTRAINDICATIONS

A number of protocols have been suggested for integrating the intraosseous infusion technique into the array of procedures available to provide vascular access in children. The primary indication is the unmet need for venous access in a patient with a life-threatening emergency medical condition.

Blood products, fluids, and a wide variety of pharmacological agents have been administered through the marrow cavity.

Although it is not typically a reason for establishing an intraosseous catheter, bone marrow aspirates may be obtained before fluid or drug infusion is begun and can be analyzed for blood chemistry values, partial pressure of carbon dioxide, pH, and hemoglobin level. Studies have demonstrated that the pH, P_{CO_2}, concentration of electrolytes, chemistry values, absolute white blood cell count, and hemoglobin values do not differ significantly in arterial, venous, and bone marrow samples. Samples obtained from the intraosseous site may thus be used to diagnose and begin early treatment of acid-base imbalance and electrolyte abnormalities.

The marrow aspirates can be cultured instead of peripheral blood samples and may be used for typing and crossmatching. Differences in the white blood cell differential and red blood cell morphology caused by displacement of bone marrow contents into the general circulation during intraosseous infusion have been documented, however. The white blood cell differential and red blood cell morphology thus may not be reliable in samples obtained from the intraosseous site and may not coincide with findings based on peripheral blood samples.

There are few absolute contraindications to the use of intraosseous infusion. These include the presence of osteogenesis imperfecta or osteopetrosis and an ipsilateral fractured extremity, because subcutaneous extravasation will occur. The risk of infectious complications is increased when the needle is introduced through an area affected by cellulitis or an infected burn.

TECHNIQUE

The proximal tibia is generally accepted as the optimal site for insertion of an intraosseous needle in children. The sternum has been associated with dangerous, potentially fatal complications and is not recommended. Select a point in the midline of the medial flat surface of the anterior tibia below the tibial tuberosity (Fig. 29–1). Depending on the size of the child, the point is usually located 1 to 3 cm below the tibial tuberosity. The advantage of this site is that it provides a stable, relatively flat, and easily penetrable location for needle placement. In addition, it does not interfere with airway maintenance, mechanical ventilation, or chest compressions.

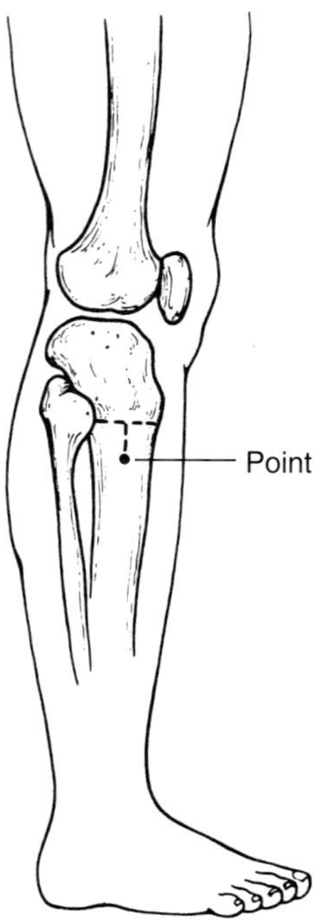

Figure 29–1 Insertion site in the proximal tibia. The tibial tuberosity and medial border of the tibia are palpated. Halfway between these points and 1 to 3 cm distally, the needle is inserted pointing away from the joint space in a caudal direction. The dashed line represents the level of tibial tuberosity.

If the proximal tibia is impenetrable, the distal tibia may be used. The cortex of the bone and tissue overlying the distal tibia are thin enough for inserting the needle proximal to the medial malleolus and posterior to the saphenous vein. This site has been used successfully in older children and adults despite the fact that the amount of marrow in the tibia in those age groups is questionable. There are other sites that can be used in an emergency (Fig. 29–2).

Investigators have demonstrated that substances injected into the bone marrow are absorbed almost immediately into the systemic circulation, even during chest compressions. Table 29–1 lists the equipment needed to place an intraosseous needle. The technique is as follows:

Restrain the patient's leg by placing it on an intravenous board or having another person hold it. Place a small sandbag behind the knee for support.

Using aseptic technique, clean the selected site with a povidone-iodine solution, and inject the skin with 1% lidocaine for anesthesia.

Insert the needle through the skin and direct it at a slight angle, 10 to 15 degrees from the vertical, while applying firm downward pressure and a twisting motion similar to that used in bone marrow aspiration and biopsy.

As the needle passes through the cortex into the marrow, a release of resistance is felt. At this point, the needle should stand without support.

Remove the stylet and connect a syringe to the needle. Proper placement is further confirmed by aspiration of bone marrow.

Flush the needle with heparinized saline and connect it to conventional intravenous infusion tubing.

Note: If aspiration of bone marrow is not obtained, and it is thought that the needle is properly placed, push in a few milliliters of saline solution while observing for soft tissue swelling. Frequently, no bloody aspirate will be present even if the needle is correctly placed; ability to infuse saline with no extravasation confirms correct placement.

Do not cover this site; this allows observation for extravasation. Observe the site repeatedly for extravasation of fluid, an indication that the placement of the needle is too superficial, the bone has been pierced, or infusion

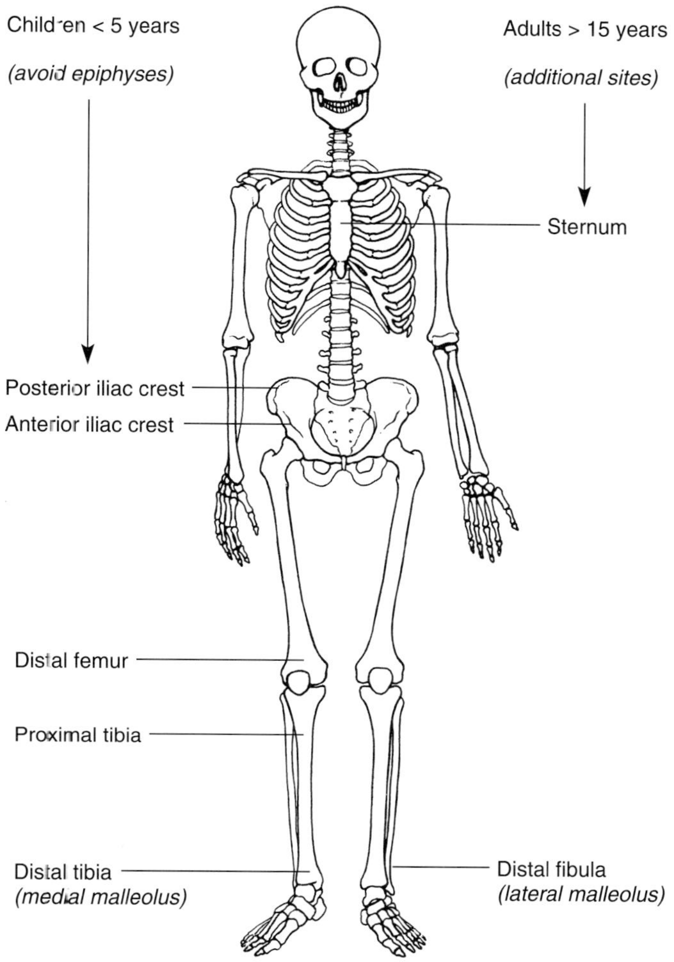

Figure 29–2 Possible sites for needle insertion.

Table 29–1 Intraosseous Infusion Equipment

For children < 18 months old, 18- to 20-gauge spinal or intraosseous needle
For older children, 13- to 16-gauge bone marrow or intraosseous needle
Lidocaine, 1% (three syringes and 25-gauge needle)
Povidone-iodine swabs
T-connector
10-ml syringes (two)
Sterile saline solution
¼-inch tape
1-inch tape
Padded board
Intravenous tubing setup
Syringe with heparinized saline
Small sandbag (place behind knee for support)

pressure is excessive. If the patient is to be transported with a leg manipulated, the leg should be splinted (Fig. 29–3).

Once another access route has been obtained, the intraosseous needle can be removed. It is not necessary to stop the infusion for a time before removing the needle. A pressure dressing is not usually needed.

Many types of cannulas are available for intraosseous infusions, including 16- or 18-gauge hypodermic needles and spinal needles with stylets that are available in most institutions (Fig. 29–4). A disadvantage of hypodermic needles without stylets is that they may become plugged with fragments of bone and marrow. Spinal needles may bend or break because of their length and narrow gauge.

Currently, several needles on the market have an inner stylet and a short shaft with a protective sheath that prevents the tip of the needle from being forced too deep into or

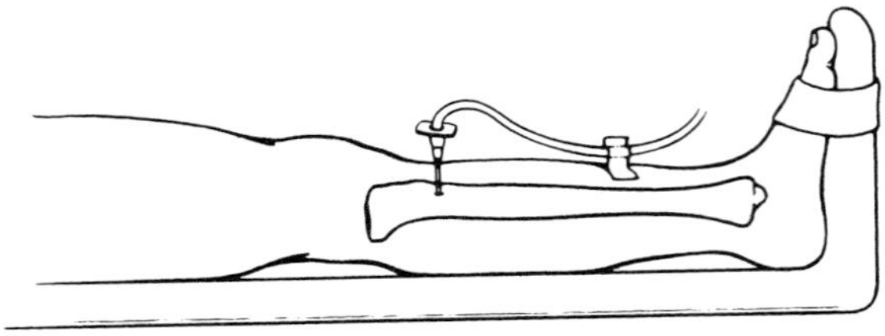

A

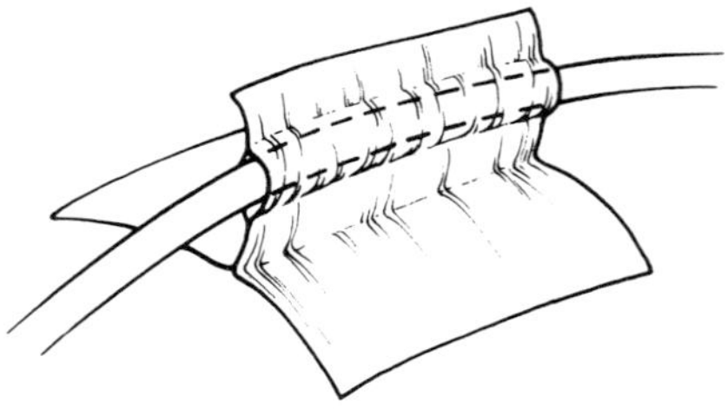

B

Figure 29–3 Stabilization and dressing for needle insertion. **A.** Footboard. **B.** Hinge-tape on the line.

through the bone. These needles include the short, large-bore Jamshidi bone marrow biopsy needle and disposable intraosseous needle kits (such as that manufactured by Cook Critical Care, Inc., Bloomington, IN).

The medications and fluids listed in Table 29–2 have been administered by intraosseous infusion. In general, the pharmacokinetics of intraosseous infusion approximate those seen with peripheral and central intravenous injection.

Intraosseous infusion of pharmacological agents should not be limited to primary and secondary resuscitation drugs. Medications that give ongoing support (i.e., antibiotics, sedatives, and narcotics) to the pediatric trauma patient as well as facilitate various stabilizing functions such as intubation can be given intraosseously.

Table 29–2 What Can Be Given by Intraosseous Infusion?*

Fluids
Blood
Contrast material
Crystalloid
Hydroxyethyl starch
Hypertonic dextrose

Advanced Cardiac Life Support Medications
Epinephrine
Atropine
Calcium chloride
Sodium bicarbonate

Antiarrhythmics
Lidocaine
Bretylium

Anticoma
Narcan
Glucose
Glucagon

Anticonvulsants
Diazepam
Phenobarbital
Phenytoin

Muscle Relaxants
Atracurium
Succinylcholine
Vecuronium

Inotropic/Vasoactive Drugs
Dopamine
Dobutamine
Isoproterenol

Narcotics
Morphine
Meperidine

Sedatives

Other Medications
Antibiotics
Insulin
Diuretics
Mannitol

*Avoid cytotoxic drugs when possible.

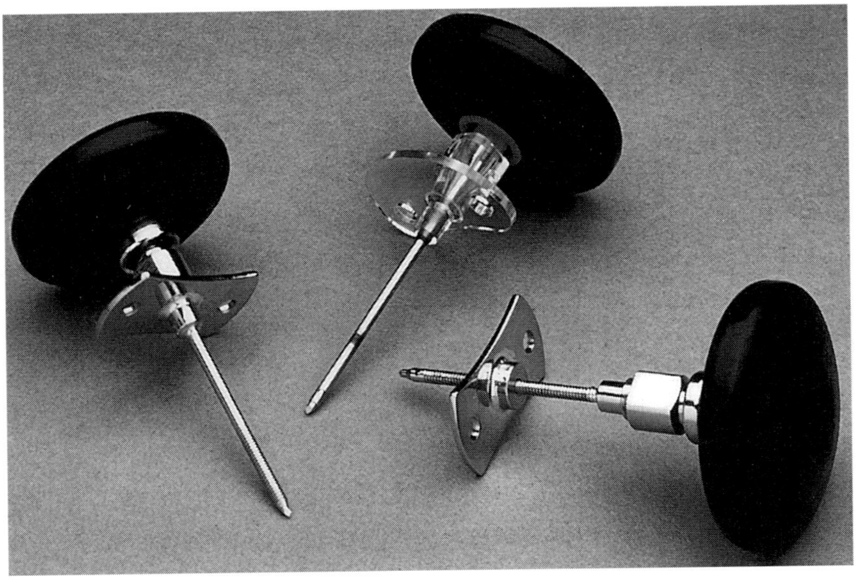

Figure 29–4 Types of cannulas available for intraosseous infusions.

Intraosseous flow rates have been reported to be determined by the flow through the bone marrow cavity rather than solely by the site of the needle. Infusion by a gravity infusion device has received infrequent mention in the pediatric literature. Goldstein et al (1990) reported that successful volume replacement usually requires bilateral intraosseous infusion with pressure infusion by pump or hand. Most experience suggests that rapid infusion of large amounts of fluid requires use of a pressure infusion device.

The flow rates achieved with intraosseous infusions vary. Tocantins et al (1941) reported an average of 1.7 ml/min (102 ml/h) with gravity infusion in the tibia of an infant. Hodge et al (1987) studied "pediatric" dogs and recorded mean flow rates by gravity of approximately 12 ml/min. Although fluids may be infused under pressure (pressurized intravenous fluid bag up to 600 mm Hg) and increased flow rate, the frequency of extravasation and pain are also increased. Shoor et al (1979) achieved flow rates of 40 ml/min (2500 ml/h) in tibial bone infusions. These data suggest that a significant volume of fluid can be delivered by intraosseous infusion and that, in some instances, the rates achieved may provide sufficient volumes for resuscitation until functional intravenous lines can be established. Some concern remains, however, that the flow rates obtained may not be adequate to provide the sole route of volume resuscitation for older children and adults. Replacement of red marrow by fat in the long bones of older children and adults may make intraosseous infusion less effective for volume replacement in children older than 5 or 6 years. It has been shown to be useful for administration of drugs, however.

Studies have shown that crystalloid, colloid, and blood products can be successfully infused by the intraosseous route for the initial resuscitation of the pediatric trauma patient in both the prehospital and emergency department settings. However, some type of pressure infusion device may be most useful with intraosseous line placement to ensure continued fluid flow during the resuscitation.

COMPLICATIONS

Intraosseous infusion is associated with a relatively low rate of complications. Rosetti et al (1985) reviewed 4270 cases in the intraosseous literature and found a 0.6% incidence of osteomyelitis, which was by far the most frequent complication. The majority of cases occurred in patients who had an intraosseous line in place for prolonged periods (up to 32 hours), in bacteremic patients, and in patients who received hypertonic infusions. A few cases of mediastinitis or sternal puncture as well as several subcutaneous abscesses were noted. Since that review, bilateral tibia fractures were reported in a 3-month-old infant, and a compartment syndrome was reported in a 5-week-old boy.

Growth plate injury, a complication that has long concerned researchers, has not been sustained by animal studies or reports from the literature. The only instances of growth plate abnormalities have been in patients with severe osteomyelitis. A second concern has been fat emboli. That fat emboli occur is not disputed, but they are not clinically relevant.

The only problem with the intraosseous technique that can have severe clinical relevance is extravasation into the subcutaneous tissues. Even well-placed intraosseous cannulas may result in microextravasation under pressurized infusion. The authors (with parental consent) placed an intraosseous infusion device into the tibia of an infant at time of death and fluoroscopically observed the infusion of radiopaque dye. Under cardiopulmonary resuscitation conditions (chest compressions), the contrast material was noted to rapidly enter the central circulation. This was a line placed by an experienced operator and placement was verified by fluoroscopy, yet extravasation is noted under pressurized infusion (Fig. 29–5).

Extravasation risk may arise from a number of technical errors (Fig. 29–6). Insertion error may result from misplacement in the soft tissue because of failure to completely penetrate the cortex or overpenetration through the opposite cortex. This may be a complication of poor operator technique from a to-and-fro motion or of excessive fluid pressure from dull needle tips due to repeated use requiring greater pressure for insertion.

Another source of error is cortical disruption. This can result when previous insertion attempts are ignored, by an unrecognized previous fracture, or by fracture of the extremity when the line is placed.

A final source of error can occur after the intraosseous cannula has been successfully placed. If the limb is not splinted, movement of the patient may result in loosening or dislodgment of the intraosseous needle. If the intravenous tubing is not adequately secured, tugging on it may again result in loosening or dislodgment of the needle. It is important to always remain alert for extravasation by monitoring the infusion site. If the site is obscured

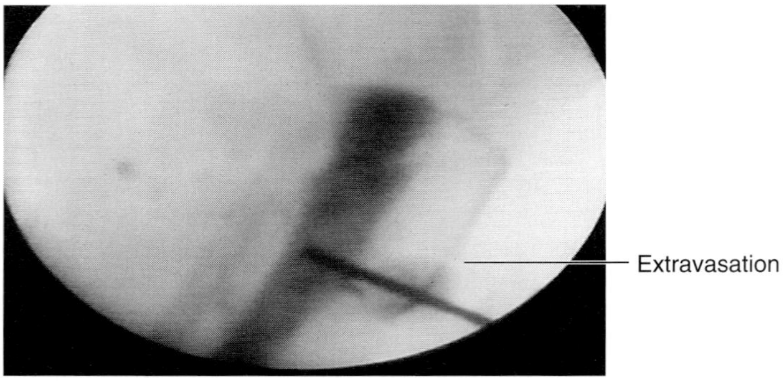

Figure 29–5 Intraosseous infusion with extravasation.

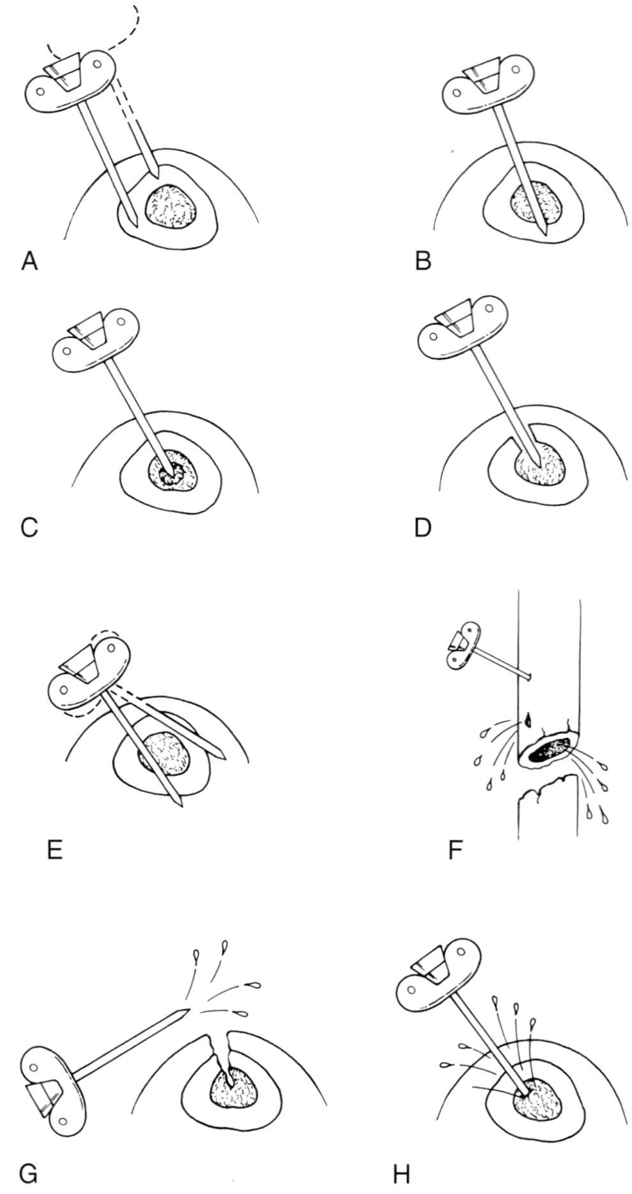

Figure 29–6 Placement complications of intraosseous infusions. **A.** Failure to completely penetrate the cortex. **B.** Penetration with re-entry into the back wall cortex. **C.** Needle lumen plugged with clot or tissue. **D.** Cortex hole larger than needle shaft. **E.** Penetration of the cortex wall after marrow entry tangential passage through the cortex into soft tissue. **F.** Infusion into fractured bone or a site of prior cortex puncture. **G.** Needle dislodged after placement in marrow. **H.** Excess pressure on fluid.

by a dressing, the risk of a significant extravasation is greatly increased.

Screw designs and improved tip and shaft material may improve shaft continence. Meanwhile, the following modifications should be considered:

1. Use sharp needles requiring less pressure for cortical perforation.
2. Use needles with strong metal resistant to damage during penetration efforts.
3. Emphasize rotary motion with stabilizing fingertips on insertion surface, rather than downward pressure with high shaft center of gravity.
4. Avoid direct aspiration/infusion syringe tests of placement (use injection sites of intravenous tubing).
5. Avoid dressing on site.
6. Stabilize tubing and limb (not needle shaft) to minimize accidental dislodgement or traumatic loosening.
7. Continuously monitor for signs of extravasation and other complications of infusion (Table 29–3).
8. Discontinue infusion on accomplishing other venous access.

CONCLUSIONS

Every health care professional involved in the care of acutely ill or injured children should be familiar with the lifesaving technique of intraosseous infusion. It provides reliable, reasonably rapid vascular access for children suffering cardiopulmonary arrest, shock, burns, and life-threatening status epilepticus and status asthmaticus. It has a number of advantages over other techniques that may be used to obtain emergency vascular access in the pediatric patient. These advantages include a high success rate when the technique is done properly, few contraindications or restrictions, and a low complication rate. Training in the technique of intraosseous infusion is available as part of the pediatric advanced life-support course sponsored by the American Academy of Pediatrics and the American Heart Association. Intraosseous infusion may be one of the few interventions in the prehospital setting that may have an impact on morbidity and mortality. It is a skill easily obtained with little technical difficulty.

Table 29–3 Infusion Monitoring

Inspect for extravasation (swelling)
If cytotoxic drugs are being used, discontinue them and restart at another site
Maintain patency with flow (pressurized bag or push normal saline bolus)
Maintain site immobilization (avoid needle wobble)
Note pain sensitivity to pressurized infusion!

References

Drinker CK, Drinker KR: A method of maintaining an artificial circulation through the tibia of the dog with a demonstration of the vasomotor control of the marrow vessels. *Am J Physiol,* 41: 514–521, 1916.

Glaeser PW: Five-year experience in prehospital intraosseous infusions in children and adults. *Ann Emerg Med,* 22:1119–1124, 1993.

Goldstein B, Doody D, Briggs S: Emergency intraosseous infusion in severely burned children. *Pediatr Emerg Care,* 6:195–197, 1990.

Hodge D, Delgado-Paredes C, Fleisher G: Intraosseous infusion flow rates in hypovolemic "pediatric" dogs. *Ann Emerg Med,* 16:305, 1987.

Josefson A: A new method of treatment: intraosseal injections. *Acta Med Scand,* 81:550, 1934.

Rosetti VA, Thompson BM, Miller J, et al: Intraosseous infusion: an alternative route of pediatric intravascular access. *Ann Emerg Med,* 14:885, 1985.

Shoor PM, Berryhill RE, Benumof JL: Intraosseous infusion: pressure-flow relationship and pharmacokinetics. *J Trauma,* 19:772, 1979.

Tocantins LM: Rapid absorption of substances injected into the bone marrow. *Proc Soc Exp Biol Med,* 45:292, 1940.

Tocantins LM, O'Neill JF, Jones HW: Infusions of blood and other fluids via the bone marrow. *JAMA,* 117:1229, 1941.

Bibliography

Fiser DH: Intraosseous infusions. *N Engl J Med,* 322:1579, 1990.

Guy T, Haley K, Zuspan S: Use of intraosseous infusion in the pediatric trauma patient. *J Pediatr Surg,* 28:158, 1993.

Hodge D: Intrasseous infusions: a review. *Pediatr Emerg Care,* 1:215, 1985.

Miner WF, Corneli HM, Bolte RG, et al: Prehospital use of intraosseous infusion by paramedics. *Pediatr Emerg Care,* 5:5, 1989.

Simmons CM, Johnson NE, et al: Intraosseous extravasation complication reports. *Ann Emerg Med,* 23:363, 1994.

Spivey WH: Intraosseous infusions. *J Pediatr,* 111: 639, 1987.

Appendix

American Academy of Pediatrics Endorsement of Intraosseous Infusion*

The American Academy of Pediatrics Committee on Pediatric Emergency Medicine issued a policy statement endorsing intraosseous infusion (IOI) as "a livesaving alternative to IV [intravenous] infusion when resuscitation must proceed rapidly" in critically ill or injured infants and young children. The statement hails IOI as a "safe, rapid, and reliable" route of vascular access, particularly for very young children in whom vascular access is especially difficult.

The AAP urges that "every physician caring for infants and small children should become educated in the indications, contraindications, risks, potential sites of insertion of IO lines, and techniques of IOI. Pediatricians and other physicans concerned with child health should actively promote the use of IOI in prehospital and emergency care protocols and training programs."

*American Academy of Pediatrics Committee on Pediatric Emergency Medicine: Policy statement: intraosseous infusion. *AAP News,* March 1992:16.

The committee made the following recommendations:

- In all resuscitation efforts, attention to ensuring adequate oxygenation and ventilation should precede any attempt to establish vascular access.
- Intraosseous infusion should be reserved for situations in which immediate vascular access is needed and in which peripheral or central venous access cannot be established rapidly, as in cases of shock, status epilepticus, or any form of cardiac arrest.
- In most cases, peripheral venous access should be attempted before placement of an IO line, although such efforts should continue for no longer than several minutes.
- In a child with full cardiopulmonary arrest, it may be appropriate to insert an IO line as the first attempt at vascular access.
- Once IOI is under way, ongoing attempts should be made to establish peripheral or central venous access. The IO needle should be removed when functional IV lines are in place and the patient is medically stable.
- Intraosseous infusion can be used in both

the prehospital setting (ground and aeromedical transport) and the emergency department.

The statement also noted several limitations:

- Flow rates with IOI do not approximate those of an IV line of similar caliber, which may limit the usefulness of IOI in severe shock or exsanguinating hemorrhage.
- Intraosseous lines cannot be inserted in a recently fractured bone.
- Replacement of red marrow by fat in the long bones limits the use of IOI in the tibia or femur of children older than 5 or 6 years of age.

Chapter 30

Pediatric Trauma and Musculoskeletal System Procedures

Robert W. Frenck, Jr., and E. Stephen Buescher

EMERGENCY ASSESSMENTS AND MANAGEMENT PRIORITIZATION

Trauma, the leading cause of death in children older than 1 year of age, accounts for 25,C00 deaths annually in the pediatric age range. Ninety percent of life-threatening injuries are related to blunt trauma as seen with automobile accidents, and more than 80% of severe blunt trauma has accompanying head injury. It is therefore critical for the pediatrician to have the understanding and skill to care for the injured child.

The assessment and management of the patient who has suffered multiple trauma involves three steps. The first and most important is to determine whether a risk to survival exists and what short-term interventions must be instituted to minimize the chance of the patient's dying of the injury.

Step One

Acute threats to survival always involve depression of the vital signs; a simple mnemcnic routinely applied to this situation is the ABCs:

AIRWAY ESTABLISHMENT: Having the patient talk is a simple and rapid way to assess the airway. A patient unable to talk should be assumed to have an inadequate airway. A first step in establishing the airway is to reposition the head, using in-line traction if a cervical injury is suspected. Next, all *visible* foreign material (vomitus, food, teeth, blood) should be removed from the airway. *Blind sweeps* of the mouth *are not recommended* for young infants. When aspiration is witnessed or strongly suspected, a Heimlich maneuver may be attempted in children older than 1 year. The next level of intervention is use of a mechanical airway. If the patient has adequate respiratory effort and is *not conscious*, an *oral airway* may be used. Otherwise, a nasal airway must be employed. If these measures still do not establish an airway or an *inadequate respiratory effort* exists, *endotracheal intubation* is needed to secure the airway.

BREATHING SUPPORT: When a patient is unable to maintain adequate spontaneous ventilation, steps must be initiated to assist the patient. Temporarily, mouth-to-mouth resuscitation may be used, but at most this provides 17% FIO_2. Humidified 100% oxygen should be administered to the patient as soon as possible. A bag-valve-mask system can be used initially; this can then be converted to a bag-valve-endotracheal tube if necessary. A soft, clear plastic mask should be used because it seals well and allows the physician to observe for cyanosis or the presence of vomitus. If prolonged ventilation will be required, the patient should be intubated. Before intubation, the patient should be preoxygenated with 100% oxygen by mask. If attempts at intubation are not successful within 20 seconds, mask ventilation should be resumed before another attempt is made. Holding your own breath during attempts at intubation is a good gauge for when mask ventilation should be resumed. If you are feeling short of breath, so is the patient! Patients with crush injuries of the chest or flail chest injuries should be placed on positive-pressure ventilation immediately, with particular attention paid to development of tension pneumothorax.

CIRCULATION SUPPORT: As the airway is being secured, other members of the team should be establishing circulation. If the pulse is absent, the patient is placed on a hard surface and chest compressions are begun. *Intravenous access is critical*; the goal is to establish access in less than 2 minutes if the child is hypotensive. *Upper extremity access is preferable*, but lower extremities may be used if there is no evidence of abdominal trauma. Peripheral venous catheterization is often not possible, and other routes need to be used. Femoral vein access, saphenous vein cutdown, and intraosseous infusion in the tibia are the preferred alternative routes for vascular access if access in an extremity is difficult. An intraosseous infusion is often the fastest and easiest method and is recommended for children younger than 3 years. As vascular access is being established, the cause of hypotension/hypovolemia needs to be considered before replacement therapy is begun. Patients with acute blood loss and shock require large amounts of fluids, whereas patients with head injuries, for example, may be harmed by aggressive fluid replacement therapy. Rapid volume expansion is best accomplished with isotonic crystalloid solutions such as normal saline or Ringer's lactate administered by bolus at 20 ml/kg. If little response is seen with the first bolus, it can be repeated. If little response is seen after the second bolus, packed red blood cells (10 ml/kg) should be considered. Occasionally, inotropic and pressor agents such as dopamine, dobutamine, and epinephrine are required to re-establish the pulse and blood pressure.

SPINE/CENTRAL NERVOUS SYSTEM EVALUATION: Because 80% of major trauma in children has accompanying head injury, care of the cervical spine is crucial. Whenever a child has sustained major trauma to the clavicle or higher, a cervical injury should be presumed. The patient's neck should therefore be immobilized until radiographs have either confirmed or ruled out a neck injury.

As part of the initial resuscitation, a nasogastric tube is placed unless a cribriform plate fracture is possible (suggested by the presence of clear fluid from the nose or ears). In this case, an orogastric tube is used. A urinary catheter should also be placed to gauge the efficiency of fluid resuscitation (unless blood at the urethral meatus or a scrotal hematoma is present, either of which may indicate urethral injury).

Step Two

TRAUMA: After the patient is stabilized, the second step is to determine the extent of trauma suffered by the patient. This is best approached by a systematic physical examination, also referred to as the secondary survey. Each area of the body needs to be visualized, palpated, and auscultated as appropriate. The importance of this detailed examination cannot be overemphasized, because unrecognized injuries may pose great risk to the patient. With specific types of trauma, certain points should always be considered and examined.

Head Trauma: Level of consciousness; cranial, motor, and sensory nerve function; the possibility of cervical spine injury or instability. The Glasgow Coma Scale (Table 30–1) provides an objective assessment of the patient with central nervous system injuries (Teasdale and Jennett, 1974). Scores of 5 or below are associated with a high probability of mortality or permanent neurological injury.

Thoracic Trauma: Loss of thoracic rigidity (flail chest); presence of hemothorax or pneumothorax; presence of bone fractures; great vessel laceration, penetrating (sucking) chest wounds; pulmonary contusion.

Blunt Abdominal Trauma: Unrecognized intra-abdominal bleeding (lacerated liver, spleen, or kid-

Table 30–1 The Glasgow Coma Scale

	Score*
Eye Opening	
Spontaneous	4
To speech	3
To noxious stimulation	2
None	1
Best Motor Response	
Obeys commands	6
Localizes stimuli	5
Withdraws	4
Abnormal flexion	3
Extensor response	2
None	1
Verbal Response	
Oriented	5
Confused conversation	4
Inappropriate words	3
Incomprehensible sounds	2
None	1

*The coma score is the sum of individual scores (eye opening + verbal + motor) and equals 3 to 15.

ney; visceral hematomas) or ruptured viscus. Although intra-abdominal injuries occur in only 10% of cases, exsanguination from unrecognized bleeding into the abdomen is the second leading cause of death in childhood trauma.

Extremity Trauma: The adequacy of perfusion; presence of deformities; altered or absent function of the extremities. If not treated promptly, these injuries can result in permanent disfiguration or loss of limbs. Angulation, shortening, swelling, or bruising of extremities should be noted. Palpate for point tenderness or crepitance. Presence of inordinate pain or cool extremities should alert one to the possibility of compartment syndrome or vascular injury. If indicated, tetanus prophylaxis should be administered.

Step Three

The third step is to design and implement the management plans for each injury and the involved organ systems. These management plans may involve outpatient management, hospitalization, or transfer or referral for specialized care. Various aspects of outpatient management of musculoskeletal trauma are addressed later in this chapter. If transfer or referral is considered appropriate, the following points must be ensured:

1. Vital signs are stable.
2. A stable airway is established.
3. Vascular access is established.
4. Existing spinal cord injury has been stabilized.
5. Appropriate personnel are available to accompany the patient.

MINOR SURGICAL PROCEDURES

Numerous minor surgical procedures are appropriately performed on children by the general pediatrician. The reasons for this include experience with addressing concerns unique to children (pain, separation from parents, levels of cooperation), everyday experience with technically demanding procedures (phlebotomy, lumbar puncture, intubation), and perhaps most important, general empathy for the injured child. Technical competence is only one facet of performing minor procedures on children. Others that at times are even more important are preparedness, anticipation, and patience. Most children should be advised of expected discomfort and the ways that it will be alleviated. Older children often expect a detailed explanation before and sometimes even during procedures.

Restraint

It is not always reasonable to depend on a child's willing cooperation. Knowledge of efficient, effective ways to restrain appropriate body parts is an indispensable asset for the pediatrician. Use of restraints, and loosening them during the procedure if they are no longer indicated, is much easier than trying to initiate restraints after the procedure is under way.

With smaller children, it is often necessary to maintain whole-body restraint to immobilize an extremity effectively. A number of specialized "papoose boards" are available for this purpose, but the same effect can also be achieved by "bundling" the child with a bed sheet (Fig. 30–1).

To restrain extremities for intravenous line placement or minor procedures (suturing, biopsy), handboards, armboards, or footboards (leaving the procedure field unobstructed) are often useful. As a general rule,

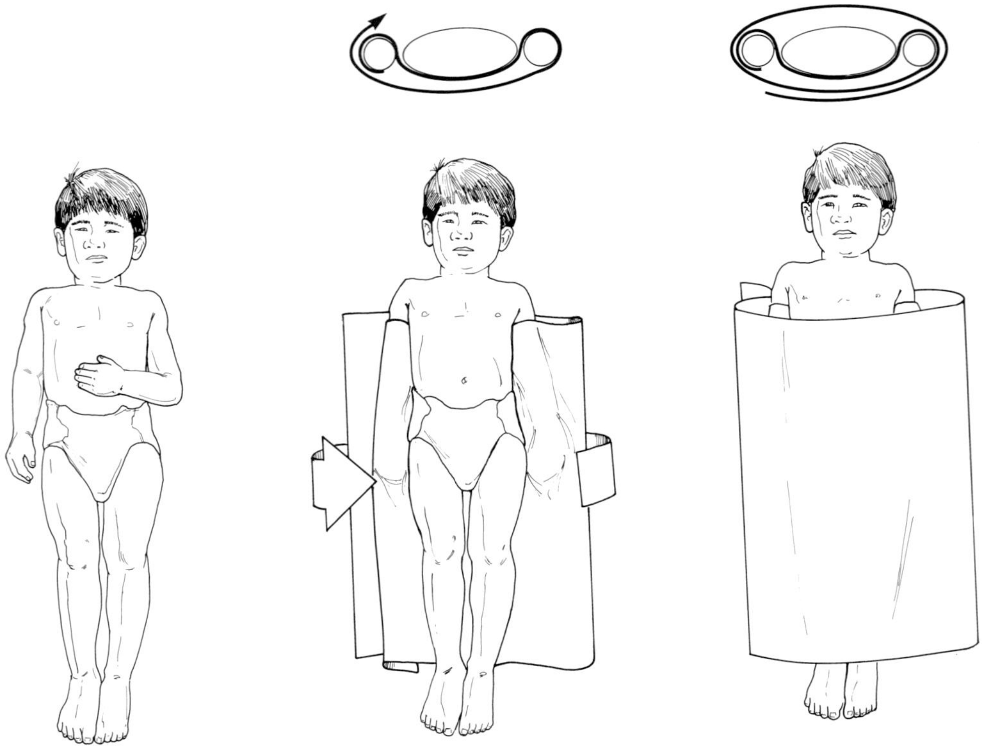

Figure 30–1 Method for whole-body restraint of a small child by "bundling." Figures at the top show the path followed by the bundling material when the patient is viewed from below.

immobilization that includes one joint above and below the site (as is prescribed for casting or splinting) ensures adequate restraint and control of the site of interest. For procedures in some toddlers, it is often of benefit to have an assistant restrain the shoulder or hip joint if immobilization of the relevant extremity is necessary. This assistance minimizes movement of the extremity caused by twisting of the axial skeleton. Armboard and footboard restraints must be placed securely to perform their intended functions; but at the same time, care must be taken to ensure that the restraining board does not obstruct vascular flow, compress neural tissue, or cause pressure necrosis. In addition, keep in mind that restraint does not obviate the need to minimize pain while performing procedures. Figures 30–2 and 30–3 illustrate methods for immobilizing a hand or foot for minor procedures.

Pain Control

A major concern of every child being prepared for a procedure is, will it hurt? As physicians, we are supposed to alleviate pain and suffering, and so the standard answer is no, with the unspoken qualification "I hope." Adult patients are more able to accept the subtleties of this answer, but a child interprets the response of no as concrete and guaranteed. Failure to achieve the promise ensures mistrust and loss of cooperation. The pediatrician, therefore, should be effective in controlling pain and the anxiety that accompanies and contributes to it.

Three main categories of agents are useful in pain and anxiety management. Anesthetics are agents that remove sensation, particularly pain sensation, which is needed for surgery to be performed. Analgesics relieve pain but do not cause loss of sensation. Sedatives calm the patient but do not relieve pain. Soporifics induce sleep but do not cause loss of sensation, relief of pain, or true sedation. No one drug or combination of drugs fulfills every need for ideal pain control. The agents used are best individualized to each patient's needs on the basis of the patient's age, the procedure to be done, and the patient's psychological state.

Orally administered agents are the least in-

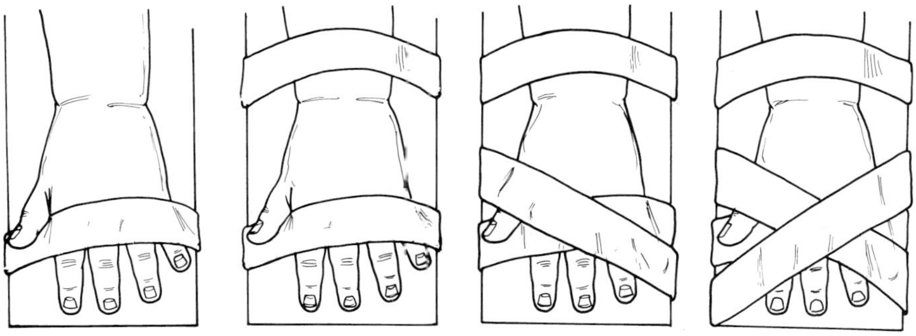

Figure 30–2 Method for restraining a hand using a handboard.

vasive, but their onsets are typically slow and unpredictable. Intramuscular agents are rapid and predictable but have the disadvantage of pain during administration. Intravenous agents have the initial pain and trauma associated with obtaining venous access. However, once access is obtained, further sedation or analgesia is painless. Therefore, if repeated or prolonged sedation or analgesia is necessary, intravenous agents are probably best.

The categories of agents used depend on the effect that is to be achieved. If a procedure is not inherently painful (e.g., computed tomography), sedation or soporific effect may be all that is needed. If pain control is necessary, combination of agents with anesthetic or analgesic and sedative effects is usually appropriate. Guidelines for the monitoring and management of pediatric patients during and after analgesia/sedation for procedures have been suggested (Guidelines for monitoring and management of pediatric patients during and after sedation for diagnostic and therapeutic procedures, 1992). These guidelines outline the appropriate candidates for sedation, the facilities and emergency back-up services necessary, the necessary on-site equipment, the responsible personnel, and the necessary documentation for outpatient sedation procedures.

The following agents are commonly used in pediatrics for sedation and pain control.

Sedatives

BARBITURATES: These agents depress the central nervous system, producing sedation or sleep. At sedative doses, these medications have little effect on the respiratory drive or cardiovascular system. However, overdoses may produce apnea, depress respiratory drive, and have cardiovascular effects. Barbiturates have *no analgesic effect*. Commonly used barbiturates include the following.

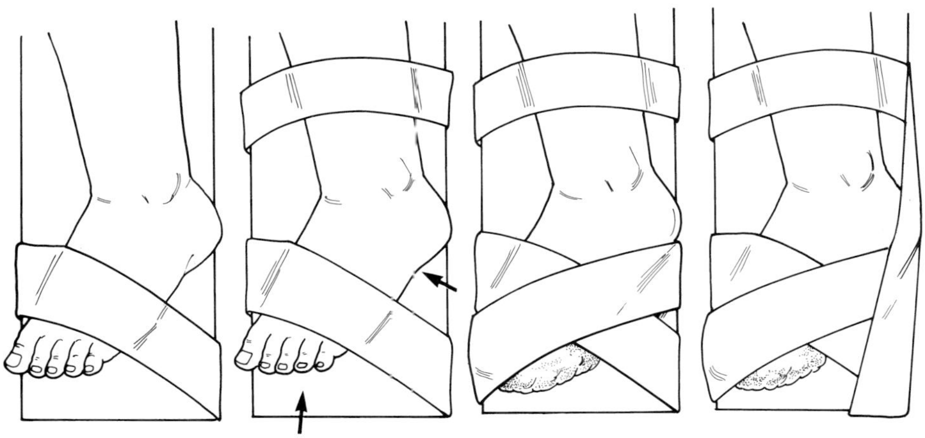

Figure 30–3 Method for restraining a foot using a footboard. The arrows show locations where gauze or cotton padding is placed to support the heel and distal foot as the restraint is being placed.

Thiopental (Pentothal): Administration in children is typically per rectum (25–45 mg/kg) or intravenously (1–1.5 mg/kg/dose). The onset of sedation is rapid, occurring in less than 1 minute after intravenous administration, and the period of sedation is short. Some children may require additional sedation after rectal administration (25–45 mg/kg) owing to defecation of drug after administration (Burckert et al, 1980).

Pentobarbital (Nembutal): Administration is either intramuscularly (5–6 mg/kg) or intravenously (2–6 mg/kg), but intravenous administration may be more reliable. Onset of sedation is slower than with thiopental.

BENZODIAZEPINES: These agents produce sedation, decrease anxiety, and produce skeletal muscle relaxation. In some instances, they may also produce antegrade amnesia. Sedative doses have minimal respiratory depression and cardiovascular function effects. These agents *have no analgesic effect.*

Midazolam (Versed): A relatively new agent, midazolam has become the benzodiazepine of choice for many pediatricians. It has the favorable characteristics of being water soluble and rapid acting (usually 10–20 minutes) with a short duration (typically 40–60 minutes). Additionally, midazolam may be administered intramuscularly, intravenously, orally, intranasally, or rectally. When used in conjunction with a local anesthetic, midazolam is an effective sedative for children undergoing laceration repair, bone marrow aspiration, or lumbar puncture (Latson et al, 1991; Sandler et al, 1992). Deaths due to respiratory depression have been reported, especially when midazolam is used in conjunction with opioids. Therefore, careful monitoring during sedation is warranted. Typical doses are 0.035 mg/kg intravenously in a 1 to 2 minute period, repeated prn; 0.08 mg/kg intramuscularly; 0.04 mg/kg intranasally; and 0.3 mg/kg rectally.

Diazepam (Valium): Diazepam is a commonly used benzodiazepine with good oral absorption. Intramuscular and intravenous administration should be avoided because the drug is painful when administered this way. Typical dosages: oral 0.12 to 0.8 mg/kg/24 h divided every 6 to 8 hours; IM or IV 0.04 to 0.2 mg/kg every 2 to 4 hours.

Soporifics

CHLORAL HYDRATE: This is still the most commonly used sedative in pediatrics, due possibly to habit more than to science. It produces *somnolence but no analgesia.* The proper dose is debated but ranges from 30 to 100 mg/kg with a maximum dose of 2 to 3 g. It has a disagreeable taste, often making oral administration difficult. Chloral hydrate has been effectively used for electroencephalography, computed tomography, and magnetic resonance imaging scans. However, it may be less effective in children older than 48 months (Greenberg et al, 1993). The main advantage of chloral hydrate is its safety; however, deaths after chloral hydrate administration have been reported.

Analgesics

NON-NARCOTIC ANALGESICS: Although not a single chemical class of agents, non-narcotic analgesics have in common that they are not usually sedating at analgesic doses.

Acetaminophen (Tylenol): Acetaminophen has analgesic and antipyretic effects but essentially no anti-inflammatory activity; it is more useful for postprocedure pain. Doses are 10 to 15 mg/kg given every 4 hours with a maximum of five doses per 24 hours.

Aspirin: Aspirin is effective for mild to moderate pain, particularly pain of inflammatory origin (bone, joint), but is less popular because of epidemiological association with Reye's syndrome. Analgesic doses are 10 to 15 mg/kg given every 4 hours; anti-inflammatory doses are 60 to 100 mg/kg/d, divided every 4 hours.

Ibuprofen: A nonsteroidal anti-inflammatory agent with potent antipyretic effects equal or superior to acetaminophen, ibuprofen is especially useful for pain of inflammatory origin. Gastritis has been associated with repeated use, so administration with meals is advised. Doses of 30 to 70 mg/kg/24 h, divided every 6 to 8 hours, are needed for analgesia.

Ketamine: Ketamine produces a state of consciousness termed "dissociative anesthesia." Patients have significant analgesia but appear only mildly sedated. Patients may move or talk but are amnestic to the procedure. The onset of action is rapid, and patients typically recover within 2 hours. Respiratory depression is rare. The main side effect is postemergence delirium with hallucinations that may occur in up to 30% of patients. In cancer patients undergoing painful procedures, oral ketamine (10 mg/kg) is effective and side effects are rare (Tobias et al, 1992). Intravenous dose is 0.5 mg/kg; if necessary, this may be followed by a 0.01 to 0.02 mg/kg/min infusion for longer procedures. Intramuscular dose is 0.5 to 1 mg/kg. Oral dose is 10 mg/kg.

NARCOTIC ANALGESICS: This analgesic class has notable sedative and soporific effects in addition to analgesic effects.

Codeine: This opioid is usually administered orally, and used for postprocedure pain; nausea, vomiting, or dizziness is often seen. The dose is 0.8 to 1.5 mg/kg orally every 4 hours.

Meperidine (Demerol): Meperidine is a semisynthetic opioid with duration of effect slightly shorter than that of morphine. It can cause hypotension and respiratory depression. Intravenous dose is 0.8 to 1 mg/kg every 2 hours. Intramuscular/subcutaneous dose is 0.8 to 1.3 mg/kg every 3 to 4 hours.

Morphine: Morphine is the original opioid analgesic effective for moderate to severe pain against which others are compared; it causes respiratory depression and vasodilation (hypotension). Starting doses are 0.1 mg/kg intravenously every 2 hours or 0.1 to 0.15 mg/kg intramuscularly or subcutaneously every 3 to 4 hours; tolerant patients require larger doses.

Fentanyl: Fentanyl has shorter action of effect than morphine with less vasodilation effects. The drug is lipophilic, so it can be administered mucosally or transdermally. Itching and rash are common side effects of intravenous administration but rarely require treatment. There is the potential for potent respiratory depression with this medication, so close monitoring is mandatory and resuscitation equipment must be available. Dosing usually starts at 2 μ/kg intravenously with a maximum dose of 4 μ/kg. Doses may be increased by increments of 0.5μ/kg every 1 to 2 minutes as needed.

Analgesic/sedative drug combinations

DPT/LYTIC COCKTAIL: Meperidine (*D*emerol) 2 mg/kg plus promethazine (*P*henergan) 1 mg/kg plus chlorpromazine (*T*horazine) 1 mg/kg (maximum meperidine dose of 50 mg) is a dependable and commonly used analgesic/sedative combination (Cook et al, 1992; Zeltzer et al, 1989). Given by intramuscular injection, with all medications in one syringe, it provides potent analgesia and sedation and is soporific. Because of its potential for respiratory depression, half the dose is used in patients with cyanotic congenital heart disease, sick children, or small infants. Because of the high frequency of side effects, slow onset (30–40 minutes), and the often prolonged sedation (may last up to 7 hours), it may be replaced by other medications in the future (Snodgrass and Dodge, 1989).

INTRAMUSCULAR MEPERIDINE: Intramuscular meperidine (Demerol) 1 mg/kg alone or in combination with hydroxyzine (Vistaril, Atarax) 0.5-1 mg/kg provides effective analgesia and sedation. Use local anesthetic at the procedure site. Intramuscular meperidine can be associated with respiratory depression and is irritating; local soreness at the injection site for several days is to be expected.

Anesthetics

LOCAL ANESTHETICS: These agents are used locally to eliminate pain sensation and can be grouped as topically applied and injectable.

Topical: Topical local anesthetics can be used alone for anesthesia, can be used to minimize the pain associated with the administration of injectable local anesthetics, or can be used to augment the effects of injectable local anesthetics.

Ethylene chloride spray is rapid and inexpensive, but because of the brief duration of anesthesia, its major use is as a topical anesthetic before injectable anesthetic infiltration (and the injectable anesthetic must be infiltrated promptly).

A formulation of tetracaine-epinephrine (Adrenalin)-cocaine (TAC: 0.5% tetracaine, 0.05% epinephrine, 11.8% cocaine), prepared by the hospital pharmacy, has been well tolerated by children as either sole local anesthesia or to augment injectable anesthetic effects. Starting with about 5 ml, some of the TAC solution is dripped directly into the wound. The rest is soaked in a gauze pad and held in place over the wound by a gloved hand. This is necessary because the compound has potent vasoconstrictive effects even on normal skin. Full effects are seen after 5 to 10 minutes and are approximately equivalent to infiltration with 1% lidocaine (Bonadio and Wagner, 1988). TAC is specifically useful for face and scalp lacerations and provides adequate anesthesia for extremity wounds (Anderson et al, 1990). Use of the agent is contraindicated in areas where epinephrine cannot be used. Systemic absorption of cocaine can occur after the application of TAC, which may result in a positive urine drug screen response.

EMLA is the trade name of an oil/water emulsion of lidocaine and prilocaine. In pediatric oncology patients, it is useful as an anesthetic for needle puncture procedures, such as bone marrow aspirations, lumbar punctures, and intravenous line placement (Halperin et al, 1989; Young et al, 1987). To be effective, it must be applied at least 1 hour before the procedure and covered with an occlusive, semipermeable dressing. Currently, a drawback to EMLA is its high cost, but this may change in the future. Because it is often not practical or possible to wait the 60 minutes necessary for EMLA to work, local anesthesia is more typically achieved by anesthetic infiltration into the tissues or by nerve blockade. A method for tissue infiltration of local anesthetic is given in the following.

Injectable: A variety of injectable local anesthetics used by infiltration are available:

1. Bupivacaine hydrochloride, 0.25% to 0.5% with or without 1:200,000 epinephrine*; maximum subcutaneous dose, 3 mg/kg; duration of effect up to 6 hours.
2. Lidocaine hydrochloride, 0.25% to 2% with 1:200,000 epinephrine; maximum subcutaneous dose, 7 mg/kg; duration of effect, 30 to 60 minutes; buffering lidocaine with sodium bicarbonate (0.1 mEq/ml) makes local infiltration almost painless (McKay et al, 1987) but decreases the stability of the lidocaine when stored.

These injectable agents are used similarly. After 1 to 2 ml of anesthetic is drawn into a sterile syringe, a short, fine needle (25- to 27-gauge, 0.5 to 1 inch) is attached. If a wound is being infiltrated for suturing, the subcutaneous tissue is entered through the wound itself, and the anesthetic is slowly injected under the entire wound edge. As anesthesia is achieved at the wound edge, the needle is advanced deeper into the surrounding subcutaneous tissues, and the anesthetic is injected slowly as the needle is advanced. Anesthesia should be achieved in 5 to 10 minutes. If skin is being prepared for an incision or puncture, a small intradermal bleb of anesthetic is raised, which will typically cause a burning sensation. The needle is removed, and after the skin patch has lost sensation, the needle is reinserted through the anesthetic area into the deeper tissues; anesthetic is injected slowly until the degree of local anesthesia needed is obtained. Rubbing the skin proximal to the injection site immediately before injection may help decrease the pain of injection by blocking nerve fibers that sense pain.

Effective local anesthesia relieves pain sensation, but the patient often continues to sense pressure or tugging. Informing the child of this often helps to alleviate the anxiety that feeling the tugging/pulling sensations may cause.

*As a local vasoconstrictor, epinephrine increases the duration of action of the anesthetic; but it should not be used on distal body parts, like the nose, penis, digits, nipples, or ears.

WOUND CLOSURES

Wound Cleaning

Superficial lacerations are common injuries in children and heal most rapidly when they remain uninfected and the wound edges are apposed. Lacerations result from a wide variety of causes, most of which also result in some degree of wound contamination. Cleaning the contaminating materials from the wound is the first and most important step in minimizing the risk of infection.

For wound cleaning, a sterile bowl, 1% povidone-iodine solution (Betadine), irrigating syringe, 16- to 18-gauge intravenous catheter, sterile irrigating saline, sterile 4×4 gauze pads, and sterile gloves are needed.

If possible, immerse the wound in the povidone-iodine solution and soak it for 10 to 20 minutes. Use the irrigating syringe/intravenous catheter and 4×4 pads soaked in povidone-iodine solution to clean the wound and remove contaminating debris. A high-pressure jet of either irrigating saline or povidone-iodine solution directed into all areas of the wound by syringe/intravenous catheter works well. The amount of fluid used is important: for an average wound, 500 ml of irrigation is appropriate. Because washing and irrigating wounds is painful, use of local anesthesia before washing may be appropriate to minimize pain and allow wound cleaning to be done more thoroughly. After cleaning, explore the wound for injuries to deep tissues or structures and remove any foreign bodies. If doubt exists about the presence of foreign bodies, radiographs may be needed.

Prolonged contact of the skin with povidone-iodine can damage tissue. It is therefore important to rinse the surgical scrub from the wound with the saline irrigation. The wound can then be gently dried with sterile 4×4 gauze pads.

Wounds that are more than 8 to 12 hours old or those that have a high risk of contamination, such as animal bites, should not be sutured. A possible exception to this is a facial laceration; facial wounds older than 8 to 12 hours may be cleaned extensively and then closed in an attempt to minimize scarring. When this is done, close and careful follow-up is mandatory to watch for signs of infection.

Puncture wounds can present problems for effective wound management. These wounds should be irrigated by insertion of either a needle or plastic intravenous catheter down the track with vigorous expulsion of irrigating solution.

Tetanus immune status must be considered with every wound. If any doubt exists, it is best to administer appropriate tetanus prophylaxis.

Wound Closure

Considerations regarding wound closure include the age and type of wound as well as the methods for closure and techniques available. Because primary closure of old or infected wounds interferes with effective local care and drainage, it often results in local tissue destruction and other morbidities. Delayed primary closure may be possible, however, if the wound appears clean after 4 or 5 days. Puncture wounds are not typically closed. If infection is present in a wound, it should be treated with appropriate antibiotics and local care/drainage.

Suture and nonsuture methods exist for wound closure. Whereas different suture materials are available, monofilament is now the preferred suture for skin closure. Absorbable sutures are less likely to cause scarring and do not require removal; but because of lack of tensile strength, they are mainly used for deep tissue suturing. Nonsuture methods include surgical staples and sterile skin bandage closure. Surgical staples have the advantage of speedy placement but require specialized devices for both placement and removal. Sterile skin bandage closures work well on smaller, more superficial wounds but require undisturbed placement for 10 to 14 days, something that can reasonably be expected only of older, cooperative children.

Suture closure of wounds

Necessary materials include sterile drapes, sterile gloves, sterile suture material with needle attached, sterile needle driver, sterile mosquito hemostat, sterile scissors, sterile 4×4 gauze pads, and bandage tape. Monofilament suture (5–0 or preferably 6–0) should be used for facial lacerations. Heavier suture material (4–0) is sufficient for most other wounds, but 3–0 may be needed on the feet or hands.

After local anesthesia is attained, the area is draped and the best way to approximate the wound edges is determined. If the wound is short and linear, one or two superficial stitches will accurately approximate the edges. If the wound is curved with gapes, a temporary stay suture can be placed at the middle of the wound to roughly approximate the edges while the working sutures are placed (Fig. 30–4). If the wound is deep and superficially placed sutures roll the edges under, a temporary mattress suture can be used to bring the wound base together while the superficial sutures are placed (Fig. 30–5). Alternatively, deep placement of absorbable suture material may be necessary to allow approximation of the wound edges. If the wound is jagged or angulated, placement of several temporary stay sutures to align the gaping segments may aide in achieving wound edge approximation and alignment.

The tissue at the wound edges is edematous, and as the edema resolves, the sutures placed acutely will loosen. To compensate for this, su-

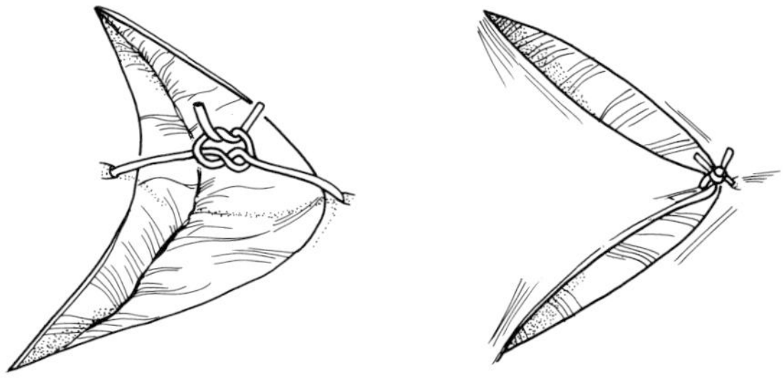

Figure 30–4 Placement of a temporary stay suture in an irregular/angulated laceration to facilitate edge approximation.

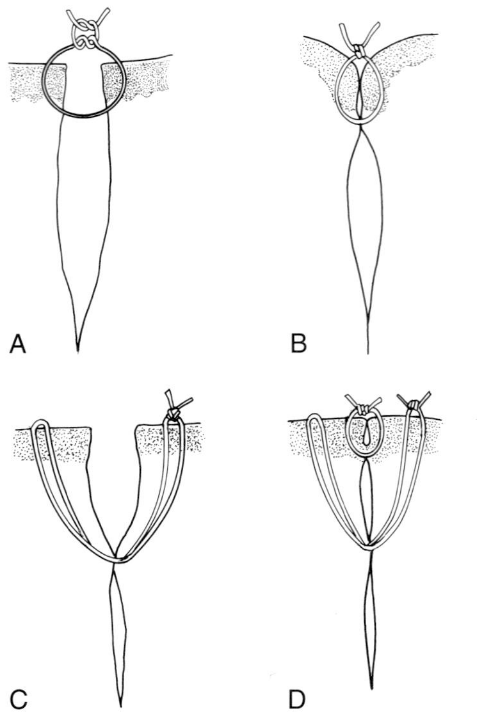

Figure 30–5 Placement of a temporary mattress suture to prevent wound edge rolling. **A** and **B** show the effects of closing a deep laceration using superficial sutures without approximating the deep wound edges first. **C** and **D** show the effect of placing a temporary deep mattress suture to approximate deep wound edges before superficial suture placement.

tures should be pulled and tied slightly tighter than is needed simply to approximate the wound edges. As the edema resolves, this should leave the sutures at the appropriate tension. After all sutures have been placed, the surface of the closed wound is cleansed with sterile saline and dried; the suture line is covered with an appropriate bandage for at least 24 hours.

The timing of suture removal varies with the wound location and cosmetic concerns. Sutures on the head or face can be removed after 3 to 5 days to minimize suture scars and, if possible, should be replaced with surgical tapes for an additional 3 to 5 days. At other sites, where mechanical strength is more important than cosmetic appearance, sutures are removed after 7 to 10 days.

Sterile skin bandage closure of wounds

Local anesthesia may or may not be necessary. After the cleaned wound is draped and the best way to approximate the wound edges is determined, the first set of bandages is placed perpendicular to the axis of the wound (Fig. 30–6). Each bandage strip is attached to one side of the wound, and traction is applied to bring the wound edges together, the free end of the bandage is attached to the skin on the other wound edge. The second set of bandages is applied diagonally across the axis of the wound, overlying the first set of closures. The third set of bandages is applied at right angles to the second set. The final two bandage strips run parallel to the wound, one on each side. Each strip runs the length of the wound and is used to cover and anchor the ends on the three previously applied layers of bandage strips.

The skin around wounds closed with ban-

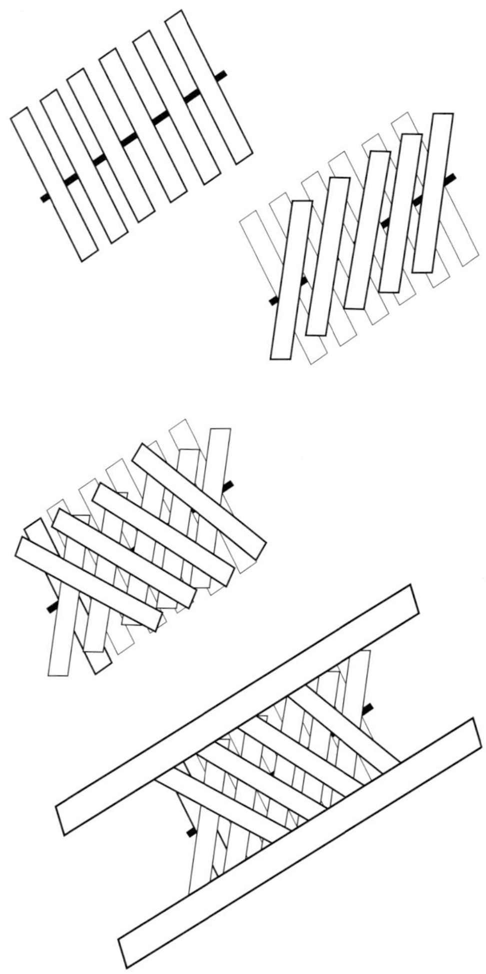

Figure 30–6 Method for placement of sterile skin closure bandages. The first course of bandages is placed perpendicular to the wound. The second and third are placed diagonally, and the last pieces are placed parallel to the wound to anchor the ends of the first three courses.

dage strips must be kept clean and dry to ensure that the layers of bandage remain adherent to the skin. Tincture of benzoin applied to the skin before bandage placement may aide in maintaining skin attachment.

Special considerations

BITE WOUNDS: Bite wounds, both human and nonhuman, are common in children. Most of these are minor, but even innocuous-appearing bites have potential for serious infection. Dog and cat bites account for about 90% and 10% of animal bites, respectively. These wounds are often heavily contaminated with the oral flora of the animal and the skin flora of the patient. The common organisms, *Staphylococcus aureus*, *Streptococcus* species, anaerobic cocci, and *Bacteroides* species, as well as *Pasteurella multocida* (common mouth flora in dogs and cats) can cause serious infection. The *foundation of care* for all bite wounds is *extensive cleaning* as described in the section on wound closure. Whether bite wounds should be closed primarily is an area of controversy. If the wound does not appear infected and is treated within 8 hours, it may be sutured or closed with tape after irrigation is completed. Bite wounds (both animal and human) that appear infected or are older than 8 hours should be packed open with either saline-soaked sterile gauze or petrolatum gauze and covered with a bulky dressing. For the first several days, the wound should be inspected frequently and the packing removed and replaced as needed. If the wound is large or in a cosmetically important area, delayed closure may be considered if the wound remains uninfected at 4 to 5 days.

ANTIBIOTIC PROPHYLAXIS: Prophylactic antibiotics are probably indicated for wounds with a high risk for infection. These wounds include cat bites, non-minor human bites, dog bites more than 8 hours old, deep puncture wounds, hand wounds, and wounds that have potential for delayed primary closure. Currently, the best broad-spectrum antibiotic for bites is amoxicillin–clavulanic acid. Erythromycin may be used in the penicillin-allergic patient. Under no conditions, however, should antibiotic treatment be considered a substitute for careful, extensive cleaning of the wound.

TETANUS AND IMMUNIZATION: Tetanus toxoid administration should be given if indicated. The need for rabies prophylaxis depends on the biting animal and area of the country. Consultation with the local public health department for advice is recommended.

PENETRATING BITE/TOOTH INJURIES: Penetration of bite or tooth injuries into deep spaces, joints, or bone should be regarded as particularly serious and susceptible to infection. These injuries should be referred for specialist management.

BARBED OBJECTS: Wounding by barbed objects such as fishhooks is common and presents the problem of how best to remove them. Many removal methods are described, but the simplest is to continue to pass the embedded barbed tip through the skin, remove the tip with wire cutters, and then back the remaining shaft out of the original puncture wound.

SPECIAL TISSUES: Most lacerations of the tongue or palate do not need to be closed because they will heal rapidly on their own. If bleeding is difficult to control or the injury creates a tissue flap that will interfere with eating, one or two stitches can be used to approximate the edges of the wound.

Lacerations of the free margin of the eyebrow, the eyelid, the vermilion border of the lip, and the pinna of the ear require particular care regarding alignment and closure technique. Eyebrows should not be shaved (they grow slowly), and the wound edges should be aligned and approximated with a temporary "tacking" skin suture before repair of the deep layers. Likewise, lacerations through the vermilion border are first aligned by tacking the skin, then repaired from bottom to top. In tissues containing cartilage, lacerated cartilage must first be reapproximated and closed with use of minimal numbers of absorbable sutures, followed by a layered closure of other tissues. Hematomas from either lacerations or blunt trauma must be evacuated to prevent significant perichondrial scar fibrosis (see Chapter 40). Lacerations on the face, particularly the forehead and chin in small children (1–4 years), often result from falls, and these injuries, despite superficial appearances, are usually deep. Such injuries require careful examination to determine the degree of injury, complete cleaning, and removal of foreign materials. Because the face contains specialized anatomy, complex lacerations involving specific structures (facial nerve, parotid gland) or loss of significant amounts of tissue are best referred for specialized care.

JOINT ASPIRATIONS

For most swollen joints, examination of the joint fluid is necessary for proper diagnosis and management. Because of the complex local anatomy of the hip and shoulder, aspiration of these joints is usually done by a consultant orthopedist. However, the other extremity joints are readily accessible to the pediatrician's needle if the proper approach is taken. The materials needed for joint aspiration are povidone-iodine (1%) solution, sterile drapes, sterile gloves, 16-gauge 1-inch needle, 18- or 20-gauge 1-1/2-inch needle on a 10-ml sterile syringe, 3-ml syringe with 1-1/2-inch 22-gauge needle and local anesthetic, 25-gauge 5/8-inch needle, 4 × 4 sterile gauze pads, and appropriate specimen tubes for joint fluid analysis. After the appropriate anatomical landmarks are identified, the puncture site is marked with either gentle pressure from a fingernail or with a surgical marker. The skin is prepared with povidone-iodine solution and draped for a sterile field. With use of the small needle (25-gauge, 5/8 inch), an intradermal bleb of local anesthetic is raised; after loss of sensation, local anesthetic is infiltrated along the predicted needle track. Emla cream is an alternative to intradermal anesthesia if time permits (see pain control section for details on use of Emla). The sterile 16-gauge needle is used to create an open path through the skin and is then removed. The 18- or 20-gauge needle is attached to a 10-ml syringe, and this needle is passed through the skin opening and along the anesthetic track. As the needle approaches the joint space, slight negative pressure is applied to the syringe, and the needle is advanced into the joint space.

A volume of joint fluid appropriate for the necessary tests is aspirated from the joint, and the needle is removed from the joint in one smooth motion. Pressure is applied to the puncture site with a sterile 4 × 4 gauze pad for 2 to 5 minutes.

Site for Elbow Aspiration

With the forearm extended to about 120 degrees and the hand *supinated*, the lateral humeral epicondyle and the radial head are identified by palpation. Once they are located, the hand is pronated and the needle is introduced from the lateral aspect at a point between these two landmarks (Fig. 30–7).

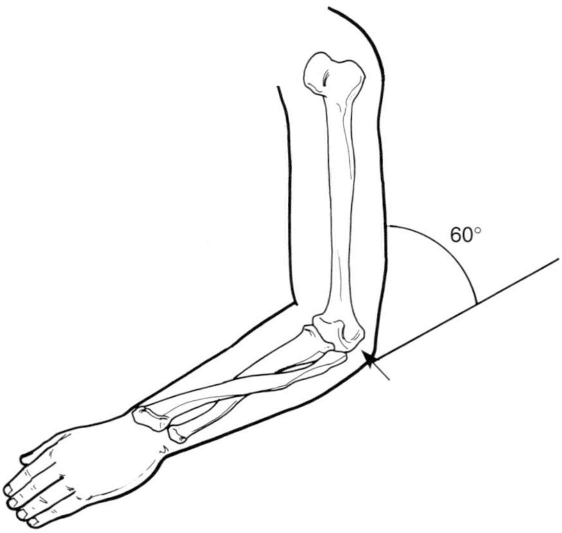

Figure 30–7 Elbow aspiration site *(arrow).*

Sites for Wrist Aspiration

Because of its complex bone structure, there are several possible sites for arthrocentesis in the wrist joint: medial, lateral, and middle (Fig. 30–8). The route chosen is dictated by the orientation of distention in the joint. The important landmarks are Lister's tubercle (a palpable bone prominence on the distal dorsal radius) and the styloid process of the radius (the pointed prominence on the lateral aspect of the distal radius). The hand is placed in pronation

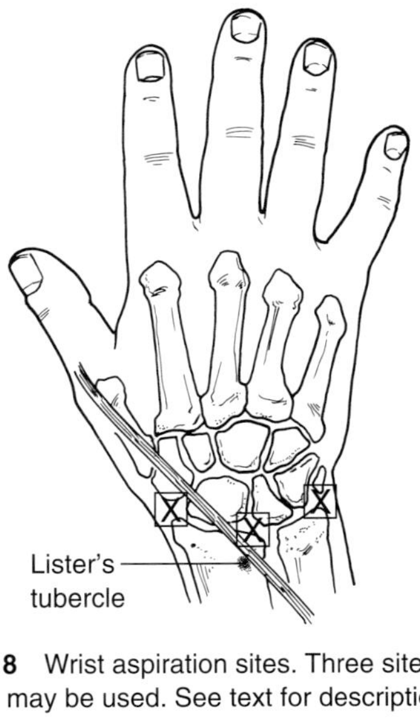

Figure 30–8 Wrist aspiration sites. Three sites (denoted by X) may be used. See text for descriptions.

with slight ulnar deviation; the middle site for needle entry is approximately 1 cm distal to Lister's tubercle even with the styloid process of the radius. The tendon of the extensor pollicis longus is to the radius side of the site. The lateral aspiration site is distal to the styloid of the radius and slightly dorsal, to avoid the radial artery. The medial aspiration site is just distal to the ulnar styloid but dorsal to the pisiform bone with the needle passing between the extensor carpi ulnaris and flexor carpi ulnaris.

Site for Finger Aspiration

Aspiration of the interphalangeal joints or the metacarpophalangeal joints uses a dorsal approach with a slight medial or lateral shift to avoid the extensor tendon (Fig. 30–9). The needle is inserted at approximately 15 degrees to the axis of the finger with slight traction to help widen the joint space.

Sites for Knee Aspiration

Several sites can be used (Fig. 30–10) to aspirate the knee. For an anterior approach, the knee is flexed to 90 degrees over a table edge; the needle is inserted through the patellar tendon, in the midline, about 1 cm distal to the lower pole of the patella. After passing through the tendon and infrapatellar fat pad, the needle will enter the intercondylar notch. This approach is said to be useful when the joint effusion is small. With noticeable effusions, a lateral approach can be used. The knee is extended and the needle is placed just below the superolateral corner of the patella, well proximal to the femoral-tibial joint line. Alternatively, a medial site can be used. With the knee flexed to 90 degrees, the needle entry site is located within the triangle formed by the patellar tendon, medial tibial plateau, and medial femoral condyle.

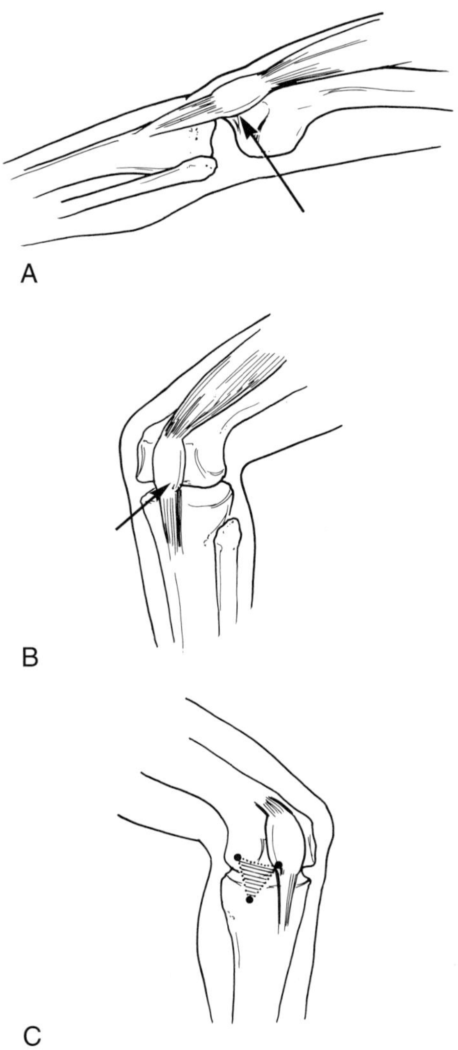

Figure 30–10 Knee aspiration sites. **A.** The lateral site below the superior lateral edge of the patella *(arrow)*. **B.** The infrapatellar tendon site *(arrow)*. **C.** Area of the medial site within the triangle formed by the infrapatellar tendon, the medial plateau of the tibia, and the medial femoral condyle.

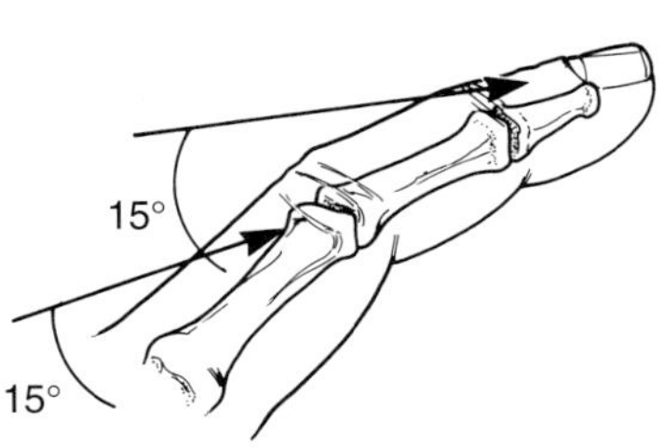

Figure 30–9 Method for finger joint aspiration. The aspirating needle is angled at about 15 degrees to the long axis of the extended finger to enter the skin on either side of the midline, avoiding the extensor tendon.

Sites for Ankle Aspiration

The ankle can be approached anteriorly from either the medial or lateral aspects (Fig. 30–11). An anteromedial approach is most common, using the site approximately 1 cm cephalad and lateral to the tip of the medial malleolus. The needle is introduced into the

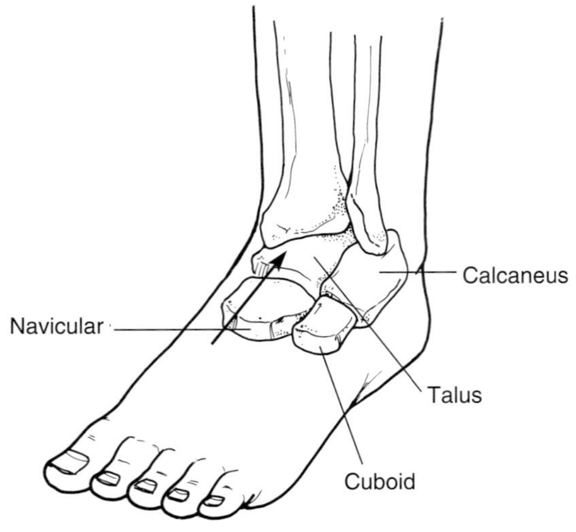

Figure 30–11 The anteromedial ankle aspiration site. The needle is placed into the sulcus between the talus and the distal tibia *(arrow)*.

space between the tibia and the talus from an angle perpendicular and directly anterior to the tibia. The needle should pass just medial to the tibialis anterior tendon. Dorsiflexion of the foot with inversion of the ankle allows this site to be easily located. The anterolateral aspiration site is 1 cm medial and cephalad of the lateral malleolus so that the needle, coming from directly anterior, enters the lateral sulcus between the articular surfaces of the talus and distal fibula.

Site for Toe Aspiration

As with fingers, a dorsal approach with either medial or lateral shift to avoid the extensor tendons is used.

SKIN BIOPSY

A simple way to perform a skin biopsy is with a punch biopsy device. These are available in a range of diameters (1–6 mm) as disposable devices. The materials needed are a sterile skin biopsy punch, povidone-iodine (1%) solution, sterile saline or 70% alcohol, local anesthetic, two 23- to 25-gauge 5/8-inch needles, 3-ml syringe, sterile 4 × 4 gauze pads, sterile specimen cup, fine sterile forceps, fine sterile scissors, suture material/needle, needle driver, and bandage tape.

After the area for biopsy is cleaned with povidone-iodine, residual solution is removed with either sterile saline or 70% alcohol. The site is anesthetized by slowly raising a small intradermal bleb to the side of the intended biopsy site (to minimize distortion of the skin's histological features by injected anesthetic), followed by infiltration of the subcutaneous tissues below the biopsy site. After cutaneous insensitivity has appeared at the biopsy site, the biopsy punch is inserted with a "screwing" motion into and through the skin to the depth of the flange at the base of the cylindrical blade. The biopsy punch is removed, and the circumscribed skin plug is elevated up and out of the wound with forceps. The pedicle of the plug is then snipped with fine sterile scissors. The biopsy specimen is then placed in a sterile specimen cup and processed as appropriate. If a 4- to 6-mm biopsy punch is used, a single suture is placed to close the wound followed by application of a sterile bandage.

INJECTIONS

The routine health care of the normal child continues to require both intramuscular (vaccinations and occasionally antibiotics) and intradermal (Mantoux test) injections. Although injections are not frequently performed by the pediatrician, the questions about how, why, where, and when almost always come back to the physician for answers.

Sites for Injections

Whereas any muscle group can theoretically be used for intramuscular injections, in practice, three areas are routinely used: the deltoid muscle, the quadriceps muscle group of the anterolateral thigh, and the gluteus muscle group in the buttock. Typically, the deltoid muscle has little overlying fat or subcutaneous tissue, which makes intramuscular injection of materials relatively easy. In some instances, failure to deposit injected materials intramuscularly (as with hepatitis B vaccine) has led to immunization failure. The quadriceps muscle group is the area often used in children or uncooperative patients. Injecting the quadriceps muscles minimizes the risk of either intravenous injection or striking the femur with the needle. The gluteus group also presents a large muscle mass for use, but the variable amounts of fat and subcutaneous tissue that frequently overlie it make intramuscular deposition less predictable. With the gluteus group, care must also be taken to avoid the vascular and neural anatomy of the region, especially in young children.

Pain with Intramuscular Injections

Pain at injection sites can be either immediate or delayed. Immediate pain can be the result of mechanical trauma caused by needle penetration of the tissue or sudden distention of tissue by injected fluid. These mechanical traumas can be minimized by using a sharp needle of the smallest diameter that will allow fluid flow, by ensuring that no material for injection is in the needle at the time of injection, by using a minimal volume for injection (≤ 2 ml at any single injection site), and by avoiding rapid injection of material. Abnormal tissue sensitivity due to diseased muscle or previous injection into the same area can also cause immediate pain. Use of alternative injection sites for subsequent injections minimizes pain. Injection of materials that are irritants can also cause acute, immediate pain during an intramuscular injection. Failure to remove antiseptic (e.g., alcohol) from the injection site or administration of materials with acid or alkaline pH, hypertonicity or hypotonicity can result in acute pain. Awareness of the irritant qualities (Table 30–2) of some injected materials is useful to both parent and pediatrician for anticipating complaints about pain.

Delayed pain occurring some time after an injection has been given can be the result of local infection, sterile inflammation or necrosis, antigen-antibody reactions, or local muscle sensitivity or spasm.

There are many potential complications of injections: inadvertent intra-arterial or intravenous injection; infection from contaminated injection material; neural injury (typically the sciatic nerve after gluteal injections); local atrophy; local necrosis or calcification due to injection of irritants. To minimize the risk of complications, the following points (Hughes and Buescher, 1980) should be considered.

1. Select the safest agent for injection.
2. Choose the proper injection site.
3. Establish the anatomical landmarks.
4. Place therapeutic efficacy and safety above modesty and convenience.
5. Cleanse the skin thoroughly.
6. Alternate sites for subsequent injections.
7. Aspirate before injection.
8. Avoid tracking the drug into superficial tissues.
9. Use a needle of adequate length to reach the intended injection site.

Intramuscular Injections

The materials needed include skin cleanser (70% alcohol, benzalkonium chloride [Zephiran]), 22-gauge 1-inch needle, 2×2 sterile gauze pads or cotton, and a sterile 3-ml syringe. Three sites are usually considered for intramuscular injection: the gluteal muscles, either ventral gluteal (von Hochstetter's site) or dorsogluteal (Figs. 30–12 and 30–13); the

Table 30–2 Medications Associated with Local Irritation/Pain at the Injection Site

Meperidine
Erythromycin
Tetracyclines
Calcium gluconate
Benzathine penicillin
Hydroxyzine
Cephalosporins (first generation)
Prochlorperazine
Calcium chloride
Diphenhydramine HCl
Ceftriaxone
Varicella-zoster immune globulin
Thiopental sodium
Thiamine HCl

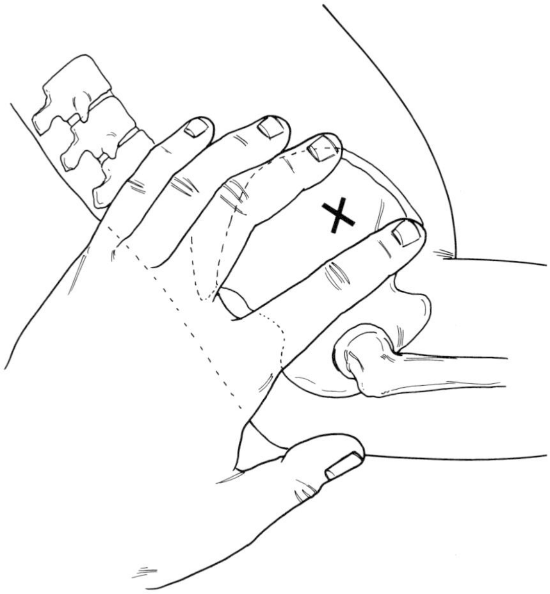

Figure 30–12 Ventral gluteal muscle site for intramuscular injection. X denotes the injection site within the triangle formed by the fingers on the anterior superior iliac tubercle and the superior iliac crest.

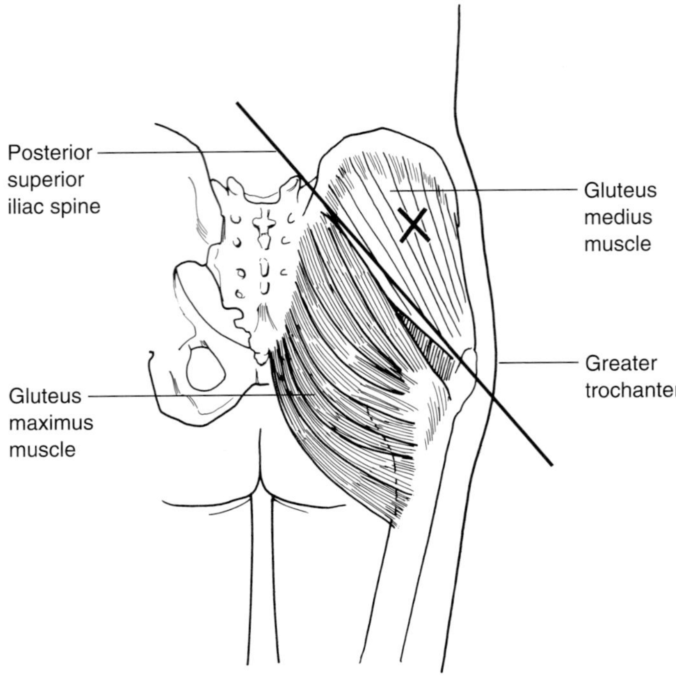

Figure 30–13 Dorsogluteal intramuscular injection site. X denotes the injection site in the gluteus medius muscle.

deltoid muscle (Fig. 30–14); or the vastus lateralis muscle (Fig. 30–15). The ventral gluteal muscle site is in the middle of the triangle formed by placing the index finger on the anterior superior iliac tubercle and the middle finger on the superior iliac crest. The dorsogluteal site is located in the upper outer region of the buttock (the region above the line between the posterior superior iliac spine and the greater trochanter). The injection is made perpendicular to the table or bed, with the patient in a full prone position. The deltoid muscle injection

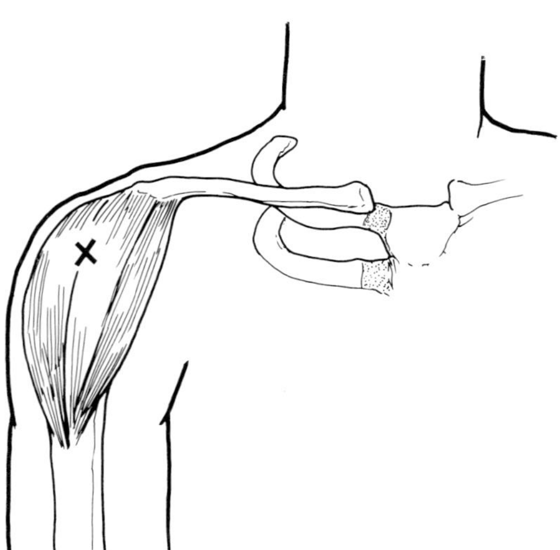

Figure 30–14 Deltoid muscle site for intramuscular injection. X denotes the injection site in the proximal third of the muscle.

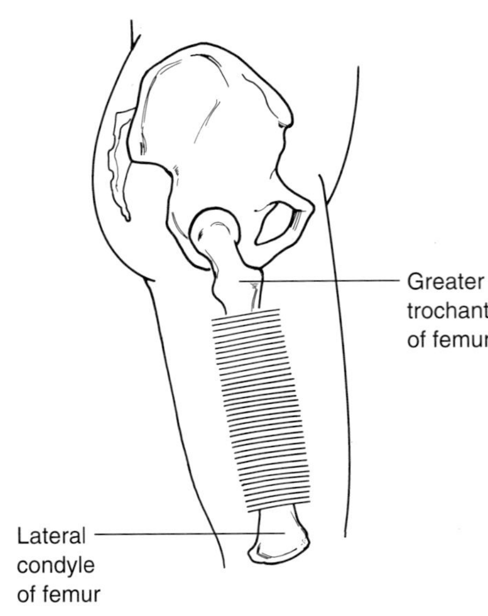

Figure 30–15 Vastus lateralis site for intramuscular injections. Hatched area shows the region used for injections.

site is in the upper third of the muscle, about two fingerbreadths below the acromion. The quadriceps muscle site is in the vastus lateralis in a narrow (finger-breadth) strip at the middle third of the femur, along the line between the greater trochanter and the lateral femoral condyle. Which site is used is based on the patient's cooperativeness, age, habitus, and number of injections given. In infants and small children, the deltoid and gluteus muscles are relatively underdeveloped, so the lateral quadriceps site is typically used.

After the skin is cleaned with antiseptic and allowed to dry, the belly of the target muscle is secured between the thumb and forefinger if possible. The needle is then plunged perpendicularly through the skin with a single quick motion to a depth of about 2 to 3 cm for the deltoid, 2 to 4 cm for the vastus lateralis or gluteus. The plunger is withdrawn slightly to ensure that the needle tip is not in a vascular space. If return of blood is noted, remove the needle without injecting, change the injecting needle, and choose a new site for injection. The material is injected with steady pressure for 3 to 5 seconds. After injection, the needle is withdrawn in a single movement and pressure applied with a sterile gauze or cotton pad.

Subcutaneous Injections

For subcutaneous injections, the method is similar. After the skin is prepared aseptically, it is pierced with a 1-inch needle held at a 30- to 45-degree angle for a distance of about 1 cm with a single smooth motion. The syringe plunger is withdrawn a bit to check for return of blood; if no return is seen, the material is injected with steady pressure for 3 to 5 seconds. The needle is then withdrawn in a single smooth motion, and pressure is applied to the site with a sterile gauze pad or cotton ball.

Intradermal Injections

After the skin is aseptically prepared, the material for injection (typically a 0.1-ml volume) is drawn into a tuberculin syringe and a 25- to 27-gauge 5/8-inch needle is attached. Because of its size and design, the tuberculin syringe is optimal for generating the pressure needed to inject materials intradermally. Use of other syringe sizes for this procedure dramatically increases the difficulty in getting the injection into the intradermal space. When the syringe and needle are held almost parallel with the skin (bevel up), the skin is just barely picked up with the needle tip, and the needle is advanced slowly until the bevel has fully entered the skin. Steadily inject the material for 3 to 5 seconds (there will be significant resistance), then withdraw the needle. A true intradermal injection often burns slightly as it splits skin layers to produce a "peau d'orange" pattern at the injection site.

FRACTURES, CASTS, AND TRACTION

Although nearly all management of skeletal fractures has become the responsibility of the orthopedic specialist, fractures, casts, and traction are common enough in children that a working knowledge of some of their aspects is appropriate for the pediatrician.

Children's bones often fracture differently from those of adults (greenstick and torus fractures, plastic deformities) and show rapid healing and greater remodeling ability. Fractures in childhood have a broad spectrum of severity and complication. On one hand, simple closed fractures without displacement or neurovascular compromise require only immobilization to allow complete healing. On the other, open, comminuted fractures with bleeding, tissue devitalization, or neurovascular compromise require an integrated, comprehensive approach to treatment and management to optimize outcome. Casts are the mainstay of simple fracture management, providing an "exoskeleton" for the immobilization, splinting, and protection of the fracture. For effective immobilization, the cast must extend a joint above and below the fracture. The interior should be padded to prevent friction injury. To apply a cast, the plaster of Paris bandage is wound evenly around the limb, overlapping half of the previous bandage strip, with the same tension applied throughout. Four layers of plaster in a circular cast are usually adequate for a non–weight-bearing cast. The circulation in the limb should be examined immediately after casting and repeatedly in the following 24 hours. Complaints consistent with neurovascular compromise should be evaluated carefully: pain (either spontaneous or on passive motion) or paresthesia, the appearance of pallor, loss of pulse, or the appearance of paralysis. If emergency cast removal at home is indicated, plaster casts can be softened by soaking in water and removed by either unrolling or cutting the bandage. With time, as edema decreases or muscle mass wastes, casts can loosen. Loose casts do not perform their intended function of immobilization and should be removed and replaced rather than wedged or shimmed, which can result in pressure sores.

Traction is used to achieve alignment and prevent rotation or angulation of fragments. Skin traction, applied by bandaging over intact skin, has the major danger of circulatory embarrassment. Injury from tight bandages can range from superficial decubitus ulcers to ischemic myonecrosis. Complaints of pain, cyanosis, swelling, or pallor require prompt removal of the skin traction bandages and inspection of the skin. Skeletal traction, using either osseous transfixion wires or pins, carries the risk of infection at the pin site unless lateral movement of the wire/pin is prevented and the site is protected from manipulation by the child. Use of either skin or skeletal traction has the disadvantage of requiring prolonged hospitalization. Not surprisingly, alternatives to traction are being examined. Some alternatives include early spica cast placement in the situation of femoral shaft fractures and the use of internal or external fixation devices in a variety of fractures. Whereas some of these treatments require open procedures, the costs of surgery plus several days of recuperation are still less than the costs of traction, and the results and complication rates appear to be similar.

LOCAL CARE

Support/Bandaging

For the pediatrician, the bandage is a way to keep dressings in place, cover unprotected or healing wounds, minimize body part movement, or maintain pressure at an anatomical site. For children, it is a mark of distinction and courage. For any of these purposes, it should be neatly, efficiently, and professionally applied. Generally, four types of materials are used in bandaging. Sterile gauze pads are used to keep the wound clean, absorb drainage, and cushion the wound. Porous gauze wrapping, either nonstretching (Kling gauze) or somewhat elastic (Kerlix gauze), is used to keep gauze pads in position. Elastic bandage material (Ace bandage, Elastoplast bandage) provides support or pressure, and tape (adhesive tape, paper tape) is needed to keep everything in place. Bandaging is as much an art form as a science. The methods described here are only examples of how specific body parts can be bandaged.

Forearm sling

The traditional arm sling can be fashioned by diagonally folding a square sheet of cloth or sheeting into a triangle (Fig. 30–16). The midpoint of the diagonal fold is placed un-

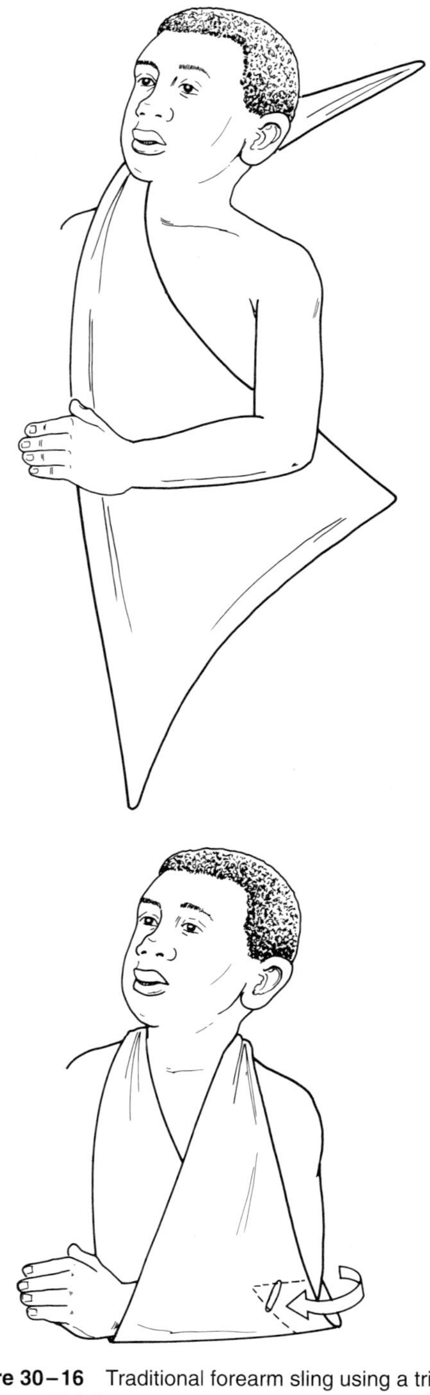

Figure 30–16 Traditional forearm sling using a triangular piece of fabric.

der the wrist, and its free ends are carried behind the neck and tied. The point of the triangle at the elbow is folded over anteriorly and pinned to the front of the sling.

Alternatively, a sling that both supports the forearm and holds it relatively immobilized against the lower chest can be fashioned from stockinette (Fig. 30–17). Starting with a 5- to 6-foot length of stockinette, an opening is made about 2 feet from one end and a second opening is placed farther along the stockinette, at about the patient's shoulder-wrist length. The arm to be supported is passed through the first hole and through the stockinette until the hand passes out of the stockinette through the second hole. The stockinette that extends beyond the hand and wrist is carried around the waist and attached to the stockinette covering the distal upper arm. The empty length of stockinette above the shoulder is carried around the back of the neck and down the chest to be attached to the stockinette covering the wrist.

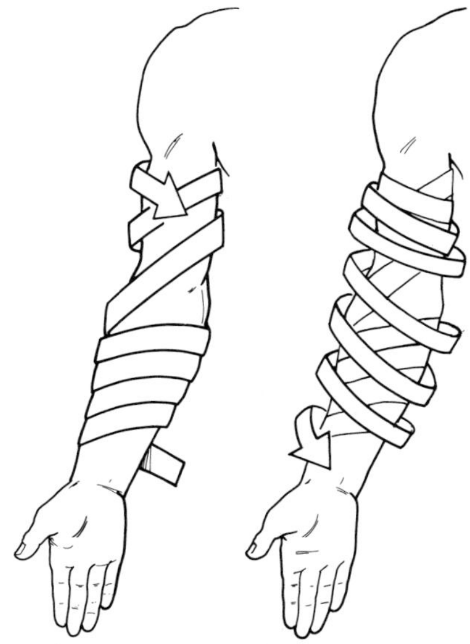

Figure 30–18 Method for applying a bandage to the elbow and arm.

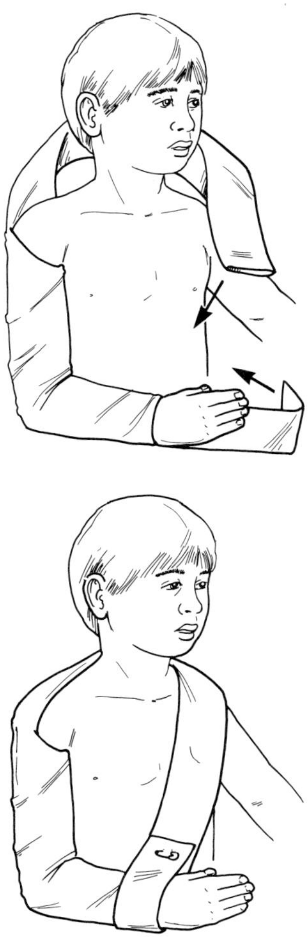

Figure 30–17 Stockinette forearm sling that can be used for both forearm support and limitation of movement.

Elbow bandage

Using 1- to 2-inch-wide gauze bandage, wrap the forearm in a spiral from wrist to elbow, cross the antecubital fossa diagonally, and continue the spiral up to the axilla (Fig. 30–18). At the axilla, reverse the spiral down the arm, cross the antecubital fossa on the opposite diagonal, and continue the spiral wrap to the wrist. Repeat the wrap up and down the arm until it is covered. Reinforce with bandage tape.

Hand and wrist bandage

Using 1- to 2-inch-wide gauze, begin the wrap over the dorsum of the hand, across the palm, over the dorsum, and spiral up over the wrist and distal forearm (Fig. 30–19). Reverse direction at the midforearm and spiral back down to the starting point. Repeat the wrap until the wrist is covered and then secure with tape.

Finger bandage

Effective finger bandaging can be achieved with either gauze wrapping or tubular gauze. If gauze wrap is used (Fig. 30–20), bring 0.5-inch gauze bandage under the wrist, over the dorsum of the hand, down the length of the injured finger, over the fingertip, and back up the

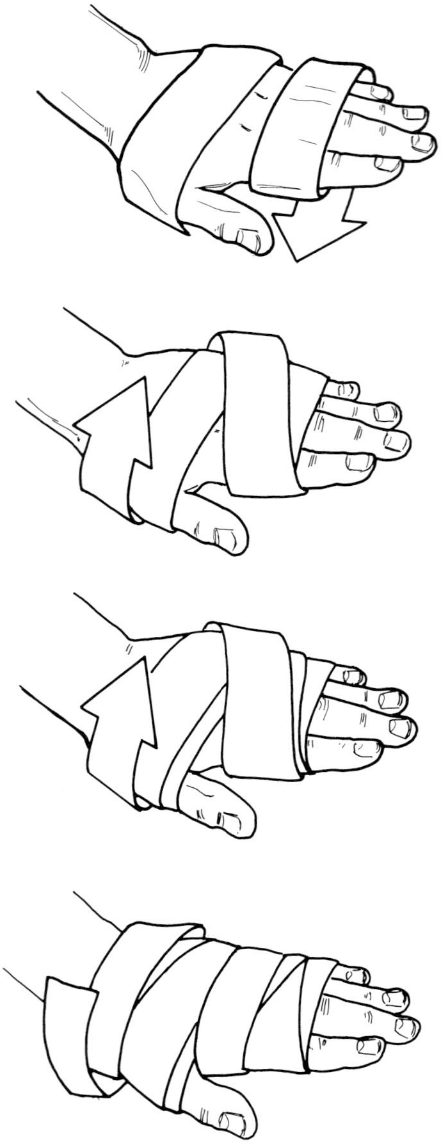

Figure 30–19 Method for applying a bandage to the hand and wrist.

palmar surface of the finger to the base. Spiral wrap the gauze from the base of the finger to the tip and back down, then over the dorsum of the hand and around the wrist. Tie the free ends to keep the bandage in place.

If tubular gauze is to be used (Fig. 30–21), slip 8 to 10 finger lengths of tubular gauze over the cylindrical applicator (almost any cylindrical tube that is about three times the finger diameter can be used if an applicator is not available). Place the applicator and gauze over the finger, slip the free edge of the gauze onto the base of the finger, and withdraw the cylinder. As the cylinder is removed, the gauze is fed onto the finger. At the fingertip, twist the cylinder tube 180 to 360 degrees around the axis of the finger and advance the cylinder down the finger again to cover it with a second layer of gauze. At the finger base, twist 90 to 180 degrees and withdraw the cylinder over the finger again. Repeat the process three or four times. With the applicator at the finger base, remove the remaining gauze from the applicator. Cut the remaining gauze on opposite sides along its long axis to form two tails, carry the free ends around the wrist, and tie them together to secure the bandage.

Thigh bandage

Encircle the distal thigh once or twice with 1- to 2-inch gauze wrap and spiral it up the thigh

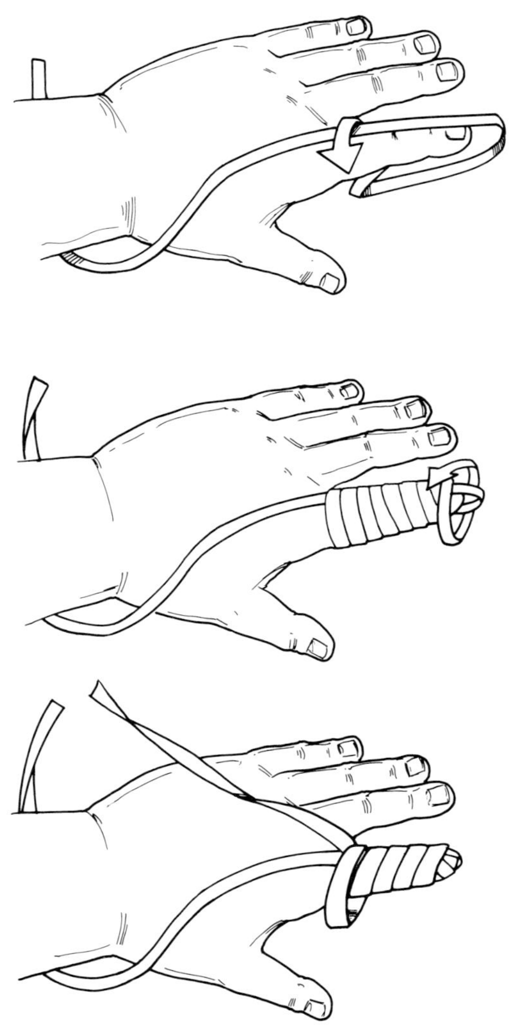

Figure 30–20 Method for applying a gauze wrap bandage to a finger.

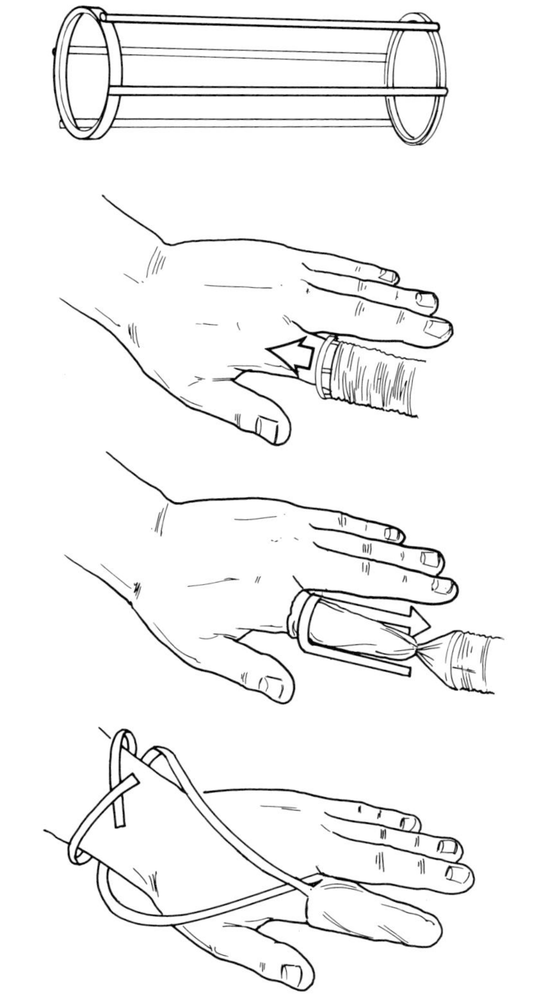

Figure 30–21 Method for applying a tubular gauze bandage to a finger. The device shown at the top is used to hold tubular gauze during application.

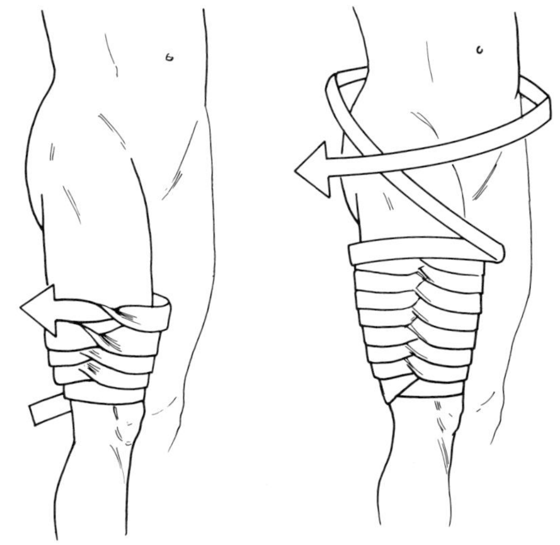

Figure 30–22 Method for applying a bandage to the thigh.

to the groin (Fig. 30–22). With every or every other wraparound, twist the gauze wrap 180 degrees to create reverse turns along the way. At the groin, extend the bandage to wrap around the waist several times and secure the free end with tape for anchorage.

Knee bandage

Using 1- to 2-inch gauze, begin a spiral wrap below the knee, carry it diagonally across the knee (below the patella), and continue the spiral wrap to the midproximal femur (Fig. 30–23). Reverse the direction of the wrap, cross the knee on the opposite diagonal below

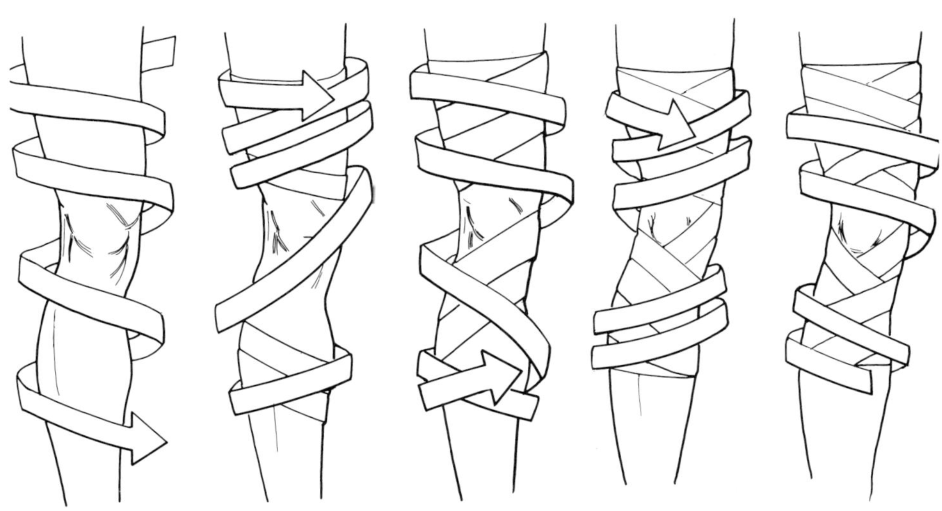

Figure 30–23 Method for applying a knee bandage.

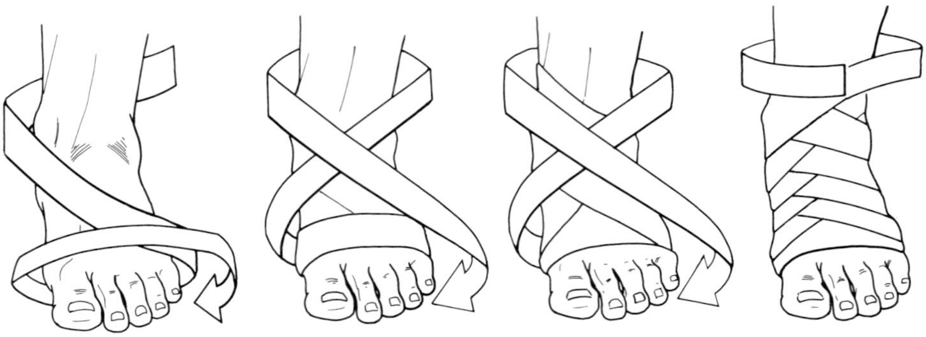

Figure 30–24 Method for applying a foot bandage.

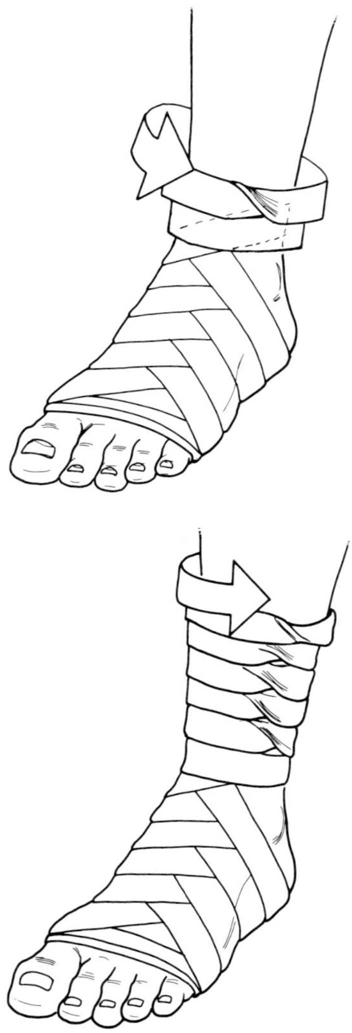

Figure 30–25 Method for applying a bandage to the ankle and calf. This bandage is an extension of the foot bandage shown in Figure 30–24.

the patella, and continue down to the starting point. Repeat the process again, this time crossing the knee above the patella both on the way up and (on the opposite diagonal) on the way down.

Foot bandage

Using 1- to 2-inch gauze, begin behind the ankle, cross the medial ankle, and pass the bandage diagonally across the dorsum of the foot toward the toes (Fig. 30–24). Next, wrap under the sole, over the base of the phalanges, back under the sole, across the dorsum on the reverse diagonal, and around the back of the ankle to the end. Repeat the process, but with each cycle, advance the wrapping from toes to heel until the area is covered.

Ankle and calf bandage

Bandage the foot as in Figure 30–24, but extend the bandage above the ankle and up the calf with a spiral wrap. At every or every other wraparound, half-twist the bandage to allow contour changes (Fig. 30–25).

Chest and abdomen bandage

Wounds of the chest or abdomen are best covered with noncircumferential bandages. Use short pieces of elastic adhesive tape, applied perpendicular to the long axis of the body, with each overlapping about half of the previous strip (Fig. 30–26).

Rib bandage

To bandage/support a fractured rib, drape a piece of muslin over one shoulder and diagonally across the back and chest as a founda-

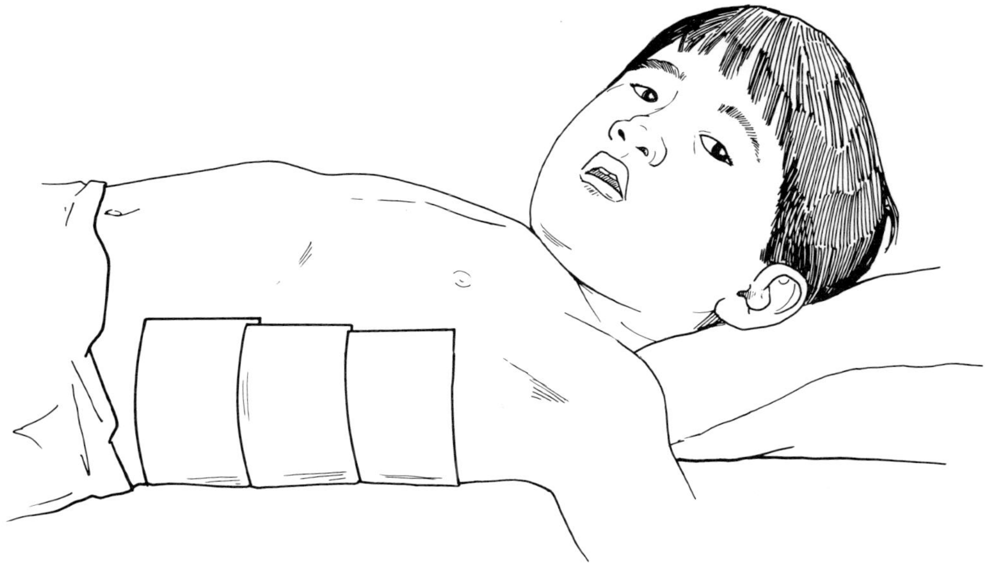

Figure 30–26 Method for applying a chest/abdomen bandage.

tion. Wrap over the muslin with elastic bandage, making sure not to compromise respiration. Start above the muslin and work down with about 50% overlap of each spiral. Secure the spiral wrap to the muslin foundation with safety pins both front and back (Fig. 30–27).

Scalp bandage

To bandage the scalp (Fig. 30–28), pass the bandage material from side to side over the crown of the head, beginning anteriorly and progressing rearward. Each side-to-side pass should overlap the previous one by about half. After the crown is covered, encircle the head (forehead to occiput) several times with bandage material, securing the ends of the side-to-side strips under the encircling bandage. Attach the end of the encircling bandage with tape.

Eye bandage

Place a sterile, soft gauze pad over the socket and hold in place either with tape (do not shave eyebrows) or by wrapping around the head with gauze bandage. Avoid applying pressure to the globe.

BURNS

Burns occur commonly enough in children that familiarity with the proper procedures for burn care is appropriate for every pediatrician. Determining whether referral for specialized care of a burn is necessary depends on the severity, extent and location of the burn. For children, second-degree burns over more than 10% body surface area or any third-degree burns are considered severe injuries. They usually require hospitalization and large-volume intravenous fluid resuscitation. Therefore, burns of this magnitude are usually referred for specialized care. "Minor" burns, such as large first-degree burns (e.g., severe sunburn) or small (< 10% body surface area) second-degree burns (blistering) can usually be handled in the outpatient setting and do not typically require intravenous fluid resuscitation. However, if such minor burns involve the hands, feet, face, perineum, major joints, or genitalia, referral for specialized management is usually appropriate.

The care of a minor burn requires sterile saline, a sterile 10-ml syringe with a 22-gauge 5/8-inch needle, povidone-iodine or silver sulfadiazine (Silvadene) ointment, petrolatum gauze bandage, sterile 4 × 4 gauze pads, and rolled gauze mesh. Cold should be applied to the burned area as soon as possible after the injury to minimize extension. After the burn has cooled, it is cleaned gently with sterile saline, rinsed, and dried. If intact blisters are present, they should be left undisturbed. Opening or aspirating blisters only increases the risks for development of infection. If the burn

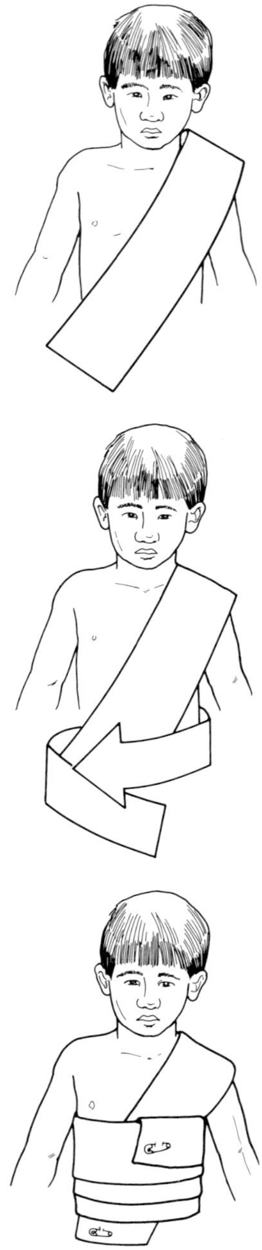

Figure 30–27 Procedure for applying a bandage for rib support.

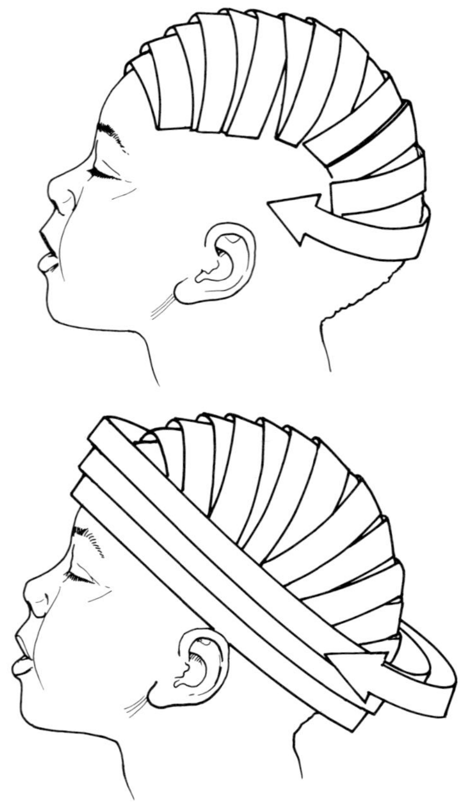

Figure 30–28 Procedure for applying a scalp bandage.

is denuded, the area is covered with petrolatum gauze (after the excess petrolatum is removed by wringing the gauze between sterile gauze pads). Alternatively, a thin layer of silver sulfadiazine ointment can be applied over the burn to keep the overlying bandage from drying and sticking to the burn surface. Silver sulfadiazine is a mild antibiotic and therefore decreases the risk of infection. After the petrolatum gauze or ointment is applied, the burn is covered with loose gauze mesh (4 × 4 gauze pads opened out and trimmed to size), which is secured with a bulky wrapping of rolled gauze (for an extremity) or by taping 4 × 4 pads over the mesh. If blisters have ruptured and are fragmented, they should be gently debrided before petrolatum gauze or silver sulfadiazine ointment is applied. The dressing should be changed and the wound site inspected daily for evidence of infection. Some experts recommend a brief (2- to 3-day) course of oral penicillin treatment to minimize the risk of streptococcal infection (Phillips et al, 1989).

References

Anderson AB, Colecchi C, et al: Local anesthesia in pediatric patients: topical TAC versus lidocaine. *Ann Emerg Med,* 19:519–522, 1990.

Bonadio WA, Wagner V: Efficacy of TAC topical anesthetic for repair of pediatric lacerations. *Am J Dis Child,* 142:203–205, 1988.

Burckert GJ, White TJ, Siegle RL: Rectal thiopental

versus an intramuscular cocktail for sedating children before computerized tomography. *Am J Hosp Pharm,* 37:222–224, 1980.

Cook BA, Bass JW, et al: Sedation of children for technical procedures: current standard of practice. *Clin Pediatr,* 31:137–142, 1992.

Greenberg SB, Faerber EN, et al: High-dose chloral hydrate sedation for children undergoing MR imaging: safety and efficacy in relation to age. *AJR,* 161:639–641, 1993.

Guidelines for monitoring and management of pediatric patients during and after sedation for diagnostic and therapeutic procedures. *Pediatrics,* 89: 1110–1115, 1992.

Halperin DL, Koren G, et al: Topical skin anesthesia for venous, subcutaneous drug reservoir and lumbar punctures in children. *Pediatrics,* 84: 281–284, 1989.

Hughes, WT, Buescher, ES: Injections. In *Pediatric Procedures.* Philadelphia, WB Saunders, 1980, p 149.

Latson LA, Cheatham JP, et al: Midazolam nose drops for outpatient echocardiography sedation in infants. *Am Heart J,* 121:209–210, 1991.

McKay W, Morris R, Mushlin P: Sodium bicarbonate attenuates pain on skin infiltration with lidocaine, with or without epinephrine. *Anesth Analg,* 66:572–574, 1987.

Phillips LG, Robson MC, Heggers JP: Treating minor burns: ice, grease or what? *Postgrad Medicine,* 85:219–231, 1989.

Sandler ES, Weyman C, et al: Midazolam vs. fentanyl as premedication for painful procedures in children with cancer. *Pediatrics,* 89:631–634, 1992.

Snodgrass WR, Dodge WF: Lytic/“DPT” cocktail: time for rational and safe alternatives. *Pediatr Clin North Am,* 36:1285–1291, 1989.

Teasdale G, Jennett B: Assessment of coma and impaired consciousness: a practical scale. *Lancet,* 2:81–84, 1974.

Tobias JD, Phipps S, et al: Oral ketamine to alleviate the distress of invasive procedures in pediatric oncology patients. *Pediatrics,* 90:537–541, 1992.

Young AC, Shorthall A, et al: Lignocaine-prilocaine cream for lumbar puncture. *Lancet,* 2: 1533–1534, 1987.

Zeltzer LK, Jay SM, Fisher DM: The management of pain associated with pediatric procedures. *Pediatr Clin North Am,* 36:941–996, 1989.

Chapter 31

Sexual Abuse

Kevin Coulter

In the past decade, the sexual abuse of children and adolescents has become a more frequently recognized form of child abuse. As recognition has increased, there is greater pressure on health care providers to examine alleged victims to uncover evidence that, indeed, abuse has occurred. Sexual abuse is a complex phenomenon with serious social, legal, and medical implications. The approach to the victim of sexual abuse, therefore, must be multidisciplinary. A coordinated team composed of individuals from social services, the local child protection agency, the police department, the district attorney's office, and medicine can ensure that an allegation of sexual abuse is fully and efficiently investigated with a minimum of trauma to the child and family. In many locales, these teams have been centralized around child abuse referral centers where individuals with special training conduct an investigation as well as provide counseling for the victim.

The elements of the medical evaluation of sexually abused children are the

1. medical interview
2. physical examination
3. evaluation for sexually transmitted diseases (STDs)
4. evidence collection
5. treatment (e.g., injuries, STDs)
6. documentation of findings
7. provisions for medical follow-up and counseling

INDICATIONS

Sexual abuse can present in many different ways and settings. The need for and the extent of a medical evaluation should be individualized to the particular patient. For example, an adolescent who alleges a recent sexual assault should be promptly interviewed, examined, and offered prophylaxis against STDs and pregnancy. A toddler, however, may be brought to a physician's office because a certain "sexualized" behavior raises concerns of prior sexual molestation. Observation of the child's play by a therapist and further evaluation of the family may be necessary before the need for an examination is known.

Children should be referred to local physicians or nurse practitioners with experience in examining sexual abuse victims. These examiners need to be available on an on-call basis to manage emergency cases. A reasonable triage system for determining which cases require immediate attention is as follows:

Immediate evaluation indicated:

1. Sexual assault occurred within 72 hours of reporting.
2. Complaints suggest genital injury (pain, bleeding, discharge).
3. The safety of the child from further abuse cannot be ensured.

Evaluation can be deferred to a scheduled appointment:

1. Sexual assault occurred more than 72 hours before reporting.
2. No signs or symptoms of genital injury are observed.
3. The child is safe from further abuse.

EQUIPMENT/SUPPLIES

The examination of a child resulting from suspicions of sexual abuse should take place in a setting that is comfortable for the child. Busy, impersonal emergency departments are not conducive to interviewing and examining already frightened and traumatized children. Specified areas for the evaluation of sexual abuse victims that are quiet, contain toys and art equipment, and have two-way mirrors for observing interviews have proved to be helpful in comforting children during a difficult process.

Children undergoing an examination because of sexual abuse require a full general examination, and thus the usual instruments for such are required (stethoscope, otoscope, ophthalmoscope).

A detailed examination of the prepubertal girl's genitalia and of the anus in all children requires adequate lighting and magnification. This can be adequately achieved with an otoscope. Many child abuse centers employ the use of a colposcope for examination of the anus and the external female genitalia. This instrument provides excellent lighting and magnification, and a camera attachment allows photographic documentation of genital and anal injury.

The following supplies necessary for detecting the presence of STDs should be available:

1. Calcium alginate (nasopharyngeal) swabs for culturing
2. Culture media for the detection of *Neisseria gonorrhoeae, Chlamydia trachomatis*, and herpes simplex
3. Gram stain, saline, and potassium hydroxide for the microscopic evaluation of anogenital discharge

Some examiners employ a special dye, toluidine blue, to look for occult genital injury. This dye can detect previously unobserved abrasions by staining the nuclei of cells in the subepidermal layers of the skin.

In cases of acute sexual assault, the examiner may need to collect specimens for forensic analysis. Most hospitals have "rape kits" that contain the swabs, combs, and envelopes necessary to collect and package these specimens so that a proper chain of evidence is maintained. An air dryer is necessary to dry swabs collected for seminal fluid analysis before sealing in an envelope. Health care providers conducting sexual assault examinations must familiarize themselves with evidentiary collection protocols required by the local crime laboratory.

PREPARATION OF THE FAMILY AND PATIENT

A disclosure of sexual abuse by a child usually results in great anxiety and turmoil within the victim and family. An empathic and supportive approach on the part of the health care provider is key to a thorough medical evaluation.

The child and family should be given a careful explanation of the interview and the examination. Allowing young children to see and feel the culture swabs can help allay their fears of intrusive procedures. Children should be given a sense of control by reassuring them that they have the right to stop the examination if they are frightened or uncomfortable.

Consent for the examination from the family is required, unless a parent is thought to be the perpetrator. Children older than 12 years in most states have the right to give consent for their own examinations. The family should be ensured privacy and an explanation given them as to which agencies receive the results of the examination.

METHODS

Medical Interview

The interview of a child about whom there are concerns of sexual abuse should include a general history as for any other patient. A history of previous anogenital trauma, surgery, or disease should be sought. Adolescent patients should be asked for a careful menstrual history as well as any history of STDs, pregnancy, and contraception, and the date of the last consensual intercourse is noted.

The medical interview is a critical component of the evaluation of sexual abuse. The interviewer must be comfortable with children and knowledgeable in conducting forensic interviews. Whereas a complete discussion of the art of interviewing abused children is beyond the scope of this chapter, the following points are emphasized:

1. The interviewer's questions should proceed from general to specific. In attempting to elicit the actual sexual acts that occurred, the use of drawings of human figures or anatomically correct dolls may be a more comfortable way for children to demonstrate how they were touched.
2. Questions should generally be open ended and nonleading, although this is not always practical with young children.
3. The interviewer should appear calm and interested in the child but not shocked at what the child divulges. Acknowledging how difficult it is to discuss sexual acts and providing assurance that the child will be kept safe in the future are appropriate in supporting the child.
4. Accurate documentation of the interview is essential. Audio or video tapes of interviews are helpful because they more reliably capture the emotional state of the child.

The reader is referred to the bibliography at the end of this chapter for more complete discussions of interviewing.

Physical Examination

The timing of the physical examination depends on the need for collecting physical evidence and the medical condition of the child. Those patients who are victims of recent sexual assault (within 72 hours) or who have signs or symptoms of anogenital injury should be evaluated immediately.

Sexual abuse examinations include a complete examination of the body. Careful inspection for signs of nongenital injury are important in the care of the patient as well as for establishing the nonconsensual nature of the act in the adolescent patient.

The examiner should be familiar with the range of normal findings of the prepubertal female genitalia and the anus of children in general. The reader is referred to the studies of McCann et al and Berenson et al in the bibliography for further details.

The genitalia of the prepubertal girl should be examined in both the supine and knee-chest positions (Fig. 31–1). Examine the inguinal areas for abnormal adenopathy. Examine the perineum and labia for any injuries or signs of infection (e.g., condylomata acuminata).

In the supine position, gentle traction on the labia majora with thumb and forefinger exposes the hymen, vaginal opening, and distal portion of the vagina. If the child is too anxious on separation from a parent for the examiner to adequately visualize the genitalia, the child can be examined in the parent's lap. The parent can gently abduct the child's hips and

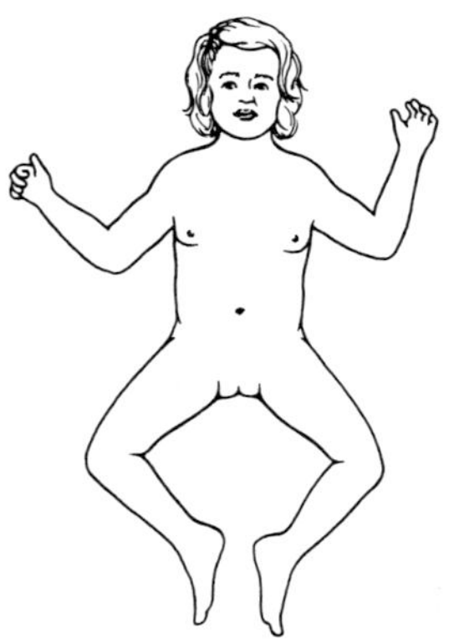

A

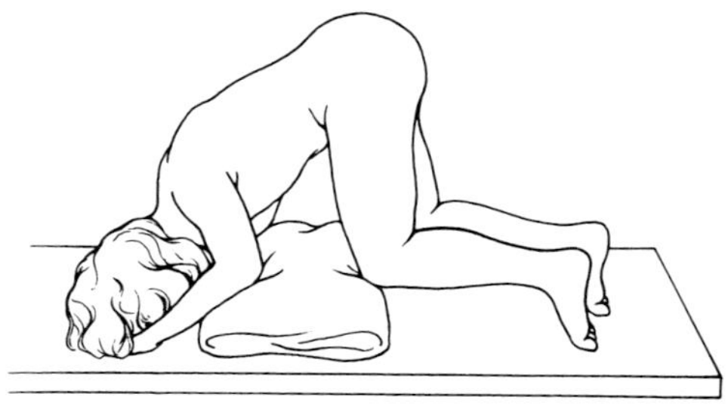

B

Figure 31–1 **A.** Supine position for genital examination. **B.** Knee-chest position for genital examination. (Redrawn from Grossman M, Dieckmann R [eds]: *Pediatric Emergency Medicine: A Clinician's Reference.* Philadelphia, JB Lippincott, 1991, p 591.)

Table 31-1 Medical Findings in Sexually Abused Children

Female Genitalia
Acute
Ecchymoses; abrasions; lacerations of perineum, labia, vestibule, hymen
Chronic
Focal loss of hymenal tissue along posterior rim of hymen
Diffuse loss of hymenal tissue ("absent hymen")
Scar tissue on hymen, labia, perineum
Male/Female Anus
Acute
Perianal swelling, erythema, abrasions, lacerations, bruises
Chronic
Patulent anal sphincter, perianal scarring
Male Genitalia
Acute
Bruising, erythema, lacerations, bite marks on penis or scrotum
Other
Presence of seminal fluid or sperm on or within children

even retract the outer labia. The hymen can then be examined for any signs of acute or old trauma (Table 31–1). In some prepubertal girls, further examination in the knee-chest position is necessary to evaluate suspicious findings. In this position, the child rests her head on her arms and, with her buttocks in the air, allows her abdomen to relax downward. The gluteal folds are then pressed upward and laterally to expose the hymen. Some children may be too anxious in this position and can be examined in the lateral recumbent position. Abnormal findings can then be photographed through a colposcope for documentation.

In prepubertal girls, an external genital examination is usually adequate. If there is concern of intravaginal injury that may require treatment (e.g., laceration, perforation), an internal examination under general anesthesia is indicated. Adolescent patients should routinely have a speculum examination after sexual assault.

The anus and perianal tissue can best be examined in the knee-chest or lateral recumbent position. As in the examination of the hymen, the examiner must be familiar with acute and chronic injuries that can occur after anal penetration during sexual abuse (Table 31–1). Rarely, proctoscopy may be necessary if there is rectal bleeding without an easily visible source after a sexual assault. As in the genital examination, abnormal anal findings can be photographed through a colposcope.

Evaluation for Sexually Transmitted Diseases

An evaluation for the presence of STDs is a major component of the examination of the sexually abused child or adolescent. The finding of an STD in a child may indicate prior sexual contact and thus has both medical and legal implications. Table 31–2 lists the recommended tests for STDs in sexually abused children. Not every child in whom suspicions of sexual abuse are raised requires STD testing. Children who give a history of or are suspected of having had genital-genital, oral-genital, or oral-anal contact or who have any symptoms of an STD should be tested. Obviously, in many children, particularly those who are preverbal, the examiner cannot ascertain the true risk of an STD. One should be more conservative, therefore, in testing preverbal children.

The timing of the examination also determines the need for STD testing. In the preadolescent child, if the examination occurs within 1 to 2 days of a single episode of sexual abuse, STD testing can be postponed for 1 to 2 weeks to allow completion of the various incubation periods. This may also be done in the adolescent who has not had prior sexual contact. The

Table 31-2 Laboratory Tests in the Diagnosis of Sexually Transmitted Diseases in Sexually Abused Children

Wet mount of vaginal discharge for presence of *Trichomonas* or clue cells (bacterial vaginosis)
Gram's stain of vaginal, urethral, or rectal discharge for gram-negative diplococci (*Neisseria gonorrhoeae*)
Culture of oropharynx, vaginal (prepubertal girls), cervix (adolescent girls), urethra (symptomatic boys), and rectum for *N. gonorrhoeae*
Culture of vagina (prepubertal girls), cervix (adolescent girls), and urethra (symptomatic boys) for *C. trachomatis*
Culture of lesions suspicious for herpes simplex
Serological studies for syphilis, hepatitis B, and human immunodeficiency virus infection, if indicated

adolescent who has been sexually active before the sexual assault should be tested at the first examination for pre-existing STDs.

C. trachomatis and *N. gonorrhoeae* infect the vaginal epithelium of preadolescent girls, and thus vaginal swabs are sufficient for culturing. Vaginal, rectal, and urethral cultures can be obtained with calcium alginate swabs moistened in nonbacteriostatic saline. The preadolescent girl easily tolerates a vaginal culture if the swab has minimal contact with hymenal tissue. The swab must be rubbed against the mucosal surface because epithelial cells are required for successful isolation of *C. trachomatis*. Because urethral infections with STDs in preadolescent boys are rare, the male urethra should be cultured only if there are signs or symptoms of infection.

Fluorescent antibody or antigen tests for detecting chlamydial infection or gonorrhea are contraindicated in the evaluation of sexually abused children because of their unacceptably high rate of false-positive results. Gram's stains of genital or anal secretions can also be misleading, and thus the examiner must await culture results before making a diagnosis of gonorrhea.

Serological testing for syphilis, hepatitis B, and human immunodeficiency virus (HIV) infection should be considered for all sexually abused children. A VDRL test should be obtained for children with an STD, those who have an abnormal genital examination, or those who give a clear history of sexual contact. Serological testing for hepatitis B virus and HIV should be considered for children who have an STD, when the child has been molested by a stranger or multiple assailants or an individual known to be at risk for such infections, or if the parents or victim request testing to allay anxiety. Testing should occur at the time of the examination and 3 months later (and again at 1 year for HIV).

Evidence Collection

The examiner has a dual role, forensic and medical, in evaluating sexually abused children. The collection of specimens for detecting the presence of seminal fluid, saliva, or hair belonging to the perpetrator is indicated when a victim is seen acutely after a sexual assault. The examiner must be familiar with the techniques of collection as well as proper labeling and packaging of evidence to preserve chain of custody. Evidence should be securely stored, and a written record of every person-to-person transfer is maintained between the physician and the forensic laboratory.

Collect the clothing worn during the assault by having the patient undress over a large piece of paper. The clothing can then be wrapped, packaged, and sent to the forensics laboratory.

If the victim scratched the assailant, rub a toothpick under the fingernails. Material collected is analyzed for the assailant's blood.

Comb the victim's pubic hair over a piece of paper. Wrap the comb in the paper and send it for detection of the perpetrator's hair. Samples of the victim's hair can be separately obtained by cutting or plucking for comparison.

Carefully examine the patient for any injuries. Bruises and bite marks should be accurately described and measured. Photograph injuries with a good-quality camera. A ruler for reference as well as a card with the date and the victim's name clearly legible should be placed in the photographic field.

Trace evidence such as hair, grass, or lint should be collected and packaged.

Scan the victim's body with a Wood's lamp. Areas that fluoresce may represent seminal fluid. These areas should be swabbed with a moistened cotton swab.

Collect oral, vaginal, and rectal swabs for seminal fluid analysis. In the mouth, swab the gingival sulci, under the tongue, and over the tonsillar pillars and posterior pharynx. Moistened vaginal swabs can be obtained in prepubertal girls. In adolescents, swab the posterior fornix during the speculum examination.

Swab bite marks with moistened cotton swabs. These can be analyzed for the presence of genetic markers present in saliva.

A saline wet mount of vaginal secretions should be examined immediately after the physical examination for the presence of sperm, trichomonads, and clue cells.

Before swabs are packaged for transport to the forensics laboratory, they should be air dried in a dryer. Drying greatly increases the sensitivity of forensic analysis for the presence of semen and saliva.

Treatment

Traumatic injuries should be treated as necessary. Consultation with a gynecologist may be necessary for complete evaluation and treatment of vaginal injuries.

Guidelines for the treatment of STDs are outlined in Table 31–3. Some experts recommend empirical therapy of adolescents for

Table 31-3 Treatment Guidelines for Sexually Transmitted Diseases in Children

Neisseria Gonorrhoeae
< 45 kg body weight
Ceftriaxone 125 mg IM as single dose
> 45 kg body weight
Cefixime 400 mg PO as single dose
or
Ceftriaxone 250 mg IM as single dose
Chlamydia Trachomatis
< 8 years old
Erythromycin base 50 mg/kg/d PO for 7 days
or
Sulfisoxazole 120–150 mg/kg/d PO for 14 days
> 8 years old
Doxycycline 100 mg PO bid for 7 days
or
Tetracycline 500 mg qid for 7 days
Bacterial Vaginosis
Metronidazole 15 mg/kg/d PO for 7 days (max. 500 mg bid)
or
Amoxicillin–clavulanic acid 20–40 mg/kg/d PO for 7 days (max. 250 mg tid)
Trichomonas Vaginalis
Children: metronidazole 30 mg/kg/d for 7 days (max. 250 mg tid)
Adolescents: metronidazole 2 g PO as a single dose
Syphilis
Incubating: ceftriaxone (see dosage for *N. gonorrhoeae*)
Early acquired (< 1 year): benzathine penicillin G 50,000 U/kg IM (max. dose 2.4 million units)
Herpes Simplex
Acyclovir 200 mg 5 times daily PO for 10 days
Human Papillomavirus
Various options, including laser therapy, cryosurgery, surgical excision, or application of podophyllum resin or trichloroacetic acid

bid, twice daily; qid, four times a day; tid, three times a day; IM, intramuscularly; PO, orally.

chlamydial infection and gonorrhea rather than awaiting culture results. Empirical therapy is not indicated in prepubertal children because the incidence of STDs in these patients is low. Treatment should await the results of definitive tests. Obtain repeated cultures for *C. trachomatis* and *N. gonorrhoeae* 1 week after therapy to ensure cure.

Routinely screen adolescent rape victims for pregnancy. If a urine pregnancy test result is negative, offer prophylaxis against pregnancy with ethinyl estradiol (Ovral), two pills at the time of the examination and two pills 12 hours later.

Documentation

The medical chart is also a legal document. Handwriting should be clear and legible. Describe the location, shape, size, and color of injuries. Drawings are useful for documentation, but photographs are most helpful for conveying the true appearance of injuries. All tests, medical procedures, and treatment should be documented. Ensure that test results are present in the medical record. Many locales have specific child abuse forms for documentation that also act as reminders to examiners for the necessary elements of the abuse evaluation.

Medical Follow-up and Counseling

The examiner must ensure appropriate follow-up for the patient. Repeated appointments may be necessary for the follow-up of injuries, repeated STD cultures and serological testing, and psychological counseling. Family members may also require counseling, particularly in cases of incest.

Bibliography

Adams J, et al: Examination findings in legally confirmed child sexual abuse: it's normal to be normal. *Pediatrics,* 94:310–317, 1994.

Bays J, Chadwick D: Medical diagnosis of the sexually abused child. *Child Abuse Neglect,* 17:91–110, 1993.

Berenson AB, et al: Appearance of the hymen in prepubertal girls. *Pediatrics,* 89:387–394, 1992.

Berkowitz C: Sexual abuse of children and adolescents. *Adv Pediatr,* 34:275–287, 1987.

Heger A, Emans J: *Evaluation of the Sexually Abused Child.* New York, Oxford University Press, 1992.

McCann J, et al: Genital findings in prepubertal children selected for non-abuse: a descriptive study. *Pediatrics,* 86:428–439, 1990.

Paradise J: The medical evaluation of the sexually abused child. *Pediatr Clin North Am,* 37: 839–862, 1990.

Chapter 32

Pediatric Toxicology Tests and Procedures

Ernest G. Bertha and E. Stephen Buescher

In the United States, between 1 and 2 million reported poison exposures occur yearly, 60% of these in individuals younger than 6 years (Cunningham, 1992). In addition, an estimated 2 to 3 million exposures go unreported. In children, approximately 40% of exposures involve pharmaceutical products. The remaining 60% of exposures involve cosmetics and personal care products, cleaning substances, plants, pesticides, paints and solvents, and hydrocarbon by-products. The majority of pediatric exposures involve nontoxic or minimally toxic materials. Only a small percentage have major or life-threatening intoxications that require emergency department and hospital inpatient medical, social, and psychiatric care. Typically, children presenting with exposures are younger than 6 years and have ingested a substance in the home. True "accidental" poisoning by children older than 6 years is uncommon and should be regarded with suspicion. Emergency personnel must be aware that child abuse in younger children, and attempted suicide in older children and teen-agers, may present as accidental ingestions. Whether an ingestion episode represents an accident, a plea for help, or a true attempt at taking one's own life will change the medical, social, and psychiatric management of the patient. Parents, sitters, or friends are often aware of the type and amount of substance ingested as well as the time since the ingestion occurred. This information is often crucial for the proper management of the patient and is typically available. Ancillary support in the form of social services, child protective services, police, and psychiatric support needs to be considered after initial stabilization efforts. Often, these types of services take time to mobilize, but they should be involved in the care of the child as early in the treatment process as possible.

APPROACH TO THE POISONED PATIENT

The procedures and tests relevant to the poisoned child can be grouped into those procedures appropriately performed at home, those performed in the emergency department, and those performed on hospitalized patients (Fig. 32–1). The procedures that need to be performed are individualized to each patient and depend on the patient's age; the underlying

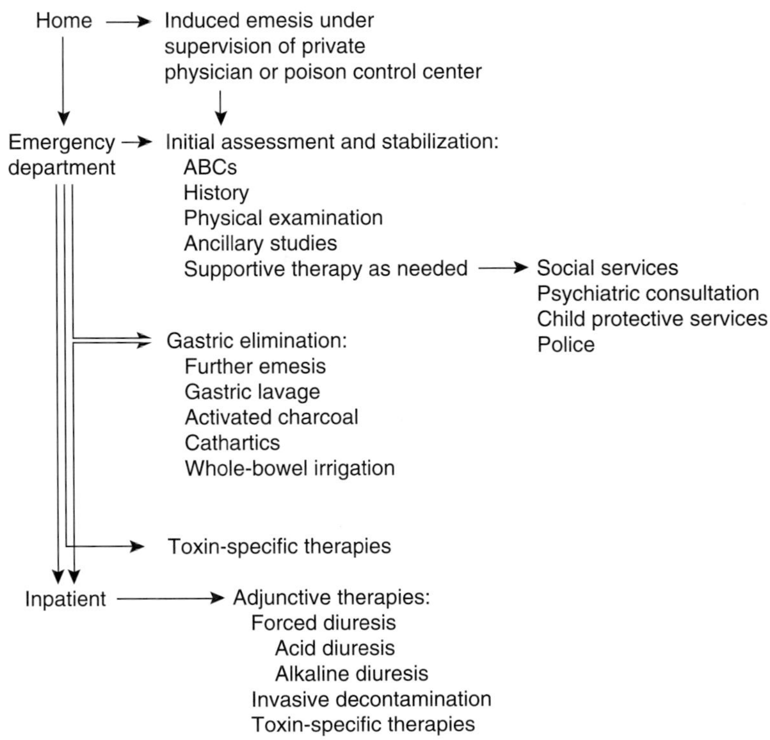

Figure 32–1 Schema for application of procedures and tests for poisoning in children.

medical and physical condition; and the type, form, and amount of toxin consumed. In some types of poisoning, home administration of syrup of ipecac to induce emesis may be appropriate. In others, full physiological support and invasive decontamination may be necessary. Once the patient arrives in the emergency department, the management of the poisoned child can be outlined as follows.

Stabilization of the Patient

Evaluate and address airway status, breathing, and circulation. Provide oxygen if necessary and assess neurological status.

Surface Decontamination

Remove all residual poisons (if it is a surface exposure) by removing clothing and flushing skin, mucous membranes, and eyes with appropriate fluids (water, saline).

Evaluation of the Patient

History

Obtain basic information, such as age, weight, type and amount of toxin, time since exposure, and route of exposure.

Record any change in physical or neurological condition from before the ingestion or the time of initial presentation to the time of evaluation in the emergency department. If changes have occurred, determine when and at what rate they have occurred.

Record attempted remedies or decontamination measures administered before arrival in the emergency department.

These pieces of information assist in the choice, prioritization, and combination of specific treatment types or therapies.

Physical examination

Include notation of odors (gasoline, alcohol) that may help identify the poisoning agents, the patient's mental status, and any associated injuries.

In patients with altered mental status, stabilization of the cervical spine should be ensured immediately and maintained until the integrity of the cervical vertebrae is confirmed by appropriate radiographic studies. Oxygen, naloxone, and dextrose (and possibly thiamine) should be available and considered for administration if indicated.

Ancillary studies

Specimens for toxicological analysis should include blood, urine, and gastric contents. The urine toxicology screen is easiest to analyze and has the most rapid turnaround time. If a specific drug has been ingested and blood level determinations are available for the drug, the specific blood level assay should be ordered in addition to the general blood toxicology screen.

Other laboratory studies to be considered include electrocardiography (looking for conduction or rhythm disturbances), chest radiograph (looking for evidence of aspiration or pulmonary edema), electrolyte levels and blood pH (looking for the presence of metabolic imbalance or acidosis/alkalosis), and serum osmolality (to determine whether a difference exists between measured and calculated values).

Initiate Treatment

1. Begin treatment to decrease absorption of the toxin or enhance its excretion and elimination (see later).
2. Administer antidote or specific therapy, if available (see later).
3. Maintain general physiological support.

During the emergency department evaluation, physicians should be prepared for guilt, defensiveness, and fear of punishment from the patient and the patient's family and friends. The physician must be patient, ensure confidentiality, and avoid being judgmental.

PROCEDURES TO DECREASE GASTROINTESTINAL ABSORPTION

When an ingestion occurs, the first intervention is to prevent absorption of the poison from the gastrointestinal tract. Several different approaches are available.

Forced Emesis

By inducing vomiting, ingested toxin still present in the stomach can be purged from the body. Historically, this has most often been accomplished by the administration of syrup of ipecac. Syrup of ipecac contains alkaloids that induce vomiting by both central stimulation and local gastric irritation. Although ipecac has been popular with generations of pediatricians, its use has decreased significantly in recent years (Hoffman, 1992) because it is now realized that gastric emptying after ipecac-induced emesis is not as complete as previously thought (only about 50% of stomach contents is removed) (Tandberg and Murphy, 1989). This is not to say that there is not a continued role for ipecac: it continues to be an appropriate initial therapy that can often be initiated by parents at home under the telephone supervision of a physician or poison control center. Once the child arrives in the emergency department, other methods are more effective at preventing absorption of toxins with less morbidity. Drawbacks to the use of ipecac include the delay of 15 to 30 minutes between administration and emesis, which potentially allows continued absorption of ingested toxin in that time. In addition, prolonged emetic effects for a period of several hours after its administration may interfere with the application of more effective types of decontamination therapy, such as activated charcoal administration (Harris and Kingston, 1992). Forced emesis may actually drive stomach contents and ingested toxins from the stomach into the small intestine more quickly.

Contraindications against syrup of ipecac use are age younger than 1 year; the presence of risks for aspiration (as in patients with stupor, impending coma, convulsions, or absent gag reflexes); ingestion of caustic substances, strychnine, or hydrocarbons; ingestion of foreign bodies or sharp objects; or ingestion of substances with unpredictable onset of symptoms (e.g., tricyclic antidepressants, barbiturates).

The dose of ipecac used is based on the patient's age. For children 1 to 7 years of age, a dose of 15 ml followed by several cups of water is given. For children older than 7 years, the dose is 30 ml. Some experts recommend the 30-ml dose for all pediatric patients, citing increased efficacy and more rapid onset of vomiting (Krenzelok and Dean, 1987). In all cases, if vomiting has not occurred within 20 to 30 minutes of administration, a second dose may be given. After ipecac administration, the child should be kept in an upright or seated position to prevent aspiration when vomiting begins. Syrup of ipecac is available without a prescription and is supplied in 15- and 30-ml doses.

Apomorphine hydrochloride has also been recommended for induction of vomiting; however, it is difficult to prepare and unpredictable in efficacy. Apomorphine hydrochloride is a dopaminergic agonist that causes vomiting by directly stimulating the chemoreceptor trigger zone. It is available in 6-mg tablets and must be dissolved in a sterile lactose solution before subcutaneous administration. Adverse reactions include central nervous system changes, restlessness, and tremors. Overdosage can result in violent vomiting, cardiac depression, acute circulatory failure, and death. The usual dose in pediatric patients is 0.1 mg/kg given one time only. Effects are usually seen within 5 to 10 minutes but can be prolonged, thus preventing the initiation of other therapies. The effects of apomorphine hydrochloride can be reversed by a narcotic antagonist such as naloxone.

Gastric Lavage

This technique mechanically removes toxins from the stomach. It involves placement of either a nasogastric tube or, more commonly, a large-bore orogastric tube (34–40 French) and irrigation of the stomach. Its use is preferred in patients in whom vomiting cannot be safely induced, such as those with altered mental status. In some cases, placement of a cuffed endotracheal tube to protect the airway before lavage is necessary. Like ipecac-induced forced emesis, gastric lavage is unpredictable in its effectiveness at gastric emptying (10% to 40% effective) (Tenenbeim, 1985). It is contraindicated in ingestions of sharp objects, acids, alkali, and most hydrocarbons. When lavage is performed, the patient must be maintained in the left lateral decubitus position, with the head down slightly. The fluid should be warm; this aids in decreasing peristalsis and gastric emptying. Typically, 0.9% saline is used in 20 to 50-ml aliquots per pass. Lavage is continued until the gastric return is clear. In some instances, the first-pass return can be sent to the laboratory for toxicological examination.

Whether gastric emptying is accomplished by forced emesis or by gastric lavage, activated charcoal is administered as soon as possible to further retard absorption of the ingested toxin from the gastrointestinal tract.

Activated Charcoal Administration

Activated charcoal is extremely fine powdered charcoal whose tremendous surface area (approximately 10^3 m^2/g) effectively adsorbs a wide variety of toxins. It is used to bind ingested materials in the intestinal lumen and is typically administered in combination with, or followed by, a cathartic. A dose of 1 g/kg charcoal is given as a slurry (either in water or 70% sorbitol [25 g/120 ml]). Sorbitol as the slurry carrier increases the sweetness of the mixture and hides the gritty texture of the charcoal. If sorbitol is not used in the slurry mixture, the taste and grittiness can be disguised somewhat by adding cola or chocolate syrup.

Activated charcoal should *not* be used if intestinal obstruction is suspected or if the ingested material will not be adsorbed to it. Whereas charcoal adsorbs many toxins, there are several on which charcoal has no effect (Table 32–1). Repeated doses of charcoal given every 4 to 6 hours (without sorbitol) have been shown to be effective in removing time-release or long-acting substances and in decreasing enterohepatic circulation of several toxins and their metabolites (McLuckie et al, 1990). A dose of 0.5 to 1 g/kg is given every 4 to 6 hours for 12 to 24 hours. Plain activated charcoal is constipating, and repeated administration of a cathartic may be necessary after several doses of charcoal. Signs of developing abdominal obstruction or electrolyte imbalance must be investigated and addressed as they are noted. Activated charcoal is extremely messy and can stain clothing. Gloves and gowns protect staff and family during administration and during the hours after administration, when emesis is common.

Whole-Bowel Irrigation

Adaptation of whole-bowel irrigation to gastrointestinal decontamination is based on its ability to clear the bowel of material. It may also promote "gut dialysis," with back-diffusion of previously absorbed toxins into the bowel (Tenenbeim et al, 1987). This therapy may be especially useful for ingested toxins

Table 32–1 Ingested Substances with Minimal to No Adsorption to Activated Charcoal*

Alkali	Ethanol	Methyl carbamate
Boric acid	Ferrous sulfate	Mineral acids
Chlorpropamide	Isopropanol	Potassium hydroxide
Cyanide	Lithium	
DDT	Methanol	Sodium metasilicate
Common electrolytes	Solvents	Water-insoluble compounds

*This is not a complete list.

that cannot be removed by emesis or lavage, as with sustained-release capsules or ferrous iron tablets, which may form concretions in the intestine.

The solution used is a polyethylene glycol/ electrolyte mixture (e.g., GoLYTELY [Braintree], Colyte [Reed and Carnrick]) that is not absorbed and does not alter electrolyte balance. The dose is 25 to 40 ml/kg/hr for small children and 2 L/h for adolescents and adults given until the fecal effluent is clear (usually 4 to 6 hours). This mode of therapy appears to be safe and effective in children. It can be paired with activated charcoal therapy after emesis or gastric lavage or used as primary therapy, depending on the ingested toxin.

Cathartics

These agents mediate gastrointestinal decontamination by causing diarrhea. Five classes of cathartics exist: bulk-forming agents, irritants/stimulants, osmotic agents, lubricants, and softeners. The most common class used in ingestions is the osmotic agents, such as magnesium citrate, magnesium sulfate, and sorbitol. Doses for these are provided in Table 32–2. Of these, sorbitol is preferred because it has the shortest gastrointestinal transit time (about 1 1/2 hours) and is associated with fewer electrolyte abnormalities. It can, however, also cause liquid stools and some abdominal distress. Repeated doses of sorbitol in younger children can lead to osmosis-related fluid loss and, in turn, hypotension and hypovolemic shock. Magnesium citrate and magnesium sulfate are less likely to cause abdominal discomfort, but their gastrointestinal transit times are longer (4–16 hours). The most commonly used preparation is a slurry of activated charcoal in sorbitol. This preparation has the advantage of combining a potent cathartic with the adsorptive properties of activated charcoal. It also reduces the constipating tendencies of charcoal given alone. Cathartics are contraindicated in adynamic ileus, abdominal trauma, renal failure, and pre-existing severe diarrhea. Irritant cathartics such as cascara oil are never indicated in the treatment of toxic ingestions.

Table 32–2 Recommended Dosages for Selected Cathartics

Magnesium citrate	4 ml/kg up to 200 ml
Sorbitol (70%)	2.8 ml/kg or 2 g/kg to a maximum of 50 g. It can also be used as 35% solution by diluting the standard solution 1 : 1 with water.

PROCEDURES TO INCREASE TOXIN ELIMINATION AFTER ABSORPTION

If absorption cannot be prevented by use of the methods discussed in the preceding, enhancing the elimination of the toxin or its metabolites from the body is an alternative approach. Depending on the toxin ingested, enhanced elimination may be accomplished by forced diuresis or by invasive decontamination procedures such as plasmapheresis, exchange transfusion, dialysis, and hemoperfusion. The invasive methods of decontamination require in-depth consideration before their application because they are associated with higher morbidity and mortality risks than the gastrointestinal decontamination procedures are. Indications for their use are limited, and these methods are not equally effective. Depending on the type of poison, the time between ingestion and treatment, the effectiveness of gastric decontamination, and the availability of specific antidotes, some methods may be more effective in preventing more serious sequelae from the poisoning.

Forced Diuresis

If the ingested toxin or its metabolites are renally excreted, forced diuresis may enhance their elimination and decrease toxic effects. Numerous techniques are described, with specific applications depending on the toxin ingested. Typically, therapy begins with one to two intravenous boluses of 20 ml/kg of normal saline or lactated Ringer's solution (isotonic solutions only) followed by appropriate solutions at 1 1/2 times maintenance fluid administration. Urine output of 1 to 3 ml/kg/h should result and can be confirmed by the appearance of urine with specific gravity less than 1.003. Forced diuresis is not usually regarded as primary therapy but is accepted as effective adjunctive therapy in poisonings with agents that are primarily excreted by the kidneys or when secondary or tertiary toxic metabolites, also excreted in the urine, are produced.

Forced diuresis is contraindicated in renal failure, cardiac compromise, or the absence of critical care monitoring facilities. It is also relatively contraindicated in pulmonary edema, cerebral edema, or the syndrome of inappropriate antidiuretic hormone secretion.

Acid Diuresis

Acid diuresis increases the renal clearance of weak bases and may be beneficial with ingestion of amphetamines, phencyclidine hydrochloride (PCP), and strychnine. It is accomplished by giving ammonium chloride, 75 mg/kg/d, intravenously or orally in divided doses every 6 hours. Urinary acidification to a pH of 5 to 5.5 is the objective. Urine output of at least 3 ml/kg/h must be maintained. Ascorbic acid is *not* an effective agent for acid diuresis. In situations in which metabolic acidosis and rhabdomyolysis are caused by the ingested agent, acid diuresis may worsen both. Acid diuresis is potentially dangerous and has been recommended less in recent years. Appropriate specialty consultation (nephrology or intensive care) should be sought prior to initiating this type of forced diuresis.

Alkaline Diuresis

Alkaline diuresis increases the renal clearance of weak acids and may be effective with ingestions of salicylates, phenobarbital, and possibly isoniazid. Sodium bicarbonate is given in an initial intravenous bolus of 2 mEq/kg, followed by an infusion of 1 mEq/kg/h. The aim of therapy is urinary alkalinization to pH 7.5 or above. Urine output of at least 3 ml/kg/h must be maintained. Careful monitoring of serum potassium concentration for hypokalemia secondary to systemic alkalosis should be performed when this mode of therapy is used.

Acetazolamide (Diamox) is *not* a true urinary alkalinizing agent and should not be used for alkaline diuresis. Although administration of acetazolamide does result in alkalinization of the urine, it also creates systemic acidosis.

Hypertonic Diuresis with Mannitol

Hypertonic diuresis decreases proximal tubule reabsorption of solute owing to increased water excretion, thereby decreasing the tubule concentration of toxin. It can be induced by administering a sterile 23% solution of mannitol intravenously at a dose of 0.5 g of mannitol per kilogram. In general, loop diuretic administration to force diuresis is not as effective as hypertonic diuresis because there is no effect on absorption in the proximal tubule.

With all types of forced diuresis, careful attention must be paid to fluid and electrolyte status. Hyponatremia, water intoxication, pulmonary edema, cerebral edema, and severe acid-base derangements may result from efforts to enhance diuresis.

Invasive Decontamination Methods

Depending on a number of variables (the type of toxin ingested, the length of time between ingestion and medical attention, the effectiveness of decreasing toxin absorption, the availability of specific antidotes), invasive types of toxin decontamination may also be considered in selected, severely poisoned patients.

Plasmapheresis

This procedure selectively removes plasma from blood obtained by phlebotomy, returning only the cellular elements to the patient. It is in theory best applied in the removal of toxins that are highly protein bound. The most promising application for this procedure in poisonings is in the treatment of thyroxine overdosage (Jones and Dougherty, 1986). In reality, plasmapheresis is rarely used as adjunctive therapy for poisonings.

Exchange transfusion

In this procedure, whole blood is removed by phlebotomy and replaced with donor whole blood. Because of the amounts of blood required, this procedure is only practically considered in infants or children whose total blood volume is small. It has been successfully used in patients poisoned with chloral hydrate, chloramphenicol, iron, pentachlorophenol, lithium, vincristine, and quinine as well as in treatment of severe methemoglobinemia (Pond, 1991). Like plasmapheresis, exchange transfusion is not commonly used to treat poisonings.

Hemodialysis/peritoneal dialysis

Dialysis exposes blood to either manmade or natural semi-permeable membranes to remove low-molecular-weight materials. Hemodialysis is theoretically best applied to toxins that are relatively small (< 1 kd) and that do not bind well to plasma components. Such substances include ethylene glycol and other alcohols, lithium, salicylates, and procainamide (Pond,

1991). Peritoneal dialysis has only limited applications because of its only minor effect on enhancing drug or toxin clearance.

Hemoperfusion

Hemoperfusion passes plasma over or through an adsorbent column (usually activated charcoal) to extract protein- or lipid-bound materials. It is ineffective for intracellular toxins. Beneficial effects of this procedure in ingestions of carbamazepine, phenobarbital, salicylates, xylene, phenacetin, and theophylline have been reported.

Indications for invasive decontamination

Before invasive decontamination procedures are used, specific indications for their use should be present (Pond, 1991). These indications include the following:

1. A patient who is deteriorating despite full supportive care. Clinically, this includes persistent hypotension, hypoperfusion of vital organs, and cardiac dysrhythmias.
2. A patient in whom clearance of the toxic compound is impaired. This may result from saturated metabolic or excretion pathways, congenital metabolic defects, preexisting hepatic or renal damage, or damage induced by the toxin itself.
3. A patient who has ingested a dose of toxin that will cause serious morbidity or death, and supportive care is ineffective or impractical. These substances could include salicylates, alcohols, lithium, and theophylline.
4. A patient who is more susceptible to the effects of the toxin because of concurrent disease states or age (very young or very old).

As these indications suggest, the applications for invasive decontamination are limited. Patients who have ingested the compounds noted in item 3 are most likely to benefit from these types of procedures.

Complications

Complications of the invasive decontamination procedures can be divided into four types: those related to altered coagulation, to infection, to fluid or electrolyte loss or replacement, and to the gaining of peripheral vascular or peritoneal access. Plasmapheresis, hemodialysis, and hemoperfusion all require anticoagulation to prevent extracorporeal clotting. Too much or too little anticoagulation results in problems with hemorrhage, coagulation factor consumption, or embolic events. All methods require access to the circulation, which carries with it an infection and clotting risk. Finally, these therapies may result in hypovolemia, fluid overload, unexpected fluid shifts, or electrolyte imbalance.

SPECIFIC ANTIDOTE THERAPY

The origins of the word "antidote" are Greek: *anti*, against, *dotos*, what is given. An antidote in toxicology is defined as an agent that neutralizes or counteracts a poison or its effects. Unfortunately, there are only a few true antidotes. Symptomatic support such as gastrointestinal decontamination, enhanced elimination, or, in some cases of severe poisoning, invasive decontamination remains the mainstay of therapy. Nonetheless, several types of poisonings respond to specific, antidote-like therapies. Table 32–3 summarizes the poisonings that can be treated with specific antidotes or therapies (Howland, 1990). These treatments are usually part of the total treatment plan for the poisoned patient and, as such, should be combined with methods to minimize absorption, hasten excretion, or block toxic effects of the poison and its metabolites.

INFORMATION RESOURCES

The number of pharmaceutical or household agents that can poison a child is so large that keeping current with the appropriate management for each agent is impossible. Physicians faced with this problem have several resources at their disposal. These include local or regional poison control centers, accessible by telephone, and textbooks on toxicology and poisoning. These references are excellent in their coverage of poisoning agents, the effects of specific agents, and appropriate management of exposures or ingestions. In addition, some poison control centers coordinate emergency services and transport of patients. Poison control centers are located throughout the United States and are staffed by nurses or other specially trained personnel with access to detailed information on toxic agents and appropriate management of the patient. The nearest poison control center can be reached by dialing the telephone number directly if it is known, by contacting the local operator, or by calling 911. Detailed information and references are also available in a number of toxicology texts. Three recent and particularly extensive texts are listed in the bibliography.

Table 32–3 Toxic Ingestions and Their Specific Antidotes/Therapies

Toxin	Antidote	Dosage
Acetaminophen	*N*-acetylcysteine	140 mg/kg as a loading dose, then 70 mg/kg IV every 4 h for 17 doses
Narcotics	Naloxone	0.1 mg/kg IV, IM, or SC; may require a continuous IV infusion
Benzodiazepines	Flumazenil	0.2 mg initially, then 0.5 mg every minute; maximum dose of 3 mg
Digoxin	Digoxin immune Fab	Equimolar to the amount of digoxin ingested. Calculate as follows: 1. Digoxin ingested (mg) × 0.8 (expect 80% absorption) = Fab (mg) to be administered 2. $\frac{\text{Digoxin level (ng)} \times 5.6 \text{ (volume of distribution for digoxin)} \times \text{patient's weight (kg)}}{1000}$ = Fab (mg) to be administered in a 30-minute period (unless in cardiac arrest, then give as a bolus)
Carbon monoxide	Oxygen	Administer 100% FiO_2; severe cases require hyperbaric oxygen therapy
Cholinesterase inhibitors (organophosphate and carbamate insecticides)	Atropine	0.01 mg/kg; minimum dose 0.15 mg, maximum dose 2.0 mg
Methemoglobinemic agents (nitrites, nitrates, aniline dyes, phenacetin, sulfonamides)	Methylene blue 1%	1–2 mg/kg IV in 5-minute period
Cyanide	Sodium nitrite (3%)/ sodium thiosulfate (25%)	Dependent on hemoglobin (Hgb) concentration

Hgb	Initial dose 3% sodium nitrite IV*	Initial dose 25% sodium thiosulfate IV
8 g	0.22 ml (6.6 mg)/kg	1.10 ml/kg
10 g	0.27 ml (8.7 mg)/kg	1.35 ml/kg
12 g	0.33 ml (10 mg)/kg	1.65 ml/kg
14 g	0.39 ml (11.6 mg)/kg	1.95 ml/kg

*Sodium nitrite should not exceed the recommended dosage; fatal methemoglobinemia may result.
IM, intramuscular; IV, intravenous; SC, subcutaneous.

Bibliography

Ellerhorn MJ, Barceloux DG (eds): *Medical Toxicology: Diagnosis and Treatment of Human Poisoning.* New York, Elsevier Science Publishing, 1988.

Goldfrank LR, Flomenbaum NE, et al (eds): *Goldfrank's Toxicologic Emergencies.* Norwalk, CT, Appleton & Lange, 1990.

Haddad LM, Winchester JF (eds): *Clinical Management of Poisoning and Drug Overdosage.* Philadelphia, WB Saunders, 1990.

References

Cunningham SJ: Overview of toxic ingestions. *Emerg Pediatr,* 5:97–98, 1992.

Harris CR, Kingston R: Gastrointestinal decontamination: which method is best? *Postgrad Med,* 92:116–128, 1992.

Hoffman R: Induced vomiting in poisoning management—yes or no? *Emerg Pediatr,* 5:95–96, 1992.

Howland MA: A quartet of antidotes. *Emerg Med,* 2/15:144–165, 1990.

Jones JS, Dougherty J: Current status of plasmapheresis in toxicology. *Ann Emerg Med,* 15: 474–482, 1986.

Krenzelok EP, Dean BS: Effectiveness of 15 mL versus 30 mL doses of syrup of ipecac in children. *Clin Pharmacol,* 6:715–717, 1987.

McLuckie A, Forbes AM, Ilett KF: Role of repeated doses of activated charcoal in the treatment of acute intoxications. *Anaesth Intensive Care,* 18:375–384, 1990.

Pond SM: Extracorporeal techniques in the treatment of poisoned patients. *Med J Aust,* 154: 617–622, 1991.

Tandberg D, Murphy LC: The knee-chest position does not improve the efficacy of ipecac-induced emesis. *Am J Emerg Med,* 7:267–270, 1989.

Tenenbeim M: Inefficacy of gastric emptying procedures. *J Emerg Med,* 3:133–136, 1985.

Tenenbeim M, Cohen S, Sitar DS: Whole bowel irrigation as a decontamination procedure after acute drug overdose. *Arch Intern Med,* 147: 905–907, 1987.

Chapter 33

Outpatient Minor Surgical Procedures

Yvonne Brouard and Lubna Hasanain

Primary care physicians are called on to carry out a variety of minor surgical procedures on children. The principles of preparation of the parent and patient, conscious sedation, and local pain relief pertain here, as they do for most procedures discussed in this text.

INCISION AND DRAINAGE

Incision and drainage allows cleansing of a contained infection and healing of the tissue by secondary intention. Drainage is required for any pocket of pus that is unlikely to drain spontaneously. Sometimes fullness is felt without demonstrable fluctuance. In these cases, purulence should be sought with needle aspiration. If pus is obtained, a formal incision and drainage should follow.

Contraindications and precautions include abscesses on the face and neck; deep rectal abscesses; or abscesses with extension, especially in the hand. These need surgical referral and drainage in the operating room. Children with immune deficiencies should have incision and drainage carried out in the operating room. The frequency of bacteremia after incision and drainage of cutaneous abscesses is approximately 30%. Such bacteremia is usually transient and does not lead to systemic infection. However, patients at risk for endocarditis, especially those with indwelling vascular devices, should receive antibiotic prophylaxis.

Equipment and Supplies

Local anesthetic (e.g., 1% lidocaine)
6-ml syringe
25-gauge needle
Povidone-iodine solution
Sterile gloves
Sterile gauze pads
Cotton-tipped culture swab
No. 11 scalpel blade
Scalpel handle
Blunt-tipped clamp
Saline irrigation solution
5 French catheter or intravenous tubing—sterile
Ribbon gauze 1 to 1 1/2 inches in width

Procedure

- Prepare the area with povidone-iodine and administer local anesthesia.

- Don sterile gloves and drape the area as a sterile field.
- Make an incision with the scalpel in a skin line over the abscess (Fig. 33–1).
- Take a culture specimen of the pus at the time of incision.
- Probe the cavity with a clamp and gently spread the clamp in all four quadrants to open all pockets of infection. A fingertip often works well to break the loculi.
- Remove the remaining pus and tissue by irrigation with normal saline under pressure from a syringe through the plastic intravenous catheter.
- Pack the cavity with plain ribbon gauze to allow continuous drainage. Packing should be placed into all recesses of the abscess cavity and then out through the incision. Packing should be removed in 24 to 48 hours. If purulence recurs, the wound should be explored, irrigated, and packed again. When the wound is dry and without pus, packing is not necessary.

Antibiotics are not prescribed routinely except in the following cases:

- Underlying immunodeficiency
- Systemic intoxication
- Failure to respond to incision and drainage
- Involvement of high-risk areas, such as the face or perirectal region

Choice of antibiotic is based on the likely pathogen. Extremity and trunk abscesses are usually caused by staphylococci and streptococci, for which dicloxacillin or cephalexin provides good coverage. Perioral abscesses may contain mouth flora, such as anaerobes, for which penicillin provides good coverage. Perirectal abscesses contain gram-negative rods and fecal anaerobes.

PARONYCHIA

This condition represents nail fold infection (Fig. 33–2). A predisposing factor is overzealous cutting of nails. The common causative organism is *Staphylococcus aureus*. Oral antibiotic therapy may be sufficient in early infection. Nonresolution is denoted by throbbing pain that awakens the patient from sleep. In these cases, surgical drainage is indicated.

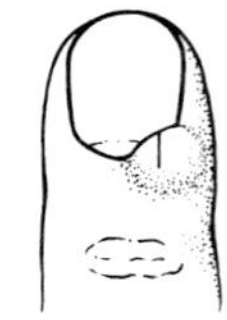

Figure 33–2 Incision and drainage of paronychia. (Redrawn from Lohr JA: *Pediatric Outpatient Procedures.* Philadelphia, JB Lippincott, 1991.)

Procedure

1. Apply digital block by creating a wheal on the skin with 1% lidocaine *without* epinephrine. At the base of the finger or toe, create a ring of local anesthesia by infiltrating around the digit from skin to bone (Fig. 33–3).
2. Make an incision at the nail fold with a No. 11 scalpel blade.
3. Evacuate the pus and place a wick soaked in povidone-iodine in place.
4. Splint the digit and instruct the patient to keep it elevated.
5. Remove the wick and re-examine the wound in 24 to 48 hours.

FELON

A felon is an abscess in the pulp of the distal finger. The causative organism frequently is *S. aureus*. There is a risk of phalangeal osteomyelitis if the telon is left untreated.

Procedure (Fig. 33–4)

1. Use a digital block.
2. Make a 1-cm-long and 1-cm-deep incision directly through the pulp of the distal digit in the midline of the palmar surface.
3. Place a wick in the wound.

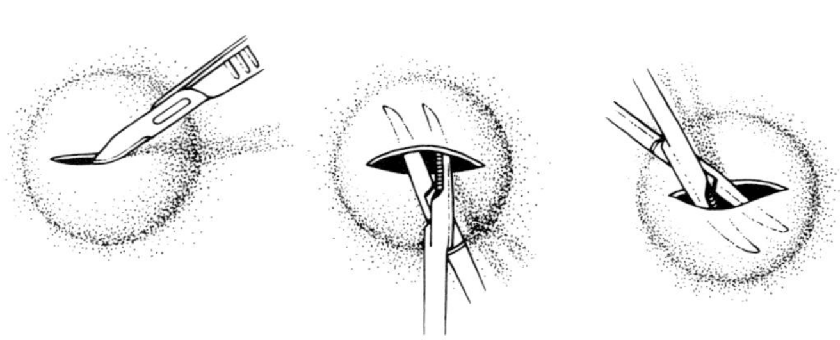

Figure 33–1 Incision and drainage of abscess. (Redrawn from Lohr JA: *Pediatric Outpatient Procedures.* Philadelphia, JB Lippincott, 1991.)

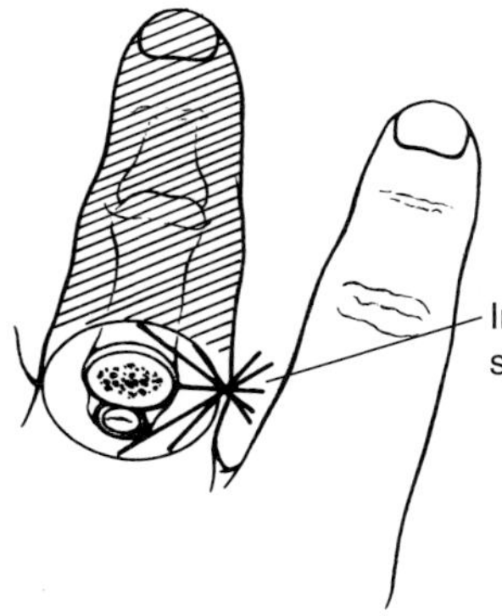

Figure 33–3 The digits are blocked with anesthesia for operations. (Redrawn from Nealon TF, Nealon WH [eds]: *Fundamental Skills in Surgery.* Philadelphia, WB Saunders, 1994.)

4. Splint and elevate the digit.
5. Re-examine and remove the packing in 24 to 48 hours.

LACERATIONS

Simple lacerations can be treated in an outpatient setting. Lacerations heal best when they are sutured within 8 to 10 hours of injury. Facial lacerations are best repaired by plastic surgeons for optimal cosmetic outcome. Absorbable sutures are used for subcutaneous suturing, as in multilayered repair of a facial wound; for mucous membrane repair, as in lip lacerations; or for superficial facial wounds in a noncooperative patient, such as a toddler. Suture thickness is denoted by number of zeroes. The more zeroes, the finer the suture: 0 (largest), 2–0, 3–0, 4–0, 5–0, 6–0 (smallest). Suture materials are described in Table 33–1.

Needles are straight, 3/8 curved (for most uses), or 1/2 curved (for web spaces of fingers and toes). Needle cross sections come in different varieties. Tapered needles are used for closure of subcutaneous tissue. Cutting needles end in a triangle, with the flat base on the outer circumference and the cutting point on the inner surface. Reverse-cutting needles also end in a triangle, with the flat base on the inner circumference and the cutting point on the outer surface. This type is commonly used for outpatient suturing situations. The picture on the needle box reflects the actual size of the needle. The letters and numbers stand for different things, depending on the manufacturer: M is a series number used with Ethicon; FS is for skin; P indicates plastic; PS denotes plastic surgeon. Larger numbers generally mean smaller needle sizes.

Needle holders come with either smooth or corrugated grasping surfaces. Smooth is best for 5–0 and 6–0 sutures. Likewise, forceps are either smooth or toothed. Toothed forceps cause less crushing of skin.

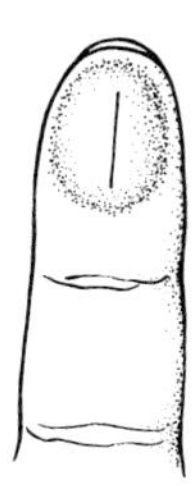

Figure 33–4 Incision and drainage of felon. (Redrawn from Lohr JA: *Pediatric Outpatient Procedures.* Philadelphia, JB Lippincott, 1991.)

Procedure

1. Examine the wound and ascertain neurovascular integrity (CMS: circulation, motor function, and sensation) before starting the procedure.
2. Check tetanus vaccine status.
3. Administer local anesthesia.
4. Irrigate the wound with normal saline through a 16- or 18-gauge angiocatheter attached to a 20-ml syringe. Wear disposable goggles when doing this to prevent accidental splashing of eyes.
5. Debride the wound, removing all foreign material and devitalized tissue. Trim irregular wound edges. This ensures better healing. Undermine at the wound edge by using scissors with blades closed, entering the subcutaneous tissue in the fascial planes, and opening the blades to dissect. Undermining helps approximate wound edges without increasing tension (Fig. 33–5).
6. Suture the wound by holding the needle at the junction of the middle and proximal thirds from the "eye" of the needle. Hold the clamp with the ring finger in a loop of the needle holder and the index finger along the shaft. Use the monofilament nylon or Prolene for skin closure. Enter the skin at 90 degrees to the skin surfaces (Fig. 33–6).

The type of wound closure depends on the location and nature of the laceration.

1. Simple interrupted suturing is used for cosmetic closures on the face and wounds with minimal tension. The instrument tie is the simplest for the novice (Fig. 33–7).

Table 33-1 Types and Characteristics of Suture Material

Suture	Absorption	Characteristics	Uses
Vicryl and Dexon	40 days; loses tensile strength in 14 days	Low rate of infection and tissue reactivity Braided, hence holds knot well	Deep facial repair (5–0) Galea (2–0) Oral mucosa and tongue (6–0)
Chromic gut	14–17 days	Slightly higher rate of infection High tissue reactivity Nonbraided Lower tensile strength than Vicryl and Dexon	
Plain gut	4 days	Infection potential like chromic gut Higher tissue reactivity Low tensile strength	Oral mucosa repair where rapid absorption is required
Fast-absorbing gut		Lowest tensile strength Most rapid absorption	Facial wounds in toddlers
Silk	Nonabsorbable	Easy to tie Braided Higher infection potential than monofilament sutures	
Nylon (Ethylon and Dermalon)	Nonabsorbable	Monofilament Harder to handle than silk Knots tend to unravel, 4–5 throws per knot are needed Low infection risk and low tissue reactivity	Face (6–0) Scalp (3–0, 4–0, 5–0) Hand (5–0, 6–0) Extremities (4–0, 5–0) Trunk (4–0, 5–0)
Polypropylene (Prolene)	Nonabsorbable	Monofilament Easier to handle than nylon	As above
Dacron	Nonabsorbable	Braided Low tissue reactivity	May be used instead of nylon or polypropylene

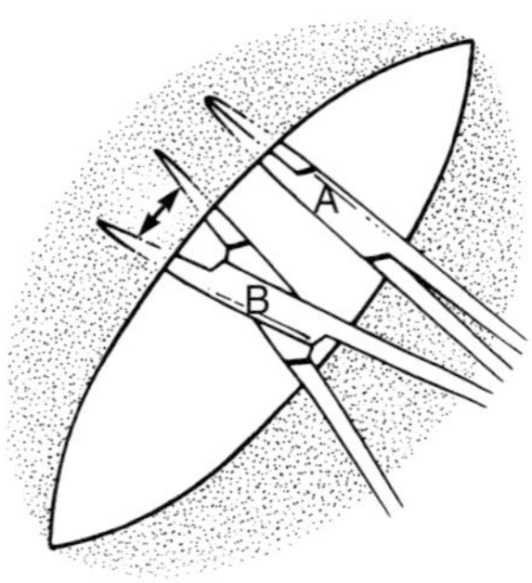

Figure 33–5 Technique of undermining using a mosquito clamp. The extent of undermining on both sides of the wound should roughly equal the gape of the wound. **A.** First the clamp enters to the desired depth. **B.** Next the blades are opened to bluntly dissect open the tissue plane. (Redrawn from Zukin DD, Simon RR: *Emergency Wound Care: Principles and Practice.* Rockville, MD, Aspen Publishers, 1987.)

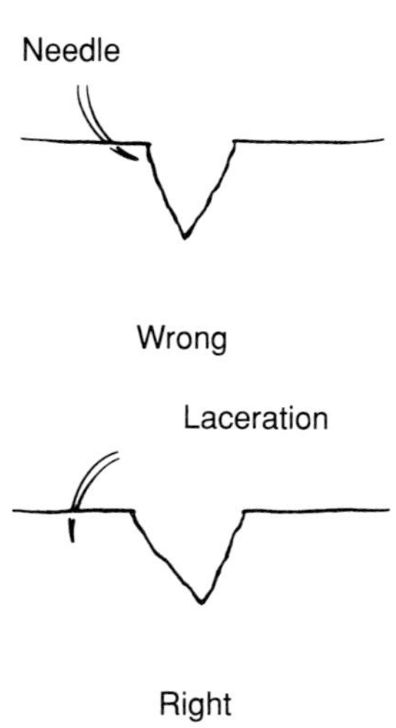

Figure 33–6 The needle should enter the skin at a 90-degree angle, then be rolled through the opposite edge of the laceration.

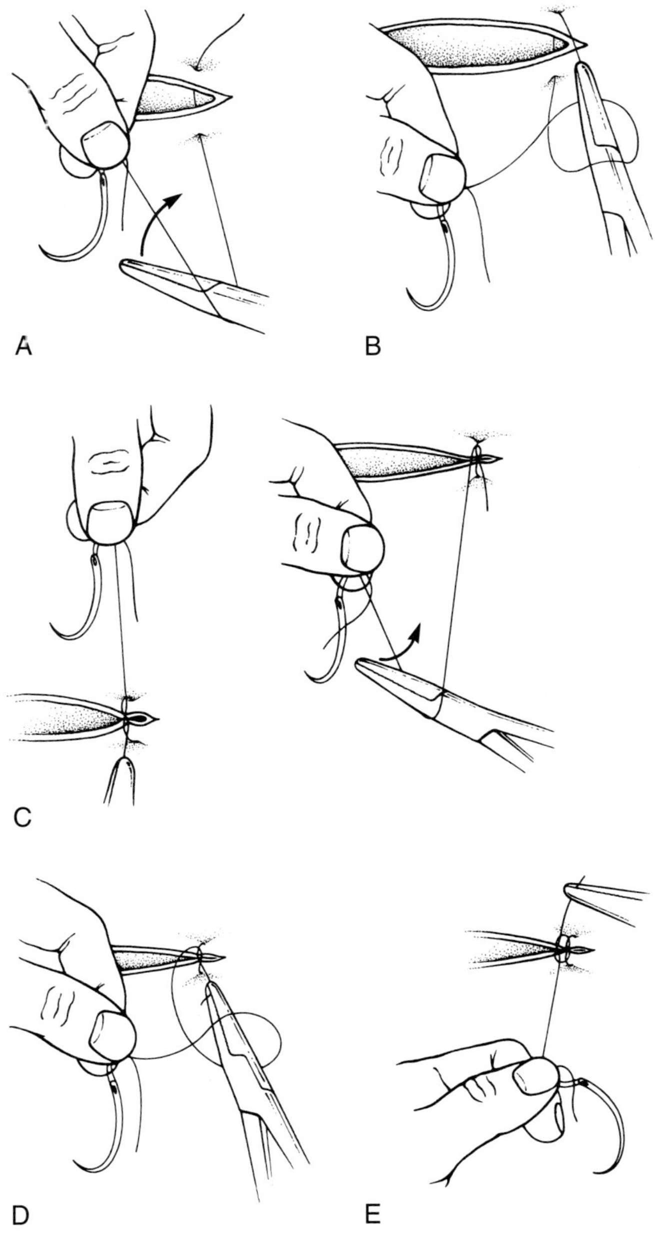

Figure 33–7 Simple interrupted suturing. **A.** The short end can be pulled short. Make a loop of the long end of the suture around the instrument, beginning with the instrument in front of the suture. **B.** Grasp the short end of the suture with the hemostat, which is placed through the loop. **C.** Pull the suture through the loop and set the knot down properly. Use only the instrument for traction. The traction must be exerted in the plane of the knot. Pull the short end toward you and the long end away. **D.** Start the second half-hitch by again wrapping the long end around the instrument, but in this instance, do it in the opposite direction. The instrument is first placed behind the long end of the suture. **E.** After you make the loop around the instrument, grasp the short end of the suture with the instrument and pull the suture through the loop. (Redrawn from Nealon TF, Nealon WH [eds]: *Fundamental Skills in Surgery*. Philadelphia, WB Saunders, 1994.)

2. Vertical mattress sutures are used for added strength and enhanced eversion of the wound margins. They are used mostly in areas of extensive skin movements or in areas where the skin is thick. Such areas include the back, soles of the feet, scalp, and palms of the hands (Fig. 33–8).
3. Horizontal mattress sutures are used in thin skin, such as lower extremities of adults (Fig. 33–9).
4. Deep closure is commonly used for facial lacerations. Layered suturing gives better cosmetic results. This occurs because the deep layer provides 6 weeks of additional support to the wound after the skin sutures are out, ensuring less widening of the wound scar. The deep layer repair avoids the development of pitting on the skin, which is caused by lack of healing in the deep portions of the wound. It also preserves integrity of the facial expression musculature. There are two main types of subcuticular stitches, running and horizontal mattress (Fig. 33–10).

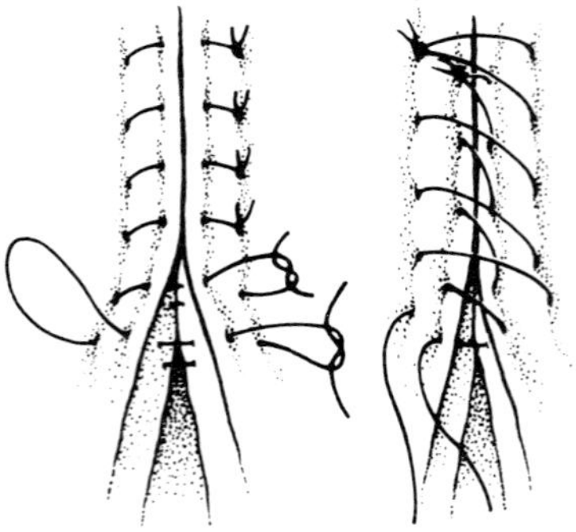

Figure 33–8 Vertical mattress suture.

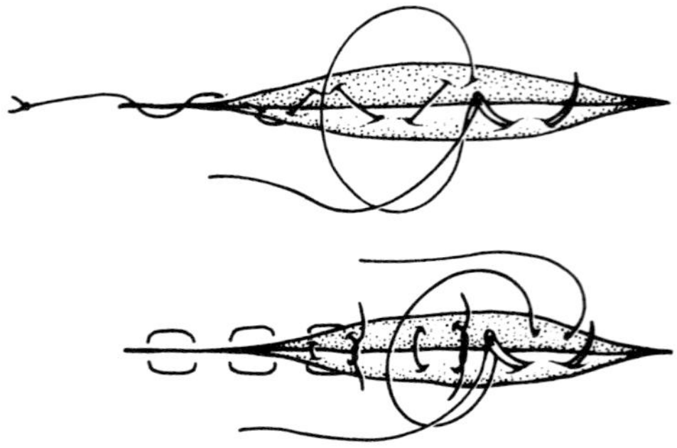

Figure 33–10 Subcuticular suture. (Redrawn from Nealon TF, Nealon WH [eds]: *Fundamental Skills in Surgery*. Philadelphia, WB Saunders, 1994.)

Skin tapes (Steri-Strips) may be applied to shallow, nongaping wounds. Skin staples are useful for small scalp lacerations.

Aftercare

Aftercare of sutures is important to ensure proper healing. Prophylaxis with antibiotics does not decrease wound infection; however, antibiotics have a place in human and certain animal bite wounds. Dressings with Xeroform have the advantage of not adhering to the wound. Adhesive bandages are useful for small wounds. Elevation of the involved area reduces edema. Lacerations overlying joints should be splinted. The patient should be seen in 24 to 48 hours to check for signs of wound infection. Suture removal is carried out according to these guidelines:

- Face: 4 days. Reinforce the wound with Steri-Strips after removal.
- Scalp: 5 to 7 days.
- Hand/extremities: 7 to 10 days; 10 to 14 days over joints. Reinforce with Steri-Strips.
- Trunk: 7 days.

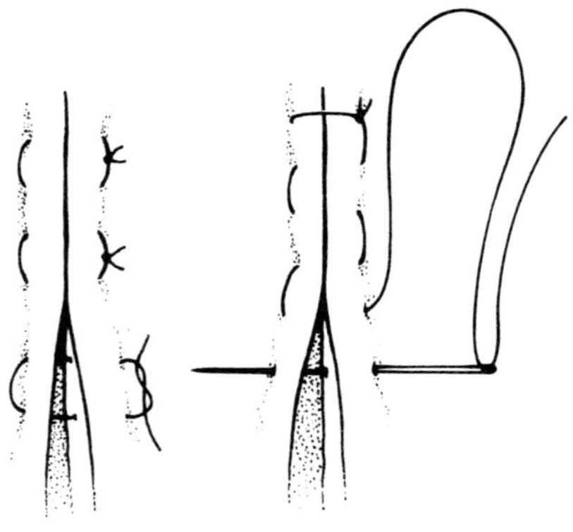

Figure 33–9 Horizontal mattress suture.

REMOVAL OF AN INGROWN TOENAIL

An ingrown toenail with or without infection is indicated by an area of tenderness with or without swelling and erythema along either edge of the great toenail. Conservative management, involving careful, repeated trimming of the nail (accompanied by oral antibiotics in the case of infection), is usually painful and often provides an unsatisfactory outcome. Whereas conservative management may be appropriate in a first episode of ingrown toenail (and is often attempted by the patient at home), removal of the affected part of the nail is indicated in recurrent or persistent cases. If a case is long-standing or has recurred after simple nail edge excision, phenolization of the germinal matrix is indicated. Infection that has progressed to cellulitis, lymphangitis, or osteomyelitis requires systemic antibiotics and possibly hospital admission and should not be treated with simple removal of the ingrown nail.

Nail Edge Excision (With or Without Phenolization of the Germinal Matrix)

(Fig. 33–11)

1. Place the patient in a comfortable supine position, with the affected foot slightly elevated.
2. Prepare the skin of the toe down to the

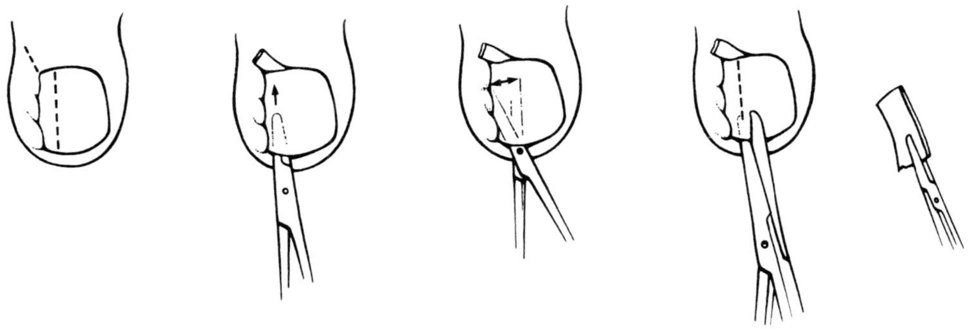

Figure 33–11 Excision of ingrown toenail. (Redrawn from Lohr JA: *Pediatric Outpatient Procedures.* Philadelphia, JB Lippincott, 1991.)

base with use of swabs and povidone-iodine.

3. Administer the digital block. Anxious patients may be helped by having a small amount of local anesthetic injected into the skin on both sides of the great toe before the administration of the digital block.
4. Apply a heavy gauge rubber band to the base of the toe (near the area of application of the digital block) as a tourniquet.
5. Test the adequacy of anesthesia by pricking the tip of the toe with a needle. Infiltrate with further anesthetic as necessary.
6. Determine the amount of nail to be removed. This should be approximately 0.5 cm in width, more if infection has spread beyond that point.
7. Undermine the edge of the nail with a straight clamp.
8. Cut the nail down its longitudinal axis by use of heavy scissors or nail cutters.
9. Work the nail edge loose and remove it with the straight clamp. Great care should be taken to remove the nail edge completely, including the area under the skin fold at the base of the nail. It may be necessary to incise the skin fold in the corner to achieve this. If fragments of nail remain, recurrence is more likely. If phenolization is indicated, continue through steps 10 and 11. If not, skip to step 12.
10. Compress the toe and dry the exposed nail bed with gauze swabs.
11. Apply 80% phenol with a cotton-tipped applicator inserted under the nail fold. Leave the applicator in place for 4 minutes. Take great care to avoid spilling phenol onto the surrounding skin because it may cause a chemical burn. Contaminated skin should be washed immediately with alcohol-soaked gauze.
12. Apply a circumferential dressing of antibacterial-impregnated gauze, followed by circumferential applications of plain gauze and finally conforming gauze. These must be applied tightly enough to provide hemostasis once the tourniquet is removed. Leave the tip of the toe visible to check for circulation.
13. Release the tourniquet by cutting the rubber band.
14. Leave the foot elevated for 10 to 15 minutes to ensure hemostasis.
15. Assess circulation at the tip of the toe. If it is inadequate, place the foot in a dependent position and reassess. If it is still inadequate, reapply the bandages more loosely until adequate circulation returns.

Aftercare

Prophylactic antibiotics are not indicated in the majority of cases. However, there is a small risk of secondary infection or persistence of infection present at the time of treatment. Therefore, the patient should be instructed to return if any signs of infection occur. There is also an increased risk of secondary infection after phenolization of the germinal matrix; therefore, these patients should receive prophylactic antibiotics. Appropriate antibiotics include those that are effective against *S. aureus* and *Strepto-*

coccus pyogenes. Adequate pain control may be achieved by use of acetaminophen with codeine for the first 24 hours, followed by acetaminophen alone. The foot should remain elevated as much as possible for the first 24 hours. Subsequently, normal walking and activity should be resumed. The dressing should remain in place for 3 days, unless it becomes wet or soiled, in which case it should be changed sooner. For removing the initial dressing, soaking in warm, soapy water may be helpful. The toe may subsequently be kept covered for a week with a simple adhesive bandage. The patient should be instructed to wear slightly loose fitting shoes and to cut nails straight across in the future.

Complications include ischemia that may be associated with the time taken for the procedure, the tightness of the bandage, and the adequacy of the patient's circulation before the procedure. Ischemia can be avoided by (1) limiting the tourniquet time to less than 30 minutes, (2) checking adequacy of circulation after the procedure and loosening the dressing, as necessary, and (3) being aware of underlying conditions that put the patient at increased risk of ischemia (such as diabetes) and avoiding tourniquet use in these cases.

Infection at the time of presentation is common. Postprocedure prophylactic antibiotics are not generally indicated; nail edge excision is usually sufficient treatment in itself, and the risk of postprocedure infection is low. However, if phenolization is performed, or if there is underlying vascular or immunological incompetence, the risk of postprocedure infection is increased, and prophylactic antibiotics are indicated.

The rate of recurrence of ingrown toenails is variable. Ensuring that the nail edge is completely removed decreases the recurrence rate, as does phenolization of the germinal matrix. Recurrences are typically manifested either by complete regrowth of the ingrowing area or by the appearance of fragments of nail growing out from the cut edge. Both should be treated with nail edge excision accompanied by phenolization.

FISHHOOK REMOVAL

The simple retrograde technique works best in cases involving unbarbed fishhooks or in any case of shallow penetration in which the barb has not penetrated the skin. The fishhook is gently backed out of the skin along the path of entry; continuous gentle tension along with downward pressure on the shank of the fishhook disengages the tip of the hook. Needle drivers may be used to manipulate the hook.

The needle cover technique may be used for removal of hooks with a single barb embedded in the skin. An 18-gauge (or larger) needle is advanced along the path of entry until the tip of the needle is covering the barb of the hook. Next, the hook and needle are backed out as a unit by the simple retrograde removal technique.

The string technique (Fig. 33–12) is quick and therefore relatively pain free and is the preferred method among fishermen. It may be used in any case appropriate for simple retrograde removal. The injured part should be resting on a firm surface. A string approximately 18 inches in length is looped around the curve of the hook, and the free ends are tied and held slightly slack in one hand of the operator. Needle drivers or forceps (or a stick or pen) may also be used to hold the free ends and may afford better leverage. The other hand of the operator is used to apply gentle downward pressure on the shank of the hook (to disengage the tip) while the string is given a quick, gentle tug to remove the hook in a retrograde fashion.

The advance and cut technique should be employed only when retrograde techniques have failed or are judged inappropriate, such as when the tip of the hook has advanced through an exit wound or when the location or depth of the hook makes success unlikely. This technique requires good local anesthesia or digital block before the procedure. It also requires that the tissue through which the hook is to be advanced contain no bone or vital structures. This may be determined by obtaining radiographs of the area in two planes. Because the hook is being advanced farther through the skin, it is wise to clean the area and the exposed parts of the hook with povidone-iodine or antibacterial soap before the

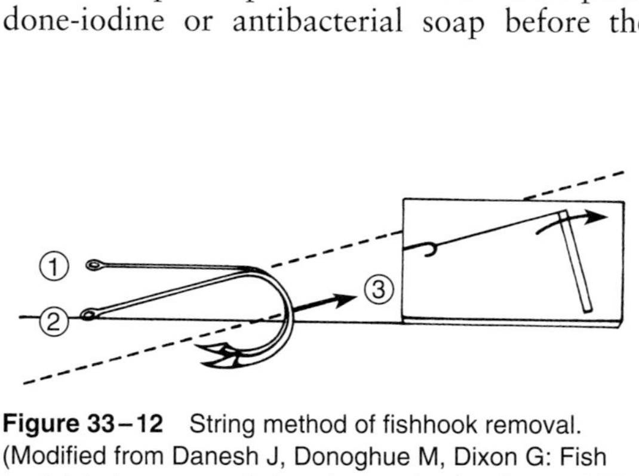

Figure 33–12 String method of fishhook removal. (Modified from Danesh J, Donoghue M, Dixon G: Fish hook injuries—wounded anglers and string theory. *N Z Med J*, 105:136, 1992.)

procedure. The fishhook is advanced through the skin by use of the needle drivers until the sharp tip of the hook has protruded through an exit wound. If the hook is unbarbed, the sharp tip is cut off with wire cutters, and the hook is subsequently removed in a retrograde fashion with the needle drivers. If the hook is barbed, the needle drivers are used to grasp the sharp tip of the hook (after it is advanced through the skin), and the shank of the hook is then removed in an anterograde fashion by use of the needle drivers.

Aftercare

All patients with fishhook injuries should be reimmunized with tetanus toxoid, unless they received a tetanus booster within the last 5 years. Infection is rare after fishhook injuries, and routine topical or systemic prophylactic antibiotics are not indicated. However, if cartilage, tendon, or oral mucosa is involved, systemic antibiotics directed against skin or oral flora may be indicated. They may also be indicated in diabetic patients or in the case of a dirty wound. Postprocedure wound care should include simple washing of the site with an antibacterial soap and the application of a simple dry dressing. Topical antibiotics do not seem to improve the outcome. Complications of both injury and treatment are rare but can include deep tissue infections, including osteomyelitis.

RELEASE OF THE ZIPPER-ENTRAPPED PENIS

This problem occurs when the skin of the penile shaft or prepuce is entrapped in a zipper after rapid or careless opening or closing of the zipper, particularly in the absence of underwear.

A simple and noninvasive method should be attempted first. This involves the liberal application of mineral oil to the zipper and entrapped skin. After a few minutes of soaking in mineral oil, it may become possible to liberate the entrapped skin with little traction. If any significant manipulation is necessary, local anesthesia is helpful. Note that attempts to manipulate the skin free or to reverse the zipper, in the absence of any lubrication, are usually unsuccessful and always painful.

In the event that this method is unsuccessful, the next approach is to divide the median bar of the zipper with wire or bone cutters (Fig. 33–13). Because of the threatening nature of this procedure, sedation or local anesthesia may be indicated.

Aftercare

Apply topical antibiotics to any skin abrasion. Ensure that the patient is able to urinate normally. If the prepuce of an uncircumcised male is involved, consider referral to a urologist for elective circumcision. Complications are rare;

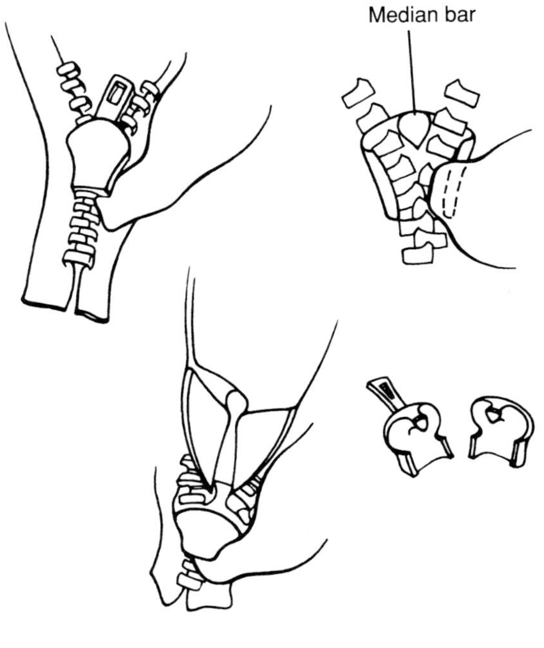

Figure 33–13 Removal of foreskin entrapped in a zipper. (Redrawn from Flowerdew R, Fishman IJ, Churchill BM: Management of penile zipper injury. *J Urol,* 117:671, 1977.)

however, in refractory cases, surgical removal of the zipper and simultaneous circumcision may be necessary.

Bibliography

Callaham ML: *Current Practice of Emergency Medicine,* Philadelphia, BC Decker.

Danesh J, Donoghue M, Dixon G: Fish hook injuries—wounded anglers and string theory. *N Z Med J,* 105:136, 1992.

David SS: Fish-hook removal. *Lancet,* 338:1463–1464, 1991.

Doser C, Cooper WL, et al: Fishhook injuries: a prospective evaluation. *Am J Emerg Med,* 9: 413–415, 1991.

Flowerdew R, Fishman IJ, Churchill BM: Management of penile zipper injury. *J Urol,* 117:671, 1977.

Grieg JD, Anderson JH, et al: The surgical treatment of ingrowing toenails. *J Bone Joint Surg Br,* 73:131–133, 1991.

Iseli A: The management of ingrown toenails. *Aust Fam Physician,* 19:1414–1419, 1990.

Kanegaye JT, Schonfeld N: Penile zipper entrapment: a simple and less threatening approach using mineral oil. *Pediatr Emerg Care,* 9:90–91, 1993.

Lantsberg L, Blintsovky E, Hoda J: How to extract an indwelling fishhook. *Am Fam Physician,* 45: 2589–2590, 1992.

Lohr JA: *Pediatric Outpatient Procedures*. Philadelphia, JB Lippincott, 1991.

Murtagh J: Ingrown toenail. *Aust Fam Physician,* 22:1022, 1993.

Nolan JF, Stillwell TJ, Sands JP Jr: Acute management of the zipper-entrapped penis. *J Emerg Med,* 8:305–307, 1990.

Wolcott MW: *Ambulatory Surgery and the Basics of Emergency Surgical Care,* 2nd ed. Philadelphia, JB Lippincott, 1988.

Zukin DD, Simon RR: *Emergency Wound Care: Principles and Practice*. Rockville, MD, Aspen, 1987.

Section F

Prenatal/Genetic/Neonatal

Chapter 34

Prenatal Assessment

Sabitha S. Sehgal

Routine clinical assessment by biochemical techniques and/or obtaining DNA from the fetus is possible for more than 100 of the thousands of possible genetic diseases at the present time. Chorionic villous sampling, amniocentesis, and fetal blood sampling are the most widely used techniques. Screening of maternal blood for fetal constituents (mainly alpha-fetoprotein or DNA) "leaked" from the intrauterine compartment is also done.

CHORIONIC VILLOUS SAMPLING

The ability to detect genetic disorders before birth has improved dramatically during the last 2 decades. In less than 5 years of widespread use, chorionic villous sampling (CVS) has rapidly emerged as a first-trimester alternative to amniocentesis. Its acceptance underscores the limitations inherent in amniocentesis, which is performed in the second trimester of pregnancy and requires up to 4 weeks for diagnostic information to be available, at which time if an abnormality is detected the methods of termination of pregnancy available are less acceptable to patients and may be associated with increased risks.

The chorionic villi are derived from the trophectoderm and rapidly proliferate to completely cover the chorion by 2 weeks after implantation. Villi on the implanting side of the gestational sac (chorion frondosum) will form the placenta; those on the opposite side (chorion laeve) will degenerate gradually during the next few weeks. By 14 weeks, a clearly defined placenta and smooth chorion is seen. Because the trophoblastic tissue has the same genetic constitution as the fetus, samples of chorionic villi should reflect the chromosomal, biochemical, and DNA status of the fetus.

Techniques

CVS is most commonly performed employing a transcervical approach using a 1.5-mm (16-gauge) polyethylene catheter with a 1-mm malleable stainless steel stylet. Under direct ultrasound guidance, the catheter is passed transcervically and is placed within the villi of the chorion frondosum. Application of 5 to 15 ml of suction to the catheter by using a 20-ml syringe allows samples of 10 to 40 mg wet weight to be obtained. The sample is then placed into culture medium, and under a dissecting microscope, the villi are separated from maternal decidual tissue. The villi can be analyzed for enzymatic activity and DNA, or they can be placed into culture for cytogenetic studies.

Indications

Couples at risk for a fetus with a chromosomal disorder are the largest group to which CVS is applicable. This group includes those at risk because of maternal age, the presence of chromosomal translocation in one parent, or the birth of a previous trisomic child. Chorionic villous samples can be assayed directly for enzyme activity to detect a number of metabolic disorders. Careful separation of the villi is mandatory for an accurate biochemical diagnosis with either enzymatic or DNA analysis techniques.

Advantages

There are several advantages to CVS in addition to the earlier timing of the procedure. The short culture time for the genetic studies and the direct assays performed from biochemical and DNA analysis result in a significantly shorter time to final diagnosis than is possible with amniocentesis.

Problems

Immediate complications of CVS are rare. A sufficient sample for diagnosis is obtained in 98% of the procedures performed. Culture failure occurs in less than 1% of cases. Immediate rupture of fetal membranes is extremely uncommon; this reflects the benefit of sonographic guidance of the catheter.

The major short-term complications of CVS are pregnancy loss and diagnostic error. An overall spontaneous abortion rate of 3.5% to 4% has been cited, but no control data on the background risk for patients of similar maternal and gestational age are available. Risk related to the procedure may be 1% or less. Preliminary data from the National Institutes of Health (NIH) collaborative study indicated that CVS has a 0.7% higher pregnancy loss rate than amniocentesis.

A second short-term complication is false, or misleading, diagnostic results. Maternal cell contamination has been a source of several diagnostic errors and appears to be related to experience. A potential source of error that is more difficult to prevent is the presence of discrepancies between the chromosomal constitution of the fetus and that of the chorionic villi. These discrepancies may be in the form of chromosomal aneuploidy confined only to the villous sample and appear to represent true mosaicism within the placenta. The incidence of this finding has ranged from 1% to 3%. Although the significance of placental mosaicism is unknown, it may be associated with an increased risk of pregnancy loss. In such cases, amniocentesis should be offered for confirmation.

A third source of error has been found when using direct chromosomal preparations only. In a small number of cases, the diagnosis of normal karyotype was made on a direct preparation, but subsequently an abnormal chromosomal constitution was found in cultured villous samples, amniocytes, or blood obtained at birth. This preliminary information on false-negative findings makes it essential that long-term cultures be performed on all patients and that the true incidence of this complication be determined.

There might be discrepancies in enzyme expression between direct assays of chorionic villi and cultured amniotic fluid cells.

There appears to be little maternal risk associated with CVS. There have been reports of maternal sepsis after the procedure, but the overall risk in larger series appears to be quite low.

Potential long-term complications could include rhesus blood factor (Rh) isoimmunization, prematurity, placental abnormalities, and birth defects. There is no information to suggest that fetal growth is affected by CVS. There may be an increased incidence of delayed membrane damage. There have been several reports of oligohydramnios detected at 16 to 20 postmenstrual weeks in patients who have had CVS. Almost all had a history of persistent vaginal spotting or wetness after the procedure.

Future Directions

Transcervical CVS has several significant limitations:

1. The time at which it can safely be performed is limited to 9 to 12 weeks' gestation.
2. Anterior and fundal locations of the placenta may be technically difficult to sample.
3. There is a small but significant risk for infection.

For these reasons transabdominal CVS is being investigated. Preliminary information indicated a higher rate of successful sampling and apparently a lower rate of fetal loss than with transcervical CVS. Transabdominal CVS has the additional benefit of allowing villous sampling in both the second and third trimesters for rapid karyotyping when fetal abnormalities are detected by ultrasound.

Despite the questions regarding infection, membrane damage, and placental mosaicism that remain to be answered, the initial experience with CVS has been quite promising. It appears to be a safe and reliable method for prenatal diagnosis.

AMNIOCENTESIS

Bevis introduced the modern era of diagnostic amniocentesis with his report of the technique of amniocentesis. Liley was the first to demonstrate its utility in assessing the severity of erythroblastosis indirectly by determining the amount of bilirubin in amniotic fluid. In 1965, it became clear that fetal cells obtained from amniotic fluid could be cultured and later karyotyped.

Techniques

Jeanty and associates reported a technique of amniocentesis that required the simultaneous use of real-time ultrasound, which allowed the operator to adjust the pathway of his/her needle to avoid the fetus, the placenta, and the umbilical cord. The most commonly used technique by obstetricians involves linear array. Generally, the operator places a needle next to the linear array transducer after choosing an insertion site that is distant from the fetus and, in most cases, away from the placenta. The needle, soon after insertion through the maternal skin, appears as a bright spot on the ultrasound monitor. The aim of the technique is to adjust the angle of the needle so that its tip runs within the ultrasound beam. Thus, the bright spot on the monitor will represent the tip, rather than the shaft, of the needle. If a sector transducer is used, the operator can position the needle and transducer in such a way as to make the entire length of the needle visible within the uterine cavity.

A twin pregnancy represents a challenge for the operator, whose task is to ensure that both sacs are being sampled. A careful ultrasound evaluation is therefore carried out to determine the exact position of the separating membranes. The most common technique to ensure that the same sac has not been entered twice requires the injection of a dye into the first sac sampled after the sample has been withdrawn. Because it is important to later identify a twin whose test results are abnormal, it is imperative that one attempt to describe the location of the fetuses at the time of amniocentesis. Although the twins can change positions, their placentas cannot.

One of the most common problems encountered in the second trimester amniocentesis is inability to penetrate the amnion. The chorion usually adheres to the uterine wall, but the amnion can float freely ahead of the needle tip. The ultrasound scan will indicate the needle tip to be in the middle of the cavity, but no fluid can be aspirated. The problem is solved by either advancing the needle tip vigorously through a fetus-free pocket of fluid or reinserting the needle into another area where the amnion is not "tented" into the cavity.

Risks of Second-Trimester Amniocentesis

Fetal loss rate

A higher total fetal loss rate occurred with amniocentesis compared with control groups of about 0.5%. These differences were not statistically significant. Since 1979, 17 studies have been published dealing with the risk of second-trimester amniocentesis, but most of these studies have no control data. The total fetal loss rate was 3.3% and the spontaneous abortion rate was 1.3%. The average loss rate to 28 weeks was 2.4%. There was a 1% difference in spontaneous abortions between the amniocentesis group and the control group. The stillbirth rate was identical. These studies underscore the fact that amniocentesis is not a completely innocuous undertaking and can result in a spontaneous abortion in up to 1% of cases.

Other risks

Infants born after a second-trimester amniocentesis had a higher rate of respiratory difficulties than did controls. The most likely mechanism for developing respiratory difficulties would be the effect on developing fetal lung from a sudden decrease in amniotic fluid volume. There may be a higher rate of hip dislocation and talipes equinovarus. The Danish randomized control trials showed no difference between the amniocentesis group and the control group. Another source of potential morbidity is placental penetration by the amniocentesis needle. Poorer outcome of pregnancy may be associated with blood-stained amniotic fluid. Another potential source of later reproductive problems is the possibility of fetomaternal hemorrhage at the time of amniocentesis, causing later sensitization to Rh and other antigens. There have been isolated reports of fetal injury, but the incidence of fetal trauma is very small. There is no difference in mental or motor development, physical growth, or orthopedic development by 6 months of age compared with the control group. A few infants may have needle marks.

First-Trimester Amniocentesis

Amniocentesis has been generally performed at 10 weeks to 14 weeks of gestation. The initial results have suggested fetal loss rates that are comparable to second-trimester amniocentesis. Of theoretical concern is the fact that more amniotic fluid proportionately is taken from the amniotic cavity in early amniocentesis than 16 weeks or later. Given the data mentioned earlier with regard to respiratory distress syndrome and pneumonia in later amniocentesis, more information is needed to assess the long-term effects of early amniocentesis. Until then, one cannot with accuracy advise patients who wish to have an early amniocentesis about the potential risks of the procedure.

FETAL BLOOD SAMPLING

Since 1972 it has been possible to obtain fetal blood during pregnancy. Before 1982, the blood sampling was performed by fetoscopy, which is a difficult and invasive technique that has significant associated fetal risks. The ability to sample pure fetal blood under ultrasound guidance has completely changed this situation and has provided ready access to new information in fetal medicine.

Technique

Fetal blood sampling (FBS) is performed on an outpatient basis without medication, either before or after the procedure. FBS rarely stimulates uterine contractions, which, if they occur, can be readily suppressed with beta-mimetic drugs. The cord insertion into the placenta must be clearly exposed without fetal interposition. The insertion of the cord into the placenta is its most fixed position; therefore, the cord can be punctured more easily at this point. When the insertion cannot be seen, it is possible, although more difficult, to puncture the abdominal insertion or to perform FBS on a loop of cord pushed against the uterine wall.

Once the cord insertion site has been chosen, the cord must remain strictly immobile and a 20-gauge, 9-cm spinal needle is introduced under aseptic conditions. The cord is entered approximately 1 cm from its insertion site. Use of a rigid needle is very important so that the operator will not have to reinsert the needle several times through the maternal abdominal wall. Depending on whether the placenta is anterior, lateral, or posterior, the cord insertion can be reached directly through the placenta without traversing the amniotic cavity, transplacentally and then transamniotically, or simply transamniotically.

FBS can be performed from 18 weeks after the last menstrual period to term, even intrapartum. A fetal blood sampling can be performed many times during the pregnancy. The lack of change in the fetal hemoglobin sampled many times confirms that the sampling procedure does not produce fetal anemia. The quantity of blood taken out during each procedure is minimal (1.5–4 ml, depending on the gestational age). The overall fetal loss rate is 1.6%, the preterm delivery rate is 3.8%, and the intrauterine growth retardation rate is 8.5%. Fetal deaths have been attributed to mechanical cord problems, major fetal malformations, or severe intrauterine growth retardation, in which a decision was made not to deliver the fetus. In a few cases fetal demise occurred less than 2 weeks after the FBS and seemed to be directly related to the procedure. On four occasions, fetuses sampled between 18 and 20 weeks gestation had severe persistent bradycardia that did not resolve, and they died within several hours of sampling. One FBS was complicated by chorioamnionitis, which produced miscarriage several days later. The apparent fetal risk is between 1% and 2%. The overall fetal loss rate due to fetal blood sampling is 3.6%, but this includes fetuses having in utero transfusions for severe anemia. There is an inherent procedural risk ranging from 0.5% to 1%.

Problems and Difficulties

The duration of the procedure is less than 5 minutes in 70% of cases and less than 10 minutes in 90% of cases. A variety of technical difficulties may be encountered. Although difficulties cannot be avoided completely, they can be reduced by use of a high resolution ultrasound system. Maternal obesity decreases the quality of the ultrasound image and necessitates the use of longer needles, which make manipulation more difficult. Similarly, oligohydramnios decreases the quality of the ultrasound image and often interferes with cord puncture. In these cases, FBS can be done on a loop of cord because the cord cannot move away from the needle. Polyhydramnios may necessitate emptying a large quantity of amniotic fluid before the procedure. When access to the cord is blocked by the fetus, it is possible to move the fetus by gentle external manipulation. Fetal movements can interfere with maintaining the needle in the vessel, and the operator has to wait for the fetal movements to stop spontaneously. Finally, cooperation and immobility of the mother are necessary for the success of the technique.

Indications for Fetal Blood Sampling

1. Infections
    - Toxoplasmosis
    - Rubella
    - Other viral
2. Karyotyping
3. Coagulation disorders
    - Hemophilia
    - Factor deficiencies
4. Platelet disorders
5. Rhesus isoimmunization
6. Hemoglobinopathies
7. Fetal welfare assessment
8. Miscellaneous

Bibliography

Chorionic Villous Sampling

Anon: Diagnostic and therapeutic technology assessment. Chorionic villous sampling: A reassessment. *JAMA*, 263:305–306, 1990.

Blakemore KJ, Mahoney MJ, Hobbins JC: Infection in chorionic villus sampling. *Lancet*, 2:339, 1985.

Bodurtha J, Redwine F, Jackson-Cook C: Three methods of fetal sampling in prenatal diagnosis. *VA Med Q*, 119:92–95, 1992.

Brambati B, Oldrini A, Ferrazzi E, et al: Chorionic villus sampling: an analysis of the obstetric experience of 1000 cases. *Prenat Diagn*, 7:157, 1987.

Doran TA: Chorionic villous sampling as the primary diagnostic tool in prenatal diagnosis. Should it replace genetic amniocentesis? *J Reprod Med*, 35:935–940, 1990.

Eichenbaum SZ, Krumins EJ, Fortune DW, et al: False-negative findings on chorionic villus sampling. *Lancet*, 2:391, 1986.

Elias S, Simpson JL, Martin AO, et al: Chorionic villus sampling in continuing pregnancies: Low fetal loss rate in initial 109 cases. *Am J Obstet Gynecol*, 154:1349, 1986.

Hogge WA, Schonberg SA, Golbus MS: Chorionic villus sampling: Experience of the first 1000 cases. *Am J Obstet Gynecol*, 154:1249, 1986.

Hook EB, Cross PK, Jackson LG, et al: Rates of 47, +21, and other cytogenic abnormalities diagnosed in first trimester chorionic villus sample (CVS): Comparison with rates from second trimester amniocentesis. *Am J Hum Genet*, 41: 276A, 1987.

Jackson LG: Fetal genetic diagnosis by chorionic villous sampling. *Semin Perinatol*, 15(Suppl 1): 43–48, 1991.

Jackson LG, Wapner RA, Barr MA: Safety of chorionic villus biopsy. *Lancet*, 1:674, 1986.

Ledbetter DH, Martin AO, Verlinsky Y, et al: Cytogenic results of chorionic villous sampling: High success rate and diagnostic accuracy in the United States Collaborative Study. *Am J Obstet Gynecol*, 162:495–501, 1990.

Mastroiacovo P, Botto LD, Cavalcanti DP, et al: Limb anomalies following chorionic villous sampling: A registry based case-control study. *Am J Med Genet*, 44:856–864, 1992.

McGovern MM, Goldberg JD, Desnick RJ: Acceptability of chorionic villi sampling for prenatal diagnosis. *Am J Obstet Gynecol*, 155:25, 1986.

McGowan KD, Blakemore KJ: Amniocentesis and chorionic villous sampling. *Curr Opin Obstet Gynecol*, 3:221–229, 1991.

Orrell RW, Lilford RJ: Chorionic villous sampling and rare side-effects: Will a randomised controlled trial detect them? *Int J Gynecol Obstet*, 32:29–34, 1990.

Perry TB, Vekemans MJJ, Lipmann A, et al: Chorionic villi sampling: Clinical experience, immediate complications, and patient attitudes. *Am J Obstet Gynecol*, 151:161, 1985.

Philip J, Smidt-Jenses S, Hilden J: The safety of chorionic villous sampling. A synthesis of literature. *Ann N Y Acad Sci*, 626:568–579, 1991.

Rhoads GG, Jackson LG, Schlesselman SE, et al: The safety and efficacy of chorionic villous sampling for early prenatal diagnosis of cytogenic abnormalities. *N Engl J Med*, 320:609–617, 1989.

Rosevear SK: Placental biopsy. *Br J Hosp Med*, 41:334, 338–344, 348, 1989.

Silverman NS, Wapner RJ: Chorionic villus sampling and amniocentesis. *Curr Opin Obstet Gynecol*, 2:258–264, 1990.

Simoni G, Fraccaro M, Gimelli G, et al: False-positive and false-negative findings on chorionic villus sampling. *Prenat Diagn*, 7:671, 1987.

Simpson JL: Chorionic villous sampling. *Semin Perinatol*, 14:446–455, 1990.

Smidt-Jensen S, Permin M, Philip J, et al: Randomised comparison of amniocentesis and transabdominal and transcervical chorionic villous sampling. *Lancet*, 340:1237–1244, 1992.

Williams J, Medearis AL, Bear MB, et al: Chorionic villus sampling is associated with normal fetal growth. *Am J Obstet Gynecol*, 157:708, 1987.

Williams J, Wang BB, Rubin CH, et al: Chorionic villous sampling: Experience with 3016 cases performed by a single operator. *Obstet Gynecol*, 80:1023–1029, 1992.

Young SR, Shipley CF, Wade RV, et al: Single-center comparison of results of 1000 prenatal diagnoses with chorionic villous sampling and 1000 diagnoses with amniocentesis. *Am J Obstet Gynecol*, 165:255–261; discussion 261–263, 1991.

Amniocentesis

Anderson RL, Goldberg JD, Golbus MS: Prenatal diagnosis in multiple gestation: 20 years' experience with amniocentesis. *Prenat Diagn*, 11:263–270, 1991.

Bowman JM, Pollack JM: Transplacental fetal hemorrhage after amniocentesis. *Obstet Gynecol*, 66:749, 1985.

Doran A: Chorionic villous sampling as the primary tool in prenatal diagnosis. Should it replace genetic amniocentesis? *J Reprod Med*, 35:935–940, 1990.

Evans MI, Koppick FC, Nemitz B, et al: Early genetic amniocentesis and chorionic villous sampling: Expanding the opportunities for early prenatal diagnosis. *J Reprod Med*, 33:450, 1988.

Finegan JA, Quarrington BJ, Hughs HE: Infant outcome following midtrimester amniocentesis: Development and physical status at age six months. *Br J Obstet Gynaecol*, 92:1015, 1985.

Hanson FW, Zorn EM, Termant FR, et al: Amniocentesis before 15 weeks gestation: Outcome risk and technical problems. *Am J Obstet Gynecol*, 156:1524, 1987.

Hanson FW, Tennant F, Hune S, et al: Early amniocentesis: Outcome, risks, and technical problems at less than or equal to 12.8 weeks. *Am J Obstet Gynecol*, 166:1707–1711, 1992.

Jeanty P, Rodesch F, Romero R, et al: How to improve your amniocentesis technique. *Am J Obstet Gynecol*, 146:593, 1983.

Johnson A, Hodmilon L: Genetic amniocentesis at 14 weeks or less. *Clin Obstet Gynecol*, 31:345, 1988.

Kappel B, Nielsen J, Broggard-Hansen K, et al: Spontaneous abortion following midtrimester amniocentesis: Clinical significance of placental perforation and blood stained amniotic fluid. *Br J Obstet Gynaecol*, 94:50, 1987.

McGowan KD, Blakemore KJ: Amniocentesis and chorionic villous sampling. *Curr Opin Obstet Gynecol*, 3:221–229, 1991.

Penso CA, Frigoletto FD, Jr: Early amniocentesis. *Semin Perinatol*, 14:465–470, 1990.

Penso CA, Sandstrom MM, Garber MF, et al: Early amniocentesis: Report of 407 cases with neonatal follow-up. *Obstet Gynecol*, 76:1032–1036, 1990.

Pijpers L, Jahoda MG, Vosters RP, et al: Genetic amniocentesis in twin pregnancies. *Br J Obstet Gynaecol*, 95:323, 1988.

Robertson AW: Amniocentesis: Indications. *Nebr Med J*, 77:263–264, 1992.

Rooney DE, MacLachlan N, Smith J, et al: Early amniocentesis: A cytogenic evaluation. *Br Med J*, 299:25, 1989.

Siverman NS, Wapner RJ: Chorionic villous sampling and amniocentesis. *Curr Opin Obset Gynecol*, 2:258–264, 1990.

Smith CV: Amniotic fluid assessment. *Obstet Gynecol Clin North Am*, 17:187–200, 1990.

Tabor A, Madsen M, Obel EB, et al: Randomized control trial of genetic amniocentesis in 4606 low risk women. *Lancet*, 1:1287, 1986.

Vyas H, Milner AD, Hopkin AE: Amniocentesis and fetal lung development. *Arch Dis Child*, 57:627, 1982.

Young SR, Shipley CF, Wade RV, et al: Single-center comparison of results of 1000 prenatal diagnoses with chorionic villous sampling and 1000 diagnosis with amniocentesis. *Am J Obstet Gynecol*, 165:255–261; discussion 261–263, 1991.

Fetal Blood Sampling

Bald R, Chatterjee MS, Gemburch U, et al: Antepartum fetal blood sampling with cordocentesis. Comparison with chorionic villous sampling and amniocentesis in diagnosing karyotype anomalies. *J Reprod Med*, 36:655–658, 1991.

Blackstone J, Young BK: Umbilical cord blood acid-base values and other descriptors of fetal condition. *Clin Obstet Gynecol*, 36:33–46, 1993.

Bodurtha J, Redwine F, Jackson-Cook C: Three methods of fetal sampling in prenatal diagnosis. *VA Med Q*, 119:93–95, 1992.

Boulot P, Deschamps F, Lefort G, et al: Pure fetal blood sampling obtained by cordocentesis: Technical aspects of 322 cases. *Prenat Diagn*, 10:93–100, 1990.

Chamberlain G: ABC of antenatal care. Checking of fetal wellbeing—II. *Br Med J*, 302:900–902, 1991.

Craparo FJ, Weiner S, Ludomirski A: Fetal blood sampling. *Curr Opin Obstet Gynecol*, 2:265–267, 1990.

D'Alton ME, DeCherney AH: Prenatal diagnosis. *N Engl J Med*, 328:114–120, 1993.

Daffos F: Fetal blood sampling. *Ann Rev Med*, 40:319–329, 1989.

Daffos F, Capella-Pavlovsky M, Forestier F: Fetal blood sampling during pregnancy with the use of a needle guided ultrasound. A study of 606 consecutive cases. *Am J Obstet Gynecol*, 153:655, 1985.

Golbus MS: Fetal diagnosis and therapy: An update. *Birth Defects Orig Art Ser*, 26:19–23, 1990.

Hobbins JC, Grannum PA, Romero R, et al: Percutaneous umbilical blood sampling. *Am J Obstet Gynecol*, 152:1, 1985.

Hoskins IA: Cordocentesis in isoimmunization and fetal physiologic measurement, infection, and karyotyping. *Curr Opin Obstet Gynecol*, 3: 266–271, 1991.

Hsieh FJ, Chang FM, Ko TM, et al: Percutaneous ultrasound-guided fetal blood sampling in the management of non-immune hydrops. *Am J Obstet Gynecol*, 156:1218, 1987.

Hurley PA, Rodeck CH: Fetal therapy. *Curr Opin Obstet Gynecol*, 4:4–9, 1992.

Loukopoulos D, Hadji A, Papadakis M, et al: Prenatal diagnosis of thalassemia and of the sickle cell syndrome in Greece. *Ann N Y Acad Sci*, 612:226–236, 1990.

Maeda H, Shimokawa H, Satoh S, et al: Safety of cordocentesis under ultrasound guidance for fetal blood sampling. *Acta Obstet Gynecol Jpn*, 42: 199–202, 1990.

Martin RW, McColgin SG: Evaluation of fetal and neonatal acid-base status. *Obstet Gynecol Clin North Am*, 17:223–233, 1990.

Maxwell DJ, Johnson P, Hurley P, et al: Fetal blood sampling and pregnancy loss in relation to indication. *Br J Obstet Gynecol*, 98:892–897, 1991.

Nocolaidis P, Nicolini U, Fisk NM, et al: Fetal blood sampling from the intrahepatic vein for rapid karyotyping in the second and third trimesters. *Br J Radiol*, 64:505–509, 1991.

Schulman LP, Elias S: Percutaneous umbilical blood sampling, fetal skin sampling, and fetal liver biopsy. *Semin Perinatol*, 14:456–464, 1990.

Soothill PW: Cordocentesis: Role in assessment of fetal condition. *Clin Perinatol*, 16:755–790, 1989.

Suzumori K: The role of fetal blood sampling in prenatal diagnosis. *Early Hum Dev*, 29:155–159, 1992.

Ulm JE, Shah DM, Dev VG, et al: Counseling and decision dilemmas associated with fetal blood sampling. *Am J Med Genet*, 35:75–78, 1990.

Wax JR, Blakemore KJ: What can be learned from cordocentesis? *Clin Lab Med*, 12:503–522, 1992.

Whittle MJ: Cordocentesis. *Br J Obstet Gynecol*, 96:262–264, 1989.

Whittle MJ, Gilmore DH, McNay MB: Obstetrics aspects of prenatal diagnostic methods. *J Inherit Metab Dis*, 12(Suppl 1):97–104, 1989.

Chapter 35

Circumcision

Elena Fuentes-Afflick

Circumcision is performed annually on approximately half the male newborn infants born in the United States (Poland, 1990)—over one million in total (Wallerstein, 1985)—and represents one of the most commonly performed surgical procedures (Broecker, 1991; Elder, 1992; Kochen and McCurdy, 1980; Maxwell et al, 1987; Toffler et al, 1990). Recently, there has been debate and discussion about the relative benefits and risks of the procedure.

At birth, the inner surface of the foreskin and the surface of the glans share a common epithelium (Grimes, 1978; Weiss, 1964). Differentiation and separation of these epithelial layers occurs during infancy and early childhood in uncircumcised males (Wallerstein, 1985). At birth, only 4% of infants have fully retractable foreskins; by the age of 4 years, 90% of foreskins are completely retractable (Osborn et al, 1981). The process of differentiation and separation of epithelial layers occurs naturally and should not be subjected to forcible foreskin retraction (Wallerstein, 1985).

Child health providers often do not receive proper education and training regarding care of the penis, both uncircumcised and circumcised (Wallerstein, 1985). Parents, therefore, often receive inadequate information regarding genital care, including circumcision (Metcalf et al, 1983; Osborn et al, 1981; Shaw and Robertson, 1963), and may be unable to make an informed choice. It is important that parents understand that circumcision is an elective surgical procedure with benefits and risks (Thompson, 1983; Wiswell and Geschke, 1989).

BENEFITS

Circumcision reduces the risk of phimosis, balanitis, urinary tract infection (UTI) in infancy, and cancer of the penis (Elder, 1992). The odds of UTI in infancy are increased in uncircumcised males by a factor of 10 to 39 (Devine et al, 1992; Wiswell, 1990; Wiswell and Geschke, 1989; Wiswell and Roscelli, 1986). The incidence of UTI in uncircumcised males is reported to range from 0.98% to 4.12%, and the corresponding incidence rates of UTI in circumcised males range from 0.10% to 0.21% (Wiswell and Roscelli, 1986; Wiswell et al,

1985, 1987). This appears to be related to periurethral colonization by uropathogenic bacteria. Cancer of the penis, a rare form of cancer, is effectively prevented with neonatal circumcision (Elder, 1992; Kochen and McCurdy, 1980). The incidence of penile cancer, however, is highly variable, even in countries that do not routinely perform neonatal circumcision. This suggests that proper genital hygiene in males may greatly reduce the risk of penile cancer, regardless of circumcision (Grimes, 1978).

INDICATIONS

Medical Indications

Phimosis, paraphimosis, and balanoposthitis are often considered indications for circumcision. Phimosis may be congenital or it may occur secondary to balanoposthitis (Schlosberg, 1971). It is estimated that 2% to 10% of circumcisions are performed later in life because of phimosis (American Academy of Pediatrics, 1975; Thompson, 1983). Paraphimosis, the inability to restore a retracted foreskin to its normal position, prevents lymphatic drainage of the penis and requires rapid intervention. Infections of the glans (balanitis) and glans-foreskin unit (balanoposthitis) are caused by a variety of factors, including bacteria and chemical irritants.

Socioreligious Indications

Parents, particularly mothers, request circumcision for a wide variety of reasons (Bolande, 1969; Gellis, 1978; Grimes, 1978; Herrera et al, 1982; Maisels et al, 1983; Morgan, 1965; Patel et al, 1982; Preston, 1970; Shaw and Robertson, 1963; Wallerstein, 1985). The factors involved in the decision range from sociocultural to religious and highlight the importance of educating and informing parents so that they are aware of the benefits and risks of the procedure (Herrera and Trouern-Trend, 1979; Wiswell, 1990).

CONTRAINDICATIONS

Contraindications include most congenital anomalies of the penis (Devine et al, 1992), prematurity, neonatal illness, and coagulation defects (Cunningham et al, 1989). Congenital anomalies of the penis, including hypospadias and epispadias, represent contraindications to circumcision because the foreskin is often necessary for adequate surgical repair (Devine et al, 1992). Prematurity is a relative contraindication to circumcision caused by physiological instability. Medical centers may circumcise premature infants after problems of prematurity have resolved and the baby has attained a weight sufficient for discharge from the hospital. Neonatal illnesses, such as perinatal infection, congenital heart disease, and other conditions, are usually considered contraindications to circumcision. Coagulation defects, if known or suspected on the basis of family history, are contraindications to circumcision due to the risk of excessive hemorrhage.

TECHNIQUE

General

Circumcision involves selection of the appropriate surgical tool for the procedure, administration of analgesia, and removal of an appropriate amount of foreskin. Marking the desired amount of foreskin to be removed with a surgical pen may be useful (Broecker, 1991). Reports of inadequate or excessive circumcision are well documented.

Depending on the surgical instrument chosen for circumcision, the appropriate size may need to be selected on the basis of the size of the penis. Circumcision is usually performed with the baby restrained on a plastic molded board with the legs immobilized using Velcro straps. The process of restraint often causes a certain amount of discomfort. It is also common for neonates to remain without oral intake for approximately 2 hours prior to circumcision, which minimizes the risk of aspiration of gastric contents during vigorous crying.

Types of Circumcision

There are four general types of circumcision: dorsal slit, shield, clamp, and sleeve techniques. The shield and clamp types will be detailed because they are the methods used in neonatal circumcision. Other references are available for the dorsal slit and sleeve techniques (Broecker, 1991; Devine et al, 1992; Diaz and Kantor, 1971). The dorsal slit involves a dorsal incision in the foreskin, which allows for complete retraction without excision of foreskin (Diaz and Kantor, 1971). The sleeve technique may be used by urologists to incise the inner and outer foreskin layers at different locations, remove the foreskin, and approximate the skin layers with suture (Broecker, 1991). Sleeve circumcision is often performed in older boys and men (Broecker, 1991). Although specialized circumcision instruments, both metal and plastic, may be available in larger sizes, they should not be used in older children because the larger vascular caliber of older infants and boys prevents the clamp from achieving hemostasis, and serious hemorrhage may occur (Devine et al, 1992). The three basic steps of circumcision are freeing the foreskin from the glans, thereby surgically separating the epithelial layers of the glans and the inner surface of the foreskin; applying the surgical instrument; and removing of the foreskin.

Gomco

The Gomco is one of the two most popular surgical instruments used in the United States for neonatal circumcision (Fig. 35–1). It is composed of a series of metal pieces, which must be assembled during the circumcision. The bell of the instrument is placed over the glans, and the foreskin, drawn over the bell, is clamped into place. The clamp compresses the interposed layer of foreskin, ensuring hemostasis, and the residual foreskin is incised above the level of the clamp (Broecker, 1991).

Advantages

The primary advantage is hemostatic capability.

Disadvantages

The multiple components can be cumbersome, and excessive foreskin can be removed by overzealous traction during application of the clamp.

Plastibell

The Plastibell is the other popular circumcision device currently in use in the United States (Fig. 35–2). The plastic instrument consists of a single plastic ring with a central groove, an inverted V-shaped bridge above, and a removable stem. The foreskin is placed over the Plastibell and a suture is used to secure the Plastibell at the base of the foreskin. The suture must be tightly applied because it causes ischemic necrosis of the foreskin. Within 10 to 12 days, the remaining foreskin necrotizes and falls off with the plastic ring (Marshall et al, 1980; Rubenstein and Bason, 1968).

Advantages

The foreskin is in full view and control of the operator during the circumcision, and the risk of removing an excessive amount of foreskin is minimal. It has been reported to be more rapid and efficient than metal clamps such as the Gomco (Rubenstein and Bason, 1968).

Disadvantages

The plastic ring of the Plastibell can migrate and cause problems. If the ring is too small, it may migrate distally and produce a groove in

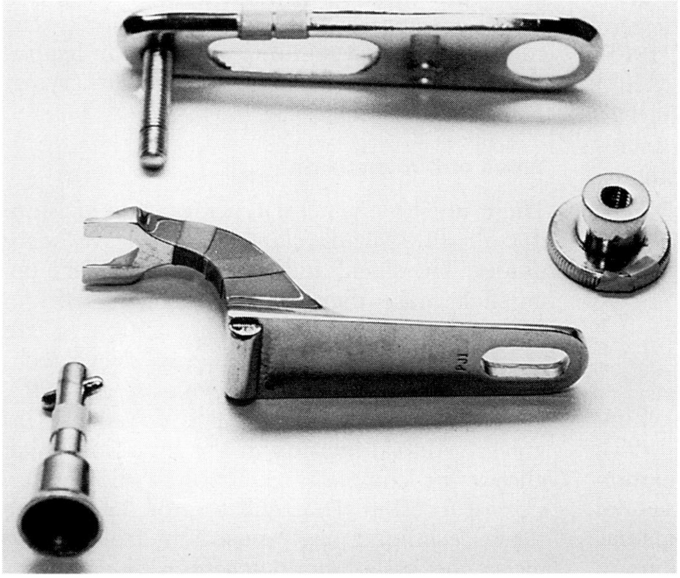

Figure 35–1 The Gomco clamp disassembled.

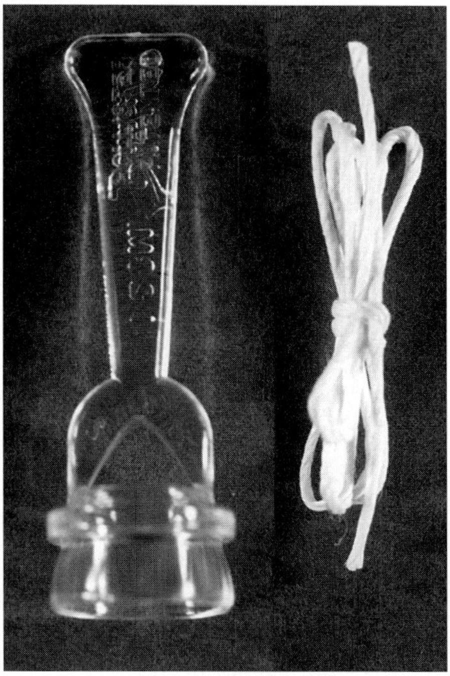

Figure 35–2 The Plastibell with ligature.

the glans, edema, or cyanosis (Gee and Ansell, 1976; Rubenstein and Bason, 1968). A larger ring may move proximally onto the shaft of the penis and make a grooved indentation (Rubenstein and Bason, 1968).

Mogen

The Mogen clamp, developed by a traditional Jewish *mohel*, or ritual circumciser, is a shield type of device used for neonatal circumcision (Fig. 35–3). It consists of a lightweight metal unit with two approximated plates separated by a narrow aperture and an arm that locks into place. The foreskin is placed into the aperture, the arm is locked across the lower edge of the clamp, and hemostasis is achieved by approximation of the metal plates. The foreskin is then removed with a scalpel. At the conclusion of the procedure, the skin layers must be carefully separated (Kaweblum et al, 1984).

Advantages

The clamp acts as a cutting surface and hemostat (Trochtenberg, 1991), thereby minimizing the risk of bleeding (Schlosberg, 1971). Few surgical instruments are necessary, and no dorsal slit is required (Kaweblum et al, 1984).

Disadvantages

The aperture of the Mogen clamp must be narrow enough to permit entry of the foreskin only, so that the tip of the glans is not inadvertently placed into the clamp.

COMPLICATIONS

Circumcision is reported to be safe, with reported complication rates from 0.06% to

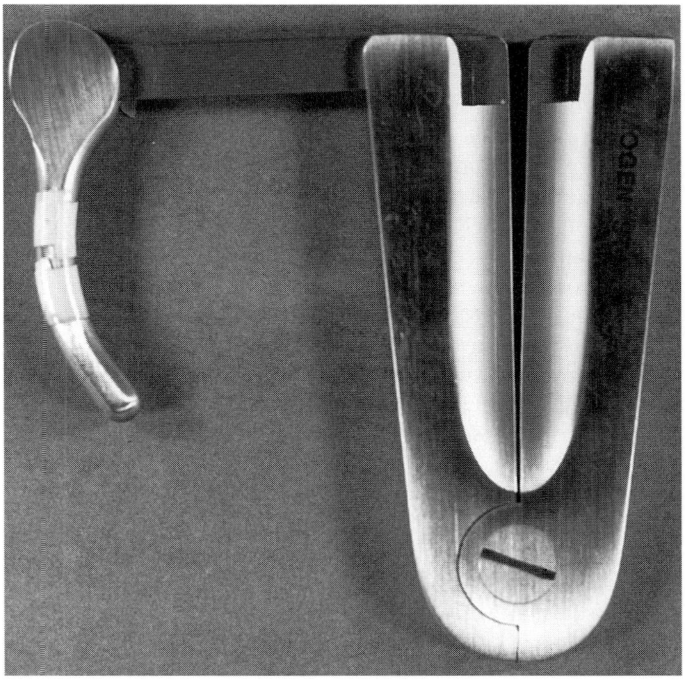

Figure 35–3 The Mogen clamp.

0.2% in large series (Wiswell, 1990). Nonetheless, circumcision should be performed by an experienced operator (Poland, 1990) who is familiar with anatomical landmarks, the circumcision procedure, and management of complications. When one is considering complications, however, the distinction should be made between minor and major.

Minor

The three most common minor complications are mild bleeding, mild infection, and surgical trauma (Devine et al, 1992; Preston, 1970). The cause of bleeding following circumcision may be inadequate hemostasis, coagulopathy, or anomalous vessels (Preston, 1970). Bleeding is usually treated with pressure dressings, suture placement, topical administration of epinephrine, or transfusion (Broecker, 1991; Devine et al, 1992; Gee and Ansell, 1976; Grimes, 1978). Mild infection may be managed with topical antibiotics or systemic therapy. It is possible that scarring, deformities, and phimosis can follow infection of the circumcised penis (Grimes, 1978). The types of surgical trauma that are considered minor complications include insufficient removal of foreskin (Broecker, 1991) and urethral trauma. The urethra may be damaged during circumcision or may become ulcerated and stenotic following circumcision (Preston, 1970; Schlosberg, 1971).

Major

Major complications, which are reported to be very rare, include hemorrhage, serious infection, surgical trauma, and death. Excessive hemorrhage may occur as a complication of circumcision or when circumcising an infant with a coagulation defect. Serious infections, including osteomyelitis, staphylococcal scalded skin syndrome, bacteremia, and death, have been reported with circumcision (Grimes, 1978). Major surgical injuries, such as denudation of the penile shaft; lacerated scrotum; bivalved, grooved, or amputated glans; concealed penis; penile necrosis; and penile loss, have also been described as a consequence of circumcision (Devine et al, 1992; Grimes, 1978). Electrocautery should never be used during circumcision because it has been reported to cause penile loss (Devine et al, 1992).

ANALGESIA

Circumcision is a painful surgical procedure, and neonates are capable of perceiving and sensing pain (Anand and Hickey, 1987). The choice of analgesic method is highly individual, but many physicians fail to provide analgesia or anesthesia, despite the variety of options (Wellington and Rieder, 1993). Increases in blood methemoglobin have been reported with analgesic agents (Mandel, 1989; Uhari, 1993); this potential risk must be considered within the broader context of pain relief.

None

There are a variety of reasons why physicians have opted against the use of analgesia during neonatal circumcision (Weiss, 1964). Physicians may be concerned about the safety and efficacy of analgesic alternatives (Masciello, 1990; Schlosberg, 1971). Physicians may also believe that the inconvenience of administering an analgesic outweighs its usefulness for circumcision. Lack of familiarity with anesthetic alternatives is also reported to be common among physicians who perform circumcision (Wellington and Rieder, 1993).

Dorsal Penile Nerve Block

The dorsal penile nerve block (DPNB) technique was reported by Kirya and Werthmann in 1978 as a means of anesthetizing the foreskin for circumcision. The dorsal penile nerves, which provide sensory innervation to the penis and foreskin (Fontaine and Toffler, 1991), branch approximately 1 cm distal to the penile root, and the goal is to anesthetize the nerves proximal to the branching (Kirya and Werthmann, 1978). Lidocaine (1%) without epinephrine is injected with a fine needle and a 1-ml tuberculin or insulin syringe (Fontaine and Toffler, 1991; Maxwell et al, 1987). No more than 0.8 ml should be injected, and aspiration of the syringe prior to infusion of the lidocaine will minimize the chance of intravascular administration. Following administration of the penile block, 2 to 5 minutes should elapse before proceeding, to allow the anesthetic agent to take effect (Fontaine and Toffler, 1991; Kirya and Werthmann, 1978). The duration of the anesthetic effect is 1 to 2 hours (Fontaine and Toffler, 1991). DPNB has been reported in multiple studies to ameliorate the pain and discomfort experienced by neonates undergoing circumcision (Holve et al, 1983; Maxwell et al, 1987; Stang et al, 1988; Williamson and Williamson, 1983).

The success rate for DPNB is reported to be 70% to 93% (Kirya and Werthmann, 1978; Mintz and Grillo, 1989; Toffler et al, 1990). Sometimes partial or unilateral anesthesia is achieved with DPNB (Fontaine and Toffler, 1991). This may be attributed to inadequate infusion of the anesthetic or an inexperienced operator, or it may represent an idiosyncratic reaction. The ventral surface of the foreskin, innervated by the ventral frenular penile nerve, may be only partially anesthetized with DPNB (Williamson and Williamson, 1983). Epinephrine should not be used because vasoconstriction may cause compromise of tissue perfusion (Fontaine and Toffler, 1991).

Caveats

Small or premature infants may require less volume for anesthesia (Fontaine and Toffler, 1991).

Advantages

The DPNB is a simple procedure that is easily taught (Maxwell et al, 1987; Stang et al, 1988). It is reported to prolong the time of circumcision by no more than 1 minute in experienced hands and seems to be safe for neonatal circumcision when administered properly (Fontaine and Toffler, 1991). The dose of lidocaine recommended for use in DPNB (no more than 0.8 ml of 1% lidocaine without epinephrine) is considered safe (Fontaine and Toffler, 1991; Maxwell et al, 1987).

Complications

The major complications of DPNB are localized bleeding and accidental puncture of the superficial vein of the penis, causing a visible hematoma (Fontaine and Toffler, 1991; Kirya and Werthmann, 1978). These complications resolve without further intervention. A theoretical concern is necrosis of the penis secondary to excessive pressure due to the infused lidocaine at the base of the penis (Kirya and Werthmann, 1978). The volume limitation of 0.8 ml is intended to minimize this risk.

Local Infiltration

Local infiltration of lidocaine (1%) without epinephrine into the foreskin at the level of the corona has been reported to be effective for circumcision analgesia (Masciello, 1990). The author of the reported study suggested that the ventral surface of the foreskin is more effectively anesthetized with local infiltration. The injection of the anesthetic agent in this location is unlikely to cause hematomas secondary to disruption of vascular structures.

EMLA

The eutectic mixture of local anesthetics (EMLA) consists of prilocaine and lidocaine hydrochloride bases in a 1:1 oil-water emulsion (Fontaine and Toffler, 1991). This preparation has been used for heel stick sampling, immunization, lumbar puncture, skin grafting, and venipuncture (Benini et al, 1993; Uhari, 1993) and has been studied for circumcision (Benini et al, 1993). For circumcision, Emla is applied to the external foreskin with a cotton-tipped applicator and is covered with an occlusive dressing. It has been demonstrated to diminish physiological measures of pain during neonatal circumcision (Benini et al, 1993).

Advantage

The primary advantage of Emla is its ease of administration. The mixture is easily applied to the external foreskin and must be covered with an occlusive dressing.

Disadvantages

The primary disadvantage is the length of time, 45 to 120 minutes, required for proper absorption of the topical anesthetics (Benini et al, 1993; Uhari, 1993). The pharmacokinetics of anesthetic absorption have not been well described, and the minimum amount of time required for anesthetic effect has not yet been defined for circumcision (Benini et al, 1993).

Topical Lidocaine

Topical lidocaine has been reported to be beneficial for neonatal circumcision (Weatherstone et al, 1993). The preparation, consisting of 30% lidocaine in an acid mantle cream and applied 20 minutes prior to circumcision, was found to significantly diminish the physiological and endogenous opioid response to the pain and stress of circumcision. Serum lidocaine levels were measured and found to be well within the range of safety.

Acetaminophen

Acetaminophen is commonly used in pediatrics for its analgesic properties and accepted safety profile, even in young infants. It is used as a systemic analgesic (Ipp et al, 1987) but has not yet been studied for relief of circumcision pain (Wellington and Rieder, 1993).

Sucrose

Sucrose, either in the form of an oral sucrose solution or a pacifier dipped in such a solution, has been demonstrated to provide analgesia during neonatal circumcision (Blass and Hoffmeyer, 1991). It has nociceptive properties, which may be mediated through opioid pathways in the central nervous system. Additionally, the latency period for action is short, which is advantageous for neonatal circumcision.

Ethanol

The "whiskey nipple" is a time-honored but unevaluated method for circumcision analgesia and is in current use. The anesthetic effect is mediated systemically (Wellington and Rieder, 1993). Theoretical complications include apnea and hypoglycemia.

References

American Academy of Pediatrics: Report of the Ad Hoc Task Force on Circumcision. *Pediatrics*, 56:610–611, 1975.

Anand KJS, Hickey PR: Pain and its effects in the human neonate and fetus. *N Engl J Med*, 317:1321–1329, 1987.

Benini F, Johnston C, Faucher D, et al: Topical anesthesia during circumcision in newborn infants. *JAMA*, 270:850–853, 1993.

Blass EM, Hoffmeyer LB: Sucrose as an analgesic for newborn infants. *Pediatrics*, 87:215–218, 1991.

Bolande RP: Ritualistic surgery—Circumcision and tonsillectomy. *N Engl J Med*, 280:591–596, 1969.

Broecker BH: Circumcision. In Glenn JF (ed): *Urologic Surgery,* 4th ed. Philadelphia, JB Lippincott, 1991, pp 841–844.

Cunningham FG, MacDonald PC, Gant NF (eds): *Williams Obstetrics,* 18th ed. Norwalk, CT, Appleton & Lange, 1989, p 243.

Devine CJ, Jordan GH, Schlossberg SM: Surgery of the penis and urethra. In Walsh PC (ed): *Campbell's Urology,* Vol. 3, 6th ed. Philadelphia, WB Saunders, 1992, pp 2972–2973.

Diaz A, Kantor HI: Dorsal slit. *Obstet Gynecol*, 37:619–622, 1971.

Elder JS: Congenital anomalies of the genitalia. In Walsh PC (ed): *Campbell's Urology,* Vol 2, 6th ed. Philadelphia, WB Saunders, 1992, pp 1921–1922.

Fontaine P, Toffler WL: Dorsal penile nerve block for newborn circumcision. *Am Fam Physician*, 43:1327–1333, 1991.

Gee WF, Ansell JS: Neonatal circumcision: A ten-year overview: With comparison of the Gomco clamp and the Plastibell device. *Pediatrics*, 58:824–827, 1976.

Gellis SS: Circumcision. *Am J Dis Child*, 132: 1168–1169, 1978.

Grimes DA: Routine circumcision of the newborn infant: A reappraisal. *Am J Obstet Gynecol*, 130:125–129, 1978.

Herrera AJ, Hsu AS, Salcedo UT, Ruiz MP: The role of parental information in the incidence of circumcision. *Pediatrics*, 70:597–598, 1982.

Herrera AJ, Trouern-Trend JBG: Routine neonatal circumcisions [letter]. *Am J Dis Child*, 133: 1069–1070, 1979.

Holve RL, Bromberger PJ, Groveman HD, et al: Regional anesthesia during newborn circumcision. *Clin Pediatr*, 22:813–818, 1983.

Ipp M, Gold R, Greenberg S, et al: Acetaminophen prophylaxis of adverse reactions following vaccination of infants with diphtheria-pertussis-tetanus toxoids-polio vaccine. *Pediatr Infect Dis J*, 6:721–725, 1987.

Kaweblum YA, Press S, Kogan L, et al: Circumcision using the Mogen clamp. *Clin Pediatr*, 23:679–682, 1984.

Kirya C, Werthmann MW: Neonatal circumcision and penile dorsal nerve block—A painless procedure. *J Pediatr*, 92:998–1000, 1978.

Kochen M, McCurdy S: Circumcision and the risk of cancer of the penis. *Am J Dis Child*, 134: 484–486, 1980.

Maisels MJ, Hayes B, Conrad S, et al: Circumcision: The effect of information on parental decision making. *Pediatrics*, 71:453–454, 1983.

Mandel S: Methemoglobinemia following neonatal circumcision (letter). *JAMA*, 261:702, 1989.

Marshall RE, Stratton WC, Moore JA, et al: Circumcision I: Effects upon newborn behavior. *Infant Behav Dev*, 3:1–14, 1980.

Masciello AL: Anesthesia for neonatal circumcision: Local anesthesia is better than dorsal penile nerve block. *Obstet Gynecol*, 75:834–838, 1990.

Maxwell LG, Yaster M, Wetzel RC, et al: Penile nerve block for newborn circumcision. *Obstet Gynecol*, 70:415–419, 1987.

Metcalf TJ, Osborn LM, Mariani EM: Circumcision. A study of current practices. *Clin Pediatr*, 22:575–579, 1983.

Mintz MR, Grillo R: Dorsal penile nerve block for circumcision. *Clin Pediatr*, 28:590–591, 1989.

Morgan WKC: The rape of the phallus. *JAMA*, 193:123–124, 1965.

Osborn LM, Metcalf TJ, Mariani EM: Hygienic care in uncircumcised infants. *Pediatrics*, 67: 365–367, 1981.

Patel DA, Flaherty EG, Dunn J: Factors affecting the practice of circumcision. *Am J Dis Child*, 136: 634–636, 1982.

Poland RL: The question of routine neonatal circumcision. *N Engl J Med*, 322:1312–1315, 1990.

Preston EN: Whither the foreskin? *JAMA*, 213: 1853–1858, 1970.

Rubenstein MM, Bason WM: Complication of circumcision done with a plastic bell clamp. *Am J Dis Child*, 116:381–382, 1968.

Schlosberg C: Thirty years of ritual circumcisions. *Clin Pediatr*, 10:205–209, 1971.

Shaw RA, Robertson WO: Routine circumcision. *Am J Dis Child*, 106:130–131, 1963.

Stang HJ, Gunnar MR, Snellman L, et al: Local anesthesia for neonatal circumcision. *JAMA*, 259:1507–1511, 1988.

Thompson HC: The value of neonatal circumcision. *Am J Dis Child*, 137:939–940, 1983.

Toffler WL, Sinclair AE, White KA: Dorsal penile nerve block during newborn circumcision: Underutilization of a proven technique? *J Am Fam Physician*, 3:171–174, 1990.

Trochtenberg DS: Neonatal circumcision [letter to the editor]. *N Engl J Med*, 323:1206, 1991.

Uhari M: A eutectic mixture of lidocaine and prilocaine for alleviating vaccination pain in infants. *Pediatrics*, 92:719–721, 1993.

Wallerstein E: Circumcision: The uniquely American medical enigma. *Urol Clin North Am*, 12: 123–132, 1985.

Weatherstone KB, Rasmussen LB, Erenberg A, et al: Safety and efficacy of a topical anesthetic for neonatal circumcision. *Pediatrics*, 92:710–714, 1993.

Weiss C: Circumcision in infancy. *Clin Pediatr*, 3:560–563, 1964.

Wellington N, Rieder MJ: Attitudes and practices regarding analgesia for newborn circumcision. *Pediatrics*, 92:541–543, 1993.

Williamson PS, Williamson ML: Physiologic stress reduction by a local anesthetic during newborn circumcision. *Pediatrics*, 71:36–40, 1983.

Wiswell TE: Routine neonatal circumcision. A reappraisal. *Am Fam Physician*, 41:859–863, 1990.

Wiswell TE, Enzenauer RW, Holton ME, et al: Declining frequency of circumcision: Implications for changes in the absolute incidence and male to female sex ratio of urinary tract infections in early infancy. *Pediatrics*, 79:338–342, 1987.

Wiswell TE, Geschke DW: Risks from circumcision during the first month of life compared with those for uncircumcised boys. *Pediatrics*, 83:1011–1015, 1989.

Wiswell TE, Roscelli JD: Corroborative evidence for the decreased incidence of urinary tract infections in circumcised male infants. *Pediatrics*, 78:96–99, 1986.

Wiswell TE, Smith FR, Bass JW: Decreased incidence of urinary tract infections in circumcised male infants. *Pediatrics*, 75:901–903, 1985.

Bibliography

Bigelow J: *The Joy of Uncircumcising!* Aptos, CA, Hourglass Book Publishing, 1992.

Ritter TJ: *Say No to Circumcision!* Aptos, CA, Hourglass Book Publishing, 1992.

Chapter 36

Well Infant and Child Procedures

Myles B. Abbott and Moses Grossman

An ounce of prevention is worth a pound of cure. — *T.C. Haliburton*

Prevention is the cornerstone of medical care for children. Regular health care examinations, which include immunizations and selective laboratory testing, have significantly decreased pediatric morbidity and mortality over the last half-century. These preventive examinations are most effective when conducted or directed by physicians well trained in pediatrics who have an ongoing relationship with their patients and their families.

Table 36–1 lists the ages at which pediatric patients should be seen for preventive care. This table is based on the National Guidelines for Health Supervision of Infants, Children and Adolescents (The Bright Futures Report, 1994), which has been endorsed by the American Academy of Pediatrics (AAP).

Certain procedures should be performed at each preventive care visit, whether an initial or interval visit: a complete physical examination, including vision, hearing, height, and weight; developmental/behavioral assessment; and anticipatory guidance. Head circumferences should be measured and plotted routinely until 24 months, and blood pressure should be recorded at each visit beginning at age 3 years. A routine hearing screen for all newborns has been suggested, but the technology is not available at the present time. Therefore, the child's ability to hear should be questioned and observed at all visits until 4 years of age. Objective, standardized testing of hearing and vision should begin at age 4.

Anticipatory guidance should be an integral part of each health care visit. It should be age specific and incorporate health education on safety, nutrition, and developmental/behavioral topics. An abbreviated and adapted age-specific anticipatory guidance schedule, as suggested in Chow et al (1984), is listed in Table 36–2. The age of the child dictates when routine laboratory procedures should be performed (Table 36–3).

LEAD SCREENING

The current recommendations for lead are universal screening at 9 to 12 months of age and, if possible, again at 24 months. Many pediatricians, however, believe that routine lead screening is not necessary or cost effective, except in children at high risk for lead exposure.

Table 36–1 Ages for Preventive Pediatric Health Care Visits

Childhood Period	Age
Infancy	Prenatal; newborn; first week; 1, 2, 4, 6, and 9 months
Early	12, 15, and 18 months; 2, 3, and 4 years
Middle	5, 6, 8, and 10 years
Adolescence	Yearly from 11 to 21 years

Table 36–2 Age-Specific Anticipatory Guidance

Infancy	Safety: car seat, falls Breast vs. bottle feeding; introduction of solids Sleeping position/patterns Fussiness/colic Teething Separation anxiety Exploration Locomotion
Early childhood	Safety: car seat, falls, drowning, poisoning, choking, burns Decreased appetite Setting limits/discipline Toilet learning Normalcy of masturbation Night terrors Self-care activities Verbal, visual, and tactile stimulation
Late childhood	Safety: seat belts, bike helmets, swimming Nutrition Educational stimulation Daily hygiene Controlled use of TV Peer activities Increasing self-esteem Sibling rivalry
Adolescence	Safety: driving, smoking, alcohol and drugs, guns Nutrition Physical and mental body changes Problem-solving techniques Relationship development Scholastic achievement Confidentiality Sex education

Table 36–3 Routine Laboratory Testing by Age

Metabolic screening*	Newborn
Hematocrit or hemoglobin	Once during each childhood period†
Urinalysis	Once during each childhood period†
Lead	9–12 months and, if possible, 24 months
Tuberculosis	See recommendations in text

*Metabolic screening (e.g., thyroid, PKU, galactosemia, hemoglobinopathy) should be done according to state law.
†See Table 36–1 for childhood periods.

TUBERCULIN TESTING

A screening tuberculin test in a healthy child determines whether the child has an inapparent infection with *Mycobacteria tuberculosis*. A positive reaction, meaning the presence of infection, would require prophylactic treatment and an epidemiological search for contacts, usually within the family. As the disease has become less frequent in the United States, an annual test is no longer recommended for all children.

- Children at high risk of infection (Table 36–4) should receive annual tuberculin tests.
- Children who live in high-prevalence areas, or for whom the degree of risk cannot be ascertained, should be tested periodically. A reasonable schedule is testing at ages 1, 5, and between 11 and 16 years. Many school districts require a tuberculin test prior to school entry.
- Children with no risk factors need not be tested unless there is a suspicion of clinical disease.

Two methods of tuberculin testing are available, the multiple puncture test (e.g., Tine, Aplitest, Mono-Vac) and the intradermal or Mantoux test. The Mantoux is recommended.

Mantoux Test

Five tuberculin units of protein purified derivative (PPD) are injected intradermally on the volar surface of the forearm using a tuberculin syringe and a 27-gauge needle. This should produce a 6- to 10-mm wheal. If the wheal does not appear, the likelihood is that the injec-

Table 36–4 Children at High Risk for Tuberculosis Infection

Contact with infected adults
HIV seropositivity or other immunosuppression
Living in homeless shelters or jails
Coming from, having parents from, or travel to countries with high prevalence of tuberculosis
Medical risk factors, e.g., malnutrition, malignancy, chronic renal failure
Frequent exposure to high-risk adults

Adapted from American Academy of Pediatrics: Report of Committee on Infectious Diseases. Red Book. Elk Grove Village, IL, 1994, AAP.

tion was too deep. In that case the test should be immediately repeated using the other arm.

In 48 to 72 hours, the child's arm is checked for induration by inspection and palpation. The area of induration should be measured in millimeters. It is only the induration, not the redness or edema, that counts.

A negative test (< 5 mm of induration) means that the child has not had a tuberculous infection. However, it could also mean that the child is anergic or that it is so early in the course of infection that delayed hypersensitivity has not yet developed (< 6–10 weeks)

An induration of greater than 5 mm is considered positive in the following groups of children:

- Those suspected to have disease, clinically or radiologically
- Those with human immunodeficiency virus (HIV) or otherwise immunosuppressed
- Those who have had close contact with an infectious adult

An induration of greater than 10 mm is considered positive for the following groups:

- Children younger than 4 years
- Children at increased risk because of environmental exposure
- Children at increased risk because of underlying medical conditions

An induration of greater than 15 mm is considered positive in all children.

IMMUNIZATIONS

Routine immunization of all children against common diseases of childhood is an important part of health care supervision. Table 36–5 lists the diseases we immunize against and the vaccines used.

Table 36–5 Childhood Immunizations

Disease	Vaccine
Diphtheria	Diphtheria toxoid
Hepatitis B	Hepatitis B recombinant vaccine
Haemophilus influenzae (type b)	*Haemophilus influenzae* conjugated vaccine
Measles	Measles attenuated vaccine
Mumps	Mumps attenuated vaccine
Pertussis	Pertussis killed whole cell and acellular vaccines
Poliomyelitis	Poliomyelitis polyvalent attenuated vaccine (Sabin)*
Rubella	Rubella attenuated vaccine
Tetanus	Tetanus toxoid
Varicella	Varicella attenuated vaccine

*Polyvalent killed vaccine (Salk) is used for immunosuppressed children.

Schedules

Table 36–6 provides a suggested immunization schedule for normal infants and children. This schedule is adapted from the recommendations of the Advisory Committee on Immunization Practices (ACIP) of the Centers for Disease Control and Prevention (CDC) (1994) and those of the AAP (1994). Infants born prematurely, regardless of birth weight, should be vaccinated at the same chronological age as full-term infants and children. The one exception to this recommendation is that small premature infants who remain in the nursery should receive their first hepatitis B injection at the time of nursery discharge. Children of hepatitis B surface antigen–positive mothers should receive hepatitis B immune globulin (HBIG) at birth along with the first dose of hepatitis B vaccine.

Contraindications

It is important to immunize children in a timely fashion and not to delay immunizations because of inappropriate contraindications. Table 36–7 provides a list of both appropriate and inappropriate contraindications compiled

Table 36-6 Recommended Schedule for Immunization of Normal Infants and Children

Age	Vaccine	
Birth	Hepatitis B vaccine (HBV)	
2 months	Diphtheria, tetanus, pertussis (DTP) and conjugated *Haemophilus influenzae* type b (HbCV) Oral polio vaccine (OPV) HBV	These four vaccines are available as a single preparation (DTPH)
4 months	DTPH OPV	
6 months	DTPH HBV	
6–18 months	OPV	
12–15 months	Measles, mumps, rubella (MMR)	
15–18 months	Varicella DTPH*	
4–6 years	DTP or diphtheria, tetanus, and acellular pertussis (DTaP) MMR OPV	
14–16 years	Tetanus + adult (attenuated) diphtheria (Td)	

Adapted from the American Academy of Pediatrics and the Advisory Committee on Immunization Practices. Report of Committee on Infectious Diseases. Red Book, Elk Grove Village, IL, 1994 AAP.
*The pertussis vaccine may be given as an acellular vaccine at this age.

by the AAP and the ACIP. We call attention to the meaning of precautions as noted in the footnote.

Patient Information

Informed parental consent is essential. The public provider is required to provide the family with pamphlets developed by the CDC about three immunizing agents—diphtheria, tetanus, pertussis (DTP); oral polio vaccine (OPV); and measles, mumps, rubella (MMR)—and to answer questions about the procedure.

Administration

Care must be exercised in storage and handling of vaccines. Many of them contain live attenuated viruses. Accidentally killing the virus (e.g., by storage at room temperature) will destroy the immunizing property of the vaccine. Attention must also be paid to the proper route of administration.

Subcutaneous injections are usually administered into the thigh of infants and into the deltoid area of older children. The needle should be gauge 23 to 25 and 5/8 to 3/4 inch long. Intramuscular injections are usually administered into the anterolateral aspect of the upper thigh in infants, and into the deltoid muscle of the arm in children. The buttock should not be used. In infants, the needle should be long enough to reach the muscle. After 4 months of life, a 22- to 25-gauge needle, 7/8 to 1 inch long, is usually optimal. A small infant with little subcutaneous tissue may require a smaller needle. Toddlers may require a slightly longer needle (1 1/4 inch). When multiple injections are given at the same visit, it is best to use separate anatomical sites for the injections.

Medical Records

It is particularly important to provide a record of the immunizations to the family and to keep an accurate office record. This record must include the date the vaccine was administered; the vaccine manufacturer; the vaccine lot number; and the name, address, and title of the person administering the vaccine.

Reporting of Adverse Reactions

Health care providers are required to report adverse events following the administration of vaccines to the Vaccine Adverse Events Report-

Table 36–7 Guide to Contraindications and Precautions for Vaccinations[1]

True Contraindications and Precautions	Not Contraindications (Vaccines May Be Administered)
General for all vaccines (DTP/DTaP, OPV, PIV, MMR, Hib, Hepatitis B)	
Contraindication Anaphylactic reaction to a vaccine Contraindicates further doses of that vaccine Anaphylactic reaction to a vaccine Constituent contraindicates the use of vaccines containing that substance Moderate or severe illnesses with or without a fever	***Not contraindications*** Mild to moderate local reaction (soreness, redness, swelling) following a dose of an injectable antigen Mild acute illness with or without low-grade fever Current antimicrobial therapy Convalescent phase of illnesses Prematurity (same dosage and indications as for normal, full-term infants) Recent exposure to an infectious disease Allergy to penicillin, other nonspecific allergies, or family history of such allergies
DTP/DTaP	
Contraindication Encephalopathy within 7 days of administration of previous dose of DTP ***Precaution*** Fever of >40.5°C (105°F) within 48 hr after vaccination with a prior dose of DTP Collapse or shocklike state (hypotonic-hyporesponsive episode) within 48 hr of receiving a prior dose of DTP Seizures within 3 days of receiving a prior dose of DTP Persistent, inconsolable crying lasting > 3 hr within 48 hr of receiving a prior dose of DTP	***Not contraindications*** Temperature of < 40.5°C (105°F) following a previous dose of DTP Family history of convulsions Family history of sudden death syndrome Family history of an adverse event following DTP administration
OPV	
Contraindications Infection with HIV or household contact with HIV Known altered immunodeficiency (hematologic and solid tumors, congenital immunodeficiency, and long-term immunosuppressive therapy) Immunodeficient household contact ***Precaution*** Pregnancy	***Not contraindications*** Breastfeeding Current antimicrobial therapy Diarrhea
IPV	
Contraindication Anaphylactic reactions to neomycin or streptomycin ***Precaution[2]*** Pregnancy	
MMR[3]	
Contraindications Anaphylactic reactions to egg ingestion and to neomycin[4] Pregnancy Known altered immunodeficiency (hematologic and solid tumors, congenital immunodeficiency, and long-term immunosuppressive therapy) ***Precaution[6]*** Recent immune globulin administration	***Not contraindications*** Tuberculosis or positive PPD skin test Simultaneous TB skin testing[5] Breast-feeding Pregnancy of mother of recipient Immunodeficient family member or household contact Infection with HIV Non-anaphylactic reactions to eggs or neomycin

Table 36-7 Guide to Contraindications and Precautions for Vaccinations[1] *Continued*

True Contraindications and Precautions	Not Contraindications (Vaccines May Be Administered)
Hib	
Contraindication	***Not a contraindication***
None identified	History of Hib disease
Hepatitis B	
Contraindication	***Not a contraindication***
Anaphylactic reaction to common baker's yeast	Pregnancy

From Centers for Disease Control: Advisory Committee on Immunization Practices (ACIP) General recommendations on immunizations. *MMWR,* 43:RRI 1–38, 1994.

[1]This information is based on the recommendations of the Advisory Committee on Immunization Practices (ACIP) and those of the committee on Infectious Diseases (Red Book Committee) of the American Academy of Pediatrics (AAP). Sometimes these recommendations vary from those contained in the manufacturer's package inserts. For more detailed information, providers should consult the published recommendations of the ACIP, AAP, and the manufacturer's package inserts.

[2]The events or conditions listed as precautions, although not contraindications, should be carefully reviewed. The benefits and risks of administering a specific vaccine to an individual under the circumstances should be considered. If the risks are believed to outweigh the benefits, the vaccination should be withheld; if the benefits are believed to outweigh the risks (for example, during an outbreak or foreign travel), the vaccination should be administered. Whether and when to administer DTP to children with proven or suspected underlying neurological disorders should be decided on an individual basis. It is prudent on theoretical grounds to avoid vaccinating pregnant women. However, if immediate protection against poliomyelitis is needed, OPV is preferred, although IPV may be considered if full vaccination can be completed before the anticipated imminent exposure.

[3]Acetaminophen given before administered DTP and thereafter every 4 hours for 24 hours should be considered for children with a personal or family history of convulsions in siblings or parents.

[4]No data exist to substantiate the theoretical risk of a suboptimal immune response from the administration of OPV and MMR within 30 days of each other.

[5]Persons with a history of anaphylactic reactions following egg ingestion should be vaccinated only with caution. Protocols have been developed for vaccinating such persons and should be consulted. (Herman et al, 1983; Greenberg and Birx, 1988).

[6]Measles vaccination may temporarily suppress tuberculin reactivity. If testing cannot be done the day of MMR vaccination, the test should be postponed for 4–6 weeks.

DTP, diphtheria, tetanus, pertussis; DTaP, diphtheria, tetanus, acellular pertussis; OPV, oral polio vaccine; PIV, parainfluenza virus; MMR, measles, mumps, rubella; Hib, *Haemophilus influenzae* type b; HIV, human immunodeficiency virus; TB, tuberculosis; PPD, purified protein derivative (tuberculin).

ing System. Among other benefits of reporting, such reports will enable the family to claim compensation for any injuries suffered as a result of immunization. The address and phone for communicating about these reports is

National Vaccine Injury Compensation Program
Health Resources and Services Administration
Parklawn Building, Room 8-05
5600 Fisher's Lane
Rockville, MD 20857
Telephone: (800) 338-2382

References

American Academy of Pediatrics. Report of Committee on Infectious Diseases. Screening for tuberculosis in infants and children. *Pediatrics,* 93:131–134, 1994.

Bright Futures. *National Guidelines for Health Supervision of Infants, Children and Adolescents.* Arlington, VA, National Center for Education in Maternal and Child Health, 1994.

Centers for Disease Control: Advisory Committee on Immunization Practices (ACIP) General recommendations on immunizations. *MMWR,* 43:RR1 1–38, 1994.

Chow MP, Durand BA, Feldman MA, et al: *Handbook of Pediatric Primary Care,* 2nd ed. New York, John Wiley & Sons, 1984.

Greenberg MA, Birx DL: Safe administration of mumps-measles-rubella vaccine in egg-allergic children. *J Pediatr,* 113:504–506, 1988.

Herman JJ, Radin R, Schneiderman R: Allergic reactions to measles (rubeola) vaccine in patients hypersensitive to egg protein. *J Pediatr,* 102: 196–199, 1983.

Bibliography

Ad Hoc Working Group Standards for Pediatric Immunization Practices. *JAMA,* 269:1817, 1993.

American Academy of Pediatrics. Report of Committee on Infectious Diseases. Red Book. Elk Grove Village, IL, 1994.

American Academy of Pediatrics. Report of Committee on Environmental Health. Lead poisoning: From screening to primary prevention. *Pediatrics*, 92:176–183, 1993.

Bess FH, Paradise JL: Universal screening for infant hearing impairment: Not risk free, not necessarily beneficial, and not presently justified. *Pediatrics*, 93:330–334, 1994.

Harvey B: Should blood lead screening recommendations be revised? *Pediatrics*, 93:201–204, 1994.

Huebner RE, Schein MF, Bass JB: The tuberculin skin test. *Clin Infect Dis,* 17:968, 1993.

NIH Consensus Statement: *Early Identification of Hearing Impairment in Infants and Young Children*. Bethesda, MD, National Institutes of Health Office of Medical Applications of Research, 1993.

Chapter 37

Diagnostic Ultrasound Screening of Infants

Frans J. Walther and John O. Leighton

Ultrasound equipment has become smaller and more mobile and is now widely available in most clinical settings, providing the interested pediatrician with the opportunity to perform ultrasound examinations. Although ultrasound is highly operator dependent and may be perplexing, screening examinations of various organ systems are now possible for pediatricians, who can rely on back-up by a radiologist or cardiologist with specific training in diagnostic ultrasound. This chapter focuses on major neonatal and pediatric anomalies that may be readily imaged by two-dimensional and Doppler ultrasonography.

Ultrasonography uses a transducer equipped with a piezoelectric crystal that converts electrical energy into mechanical sound waves. The usual frequencies for transducers used in infants and children are 5 and 7.5 MHz. With the transducer applied to the skin, the sound waves enter the tissue and are reflected at interfaces with different acoustic properties. The reflected echo is received by the transducer and converted to an electrical signal that is displayed. Two types of transducers are used in ultrasonography. The *linear array scanner* has a transducer that contains multiple crystals in a linear arrangement and produces a rectangular image as wide as the transducer but is too large to fit into the anterior fontanel or the intercostal spaces of infants. The *sector scanner* produces a triangular image by rotating its crystals with an electric motor (mechanical sector scanner) or by electrical phasing (phased array sector scanner). Higher-frequency or short-focus sector scanners provide better axial and lateral resolution and sharper images and are preferred over the lower-frequency, long-focus phased array sector scanners. Most of the images presented in this chapter were obtained with a high-frequency (7.5 MHz) mechanical sector scanner that provides superb resolution in the near field (0–3 cm). A limitation of ultrasound imaging is that air-filled lungs and gas-filled bowel loops are impenetrable to ultrasound. However, ultrasound does not produce ionizing radiation, is biologically safe, and does not require sedation. Portable equipment allows for quick noninvasive bedside examinations in sick infants without deterioration in their condition.

Doppler ultrasound detects the shift in

transmitted frequency of blood cells in motion and provides direct measurements of blood flow direction and velocity. Color Doppler imaging shows blood flow toward the transducer as a red flow area and shows blood flow away from the transducer as a blue flow area, with lighter colors representing higher velocities. Measurement of blood flow velocities and vessel diameter allows for the calculation of blood flow; for example, cardiac output can be quantified from the blood flow in the ascending aorta. (For more discussion on physical principles, see Chapter 24.)

Though instrumentation varies, the steps when beginning an ultrasound examination are standard. After switching on the power of the ultrasound equipment, select and activate a 5.0- or 7.5-MHz transducer. Check which transducer is active by placing the gel on the transducer and touching it with a finger; then select the two-dimensional mode and make sure you are not in freeze frame. Use plenty of gel between the transducer and the skin, as any air produces unwanted shadowing. Gain and output are usually preset; however, we prefer to vary the gain using both high and low settings during the study. Gain amplifies the returning signal, and increasing the gain will make the image whiter and may cause blurring if set too high. The lower the output, the better the resolution of the two-dimensional image; therefore, we try to use low-output settings between 25% and 50%. Changes in the depth settings will augment or reduce the size of the image. Vary the size of the image so that the whole organ may be imaged, and use magnification for areas of interest. The ultrasound signal becomes weaker with increasing depth. The time gain compensator allows stronger signals at greater depths and looks like a stereo equalizer. Use the slide-pods of the time gain compensator to suppress some of the near-field (first 2–3 cm) echoes and enhance the far-field (> 3 cm) echoes. Record the images on videotape for later playback or hit the freeze button and produce a hard copy.

BRAIN

The most common reason to perform cranial ultrasound in premature newborns is the suspicion of an intracranial hemorrhage. The four major varieties of neonatal intracranial hemorrhages are subdural hemorrhage, primary subarachnoid hemorrhage, intracerebellar hemorrhage, and periventricular-intraventricular hemorrhage (PV-IVH). Subdural hemorrhages in the newborn infant are almost exclusively traumatic in origin and uncommon. Primary subarachnoid hemorrhages are relatively common and relate to trauma in term infants and to hypoxic-ischemic events in premature infants but are usually not of major clinical importance. Intracerebellar hemorrhages have been described in retrospective autopsy studies in 15% to 25% of small premature infants.

PV-IVH is pre-eminent in terms of frequency and clinical importance in premature infants. Seventy-five to 90% of PV-IVHs originate in the subependymal germinal matrix at the level of the foramen of Monro (i.e., the more anterior portion of the frontal horn of the lateral ventricle) and the head of the caudate nucleus, where the terminal, thalamostriate, and choroidal veins come together to form the internal cerebral vein. Rupture of these small vessels, secondary to hypoxia and/or hyperperfusion, initiates the hemorrhagic process. Fifty percent of premature infants with PV-IVH have onset of their hemorrhage on the first day, an additional 25% on the second day, and an additional 15% on the third day after birth. In 20% to 40% the lesions progress and reach a maximal extension within 3 to 5 days of the initial positive exam. Therefore, we routinely screen newborn infants younger than or equal to 32 weeks of gestation on the first day of life and repeat the exam daily until day 5 to 7, when most cranial hemorrhages have occurred, and on day 14, when ventricular dilatation secondary to post-hemorrhagic hydrocephalus can be diagnosed. If the infant suddenly becomes unstable or has an unexplained drop in hematocrit, exhibits a sudden change in neurological status such as irritability or seizures, has a bleeding disorder, or develops apnea, ultrasound studies may be done on an emergency basis.

At the beginning of the cranial ultrasound examination, the anterior fontanel is palpated to determine its size and to gain an impression of the intracranial pressure. The transducer is then held steadily over the fontanel (which functions as an acoustic window), as bone does not allow passage of ultrasound waves. By placing the transducer in the coronal plane, perpendicular to the calvarium in the center of the anterior fontanel, a part of the ventricular and parenchymal system can be imaged (Fig. 37–1). By angling the transducer back and forth from the eyes (anterior tilt) to the occipital area (posterior tilt), most of the cerebral tissue can be imaged (see Fig. 37–1). By rotating the transducer 90 degrees to the sagittal plane and tilting it to-

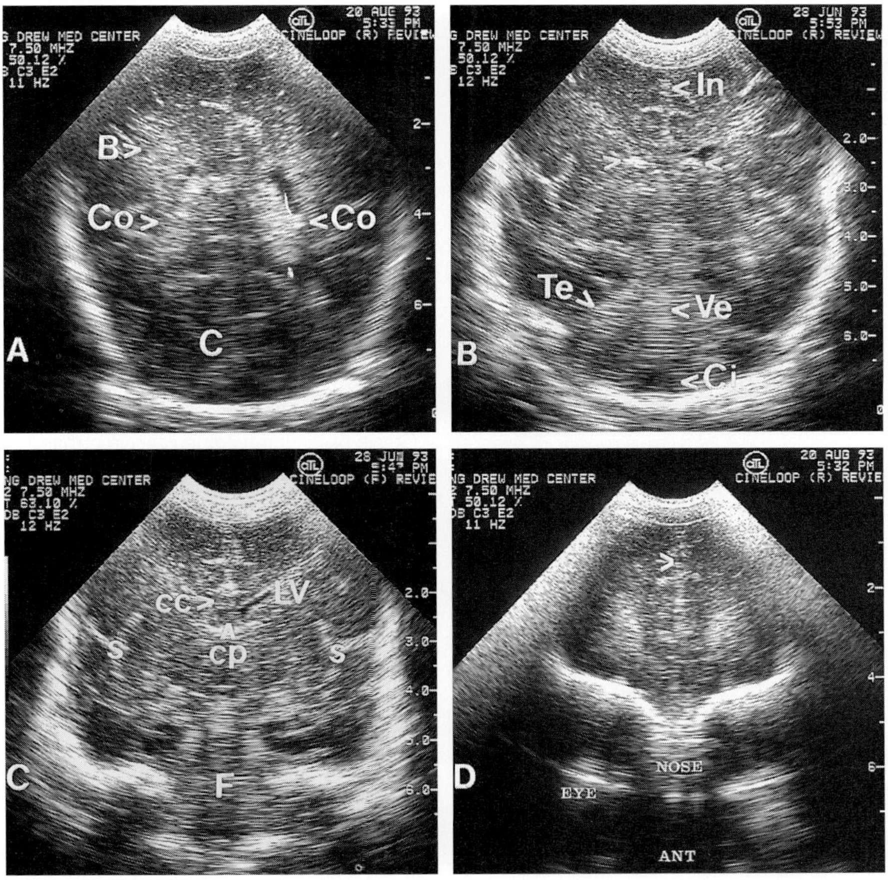

Figure 37–1 Four coronal views through the anterior fontanel. **A**. Coronal view through the trigone of the ventricle. The lateral ventricles diverge laterally, and the choroid plexuses (Co) show as highly echogenic structures. The cerebellum (C) can be identified, and a normal periventricular blush (B) is seen. **B**. Coronal view through the body of the lateral ventricles and the cerebellar vermis (Ve). The tentorium cerebelli (Te) forms an echo-free V-shaped area, beneath which the cerebellum is seen. The interhemispheric fissure (In) and cisterna magna (Ci) can be identified. The unlabeled arrows indicate the heads of the choroid plexuses seen along with the lateral ventricles. **C**. Coronal view at or just anterior to the foramen of Monro. The connection of the lateral ventricles to the slitlike third ventricle via the foramen of Monro is seen. The corpus callosum (cc) is seen between the superior portions of the lateral ventricles (LV). The cavum septi pellucidi (cp) is seen as a space between the lateral ventricles. Sylvian fissures (s) and foramen magnum (F) can be identified. **D**. Coronal view toward the eyes and the bridge of the nose provides a view of the frontal lobes. The unlabeled arrow indicates the midline.

ward one ear, the entire body of the lateral ventricle on that side can be studied (Fig. 37–2). Using both coronal and (para)sagittal cuts, it is possible to divide PV-IVH into four grades, from a localized subependymal hemorrhage in the germinal matrix to a major intraventricular hemorrhage with ventricular dilatation and parenchymal involvement (Table 37–1).

On a coronal scan a germinal matrix hemorrhage is visualized as a well-defined area of echogenicity inferolateral to the body of the lateral ventricles or to the floor of the frontal horn. On a parasagittal view a germinal matrix hemorrhage produces strong echoes anterosuperior to the foramen of Monro. The normal choroid plexus is vascular and echogenic and therefore is easily mistaken for a hemorrhage. However, any echogenicity anterior to the foramen of Monro is abnormal and cannot be caused by the choroid plexus, which is attached to the medial side of the ventricular floor and passes through the foramen to the roof of the third ventricle. When compared with a grade IV PV-IVH, which has parenchy-

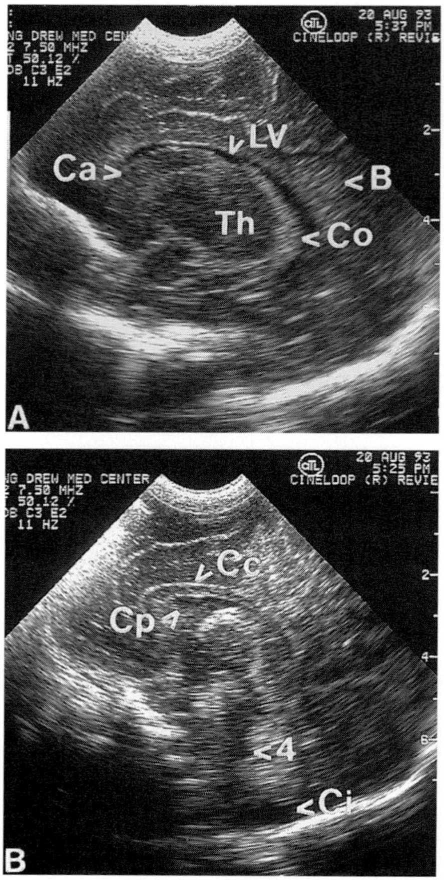

Figure 37–2 Sagittal cranial ultrasound scans through the anterior fontanel. **A**. Parasagittal scan through the body of the lateral ventricle (LV). Note the periventricular blush (B) around the trigone and the tip of the frontal horn of the lateral ventricle. The head of the caudate nucleus (Ca) and the thalamus (Th) can be identified. The choroid plexus (Co) has a normal appearance. **B**. Sagittal scan through the midline structures. The cavum septi pellucidi (Cp) remains sometimes as a triangular space between the lateral ventricles and can be visualized. 4, fourth ventricle; Ci, cisternal magna; Cc, corpus callosum.

mal involvement, the difference of an echogenic choroid plexus is readily apparent (Fig. 37–3). Lesser degrees of PV-IVH may be difficult to differentiate, but dilated lateral ventricles with large echogenic clots well within the body of these ventricles are indicative of PV-IVH grade III (Fig. 37–4). Smaller ventricles with small amounts of blood (grade II PV-IVH, Fig. 37–5) may be indistinguishable from a germinal matrix hemorrhage (grade I PV-IVH, Fig. 37–6). About 1 week after the occurrence of PV-IVH, the ventricles may develop very echogenic margins caused by a chemical ventriculitis in response to the presence of blood. Ventricular dilatation, especially prominent in PV-IVH grades III and IV, may progress to frank hydrocephalus (Fig. 37–7), which is usually secondary to an obliterating arachnoiditis in the posterior fossa and, less commonly, to obstruction at the aqueduct by blood clots.

Table 37–1 Grading of Periventricular-Intraventricular Hemorrhages in the Premature Infant

Grade	Description
Grade I	Germinal matrix hemorrhage with no or minimal intraventricular hemorrhage occupying < 10% of the ventricular area
Grade II	Intraventricular hemorrhage occupying 10–50% of the ventricular area, but no ventricular dilatation
Grade III	Intraventricular hemorrhage occupying > 50% of the ventricular area, usually with ventricular dilatation
Grade IV	Intraventricular hemorrhage with ventricular dilatation and parenchymal involvement

Data from Grant, 1986; Papile et al, 1978; and Volpe, 1987.

Clinically important subdural and subarachnoid hemorrhages are diagnosed by the presence of midline shifts on cornonal views (Fig. 37–8). Though intracerebellar hemorrhage is rare, any posterior fossa hemorrhage is serious because increased pressure within a confined space may lead to pressure on critical structures within the brain stem. The normal cerebellum is divided by the vermis, with the tentorium forming a superior roof; both can be quite echogenic. One has to carefully search for echodensities and cystic areas in the parenchyma of the cerebellum.

Periventricular leukomalacia (PVL) represents an infarction in the watershed area of the neonatal brain, between the branches of the deep penetrating arteries. It occurs most often lateral to the frontal horns and in the occipital radiations at the trigone of the lateral ventricles and is in 25% of cases accompanied by a hemorrhage in the affected area. Ultrasound findings include marked echogenicity due to localized edema, infarction, and hemorrhage on parasagittal scans. As these densities resolve, the areas become necrotic and develop into a series of small cysts (Fig. 37–9). If the PVL extends into the motor tracts, it is often associated with spastic diplegia or hemiparesis. The diagnosis of PVL by ultrasound alone should

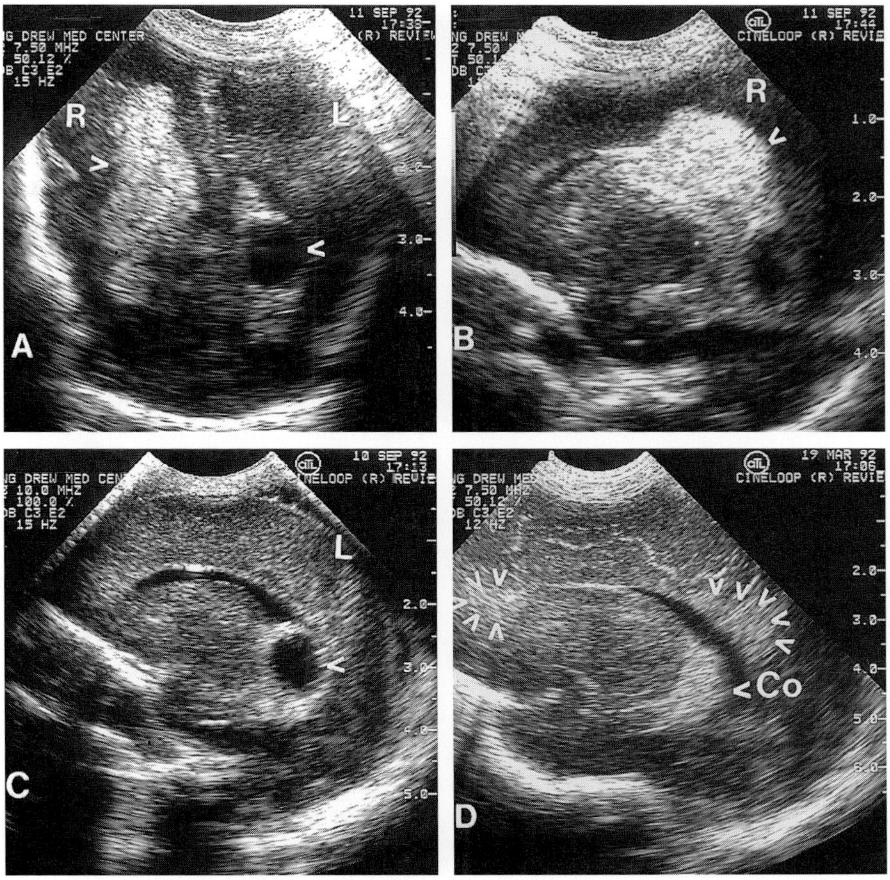

Figure 37–3 Coronal **(A)** and sagittal **(B** to **D)** views of a right-sided grade IV and a left-sided grade III periventricular-intraventricular hemorrhage in a premature infant (*arrows*). **A** and **B**. The right lateral ventricle is dilated and completely filled with blood, and the hemorrhage has extended into the periventricular area. **C**. The hemorrhage in the left lateral ventricle shows an echolucent center secondary to liquefaction. **D**. Intraventricular blood may resemble and be confused with a prominent but normal choroid plexus (Co), and periventricular blood should not be confused with a periventricular blush (*multiple arrows*).

be made with caution. On parasagittal scans of the normal premature infant, a periventricular blush around the trigone of each lateral ventricle and the tip of the frontal horns is produced by reflections from radiating neuronal fibers and accompanying blood vessels of the corona radiata (see Fig. 37–2). These periventricular echodensities should therefore be interpreted as normal findings and not as signs of PVL, especially in the absence of an intraventricular hemorrhage. If the periventricular echodensities are clearly asymmetrical, coarse, irregular in outline, or larger than 1 cm in diameter, they may be considered as warning signs of PVL. Even then, studies using orthogonal planes should be repeated over time to establish if these echogenicities fade and disappear, or cavitate with gradual development of a cystic area. Caution must be exercised as the echogenicity of the radiating neuronal fibers may vary with different equipment, transducer selection, and gain settings.

In addition to screening for intracranial hemorrhage and PVL, cranial ultrasound is worthwhile to screen for congenital brain anomalies, such as holoprosencephaly (Fig. 37–10), hydranencephaly (Fig. 37–11), calcifications secondary to cytomegalovirus or toxoplasmosis infection (Fig. 37–12), Dandy-Walker cyst, and arteriovenous malformation.

Though imaging of a clinically significant intraventricular hemorrhage is fairly straightforward in the presence of a dilated ventricle filled with an echogenic mass, confusing images are not uncommon in calamities such as severe asphyxia or massive bleedings, when

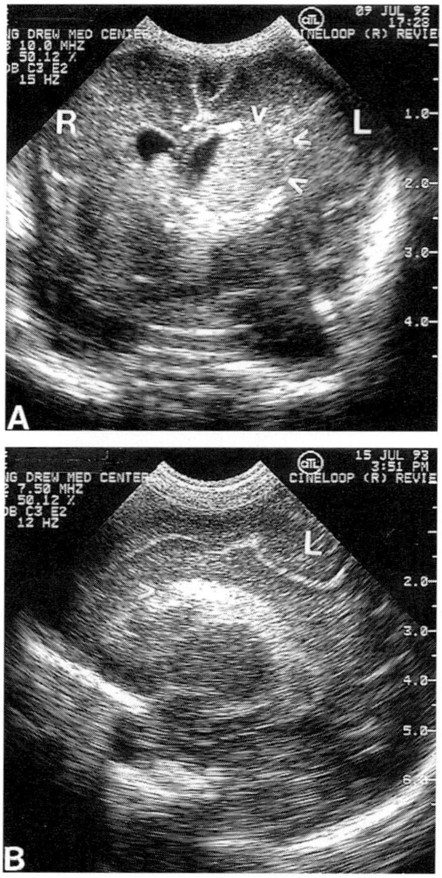

Figure 37–4 Coronal **(A)** and parasagittal **(B)** views of a left-sided grade III intraventricular hemorrhage. The coronal view shows an echogenic cast in the left-sided lateral ventricle typical for a grade III intraventricular hemorrhage (*arrows*). The arrow on the parasagittal view points to an abnormal echogenic area compatible with a grade II or III intraventricular hemorrhage.

echogenicities throughout the brain tissue may lead to a so-called bright brain image (Fig. 37–13).

CONGENITAL HEART DISEASE

Echocardiography encompasses visualization of the heart, the pericardial space, and the great vessels. A screening examination will probably concentrate on the possible presence of a congenital heart defect, cardiac function, and patency of the ductus arteriosus. Ultrasound examination of the beating heart is more complicated than visualization of the static brain structures and is full of pitfalls because of the diversity of views and anatomical structures presented in quick succession. (For an expanded discussion of echocardiography, see Chapter 24.)

The standard (apical) or modified (parasternal) *four-chamber view* is very helpful to screen for congenital heart defects. The four chambers of the heart can be visualized by placing the transducer in a transverse plane over the precordium, between the sternum and midclavicular line in the fifth or sixth intercostal space, and tilting it toward the head (superior tilt) (Fig. 37–14A). This modified apical four-chamber view is considered technically adequate when both the mitral and the tricuspid valves are visualized opening and closing simultaneously and look like two sets of clapping hands (Fig. 37–14A). The right atrium and right ventricle tend to be slightly larger than the left atrium and ventricle in the newborn infant. The ventricular septum should be detected easily, while the atrial septum may drop out due to poor ultrasound reflection or the presence of a patent foramen ovale. Marked enlargement of the right atrium and ventricle suggests the presence of congenital heart disease, such as total anomalous pulmonary veins (Fig. 37–14B), coarctation, Ebstein's anomaly, and hypoplastic left heart (Fig. 37–15). Unfortunately, severe pulmonary hypertension may also cause enlargement of the right heart. If the right heart is unusually small, this would be consistent with hypoplastic right heart syndrome, which is associated with pulmonary and tricuspid atresia. Inability to visualize the ventricular septum in multiple, orthogonal planes suggests a single ventricle (Fig. 37–15). Inability to visualize a mitral or tricuspid valve suggests mitral or tricuspid atresia. To be sure of left-right orientation, place the gel on the scan head and touch the left and right edges. The right ventricle can be recognized by the presence of a moderator band and a slightly more apical insertion of the tricuspid than the mitral valve (see Fig. 37–14). Contractility of the left ventricle can also be assessed. Poor contractility is associated with asphyxia, cardiomyopathy, anomalous coronary artery, left heart obstructive lesions, aortic stenosis, and coarctation of the aorta. When combined with auscultation, four-extremity blood pressure measurements, hyperoxia challenge, a chest radiograph, and an electrocardiogram, the four-chamber view will help to limit the potential lesions in the differential diagnosis. If the apical four-chamber view is of poor quality, subcostal views may be helpful. However, these views are considerably more difficult to interpret.

Parasternal long- and short-axis views of the heart are used to investigate the size and

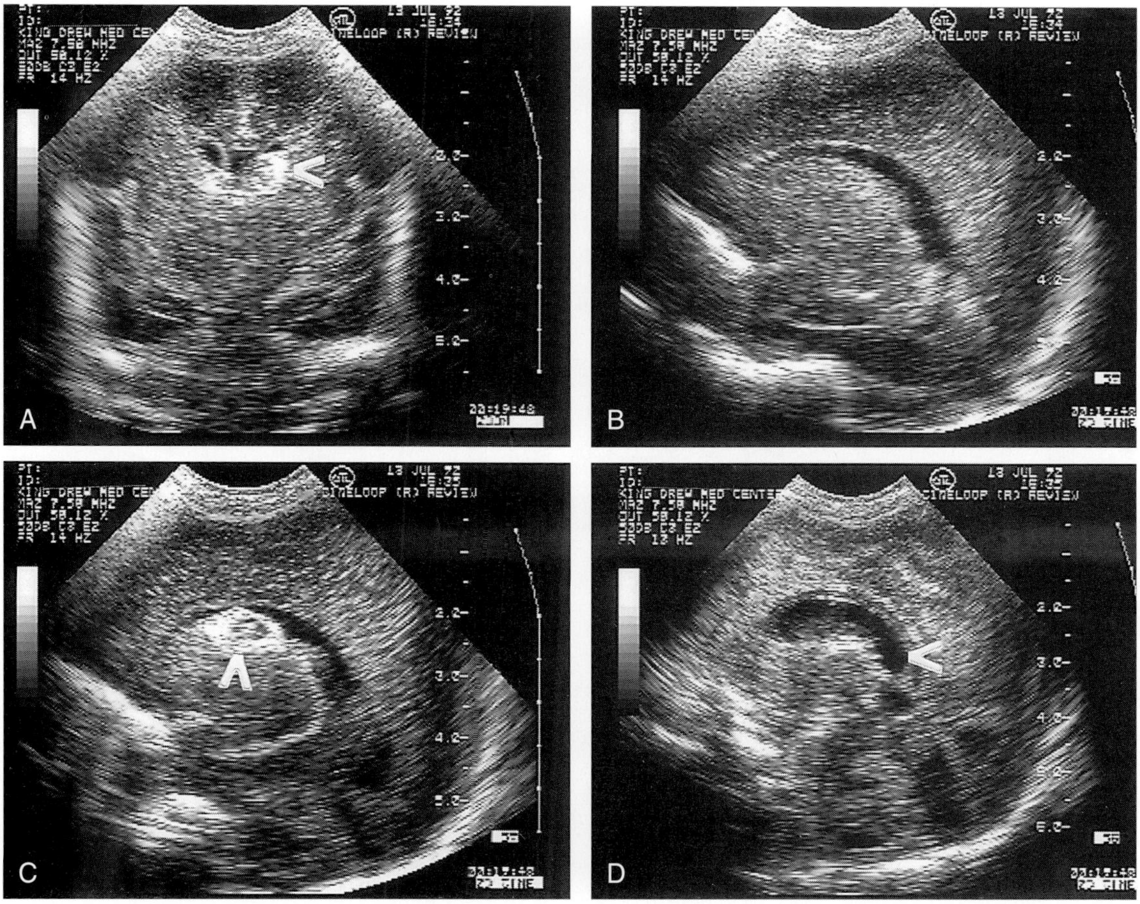

Figure 37–5 Coronal **(A)** and parasagittal **(B** to **D)** views of a left-sided grade II intraventricular hemorrhage. **B** and **C** are right and left parasagittal views. The arrows in **A** and **C** indicate a bleed with a large clot. **D** is a midline view, as indicated by the presence of midline structures like the cavum septi pellucidi (*arrow*).

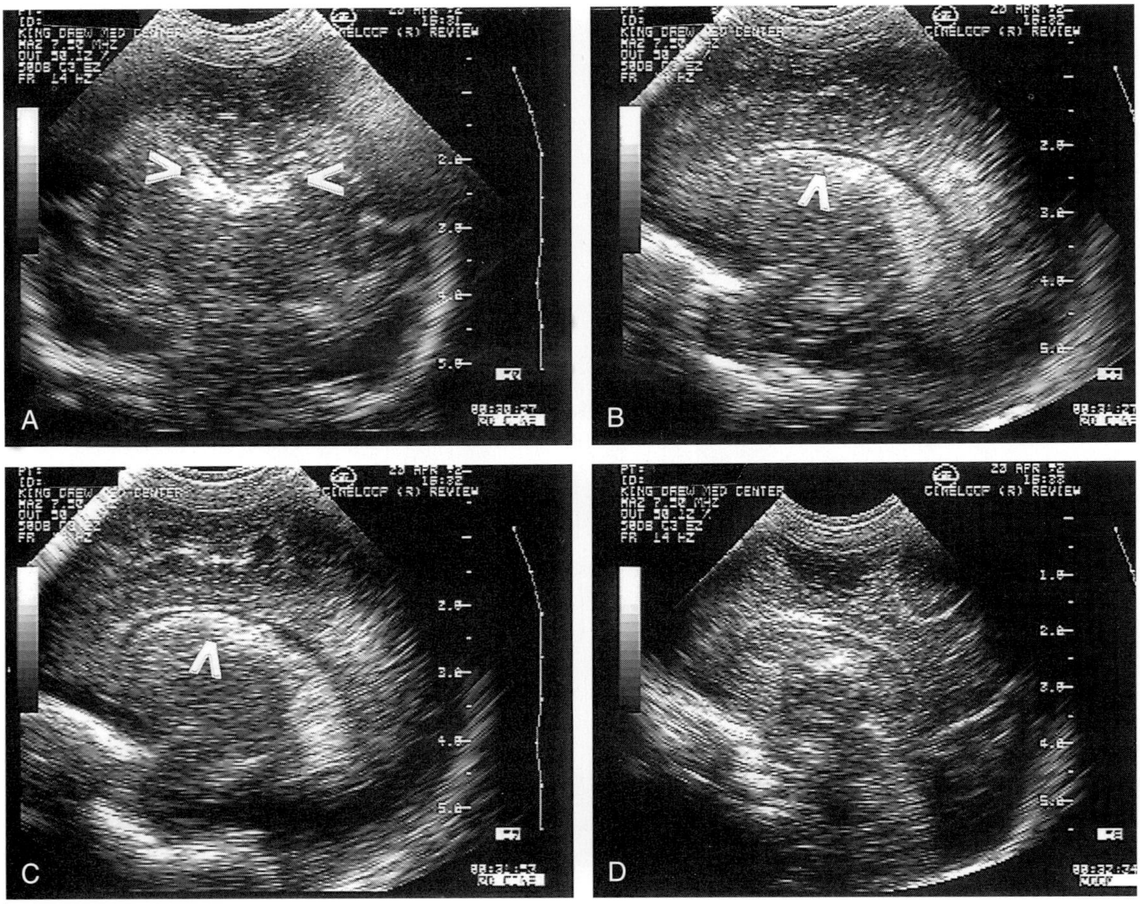

Figure 37–6 Coronal **(A)** and parasagittal **(B** to **D)** views of a bilateral grade I intraventricular hemorrhage. The arrows indicate a subependymal bleed without blood in the ventricles or ventricular dilatation. The cavum septi pellucidi in **D** is small and collapsed.

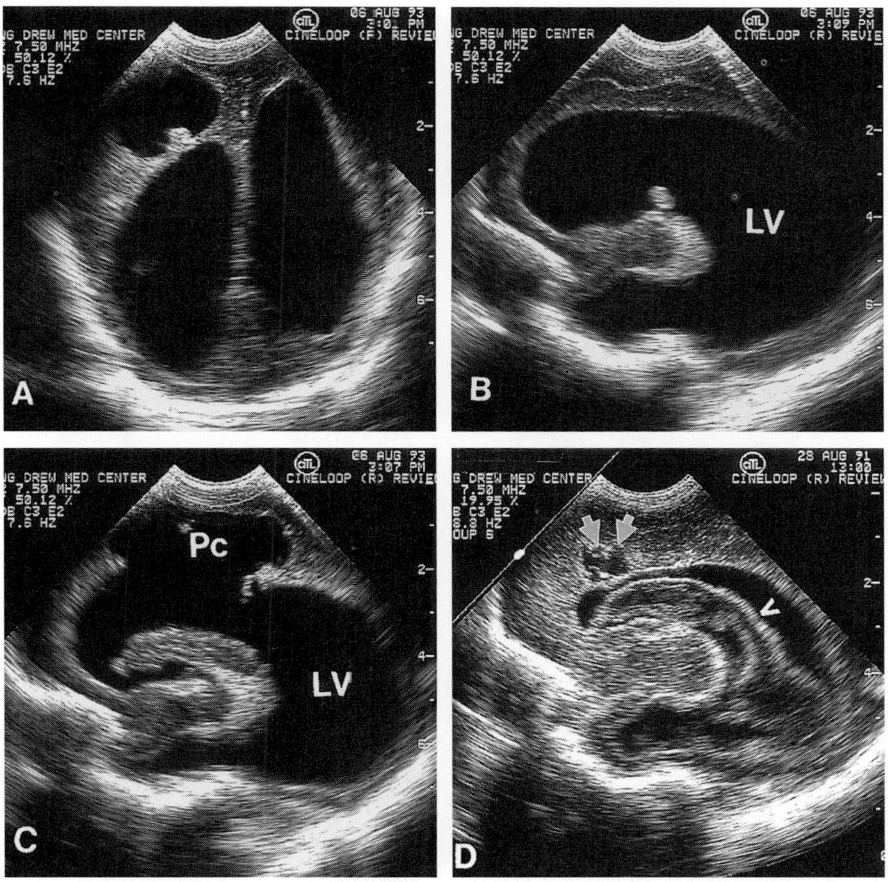

Figure 37–7 Coronal **(A)** and right parasagittal **(B** and **C)** views of a posthemorrhagic hydrocephalus with a communicating porencephalic cyst (Pc) shown in **C**. LV, lateral ventricles. **D**. Parasagittal view of the lateral ventricle from a different patient with a porencephalic cyst (*arrows*) and a large clot (*single arrow*), shaped like a cast of the original ventricle, that is liquefying from the center.

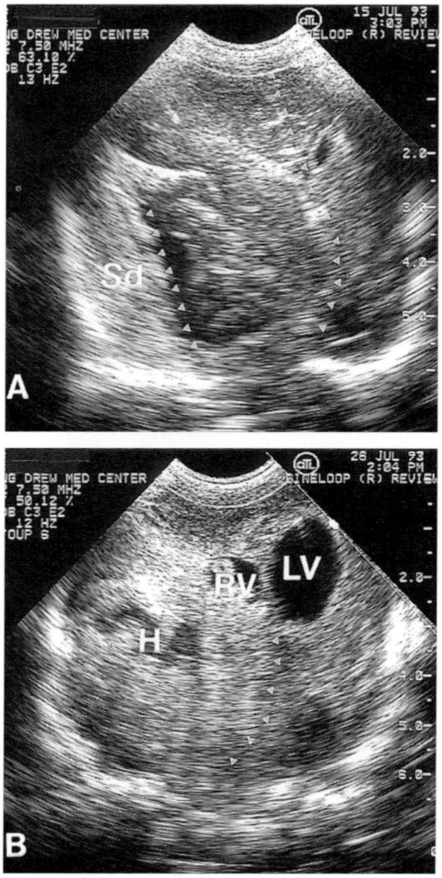

Figure 37–8 Midline shift secondary to a right-sided subdural hemorrhage **(A)** and a massive grade IV periventricular-intraventricular hemorrhage **(B).** Left line of arrows in **A** indicates subdural hemorrhage (Sd); right line of arrows depicts midline. Arrows in **B** indicate large parenchymal hemorrhage (H). RV and LV, right and left lateral ventricles.

structure of the aorta and pulmonary artery and their relationship to their respective ventricles. A long-axis view of the heart is obtained by placing the transducer perpendicular to the chest wall in a transverse plane in the third or fourth intercostal space along the left sternal border and rotating it clockwise (about 45 to 60 degrees) to a plane running from the right shoulder to the left hip. The aorta should appear as a long tube with the mitral and aortic valves seen simultaneously (Fig. 37–16). Check to see if the ventricular septum is continuous with the anterior wall of the aorta. In this view a large malalignment ventricular septal defect may be seen associated with tetralogy of Fallot, truncus arteriosus, and a double outlet of the right ventricle. The short-axis view is orthogonal to the long-axis view, and a 90-degree counterclockwise rotation of the transducer will change the long tube into a circle. Tilt the transducer toward the aortic valve until all three aortic leaflets are seen (resembling the Mercedes-Benz logo) (Fig. 37–17). The aorta and pulmonary artery should be approximately equal in size. Above and lateral to the aortic valve the pulmonary artery is seen "crossing over" the aorta. This view rules out transposition of the great arteries. In transposition of the great arteries, the arteries are parallel and have the appearance of two circles in the short-axis view. To further confirm the presence of transposition of the great arteries, find the vessel that comes to a dead end and bifurcates into right and left pulmonary arteries, and trace it to its ventricle of origin, remembering that the left ventricle is posterior in this view. Similarly, the vessel that arches and gives rise to head and neck vessels may be traced. A high right parasagittal view from the first or second intercostal space will aid in visualization of the aortic arch. If the circular aortic valve is seen and no pulmonary artery or valve can be found after considerable searching, a diagnosis of pulmonary atresia may be considered.

Figures 37–18 and 37–19 show how the described views can be used to diagnose major cardiac problems. The long-axis view in Figure 37–18 reveals hypertrophy of the interventricular septum in the presence of otherwise normal cardiac structures and is typical for infants of diabetic mothers. The four-chamber view in Figure 37–19 shows an arteriovenous canal or endocardial cushion defect in a Down syndrome infant with a heart murmur and an electrocardiogram with extreme right axis deviation.

ABDOMEN

Examination of the genitourinary system includes identification of both kidneys, both adrenal glands, and the bladder. Normal ureters are not seen by ultrasound. Doppler examination of the renal vessels may detect arterial stenosis and arterial or venous thromboses. Ultrasound scanning of the abdomen further allows for the identification of fluid in the peritoneal cavity, such as ascites, and the presence of liver pathology, such as hepatic cysts, abscesses, and pneumobilia.

Palpation of the kidneys provides a reference to renal morphology and to transducer placement. By holding the transducer in a coronal plane and sliding it anterior and posterior along

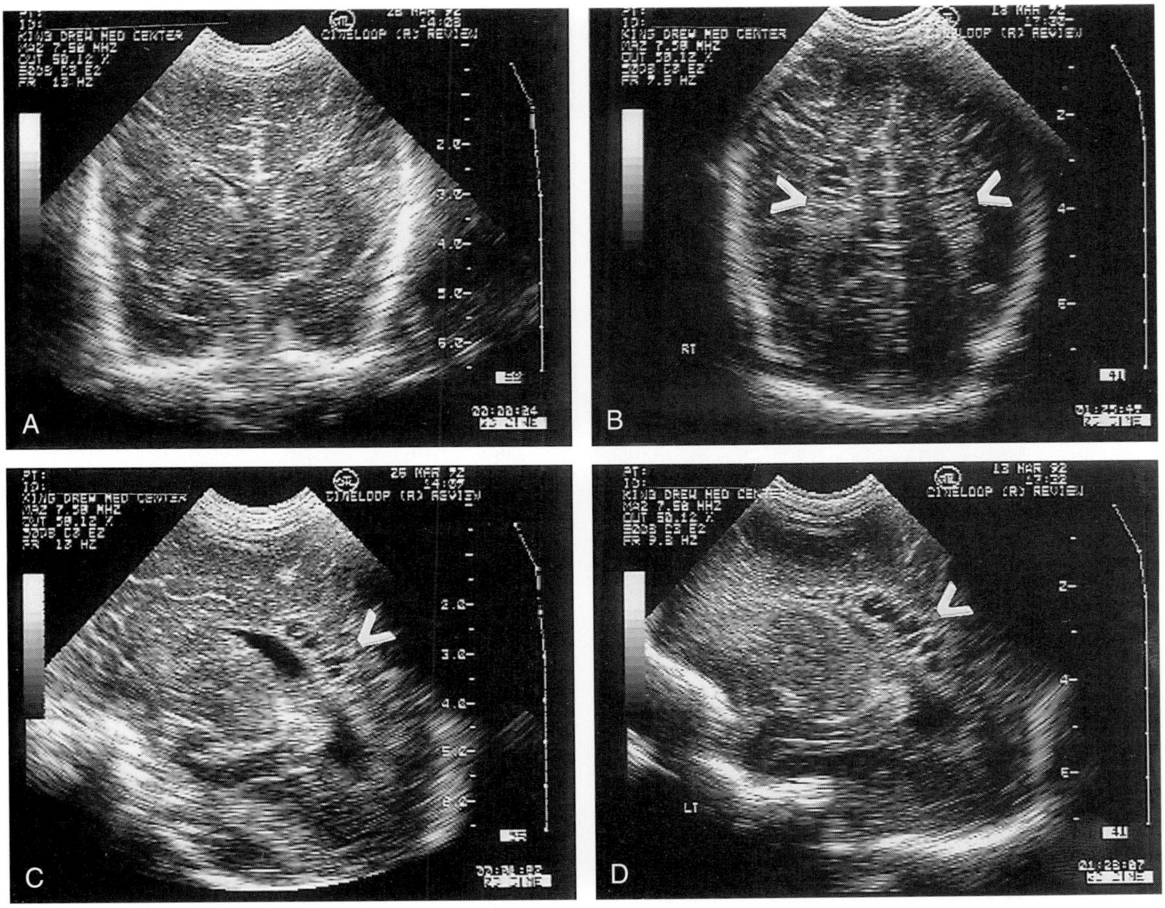

Figure 37–9 Bilateral cystic periventricular leukomalacia. **A** and **B**. Coronal views. **C**. Right parasagittal views. **D**. Left parasagittal view. Note the extensive cystic changes above the occipital horns of the lateral ventricles (*arrows*).

the right flank, the right kidney may be visualized (Fig. 37–20). Some searching may be necessary, as bowel gas may obscure the image. The right kidney is much easier to image than the left kidney, as the latter is more likely to be obscured by gas in the stomach and bowels. The neonatal kidney shows a different ultrasound picture from that of the older child. The renal cortex is echogenic, the medullary pyramids are relatively echolucent and slightly enlarged (mimicking cystic structures), and there is a lack of perirenal fat. The increased echogenicity of the renal cortex, seen in premature and term infants, is due to a larger number of glomeruli, increased cellular content of glomerular tufts, and the presence of loops of Henle within the cortex, all leading to an increased number of cellular interfaces with resulting greater echogenicity. This ultrasound finding should therefore not be confused

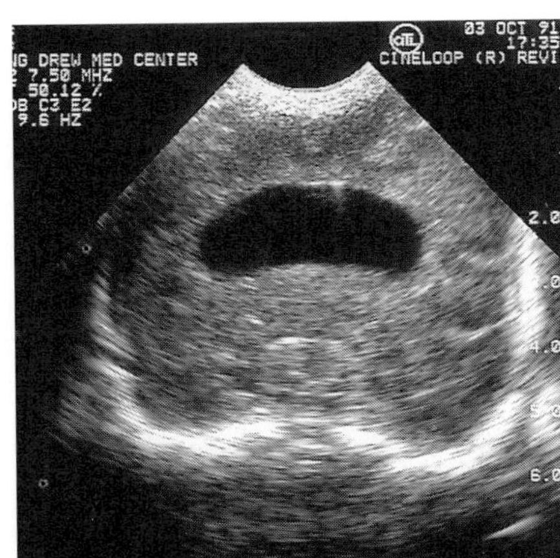

Figure 37–10 Coronal view of holoprosencephaly. The prosencephalon has failed to cleave in two, resulting in a single-sphered cerebral structure with a common ventricle that surrounds the fused thalami.

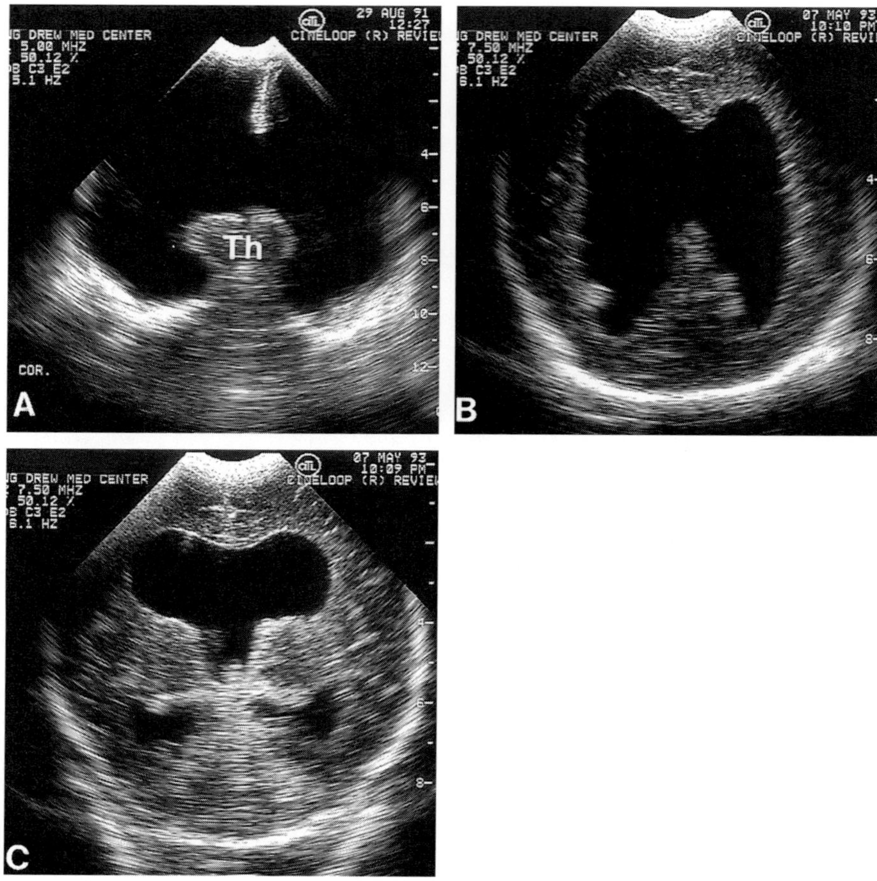

Figure 37–11 Coronal views of hydranencephaly and hydrocephalus. **A**. In hydranencephaly, both cerebral hemispheres are reduced to fluid-filled sacs of cerebrospinal fluid. Th, thalamus. **B** and **C**. In hydrocephalus, one or more ventricles are dilated, but various amounts of brain parenchyma are still visible.

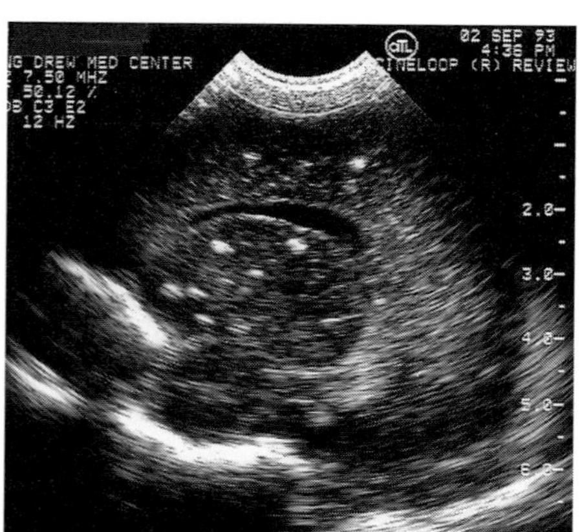

Figure 37–12 Intracranial calcifications.

with renal parenchymal disease. Three to 6 months after birth, this neonatal pattern is gradually replaced by decreased echogenicity. Premature infants receiving chronic furosemide therapy are at high risk for developing medullary nephrocalcinosis and kidney stones, which produce strong echoes and distinct acoustic shadows.

Congenital hydronephrosis and multicystic dysplastic kidneys are the most common abdominal masses of renal origin identified during the neonatal period. Transient mild hydronephrosis is common in sedated and paralyzed infants and should not be mistaken for cystic renal disease or more severe obstructive uropathies (Fig. 37–21). Congenital hy-

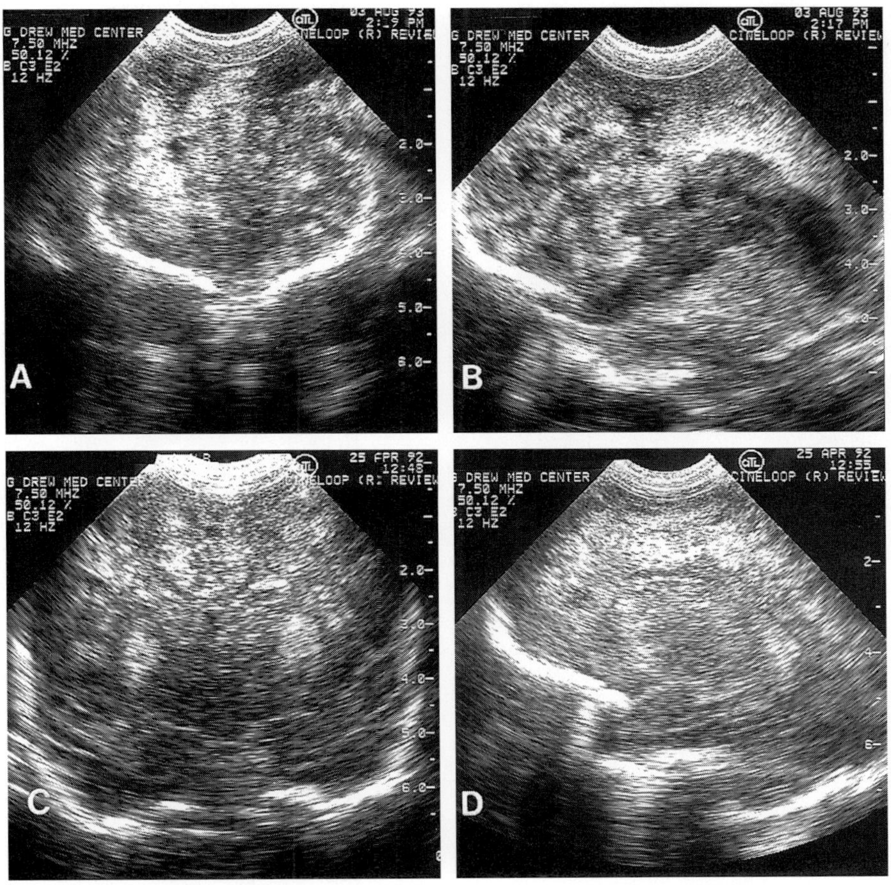

Figure 37–13 Cranial ultrasound scans of a preterm infant with a massive intracranial hemorrhage **(A** and **B)** and of a term infant who experienced severe asphyxia and brain damage **(C** and **D).** Normal structures have vanished, and bright echogenicities are seen throughout the brain, the so-called bright brain image.

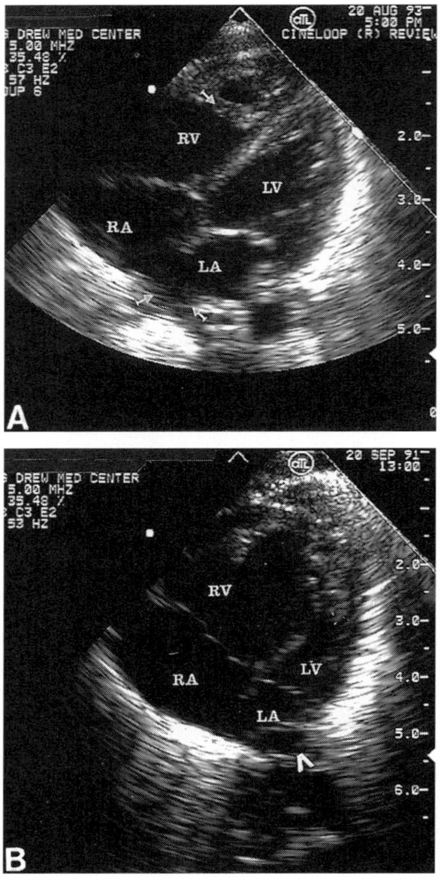

Figure 37–14 **A**. Standard apical four-chamber view. Note the moderator band in the right ventricle (*single arrow*) and the pulmonary veins entering the left atrium (*double arrows*). Both the mitral and tricuspid valves are visualized opening and closing simultaneously, like clapping hands, on this apical four-chamber view. **B**. Marked enlargement of the right atrium and right ventricle suggests the presence of congenital heart disease, in this case total anomalous pulmonary veins. In **B**, a pulmonary venous confluence (*arrow*) can be seen. LV, left ventricle; RV, right ventricle; LA, left atrium; RA, right atrium.

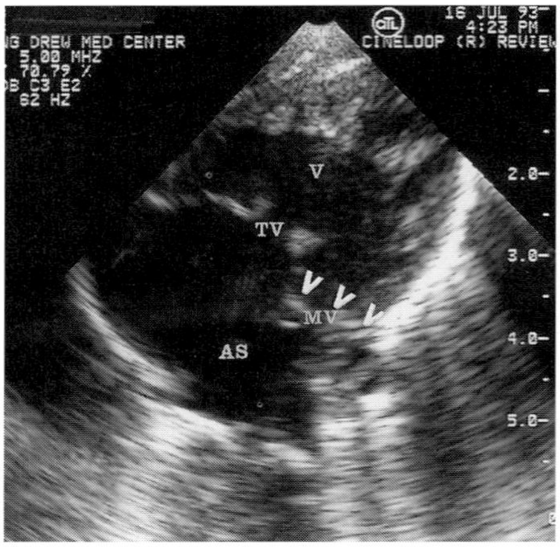

Figure 37–15 Ultrasound scan of hypoplastic left heart syndrome. Note the massive enlargement of the right side of the heart, a single ventricle (V), a functional tricuspid valve (TV), an atretic mitral valve (*arrowheads,* MV), and a normal atrial septum (AS). The left side of the heart was small and not seen in this view.

dronephrosis of the Finnish type is associated with slightly enlarged kidneys with a poor delineation between cortex and medulla, and ascites. Multicystic kidneys show many noncommunicating cysts of various sizes, and renal parenchyma is hardly if at all identifiable (Fig. 37–22). Polycystic kidneys, seen in autosomal recessive polycystic kidney disease, are both striking in their large size and very echogenic, with many small and echolucent cysts originating from dilated collecting tubules. Polycystic kidney disease is associated with congenital hepatic fibrosis and biliary ectasia, leading to biliary hepatic cysts.

In Potter's syndrome with renal aplasia, a

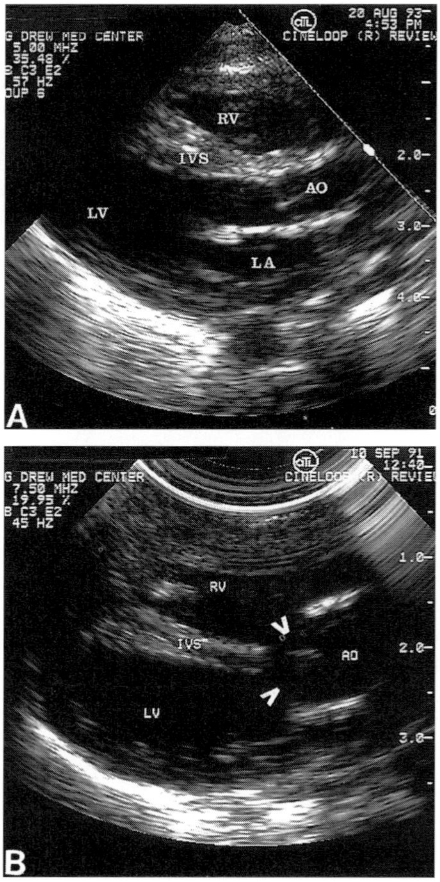

Figure 37–16 **A**. Normal long-axis view of the heart. **B**. A defect in the perimembranous portion of the ventricular septum and an overriding aorta (*arrows*), are seen in a case of a tetralogy of Fallot (the diagnosis in this case), truncus arteriosus, or double outlet of the right ventricle. LV, left ventricle; RV, right ventricle; LA, left atrium; AO, aorta and aortic valve; IVS, interventricular septum.

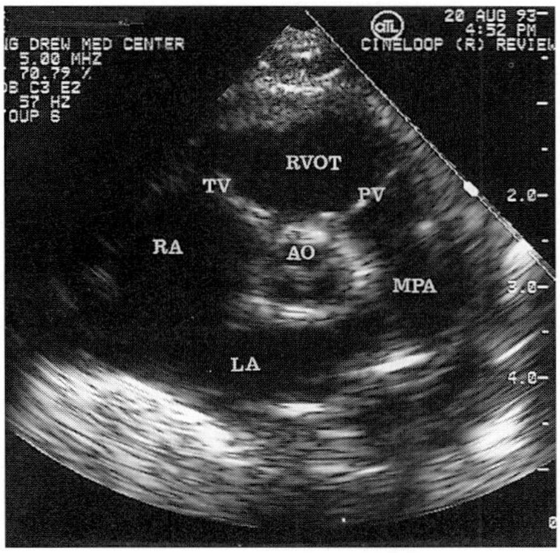

Figure 37–17 Standard short-axis view of the heart. RA, right atrium; LA, left atrium; AO, aorta and aortic valve; TV, tricuspid valve; PV, pulmonary valve; RVOT, right ventricular outflow tract; MPA, main pulmonary artery.

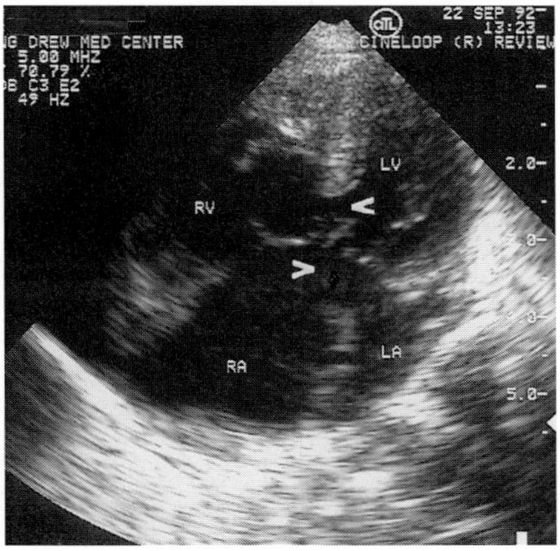

Figure 37–19 Ultrasound scan of endocardial cushion defect (*arrows*) in infant with trisomy 21. Note the simultaneous visualization of a primum atrial septal defect and a ventricular septal defect and the common atrioventricular valves. RV, right ventricle; LV, left ventricle; RA, right atrium; LA, left atrium.

long, thin adrenal gland may be mistaken for a normal kidney. An echogenic line representing the adrenal medulla surrounded by an echolucent cortex will aid in the distinction (Fig. 37–23). In renal duplication, both kidneys are on the same side and occasionally leave an adrenal gland on the contralateral side, mimicking renal agenesis. The duplicated kidney generally has hydronephrosis of the upper pole and is easily palpated. It should be noted that inability to visualize the kidneys generally indicates a poor scanning technique and not renal agenesis, and that to the novice the normal renal pyramids may appear to be cysts.

The neonatal adrenal glands can be identified as triangular structures that cap the superior poles of the kidneys. Their cortex is echolucent or anechoic, and their medulla forms an echogenic line (see Fig. 37–23). In adrenal hemorrhage a large mass in the adrenal gland with multiple cystic areas may be seen (Fig. 37–24). At resolution the mass decreases and may calcify.

The routine use of arterial umbilical catheters has increased the incidence of renal thromboembolism and subsequent renovascu-

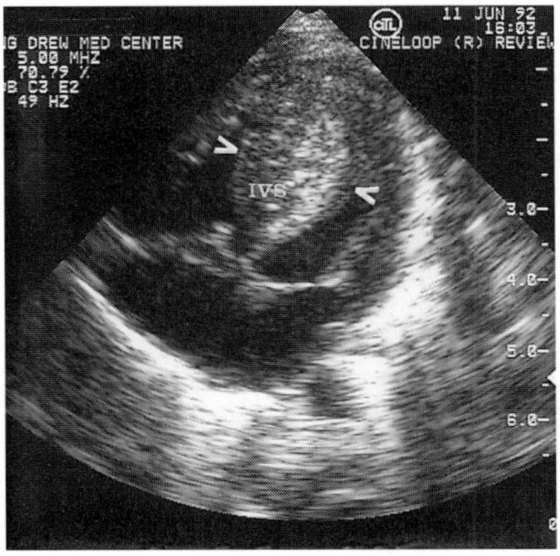

Figure 37–18 Heart of an infant of a diabetic mother. Note the hypertrophy (*arrows*) of the interventricular septum (IVS), that is, 2.5 times the normal size.

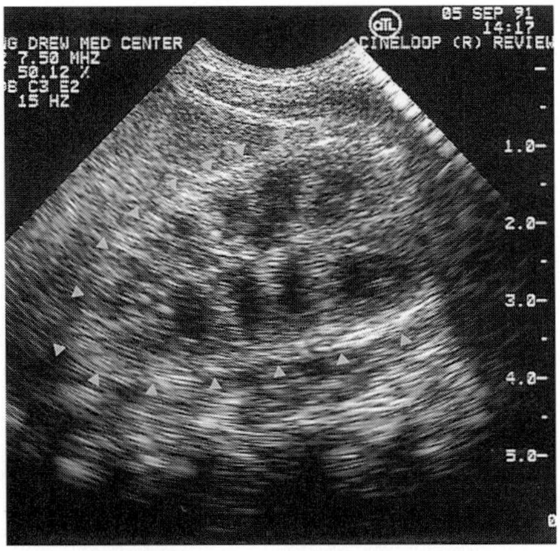

Figure 37–20 Coronal scan of the right kidney (*arrows*) in a term infant showing the characteristic neonatal features: the renal cortex is echogenic, the medullary pyramids are relatively echolucent and slightly enlarged, and there is a lack of perirenal fat.

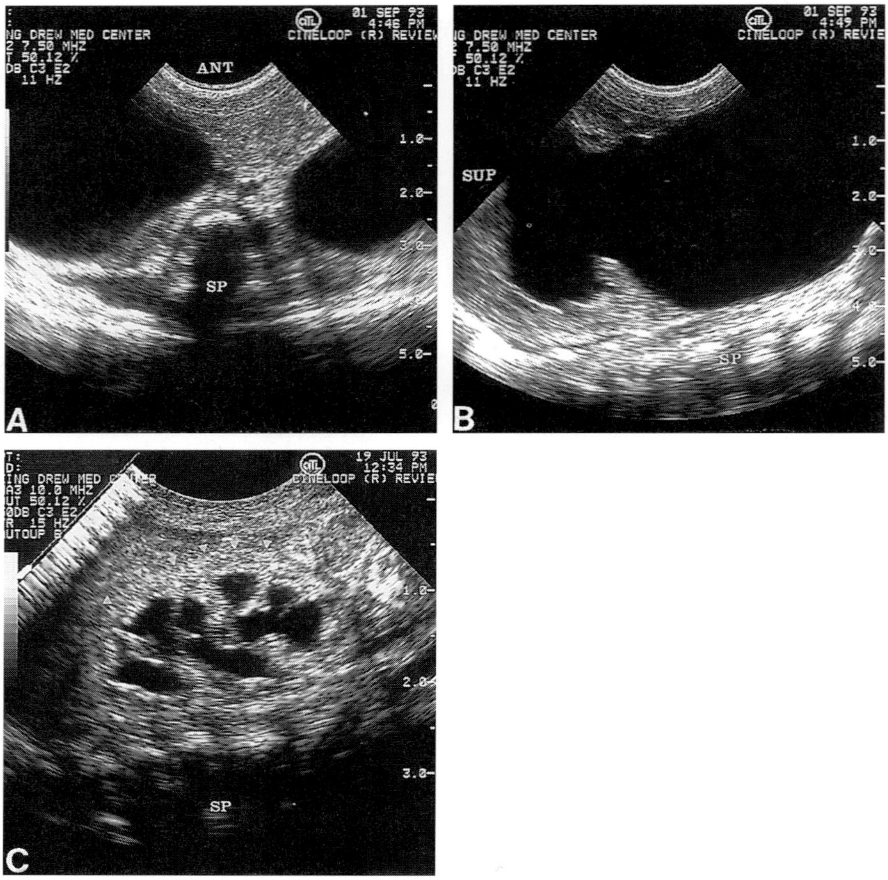

Figure 37–21 **A** and **B**. Ultrasound of severe hydronephrosis in an infant with prune-belly syndrome. **C**. Kidney (*arrows*) with mild hydronephrosis. ANT, anterior; SP, spine; SUP, superior.

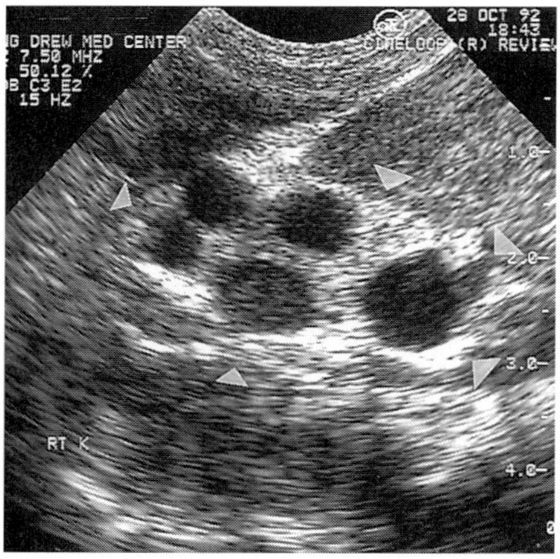

Figure 37–22 Ultrasound scan of multicystic kidney disease. The kidney (*arrows*) shows many noncommunicating cysts of various sizes, and renal parenchyma is hardly identifiable.

lar hypertension. Clinically evident thrombotic complications occur in 5% of the infants who undergo arterial umbilical catheterization. Investigation of renal blood flow by Doppler imaging is best left to an experienced vascular sonographer.

When the bladder is full, it can be visualized in the transverse and/or sagittal planes with the transducer held perpendicular to the abdomen between the umbilicus and the pubic symphysis. Palpation of the bladder will aid in transducer placement. A distended bladder (Fig. 37–25) may be useful in estimating urine output and assessing the etiology of hydronephrosis. In infants with hematuria, clots may occasionally be seen in the urinary bladder (Fig. 37–26). Urinary ascites may result from rupture of the bladder secondary to posterior urethral valves (Fig. 37–27). Diagnosis of ascites

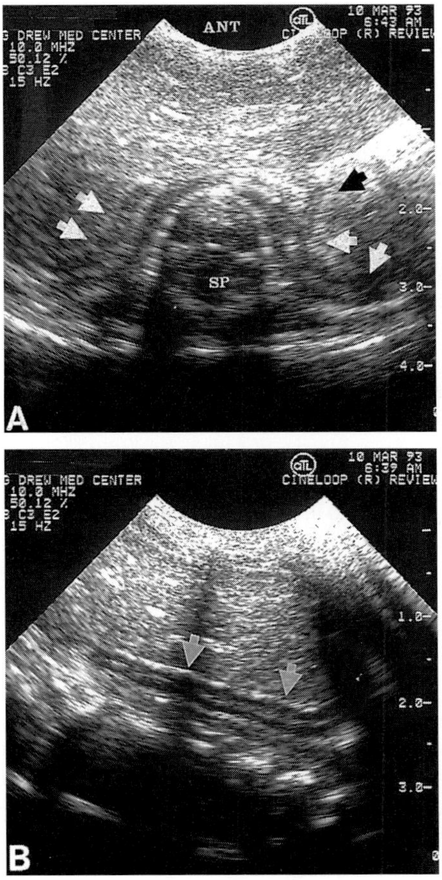

Figure 37–23 Ultrasound scan of Potter's syndrome with aplastic kidneys. **A**. Transverse view. **B**. The long, thin adrenal gland in the coronal view is easily mistaken for a kidney. The presence of an echogenic line representing the adrenal medulla surrounded by an echolucent cortex (*arrows in* **A** *and* **B**) aids in the distinction. ANT, anterior; SP, spine.

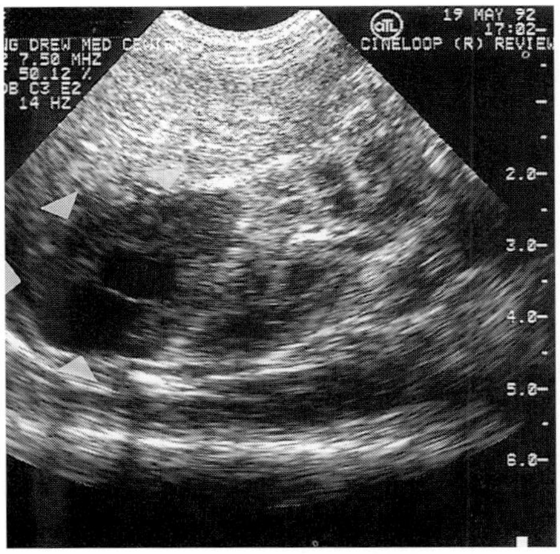

Figure 37–24 Ultrasound scan of adrenal hemorrhage shown as a large mass in the adrenal gland (*arrows*) with multiple cystic areas. The adrenal gland is superior to the kidney, shown on the right.

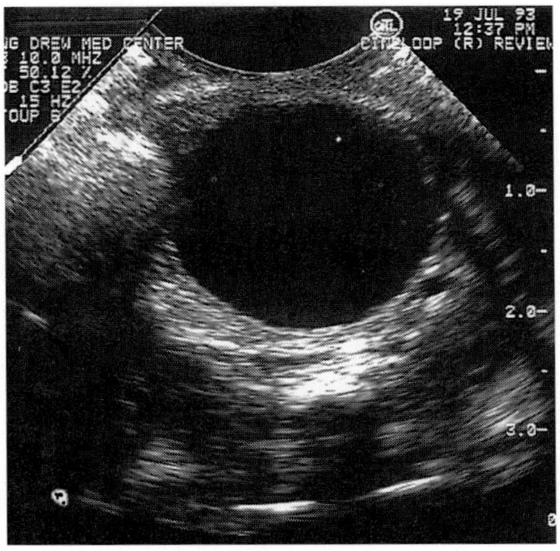

Figure 37–25 Ultrasound scan of distended urinary bladder filled with urine is seen on a transverse lower abdominal scan in an infant with transient hydronephrosis.

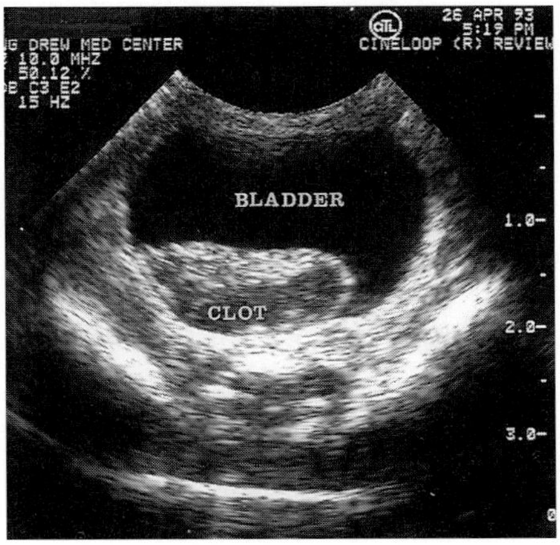

Figure 37–26 In infants with hematuria, clots may be seen in the urinary bladder.

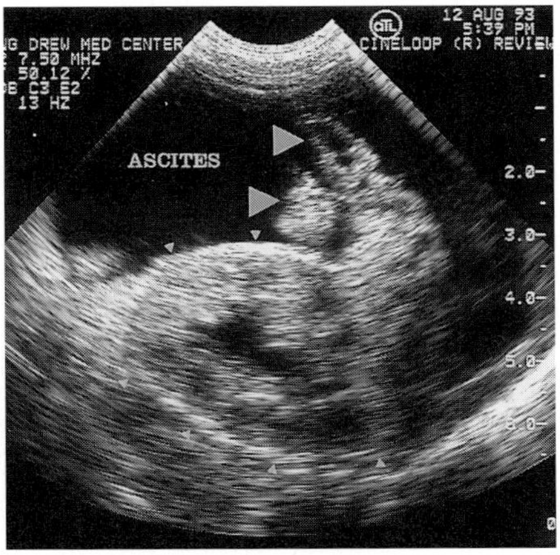

Figure 37–27 Ultrasound scan of ascites resulting from rupture of the bladder secondary to posterior urethral valves. Note the undulating peritoneal membrane (*large arrows*) and kidney (*small arrows*).

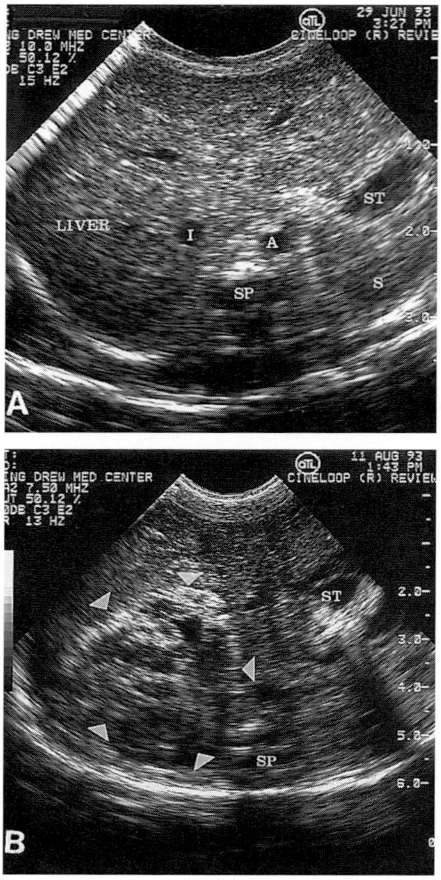

Figure 37–28 Ultrasound scan of hepatic abscess after bowel perforation. **A**. The normal anatomy seen on scanning of the upper abdomen. **B**. An abscess in the liver (*arrows*). SP, spine; S, spleen; ST, stomach; I, inferior vena cava; A, aorta.

is aided by the presence of undulating peritoneal membranes, as seen in Figure 37–27. Scanning of the liver may reveal a hepatic abscess (Fig. 37–28).

INTRAVASCULAR CATHETERS

Vascular access in the newborn infant often necessitates the insertion of arterial or venous lines, and ultrasound has been shown to be useful as a quick check, both to confirm that the line is in fact arterial and to assess the position of the line. By placing the transducer perpendicular to the abdomen in the subxiphoid area (using some pressure), first in the transverse and then in the sagittal plane, the abdominal aorta may be identified as a pulsatile round or tubular structure to the left of the spine. As foreign bodies produce strong echoes with reverberations, the umbilical artery catheter may be readily seen (Fig. 37–29). Moving the catheter or flushing the line under ultrasound may further confirm its presence in the abdominal aorta. Unfortunately, the actual tip of the catheter may be difficult to visualize. Using a sagittal view, umbilical venous catheters may be seen passing through the liver into the heart. The previously mentioned four-chamber view may be used to see if the catheter has passed from the right atrium into the left atrium via the foramen ovale (Fig. 37–30), a finding accompanied by unusually high venous oxygen saturations. Under ultra-

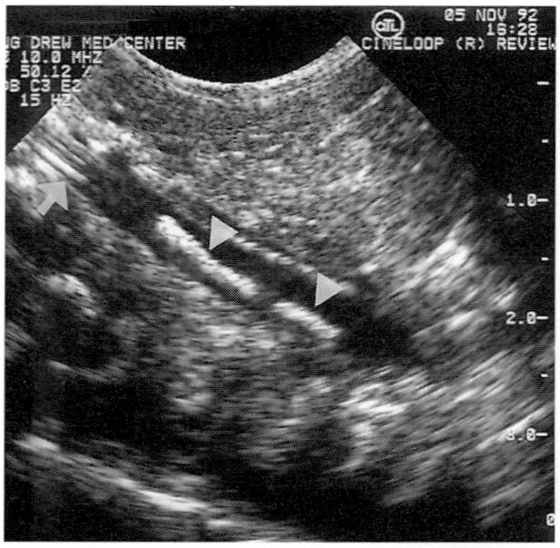

Figure 37–29 Ultrasound scan showing the location of the tip of the catheter. On this longitudinal scan of the abdominal aorta, the tip of an umbilical arterial line is detected in the abdominal aorta, its tip sending off reverberations (*arrow*). A clot at the tip of the catheter is seen on the right, just above the aortic bifurcation (*arrowheads*).

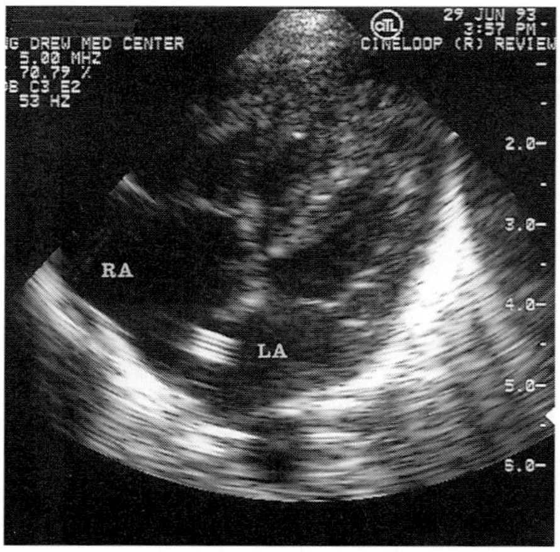

Figure 37–30 Four-chamber view of the heart showing a percutaneous line that passes from the right (RA) into the left atrium (LA).

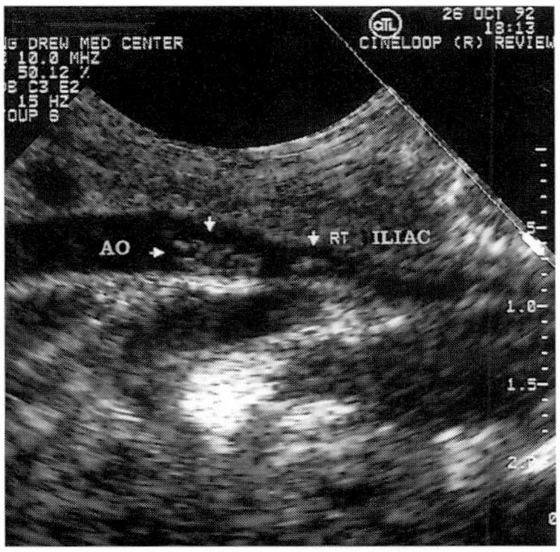

Figure 37–31 This coronal view from the side of the abdomen shows clots (*arrows*) at the bifurcation in the lower abdominal aorta (AO) and in the right iliac artery.

sound guidance, the catheter may be pulled back into the right atrium. Blood gases from this position may be extremely helpful in ruling out the presence of total anomalous pulmonary venous return. Clots may be seen on the tip of a catheter, along the aortic wall, or at the bifurcation of the aorta (Fig. 37–31). However, because catheters are reflective and cause reverberations, they also may obscure clots.

Bibliography

Grant: *Neurosonography of the Pre-term Neonate*. New York, Springer-Verlag, 1986.

Long WA: *Fetal and Neonatal Cardiology*. Philadelphia, WB Saunders, 1990.

Papile LA, Burstein J, Burstein R, et al: Incidence and evolution of subependymal and intraventricular hemorrhage: A study of infants with birth weights less than 1,500 gm. *J Pediatr*, 92:529, 1978.

Schulz RD, Willi UV: *Atlas of Pediatric Ultrasound*. Stuttgart, Georg Thieme Verlag, 1992.

Siegel MJ: *Pediatric Sonography*. New York, Raven Press, 1991.

Silverman NH: *Pediatric Echocardiography*. Baltimore, MD, Williams & Wilkins, 1993.

Snider AR, Serwer GA: *Echocardiography in Pediatric Heart Disease*. Chicago, Year Book Medical, 1990.

Teele RL, Share JC: *Ultrasonography of Infants and Children*. Philadelphia, WB Saunders, 1991.

Volpe JJ: *Neurology of the Newborn*, 2nd ed. Philadelphia, WB Saunders, 1987.

Section G

Central Nervous System

Chapter 38

Central Nervous System

Donna Ferriero and E. Stephen Buescher

A number of procedures are available to evaluate the central nervous system (CNS) in children. Lumbar puncture (LP), transillumination, computed tomography (CT), and magnetic resonance imaging (MRI) are done frequently. In some situations, more sophisticated or invasive procedures are warranted, such as continuous electroencephalographic recording (cEEG), intracranial pressure monitoring, and ventricular drainage.

PHYSICAL EXAMINATION

The neurological examination is always preceded by a general physical examination with special attention to the size and shape of the head, the location of neurocutaneous stigmata, the integrity of the spine, and the size of the liver and spleen. In some emergency situations, time allows only the briefest examination before procedures are performed. For example, the funduscopic examination should be performed prior to LP when increased intracranial pressure is suspected.

An assessment of the mental status appropriate for age should be made, with documentation of the degree of awareness, wakefulness, and cognition. The cranium is inspected for prominence of the sutures and fontanels (in the young infant) and examined for the presence of bruits. Transillumination should be performed when the infant's head is abnormally shaped or large. The cranial nerve examination begins with an assessment of vision, including visual fields by confrontation. Pupil reactivity, which is present by 30 weeks' gestation, should be assessed and fundi seen to rule out cataracts and anterior visual pathway abnormalities such as optic nerve hypoplasia or atrophy. Retinal hemorrhages, which are common in the newborn, are the sine qua non of nonaccidental head trauma in the older infant and child. Extraocular movements are observed for symmetry. The doll's eye maneuver, present in awake newborns, is seen normally only in the sleeping or comatose child.

Hearing is assessed by acoustic blink in the neonate and head turn to sound, present at 4 months of age. Vestibular integrity can be assessed in the infant by rotating the child from left to right. Facial asymmetry can be appreciated by inspection or by instructing the older child to smile, show teeth, and blow bubbles. Seventh nerve palsies will affect the entire face on the ipsilateral side, whereas central seventh nerve lesions will not involve the forehead on the contralateral side. In the nursery, it is not uncommon for asymmetrical crying facies to be mistaken for a peripheral seventh nerve lesion. Asymmetrical crying facies or cardiofacial syndrome is caused by absence of the angularis depressor oris muscle, which results in absence of depression of the affected side of the mouth when the infant cries or smiles. The bulbar cranial nerves (IX, X) can be assessed in the newborn by the gag reflex and in the older child by sounding "kee-kee." The sounds will be indistinct or garbled if there is lower cranial nerve dysfunction. Fasciculations of the tongue are seen commonly in the neonate but are abnormal otherwise.

The motor examination should be done when the child is as relaxed as possible. In the infant, tone is assessed by observation and by manipulation. Truncal tone is examined in ventral suspension and pull-to-sit in the infant and, in the older child, by grasping under the arm and lifting off the examination table. Tone in the extremities (appendicular tone) is assessed by passively moving the limb around the joint. Increased tone in the extremities can be either spastic or rigid. Spasticity produces a "catch" in the examined extremity, and rigidity is perceived as tightness in both flexion and extension on passive range of motion. Strength is assessed by inspection and individual muscle testing. The Gower sign or "tripoding" is seen when proximal muscle strength is impaired—the child will use the upper extremities to raise the trunk off the floor from a seated position. The presence of a *pronator drift* (pronation of the outstretched supinated arm after 1 minute) indicates a lesion somewhere in the upper motor neuron pathway. Coordination is assessed by having the child reach for and manipulate objects. Gait should be observed for limp, circumduction, footdrop, or ataxia. Reflexes (Table 38–1) in the upper extremities are assessed with the child sitting, and reflexes in the lower extremities with the child supine. A Babinski response should disappear by 2 years of age and should never be asymmetrical. In the neonate, caution should be taken to avoid obtaining a plantar grasp, which is often confused with a negative Babinski by stroking only the very lateral aspect of the foot or the anterior aspect of the shin.

The CNS is protected by the surrounding bony anatomy. Hence, without the use of sophisticated imaging techniques, little of the CNS can be directly visualized; only the retinas are available for easy examination. The relationship between specific parts of the CNS and surface anatomy must often be used to determine the best site for performance of specific procedures.

Table 38–1 Primitive Reflexes

Reflex	Appearance	Disappearance
Grasp—palmar	28 weeks' gestation	5 months
Grasp—plantar	32 weeks' gestation	1 year
Moro	30 weeks' gestation	5 months
Vestibulo-ocular response	32 weeks' gestation	4 months
Root, suck	34 weeks' gestation	3 months
Tonic neck	Neonate	6 months
Parachute	6 months	—
Landau	10 months	2 years

LUMBAR PUNCTURE

At birth, the tip of the spinal cord (conus medullaris) is located adjacent to the body of the third lumbar vertebra, with the cauda equina extending distally. As growth occurs, the bony spinal column elongates faster than the cord, so that by adulthood, the inferior end of the cord has moved rostrally to the lower edge of the first lumbar vertebra. In both children and adults, the L3–L4 interspace is the preferred site for LP, but the L2–L3 and L4–L5 interspaces can also be used. In newborns, because the conus medularis is low, only the L4–L5 interspace is considered a safe alternative to the standard L3–L4 site. Identification of these sites is based on surface anatomy. In adults, a transverse line between the highest point of the iliac crest and the posterior process of the fourth lumbar vertebra identifies the L3–L4 interspace. In newborns and young children, this line passes at the level of the fifth lumbar vertebra or the L5–S1 interspace (Busoni and Messeri, 1989) so that either intervertebral space above this site can be used.

Lumbar puncture is probably the most commonly performed CNS-related procedure in children. Initially described by Quincke in 1891, LP is the standard method for obtaining cerebrospinal fluid (CSF) for examination and for medication/anesthesia administration in some instances. In children, LP is stressful because the child is sometimes awake. For this reason, local anesthesia with 1% lidocaine at the LP site and conscious sedation with midazolam or another short-acting benzodiazepine administered sublingually or by the intravenous route (Friedman et al, 1991) should be used to minimize discomfort.

Materials

An LP kit, which contains a sterile LP needle with a stylet, 1% povidone-iodine antiseptic, 70% alcohol, 1% lidocaine local anesthetic, a 22-gauge, 1-inch needle, a 3-ml syringe, sterile gauze pads, sterile surgical drapes, and sterile tubes (three or four) for CSF collection, is needed. Many pediatric LP trays do not contain manometers. Check the kit before preparing the patient so that the manometer is available for obtaining opening and, if necessary, closing pressures.

Contraindications

1. Evidence of increased intracranial pressure that is obstructive (focal neurological examination with papilledema) and would cause herniation if the procedure is performed. This condition rarely exists in young children because of the compliance of the cranium (open sutures).
2. Superficial infection at the LP site.

Procedure

An assistant should be present to help with patient positioning and nonsterile handling of tubes and the manometer.

1. Place the patient in an appropriate position (Fig. 38–1) so that the back is arched and the hips are flexed. If the patient is seated, opening pressure should not be measured.
2. Locate the L3–L4 interspace via the superficial landmarks noted above and mark the site in the midline with either a surgical marker or iodine.
3. Prepare the site with povidone-iodine solution, working from the spinal site outward with circular movements. Put on sterile gloves at this time and remove residual scrub solution with 70% alcohol after a drying period of 30 seconds.
4. Raise a small wheal of anesthetic at the marked site. After 1 to 2 minutes, infiltrate the deeper tissues with local anesthetic. Select an appropriate-sized spinal needle (Table 38–2).
5. After 1 to 2 minutes, insert the spinal needle through the anesthetic wheal in the midline and advance it with the stylet in place. Angle the needle slightly cephalad but always in the midline. Remove the stylet frequently and observe the needle hub for CSF. If none is seen, replace the stylet and continue advancing the needle in small (2- to 3-

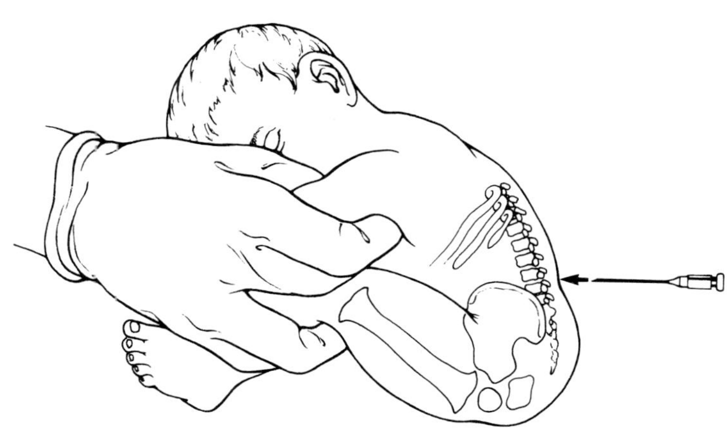

Figure 38–1 Site for lumbar tap illustrated with the infant in a sitting position. (Redrawn from Hughes WT, Buescher ES: *Pediatric Procedures*. Philadelphia, WB Saunders, 1980.)

Table 38–2 Spinal Needles for Lumbar Puncture

Patient Age	Needle Gauge	Needle Length
Newborn	21–23 gauge*	1 1/2 in
Infant	20–21 gauge	1 1/2 in
Child	20 gauge	1 1/2 –3 in
Adolescent	20 gauge	3 in

*A 24-gauge butterfly needle with the tubing cut to 2 inches can be used for the very small premature infant.

Table 38–3 CSF Drop Count Measure of CSF Pressure

	Counting Period in Seconds with Various Patient Temperatures	
Needle Size	< 40°C	> 40°C
22 gauge, 1 1/2 inch	21 sec	20 sec
22 gauge, 3 1/2 inch	39 sec	37 sec
20 gauge, 3 1/2 inch	12 sec	11 sec

mm) increments. In some instances, penetration of the dura can be appreciated as a sudden loss of resistance or a palpable "pop." If hard resistance to needle passage is felt, vertebral bone has usually been encountered. Withdraw the needle about halfway and reorient the needle (remaining in the midline) approximately parallel with the spinous processes of the vertebra above and below, and re-advance the needle.

6. As soon as CSF is seen in the hub, manometry is performed. The manometer tube is attached to a stopcock, an open port of the stopcock is attached to the hub of the LP needle, and the CSF is allowed to rise up the graduated manometer. The CSF pressure (cm H_2O) is read when the oscillations of fluid in the manometer are equal in both directions. An assistant can hold the top of the manometer so that the LP needle does not tear the skin. The stopcock is then closed and removed from the needle hub. In infants, manometry is difficult and rarely reliable (Milhorat, 1978). However, normal CSF pressures in this age group are usually 7.5 to 12.5 cm H_2O. Recording lower pressures raises questions of adequacy of technique. In normal children who are awake but relaxed, the average CSF pressure is 15 to 18 cm H_2O. Pressures between 18 and 20 cm H_2O are questionable and depend on body size and weight, and pressures greater than 20 cm H_2O are usually abnormal. If manometry equipment is not available, the CSF pressure can be estimated based on the rate of CSF flow through the LP needle (Ellis et al, 1992). In Table 38–3, the number of drops of CSF counted during the time period indicated approximates the CSF pressure in centimeters of water.
7. CSF is allowed to drain dropwise from the needle hub and is collected in 0.5- to 1-ml aliquots into sterile, screw-cap specimen tubes. Tubes 1 and 4 should be sent for cell count, especially when the procedure is traumatic and yields bloody fluid. If blood is present, one tube should be spun and analyzed for the presence of xanthochromia. The yellow pigment (bilirubin) is present when serum bilirubin is elevated and when red blood cells hemolyze. Xanthochromia takes 2 hours to appear after an acute hemorrhage, 2 days to reach peak color, and 2 weeks to clear completely from the subarachnoid space. Alternatively, bloody CSF can be differentiated from venous blood by allowing a drop of CSF to fall onto filter paper. Bloody CSF will form a "water ring" around a central patch of erythrocytes.
8. Medications administered intrathecally are usually delivered by barbotage. After adequate CSF has been collected dropwise, the syringe containing the medication is attached to the spinal needle hub and a small amount of medication (0.25–1.0 ml) is slowly injected. After a brief pause, about half this volume of CSF is gently aspirated into the syringe to mix and another volume is slowly injected. By repeating this process over and over, the medication is administered slowly and is diluted with CSF as it is given. Administration of medications by barbotage into the lumbar CSF space will not reliably expose the ventricular system to the medication because there is no direct communication between the subarachnoid space and the ventricles. If medication is needed in the ventricular system to treat a shunt infection or ventriculitis, a ventriculostomy tube should be placed by the neurosurgeon.
9. After CSF collection is complete, the stylet is replaced in the spinal needle and the needle/stylet combination is removed in a single motion. Local pressure applied for 3 to

5 minutes to the puncture site will minimize the risk of CSF leakage to the surface.

Complications

1. Headache from persistent CSF leak; an autologous blood patch can be performed by the anesthesiologist to treat this condition
2. Infection from nonsterile conditions
3. Persistent bleeding in patients with an underlying coagulopathy

TRANSILLUMINATION

Transillumination (Fig. 38–2) is based on the observation that light refects from the internal surface of fluid- or air-filled space. In adults, its application is limited because scalp-covered calvarium thicker than 2.5 mm will not transmit light. In infants whose calvarial bone is thin enough to allow transmission of light, transillumination can be used to diagnose subdural or epidural effusions (Snedeker et al, 1990), Dandy-Walker cysts, and hydranencephaly. When a standard flashlight is used, transillumination is observed only with a cortical mantle thickness of less than 1 cm. Specially designed instruments that provide intense but relatively cool light for transillumination are optimal and commercially available. These units are designed to efficiently direct heat generated by the illuminating lamp away from the patient; some use fiberoptic systems to separate the patient from the light source. Transillumination can also be performed with very simple tools, such as an appropriately modified flashlight. It is important to realize that an intense light source used in a dark ambient environment will yield better transillumination.

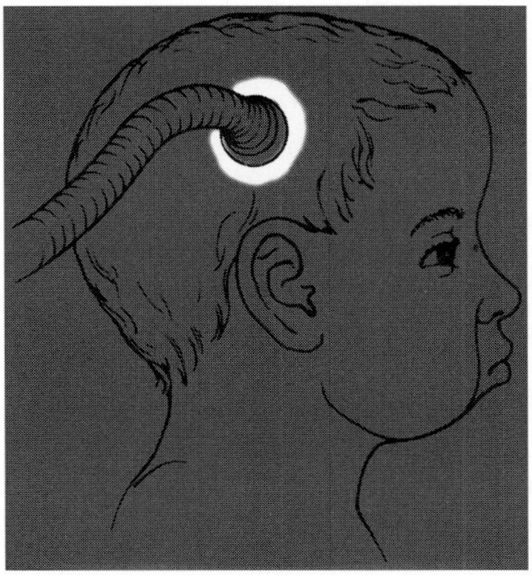

Figure 38–2 Distribution of light "ring" with transillumination of the skull. (Redrawn from Hughes WT, Buescher ES: *Pediatric Procedures.* Philadelphia, WB Saunders, 1980.)

Materials

A transillumination light source or a D-cell battery flashlight with fresh batteries is needed. If a flashlight is used, the front of the flashlight surrounding the lens must be modified to make it opaque. The typically red, translucent plastic around the flashlight lens can be opacified with several layers of black electrical tape. The tip of the flashlight should seal tightly enough against the infant's skin to prevent escape of stray light. A thin cardboard roll can be placed on the edge of the lens to form the seal.

Procedure

1. Transfer the infant to an area that is darkened as much as possible. With the help of an assistant who will hold the baby and immobilize the head, place the transilluminating instrument on the examiner's forearm to determine how long the beam can be comfortably applied to the skin. This time period should then be used as the maximum time the transilluminator will be held in contact with the infant's skin.
2. Apply the transilluminator to the lateral aspect of the head. With the free hand, make sure there is a tight seal against the infant's scalp.
3. Turn on the transilluminator and note the radius of the corona of light from the transilluminator outward. Apply the transilluminator to the same area on the opposite side of the head and note the corona size.
4. Transilluminate over the frontal, parietal, and occipital lobes, noting the size of the transilluminated coronae and whether they are symmetrical from side to side. Asymmetry or excessive size is abnormal.
5. Normal transillumination values vary somewhat depending on the type of light source used. When a standard flashlight is used, transillumination normally extends 1 to 2 cm beyond the rim of the flashlight (Swick et al, 1976). When a Chun gun light source is used, the maximum normal transillumination distance is 3 to 4 cm (Cheldelin et al, 1975).
6. Conditions affecting the dermis or supracalvarial structures, such as cephalohematoma,

caput succedaneum, or intravenous fluid infiltration, may interfere with transillumination of the skull.

CENTRAL NERVOUS SYSTEM IMAGING TECHNIQUES

The most frequently used methodologies for imaging the CNS in infants and children are ultrasonography, CT, and MRI (Barnes, 1992). Because of the noninvasiveness of these tests, they have replaced procedures such as angiography, myelography, cisternography, and ventriculography, except under very special circumstances.

Ultrasonography

Sonographic imaging is used primarily in the imaging of the CNS in newborns and infants. Its application is limited to this patient group because it requires an open fontanel for transmission of the ultrasonic signal. It is a screening tool but can be applied to the detection of spinal dysraphism, CNS hemorrhage, ventriculomegaly, intracranial malformations, and cysts.

Computed Tomography

CT has become an indispensible tool for noninvasive examination of the CNS. It is a sophisticated x-ray–based methodology, allowing visualization of all tissues with radiographic density (from bone to air) by electronic manipulation of image contrast. In addition, use of parenteral water-soluble radiographic contrast material during CNS imaging allows definition of vascular structures and identification of areas of hyperemia, such as might occur during inflammation. Use of intravenous contrast materials carries a small risk of idiosyncratic or drug-reaction hypervolemia because of an osmotic effect while the contrast agent is in the vascular space, and of hypovolemia due to osmotic diuresis as the contrast material is eliminated. CT without contrast injection is the method of choice for determination of acute intracranial hemorrhage, acute ischemic injury, and the presence of calcification.

Magnetic Resonance Imaging

MRI is the most recent CNS imaging technique to find widespread application in pediatrics. It is now the best method for definitive examination of the spinal neuraxis and for evaluating CNS neoplasia, vascular lesions, and occult hemorrhage. It can also aid in the evaluation of myelination, the localization of CNS inflammation, and the evaluation of neurodegenerative disease states. The signal intensities observed have little relationship to radiographic density, an important point to appreciate when interpreting the MRI. Mineralized bone is visualized poorly, whereas nonmineralized structures within bone, such as marrow or inflammatory foci, are visualized well. Conversely, MRI differentiates myelinated from unmyelinated CNS tissues with remarkable detail. To enhance the contrast in MRI studies, paramagnetic materials that shorten the relaxation times of protons with a resulting increase in the signal intensity are used. Gadolinium-DTPA, administered either orally or intravenously, is the MRI contrast enhancing agent used most frequently.

CT is the examination of choice in the emergency situation when MRI is unavailable. CT is also preferable to MRI when calcifications or bony abnormalities are being investigated, for example, in human immunodeficiency virus (HIV) infection, TORCH infection (toxoplasmosis, others, rubella, cytomegalovirus, and herpes simplex), and craniosynostosis.

Cerebrospinal Fluid Nuclide Scan

In the specific situation in which a CSF leak is suspected as the cause of recurrent meningitis in a child, this procedure is performed (often in combination with high-resolution CT scanning of the sinuses and temporal bones) to confirm the presence of an ongoing CSF leak. Prior to the scan, the nose of the patient is packed with pledgets and ^{99mx}Tc-labeled human albumin is injected via lumbar puncture into the lumbar space. Isotopic scanning is then used to follow the progress of the injected nuclide up the spinal canal and around the cerebral hemispheres, watching specifically for any asymmetrical or abnormal pooling of signal outside the CNS. Twenty-four hours after injection, the pledgets are removed from both sides of the nose (taking care to keep the left and right side packing clearly labeled) and are examined for any associated radioactivity. The presence of more than 1% to 2% of total injected radioactivity on the pledgets from either side is taken as evidence of a CSF leak, and high-resolution CT of the suspected side is then used to try to identify the bony abnormality.

Common Central Nervous System Surgical Procedures

In some situations, obtaining CSF via LP cannot be done. Following head trauma or drug ingestion or when a ventricular drainage system fails, it may be necessary to obtain CSF or another pathological fluid from the subarachnoid or ventricular space by other methods.

SUBDURAL PUNCTURE

In the child with an open fontanel, obtaining fluid from a subdural fluid collection can be done without much difficulty using the lateral aspect of the anterior fontanel as the entry site. Diagnostic subdural taps, although rarely performed currently, are done bilaterally, using separate needles for each site.

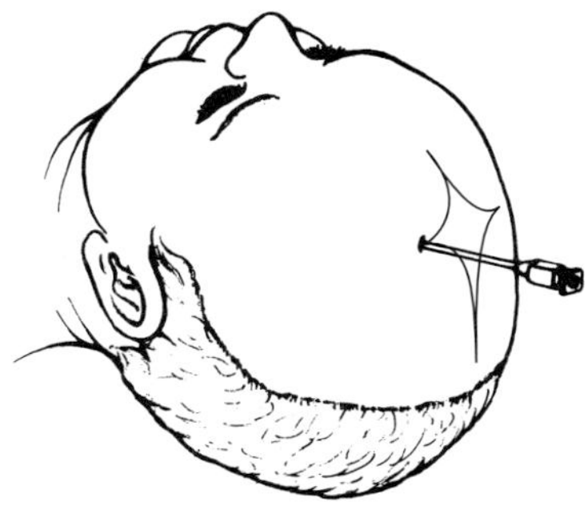

Figure 38–3 Site for subdural tap. (Redrawn from Hughes WT, Buescher ES: *Pediatric Procedures.* Philadelphia, WB Saunders, 1980.)

Materials

A 20-gauge, 1 1/2-inch spinal needle; 1% lidocaine; 10% povidone-iodine surgical scrub solution; a 3-ml syringe; a 22-gauge, 5/8-inch needle; sterile surgical gloves; surgical drapes; a sterile screw-top specimen tube; 2 × 2 sterile gauze pads; 70% alcohol; soap, warm water, and a shaving razor are needed.

Procedure

1. The patient is placed supine and administered conscious sedation. The scalp is shaved and aseptically prepared with 10% povidone-iodine solution, residual scrub solution is removed with 70% alcohol, and the site is draped to expose the anterior fontanel.
2. A small wheal of local anesthetic is raised one fingerbreadth lateral (1–1.5 cm) to the midline at the edge of the anterior fontanel. The needle is inserted perpendicular to the base of the skull (Fig. 38–3), in a plane parallel to the falx cerebri, and is advanced carefully in small increments (1–2 mm). The operator must maintain control over the needle at all times, usually with two hands: The index finger and thumb of one hand hold and stabilize the needle at the scalp surface, while the other hand advances the needle. Piercing of the dura (at a depth of 0.5–1.0 cm) is often accompanied by a palpable "pop" sensation, after which the stylet is removed and the needle hub is observed for fluid. Under normal conditions, one to two drops of fluid are obtained from the subdural space by gravity drainage (use of a syringe to aspirate fluid is dangerous and usually not indicated). If more than 3 ml of fluid is obtained, either a subdural hygroma is present or the pia-arachnoid membrane has been pierced (Milhorat, 1978).
3. In the event of traumatic bleeding during needle insertion, it is best to withdraw the needle and apply firm pressure to the puncture site for 5 minutes.
4. After completion, the stylet is replaced in the needle and the needle is removed in a single motion. Local pressure is applied to the site with a sterile gauze pad for 3 to 5 minutes.

Complications

Subdural bleeding, accidental entry into the sagittal sinus, removal of too large a fluid volume (removal of volumes more than 20–30 ml at one time may cause significant intravascular fluid shifts or bleeding in the subdural space), injury to underlying brain, and fistula formation with persistent drainage following repeated taps at the same puncture site are possible complications of this procedure.

CISTERNAL PUNCTURE

In some situations, CSF cannot be obtained from the usual lumbar sites because of the clinical situation (e.g., danger of herniation). Cisternal puncture is an alternative means of obtaining CSF by passing the needle through the foramen magnum into the cisterna magna. Cisternal puncture is more dangerous than either lumbar or ventricular puncture (Milhorat, 1978) and therefore should be performed only by an experienced operator.

INTRACRANIAL PRESSURE MONITORING

Increased intracranial pressure (ICP) following head trauma is associated with increased morbidity and mortality. Monitoring of ICP to determine the efficacy of intervention has become commonplace in pediatric intensive care units. ICP can be monitored in a number of ways. It is generally accepted that the most invasive monitoring, via an intraventricular catheter, gives the most accurate estimate of ICP and provides a means for quickly lowering ICP by ventricular fluid withdrawal when necessary. This procedure has the highest frequency of infection, approximately 20% (Aucoin et al, 1986). Intraparenchymal pressure monitoring (Tasker and Matthew, 1991) via catheter allows pressure to be measured accurately but does not allow CSF withdrawal. Subdural catheter placement reflects less well the intraparenchymal and intraventricular pressures, while subdural "bolt" devices, the tip of which just passes the inner table of the calvarium, are the least traumatic, have the lowest frequency of infection (about 8%), and are probably the least dependable for detecting increased ICP, especially in young children who have thin calvaria (Miller et al, 1986; Woster and LeBlanc, 1990). All of these pressure monitoring devices require the placement of a calvarial bur hole for access to the CNS and for stabilization of the monitoring device. It is recommended that alternation of sites be done to minimize the risk of infection (Narayan et al, 1982; Woster and LeBlanc, 1990).

VENTRICULAR PUNCTURES, DRAINAGE, AND SHUNTS

Cerebrospinal fluid is produced by the choroid plexus located in the roof of the third ventricle and both lateral ventricles. It normally passes in a caudal direction through the cerebral aqueduct to the fourth ventricle and then into the subarachnoid space via the foramina of Luschka and Magendie. For pathological conditions in which CSF flow is obstructed or brain edema occurs, placement of a catheter or needle into either lateral ventricle provides a means of relieving obstruction to CSF flow and/or monitoring and manipulating ICP.

Ventricular shunting is a more permanent ventricular drainage procedure in which the distal draining end of the tubing attached to the catheter is placed in a serosal cavity (peritoneum, pleura) to allow internal drainage of CSF. Often performed in premature infants who have experienced intraventricular hemorrhage or in children born with spinal dysraphism, ventricular shunting prevents some of the complications of hydrocephalus. The peritoneum is usually the preferred site for ventricular shunting (called ventriculoperitoneal [VP] shunts) because it presents a large surface for absorption of the CSF. Ventriculoatrial (VA) shunting has become less popular because the complications of VA shunt infections are more severe (sepsis, embolic stroke, and glomerulonephritis) when the shunt drains directly into the vascular space. Ventricular shunts are placed as operative procedures using general anesthesia; the ventricular catheter is placed and the drainage tubing is tunneled subcutaneously from the catheter site down the neck and chest to the abdomen, where the draining tip sits within the peritoneum.

EMERGENCY PROCEDURES FOR CERVICAL SPINE INJURIES

With the growing participation of children in contact sports, the pediatrician ("team physician") should be aware of the procedures used for initial care and transport of children or adolescents with suspected cervical spine injury (Vegso and Lehman, 1987; Watkins, 1986). The major objective of these procedures is to prevent further cervical spinal cord injury from occurring as the child is moved. Achieving this objective requires a team approach involving at least three people for the child and as many as five for the adolescent. In every situation, one person is designated to immobilize the head and neck and to dictate action. The leader does not participate in lifting the child. If the child is prone, the first group action is to get the child supine so that the lifesaving ABCs can be performed. The leader supports the child's head and neck with the forearms crossed so that as the child is rolled, his or her forearms will unwind. The other team members slowly and deliberately log-roll the child onto a flat, hard surface (backboard) that can be used to carry the child. If the child is prone, the head is gently brought to a neutral position if possible and the head and neck are cradled in the leader's palms and forarms for immobilization. The other team members reach under the child, clasp hands, and lift the child onto a backboard. If a helmet is worn, it is left on the child unless it interferes with the establishment of an airway. The child is transported supine on the backboard from the playing field. While the child is carried on the backboard, the leader continues to support the head and neck by cradling them between the palms and forearms. The leader's hands can be replaced with a cervical collar of appropriate size. The leader maintains the child's head and neck immobile until appropriate immobilization devices can be applied.

EMERGENCY MANAGEMENT OF SEIZURES

Pentobarbital Anesthesia for Status Epilepticus

The following is an adaptation of a protocol used for refractory seizures in adults (Lowenstein et al, 1988):

1. Intubate and ventilate the patient, admit to a neurological intensive care unit or pediatric intensive care unit, place an arterial line (central venous pressure line).
2. Perform an electroencephalogram (EEG) for monitoring control of seizures and level of anesthesia (check every 15 minutes during induction, then every 1 hour after a burst-suppression pattern is achieved on the EEG).
3. Administer a pentobarbital loading dose of 15 mg/kg over 1 hour or as tolerated hemodynamically with a maintenance infusion of 1 to 5 mg/kg/hr with additional loading doses of 5 mg/kg as needed to control seizures or attain burst suppression.
4. Give low-dose dopamine for hypotension.
5. Continue maintenance phenytoin and/or phenobarbital with monitoring of serum levels.

Stop pentobarbital at 24 hours and observe for seizure activity. If seizures recur, reinstate infusion and continue for another 24 hours before withdrawal. Repeat as necessary.

References

Aucoin PA, Kotilainen HR, Gantz NM, et al: Intracranial pressure monitors: Epidemiologic study of risk factors and infections. *Am J Med,* 80:369–376, 1986.

Barnes PD: Imaging the central nervous system in pediatrics and adolescence. *Pediatr Clin North Am,* 39:743–776, 1992.

Busoni P, Messeri A: Spinal anesthesia in children: Surface anatomy. *Anesth Analg,* 68:418–419, 1989.

Cheldelin LV, Davis PC, Grant WW: Normal values for transillumination of skull using a new light source. *J Pediatr,* 87:937–938, 1975.

Ellis RW, Strauss LC, Wiley JM, et al: A simple method for estimating cerebrospinal fluid pressure during lumbar puncture. *Pediatrics,* 89: 895–897, 1992.

Friedman AG, Mulhern RK, Fairclough D, et al: Midazolam premedication for pediatric bone marrow aspiration and lumbar puncture. *Pediatr Oncol,* 19:499–504, 1991.

Lowenstein DH, Aminoff MJ, Simon RP: Barbiturate anesthesia in the treatment of status epilepticus: Clinical experience with 14 patients. *Neurology,* 38:395–400, 1988.

Milhorat TH: *Pediatric Neurosurgery.* Philadelphia, FA Davis, 1978, pp 8–13.

Miller JD, Bobo H, Kapp JP: Inaccurate pressure readings from subarachnoid bolts. *Neurosurgery,* 19:253–256, 1986.

Narayan RK, Kishore PRS, Becker DP, et al: Intracranial pressure: To monitor or not to monitor? *J Neurosurg,* 56:650–659, 1982.

Snedeker JD, Kaplan SL, Dodge PR, et al: Subdural effusion and its relationship with neurologic sequelae of bacterial meningitis in infancy: A prospective study. *Pediatrics,* 86:163–170, 1990.

Swick HH, Cunningham D, Shield LK: Transillumination of the skull in premature infants. *Pediatrics,* 58:658–664, 1976.

Tasker RC, Matthew DJ: Cerebral intraparenchymal pressure monitoring in non-traumatic coma: Clinical evaluation of a new fiberoptic device. *Neuropediatrics,* 22:47–49, 1991.

Vegso JJ, Lehman RC: Field evaluation and management of head and neck injuries. *Clin Sports Med,* 6:1–15, 1987.

Watkins RG: Neck injuries in football players. *Clin Sports Med,* 5:215–246, 1986.

Woster PS, LeBlanc KL: Management of elevated intracranial pressure. *Clin Pharm,* 9:762–772, 1990.

Section H

Eyes/Ears/Nose/Throat

Chapter 39

The Eye

Walter T. Hughes

From birth humans are highly protective of their eyes. Immediately after they begin extrauterine life, attempts are made to pry open the newborn's eyelids and apply drops of medication. The difficulty of this maneuver whether for treatment or examination, remains a problem throughout infancy and childhood. Simple visual testing methods are further hindered in the infant by the need for cooperation and understanding. Following are some procedures useful in dealing with the eye for diagnostic and treatment purposes. They do not represent a comprehensive approach to pediatric ophthalmology, but apply primarily to the general pediatric clinic and practitioner's office.

EVERSION OF THE EYELIDS

For examination or therapy it may be necessary to evert the eyelids. If the child is cooperative, no restraint is necessary. However, for procedures in the small infant or uncooperative child, body restraint (Hughes and Buescher, 1980) can be used to limit extremity movements, and the head can be restrained manually.

Eversion of the Upper Lid

The upper lid is to be bent back on its superior tarsal margin, which is about 10 mm above the lash margin.

1. The lashes and border of the upper lid are grasped between the thumb and index finger. The lid is drawn downward and away from the globe. The patient is asked to look down (Fig. 39–1A).
2. The upper lid is indented with the operator's little finger, index finger, or a cotton tipped applicator and bent back and upward upon the indenting object (Fig. 39–1B).
3. The everted lid can be held in position by gently pressing the lashes and margin against the superior bony orbit.

Supported in part by National Cancer Institute Cancer Center Support (CORE) Grant P30CA21765 and American Lebanese Syrian Associated Charities.

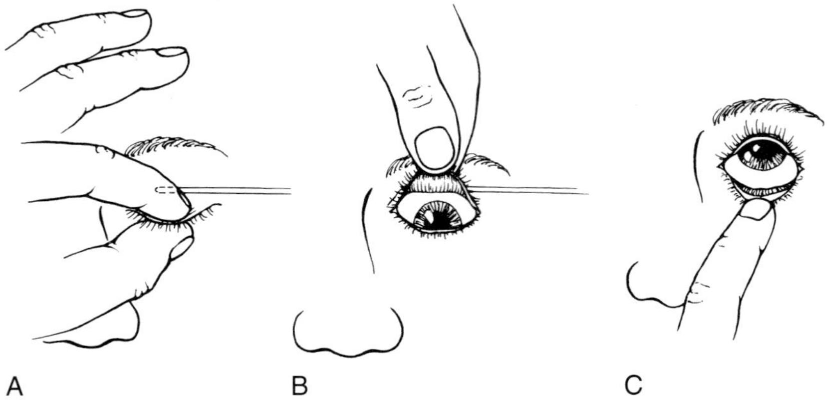

Figure 39–1 Eversion of the eyelids. (Redrawn from Hughes WT, Buescher ES: *Pediatric Procedures.* Philadelphia, WB Saunders, 1980.)

Eversion of the Lower Lid

The conjunctiva of the lower lid is exposed by placing the thumb or a finger near the margin of the lower lid and pushing downward and backward while the patient looks up (Fig. 39–1C).

EXAMINATION OF THE NEWBORN'S EYES

Jones (1968) described a satisfactory method for exposing the eyeball of the small infant. Two cotton-tipped wooden applicators are dampened with sterile water. The cotton-tipped ends of the applicators are placed in parallel, one on the upper eyelid and one on the lower, as shown in Figure 39–2. The applicators are slowly separated with some downward pressure, pulling the eyelids open and exposing the globe.

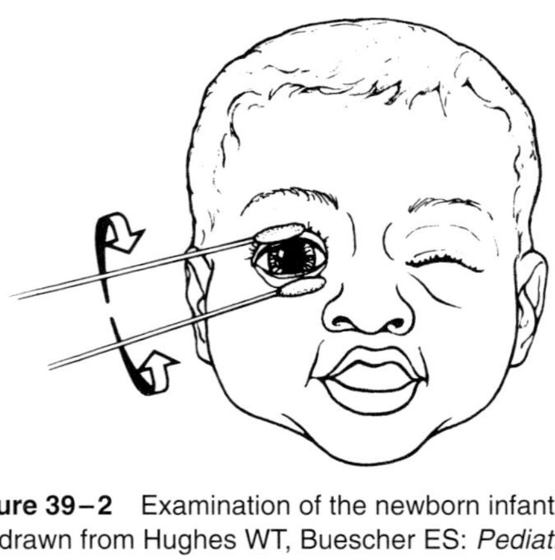

Figure 39–2 Examination of the newborn infant's eye. (Redrawn from Hughes WT, Buescher ES: *Pediatric Procedures.* Philadelphia, WB Saunders, 1980.)

METHODS FOR LOCAL APPLICATION OF MEDICAMENTS TO THE EYE

People blink by reflex to prevent the contact of minute particles or bright light. Tiny foreign bodies that cannot be felt or seen on other parts of the body can be excruciatingly painful on the conjunctival surface. It is understandable, then, that the child is extremely fearful of any procedure involving the eyes.

The medications that physicians apply topically to the eye are not pain provoking and are usually soothing. Explanation of this fact to the child and parents should be a ritual. However, regardless of how persuasive or prolonged the explanation is, it will not relieve all fears and anxiety.

A few general comments can be made relative to the instillation of medication into the conjunctival sac.

1. Drugs placed in the conjunctival sac undergo absorption by the cornea and the conjunctiva. Only the portion absorbed by the cornea enters the interior of the eye. Loosening of the epithelial barrier by disease or by the use of topical anesthetic compounds increases the absorption of drugs by the cornea.
2. Solutions are usually placed in the lower fornix of the conjunctival sac. However, if greater absorption is desired, the solution is put on the upper portion of the cornea and allowed to drain downward toward the fornix.
3. Solutions placed in the conjunctival sac are diluted with tears and follow the flow into lacrimal passages, where most of the absorption into periorbital structures occurs.
4. If pressure is exerted with the finger over

the region of the lacrimal sac, the presence of the drug in the conjunctival sac will be prolonged if the patient is not producing an overflow of tears.
5. Drying increases tear production, which in turn dilutes the medication. If tears overflow onto the face, medication will then be reduced in the eye.
6. Ointments and oily medication remain in the sac longer than aqueous preparations, a point of considerable merit in selecting medication for a child.
7. The tip of the medicine dropper must be round and smooth.
8. Usually only one drop of the medication is needed if properly applied.

Instillation of Solutions into the Conjunctival Sac

Solutions are introduced into the lower fornix with a medicine dropper. The patient should be in the supine position. No restraint is necessary for the older, cooperative child; body restraint is used for the uncooperative infant.

Method

1. Separation of the lids is usually accomplished with the thumb and index finger, using traction to hold the lids apart.
2. The dropper is filled with slightly more than the desired amount of solution. The solution should not be cold or hot, but at room temperature.
3. The dropper tip is held a few millimeters above the lower fornix, and the medication is expressed onto the conjunctival surface. Do not spatter the drops directly over the cornea. The solution can also be instilled in the upper fornix while the patient looks downward.
4. After the medication has been instilled, the patient should maintain the supine position with the face upward for 5 minutes. Tears usually pool at the inner canthus and should not be wiped away.

Introduction of Ointments into the Conjunctival Sac

Various ophthalmic ointments are available in collapsible tubes with long, slender nozzles.

Method

1. The conjunctiva of the lower lid is exposed by placing the thumb near the margin of the lower lids and pressing inferiorly and backward.
2. The patient is asked to look upward. A thin strip of the ointment is applied in the exposed gutter and traction on the lid is released.

Irrigation of the Conjunctival Sac

Loose debris and foreign bodies may be removed by flushing fluid over the conjunctival surface. This is best done with a soft rubber bulb syringe filled with a warm irrigating solution. A stream of fluid is gently directed into the lower fornix as the patient looks upward and then into the upper fornix as the patient looks downward. The irrigating solution drains out over the side of the face into a collection pan.

HYDROSTATIC NASOLACRIMAL MASSAGE

Management of congenital nasolacrimal duct obstruction may require daily massage of the area with or without probing by the ophthalmologist. The following maneuver can be taught to parents: The operator places an index finger over the common canaliculus to block the exit of material from the puncta and strokes continuously downward to increase the hydrostatic pressure within the nasolacrimal sac. Usually about five strokes twice daily are recommended.

ASSESSMENT OF VISUAL ACUITY

The accuracy of visual acuity measurements is inversely proportional to age for preschool-age children. However, by 6 years of age most children can be tested satisfactorily, and reasonable estimates can be made of how well infants and smaller children can see. The following test procedures may be used in the physician's office or clinic to estimate visual acuity.

Evaluation of Infants and Children Younger than 3 Years of Age

In newborn infants, vision may be roughly estimated for light perception by directing a beam from a penlight into the infant's eyes. Light perception may be evidenced by blinking, following the light upon its movement from lateral to midline, or closing the eyes, or by evidence of irritability. Infants often stare at the mother's face, especially while nursing. Inquiry about this experience may provide the physician with the earliest hint of severe visual problems.

For infants from about 6 months to 2 years of age, the "fixation-and-following" method can be used. Place the patient in a well-lighted room and at a time when cooperation in play is possible (parents may assist). Have the patient focus on an object, such as a toy, fixed about arm's length from the eye. Move the object slowly and observe the eyes for following. After satisfactory responses with both eyes open, the test may be repeated with one eye covered. Another test involves the placement of a small object, such as a small piece of candy or a coin, on a flat surface about 5 feet away from the infant. If the infant attempts to reach the object, the vision is estimated as at least 20/50 vision. Special tests for visually evoked potentials, optokinetic nystagmus, and forced-choice preferential looking may be used by ophthalmologists and neurologists to assess special cases.

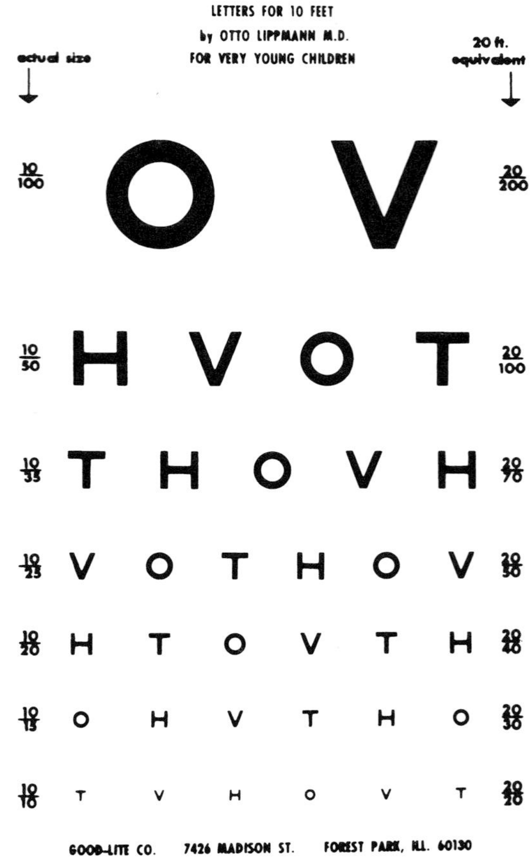

Figure 39–3 The Snellen alphabet chart. (From Harley RD: *Pediatric Ophthalmology,* 2nd ed. Philadelphia, WB Saunders, 1983. Courtesy of Good-Lite Co., Forest Park, IL.)

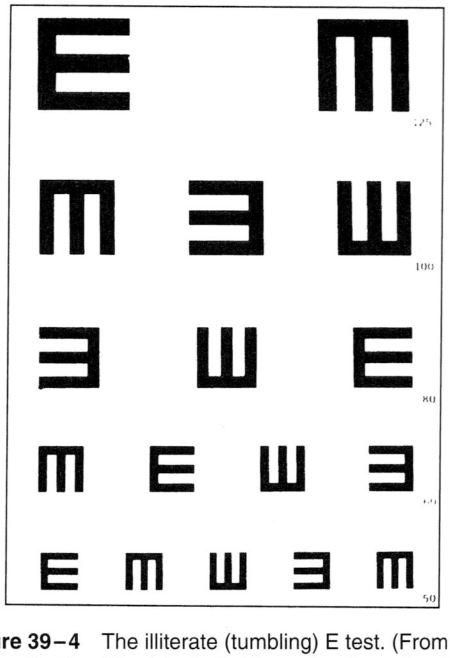

Figure 39–4 The illiterate (tumbling) E test. (From Trobe JD: *The Physician's Guide to Eye Care.* San Francisco, American Academy of Ophthalmology, 1993.)

Evaluation of Children Older than 3 Years of Age

By about 3 years of age most children can be tested by one of the visual acuity charts. Several Snellen-type charts are available and may be applied to certain age groups. Three of the charts in common use are as follows:

1. Standard Snellen alphabet chart
2. Picture optotypes
3. Illiterate (tumbling) E test

The Snellen alphabet test is used for individuals knowledgeable of the alphabet, usually older than 6 years. The other charts may be used to test younger children.

Snellen alphabet chart

The Snellen chart is made of lines of letters in decreasing size (Fig. 39–3). Each line is given a numerical designation based upon the line of letters that can be read by an individual with normal vision. The numerical fraction located at the end of each line of letters is used to describe the visual acuity. The numerator is the distance in feet the child is from the chart. The denominator (bottom number) is the distance at which an individual with normal vision can read these letters. For example, a 20/40 acuity means the patient can read at 20 feet what a normal individual can read at 40 feet. The greater the denominator, the poorer the visual acuity.

The assessment is made as follows:

1. The patient is placed 20 feet from the Snellen chart. The chart and room must be well illuminated.
2. Test one eye with the other one covered. The covered eye should not be compressed by the covering.
3. Start with line 20/40 and move higher or lower depending on the response.
4. The reading is taken as the smallest line of print in which the patient can correctly read the majority of the letters.

Illiterate (tumbling, Snellen) E test

The E chart (Fig. 39–4) is usually used with children between 3 and 5 years of age. It is generally more accurate than the picture chart test and may be used for non–English-speaking and illiterate individuals. With the Snellen E test, the child indicates which direction the E is pointed. The directions are up, down, right, and left. The patient is asked to point the direction of the E with his or her fingers. The Denver Eye Screening Test (DEST) uses a single card (20/30) held 15 feet from the patient.

Picture chart

The picture chart (Fig. 39–5) is used for children who cannot be tested with the E chart. The child may or may not be more cooperative with the picture chart than with the E chart. The picture test can best be presented as a game and is generally applicable to children from 2 to 4 years of age. The charts are available for distance and near testing (14 inches). For distance testing the patient is placed 20 feet from the chart (see Fig. 39–5). As with the other Snellen-type tests, the patient is asked to identify the smallest objects visible and the scoring is recording as with the Snellen alphabet test.

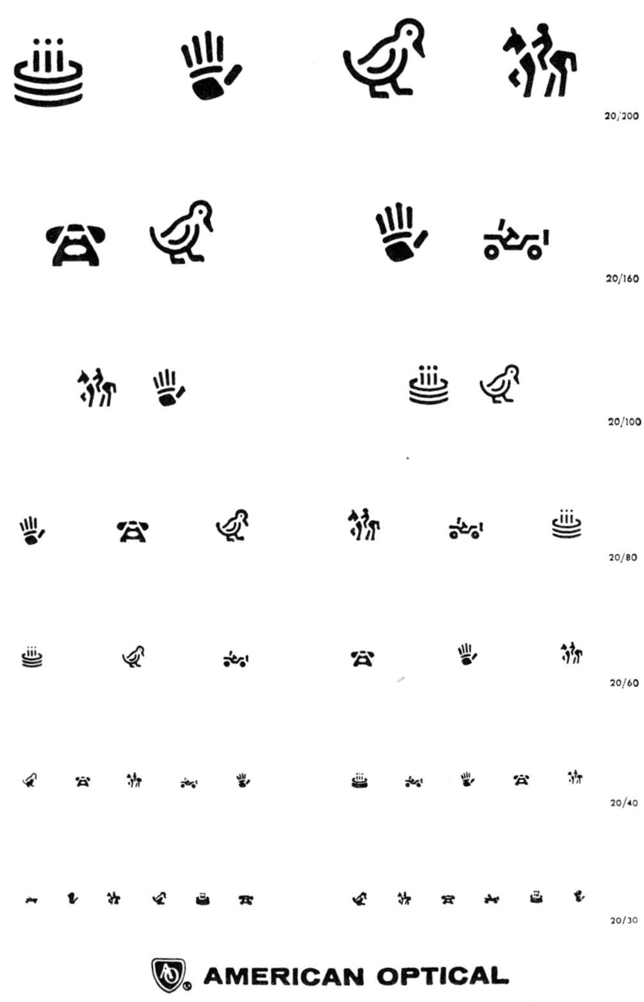

Figure 39–5 The picture chart. (From Harley RD: *Pediatric Ophthalmology,* 2nd ed. Philadelphia, WB Saunders, 1983. Courtesy of American Optical.)

References

Harley RD: *Pediatric Ophthalmology*, 2nd ed. Philadelphia, WB Saunders, 1983.

Hughes WT, Buescher ES: *Pediatric Procedures,* 2nd ed. Philadelphia, WB Saunders, 1980.

Jones JA: Examining the newborn's eyes; a satisfactory method. *Clin Pediatr*, 7:124, 1968.

Trobe JD: *The Physician's Guide to Eye Care*. San Francisco, American Academy of Ophthalmology, 1993.

Whaley LF, Wong DL: *Nursing Care of Infants and Children*, 4th ed. St. Louis, Mosby–Year Book, 1991.

Bibliography

Harley RD: *Pediatric Ophthalmology*, 2nd ed. Philadelphia, WB Saunders, 1983.

Trobe JD: *The Physician's Guide to Eye Care*. San Francisco, American Academy of Ophthalmology, 1993.

Whaley LF, Wong DL: *Nursing Care of Infants and Children,* 4th ed. St. Louis, Mosby–Year Book, 1991.

Chapter 40

Pediatric Ear, Nose, and Throat Procedures and Tests

Craig S. Derkay and E. Stephen Buescher

Every child seen by the pediatrician has an ear, nose, and throat examination. Children's ears, noses, and throats are often the sites of diagnostic or therapeutic procedures. Not surprisingly, some of the procedures performed are preparatory (cerumen removal), some diagnostic (pneumatic otoscopy, nasopharyngeal or throat swab, sinus transillumination), and some therapeutic (tympanocentesis, foreign body removal).

Procedures Related to the Ear

CLEANING THE EXTERNAL CANAL

The external auditory canal is the only body cul-de-sac that is lined with skin. Cerumen, a mixture of apocrine sebaceous gland secretions and desquamated keratinized cells, provides a water-repellent coating for the skin of the external canal. Its probable role is to decrease the impact of repeated, short-term water exposures on the external canal, but retention of cerumen can lead to obstruction (the most commonly treated condition of the external ear). Although not often a pathological condition in children, external canal obstruction can preclude proper visualization of the tympanic membrane. Cerumen can be removed from the external canal in several ways: manually, mechanically (by irrigation or suction), or by dissolution/softening.

Manual removal requires an ear curet/cerumen spoon (Fig. 40–1) or a similar improvised

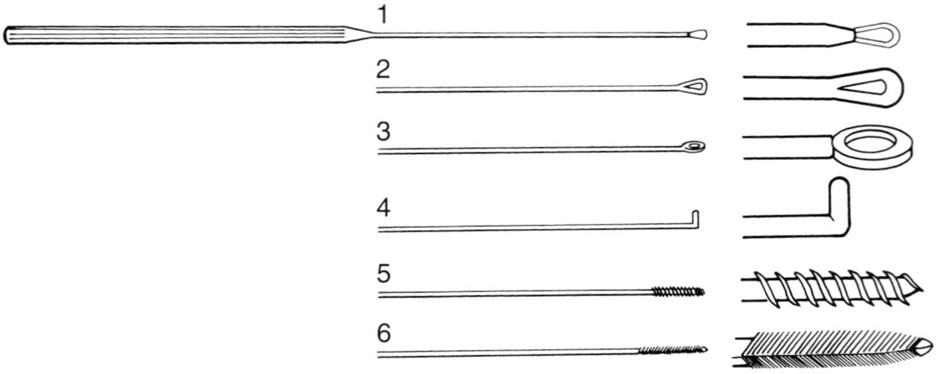

Figure 40–1 Types of applicators used for procedures in the external ear and nose. Magnified views of applicator tips are shown at right. 1 to 3, ear curets/cerumen spoons; 4, right-angle hook; 5 and 6, applicators used for cotton-tipping.

tool. With the aid of an otoscope, the operator removes the cerumen bit by bit until the canal is no longer occluded. Manual cerumen removal requires the operator's patience and the patient's cooperation to be performed successfully. It can reasonably be tried in older children, whereas in younger children, removal by irrigation, suction, or softening/dissolution may be more practical. Irrigation of the external canal can be performed with an ear syringe, an ear bulb, or a water jet device. During irrigation of the ear to clear the external canal, the irrigating water should be warm, and care must be taken not to occlude the external canal with the tip of the syringe or water jet. Because water jet devices can generate pressures as high as 500 kph at full power (Dinsdale et al, 1991) and perforation of the tympanic membrane has been reported to occur at 172 kph (range 97–227 kph) (Keller, 1958), care must be taken to use these devices at low-power settings and to avoid aiming the water jet directly at the tympanic membrane (Dinsdale et al, 1991). In adults, complications from ear syringe irrigation require referral for specialist care in about 1 of 1000 irrigations (Dinsdale et al, 1991). Of course, external ear canal irrigation is contraindicated in instances of tympanic membrane perforation or in the presence of a myringotomy tube. Softening of cerumen in the external canal can be achieved with either commercially available preparations (trolamine polypeptide oleate-condensate [Cerumenex]) or solutions of hydrogen peroxide (1%–3%) or sodium bicarbonate (5%–10%), which are cerumenolytic (cause cerumen disintegration) in a 2- to 3-hour period in vitro (Robinson and Hawke, 1989).

Cleaning the external canal in a child with external otitis (swimmer's ear) can be especially challenging. Because of the edema, tenderness, and distorted landmarks, great care must be taken in removing the debris. Cotton-tipped applicators for this purpose can be either "homemade" or of the commercial variety (Calgiswab). Direct visualization through either a fiberoptic headlight, if one is available, or an otoscope aids in the removal of the canal debris. After removal of debris, a "wick" (Pope Ear Wick, Merocel Corp, Mystic, CT; or cotton pledget dipped in coal tar) can be inserted into the external canal to maintain the lumen and convey the antibiotic drops down the length of the swollen canal. The wick can be removed by parents in 48 to 72 hours with a pair of tweezers.

Children with craniofacial anomalies such as trisomy 21 (Down's syndrome) have congenitally narrow ear canals and often require referral to the otolaryngologist for aural hygiene. In these children, external canal cleaning can best be accomplished with the use of an otoscopic microscope, gentle suction, fine ear curets, or alligator forceps. A general anesthetic may occasionally be necessary to allow full cleaning of the ear canal and establish the condition of the tympanic membrane and middle ear space.

In cleaning the ear canal of a child with a draining ear, tympanic membrane perforation, or myringotomy tube, the key is to evacuate the mucoid material so that antibiotic eardrops can be administered into the middle ear space. This requires either an otoscopic suction catheter (No. 3, 5, or 7) (Fig. 40–2) or a cotton-tipped applicator and direct visualization with a head-

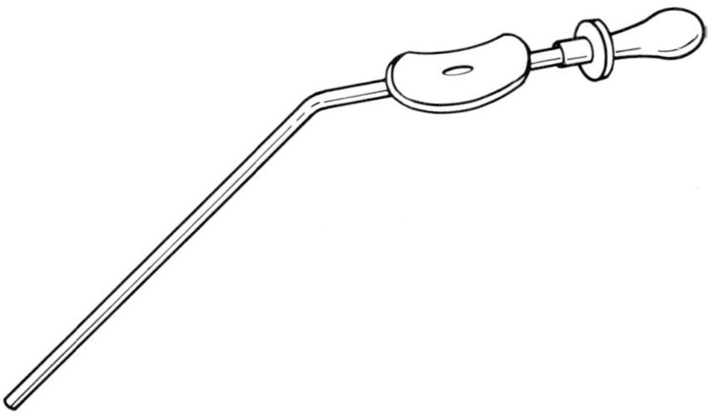

Figure 40–2 Otoscopic suction catheter.

light, microscope, or hand-held otoscope. After the ear canal is cleaned to the level of the tympanic membrane, antibiotic eardrops can be administered directly or by an otic wick.

EARDROP ADMINISTRATION

Procedures for administering eardrops are usually simple. The patient is positioned so that the external canal is roughly in the vertical plane. The child can be positioned on the examining table or on the parent's lap. The child's ear is gently pulled posteriorly and superiorly to straighten the external canal. The drops are applied to the mouth of the canal and allowed to drain into the canal by gravity. After the drops have entered the canal, some practitioners gently massage the tragus for several seconds to assist spread throughout the canal and place a cotton ball at the external meatus to keep the drops from staining clothing should they run out.

Although this procedure sounds simple, it has been noted that eardrop penetration into the canal is extremely variable and is usually worse in diseased ears; materials with water viscosity are superior to higher-viscosity materials (Wilson et al, 1991). In some instances, placement of an otic wick into the external canal increases contact between the canal wall and the applied medication. Before placement, the dry otic wick may need to be trimmed to about half the length of the ear canal. It is then placed into the canal by use of Hartman forceps or tweezers and moistened with the eardrops. On moistening, the wick expands and brings its moist surface into contact with the walls of the ear canal. As an alternative to commercially available wicks (Pope Ear Wick), some physicians prefer to make their own wicks out of a cotton ball rolled into a cigarette shape and impregnated with coal tar.

PNEUMATIC OTOSCOPY

In pediatrics, all routine otoscopic examinations should assess the mobility of the tympanic membrane by pneumatic otoscopy. To perform this procedure, the otoscope head must be capable of an airtight seal and have a port for attachment of pneumatic tubing. A speculum wide enough to press against the wall of the external canal or a smaller speculum with a short segment of soft rubber tubing around its tip must be used to seal the external canal. A length of tubing is attached to the otoscope head, and a small bulb or the operator's mouth is used to apply gentle, insufflating pressure while the tympanic membrane is observed. The operator's mouth as the pressure source has two advantages: the pressure applied can be controlled easily (only gentle pressure is required), and one of the operator's hands is left available to apply traction to the pinna. The normal tympanic membrane moves back and forth easily with slight pressure changes; immobility of the tympanic membrane detected by pneumatic otoscopy is as predictive of a middle ear effusion as an abnormal tympanogram is (Toner and Mains, 1990) and much less expensive.

Procedure

1. Position the patient so that head movement will be minimal. Cooperative children can be sitting down or lying on the examining table. Younger children who require immobilization can be examined in the sitting position in their parent's arms. The child's back is placed to the parent's front, and the child's legs are immobilized between the parent's thighs. One of the parent's hands holds both of the child's hands against the child's waist. The other hand holds the child's head, above the ear, against the parent's chest (Fig. 40–3). Alternatively, the child is positioned supine on the examining table with arms extended along both sides of the head (behind the ears). A parent restrains the arms; the operator's upper body and axilla restrain the child's upper chest, with both hands left free for otoscopy (Fig. 40–4).
2. With the otoscope in one hand, the operator holds the mouthpiece of the pneumatic otoscope head between the teeth (or holds the pneumatic bulb against the base of the otoscope) and uses the free hand to retract the pinna up and back, straightening the external canal. The hand holding the pinna

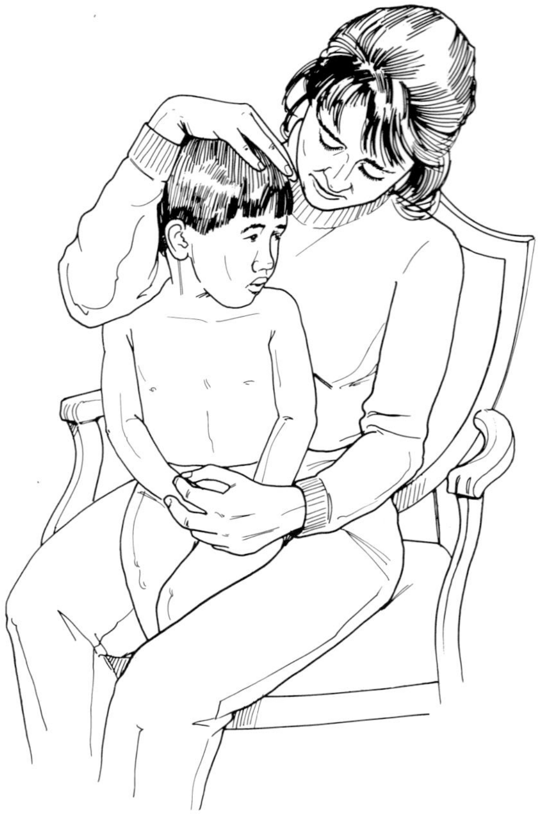

Figure 40–3 Position for restraining a child during the ear examination. The child's hands and head are restrained by the parent's hands; the child's legs are restrained between the parent's thighs.

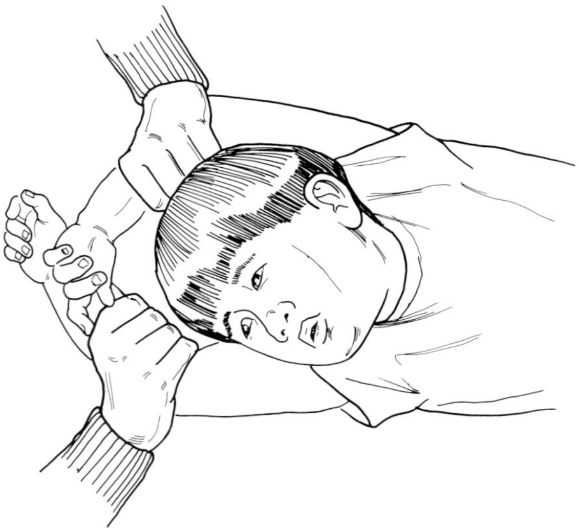

Figure 40–4 Alternative positioning for child restraint during ear examination. The child is placed supine with the arms restrained along each side of the head by the parent. The examiner positions the head and restrains the child's chest with the upper body.

should rest on the patient's head to assist in immobilization; should any accidental head movement occur, the pinna will move appropriately with the head.

3. The tip of the otoscope speculum is placed in the external canal and advanced gently until the tympanic membrane is visualized. The hand that is holding the otoscope should rest against the patient's head. With the tympanic membrane visualized, the pressure in the external canal is changed gently, and the tympanic membrane is observed for movement.

Hand-held tympanometers that use acoustic reflectometry to assess middle ear pressure are now commercially available for screening children for middle ear effusions. These should function as adjuncts to the physical examination and are not a substitute for visualization of the tympanic membrane and pneumatic otoscopy.

FOREIGN BODY REMOVAL

A wide variety of foreign objects find their way into the ears of children. The symptoms resulting from their presence vary, depending on their size, location, composition, and duration in the ear. As a general rule, organic foreign bodies cause more reaction and inflammation than do inorganic ones (Stool and McConnel, 1973), and their associated moisture predisposes the ear to infection and further inflammation. One must remember that any attempt to remove a foreign body that does not succeed will make a bad situation worse (Stool and McConnel, 1973). Because few foreign bodies require emergency removal, taking the time to make the proper preparations and obtain the necessary equipment is wise and benefits both the patient and the physician. The aural foreign body that requires the most urgent management is the button-type battery that is used in some hand-held calculators, hearing aids, and watches. Because they can leak mercury, potassium hydroxide, or other caustic contents after lodgment, these batteries can result in a severe ear canal or tympanic membrane burn and permanent damage to the tympanic membrane. They should be removed expeditiously by the most skilled practitioner available. One should not hesitate to administer an anesthetic and attempt removal in the operating room if an initial attempt at removal is unsuccessful.

If the foreign body is irregular, an ear suction, alligator, or Hartmann forceps (Fig. 40–5)

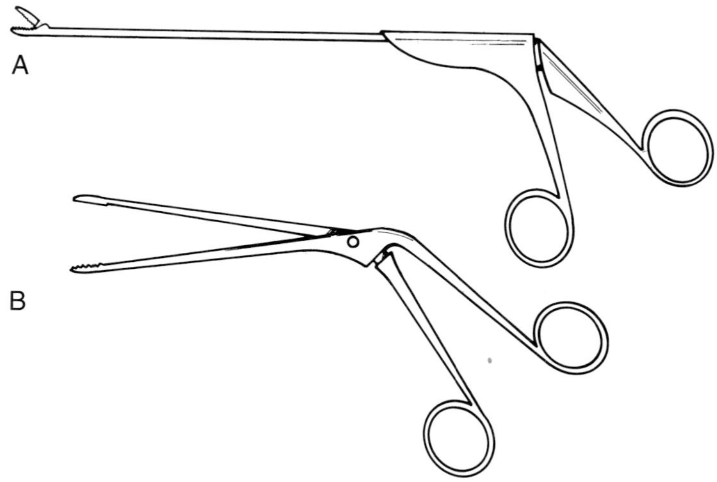

Figure 40–5 Forceps used for removal of foreign bodies from nose or ear. **A.** Alligator forceps. **B.** Hartmann forceps.

passed through a wide-mouth otoscope speculum can be used to grasp and remove it. An otoscopic microscope, if available, can be used for improved visualization and removal of the foreign body. Alternatively, a fiberoptic headlight can be used in combination with otoscopic specula to stent the opening of the ear canal and localize the foreign body. The fiberoptic headlight allows binocular vision, improved depth perception, and easier manual dexterity.

If the foreign body is of ferrous material, a magnet may be helpful in removal. In some instances, irrigation with warm water or saline can float a foreign body out of the canal. When a live insect is found in a child's ear canal, the best approach to its removal is drowning it in antibiotic eardrops and suctioning the drops and insect out after a few minutes. When the foreign body is round, smooth, and hard, such as a necklace bead or small marble, attempts to grasp the foreign body often only advance it deeper into the external canal, making removal more difficult and potentially endangering the tympanic membrane. These are the most common objects to require a general anesthetic and removal in the operating room by an otolaryngologist. A hook or loop must be passed beyond and behind this type of object, and then it is withdrawn. An alternative approach is to use a small dab of cyanoacrylate adhesive ("superglue") on the tip of an applicator stick or suture material. By touching the glue to the foreign body and allowing it to set, a handle is created with which the foreign body can be extracted (Pride and Schwab, 1989).

Care needs to be taken to re-examine the ear and eardrum after removal of any foreign body to ascertain the status of the tympanic membrane and the need for intervention with antibiotic eardrops.

TYMPANOCENTESIS

In some clinical situations, it is necessary to obtain fluid from behind the tympanic membrane for examination or culture. This can be done either by myringotomy (incision of the tympanic membrane for drainage) or by tympanocentesis (puncture of the tympanic membrane to obtain fluid). Myringotomy is usually used in the setting of a subperiosteal mastoid abscess; tympanocentesis can be performed to help direct antibiotic management in a complicated case of acute otitis media.

Cerumen is removed from the ear canal through an otoscope or a portable operating microscope, if one is available, and the tympanic membrane is identified. The anterior-inferior quadrant of the tympanic membrane is noted (Fig. 40–6). This quadrant is preferred for tympanocentesis because it avoids the ossicles and chorda tympani nerve, and it is less vascular and less innervated than other quadrants. Several different devices are available for performing a tympanocentesis:

1. Commercially available, disposable tympanocentesis sets include all the necessary materials.
2. If tympanocentesis is performed in a hospital, a Centuri trap device can be obtained from the operating room and attached to wall suction (Fig. 40–7). This is then attached to an 18- or 21-gauge, 3 1/2-inch

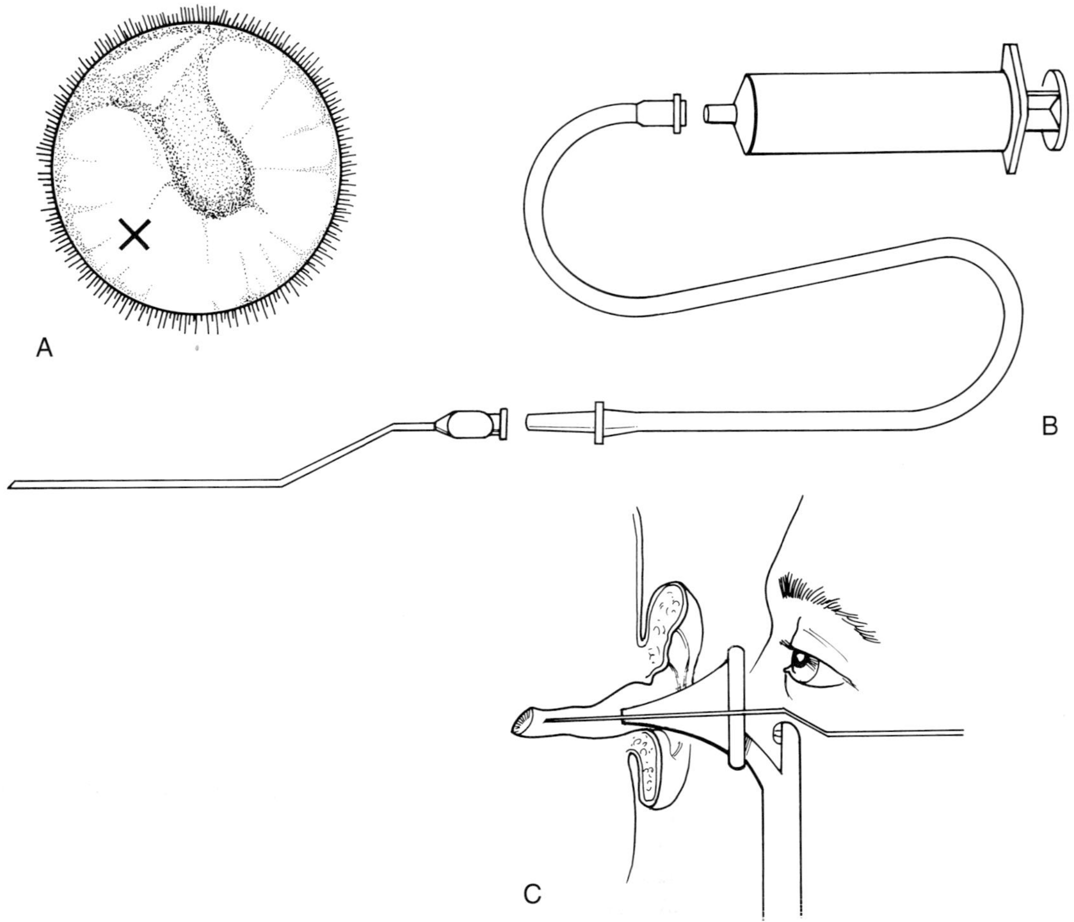

Figure 40–6 Procedure for tympanocentesis. **A.** The site on the tympanic membrane where tympanocentesis is performed. **B.** The assembly of the tympanocentesis device. **C.** The procedure for tympanocentesis.

straight spinal needle and directed through the otoscope or speculum to puncture the tympanic membrane.

3. A short-bevel, 21- or 22-gauge, 3 1/2-inch spinal needle (see Fig. 40–6) (or, alternatively, the central stylet of an "over-the-needle" intravenous catheter) is carefully bent to 30 to 45 degrees at midshaft. A second bend of 30 to 45 degrees in the opposite direction is made just above the needle hub to approximate a flattened sigmoidal shape. A length of intravenous extension tubing is attached to the needle hub, and a 10-ml syringe is attached to the distal end of the extension tubing. With this device, the operator directs the needle for the puncture, and an assistant, when instructed, applies aspirating back-pressure with the syringe.

Materials

Topical anesthetic (lidocaine, phenol, cocaine)
70% alcohol
Tympanocentesis device as appropriate
Culture tubes
Nonbacteriostatic saline
2 × 2 gauze pads
Otoscope
Suction catheter
Antibiotic eardrops

Procedure

1. Restrain the patient as necessary. For infants, hand restraint by an assistant may be all that is necessary. In older children, cooperation may be adequate to allow the proce-

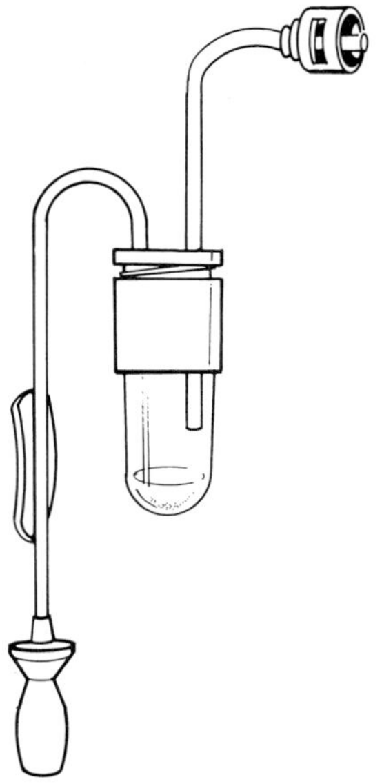

Figure 40–7 Centuri trap device used for applying suction during tympanocentesis. The metal bulb at lower left is attached to continuous suction, with occlusion of a vent in the finger plate at left used to apply suction.

dure to be done without restraint or with some sedation. In the preschool child, total body immobilization is usually necessary. If it cannot be ensured, brief general anesthesia or heavy sedation should be considered.

2. With use of the largest otoscope speculum that will comfortably fit the external canal, cerumen is cleared from the external canal, and the tympanic membrane and the anterior-inferior quadrant are visualized. In younger children and infants, a few drops of topical anesthetic are placed into the external canal after removal of the speculum. Make sure that they contact and cover the tympanic membrane and wait 5 to 10 minutes for the anesthesia to take effect. Alternatively, the iontophoresis device can be used to distribute the lidocaine, but this is somewhat cumbersome and takes more time. In the older child, phenol can be applied topically to the proposed puncture site with a cotton-tipped applicator. This produces excellent topical anesthesia as well as hemostasis and requires less than a minute to take effect.
3. If the topical antibiotic drops are used, they can be removed with a cotton-tipped applicator or suction. The external canal is sterilized with 70% alcohol, and an ear canal culture specimen of normal flora is obtained for comparison with the middle ear culture. Residual alcohol is removed with a cotton-tipped applicator or suction catheter.
4. Reinsert the speculum and revisualize the anterior-inferior quadrant. Insert the tympanocentesis needle until it is just short of the tympanic membrane. With the operator's hand steadied against the patient's head, the needle is pushed just through the tympanic membrane, the middle ear is quickly aspirated, and the needle is promptly withdrawn. The puncture motion should be linear, to produce a discrete puncture site in the plane of the tympanic membrane.
5. Clean any residual middle ear drainage or blood from the external canal and instill antibiotic eardrops.
6. The quantity of material aspirated is typically small and is often caught in the needle hub or tubing/syringe barrel attached to the needle. To retrieve the sample, gently flush a small volume of nonbacteriostatic saline through the tubing/syringe and needle and into the culture medium.

AURICULAR HEMATOMA

Blunt trauma to the external ear may disrupt the fragile blood supply to the pinna that is supplied by its perichondrium. This type of injury is common among wrestlers and boxers and can produce a hematoma that deprives the cartilage of its nutrients and results in necrosis. This is especially likely if the perichondrium on both sides of the cartilage is elevated or if the overlying skin is lacerated. The resulting "cauliflower ear" is avoidable if prompt action is taken.

Materials

1% lidocaine
No. 15 scalpel
4–0 nylon suture
Dental rolls (3)
Antibiotic ointment
Suction catheter
Sterile setup
Povidone-iodine (Betadine) solution
Sterile saline solution

Procedure

1. After the area is prepared with povidone-iodine solution and sterile towels, the skin

overlying the hematoma is anesthetized with 1% lidocaine.
2. With a No. 15 scalpel, an incision is made over the hematoma in a plane parallel with the natural skin fold (Fig. 40–8). By use of the suction catheter, the hematoma is evacuated, and the cavity is irrigated with sterile saline.

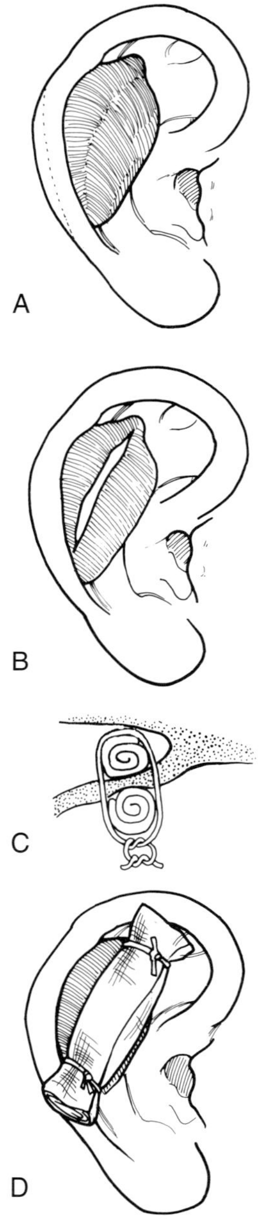

Figure 40–8 Procedure for draining an auricular hematoma. **A.** Auricular hematoma. **B.** The hematoma is incised and blood is evacuated. **C.** Arrangement of dental packs on both sides of the auricular cartilage as viewed from above. **D.** Dental packs are secured in place to prevent reaccumulation of blood.

3. A 4–0 nylon suture is then passed through and through the ear, traversing the skin, cartilage, and skin as it passes to the opposite side of the ear. The suture is passed around an antibiotic ointment (e.g., bacitracin)–impregnated dental roll on the side opposite the incision and then back through the skin, cartilage, and skin. The suture is then tied around a second dental roll overlying the incision. A second suture is placed and tied in an identical fashion at the other end of the dental roll. A third roll can be placed in the concha bowl if the hematoma extends that far.
4. An antistaphylococcal antibiotic (oxacillin, nafcillin) is prescribed for 7 days.
5. The dental rolls are removed after 1 week. They prevent reaccumulation of blood or serum in the hematoma-evacuated potential space.

HEARING TESTS

Hearing in children is of crucial importance for environmental orientation, psychological security, and the development of normal speech and language. The child who cannot hear spoken words will not develop normal expressive or receptive language, a handicap that can affect all aspects of the child's development. Screening of hearing in newborns and young children is mandated by most states and supported by the National Institutes of Health (1993) and the federal government. Guidelines for neonatal screening and infant hearing assessment have been issued by the Joint Committee on Infant Hearing, the American Speech-Language-Hearing Association, the American Academy of Otolaryngology–Head and Neck Surgery, and the American Academy of Pediatrics. These guidelines are intended for early identification of those infants thought to be at high risk for hearing loss (Tables 40–1 and 40–2). Virginia has taken the lead in recommending hearing screenings of all newborns. Whereas most high-risk babies receive their hearing screening within the hospital environment by auditory brain stem potential response (ABR) testing or otoacoustic emissions screening, any program that broadens the guidelines for testing will require the pediatrician to take an active role in hearing screening.

Hearing assessment in the older (older than 5 years), cooperative child requires some form of deliberate signal from the patient for determining whether the child hears pure tones pre-

Table 40-1 Risk Criteria for Hearing Loss from Birth to 1 Month (Corrected Age)

Family history of childhood SNHL
Congenital infection believed to be associated with SNHL
Craniofacial anomalies
Birth weight less than 1500 g
Hyperbilirubinemia
Ototoxic medication given for 5 days or more
Meningitis
Anoxia at birth (low Apgar scores)
Ventilation for 10 days or more
Stigmas of syndromes associated with SNHL

SNHL, sensorineural hearing loss.

sented over a range of frequencies (125–8000 Hz) at different intensities (0–110 dB). In younger children, auditory testing is more complex. Hand clapping, loud sounds, and loud speech produce high-intensity, broad-frequency spectrum sounds that are sufficient only to identify severe-profound hearing loss. They are unlikely to draw attention to less severe (but developmentally significant) deficits. Approaches that do not require a deliberate signal to denote response to sound have been developed to examine the hearing of infants and young children. These include modified behavioral methods and objective neural activity methods.

Several types of behavioral audiological test methods can be used in young children. Behavioral observation audiometry uses any of a number of behavioral responses (Moro reflex, alerting responses, scanning responses, localization, increase in activity, change in sucking pattern to presented sounds) to assess hearing sensitivity. Visual reinforcement audiometry uses operant conditioning with visual reinforcement (e.g., a blinking light or moving toy) of an infant's head-turning response toward a sound source that can be varied in intensity and pitch. Conditional play audiometry associates some playing activity (putting blocks in a box, putting rings on a peg) with sound and then systematically varies the sound stimulus and identifies the minimal level for the conditioned playing response. This type of behavioral audiological testing must use a playing activity that is within the developmental capabilities of the child.

The most frequently used objective audiological test, measurement of the ABR, does not require any active participation of the patient and is therefore applicable to the young infant or the uncooperative patient. A pretesting sedative such as chloral hydrate at 50 mg/kg is administered to the child older than 6 months. A series of recording electrodes are placed on the vertex of the head, the forehead, and the mastoid process of the ear to be tested. Acoustic clicks are presented to the ear at decreasing intensities, and the pattern of the electrical potential occurring in the first 10 msec after each stimulus is recorded. Click stimuli are presented quickly so that a complete set of stimuli at a given intensity is completed in 1 to 2 minutes; complete testing of both ears requires approximately an hour. By comparing the latency (time between the application of the stimulus and the peak response of specific electrical potential waves) with the intensity of the click applied and comparing it with standard curves, the infant's hearing threshold can be determined within approximately 10 to 20 dB of behavioral thresholds for higher frequencies. In addition, information about the existing auditory neural pathways through the brain stem can be obtained by close examination of the waveform latencies. Both prematurity and otitis media significantly affect absolute wave latencies. Neonates who fail an initial screening should have an ear examination with removal of vernix and cerumen and an assessment for possible middle ear effusion. Screening should be at 35 to 40 dB to "pass" most infants with transient middle ear dysfunction while still "failing" those with significant hearing loss.

Table 40-2 Risk Criteria for Hearing Loss from 1 Month to 2 Years

Parental concern regarding hearing, speech, language, or developmental delay
Neurodegenerative disorders
Neonatal risk factors associated with progressive SNHL
Postnatal head trauma
Stigmas of syndromes associated with SNHL
Ototoxic medication for 5 days or more
Neurodegenerative disorders
Childhood infectious disease known to be associated with SNHL (mumps, measles)

SNHL, sensorineural hearing loss.

Commercially available automated ABR screening units are currently in use in hospital nurseries (ALGO-1). They are said to require the same sophistication for operation as a toaster and can be administered by a trained volunteer (non-nursing personnel) under the direction of an audiologist. Children who fail ABR screening on two occasions beyond 40 weeks' gestation should be referred for a complete audiological assessment and otological examination by otolaryngologist before 6 months of age and preferably by 3 months of age.

TYMPANOMETRY

Measurement of acoustic impedance of the middle ear with tympanometry is used to objectively assess the integrity and function of the "peripheral" (middle ear and tympanic membrane) auditory mechanism in children. Put simply, sound is echoed off the tympanic membrane as the membrane is pulled or pushed by pressure in the external canal; the pattern of sound pressure levels observed across a range of external canal pressure conditions reveals information about tympanic membrane compliance and the functional status of the middle ear. When applied to a normal ear, the tympanogram pattern shows maximal tympanic membrane compliance when no pressure is applied to the external canal and decreasing compliance as either positive or negative pressures are applied progressively to the external canal. The overall pattern mimics an inverted V. Specific aberrations from this pattern can be indicative of a thickened (scarred) or flaccid (disarticulation of the ossicles) tympanic membrane, eustachian tube dysfunction, or middle ear effusion.

In addition, the acoustic reflex can be examined with tympanometry. This reflex, contraction of the stapedius muscle caused by a loud sound, increases the stiffness of the ossicular chain with an associated decrease in tympanic membrane compliance. Although interpretation of the effect of the acoustic reflex on the tympanogram is complex and to some degree age related (acoustic reflexes in newborns or young infants are sometimes difficult to measure), the presence of an acoustic reflex demonstrates an intact facial nerve distal to the geniculate ganglion.

Procedures Related to the Nasopharynx and Sinuses

NASAL AND NASOPHARYNGEAL EXAMINATION

Examination of the nose in the cooperative older child is straightforward; examination in the younger child and infant is more of a problem. Visualization of the nasal passages in infants and toddlers can be facilitated by use of an otoscope and speculum instead of a small flashlight. When available, a nasal speculum combined with a headlight may enhance visualization of the nasal cavity. Small flexible fiberoptic nasopharyngoscopes, such as those used by pulmonologists, anesthesiologists, and otolaryngologists, can be passed with minimal discomfort after topical anesthesia and decongestion in children of all ages. These instruments allow visualization of the posterior nasal cavity, nasopharynx, hypopharynx, and larynx and are useful in identifying the level of obstruction. They can be combined with a video monitor (TV screen) to demonstrate the findings to the parents as well as the child.

Adequate visualization of the pharynx is also relatively easy in the cooperative patient. In the child old enough to understand the command to open his or her mouth but unable to say *ah*, getting the child to yawn with the mouth open will widely expose the pharynx without the use of a tongue blade–induced gag reflex.

INSTILLATION OF NOSE DROPS

For intranasally applied medications to be effective, they must come into contact with the proper surface at the proper concentration. It follows, then, that before intranasal medications are administered, the nasal passages

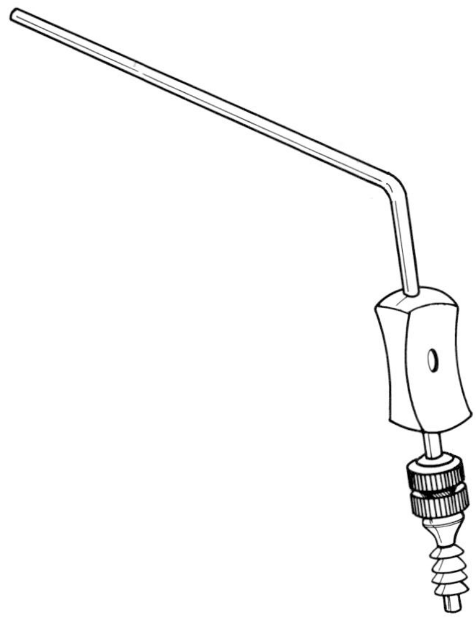

Figure 40–9 Frazier nasal suction catheter.

should be cleared of mucus or exudate that might interfere with the medication's contact or concentration. In younger children, this is achieved with bulb syringe aspiration of the nasal passages; in older children, it can be achieved by blowing the nose. If available, a nasal suction catheter (Frazier suction catheter, No. 6) (Fig. 40–9) can be used along with a headlight in the cooperative older child.

Younger children are positioned supine on the sitting parent's lap with their legs extended along each side of the parent's waist. The patient's head can be supported either by the parent's lap or by the parent's free hand (Fig. 40–10). With the child in this position, the dropper tip is placed just inside the nostril, and the medication is administered. After both sides have been treated, the patient is kept in this supine position for several minutes to allow movement into the nasopharynx by gravity.

In older children, the position used for nose drop administration depends on the intended site of the medication's effect. The Proetz technique (Fig. 40–11) optimizes contact of the medication with the ostia of the ethmoid and sphenoid sinuses; the patient lies supine with the head over the edge of the bed and the neck hyperextended, chin directed toward the ceiling. The Parkinson technique (Fig. 40–12) optimizes contact with the ostia of the frontal and maxillary sinuses. The patient lies on the

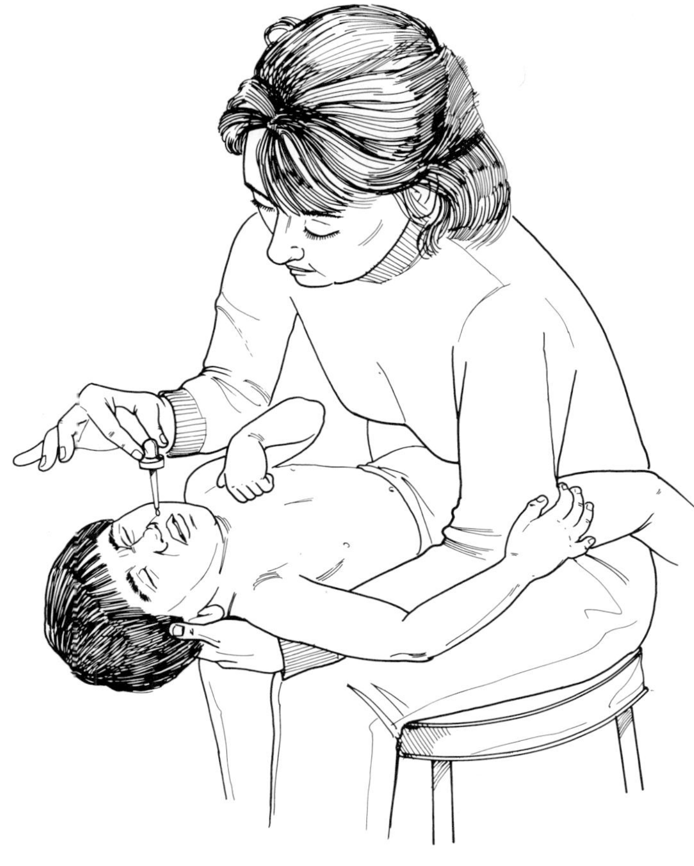

Figure 40–10 Positioning of a small child for nose drop instillation.

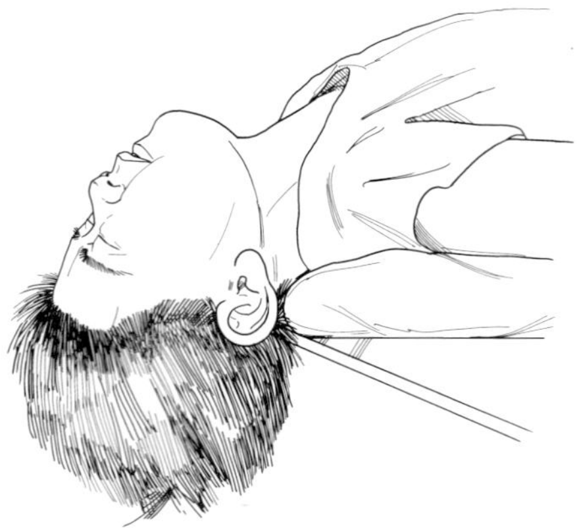

Figure 40–11 Positioning for the Proetz technique for nose drop administration. This position maximizes nose drop contact with the ostia of the ethmoid and sphenoid sinuses.

side with the lower shoulder elevated slightly with a folded sheet or blanket. The head is bent to a lateral head-low position, and drops are administered into the inferior nostril. The patient's position is then reversed so that the other shoulder is slightly elevated by the sheet, and the drops are administered into the other nostril.

PROCEDURES TO CONTROL EPISTAXIS

In the situation of persistent epistaxis, nasal packing may be necessary. Packing is performed anteriorly, posteriorly, or both. Anterior packing is used to tamponade epistaxis originating in the anterior nasal cavity (most frequently due to bleeding from Kiesselbach's venous plexus in the anterior nasal septum). Simple cautery with silver nitrate sticks should be attempted before resorting to placement of an anterior nasal pack. This is accomplished after first placing a large cotton pledget impregnated with 1% phenylephrine hydrochloride (Neo-Synephrine) and 2% tetracaine into the anterior naris for vasoconstriction and topical anesthesia. With use of a nasal speculum, headlight, and several silver nitrate sticks, the prominent vessels in Kiesselbach's area responsible for the bleeding can be identified and cauterized. Bacitracin ointment is then applied to the raw surface, and the patient is instructed to avoid nose blowing and internal and external nasal trauma for the next several days.

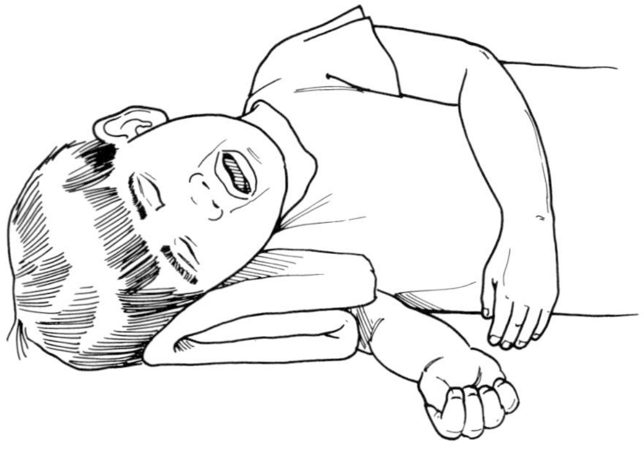

Figure 40–12 Positioning for the Parkinson technique for nose drop administration. This position maximizes nose drop contact with the ostia of the frontal and maxillary sinuses.

If this maneuver is unsuccessful, placement of an anterior nasal pack can be attempted. Many materials are available for nasal packing. The most commonly used is petrolatum gauze generously impregnated with antibiotic ointment. Other materials available to place against the septum and especially useful in children with bleeding dyscrasias are surgical Gelfoam, topical thrombin, and Avitene (which can be mixed into a slurry and painted onto the septum and compressed with the gauze pack).

Children with posterior epistaxis need to be referred to an otolaryngologist for management. The placement of a Foley catheter with the balloon inflated in the nasopharynx or a commercially available inflatable nasal tamponade device can be helpful in this situation until a specialist arrives.

Materials

Anterior pack: 1-cm-wide antibiotic-impregnated petrolatum gauze
Long bayonet-type nasal forceps
Bandage tape
Nasal speculum
Suction
Headlight

Procedure

1. Insert the nasal speculum to allow access of the bayonet forceps.
2. Insert the end of the antibiotic-impregnated petrolatum gauze into the posterior nasal cavity (*beyond* the site of bleeding) using the bayonet forceps. Place it in the posterior-inferior part of the nasal cavity and layer several accordion folds of gauze over themselves to form a base.

3. Pack the posterior-inferior region, then the posterior-superior and anterior-inferior regions with the petrolatum gauze, folding the gauze over on itself repeatedly.
4. The free distal end of the gauze strip is attached to the nose with a small piece of bandage tape; alternatively, a silk suture can be placed through the distal end to identify it.
5. Anterior packing is usually left in place for 24 to 72 hours.
6. Complications of nasal packing include obstruction of nasal ostia, which may predispose to sinusitis and transient eustachian tube dysfunction. The use of antibiotic ointment on the packing and systemic antibiotics for nasal flora and gram-negative bacilli seems to decrease this likelihood (Derkay et al, 1989). Toxic shock syndrome has also been reported to occur with nasal packing.

NASOPHARYNGEAL CULTURE

When material must be obtained from the nasopharynx for culture, it is obtained by use of a fine cotton-tipped wire applicator (wooden shaft cotton-tipped applicator sticks are too large and rigid for small children). Such applicators are commercially available (Calgiswab) or can be constructed from fine wire, cotton-tipped at one end and with a wire loop placed as a handle at the other. A supply of these swabs can be prepared by placing each in a glass tube with the loop handle protruding through a cotton plug. After autoclave sterilization, these can be stored in a rack until used.

Procedure

1. Grasp the swab by the handle in one hand; with the other hand resting on the patient's head, elevate the tip of the nose with the thumb to reveal the vestibule and straighten the path for the swab.
2. Introduce the swab through the nostril and advance it along the floor of the nasal cavity to the posterior nasopharynx. If the swab is angled cephalad, it will not reach the posterior nasopharynx.
3. Leave the swab in place for several seconds, then remove it and place it in either a sterile tube for transport to the laboratory or the appropriate culture medium.
4. In culturing the nasal cavity, the ideal location for sampling is at the middle meatus, which lies lateral to the middle turbinate. A randomly obtained nasal culture specimen is not useful clinically. With a headlight, nasal speculum, and (if available) a rigid telescope, this is best accomplished after all pooled nasal secretions are suctioned.
5. Nasal smears can be obtained to identify eosinophils and help to establish a diagnosis of nasal allergies. These are obtained from the undersurface of the inferior turbinate by use of a cotton-tipped applicator, smeared onto a glass slide, and stained with either Wright-Giemsa or Hansel stain.

TRANSILLUMINATION OF SINUSES

Transillumination can be applied to the examination of the maxillary and frontal sinuses. Its utility is limited in the infant: only the ethmoid and maxillary sinuses exist at birth, and both are rudimentary. In the older child, however, transillumination can assist in the diagnosis of fluid accumulation, mucous membrane swelling, or polyp formation. As with transillumination of the central nervous system, a bright light source and a dark environment optimize the application of transillumination.

The maxillary sinuses are visualized by placing the light source on the patient's tongue and having the patient close the mouth around it. Both maxillary sinuses should transilluminate. Transillumination should be judged on the basis of presence (normal) or absence (abnormal) of light. Judgments regarding intensity of transilluminated light are subjective and correlate poorly with clinical disease. Alternatively, each maxillary sinus can be transilluminated individually by placing the light source over the midpoint of the inferior orbital rim with the edge of the lens sealed to the skin so that no stray light illuminates the skin. The transilluminating light passing through the hard palate is then assessed through the patient's open mouth.

To transilluminate the frontal sinuses (reliable only in children older than 10 years), the light source is pressed snugly against the medial aspect of the roof of each orbit with the light directed upward. Because of the wide range of normal regarding symmetry of the frontal sinuses, only the intensity of illumination from one side to the other is assessed.

REMOVAL OF NASAL FOREIGN BODIES

Infants and young children may occasionally place objects of fascination into their nasal cavities when they are outside the sight of their guardians. This situation comes to the attention of the pediatrician when the child presents with unilateral foul-smelling rhinorrhea. The proper removal of a nasal foreign body depends on the nature of the foreign body itself as well as on the available equipment and the level of cooperativeness of the child. Ideally, a fiberoptic headlight, nasal speculum, and wide variety of foreign body forceps will be available. Nearly all children require restraint for removal of nasal foreign bodies, and some may require sedation with chloral hydrate, midazolam, or possibly a general anesthetic. Depending on the size of the child, removal can be attempted in either the supine position or sitting upright on the parent's lap. If the supine position is used on an examining table, the child can be "bundled" in a sheet with the arms secured at the side. Because there is potential danger of airway compromise if aspiration occurs during the extraction, this procedure should be performed within a setting suitable for dealing with this emergency.

Materials

Fiberoptic headlight (or operating head otoscope)
Nasal speculum
Hartmann forceps
Alligator forceps
Bayonet forceps
Phenylephrine hydrochloride or oxymetazoline hydrochloride (Afrin) 1%
Frazier suction

Procedure

1. With the child properly restrained and sedated if necessary, the nose should be sprayed with vasoconstrictor (phenylephrine hydrochloride or oxymetazoline hydrochloride) and obstructing mucus or blood suctioned clear.
2. If the variety of foreign body is known, a duplicate model should be obtained by the parent so that the proper instrument can be chosen for its removal. For instance, if an earring is the foreign body, the duplicate earring should be brought in so that the physician can judge its dimensions and choose between the available forceps to pick the one best suited for the task.
3. Round or oval foreign bodies may best be removed with a right-angle hook passed beyond the foreign body and then rotated forward. With smaller, solid foreign bodies, the Hartmann forceps may be ideal. Vegetable matter and beans may best be removed with the Frazier suction catheter. Caustic materials and batteries should be removed urgently by the otolaryngologist in the operating room because of their potential for mucosal damage and the possible need for placement of a stent and full nasal endoscopy after their removal.

MAXILLARY SINUS PUNCTURE

In a child with complicated acute sinusitis, it is occasionally necessary to obtain a culture specimen from the maxillary sinus to direct further medical management. This is most often performed by the consulting otolaryngologist but can be accomplished by the pediatrician if sufficient equipment and expertise are available.

Materials

Fiberoptic headlight
Nasal speculum
2% tetracaine
Oxymetazoline hydrochloride or phenylephrine hydrochloride 1%
3 1/2-inch 18-gauge spinal needle
Sterile saline

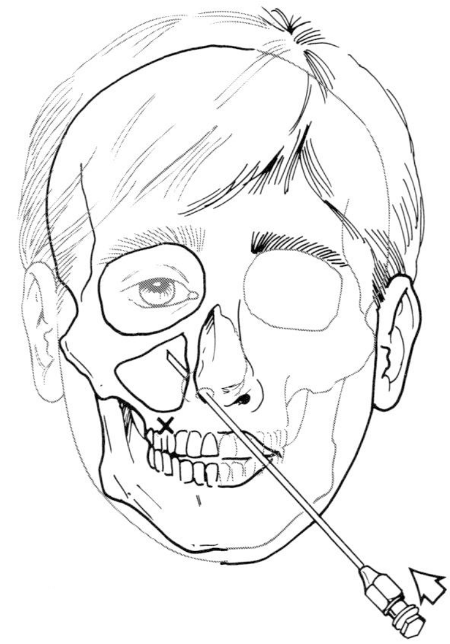

Figure 40–13 Sites used for maxillary sinus puncture. The aspirating needle is directed beneath the inferior turbinate toward the lateral canthus of the eye to enter the maxillary sinus. Alternatively, the canine fossa (X) puncture site in the maxillary gum line can be used in older children.

10-ml syringe
Frazier suction catheter No. 6
Culture swabs
Cotton pledgets

Procedure

1. In children younger than 6 years, the lack of eruption of the permanent dentition requires that the procedure be performed intranasally. In the older child and young adult, the procedure can be performed through the canine fossa in the maxillary gum line (Fig. 40–13).
2. For the intranasal approach, topical anesthesia and vasoconstrictors are applied by cotton pledgets. Most children require some degree of preprocedure sedation/analgesia in the form of chloral hydrate or midazolam, and general anesthesia may be necessary in the majority of children. Restraint is required in virtually all patients.
3. With the child supine, the spinal needle with its obturator in place is inserted beneath the inferior turbinate approximately halfway back the length of the nasal cavity and directed posterosuperiorly toward the lateral canthus of the eye (see Fig. 40–13).
4. A "pop" is felt as one enters into the maxillary sinus cavity. Aspiration is performed with a 10-ml syringe followed by instillation and aspiration with 5 ml of sterile saline solution. Material that is obtained is sent for culture, and a cotton pledget with oxymetazoline hydrochloride or phenylephrine hydrochloride is reinserted for hemostasis.

Common Procedures Involving the Oropharynx and Mouth

THROAT CULTURE

When the throat is to be cultured, a sterile cotton-tipped applicator made of wood, cardboard, or wire is used.

Procedure

1. Grasp the applicator in one hand and gently hold the patient's lower jaw with the other.
2. When the patient's pharynx is exposed to view, move the cotton swab directly to the back of the throat, avoiding contact with the tongue, buccal mucosa, or palate.
3. In one motion, draw the cotton swab laterally across the pharynx and over the surface of a tonsil. If obvious exudation is present on the pharynx or tonsils, include these areas in the swabbing.
4. Immediately place the swab in a sterile tube for transport to the laboratory, or streak the swab across appropriate culture medium.

FRENULECTOMY

Ankyloglossia is a relatively common finding in newborn children and only rarely requires correction. There is controversy concerning the benefits of releasing the tongue that is tied down to the floor of the mouth for strictly speech articulation purposes. However, in the newborn child with difficulty breast-feeding because of lack of tongue excursion, a frenulectomy can be performed in the office setting.

Materials

Topical Cetacaine (or Hurricaine spray)
Headlight or high-intensity portable surgical light
4 × 4 gauze
Sterile iris scissors
Toothed forceps (optional)

Procedure

1. The procedure is best performed with the newborn child held firmly in the mother's

or nurse's lap in a supine position. The floor of the mouth is sprayed with topical Cetacaine, and 60 seconds is allowed for the anesthesia to begin working.

2. The tongue is grasped firmly by the physician with the 4 × 4 gauze and lifted superiorly and anteriorly as far as possible. If this step proves difficult, a toothed forcep can be used to grasp the tongue, but this may cause some soft tissue trauma.
3. With the tongue elevated, the persistent frenulum is snipped along the undersurface of the tongue back to the tongue root. Care is taken to avoid any trauma to submandibular ducts at the floor of the mouth just lateral to each side of the frenulum.
4. The gauze is then used as a pressure pack for a few minutes for hemostasis.

FOREIGN BODY OF THE THROAT

The most common foreign bodies of the oral cavity in children are chicken or fish bones that become embedded in the tonsils. These can be visualized on physical examination and rarely require a visit to the operating room for removal.

Materials

Headlight
Tongue blade
Bayonet forceps
Hartman forceps
Hemostat
Cetacaine spray

Procedure

1. Removal of a tonsillar foreign body is most easily accomplished in the upright sitting position. Younger children and older noncooperative children may require restraint and light sedation.
2. The throat is sprayed with topical Cetacaine to decrease the gag reflex. A tongue blade is used to better visualize the foreign body, which is usually found "speared" into the core of one of the tonsils.
3. With a Hartman forceps, hemostat, or bayonet forceps, the foreign body is tightly gripped and pulled toward the opposite tonsil to disengage it from its embedded position. Once disengaged, it is removed swiftly.

INCISION AND DRAINAGE OF PERITONSILLAR ABSCESS

A peritonsillar abscess (or quinsy) usually occurs in older children or young adults with a history of recurrent tonsillitis. It is typically unilateral, and the pus is most often found anterosuperior to the anterior tonsillar pillar. Drainage of a peritonsillar abscess in the office setting in a child is severely limited by the amount of trismus present and the cooperativeness of the patient. In most instances, these two factors lead to a drainage procedure under general anesthesia in children. Often a "hot" tonsillectomy in which both of the tonsils are removed at the time of the drainage of the abscess may be performed. In teen-agers and cooperative older children, incision and drainage of a peritonsillar abscess can be performed in the office or emergency department.

Materials

No. 15 and No. 11 scalpel
Cetacaine spray
2% lidocaine with epinephrine 1:100,000
25-gauge and 18-gauge needles
Tonsil hemostat
10-ml syringe
Culturette swab
Yankauer suction
Fiberoptic headlight
Tongue blades (two)
Eye protection
Mask, gloves, and gown for the physician

Procedure

1. After the procedure is explained step by step to the patient, the pharynx is sprayed with topical Cetacaine, and 60 seconds is allowed for effect.
2. An 18-gauge needle and a 10-ml syringe are used to aspirate the abscess. This is most often accomplished by insertion just above the superior pole of the anterior pillar on the affected side (Fig. 40–14). Tongue blades may be needed to direct the tongue out of the way and to compensate for the trismus that is invariably present.
3. Purulent material from the aspiration is sent for culture, including culture of aerobic and anaerobic organisms and Gram's stain.
4. The area of successful aspiration is then infiltrated with the lidocaine/epinephrine local anesthetic. Either the No. 15 or No. 11 scalpel can then be used to incise the overlying mucosa in a semilunar fashion, and the

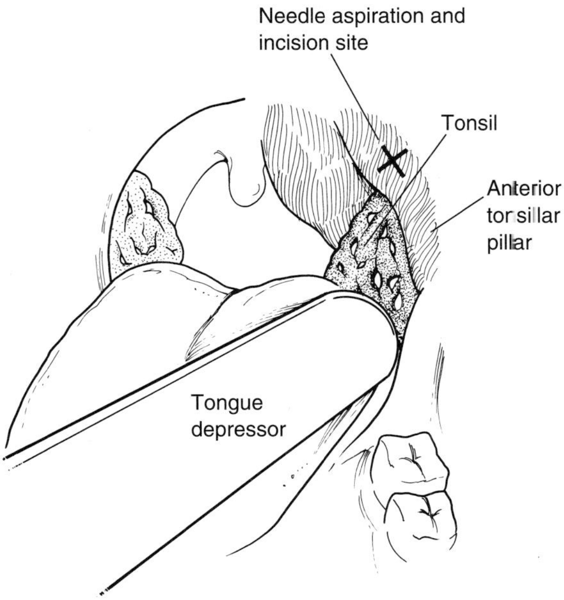

Figure 40–14 Site for needle aspiration of a peritonsillar abscess. Puncture site (X) is located on the superior pole of the anterior tonsillar pillar.

tonsil hemostat is used to spread the tissue widely. The Yankauer suction (Fig. 40–15) is then used to evacuate the blood and pus, and the patient is asked to gargle with saline.

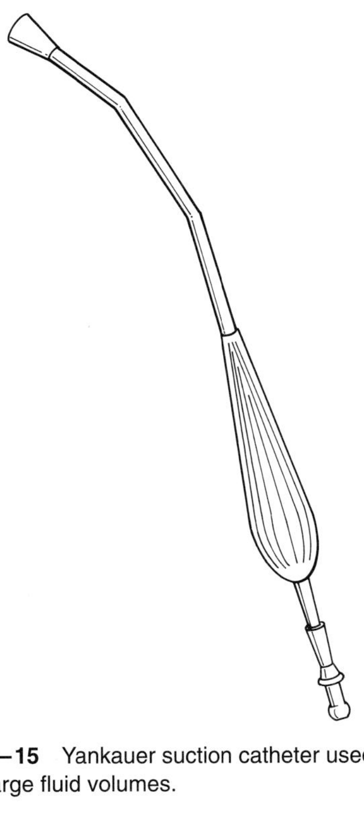

Figure 40–15 Yankauer suction catheter used for aspiration of large fluid volumes.

5. Management after drainage includes use of high-dose intravenous penicillin or a first-generation cephalosporin. Some reliable patients without signs of dehydration and with documented adequate oral intake can be sent home with oral antibiotics; the majority of patients require at least a 24-hour hospital stay to ensure reversal of dehydration and administration of antibiotics.

TREATMENT OF POST-TONSILLECTOMY BLEEDING

After removal of the tonsils, between 1% and 3% of children experience some degree of postoperative hemorrhage, usually between 5 and 10 days postoperatively. This may range from a transient amount of blood-tinged sputum to frank arterial bleeding from the tonsillar fossa that requires urgent intervention. Most older children and teen-agers with post-tonsillectomy bleeding can be managed in the outpatient center. Virtually all younger children, some older noncooperative children, and children with heavy bleeding require a trip back to the operating room.

Materials

Headlight
Yankauer suction
Tongue blades
Silver nitrate sticks
1% to 2% lidocaine with 1:100,000 epinephrine for injection
Cetacaine spray
2 × 2 gauze sponges
Eye protection, glasses, mask, and gown for the physician

Procedure

1. This procedure is best accomplished with the cooperative child sitting upright. A calm parent close at hand assists the procedure greatly.
2. The throat is first sprayed with topical Cetacaine spray, and the bleeding site is identified after gentle suctioning. The most common sites are at either the superior or inferior tonsillar pillars.
3. Lidocaine with epinephrine is then injected into the tonsillar fossa in the area of the identified bleeding site for anesthesia and vasoconstriction.
4. Successive silver nitrate sticks are then used for cauterization of the offending vessel; gentle gauze packing held in place by the patient is used for tamponade.

EMERGENCY CRICOTHYROTOMY AND TRACHEOSTOMY

Although it is preferable to perform a tracheotomy under controlled circumstances (in an operating room under sterile conditions with a trained assistant, adequate lighting, proper equipment, and an endotracheal tube in place to secure the airway), situations occasionally arise in which an emergency procedure to secure the airway is necessary and endotracheal intubation is impossible. In the setting of massive facial trauma with distorted anatomy or with advanced epiglottitis in which the larynx is obscured, an emergency cricothyrotomy may be needed acutely to establish a patent airway.

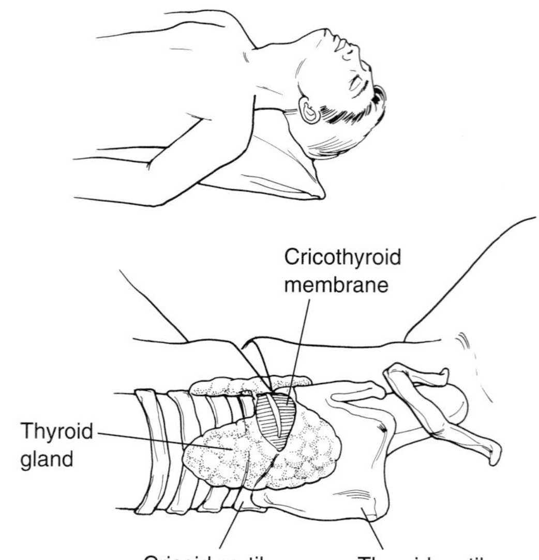

Figure 40–16 Site for emergency tracheostomy through cricothyroid membrane. Positioning of the patient is shown at top. The cricothyroid membrane is located deep to the thyroid isthmus, between the thyroid cartilage and the cricoid cartilage.

Emergency Cricothyrotomy

Materials

Headlight or high-intensity portable surgical light
No. 15 scalpel
Hemostat
Suction catheter
Tracheotomy or endotracheal tube
Shoulder roll

Procedure

1. The child is placed supine with the shoulders elevated and the neck hyperextended (Fig. 40–16).
2. The larynx and trachea are palpated. In the young child, the larynx is located relatively high in the neck, and palpation may be difficult. Palpation may also prove difficult if an expanding neck hematoma is present.
3. When the larynx is palpated, it should be held firmly in the midline with the thumb and index finger. A horizontal incision is then placed through skin and subcutaneous tissue. The cricothyroid membrane (between the lower border of the thyroid cartilage and the upper border of the cricoid cartilage) (see Fig. 40–16) is then incised from side to side.
4. A hemostat is used to enlarge the incision, and the endotracheal or tracheostomy tube is inserted. Suctioning the trachea immediately before or after insertion of the tube may be needed to clear thick secretions or blood. The tube is then connected to a supplemental oxygen source.
5. Owing to the potential for chondritis of the cricoid cartilage and subsequent development of subglottic stenosis, a cricothyrotomy should be converted to a tracheostomy in the operating room by a trained surgeon after the patient's condition has been stabilized.

Under less emergent circumstances, when appropriate equipment and personnel are available, an urgent tracheotomy can be performed in the emergency department or intensive care unit.

Tracheostomy

Materials

Tracheostomy tray
Variety of pediatric-sized tracheostomy tubes
Gowns, gloves, and masks for physicians
Headlight
Suction
2% lidocaine with epinephrine
Bovie electrocautery if available

Procedure

1. The child is positioned supine with the shoulders elevated and the neck hyperextended. An assistant (or respiratory therapist or anesthesiologist) assists the child's ventilation with bag and mask, providing supplemental oxygen and positive pressure.

An intravenous line should also be in place for administration of muscle relaxants if they are urgently needed.

2. The neck is prepared with povidone-iodine and infiltrated with the lidocaine/epinephrine along a horizontal skin crease approximately one fingerbreadth above the suprasternal notch.
3. A horizontal skin incision about 2 to 3 cm long is placed down to the fascial layer beneath the subcutaneous fat. If available, the Bovie electrocautery is useful in removing obstructing subcutaneous fat.
4. The pretracheal fascia is then incised, and the tracheal cartilage is exposed by blunt dissection. Stay sutures of 4–0 or 5–0 silk or polypropylene are placed in the trachea 1 to 2 mm lateral to the midline on both sides of the proposed vertical tracheal cartilage incision. These sutures help position the trachea in the operative field and ease placement of the tracheotomy incision. By applying traction to the stay sutures, the trachea is elevated into the wound, and a vertical midline incision is made through the third and fourth tracheal rings with a No. 15 scalpel.
5. The tracheal incision is quickly suctioned free of blood and thickened secretions, and an appropriately sized tracheostomy tube is inserted. After confirmation of adequate breath sounds by the anesthesiologist, the tube is secured in place with either tracheostomy ties alone or in combination with sutures placed through the tube flanges to the patient's skin. The skin incision is not sutured closed.
6. A postoperative chest radiograph is obtained to ascertain the exact location of the tube tip in relation to the carina.

Potential Complications

Pneumothorax, hemorrhage, placement of the tube into a "false passage," tracheoesophageal party wall injury, pulmonary edema, and respiratory arrest are potential complications of tracheostomy.

References

Derkay CS, Hirsch BE, et al: Posterior nasal packing—are intravenous antibiotics really necessary? *Arch Otolaryngol Head Neck Surg*, 115:439–441, 1989.

Dinsdale RC, Roland PS, et al: Catastrophic otologic injury from oral jet irrigation of the external auditory canal. *Laryngoscope*, 101:75–78, 1991.

Keller AP Jr: A study of the relationship of air pressure to myringorupture. *Laryngoscope*, 68: 2015–2029, 1958.

National Institutes of Health: *NIH Consensus Statement*, Vol 11, No 1:March 1–3, 1993.

Pride H, Schwab R: A technique for removing foreign bodies of the external auditory canal. *Pediatr Emerg Care*, 5:135–136, 1989.

Robinson AC, Hawke M: The efficacy of cerumenolytics: everything old is new again. *J Otolaryngol*, 18:263–267, 1989.

Stool SE, McConnel CS: Foreign bodies in pediatric otolaryngology. Some diagnostic and therapeutic pointers. *Clin Pediatr*, 12:113–116, 1973.

Toner JG, Mains B: Pneumatic otoscopy and tympanometry in the detection of middle ear effusion. *Clin Otolaryngol*, 15:121–123, 1990.

Wilson PS, Grocutt M, et al: Distribution of ear drops in normal ears. *J Laryngol Otol*, 105:359–361, 1991.

Section I

Renal

Chapter 41

Tests and Procedures for Evaluation of Renal Disorders

Elaine S. Kamil, Asha Moudgil,
Ragini K. Frederich, and Sudhir K. Anand

The types of tests or procedures used to evaluate renal disorders are based on the history and physical examination of the child. These may be simple tests (e.g., urinalysis and measurement of plasma creatinine concentration) or specialized tests (e.g., various nuclear imaging techniques and renal biopsy).

GLOMERULAR FILTRATION RATE

The filtration function of the kidney is best assessed by measurement of the glomerular filtration rate (GFR). The GFR is relatively low at birth (especially in the premature infant), even when it is corrected for surface area to adult values of 1.73 M^2. The GFR during the first 24 hours after birth in term infants is approximately 2 to 3.5 ml/min (15–25 ml/min/1.73 M^2). The GFR nearly doubles between 3 and 7 days. Thereafter, GFR continues to increase gradually so that by 1 to 2 years of age, the GFR corrected to 1.73 M^2 is the same as in an older child or an adult (Anand, 1991) (Table 41–1).

The GFR is determined by measuring the ability of the kidney to clear various endogenous or exogenous substances from plasma per unit time. The ideal substance for use of clearance as a measure of GFR is nontoxic, biologically inert, freely filtered by the glomeruli, and neither reabsorbed nor secreted by the tubules, whereby the rate at which it is cleared from plasma and excreted in the urine is the same at which it is filtered by the glomeruli. Inulin alone has been able to fulfill these criteria and has become the standard measure of GFR and the agent with which all other test markers for GFR are compared. The clearance of a substance (C) can be expressed by the equation

$$C = \frac{UV}{P}$$

where U is the concentration of the substance in urine, P the concentration in the plasma, and V the rate of urine flow.

Although inulin clearance testing has been the standard measure of GFR, the procedure is seldom used clinically because it is cumbersome, requiring urinary catheterization, constant infusion of inulin, and timed collections of urine and blood. Moreover, inulin analysis is not available in most clinical labora-

Table 41–1 Changes in Glomerular Filtration Rate and Serum Creatinine Concentration with Age

Age	Actual GFR (ml/min)	Corrected GFR (ml/min/1.73 m²)	Serum Creatinine (mG/dl)
Premature infants			
25–28 weeks	0.3–1.0	5–10	< 1.6
29–34 weeks	0.6–1.5	10–15	< 1.2
Full-term infants			
< 24 hours	2–4	15–30	0.6–1.0
3 days–2 weeks	4–8	30–50	0.5–0.6
1–2 months	10–12	60–70	0.4–0.5
3–4 months	18–20	70–80	0.3–0.4
6 months–1 year	25–30	80–100	0.3–0.5
Children			
1–2 years	30–35	90–110	0.4–0.5
2–6 years	40–60	120 ± 20	0.4–0.6
6–12 years	60–90	125 ± 20	0.5–0.8
> 12 years (male)	90–150	130 ± 20	0.6–1.4
> 12 years (female)	90–140	120 ± 20	0.6–1.1

GFR, glomerular filtration rate.

tories. Newer techniques that obviate the need for constant infusion or timed urine collections include plasma disappearance rates of chromium ^{51}Cr edetic acid, iodine ^{125}I iothalamate, and technetium ^{99m}Tc diethylenetriamine pentaacetic acid (DTPA) (Chantler and Barrett, 1972; Israelit et al, 1973; Perrone et al, 1990; Piepez et al, 1978). The disappearance of Tc-DTPA is measured by external counting over the kidneys and bladder; an added advantage of this technique is measuring of differential renal function and renal imaging. Although these techniques are reproducible and generally considered to be reliable measures of GFR, some authors have disputed their validity (Olind et al, 1985). Moreover, these tests are seldom used clinically in children (unless for renal imaging) because they are not bedside tests and there is concern about radiation exposure (even though the dose is generally limited), especially if repeated testing for follow-up is necessary. Measurements of serum creatinine concentration are sufficient for clinical evaluation of glomerular filtration, and if necessary, measurements of creatinine clearance can be added.

PLASMA CREATININE

Plasma creatinine (P_{Cr}) continues to be the most useful and simple laboratory measure for assessment of renal function (Morgan et al, 1978; Schwartz et al, 1987). Plasma creatinine values are based on GFR and muscle mass and in normal children vary with the age and build of the child (Schwartz et al, 1987) (see Table 41–1; Fig. 41–1). The values of plasma creatinine at birth reflect those of maternal plasma creatinine and may be normal even in newborns with renal agenesis. In term infants, mean plasma creatinine concentration is ap-

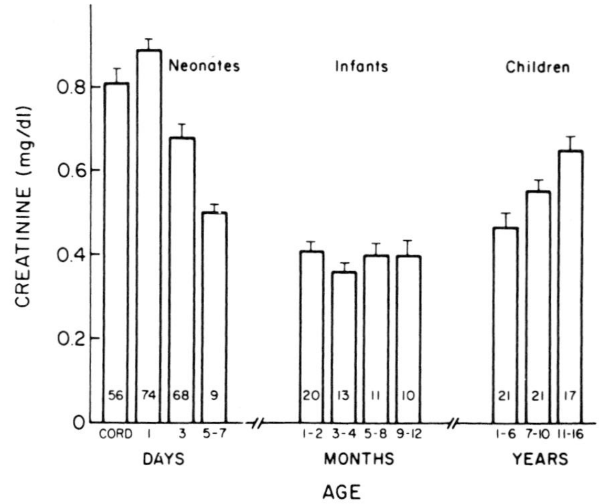

Figure 41–1 Values of serum creatinine in full-term neonates, infants, and children. (From Schwartz GJ, Feld LG, Langford DJ: A simple estimate of glomerular filtration rate in full-term infants during the first year of life. *J Pediatr,* 104:849, 1984.)

proximately 0.8 mg/dl at birth, rises to 0.9 mg at day 1, and then gradually decreases to 0.5 mg by 1 week of age. Thereafter, as GFR further increases, plasma creatinine values decrease to 0.35 mg/dl by 3 to 6 months of age. After 1 year of age, GFR remains fairly stable; however, plasma creatinine concentration gradually rises because of increasing muscle mass. Age-appropriate serum creatinine values should be used in evaluating renal function. Chemistry laboratories in most hospitals often quote normal serum creatinine values to be 0.6 to 1.4 mg/dl (adult values). However, a serum creatinine value of 0.8 mg/dl in a 1-year-old infant (with age-appropriate normal serum creatinine concentration of 0.4 mg/dl) indicates loss of 50% of kidney function. Schwartz et al (1987) have described simple estimates of GFR based on plasma creatinine concentration, body length, and age of the patient, which generally correlate with values measured by creatinine clearance (Table 41–2). However, others have questioned the validity of estimated GFR based on plasma creatinine concentration (Davies et al, 1982; Levey et al, 1988).

Although serum creatinine values gradually change with age, in any given child, serum creatinine values and daily production of creatinine do not vary from day to day. Therefore, serial measurements of plasma creatinine concentration generally provide a reasonable estimate of changes in renal function; a sudden increase in plasma creatinine concentration signifies a substantial decrease in GFR and a need for appropriate evaluation of the patient. Ketones and cephalosporin antibiotics (Levey et al, 1988; Schwartz et al, 1987) may falsely increase serum creatinine values as measured by modified Jaffé's reaction (used in autoanalyzers in most clinical laboratories).

Table 41–2 Estimation of Glomerular Filtration Rate from Serum Creatinine Values

Age	GFR Estimate
0 to 1 year (prematurely born infants)	$\frac{0.33 \times \text{length (cm)}}{P_{Cr}}$
0 to 1 year (term infants)	$\frac{0.45 \times \text{length (cm)}}{P_{Cr}}$
2 to 12 years (both sexes)	$\frac{0.55 \times \text{length (cm)}}{P_{Cr}}$
13 to 21 years (females)	$\frac{0.55 \times \text{length (cm)}}{P_{Cr}}$
13 to 21 years (males)	$\frac{0.70 \times \text{length (cm)}}{P_{Cr}}$

GFR, glomerular filtration rate; P_{Cr}, plasma creatinine.
Adapted from data of Schwartz GJ, Brion LP, Spitzer A: The use of plasma creatinine for estimating glomerular filtration rate in infants, children and adolescents. *Pediatr Clin North Am*, 34:571–590, 1987.

UREA NITROGEN

Blood urea nitrogen (BUN) concentration is another measure commonly used to assess renal function. However, values of BUN depend on several factors, including urine flow rate, state of hydration, protein intake, gastrointestinal blood loss, and tissue catabolism. Therefore, BUN measurement is much less reliable for assessment of renal function than is plasma creatinine concentration. BUN values in children usually vary between 5 and 15 mg/dl. In adults, the plasma creatinine/BUN ratio is usually 1:10, and ratios greater than 1:10 often indicate prerenal azotemia. In normal infants and children, the plasma creatinine/BUN ratio is often greater than 1:25, and only values exceeding that suggest prerenal azotemia.

CREATININE CLEARANCE

Creatinine clearance (C_{Cr}) is measured by collecting urine for a timed interval, preferably 24 hours (sometimes 12 hours or shorter intervals may be adequate) and measuring urinary creatinine (U_{Cr}) and plasma creatinine (P_{Cr}). Creatinine clearance is then calculated by the equation

$$C_{Cr} = \frac{U_{Cr}}{P_{Cr}} \times \frac{V}{1440} \times \frac{1.73\ m^2}{SA}$$

where V is the total 24-hour urine volume in milliliters and V divided by 1440 reflects per minute urine volume, SA represents surface area of the child, and 1.73 m^2 reflects adult surface area. Creatinine clearance values in normal children are generally close to GFR values measured by inulin clearance (Schwartz et al, 1987). However, in renal failure, C_{Cr} may overestimate GFR because a considerable proportion of creatinine may be secreted by renal tubules (Levey et al, 1988; Schwartz et al, 1987). Moreover, as would be apparent from the equation, accurate 24-hour collection of urine forms the basis of correct C_{Cr} measurements; in young children, this is often difficult to accomplish. Therefore, many pediatric nephrologists use serial measurements of plasma creatinine concentration as the best measure to observe the filtration function of the kidney.

URINE VOLUME

Excretion of specific urine volumes per unit time (e.g., 2 ml/kg/h) is often used as a reflection of adequate renal perfusion and function, especially in sick infants and young children admitted to intensive care units. However, in any normal person, a particular urine volume is a reflection of the fluid intake; the greater the fluid intake, the greater the urine output, and vice versa. A normal kidney can maintain homeostasis with wide variations in daily fluid intake averaging from half to 10 times the daily recommended amounts. It does so by appropriately concentrating or diluting the urine, respectively. Moreover, the so-called optimal urine volumes per unit time vary in different age groups. For an infant weighing less than 10 kg and ingesting 100 to 120 ml fluid per kilogram body weight per 24 hours, the expected urine output is 2 to 3 ml/kg/h; for a teen-ager weighing 70 kg and ingesting 2500 ml/24 h, the expected urine output is only 1 ml/kg/h (1440 ml/24 h). Urine volumes less than 30% of expected volumes for age in the presence of an adequate fluid intake suggest oliguria and require further evaluation of the patient. Excessive urine output, on the other hand, points to an inadvertent excess fluid administration, inability of the kidney to concentrate (e.g., diabetes insipidus, diuretic use, cystic kidneys), or osmotic diuresis (diabetes mellitus).

Although reduced urine output is often used as a marker for acute renal failure (ARF), 25% to 30% of children with ARF have normal urine output (nonoliguric ARF). Increasing serum creatinine concentration is a better marker for ARF than is urine volume.

URINE ELECTROLYTES AND FRACTIONAL EXCRETION OF SODIUM

Random (spot) urinary electrolyte values for sodium, potassium, and chloride are variable and depend on their daily intake and the concentration of the urine; hence, overall, they are of limited value. However, random urinary electrolyte measurement in the context of a patient with hyponatremia or hypernatremia, hypochloremia or hyperchloremia, and hypokalemia or hyperkalemia may be considerably useful; for example, spot urinary sodium values of 50 mEq/L when the serum sodium concentration is 125 mEq reflect sodium wasting and require further evaluation.

Fractional excretion of sodium (FE_{Na}) reflects the percentage of sodium excreted compared with the sodium filtered and is determined by measuring spot urinary and plasma sodium and creatinine concentrations. The value for FE_{Na} is calculated by the following equation:

$$FE_{Na} = \frac{U_{Na} \times P_{Cr}}{U_{Cr} \times P_{Na}} \times 100$$

In most children (older than 1 year) and adults with average sodium intake, FE_{Na} values are less than 1%. In dehydration and prerenal renal failure, values are also less than 1%; however, in intrinsic ARF and acute tubule necrosis, values usually exceed 3%. Caution must be used in interpreting FE_{Na} values to decide the presence of intrinsic ARF in newborn (especially premature) infants because their normal FE_{Na} may exceed 3% (Siegel and Oh, 1976). Also, in nonoliguric ARF and renal failure associated with acute glomerulonephritis, FE_{Na} values are often less than 3% and sometimes even less than 1%.

IMAGING OF THE GENITOURINARY TRACT IN CHILDREN

The last decade has seen tremendous advances in the imaging of the genitourinary tract. Not only can we obtain more detailed clinical information concerning the anatomy of the internal organs, but we are able to obtain that information with a lower radiation dose and through less invasive techniques than were used even a decade ago. With the advances in nuclear medicine technology, we are also able to gain accurate information concerning renal function and blood flow. The clinician needs to become adept at ordering the fewest number of indicated examinations to delineate the patient's problem. Figure 41–2 outlines a schema for diagnostic imaging in a child with a renal disorder.

Renal Ultrasonography

Ultrasonography is the most convenient, least invasive examination for assessment of renal anatomy. Because the machines are portable, bedside examinations can be provided even in

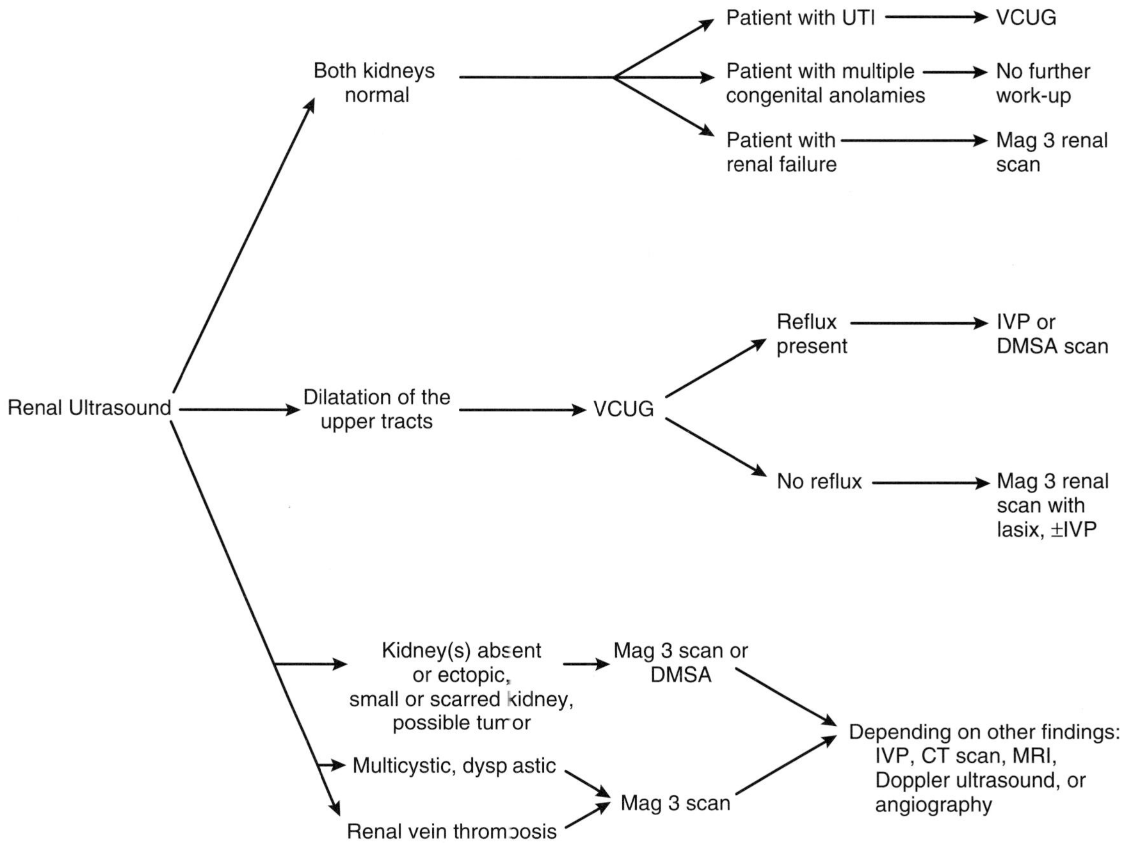

Figure 41–2 Schema for diagnostic imaging in a child with a renal mass or other renal disorder.

a critically ill patient in an intensive care unit. However, ultrasonography is operator dependent; the accuracy of interpretation depends on the skill and experience of the ultrasonographer. It is also important to have the studies performed in a center skilled in examining infants and small children because the technician must obtain the cooperation of the child, and the radiologist must be familiar with the normal variants seen in infants and small children (fetal lobulation, hypoechoic renal pyramids, differing range of renal size with growth). It is also important that the bladder be examined when a renal ultrasound study is ordered.

Renal ultrasonography is the examination of choice for screening renal anatomy. The examination can detect renal size, shape, location, and texture (e.g., "echogenicity"). When it is used in conjunction with a Doppler examination, blood flow in the main renal arteries and veins can be assessed. However, renal ultrasonography does not give information on renal function. In many instances, renal ultrasonography is the only renal imaging study indicated. When the clinician is faced with a patient with renal failure, the ultrasound examination can be used to rule out an obstruction or major malformation of the kidneys. Renal ultrasonography is ordered as the first diagnostic imaging study in the following clinical situations: hematuria (gross or microscopic), renal or abdominal mass, renal insufficiency, ARF, suspicion of abnormal renal anatomy (e.g., a child with multiple congenital abnormalities), nephrocalcinosis, nephrolithiasis, and screening for polycystic kidney disease. The presence of small, echogenic kidneys in a patient who newly presents with renal insufficiency indicates that the disease process has been prolonged and is not reversible. Ultrasonography can usually delineate the level of obstruction in the urinary tract. Patients with ureteropelvic junction obstruction show dilatation of the renal pelvis and intrarenal collecting system; ureterovesical junction obstruction demonstrates ureteral dilatation down to the level of the bladder in addition to these findings. Renal ultrasound examination is also valuable in observing patients with certain renal diseases. Renal growth can be serially monitored in children with vesicoureteral reflux, and hydronephrosis can also be serially monitored in patients with obstructive uropathies.

Voiding Cystourethrogram

When it is necessary to evaluate the urinary bladder or urethra, the voiding cystourethrogram (VCUG) is the best imaging study to order. This study provides radiographic images of the shape and size of the bladder, indicates the thickness of the bladder wall, gives some indication of bladder function, visualizes the urethra, and detects the presence of urethral abnormalities. It is always ordered in boys after a first urinary tract infection, in girls younger than 4 years with a first urinary tract infection, in girls who have had pyelonephritis, and in girls older than 4 years who have had recurrent urinary tract infections.

The VCUG is an important test to detect vesicoureteral reflux in children with urinary tract infection and to detect posterior urethral valves in boys. The study should be performed in a center that is skilled at catheterizing children. The study requires sterile urethral catheterization with a small feeding tube in an infant or a small urethral catheter in an older child. Sterile contrast material is infused by gravity from a bag held above the child until the material stops dripping or the bladder starts to leak. Fluoroscopy should be used to examine the bladder when it is full and during and after voiding. The fluoroscopic examination is critical for detecting and grading reflux, and it is critical that the posterior urethra be visualized in boys. VCUGs are also indicated in young siblings of children with vesicoureteral reflux (Buonomo et al, 1993; Jerkins and Noe, 1982; Van den Abbeele et al, 1987). The VCUG is also helpful in the evaluation of children with a suspected neurogenic bladder.

Nuclear Medicine Imaging Studies

Recent advances in nuclear medicine technology have reduced the use of conventional radiographic images, such as intravenous pyelography (IVP). Radionuclide imaging allows assessment of renal pathophysiological processes, generally with use of a dose of radiation that is a fraction of that required for conventional radiographic techniques. Nuclear medicine renal studies are particularly useful in assessing children with congenital malformations of the urinary tract, such as hydronephrosis. Clinicians should become familiar with the tracers used for nuclear medicine imaging and the studies that are most helpful for specific clinical indications. In general, dynamic scans assess renal blood flow and function (GFR); static scans help assess functional renal mass.

Dynamic scans measure several parameters of renal function. Results from dynamic scans are obtained after the intravenous injection of the radionuclide and are recorded as graphs of individual renal function and as pictures of the genitourinary system generated by the counts extracted by the kidneys that are recorded by the gamma camera (see Fig. 41–2). The parameters that are measured are the flow phase, which measures blood flow into the renal vasculature; the uptake phase, which measures the rate of uptake of the tracers by the kidneys; the transit time, which measures the time taken for the tracer to pass through the collecting system; and the excretory phase, which is the rate at which the tracer leaves the kidney (Gordon, 1987).

The two most commonly ordered dynamic scans are the ^{99m}Tc DTPA scan and the ^{99m}Tc mercaptotriacetylglycine (MAG_3) scan. Both of these tracers are labeled with ^{99m}Tc, which emits gamma radiation that is counted by the camera. ^{99m}Tc-labeled agents have advantages over radiolabeled iodine agents, including easy availability, short half-life, and reasonable cost. Both DTPA and MAG_3 scans can be used to provide an accurate assessment of renal blood flow. DTPA is eliminated rapidly from the body by glomerular filtration and can be used to determine GFR by measuring blood or urine samples for radioactivity at timed intervals after the injection of the tracer. MAG_3 measures tubule clearance; it is extracted from the blood by the renal tubule cells in a manner similar to Hippuran (Nizsche et al, 1993). The DTPA and MAG_3 renal scans are useful in assessing renal blood flow in a patient with suspected renal artery stenosis or renal artery thrombosis or embolism. Renal artery stenosis shows a delayed uptake of tracer and quantitatively less uptake of tracer in the affected kidney. Patients with hydronephrosis are best evaluated by the MAG_3 renal scan. The MAG_3 study shows a higher contrast between the urinary tract and the background than does the DTPA study (Nizsche et al, 1993). The MAG_3 study in patients with hydronephrosis should show normal blood flow, perhaps some decrease in uptake or transit, but a markedly prolonged excretory phase. The hang-up of tracer material can be clearly seen on the graph and on the pictures of the kidneys generated by the gamma counter. When hydronephrosis is seen, a dose of furosemide is given intravenously. If the collecting system is obstructed, there is continued hang-up of the contrast material with slow washout. If the collecting system is dilated but not obstructed, the tracer washes out promptly after the furosemide is given.

The most widely used static scan is the dimercaptosuccinic acid (DMSA) scan. The DMSA is injected intravenously and binds slowly to the proximal straight and convoluted tubules. The tracer is held in the kidney for several hours; therefore, the radiation dose from DMSA is greater than that experienced from a DTPA or MAG_3 scan. As a cortical imaging agent, DMSA indicates renal mass and is the most sensitive renal imaging study to show renal scarring. The DMSA images can be analyzed by single-photon emission computed tomography to generate a three-dimensional image of each kidney that can be rotated on a computer screen, allowing the nuclear medicine physician to examine the renal cortical mass from all angles (Fig. 41–3). DMSA scans are now widely used to assess renal scarring in children who have episodes of pyelonephritis and in children with vesicoureteral reflux. During episodes of acute pyelonephritis, a high proportion of children (> 90%) show filling defects on the DMSA scan; these can be a result of permanent scarring or temporary filling defects because of localized swelling (lobar nephronia) (Jakobsson et al, 1992). The DMSA scan can also be used to assess the proportion of renal function derived from each kidney.

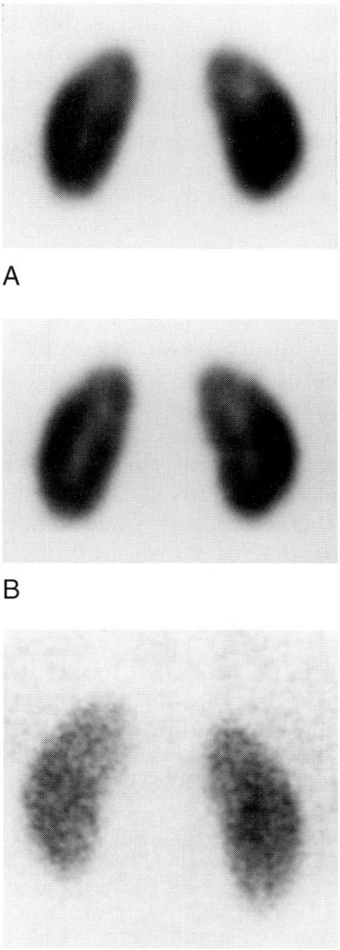

Figure 41–3 DMSA scan of a 4-year old girl with a history of recurrent, febrile urinary tract infections. **A** and **B**. Cuts done with single-photon emission computed tomography (SPECT) **C**. Planar view. Bilateral upper pole scarring is seen on the SPECT films but not easily appreciated on the planar view.

Nuclear medicine studies can also be used to evaluate children for vesicoureteral reflux. Most pediatric nephrologists and urologists use direct radioisotope cystograms to observe children who have been diagnosed as having vesicoureteral reflux by conventional VCUG. The isotope used is ^{99m}Tc pertechnetate, and it is instilled in the bladder with a urinary catheter. Images are taken during filling and voiding. The radiation exposure is a fraction of that obtained by conventional radiographic VCUG. The images obtained are not as clear as those obtained by conventional radiographic VCUG, and they cannot be used to evaluate the posterior urethra; thus, it is not recommended for children (especially boys) undergoing a first evaluation to rule out reflux. Indirect radionuclide cystography has also been used to detect vesicoureteral reflux (Gordon et al, 1990). A conventional DTPA renal scan is performed; when the upper tracts are cleared of contrast material and the remaining contrast agent is in the bladder, the child is asked to void. Images are then taken during voiding, and reflux can be detected without the need for catheterization. Indirect radionuclide cystography does require that the child be able to void on command.

Intravenous Pyelography, Computed Tomography, and Arteriography

The IVP, the renal arteriogram, and usually the computed tomographic (CT) scan require the use of intravenous or intra-arterial contrast agents. In patients with normal renal function, the uptake and excretion of these agents provide particularly good images of the renal parenchyma and collecting system. Although the contrast agents are generally well tolerated by pediatric patients, some patients are at risk for allergic reactions to the contrast material, and contrast-induced renal failure has been described in pediatric patients. CT scan and arteriography have the additional disadvantage of requiring sedation. Nevertheless, although the indications for contrast studies have narrowed in recent years, they are still important components of our diagnostic armamentarium and are the imaging study of choice in certain selected clinical situations.

The IVP was the most widely ordered examination for determination of renal anatomy and to some extent renal function. Now it is used much less frequently because ultrasonography can give accurate assessments of renal anatomy, and nuclear medicine studies provide far superior assessments of renal function. IVPs are the best examination for delineating the renal anatomy of a child with complicated urological abnormalities, such as a duplicated collecting system. They are also useful in patients with suspected nephrolithiasis, infantile polycystic kidney disease, and medullary cystic disease; a furosemide IVP may be substituted for a furosemide renal scan when more detailed anatomical information is necessary.

The CT scan with contrast enhancement is the imaging study of choice in evaluating a child for renal trauma; it not only provides excellent anatomical information on the kidney, but also provides information on the intra-abdominal organs. CT is a highly valued examination in assessing a renal or abdominal mass. Renal arteriography is an invasive procedure that demonstrates the renal arterial tree. It requires the intra-arterial injection of contrast material, and the equivalent of an IVP can also be obtained in the final stages of the arteriogram. Arteriography requires catheterization of the aorta, usually through the femoral artery, with the small risk of damage to the femoral artery or thrombosis. The procedure is done under heavy sedation. The major indication is for diagnosis of renal artery stenosis as part of the work-up of hypertension; it is the only study that can demonstrate stenosis in a branch of a renal artery. It is also helpful in planning a difficult renal surgery, such as a partial nephrectomy for a renal mass, or in evaluating renal trauma when a vascular lesion is suspected. Renal arteriography is an integral component of the procedure of renal angioplasty, whereby a renal artery stenosis is corrected by the placement and inflation of a tiny balloon in a stenotic segment of the renal artery.

In selected cases, an antegrade or retrograde pyelogram might be indicated. The antegrade pyelogram is obtained by puncturing the renal pelvis with a needle, inserting a catheter, and injecting contrast material through the catheter. It is performed in cases of hydronephrosis when the level of the obstruction cannot be ascertained by other radiographic means. The retrograde pyelogram is performed by catheterizing the ureters during a cystoscopic procedure and injecting contrast material directly into the ureter. It was formerly widely used to rule out obstruction in anuric patients but is rarely used now because the necessary clinical information can be obtained less invasively by other imaging techniques.

Magnetic Resonance Imaging

Magnetic resonance imaging (MRI) offers few advantages over CT scanning in pediatric genitourinary radiology. It is most helpful in evaluating children with retroperitoneal masses such as Wilms' tumor; MRI can often accurately demonstrate the tumor's origin, spread to other organs, and invasion of the inferior vena cava (Bisset et al, 1991). Magnetic resonance angiography is used in adults to demonstrate renal artery stenosis. This application may eventually be helpful as well in children.

RENAL BIOPSY IN CHILDREN

Percutaneous renal biopsy is accepted as a safe and practical procedure in children that enables the physician to evaluate most histopathological processes in the kidney for the purposes of diagnosis, prognosis, and evaluation of response to treatment. Its value depends on the type of disease, the adequacy and quality of preparation of the sample, and the availability of a competent pathologist. It is most useful in diseases that diffusely affect the kidney, such as most glomerulopathies, and less useful in focal disease processes, such as tumors or pyelonephritis.

Indications

Differences of opinion exist regarding indications for renal biopsy (Table 41–3); however,

Table 41-3 Indications for Renal Biopsy

Hematuria

Primary acute nephritic syndrome (hematuria, proteinuria, edema, hypertension)
- When rapidly progressive glomerulonephritis is suspected
- When impaired renal function, hypertension, and low complement (C3) persist beyond a few weeks

Systemic disorders associated with features of acute nephritis or vasculitis
- Systemic lupus erythematosus with abnormal urinalysis or impaired function
- Suspected Wegener's granulomatosis, polyarteritis nodosa with evidence of renal involvement
- Severe Henoch-Schönlein purpura

Immunoglobulin nephropathy (Berger's disease)
- With impaired renal function
- With nephrotic syndrome

Isolated gross or microscopic hematuria
- Suspected familial nephritis (Alport's syndrome)
- Parental anxiety

Proteinuria

Nephrotic syndrome
- Onset in first year or after 12 years
- Resistance to a 6- to 8-week course of steroids
- Candidate for cytotoxic drugs for treatment of the steroid-dependent or frequently relapsing patient
- Unusual clinical/laboratory features like hypertension, hypocomplementemia, gross hematuria, or persistent abnormal renal function

Asymptomatic (nonorthostatic) persistent proteinuria more than 1000 mg/24 h
- Normal renal function, if diagnosis is still uncertain after 6 months
- Impaired renal function at presentation, if diagnosis is uncertain or in the presence of microscopic hematuria or hypertension

Acute Renal Failure

When cause for renal failure is unknown
Rapidly progressive glomerulonephritis
Severe oligoanuria lasting for more than 2–3 weeks
In some cases of suspected acute interstitial nephritis
Presence of extrarenal manifestations of a diffuse renal disease

Chronic Renal Failure

If the kidney is only moderately decreased in size and the diagnosis is uncertain (not indicated if the kidney is small and shrunken)
Transplantation
Suspected allograft rejection or cyclosporine toxic effects
Recurrence of original disease
If cause is uncertain for reduced renal function

in each case, benefits to the patient must outweigh the risks involved.

Contraindications

Absolute contraindications to percutaneous biopsy occur in few circumstances. In cases of bleeding diathesis or of children receiving anticoagulant therapy, biopsy should be either postponed (by 10 days if the patient is receiving heparin) or performed after temporary correction of the bleeding disorder by appropriate factors and on-hand availability of washed red blood cells for transfusion if it becomes necessary. Open-biopsy techniques using a cup biopsy forceps have been reported to be safe in patients with clotting disorders. When indicated, open biopsy should be done in patients with marked hydronephrosis, horseshoe kidney and other disorders of fusion, renal cystic diseases, and end-stage renal disease with contracted kidneys. A patient with a solitary kidney is considered by most an absolute contraindication; however, some think that in the hands of an experienced physician, needle biopsy carries less overall risk than open biopsy.

Severe azotemia and hypertension can increase the risk of bleeding and formation of an arteriovenous fistula; therefore, hypertension needs to be controlled before biopsy. Lack of cooperation is considered a relative contraindication, especially in young children. However, with good sedation, reassurance, and technical skills, the biopsy may be performed with as much success as in older children and adults.

Evaluation and Preparation of the Patient

A thorough medical history with special stress on bleeding diathesis must be obtained. A complete physical examination, including blood pressure assessment, must be performed to rule out local and systemic signs of infection, skeletal disorders, or skin disorders that could preclude needle penetration. Routine laboratory studies should include complete blood and platelet counts, prothrombin time, partial thromboplastin time, and typing and crossmatching of a blood specimen in case transfusion is required. A baseline urinalysis should be obtained for evaluation of hematuria after biopsy.

The indications, possible value, and complications of the biopsy and an explanation of the procedure must be discussed in detail with the patient and the parents. This usually relieves anxiety in both the older child and the parents. In an older child, if the procedure is planned with use of local anesthesia that requires the patient's cooperation, the child should be trained to hold his or her breath for an adequate period of time to allow the biopsy to be performed.

The child is usually admitted on the day of the procedure; nothing is given by mouth for 8 hours for older children and 4 hours for infants. Sedation is given 30 to 60 minutes before the procedure: meperidine, diazepam, chlorpromazine, and promethazine are useful. In younger children, the procedure is performed with deep sedation, and it is strongly recommended that a pediatric anesthetist be present.

Renal Localization

Accurate localization is extremely important for the success of the biopsy. The lower pole of the right kidney is considered the preferred location for biopsy because of its distance from the major blood vessels, neighboring organs, and renal calyces. Ultrasonography, IVP, fluoroscopy, and radioisotopic scans have all been used successfully for renal localization. In a comparative study in adults, the radiation dose was calculated to be 4.4 cGy for pyelography, 3 cGy for fluoroscopy (90 seconds), and 0.34 cGy for radionuclide scan. Regardless of the technique used, the biopsy is successful in more than 95% of the children, and the complication rates are comparable. However, because of its relative simplicity, lack of exposure to radiation or contrast material, and nondependence on the level of renal dysfunction, ultrasonography is considered the method of choice (Chan et al, 1983) and is the method discussed in this chapter.

Localization by ultrasonography

The patient is placed in the prone position with a sandbag or rolled sheet placed under the upper abdomen and lower ribs to fix the kidneys to the posterior abdominal wall and thereby bring them closer to the skin. Then, by use of the ultrasound scanner with a 2.25-MHz transducer (real-time ultrasonography is found to be most useful), both kidneys are localized and scanned. The right lower pole is usually selected on the longitudinal scan and marked, and its depth and angle of entry of the needle are measured. It is advisable to make all measurements during the same phase of respiration. A special biopsy transducer that allows insertion of the biopsy needle through a fenestration in the center of the transducer crystal can be used for needle insertion under direct vision. In this case, the biopsy field is sterilized before sonography; a sterile transducer and sterile mineral oil are used.

Percutaneous Renal Biopsy Technique

The marked-out site for the biopsy is cleaned and draped with use of an aseptic technique. The biopsy site usually falls in the angle between the twelfth rib and the lateral margin of the sacrospinal muscle. At the area localized, the skin and subcutaneous tissue are infiltrated with a local anesthetic, 1% to 2% lidocaine. This is often the most uncomfortable part of the procedure, and additional sedation may be necessary.

The location and depth of the kidney are then determined by use of an exploring needle, usually a long No. 22 spinal needle that is inserted slightly cephalad and at an angle of 15 to 20 degrees. The needle is advanced a few millimeters with each breath to prevent laceration of the kidney. Occasionally, an experienced operator can feel a distinct "pop" when the renal capsule is entered. The characteristic swinging arc of the exploring needle with each breath indicates that the needle has reached the kidney capsule. The trocar of the needle is then removed, and the needle is slowly withdrawn as a small amount of local anesthetic is injected along the needle track and the depth measured. It is important that the kidney be located with reasonable certainty before insertion of the biopsy needle.

A number of biopsy needles have been used in children, including the Franklin modification of the Vim-Silverman needle (Metcoff, 1970), the disposable Tru-Cut needle modified for pediatric patients, and the Biopty System with a fine-caliber (18-gauge and 10 cm long) needle with an automatic firing device. A small skin incision is made with a No. 11 scalpel blade, and the biopsy needle is inserted along the anesthetized track to the depth measured by the exploring needle until the tip just penetrates the capsule. Depending on the type of needle being used, the subsequent steps of the procedure differ. With the modified Vim-Silverman needle, the trocar is removed, and after the next expiration, the cutting prongs are inserted to their full depth. During the next expiratory pause, the needle shaft is smoothly and quickly advanced over the prongs, and then the entire instrument is removed in one rapid movement.

When the Biopty System is used, once the tip of the needle has penetrated the kidney capsule, the automatic firing device is triggered to obtain a thin core of tissue. This particular device is highly recommended, especially in children, because the technique is easy and rapid, renal trauma is limited, and the tissue sample is usually adequate. Microscopic examination of the tissue is done by a pathologist at the procedure site to ensure an adequate number of glomeruli. Two biopsy cores are usually required for the different microscopic studies. Multiple attempts to puncture the kidney must be avoided, and if one fails after three to four attempts, it is usually wise to observe the patient for 24 hours and try again the following day or at a later date.

Postprocedure Management

A pressure dressing is placed over the biopsy site, and the child is asked to remain supine in bed for 12 to 18 hours. If the child received heavy sedation for the procedure, the child is monitored in a postoperative observation area every 15 minutes for 1 hour and then every 30 minutes for 2 hours. If the patient remains stable, the vital signs are checked less frequently. The abdomen must be examined regularly and the flanks auscultated for an arteriovenous fistula. All urine should be collected and aliquots racked for evaluation of hematuria. Pain, tachycardia, hypotension, gross hematuria, and fever must be reported to the physician. A hemoglobin and hematocrit level is obtained 4 to 6 hours after the procedure and then again before discharge. Oral intake of fluids may start as soon as the child is awake, and some physicians encourage diuresis with oral fluids to prevent obstruction with clots.

The child may be discharged the following day provided that the child's condition is stable. The patient is asked to avoid contact sports and other vigorous activity for 2 weeks but may go back to school immediately.

Complications

Percutaneous renal biopsy is a safe diagnostic procedure. When it is performed by an experienced operator in carefully selected patients, the usefulness of the procedure clearly outweighs the risks (Table 41–4) (Diaz-Buxo and Donadio, 1975; Wicker and Golper, 1982). In large series, the mortality rate is less than 0.1%.

Microscopic hematuria after biopsy and mild abdominal and flank pain occur in virtually all patients and should not be considered complications. The frequency of gross hematuria is 5% to 15%, but only 1% to 2% of all patients require blood transfusions. Nephrectomy is required in less than 0.05% of biopsies. Postoperative bleeding usually appears 1 to 8 hours after the biopsy; it usually responds to conservative management, such as bed rest, and subsides within 24 to 48 hours. If bleeding

Table 41–4 Complications of Percutaneous Renal Biopsy

Gross hematuria
Perirenal hematoma
Renal colic from passage of clots
Arteriovenous fistula
Severe abdominal and flank pain
Renal and perirenal infection
Accidental puncture or laceration of liver, spleen, gallbladder, pancreas, bowel, lungs, renal vessels

is associated with renal colic and clots, intravenous fluids are recommended. Perirenal hematomas are common; if follow-up ultrasound examination or CT scan is done, they are present in 85% of the cases. However, clinically important hematomas are present in only 0.2% to 0.3%. If bleeding is severe and persistent, blood transfusions are useful; an occasional patient may require surgical exploration to stop bleeding or for nephrectomy.

Rare complications include arteriovenous fistula; renal infection; inadvertent laceration of neighboring organs, such as the liver, spleen, gallbladder, pancreas, bowel, and lungs; and puncture of a major renal vessel.

Processing of Renal Tissue

The biopsy sample is examined under a dissecting microscope for adequacy. The glomeruli are identified as red blushes on the surface of the specimen. Ideally, a pathologist or a trained technician should be present at the time of biopsy to ensure adequacy and proper handling of the sample. The tissue is divided for light and electron microscopy and immunofluorescence; two tissue cores are usually needed for all three evaluations. While awaiting complete processing, the tissue should be covered by saline to prevent drying. If an insufficient sample is obtained, the nephrologist must choose the most important microscopic evaluation for that individual case.

PERITONEAL DIALYSIS

Peritoneal dialysis is the usual method for dialytic treatment of ARF in infants and children (Reznik et al, 1991). The development of intermittent peritoneal dialysis, continuous cyclic peritoneal dialysis, and continuous ambulatory peritoneal dialysis during the past 15 years or so has led to the application of these techniques in the care of children with end-stage renal disease (Fine, 1982). This text confines the use of peritoneal dialysis mainly to the management of ARF.

Peritoneal dialysis involves removal or addition of blood solutes in renal failure by allowing blood to equilibrate with the dialysis fluid (infused into the peritoneal cavity) across the peritoneum, which is a semipermeable membrane. Transperitoneal movement of water and solutes takes place by both diffusion and convection. The net transfer of a solute is determined by its transmembrane concentration gradient; molecular weight; charge characteristics; and membrane pore size, which may vary in different individuals. The amount of water crossing the peritoneum (ultrafiltration) is determined by the magnitude of the transmembrane osmotic gradient generated by glucose in the dialysis fluid. In addition, the flux of water and solutes is dependent on the blood flow to the peritoneum and to some extent on the rate and amount of dialysate flow to the peritoneum (Khanna and Nolph, 1989).

Indications for Acute Dialysis

Acute peritoneal dialysis is safe and effective and has been done successfully in premature neonates weighing less than 1000 g (Steele et al, 1987). It is preferred to hemodialysis because it is technically easier to perform; provides a slower, gentler, and smoother correction of uremia; and avoids rapid changes in osmolality.

The indications for dialysis in ARF are summarized in Table 41–5. However, these indications are not absolute and should be viewed as guidelines. The decision to initiate dialysis in a child must be individualized, depending on the overall clinical condition of the child, the anticipated course of ARF, and the rapidity with which metabolic changes are occurring. For example, if a child with oligoanuria and some fluid overload has severe anemia and acidosis, blood transfusion or repeated administration of bicarbonate solutions may cause worsening fluid overload and pulmonary edema. It may be safer to dialyze the child under such circumstances even though the listed indications may not yet exist. An early institution of dialysis is

Table 41–5 Indications for Dialysis in Acute Renal Failure

Fluid overload with congestive heart failure, pulmonary edema, or hypertension
Uncontrolled hyperkalemia (serum potassium > 6.5 mEq/L), despite use of ion exchange resins, especially if symptomatic
Severe metabolic acidosis
Marked hyponatremia (serum sodium < 120 mEq/L), particularly if symptomatic
Increasing blood urea nitrogen and creatinine concentrations in the presence of oligoanuria or blood urea nitrogen and creatinine concentrations 8 to 10 times above age-related normal
Symptomatic uremia, such as neurobehavioral dysfunction, gastrointestinal bleeding, and pericarditis

usually associated with a better outcome; therefore, the decision to dialyze should not be unnecessarily delayed. Peritoneal dialysis, although less effective than hemodialysis, is sometimes used to treat accidental poisonings and drug overdose in young children in whom obtaining an adequate vascular access is difficult. Contraindications to peritoneal dialysis include acute abdominal conditions (severe ileus, gut perforation, severe peritoneal bleeding), recent abdominal surgery, and lack of adequate peritoneal surface because of adhesions and inflammation.

Procedure

TYPE OF CATHETER: Two types of peritoneal dialysis catheters are available: acute and chronic. Acute catheters are designed for short-term use (preferably less than 3 days); are straight, relatively rigid, and made of nylon, polyethylene, or polyurethane; and have numerous side holes in the terminal intraperitoneal portion. Some acute catheters are advanced into the abdomen with a pointed stylet inside (e.g., Trocath); others have a pointed tip and can be introduced in the abdomen by threading over a guidewire (e.g., Cook catheter) (Nakanishi et al, 1984). We prefer the latter because of the relative ease of introduction, the lesser risk of bleeding and bowel perforation, and ease of replacement; in case of catheter blockage, a new catheter can be introduced over the guidewire through the same incision. Because there is no barrier to bacterial migration in acute catheters and they are relatively rigid, there is a higher risk of peritonitis. Therefore, some centers prefer to use chronic catheters (Tenckhoff catheters) for acute dialysis if dialysis is anticipated for more than 3 days. However, most chronic catheters require surgical placement, so the decision to use this type of catheter must be individualized on the basis of the clinical condition of the child.

CATHETER PLACEMENT: Acute peritoneal dialysis catheters are available in different sizes (5–11 French) and different lengths (5.5–20 cm). The size and length of the catheter are chosen according to the age and size of the patient. The steps of catheter introduction by the modified Seldinger guidewire technique are as follows (Nakanishi et al, 1984):

1. Catheterize the bladder.
2. Examine the abdomen and select a site for catheter insertion. The usual insertion site is in the midline below the umbilicus, one third of the distance from the umbilicus to the symphysis pubis. In premature babies, the catheter is sometimes inserted below the umbilicus, from lateral to the rectus sheath to the opposite iliac fossa, to accommodate the catheter's length. It is useful to lay the catheter on the abdomen to have an idea of catheter length in relation to the abdominal surface; on that basis, the intended site of catheter insertion is chosen.
3. Surgically prepare the skin and drape the puncture site.
4. Infiltrate local anesthetic at the puncture site and insert the introducer needle slowly into the peritoneum. Infuse 20 to 40 ml/kg of warmed dialysis solution over 5 to 10 minutes to distend the abdomen if the patient does not have ascites. The volume of the infused solution should be chosen carefully to avoid sudden respiratory embarrassment. Priming the peritoneum with the dialysis solution separates the gut from the peritoneum, minimizing gut injury during introduction of the catheter.
5. Insert the flexible end of the guidewire into the hub of the needle and advance it into the peritoneum. Remove the needle, leaving the guidewire in place.
6. Make a 4- to 5-mm skin incision with a surgical blade next to the guidewire. Introduce the catheter over the guidewire and, by holding the catheter near its tip with a firm twisting motion, advance it into the peritoneal cavity and position it into one of the iliac fossae. If necessary, predilate the track with the supplied dilator.
7. Remove the guidewire.
8. Attach the connecting tube assembly to the peritoneal catheter and the dialysate delivery tubing to the connecting tube and start infusing dialysate. The dialysis fluid should flow in a continuous stream. If the inflow is poor, the tubing may be kinked or the catheter is not positioned properly in the peritoneum. Similarly, check for outflow, which should be in a continuous stream. If inflow is good and outflow is poor, reposition the catheter. If outflow remains poor, it is probably due to wrapping of omentum around the lateral holes of the catheter, in which case the catheter will have to be removed and a new catheter introduced.
9. Treat the area with a povidone-iodine ointment.
10. Secure the retention disk to the catheter at

the skin level by tightening the pull tie positioned on its neck, and secure it to the abdominal wall with a suture.

If the dialysis fluid is blood stained, it is preferable to run one or two test cycles using a small volume of exchange and no dwell time (time dialysate is left in the peritoneum) to wash off the blood before the catheter is secured. It helps to prevent catheter blockage.

DIALYSIS PRESCRIPTION: The acute dialysis prescription should specify volume of exchange, dialysis flow rate, concentration of glucose and electrolytes in the dialysate, method of exchange (manual or automatically cycled), and duration of dialysis. The volume of the dialysis fluid used in each cycle varies between 30 and 50 ml/kg, depending on the respiratory status and degree of discomfort experienced by the patient. It should generally not exceed 2 L in an adult-sized adolescent. The choice of dialysis solution depends on the degree of hypervolemia present. In a euvolemic patient, 1.5% dextrose-containing dialysis solution is used. On the other hand, in a patient with gross fluid overload and pulmonary edema, 3.0% to 4.5% dextrose dialysate may be used until the patient becomes euvolemic. The electrolyte concentration in the commercially available dialysis solutions resembles extracellular fluid. Sodium concentration varies between 132 and 145 mEq/L, and lactate concentration ranges between 35 and 40 mEq/L. Calcium concentration varies between 3.0 and 3.5 mEq/L, and magnesium concentration ranges between 0.5 and 1.5 mEq/L. In patients with severe hypoxia and lactic acidosis and in patients with liver failure, lactate cannot be metabolized into bicarbonate, and use of standard dialysis solution may actually aggravate acidosis. In such a situation, bicarbonate-containing dialysis solution should be used in place of lactate. At the onset of dialysis, most patients are hyperkalemic, and no potassium is added to the dialysis solution. Once serum potassium concentration is normal, potassium in varying concentrations of 2 to 4 mEq/L is added to the dialysate. Heparin 500 to 1000 U/L may be added in the beginning and continued if there is evidence of bleeding or fibrin. Antibiotics are not routinely added to the dialysate.

The usual dwell time in ARF is 30 to 60 minutes. This is based on the fact that clearance of small molecules (e.g., water and potassium) is fastest and occurs early in the dialysis dwell time. In hypercatabolic states, a shorter dwell may be used (20–30 minutes) to quickly get rid of potassium and urea. Peritoneal exchanges are done by use of automated dialysis machines. Cyclers that can deliver small dialysate volumes are available and can be used in infants. However, if needed, manual exchanges can be done, particularly in small premature babies. The duration of each treatment generally varies between 24 and 72 hours. Dialysis should be continued until fluid and electrolyte disturbances, uremia, and acidosis are corrected. If it is thought that dialysis may be needed for a relatively longer time, one of the catheters designed for chronic use may be placed. At the end of dialysis, all the fluid is drained from the peritoneum, the catheter is removed, and the area is cleaned and dressed.

MONITORING: Close monitoring of the patient is important for successful dialysis. Acute peritoneal dialysis should be performed in an intensive care setting; the patient's vital signs should be frequently monitored; and weight should be recorded once a day or, in the case of neonates, preferably twice a day. A meticulous record of fluid balance should be maintained, including the amount of ultrafiltrate achieved. Serum electrolyte, glucose, BUN, creatinine, and blood gas levels should be frequently monitored; the frequency depends on the patient's clinical condition. Peritoneal fluid should be carefully watched for any turbidity; fluid should be sent for cell count, Gram's stain, and culture and sensitivity whenever there is a clinical suspicion of peritonitis.

COMPLICATIONS: Acute peritoneal dialysis may be associated with a number of complications, which may be catheter related or metabolic.

Pain: Pain during inflow and outflow may occur because of pressure of the catheter on the internal organs, administration of hypertonic and acidic dialysis solution, overdistention of the abdomen, entrapment of omentum in the catheter lumen, or peritonitis. Identification of the underlying cause is crucial for relief of pain.

Bleeding: Bleeding is usually minor and subsides after a few exchanges. Care must be taken to avoid injury to blood vessels during insertion of the catheter. In patients with a bleeding diathesis, transfusion of platelets and fresh-frozen plasma may be helpful. Catheter blockage due to clots is prevented by addition of heparin to the dialysate.

Dialysis Solution Leakage: Leakage around the catheter is the most troublesome complication. The risk of leakage increases with frequent catheter manipulations and is more frequently seen in patients with a lax abdominal wall. Excessive fluid infusion may aggravate leakage. The dialysis fluid may extravasate into the abdominal wall. During insertion of the catheter, one should make sure that all the drainage holes are intraperitoneal. Placing a purse-string suture around the catheter also helps to prevent leakage. If leakage persists or is excessive, the peritoneal catheter may need to be removed, the hole sutured, and a new catheter inserted at a different site.

Poor Drainage: Poor drainage may be due to entrapping of the terminal holes by the omentum, pressure on the catheter from the internal organs, blocking of the holes by fibrin or a clot, or intra-abdominal adhesions. Repositioning of the catheter and irrigation with heparinized saline may be useful. Reinsertion of the catheter may be necessary if these measures fail.

Organ Perforation: Organ perforation is uncommon and, if it occurs, is generally limited to the bowel. The risk of perforation is increased in patients with paralytic ileus, intestinal obstruction, or a history of previous intestinal surgery and intra-abdominal adhesions. It is diagnosed by the presence of fecal material in the dialysis effluent or by the onset of watery diarrhea. In addition, the patient may complain of sharp abdominal pain, and dialysis outflow may be poor. The perforation usually seals off within 24 hours after removal of the catheter, but surgical intervention may be necessary.

Pulmonary Complications: Respiratory compromise may occur in patients with different pulmonary problems owing to impairment of diaphragmatic movements. This is particularly true in premature neonates, who are often being simultaneously ventilated. In such babies, keeping the dialysis exchange volume small may be helpful. In addition, basal pneumonia, atelectasis, and pleural effusions may develop.

Peritonitis: Prolonged use of the acute peritoneal dialysis catheter is associated with a higher risk of peritonitis. It is suggested by abdominal pain and cloudy dialysis fluid containing more than 100 cells, predominantly polymorphonuclear leukocytes. Gram's stain and culture should be obtained and treatment instituted.

Metabolic Complications: Metabolic complications include hypoglycemia or hyperglycemia. Some patients, such as diabetics or sick neonates, may require insulin administration for correction of hyperglycemia. Hypernatremia may occur after excessive ultrafiltration using hypertonic glucose solution. It can be prevented by replacing half of the ultrafiltrate (excess fluid removed from the patient) with free water either intravenously or by mouth. Metabolic acidosis may worsen in sick, hypoxic neonates with poor peripheral perfusion and in patients with liver failure when lactate-containing dialysis solutions are used. In such circumstances, bicarbonate-containing dialysis solutions are preferable. Hypoproteinemia may be due to loss of protein in the dialysis fluid.

CONTINUOUS HEMOFILTRATION

Although peritoneal dialysis has generally become the treatment of choice for the therapy of ARF in children, the use of the peritoneal cavity is occasionally precluded by recent abdominal surgery or other concerns about a developing intra-abdominal problem. Hemodialysis may be technically difficult in small infants, requiring special equipment and staff to provide safe and effective treatment. Hemodialysis may also be complicated by hypotension, which could dictate early termination of the proposed hemodialysis treatment. Furthermore, many critically ill, oligoanuric children have continuous, significant fluid requirements for blood, plasma, and parenteral nutrition fluids. Because of its intermittent nature, hemodialysis runs the risk of maintaining such patients in cycles of fluid overload and relative intravascular volume depletion.

Continuous arteriovenous hemofiltration (CAVH) was developed in Germany in the late 1970s by Peter Kramer and was first licensed by the Food and Drug Administration for use in intensive care patients in the United States in early 1982. Since the mid-1980s, several reports have been published on the use of continuous hemofiltration in children as young as neonates (Lieberman et al, 1985; Ronco et al, 1986). Subsequent publications have demonstrated the feasibility of variations of the hemofiltration procedure in children. These variations include continuous arteriovenous hemohemodiafiltration (CAVHD), continuous venous hemofiltration (CVVH), continuous venovenous hemodiafiltration (CVVHD), and slow continuous ultrafiltration (SCUF).

All of these techniques are basically variations of the original concept that the fluid and metabolic imbalances that accompany renal failure can be modified by replacing an ultrafiltrate of plasma with intravenous fluids of a composition necessary to correct the patient's metabolic disturbances. These techniques have the advantage of offering the steady, relatively gentle removal of fluids, toxins, and electrolytes "around the clock" in an intensive care unit. The hemofiltration procedures, like hemodialysis, almost always require some degree of anticoagulation.

The original technique of CAVH is performed by use of a simple extracorporeal tubing system containing a hemofilter (Fig. 41–4). Blood enters the circuit from an arterial access and re-enters the body through a venous access. Ultrafiltration is accomplished in the filter as the patient's own blood pressure provides the driving force for ultrafiltration. Because there are no pumps in the blood circuit, there is no need for pressure detectors and bubble detectors in the circuit. The treatment can easily be monitored by an intensive care unit nurse. The ultrafiltrate of plasma drips from a tube in the hemofilter into a collection bag, and the rate of ultrafiltration can be controlled by gravity (e.g., by raising and lowering the level of the collection bag from the level of the patient toward the floor). Additional ports in the system allow the addition of heparin into the circuit before the blood reaches the filter (to prevent the filter from clotting) and allow the addition of intravenous fluids or total parenteral nutrition into the circuit after blood passes through the filter. Any substances of low molecular weight added before the blood reaches the filter are ultrafiltered, so total parenteral nutrition or medications should be added to the circuit after the filter or given though another line. Because the driving force for ultrafiltration is the patient's own blood pressure, the procedure is ineffective in patients with a mean arterial pressure of less than 60 mm Hg. Early problems included frequent clotting of the filter, poor or inconsistent ultrafiltration, and relatively inadequate clearance rates of uremic toxins in severely uremic or hypercatabolic patients. The addition of heparin and intravenous fluids before the blood reaches the filter helps alleviate the problem of the frequent clotting of the filter. Placing negative pressure on the ultrafiltration line by the use of a high-accuracy volumetric pump (such as an IVAC pump) helps achieve a reliable ultrafiltration rate and improve urea clearance.

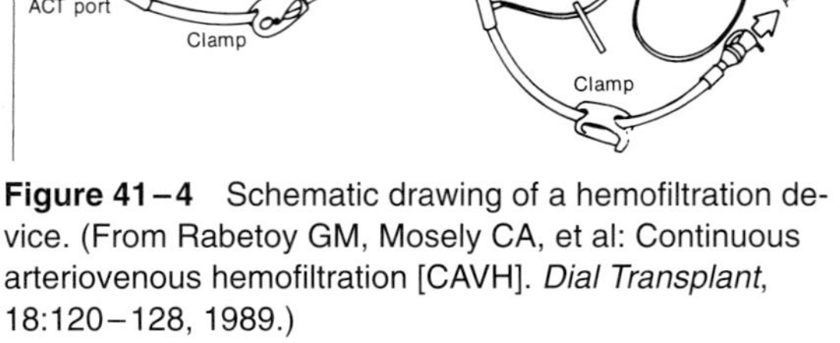

Figure 41–4 Schematic drawing of a hemofiltration device. (From Rabetoy GM, Mosely CA, et al: Continuous arteriovenous hemofiltration [CAVH]. *Dial Transplant*, 18:120–128, 1989.)

Nevertheless, clinical needs dictated the development of some improvements in the hemofiltration procedure. Because increased urea filtration was required in more hypercatabolic patients, the technique of CAVHD was developed, adding a dialysis component to the treatment. This technique uses the same setup as CAVH, but dialysate is run countercurrent through ports built into the hemofilter. Thus, the membranes carrying the patient's blood are bathed with dialysate fluid, and the uremic toxins diffuse into the dialysate. In small children, arterial cannulation can be difficult and may lead to limb ischemia. The problems of arterial access are avoided with CVVH, because access is through either a double-lumen catheter in a central vein or two catheters placed in separate large veins. Because the patient's venous blood pressure is insufficient to drive ultrafiltration, a hemodialysis machine with blood pumps, pressure monitors, and air bubble detectors is required. For larger children and adults, there is a specifically designed CVVH machine that contains the necessary pumps and safety monitors. At this writing, the machinery has not been adapted for use in the small child and infant. An additional adaptation of the hemofiltration procedure is SCUF. SCUF is performed in the same manner as CAVH with continuous, gentle fluid removal by ultrafiltration and is most helpful in those patients who mainly need fluid and not necessarily solute removal.

In summary, hemofiltration procedures provide an alternative to peritoneal dialysis or hemodialysis for the treatment of fluid overload in patients with compromised renal function or for treatment of the metabolic imbalances of uremia. The advantages of hemofiltration procedures include the capability to run continuously, the ability to remove fluid in a patient who is hemodynamically unstable provided that a mean arterial blood pressure of 60 mm Hg can be obtained, and the avoidance of invasion into the abdominal cavity. Solute clearance is adequate in most cases provided that the treatment is started early in the patient's course. Disadvantages of the procedure include the need for arterial access (in CAVH, CAVHD, and SCUF) with potential for vessel damage; the need for heparinization, which increases the risk of bleeding; and inadequate solute clearance in a severely hypercatabolic patient. The hemofiltration procedures can often be used in rotation with hemodialysis or peritoneal dialysis in patients with prolonged oliguria and changing clinical needs.

HEMODIALYSIS

In hemodialysis, blood is made to circulate extracorporeally with the help of pumps through the dialyzer, made up of a semipermeable membrane, with blood flowing on one side and dialysate flowing on the other side in the opposite direction. Blood leaves the body through the arterial limb of the catheter, circulates through the dialyzer where it equilibrates with the dialysis fluid, and returns to the patient through the venous limb. The movement of water from the blood to the dialysate (ultrafiltration) mainly depends on the hydraulic pressure differences between the blood and the dialysate. This pressure difference across the membrane is known as transmembrane pressure, which can be altered by increasing pressure in the blood compartment or by creating negative pressure on the side of dialysis flow. The movement of solutes from and to the blood depends on the difference in the concentration gradient of the solutes between blood and dialysate, the size and permeability characteristics of the dialysis membrane, and the rate of blood and dialysate flow.

Hemodialysis is much more efficient than peritoneal dialysis. Treatment duration can therefore be kept short, and the patient is free to mobilize and undergo other therapeutic or diagnostic procedures. The main disadvantages of hemodialysis are the cardiovascular effects, particularly hypotension, and the rapid changes in osmolality leading to cell edema, particularly of brain cells. It is technically more difficult to perform hemodialysis in infants and small children. Peritoneal dialysis, therefore, is considered the treatment of choice in ARF. However, at times, peritoneal dialysis may not be a feasible option, particularly in patients with abdominal catastrophes, in some patients with gross fluid overload and severe hyperkalemia, or when a relatively rapid correction is required. In such situations, hemodialysis is preferable. Hemodialysis, on occasion, may be used for treatment of acute drug intoxications and neonatal hyperammonemia. Hemodialysis is much more effective than peritoneal dialysis in these children.

Hemodialysis can be performed for either acute or chronic renal failure. For acute hemodialysis, temporary vascular catheters are placed in large veins capable of producing adequate blood flow (Uldall, 1993). Catheter placement in children should be carried out by a person well trained in such techniques. In infants and children, the vascular access sites are limited to the superior or inferior vena cava because no other veins are capable of providing adequate blood flow. The superior vena cava is the recommended site for short-term dialysis and can be approached through either the subclavian or the internal jugular vein. The inferior vena cava is approached through cannulation of the femoral vein; the choice of this site is limited to bedridden and sick patients, patients with pulmonary edema, and patients on a ventilator. Cannulation of the superior vena cava is risky in patients with pulmonary problems because of the risk of pneumothorax. However, femoral vein use is generally recommended for less than a week because of its higher chance of becoming infected. Percutaneous approach is preferred, failing which surgical exposure may be done. Finally, acute hemodialysis in newborns can be done by cannulation of the umbilical vessels. Polyurethane-reinforced Silastic catheters are available for acute hemodialysis in different sizes.

The immediate complications of subclavian and internal jugular catheters that could be life threatening include pneumothorax, hemothorax, and hemopericardium. Subclavian vein thrombosis and stenosis are the most important and disabling complications. Infection of the exit site or septicemia may occur.

Hemodialysis should be done under the supervision of personnel trained in pediatric nephrology, and its prescription is beyond the scope of this book; the reader is referred to a review by Gruskin et al (1992). In brief, hemodialysis prescription includes the size and type of dialyzer, blood flow rate, dialysate composition, dialysis flow rate, frequency and duration of treatment, estimated dry weight, ultrafiltrate to be removed, means to support the blood pressure, laboratory tests to be done before and after dialysis, and medications to be given during the treatment.

Acute hemodialysis is preferably done in an intensive care setting. Patients must be carefully monitored, and vital signs must be observed closely. Heart rate may be monitored with the help of a cardiac monitor. Blood pressure may be measured directly by an arterial transducer in critically ill children or more routinely by standard sphygmomanometer or Doppler-equipped blood pressure cuff. Oxygenation may suffer at the beginning of hemodialysis; therefore, measuring percutaneous oxygen saturation with a pulse oximeter is useful in sick children. Because critically ill infants are at risk for the development of hypothermia, core temperature should be frequently monitored during dialysis. To avoid hypothermia, dialysate is warmed to 40 to 41°C. In addition, an infrared heater may be used to keep the child warm. Weight must be carefully recorded at the beginning and end of dialysis with the help of sensitive scales. It is not generally useful to measure serum electrolyte, BUN, and creatinine levels during or immediately after dialysis because these values are not in equilibrium and tend to reflect composition of the dialysate.

References

Anand SK: Maturation of renal function. In Taeusch HW, Ballard RA, Avery ME (eds): *Disease of the Newborn.* Philadelphia, WB Saunders, 1991, p 841–847.

Bisset GS, Strife JL, Kirks DR: Genitourinary tract. In Kirks DR (ed): *Practical Pediatric Imaging. Diagnostic Radiology of Infants and Children*, 2nd ed. Boston, Little, Brown, 1991, pp 915–916.

Buonomo C, Treves ST, et al: Silent renal damage in symptom-free siblings of children with vesicoureteral reflux: assessment with technetium 99mTc dimercaptosuccinic acid scintigraphy. *J Pediatr*, 122:721–723, 1993.

Chan JCM, Brewer WH, Still W: Renal biopsy under ultrasound guidance: 100 consecutive biopsies in children. *J Urol*, 129:103–107, 1983.

Chantler C, Barrett TM: Estimation of glomerular filtration rate from plasma clearance of 51-chromium edetic acid. *Arch Dis Child*, 47: 613–617, 1972.

Davies JG, Taylor CM, et al: Clinical limitations of the estimation of GFR from height/plasma creatinine ratio: comparison with simultaneous ^{51}Cr edetic acid slope clearance. *Arch Dis Child*, 57:607–610, 1982.

Diaz-Buxo JA, Donadio JV Jr: Complications of percutaneous renal biopsy: an analysis of 1000 consecutive biopsies. *Clin Nephrol*, 4:223–227, 1975.

Fine RN: Peritoneal dialysis update. *J Pediatr*, 100:1–7, 1982.

Gordon I: Imaging the urinary tract. In Holliday MA, Barrat TM, Vernier RL (eds): *Pediatric Nephrology*, 2nd ed. Baltimore, Williams & Wilkins, 1987, pp 300–329.

Gordon I, Peters AM, Morony S: Indirect radionuclide cystography: a sensitive technique for the detection of vesicoureteral reflux. *Pediatr Nephrol*, 4:604–606, 1990.

Gruskin AB, Balurate HJ, Dabbagh S: Hemodialysis and peritoneal dialysis. In Edelman CM Jr (ed): *Pediatric Kidney Diseases*, 2nd ed. Boston, Little, Brown, 1992, pp 827–916.

Israelit AH, Long DL, et al: Measurement of glomerular filtration rate utilizing a single subcutaneous injection of ^{125}I-iothalamate. *Kidney Int*, 4:346–349, 1973.

Jakobsson B, Nolstedt L, et al: ^{99m}Technetium-dimercaptosuccinic acid scan in the diagnosis of acute pyelonephritis in children: relation to clinical and radiological findings. *Pediatr Nephrol*, 6:328–334, 1992.

Jerkins GR, Noe HN: Familial vesicoureteral reflux: a prospective study. *J Urol*, 140:119–120, 1982.

Khanna R, Nolph KD: The physiology of peritoneal dialysis. *Am J Nephrol*, 9:504–512, 1989.

Levey AS, Perrone RD, Madius NE: Serum creatinine and renal function. *Annu Rev Med*, 39: 465–490, 1988.

Lieberman KV, Nardi L, Bosch JP: Treatment of acute renal failure in an infant using continuous arterio-venous hemofiltration. *J Pediatr*, 106: 646–649, 1985.

Metcoff J: Needles for percutaneous renal biopsy in infants and children. *Pediatrics*, 46:788–789, 1970.

Morgan DB, Dillon S, Payne RB: The assessment of glomerular function: creatinine clearance or plasma creatinine. *Postgrad Med J*, 54:302–310, 1978.

Nakanishi T, Yanase M, et al: New acute peritoneal dialysis technique: wire-guide insertion and long-term dwelling of peritoneal catheter. *Nephron*, 34:128–132, 1984.

Nizsche EU, Zimmerhacki LB, et al: Correlation of ultrasound and renal scintigraphy in children with unilateral hydronephrosis in primary work-up. *Pediatr Nephrol*, 7:138–142, 1993.

Olind B, Hallgren R, et al: Is ^{125}I-iothalamate an ideal marker for glomerular filtration? *Kidney Int*, 27:9–16, 1985.

Perrone RD, Steinman TI, et al: Utility of radioisotopic filtration markers in chronic renal insufficiency: simultaneous comparison of ^{125}I-iothalamate, ^{169}Yb-DTPA, ^{99m}Tc-DPTA and inulin. *Am J Kidney Dis*, 16:224–235, 1990.

Piepez A, Denis R, et al: A simple method of measuring separate glomerular filtration rate using a single injection of ^{99m}Tc-DTPA and scintillation camera. *J Pediatr*, 93:769–774, 1978.

Reznik VM, Griswold WR, et al: Peritoneal dialysis for acute renal failure in children. *Pediatr Nephrol*, 5:715–717, 1991.

Ronco C, Brendolan A, et al: Treatment of acute renal failure in newborns by continuous arteriovenous hemofiltration. *Kidney Int*, 29:908–915, 1986.

Schwartz GJ, Brion LP, Spitzer A: The use of plasma creatinine for estimating glomerular filtration rate in infants, children and adolescents. *Pediatr Clin North Am*, 34:571–590, 1987.

Siegel SR, Oh W: Renal functional maturation in human infants. *Acta Paediatr Scand*, 65:481–485, 1976.

Steele BT, Vigneux A, et al: Acute peritoneal dialysis in infants weighing < 1500 g. *J Pediatr*, 110: 126–129, 1987.

Uldall PR: Vascular access for hemodialysis. Temporary vascular access for hemodialysis. In Nissenson AR, Fine RN (eds): *Dialysis Therapy*, 2nd ed. Philadelphia Hanley & Belfus, 1993, pp 5–10.

Van den Abbeele, Treves ST, et al: Vesicoureteral reflux in asymptomatic siblings of patients with known reflux: radionuclide cystography. *Pediatrics*, 79:147–153, 1987.

Wicker LC, Golper TA: Complications of percutaneous needle biopsy of the kidney. *Am J Nephrol*, 2:173, 1982.

Chapter 42

Renal Replacement Therapy—A Critical Care Perspective

Gary Goodman

Renal replacement therapy has found utility in the acute setting of the intensive care unit with increasing frequency. As new technology has developed and vascular access has been simplified, renal replacement therapy in one form or another has become accessible in critically ill and even unstable patients to an unprecedented degree. Renal replacement therapy can be instituted earlier and more safely for a steadily increasing number of indications.

INDICATIONS FOR RENAL REPLACEMENT THERAPY

Renal replacement therapy is indicated in a number of clinical settings. In the patient with acute renal failure, renal replacement therapy can correct fluid overload, electrolyte imbalance, metabolic acidosis, and uremia. Expanding indications for renal replacement therapy include fluid overload unresponsive to diuretics in patients with low cardiac output such as patients after cardiac surgery, tumor lysis syndrome, and unstable patients with chronic renal failure. Investigational indications include cytokine removal for patients in septic shock and adult respiratory distress syndrome/multisystem organ failure.

Absolute Indications

Uremia
Hypervolemia
Hyperkalemia
Hyperphosphatemia

Relative Indications

Hyperuricemia
Hypocalcemia
Acidemia
Tumor lysis syndrome
Hyperammonemia
Dialyzable toxic substances

Investigational

Cardiac surgery
Extracorporeal membrane oxygenation
Improved gas exchange in adult respiratory distress syndrome/multisystem organ failure
Cytokine removal for patients in septic shock.

PRINCIPLES OF RENAL REPLACEMENT THERAPY

All renal replacement therapy involves removal of water and solutes from the blood. During dialysis, a semipermeable membrane (natural or artificial) separates the blood from the dialysate and allows water and solutes to be removed selectively; larger molecules, such as proteins, protein-bound substances, and blood cells, cannot cross the synthetic membranes. The composition of the dialysate fluid determines the outcome of dialysis according to the principle of diffusion. Solute molecules diffuse according to their concentration gradients and the respective permeability of the filter or membrane. The process is regulated by varying the dialysate itself or the time period in which dialysis occurs. Glucose is used as an osmotic agent to remove water, and electrolytes are varied to adjust the serum concentrations appropriately.

Hemofiltration is an extracorporeal process that passes blood through a highly permeable membrane, which generates an ultrafiltrate that consists of plasma water and small and middle-sized unbound solutes. The ultrafiltrate is created by the hydrostatic pressure exerted across a highly permeable membrane. The obligatory ultrafiltrate is replaced with a sterile electrolyte solution (often lactated Ringer's solution) to achieve a net water loss that can be regulated to suit the clinical condition of the patient. Replacement fluid is introduced after the filter (postdilution). Dialysis solutions can also be infused in a countercurrent direction to influence the filtration process and add an element of dialysis to hemofiltration (hence the term continuous arteriovenous hemodialysis). The filtration device itself consists of plastic filters that contain highly permeable hollow fibers or plates. The filters are composed of various polymers and require minimal blood volume for priming. When the patient's own pulse pressure (with an arterial inflow catheter and venous return catheter) is used to drive blood through the extracorporeal hemofiltration circuit, the term continuous arteriovenous hemofiltration (CAVH) is used. This generally requires a mean arterial pressure of greater than 50 mm Hg. When both the inflow and return catheters are venous, a pump is used to achieve flow through the circuit, and the technique is known as continuous venovenous hemofiltration (CVVH). The dialysis component can be added to either circuit, and the general operating principles are the same.

There is thus a rapidly expanding range of options for renal replacement. The techniques vary according to the specifics of the filtering membrane, access, and technical considerations with respect to regulation of flow through the membrane (the device or dialysis machine).

Types of Renal Replacement Therapy

Extracorporeal

1. Continuous arteriovenous hemofiltration (CAVH)
2. Continuous venovenous hemofiltration (CVVH)
3. Hemodialysis

Peritoneal dialysis

The various techniques are compared and contrasted in Tables 42–1 and 42–2. Hemodialysis is less commonly used in the critical care setting because of marked hemodynamic effects and because of its intermittent application with rapid metabolic and fluid shifts. Peritoneal dialysis is useful when vascular access is difficult, in neonates, for long-term support, or when outpatient therapy is anticipated. CAVH/CVVH has found increasing utility because of the continuous flow, minimal hemodynamic effect, ease of application and adjustment, and effective water removal.

PREPARATION OF THE PATIENT AND FAMILY

The patient in renal failure will already have frequent, ongoing monitoring of multiple

Table 42–1 Filtering Membrane

Type of Renal Replacement Therapy	Dialysis Membrane
Hemodialysis	Manufactured: hemodialysis membrane
Peritoneal dialysis	Natural: peritoneal membrane
Continuous arteriovenous or venovenous hemofiltration	Manufactured: hemofilter

Table 42-2 Comparison of Dialysis Techniques

Parameter	Peritoneal Dialysis	Hemofiltration	Hemodialysis
Hemodynamics	Stable	Minimal	Significant
Dialysis	Continuous	Continuous	Intermittent
Ultrafiltration	Uncontrolled	Controlled	Uncontrolled
Training	Minimal	Moderate	Advanced
Hypotension	Uncommon	Possible	Frequent
Disequilibrium	None	None	Significant
Bleeding	Unlikely	Heparinized	Heparinized
Infection	Common	Less common	Less common

metabolic parameters as well as fluid intake and output. Fluid intake is often significantly restricted because of oliguria or anuria. With the institution of renal replacement therapy, these parameters will continue to be monitored closely. Fluid intake can often be liberalized, and there may be less protein restriction of the diet. The family needs to be informed about the surgical placement of vascular access devices or a peritoneal catheter, which may take place in the operating room. They should be educated about the risks of catheter dislodgment and the need for care when the patient is moved or turned. The patient's mobility will be restricted when dialysis is actually being performed because of the short lengths of dialysis tubing employed in the extracorporeal circuits.

METHODS

The primary role of the critical care staff is vascular access and hemodynamic support for the patient during renal replacement therapy. Other responsibilities will include dosage adjustment of medications, regulation of anticoagulation when indicated, and close physiological monitoring. The development of a dialysis team can facilitate coordination of the various aspects of renal replacement therapy. A multidisciplinary approach may include representatives from critical care, nephrology, hematology, surgery, dialysis, and critical care nursing.

Critical Care for Renal Replacement Therapy

Vascular access

Anticoagulation

Hemodynamic support

Monitoring

1. Daily weight
2. Accurate intake and output

   Native urine output
   Net water loss from dialysis
3. Hematocrit
4. Electrolytes
5. Blood urea nitrogen, creatinine

Drug disposition

1. Delayed clearance in renal failure

   Antibiotics
   Muscle relaxants
   Sedation
2. Increased clearance with dialysis

Nutritional support

Monitoring for complications

1. Thrombosis
2. Bleeding
3. Hypothermia
4. Infection
5. Vascular complications

Vascular Access

New vascular catheters have simplified vascular access for extracorporeal circuits for hemodialysis and hemofiltration (Table 42-3). As a rule, the larger the catheter lumen and the shorter the catheter length, the less resistance to flow and the more effective the filtration that can be achieved. Many of these catheters can be inserted percutaneously by use of the Seldinger technique. The femoral artery and vein, subclavian vein, and internal jugular vein

Table 42-3 Vascular Access for Extracorporeal Circuits

Mode of Renal Replacement Therapy	Vascular Access
Hemodialysis	Surgically created arteriovenous fistula (internal or external)
Continuous arteriovenous hemofiltration	Separate arterial and venous cannulas
Continuous venovenous hemofiltration	2 single or 1 double-lumen venous cannula

are all suitable sites for vascular access. In the newborn and premature infant, the umbilical vessels can also be used. Alternatively, cut-down of central veins is required to achieve adequate vascular access. The catheters can be heparin locked until they are needed for dialysis. When insufficient flow limits effective hemofiltration or causes the filter to clot frequently, it may be necessary to replace or modify the vascular access. Use of the largest-gauge catheter possible with the shortest length and avoidance of any sharp turns in the extracorporeal circuit, such as might be seen with use of a sheath-type catheter, optimize renal replacement efficiency and reduce thrombotic complications.

Peritoneal dialysis requires surgical placement of a temporary or permanent catheter in the peritoneal space. Acute peritoneal dialysis catheters are generally recommended when dialysis is anticipated for 3 days or less. A permanent catheter should be placed for longer periods of dialysis. The catheters vary in their construction and the surgical technique of placement. Acute peritoneal dialysis catheters are straight and relatively rigid and are advanced directly into the peritoneal cavity through the anterior abdominal wall. Chronic peritoneal dialysis catheters are soft, flexible catheters with an integrated extraperitoneal cuff. The catheter is surgically placed and tunneled through the anterior abdominal wall to create a barrier to infection and to discourage catheter dislodgment.

Types of peritoneal dialysis catheters

Temporary ($\leq$3 days): Trocath disposable stylet catheter
Permanent ($>$3 days): Tenckhoff permanent Silastic catheter

Anticoagulation

Patients requiring the use of extracorporeal circuits (for hemodialysis or hemofiltration) require anticoagulation to prevent the circuit from clotting as blood flows past the artificial surfaces. Anticoagulation is best accomplished with a constant heparin infusion after an initial bolus loading dose is given. A constant infusion of heparin 5 to 15 U/kg/h is titrated to maintain partial thromboplastin times or activated clotting times of 1.5 times control values. The filter itself, in the case of hemofiltration, is also flushed with heparin before use. For patients with pre-existing coagulopathy, systemic heparinization may be unnecessary. A new technique of regional heparinization has been suggested to minimize systemic anticoagulation. Heparin is infused directly into the filter through the arterial arm of the circuit, and the heparin antagonist protamine sulfate is infused through the venous arm.

Hemodynamic Support

All of the renal replacement techniques affect water balance and hence intravascular volume to a certain degree. Hemodialysis has the most dramatic effect on water balance and is capable of extremely rapid shifts in intravascular volume leading to profound hypotension. Water is removed by both osmotic and pressure gradients, which can be independently varied by the dialysis machine. Hemofiltration, on the other hand, allows meticulous regulation of water removal by balancing the ultrafiltrate with the replacement fluids. CAVH, which depends on the blood pressure gradient to maintain flow through the extracorporeal circuit, will itself become inefficient if blood pressure is low, with an accompanying risk of thrombosis of the tubing or hemofilter. CVVH, which uses a pump system, is less affected by hypotension. Systemic hypotension may initially require limiting net fluid loss with dialysis and additionally may require fluid boluses and inotropic support as appropriate. Peritoneal dialysis is the most benign of the renal replacement techniques with respect to hemodynamic compromise. Water balance and extraction are regulated by glucose concentration, dwell time, exchange volume, and cycle time.

Monitoring

The critical care staff needs to closely monitor the patient's weight and net water balance, including endogenous urine production. With hemofiltration, net water balance is determined hourly by varying the countercurrent fluid replacement. Net water balance is determined to approximate native urine production, 1 to 5 ml/kg/h. This may need to be varied, depending on the hemodynamic stability of the patient. Electrolyte, blood urea nitrogen, and creatinine levels need to be frequently monitored and appropriate adjustments made of intravenous and dialysis fluids.

Drug Disposition

For many drugs, disposition is significantly affected both by renal failure (decreased drug clearance) and by renal replacement therapy (increased clearance). Drugs or their metabolites that are normally excreted by the kidney require dosage modification. Factors that affect drug disposition include molecular size, chemical character, degree of protein binding, membrane clearance, and nonrenal metabolism. Sedation medications (especially narcotics) may also adhere to the tubing and membrane surfaces, leading to decreased bioavailability. Clearance of muscle relaxants can also be affected, leading to prolonged neuromuscular blockade; atracurium may be a good choice in the setting of renal failure because it is metabolized by an independent plasma reaction.

Drug levels, most notably of aminoglycoside antibiotics, vancomycin, theophylline, digoxin, and anticonvulsants, need to be closely monitored; dosing adjustments, in terms of both dosage and dosing intervals, will be required. Specific drugs often used in the intensive care unit that need to be adjusted for renal failure include penicillins, cephalosporins, trimethoprim-sulfamethoxazole, erythromycin, ciprofloxacin, amphotericin, flucytosine, acyclovir, cyclosporine, and radiocontrast agents. Hemodialysis has the most dramatic effect on drug removal, hemofiltration is less efficient, and in general, the clearance of most drugs by peritoneal dialysis is low.

Nutritional Support

Nutritional support of the critically ill patient is facilitated by renal replacement therapy. Removal of free water allows larger volumes of feedings or total parenteral nutrition, which increases calorie delivery. In addition, removal of nitrogen products allows increased protein supplementation without the risk of encephalopathy. In general, intralipids can be safely administered as long as triglyceride levels are monitored and maintained below 200 mg/dl. The percentage of calories as fat should not exceed 60%. It is also important to determine the nonprotein calorie to gram of nitrogen ratio, which should optimally be maintained in the range of 150 to 200:1.

Monitoring for Complications

The most frequent complications with extracorporeal circuits involve hemostasis: either systemic bleeding secondary to the required circulatory anticoagulation, or thrombosis of the circuit or filter because of insufficient anticoagulation. Hence, close monitoring of the heparin infusion and frequent measurements of partial thromboplastin time or activated clotting time are critical.

Another unique complication of the extracorporeal circuit is the propensity for heat loss and resulting hypothermia. A heating device can be applied externally around the catheter tubing to limit heat loss and maintain the patient's normothermia.

The most catastrophic complication is loss of integrity of the circuit: tubing rupture, catheter dislodgment, or disconnection of the circuit. The most frequent complication of peritoneal dialysis is infection, either of the catheter exit site and tunnel or peritonitis.

Technique-specific complications

Hemodialysis

1. Hypotension
2. Cramps
3. Febrile reactions
4. First-use syndromes
   Hypersensitivity
   Chest and back pain
5. Pruritus
6. Seizure activity
7. Arrhythmias
8. Hemolysis
9. Hypoxemia

Peritoneal dialysis

1. Infection

   Peritoneal catheter exit site and tunnel infections
   Peritonitis

2. Abdominal hernias
3. Dialysate leaks
4. Hydrothorax

Hemofiltration

1. Line disconnection
2. Accidental catheter removal
3. Arterial and venous hemorrhage
4. Thrombosis

CONTRAINDICATIONS

Peritoneal dialysis is contraindicated primarily because of absence of an adequate or intact peritoneal cavity, such as omphalocele, diaphragmatic hernia, or gastroschisis. Recent abdominal surgery is only a relative contraindication as long as there are no draining abdominal wounds.

SUMMARY

HEMODIALYSIS: Rapid, efficient dialysis in the hemodynamically stable patient with excellent vascular access; requires systemic anticoagulation; allows prompt correction of life-threatening hyperkalemia and volume overload and has the advantage of short treatment times; may be continued long term.

PERITONEAL DIALYSIS: Acute and chronic dialysis in the infant and small child with an intact peritoneum; anticoagulation is not required; hemodynamic stability is not compromised, and dialysis is smooth and steady; well suited for the newborn, especially with hyperkalemia or hyperammonemia; the technique is relatively inefficient, requiring long or continuous treatment, and there is a significant risk of peritonitis.

HEMOFILTRATION: A rapidly expanding dialysis technique; can be performed in the hemodynamically unstable patient as long as adequate vascular access can be secured; systemic anticoagulation is required; provides continuous treatment; with use of a pump system, a venovenous circuit alone suffices; excellent at water removal, which can be closely regulated; good for short-term support; not as efficient for removal of solutes (especially blood urea nitrogen and creatinine).

Suggested Indications for Renal Replacement Therapy

Hemodialysis

Ingestions
Toxins
Hyperkalemia
Chronic renal failure

Peritoneal dialysis

Hemolytic-uremic syndrome
Vascular access difficult
Newborns and premature infants

Hemofiltration

Critically ill, unstable patients with acute renal failure
Hypervolemia with oliguria
After cardiac surgery
Sepsis
Trauma
Severe burns

Bibliography

Bellomo R, Tipping P, Boyce N: Continuous venovenous hemofiltration with dialysis removes cytokines from the circulation of septic patients. *Crit Care Med*, 21:522–526, 1993.

DiCarlo JV, et al: Continuous arteriovenous hemofiltration/dialysis improves pulmonary gas exchange in children with multiple organ system failure. *Crit Care Med*, 18:822–826, 1990.

Frankenfield DC, et al: Urea removal during continuous hemodiafiltration. *Crit Care Med*, 22: 407–412, 1994.

Nahman NS Jr, Middendorf DF: Continuous arteriovenous hemofiltration. *Med Clin North Am*, 74:975–984, 1990.

Paret G, et al: Continuous arteriovenous hemofiltration after cardiac operations in infants and children. *J Thorac Cardiovasc Surg*, 104: 1225–1230, 1992.

Pascual JF, Lopez JD, Molina M: Hemofiltration in children with renal failure. *Pediatr Clin North Am*, 34:803–818, 1987.

Werner HA, Herbertson MJ, Seear MD: Functional characteristics of pediatric veno-venous hemofiltration. *Crit Care Med*, 22:320–325, 1994.

Section J

Gastrointestinal

Chapter 43

Pediatric Gastroenterology

Anthony H. Repucci

In the last 25 years, pediatric gastroenterology has become a viable subspecialty aided by the development and evolution of flexible fiberoptic endoscopy. Although some procedures are technically more difficult to perform in children, any gastrointestinal procedure possible in adults can also be safely performed in infants and children. The major and most frequently used procedures are discussed in this chapter; radiography, ultrasonography, and other imaging evaluative techniques are not. For a comprehensive discussion of pediatric gastrointestinal disease, refer to *Pediatric Gastrointestinal Disease: Pathophysiology, Diagnosis, Management* (1993) by Wyllie and Hyams.

PREPARING THE FAMILY AND CHILD FOR A GASTROINTESTINAL PROCEDURE

Infants and children require preparation for invasive gastrointestinal (GI) procedures. An endoscopy, biopsy, manometric, or pH study is a frightening and uncomfortable experience for the pediatric patient. The pediatric GI nurse lessens the child's discomfort and fear by establishing a trusting relationship with both the parent and child and by preparing them for what is to be done. The child's age, level of understanding, previous experience, and ability to cope must be considered when explaining procedures to the child.

Infants and young children are unable to comprehend or cooperate with the pediatric GI nurse and gastroenterologist. Sedation is, therefore, an essential component of successful pediatric GI procedures. Older children are less apprehensive when a procedure is explained in advance and when they are shown the procedure area ahead of time.

ANTIMICROBIAL PROPHYLAXIS

The prophylactic administration of antibiotics for the prevention of bacterial endocarditis associated with endoscopic procedures and gastrointestinal instrumentation is controversial. The incidence of bacteremia is low for most procedures, ranging from 0% to 10%; but some procedures, such as sclerotherapy, for esophageal varices and esophageal dilatation may cause bacteremia in 50% of cases (Shorron et al, 1983; Sullam et al, 1985). One study, performed prospectively in 50 children undergoing upper endoscopy or colonoscopy, revealed an incidence of bacteremia of just 2% with no serious sequelae (Byrne et al, 1982). Actual incidence of bacterial endocarditis following endoscopy is low. (Logan and Hastings, 1988; Niv et al, 1985; Rodriguez and Levine, 1984; Yin and Dellipiani, 1983).

The risk of bacterial endocarditis increases after traumatic procedures to mucosal surfaces. Enterococci (*Enterococcus faecalis* and *Enterococcus faecium*) are the organisms most frequently responsible for bacterial endocarditis after gastrointestinal tract instrumentation. Antibiotic prophylaxis therefore, is directed mainly against these organisms (Low et al, 1987). Nevertheless, bacterial endocarditis has been described in patients despite antimicrobial prophylactic therapy (Durack et al, 1983).

Despite the controversy surrounding prophylaxis for gastrointestinal instrumentation or diagnostic procedures, practical recommendations for antibiotic prophylaxis have been issued. The American Heart Association's Committee on Rheumatic Fever, Endocarditis, and Kawasaki Disease of the Council on Cardiovascular Disease in the Young (Dajani et al, 1990), and the Standards of Training and Practice Committee of the American Society for Gastrointestinal Endoscopy (Infection Control during Gastrointestinal Endoscopy: Guidelines for Clinical Application, 1988) have attempted to reach a consensus regarding antibiotic prophylaxis for gastrointestinal procedures.

Antibiotic prophylaxis is recommended for patients with (1) prosthetic heart valves, (2) previous history of bacterial endocarditis, (3) hypertrophic cardiomyopathy, (4) mitral valve prolapse with regurgitation or evidence of leaflet thickening and redundancy, (5) a surgically constructed systemic pulmonary shunt, (6) congenital heart anomaly, and (7) Marfan's syndrome (Fleischer, 1989).

Antimicrobial prophylaxis is not recommended for patients with (1) a physiological, functional, or innocent heart murmur, (2) history of Kawasaki disease, (3) mitral valve prolapse without regurgitation, (4) rheumatic heart disease or history of rheumatic heart disease without valvular dysfunction, or (5) pacemakers or implanted defibrillators. Additionally, patients who have had repair of a secundum atrial septal defect, ventricular septal defect, or patent ductus arteriosus with no residual dysfunction more than 6 months before the gastrointestinal procedure do not need prophylactic antibiotics (Neu, 1989).

It is not established whether premature infants, term infants less than 2 months of age, high-risk pediatric intensive care patients (e.g., patients with head trauma, multiple trauma, extensive burns), immunocompromised patients, or patients with prostheses should routinely receive antibiotic prophylaxis to prevent bacteremia in the absence of cardiac risk factors. Antibiotic prophylaxis should be considered, at least, in many of these patients before a procedure is performed.

Gastrointestinal procedures that require prophylaxis in patients at risk include (1) esophagogastroduodenoscopy (EGD), (2) endoscopic retrograde cholangiopancreatography (ERCP), (3) esophageal dilation, (4) sclerotherapy, (5) proctosigmoidoscopy, (6) colonoscopy, (7) polypectomy, (8) percutaneous liver biopsy, and (9) percutaneous endoscopic gastrostomy (PEG) (Fleischer, 1989). Most pediatric gastroenterologists routinely provide prophylaxis for all patients requiring PEG placement. For patients without the aforementioned risk factors, most pediatric gastroenterologists provide routine prophylaxis with cefazolin before and 6 to 8 hours after the procedure.

According to the American Heart Association's recommendations (Dajani et al, 1990), antimicrobial prophylaxis is given before the procedure and 6 to 8 hours after the initial dose:

Thirty minutes before the procedure

1. Ampicillin: 50 mg/kg intravenously or intramuscularly (maximum 2 g)
2. Gentamicin: 2 mg/kg intravenously or intramuscularly (maximum 80 mg)

Six to 8 hours after the initial dose

1. Amoxicillin: 25 mg/kg by mouth (maximum 1.5 g); 6 hours after the first dose
2. Alternatively, in patients who may be unable to take medication enterally, repeat the preprocedure parenteral regimen 8 hours after the initial dosage at half the initial dosing regimen (ampicillin: 25 mg/kg intravenously or intramuscularly).

Patients with allergy to penicillin

1. Vancomycin: 20 mg/kg intravenously; administer over a 1-hour period before the procedure
2. Gentamicin: 2 mg/kg intravenously or intramuscularly (maximum 80 mg); 30 minutes before the procedure

Eight hours after the initial dose

1. Vancomycin: 10 mg/kg intravenously; administer over a 1-hour period

Low-risk patients (patients with coronary artery disease, pacemakers, atrial septal defect, or normal heart) (Fleischer, 1989)

1. Amoxicillin: 50 mg/kg by mouth (maximum 3 g); 1 hour before the procedure
2. Amoxicillin: 25 mg/kg by mouth (maximum 1.5 g); 6 hours after the initial dose

Follow-up doses should be half the initial dosage, and the total pediatric dose should not exceed the total adult dose. Cephalosporins should not be substituted in the penicillin-allergic patient. In those patients allergic to both penicillin and vancomycin, no specific recommendations have been made, but oral or intravenous erythromycin has been suggested by Neu (1989) for adults and might apply to the pediatric patient population.

No adequate, clinical trials of antibiotic regimens to prevent bacterial endocarditis in humans have been performed. In the absence of clear scientific data, more prophylactic antibiotics for gastrointestinal procedures are used than are actually necessary. Clinicians must develop treatment plans on a case by case basis, using the available guidelines and recommendations.

ENDOSCOPY

Equipment

Both fiberoptic and video upper endoscopes are available for use in pediatric patients, although smaller outside diameter endoscopes remain exclusively fiberoptic in design (Fig. 43–1). The larger fiberoptic endoscopes are superior to video endoscopes in resolution, but resolution

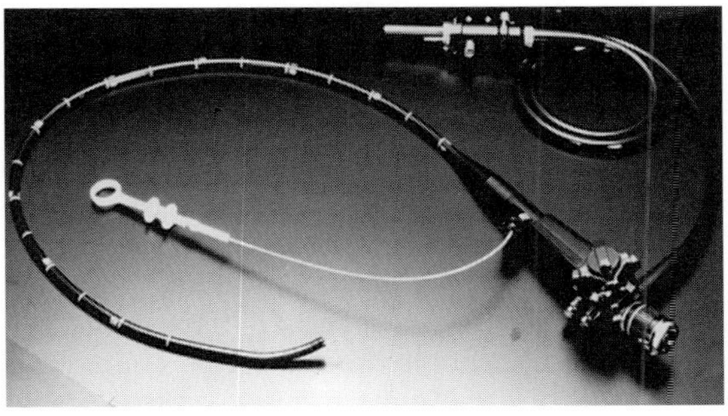

Figure 43–1 GIF × Q20 upper gastrointestinal fiberscope with biopsy forceps in biopsy channel. (Courtesy of Olympus America, Inc.)

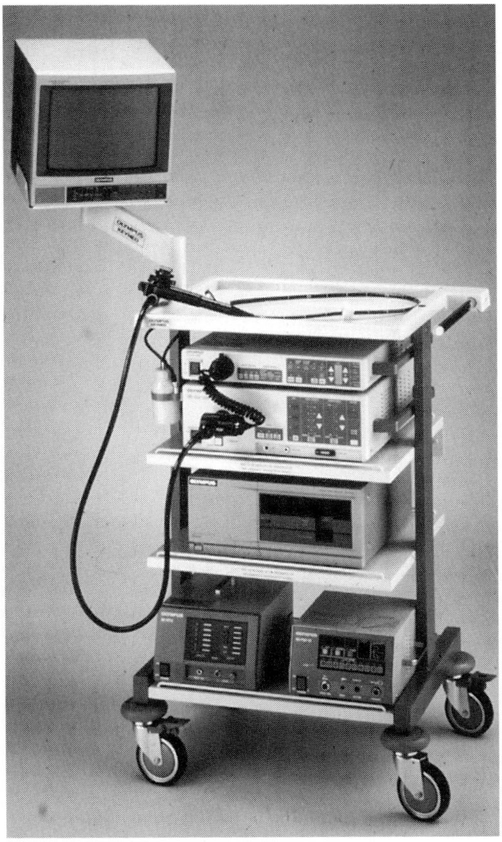

Figure 43–2 Video processor and power source for video endoscope. (Courtesy of Olympus America, Inc.)

is limited by size and number of fibers, fragility, and loss of light transmission ability over time with prolonged use. Fiberscopes require less fine tuning to control for color distortion than video endoscopes, have a longer focal range, and create less image distortion when near the mucosal surface. Many endoscopists prefer the exceptional clarity available only in the fiberoptic endoscope for the diagnosis and treatment of gastrointestinal bleeding.

Video endoscopy can be used to freeze images for instant photographic recording (Fig. 43–2). It also provides a high-quality television image with more clarity than the image obtained by connecting a television camera to a fiberoptic endoscopic eyepiece. It is the preferred system for easy storage and retrieval of data and for providing instruction. Video endoscopy units are more cumbersome than fiberscopes, however, making portability more difficult in areas outside the endoscopy unit (e.g., in the radiology department or the intensive care unit).

Pediatric upper gastrointestinal endoscopes range in outside diameter from 5.2 to 11.3 mm with a working length of 58 to 104 cm, respectively; pediatric sigmoidoscopes range in outside diameter from 12.2 to 15.4 mm with a working length of 35 to 64 cm; and pediatric colonoscopes range in outside diameter from 11.3 to 14.3 mm with a working length of 123 to 168 cm. The smaller diameter endoscopes enable the pediatric gastroenterologist to perform endoscopy safely in infants as small as 1500 g. In infants and small children, the esophagus is quite distensible and can readily accommodate an upper pediatric endoscope, but tracheal compression and respiratory compromise may occur, especially when larger instruments are used.

The endoscope is connected to a light source or video processor and a power source through a universal cord that also provides water, suction, and insufflation capabilities via fingertip control valves. The fiberscope consists of a control handle on which an eyepiece is mounted. The control handle is connected to an insertion tube through which the fiberoptic bundles pass. The videoscope, without an eyepiece, contains a sensor (video "chip") at the distal tip that relays an image to a video processor. The image is then displayed on a television monitor. Otherwise, the two endoscopic designs are functionally similar.

The endoscope is manually advanced and retrieved (Fig. 43–3). It is maneuvered by rotating the control handle, and tip deflection is controlled by two parallel dials mounted on the right side of the control handle. The medial dial controls up and down movement. The lateral, smaller dial, controls movement to the left and right. On the lower end of the control handle, a separate channel is used to grasp biopsy forceps, cytology brushes, specialized retrieval forceps and baskets, electrocautery or heater probes, sclerotherapy needles, guide wires, or polypectomy snares; air and water can be passed through this channel. The distal end of the endoscope contains an objective lens or video "chip," an air/water channel positioned to clean off the lens, two light guides, and a suction/forceps channel. Accessory equipment can provide a video record of the procedure and produce still photographs.

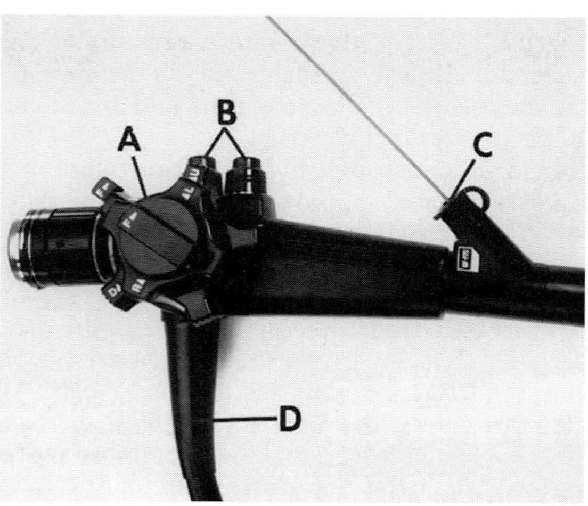

Figure 43–3 Control handle GIF P20 endoscope. **A.** Dials for directional control. **B.** Valves for suction and air-water. **C.** Biopsy channel. **D.** Universal cord. (Courtesy of Olympus America, Inc.)

Biopsy, Cytology Brushing, and Culture

Endoscopy in infants and children typically involves specimen retrieval (including polypectomy) for histopathological diagnosis, culture, or foreign body removal. Grasp biopsies are procured with a variety of forceps configurations. The size and location of the biopsies are more important than the number of biopsy samples when making a tissue diagnosis. Upon retrieval, specimens are placed in transport medium (e.g., formalin). Some pediatric gastroenterologists prefer to orient each specimen on a small square of plastic mesh (gauze) before placing it in medium. This is helpful when evaluating small intestinal villous atrophy, such as occurs in celiac disease.

The brush biopsy technique is performed by passing a sheathed cytology brush through the channel of the endoscope and brushing the suspected area several times to obtain adequate material. The brush is then withdrawn into the sheath to avoid specimen loss or contamination when retrieved through the biopsy channel. Upon removal, the brush can be stroked over a Dakin slide or the brush itself can be snipped off and placed in appropriate transport media such as a Pap smear bottle or appropriate culture media. Cytology for cancerous lesions is not routinely performed during pediatric procedures because gastrointestinal tract malignancy is rarely encountered in children (unlike in adults in whom neoplasm is always a diagnostic consideration).

Cultures can be aspirated directly through the endoscope using the air/water channel, by temporarily connecting a specimen container (sputum trap) in series with the suction tubing. Isotonic saline solution rather than sterile water instilled through the air/water channel of the endoscope enhances the recovery of organisms. Forwarding the specimen to the microbiology laboratory quickly, preferably on ice, decreases the likelihood of cell lysis. Bile or pancreatic fluid can also be obtained for analysis by the aspiration technique.

There are several types, shapes, and sizes of foreign body retrieval devices available, including rubber-tipped, rat tooth, and alligator-jaw forceps, snares, and baskets. Polypectomy snares and sclerotherapy needles (disposable or reusable) are designed specifically for use with pediatric endoscopes.

Complications for the endoscopist and endoscopy assistants can be avoided by wearing protective goggles or a face shield, a gown, and gloves; practicing good endoscopic technique; observing strict precautions against infection when handling specimens or equipment; and routine hand washing after the procedure. Nevertheless, the following are potential complications: human bite, herpetic conjunctivitis, *Helicobacter pylori* infection, hepatitis, and human immunodeficiency virus (HIV) infection (American Society for Gastrointestinal Endoscopy, 1988; Sartor, 1987).

Endoscopes and endoscopic accessories are fully immersible and should be promptly cleaned, disinfected, rinsed, and dried (inside and out) after each use. Soaking for approximately 10 minutes in a chemical disinfecting/sterilizing solution such as glutaraldehyde is necessary to achieve disinfection; manufacturer's directions should be followed (Baillie, 1992).

Upper Gastrointestinal Endoscopy: Esophagogastroduodenoscopy

INDICATIONS

The indications for upper gastrointestinal endoscopy in infants and children vary according to the age of the patient. The diagnostic sensitivity of gastrointestinal endoscopy depends on the indication. An upper gastrointestinal series may serve a complementary role in certain situations, such as in identifying a hiatal hernia, or in patients with recurrent vomiting in whom an intrinsic or extrinsic obstruction may be present. Standard pediatric upper endoscopes generally cannot visualize the small bowel beyond the second portion of the duodenum, so an upper gastrointestinal series with a small bowel follow-through may be necessary to assess the entire length of the small intestine. This is particularly important when Crohn's disease is being considered. With the advent of pediatric endoscopy, the role of an upper gastrointestinal series in the evaluation of peptic disease has diminished because direct visualization via endoscopy is not only more sensitive but also permits biopsy or therapeutic intervention when indicated.

Indications for upper gastrointestinal endoscopy are divided into diagnostic and therapeutic categories:

Diagnostic

1. Peptic ulcer disease (Fig. 43–4), which may present with any of the following: chronic periumbilical (younger children) or epigastric abdominal pain, nausea/vomiting, hematemesis, gastroesophageal reflux, heme positive stool
2. Acute abdominal pain in the epigastric or right upper quadrant (inflammation or obstruction should be considered)
3. Hematemesis, melena, or microscopic blood loss; cause may be age-related (possible toxic ingestion with concomitant liver involvement should be considered in all ages)
    a. Premature or full-term newborns—hemorrhagic disease, vascular malformation (hemangioma, telangiectasia, arteriovenous malformation), ingested maternal blood (from delivery or mother's breast), stress ulceration (e.g., premature infants in neonatal intensive care unit), milk protein allergy

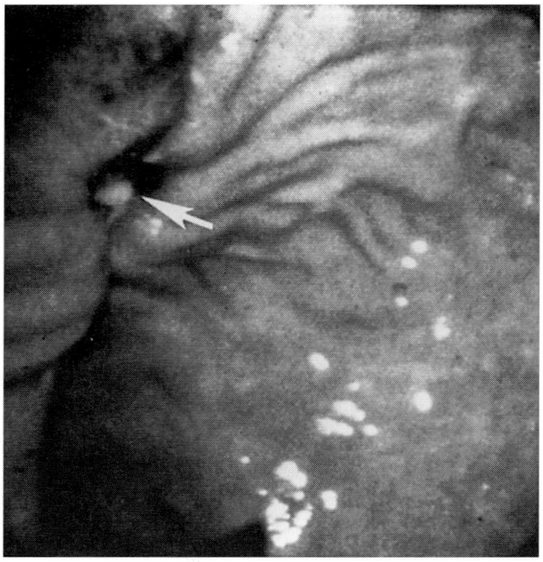

Figure 43–4 Primary peptic ulcer—proximal duodenum. (From Wyllie R, Hyams JS: *Pediatric Gastrointestinal Disease: Pathophysiology, Diagnosis, Management.* Philadelphia, WB Saunders, 1993.)

b. *Infants*—reflux esophagitis, peptic disease, vascular malformation, cow's milk/soy protein allergy

c. *Toddlers*—reflux esophagitis, peptic disease, esophageal varices, vascular malformation, cow's milk/soy protein allergy, lymphonodular hyperplasia

d. *Children and adolescents*—reflux esophagitis, peptic disease, esophageal varices, inflammatory bowel disease, lymphonodular hyperplasia

4. Dysphagia or odynophagia, which may present as irritability, regurgitation/emesis, or food refusal in infants and young children; consider anatomical obstruction or inflammation
5. Caustic or foreign body ingestion (any age)
6. Recurrent emesis, which may indicate inflammation or obstruction; central nervous system (CNS) involvement, otitis media, or urinary tract infection should be ruled out
7. Small bowel biopsy for chronic diarrhea, decreased growth velocity, foul-smelling stools, malnutrition, ascites, edema, recurrent infection (agammaglobulinemia/hypogammaglobulinemia), or abdominal pain (possible disaccharidase deficiency)
8. ERCP, which identifies a choledochal cyst, pancreas divisum, or stenosis of the sphincter of Oddi
9. Placement of antroduodenal motility catheter (to identify chronic intestinal pseudo-obstruction syndrome; signs and symptoms are often nonspecific and may occur at any age, be insidious and slowly progressive or intermittent, and include regurgitation (dysphagia, heartburn), vomiting (bile-stained; fluid/electrolyte imbalance), abdominal distention, crampy abdominal pain, constipation or diarrhea, weight loss, malnutrition, hypoalbuminemia, and edema)
10. Follow-up screening in known Barrett's esophagus or polyposis syndromes
11. Confirmation of radiological findings (e.g., ulceration, mass lesion, web, stricture)

Therapeutic

1. Coagulation with electrocautery, heater probe, or laser; bleeding ulcers; vascular malformations; antral or duodenal webs
2. Dilation of esophageal stricture
3. Dilation of lower esophageal sphincter in achalasia
4. Placement of nasojejunal feeding tube, percutaneous gastrostomy tube, or gastrojejunostomy tube
5. Sclerotherapy for esophageal varices
6. ERCP (sphincterotomy or stone removal)
7. Foreign body removal (removal of a foreign body lodged above the thoracic inlet is generally referred to an otorhinolaryngologist for removal under direct visualization)

Certain indications may require general anesthesia in infants and children because patient movement (including retching) increases the risk of perforation or aspiration. These include caustic ingestions, coagulation or sclerotherapy (especially during an active upper gastrointestinal bleed), stricture dilation, and foreign body removal. Under these circumstances, it is essential to protect the airway, which should be monitored throughout the procedure by an anesthesiologist. Also, the length or difficulty of a procedure (such as placement of an antroduodenal motility catheter) may preclude the use of conscious sedation.

CONTRAINDICATIONS

The contraindications to upper gastrointestinal endoscopy in infants and children are similar to those for adults:

Absolute

1. Shock
2. Suspected perforation of a hollow viscus
3. Peritonitis
4. Cervical spine injury
5. Atlantoaxial subluxation (e.g., may occur in Down syndrome)
6. Lack of adequately trained personnel

Relative

1. Uncooperative/combative patient
2. Coagulopathy or platelet dysfunction
3. Neutropenia
4. Patients with connective tissue disorders (e.g., Ehlers-Danlos and Marfan's syndrome) have increased risk of perforation
5. History of caustic ingestion with tight stricture
6. Partial or complete bowel obstruction
7. Recent esophageal, gastric, or bowel surgery
8. Inadvertent feeding (less than 2 to 4 hours in infants; 6 to 8 hours in children older than 2 years of age)
9. Thoracic aortic aneurysm
10. Unstable cardiac condition (arrhythmia, recent cardiac surgery, or myocardial ischemia or infarction)
11. Uncontrolled seizure activity
12. Unprotected airway for foreign body removal, active upper gastrointestinal bleeding, or sclerotherapy
13. Compromised respiratory status; severe dyspnea or hypoxemia

PATIENT PREPARATION

Preparing the patient for upper gastrointestinal endoscopy requires that the patient be fasted. Four hours in infants younger than 6 months of age is sufficient (longer periods may require intravenous glucose to prevent hypoglycemia, especially in the premature or newborn infant); 8 hours is usually necessary in children 2 years of age and older.

BIOPSY, CYTOLOGY BRUSHING, AND CULTURE

Grasp (pinch) biopsies in the esophagus can identify reflux esophagitis, Barrett's esophagus, or, although rare in the pediatric population, a malignant neoplasm. (Dahms and Rothstein, 1984; Hyams et al, 1988; Young et al, 1980). Both the normal and the immunocompromised host can acquire fungal or viral esophagitis. Biopsy, cytologic brushing, and culture for fungal and viral infections (cytomegalovirus [CMV], herpes, or *Candida*) of the esophagus collectively can contribute to reaching a diagnosis (Buss and Schary, 1979; Freedman et al, 1985; Holt, 1986). (Biopsy of the esophagus is contraindicated if the patient is to undergo esophageal dilation.)

Gastric biopsy or cytologic brushing is indicated for the diagnosis of *H. pylori*–associated gastritis, which may give a characteristic nodular appearance to the antral mucosa in the pediatric patient (Hassall and Dimmidk, 1991). *H. pylori* may be recovered from the antrum, fundus, or gastric cardia. The presence of *H. pylori* is confirmed histologically by routine hematoxylin-eosin or Giemsa staining, but a presumptive diagnosis can be made using an antral biopsy for a rapid urease test at the time of endoscopy (Czinn and Carr, 1987; Killbridge et al, 1988). Eosinophilic gastroenteritis, idiopathic granulomatous gastritis, sarcoidosis, Ménétrier's disease, autoimmune (atrophic) gastritis, lymphocytic (varioliform) gastritis, or gastric Crohn's disease can be diagnosed by biopsy (Drumm and Sherman, 1991). Infections due to CMV, herpes simplex virus, and *Candida* species are also identified in the stomach by biopsy, cytology, and culture techniques (Cronan et al, 1980; Henson, 1972; Howiler and Goldberg, 1976).

Important information can be obtained from the small bowel using the endoscopic biopsy technique. Celiac disease, intestinal lymphangiectasia, Crohn's disease, abetalipoproteinemia, agammaglobulinemia, autoimmune enteropathy, microvillus atrophy, and microvillus inclusion disease can all be identified by biopsy of the small bowel. Biopsies can be used to determine disaccharidase activity in congenital alactasia or sucrase-isomaltase deficiency in which the morphology appears normal. Infectious agents identifiable by biopsy or a wet preparation microscopic examination of a duodenal aspirate include giardiasis, strongyloidiasis, and cryptosporidiosis. Abnormal biopsy findings may be nonspecific, as with cow or soy protein allergy, transient gluten intolerance, intractable diarrhea syndrome, tropical sprue, radiation enteritis, drug-induced enteritis, malnutrition, or acquired immunodeficiency syndrome (AIDS) (Walker-Smith et al, 1991).

PROCEDURE

1. Vital signs are recorded and a pulse oximeter is connected to the patient's finger or toe before beginning the process of intravenous conscious sedation.
2. In order to minimize discomfort during introduction of the endoscope, the patient's posterior pharynx is sprayed with either a local benzocaine anesthetic (Cetacaine [Cetylite Industries, Inc., Pennsauken, NJ] or Hurricaine [Beutlich, Inc., Niles, IL]), or 1 to 2 ml of 2% lidocaine (Xylocaine) viscous solution (Astra Pharmaceutical Products, Inc., Westboro, MA) is briefly gargled and expelled. (To avoid aspiration, this step is performed before conscious sedation is employed.) Infants and young children who cannot cooperate with this step receive 1% viscous lidocaine solution mixed with lubricating jelly. This is placed on the distal end of the endoscope prior to endoscopic intubation. The child is told that the swallowing sensation will be temporarily lost but that it will return after the procedure is completed.
3. The patient is positioned on his/her left side (the side from which the procedure is routinely performed) to decrease the risk of aspiration. Infants and young children usually benefit from being wrapped in a sheet "papoose" style.
4. A protective mouthpiece is inserted and secured. This protects the patient's teeth and gums as well as the endoscope itself.
5. The lubricated distal end of the upper endoscope can be introduced. Although blind intubation of the esophagus is possible, it is best to pass the upper endoscope under direct visualization to identify the hypopharynx and avoid inadvertent laryngeal intubation or entry into the adjacent pyriform sinuses. While the assistant flexes the patient's head slightly forward, the operator flexes the tip of the endoscope approximately 60 degrees. The endoscope is then introduced under direct visualization. Some resistance is felt in the hypopharynx at the level of the cricopharyngeus (upper esophageal sphincter). If the patient can swallow, the endoscope can be passed readily. Otherwise, gentle pressure is applied to prompt the upper esophageal sphincter to open. The amount of pressure necessary to coax passage of the endoscope through the upper esophageal sphincter is learned by experience. Occasionally, passage of the endoscope is unusually difficult. A smaller diameter upper endoscope can be tried, but this is not always feasible in infants and small children. This portion of the procedure typically causes the patient to gag. Local anesthesia and a well-lubricated endoscope ensure prompt and easy entry into the esophagus.
6. The instrument is advanced through the lumen of the esophagus while the endoscopist examines the mucosa for lesions (inflammation, erosions or ulcerations, strictures, varices, webs, or hiatal hernias). In a cooperative patient in whom a sliding hiatal hernia is suspected, the position of the diaphragm can be identified when the patient sniffs. The position of the lower esophageal sphincter and of any esophageal lesions are measured and recorded as the distance from the lower incisors to the distal tip of the endoscope. Metric markings on the body of the endoscope (usually at 10-cm intervals) can then be used to calculate distance.
7. When the endoscope enters the stomach, residual gastric secretions are removed by suction before the stomach is insufflated for further inspection. It is not uncommon to see periodic peristaltic activity moving toward the pylorus.
8. The endoscope is advanced along the lesser curvature of the stomach toward the pylorus, which normally appears as a small opening with folds radiating from it.
9. The endoscope is passed through the pyloric channel into the duodenal bulb and the bulb is examined for lesions in all quadrants.
10. Further advancement of the endoscope into the second portion of the duodenum

is accomplished by torquing the scope to the right as the manual controls are simultaneously positioned down and to the right, and then quickly dialed upward. The ampulla of Vater and the duodenal mucosa are then visualized as the endoscope is withdrawn. Biopsy specimens, if necessary, are obtained in the second portion and bulb of the duodenum.

11. The endoscope is withdrawn into the stomach to inspect the antrum and pylorus more closely. Biopsy specimens, if necessary, are obtained from the body and antrum.
12. The gastric fundus and cardia are examined by retroflexion, withdrawal, and a 360-degree rotation of the endoscope as air insufflation is provided. Biopsy specimens of the fundus and cardia may be taken at this time.
13. The endoscope is then advanced into the gastric antrum again and straightened for removal. Before removal of the endoscope from the stomach, residual air and fluid are aspirated.
14. The gastroesophageal junction and, in the absence of a hiatal hernia, lower esophageal sphincter are visualized and their distance from the incisors noted as the endoscope is withdrawn into the esophagus. The gastroesophageal junction normally appears as a distinctive, irregularly shaped ridge demarcating the transition from squamous esophageal mucosa to the columnar epithelium of the gastric cardia. Biopsy specimens are usually obtained at 3 and 5 cm above the lower esophageal sphincter.
15. The endoscope is slowly retrieved as the esophageal mucosa is again inspected. At the level of the larynx, swift removal of the endoscope is best for patient comfort.

POST-PROCEDURE CARE

Upon completion of the procedure, vital signs are recorded and the patient is monitored by pulse oximetry until awake and alert. Intravenous fluids may be continued during this time. Medications used for conscious sedation, such as meperidine, may cause postprocedure nausea and vomiting in some patients. Infants and children are often hungry due to the fasting required prior to the procedure, but liquids should be limited until the patient is fully conscious. Parents should be warned that the child may experience nausea and vomiting during transport, so it is usually best if the child avoids eating until his or her return home.

The patient and family are provided with written post-procedure instructions and an emergency telephone number. Infants can be carried or placed in strollers, but larger children and adolescents are usually escorted from the hospital in wheelchairs.

COMPLICATIONS

Upper endoscopy in infants and children is considered safe, with a complication rate of 1.7%. The most common complications in a pediatric population of 6424 patients were bronchospasm, respiratory arrest, and phlebi-tis (Ament et al, 1988). In general, complications can be separated into the following categories:

Sedation-Related

1. Transient respiratory arrest
2. Phlebitis
3. Bronchospasm

Bleeding

1. Biopsy sites
2. Clot dislodgement
3. Mallory-Weiss tear induced by retching during the procedure
4. Retropharyngeal hematoma
5. Intramural duodenal hematoma
6. Tongue or lip laceration

Perforation

1. Pneumothorax
2. Pneumomediastinum
3. Spontaneous bowel perforation in patients with connective tissue disorders (e.g., Ehlers-Danlos syndrome)
4. Gastric perforation after therapeutic injection or laser therapy to control bleeding

Other

1. Aspiration
2. Infection
3. Loosened or broken teeth

Upper Endoscopy: Foreign Body Removal

Children of all ages ingest nonfood substances (Fig. 43–5). Infants and young children between the ages of 6 months and 3 years, mentally retarded older children, and older children and adolescents with psychological disturbances are especially vulnerable to foreign body ingestion (Healy, 1987; Taylor, 1987).

A history of foreign body ingestion is not always available, and signs and symptoms such as chest pain (which may be referred pain to the cervical area), drooling, choking, coughing, and gagging do not always occur (Schunk et al, 1989). Objects tend to get caught in three anatomically narrow areas of the esophagus: the hypopharynx at the level of the cricopharyngeus, the aortic arch, and the gastroesophageal junction (Byrne, 1993).

Coins are the most common objects swallowed, but small toys, buttons, bones, disk batteries, pins, and toothpicks are also common. It is unusual for foodstuffs to act as foreign body obstructions in children. When food or a small object is lodged in the esophagus, there may be an anatomical abnormality or a functional obstruction such as achalasia. Small children with foreign body ingestions have a higher incidence of lead intoxication and they should be screened for such. It is possible that a second foreign body is present in any child in whom one object has been identified.

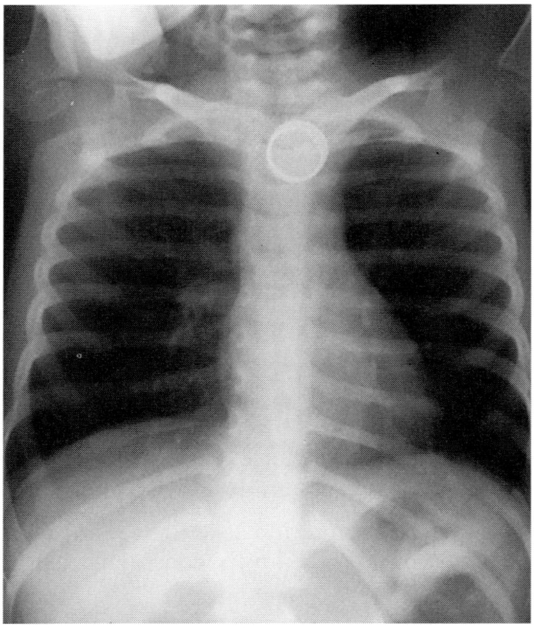

Figure 43–5 Anteroposterior view of the chest showing a bottle cap lodged in the cervical esophagus. The flat surface, as with coins, is present on the anteroposterior view. (From Wyllie R, Hyams JS: *Pediatric Gastrointestinal Disease: Pathophysiology, Diagnosis, Management.* Philadelphia, WB Saunders, 1993.)

Anteroposterior and lateral chest films (and sometimes neck films) help to identify most foreign bodies, but not all objects are radiopaque. Wood, plastic, glass, and aluminum objects are radiolucent, and a small amount of dilute barium is needed to determine their size, shape, and location. A high index of suspicion is essential to identify a radiolucent foreign body (Nussbaum et al, 1984).

INDICATIONS

Approximately 80% to 90% of foreign bodies pass spontaneously, 10% to 20% require endoscopic retrieval, and approximately 1% require surgical removal (Schwartz and Polsky, 1985). In older children and adolescents, an object more than 20 mm wide and 5 cm long usually does not pass through the gastrointestinal tract. Considerably smaller objects get caught in infants and small children (Koch, 1977). If the child is relatively asymptomatic and the object is small and carries a low risk of causing perforation (e.g., a coin or button), a period of observation may be indicated. Clear liquids and, occasionally, sedatives or glucagon (to relax the lower esophageal sphincter) are administered to assist passage of the object into the stomach (Caravati et al, 1989). If the child is symptomatic or the object carries a higher risk of causing injury, prompt removal is warranted.

Risk of complication depends on the size, shape, and composition of the foreign body. Coins larger than about 20 mm in diameter usually require retrieval. (U.S. penny equals 18 mm; dime, 17 mm; nickel, 21 mm; quarter, 24 mm). Since 1982, the composition of the U.S. penny has changed from predominantly copper to predominantly zinc, making it more corrosive (Fernbach and Tucker, 1986). Pennies in the esophagus should be retrieved after 24 hours.

Disk batteries are both foreign bodies and caustic agents (see Upper Endoscopy: Caustic Ingestion). They can be distinguished radiographically from coins by their double density and irregular contour. Smaller batteries may pass spontaneously and can be traced by sequential radiographs. Once the battery is in the stomach, cathartics or prokinetics can be given to decrease transit time. An antacid or H2 antagonist is sometimes provided to reduce gastric acidity and decrease the risk of mercury poisoning. Inducing emesis is contraindicated due to the risk of aspiration. An abdominal film is obtained after 48 hours. If the battery remains in the stomach or the child is symptomatic, the battery must be removed. Parents should be asked to look for the battery in the child's stool by straining each of the child's bowel movements. If the battery does not pass after 5 days or the child becomes symptomatic, surgical intervention is necessary (Litovitz, 1985).

Sharp objects have a greater risk of causing perforation, not only in the esophagus but also in the duodenum, ligament of Treitz, terminal ileum, ileocecal area, and sigmoid colon. They require prompt removal. Items such as small nails, thumbtacks, common pins, and closed safety pins can usually be managed conservatively because they have been shown to pass safely through the gastrointestinal tract. Although razor blades have safely traversed the gastrointestinal tract once in the stomach, they are routinely retrieved (Maleki and Evan, 1970).

When food becomes lodged in the esophagus, conservative management can be attempted in a relatively asymptomatic child. Clear liquids and sometimes sedation or glucagon can promote passage of the food into the stomach. If there is no change after 12 hours, the object should be retrieved. Forcibly attempting to push an object into the stomach risks perforation of the esophagus and should be avoided; there may be an anatomical or functional obstruction beyond the impacted food item.

Bezoars, collections of materials such as hair (trichobezoar), plant or vegetable matter (phytobezoar), or a variety of inert materials, amass in the stomach or intestines and, due to their size, generally require surgical removal rather than endoscopic retrieval. There have been reports, however, in which surgery was averted by the use of endoscopy to fragment the mass with snares and forceps, or to dissolve it with papain, acetylcysteine, or cellulase (Madsden et al, 1978; Schlang, 1970; Stanten and Peters, 1975).

SEDATION

Although endoscopic foreign body removal is sometimes performed with the patient under conscious sedation in the prone, Trendelenburg position, most pediatric gastroenterologists prefer to use general anesthesia. General anesthesia eliminates patient movement and reduces the risk of injury, perforation, or loss of the object in the hypopharynx. Intubation protects the airway from aspiration of the foreign body or its fragments.

EQUIPMENT

Specialized endoscopic accessories are designed to grasp foreign bodies of a variety of sizes and shapes under direct visualization (Fig. 43–6). Once secured, the foreign body is held against the exit port of the endoscope and is removed in tandem with the endoscope, which is withdrawn carefully. If the object is sharp or irregular, it must be removed with a protective overtube (Fig. 43–7) or a modified condom catheter fitted over the distal end of the endoscope. A Kelly or McGill forceps and a laryngoscope should be available to retrieve the object if it becomes detached from the endoscopic retrieval device as it is pulled through the hypopharynx. Glucagon (0.05 mg/kg intravenously) may be used to relax the lower esophageal sphincter, allowing objects that are impossible to retrieve from the esophagus to be advanced into the stomach.

PROCEDURE

Upper endoscopy for foreign body removal requires careful planning and manual dexterity:

1. To determine which retrieval device will work best, it is worthwhile to rehearse the endoscopy with an identical object outside of the patient's esophagus or stomach. It should be determined whether a sharp or irregularly shaped object can be easily pulled into the protective overtube or whether a modified condom catheter is needed. A radiograph taken before the procedure helps to identify the exact location of the object.
2. The hypopharynx is intubated under direct visualization and the endoscope is carefully

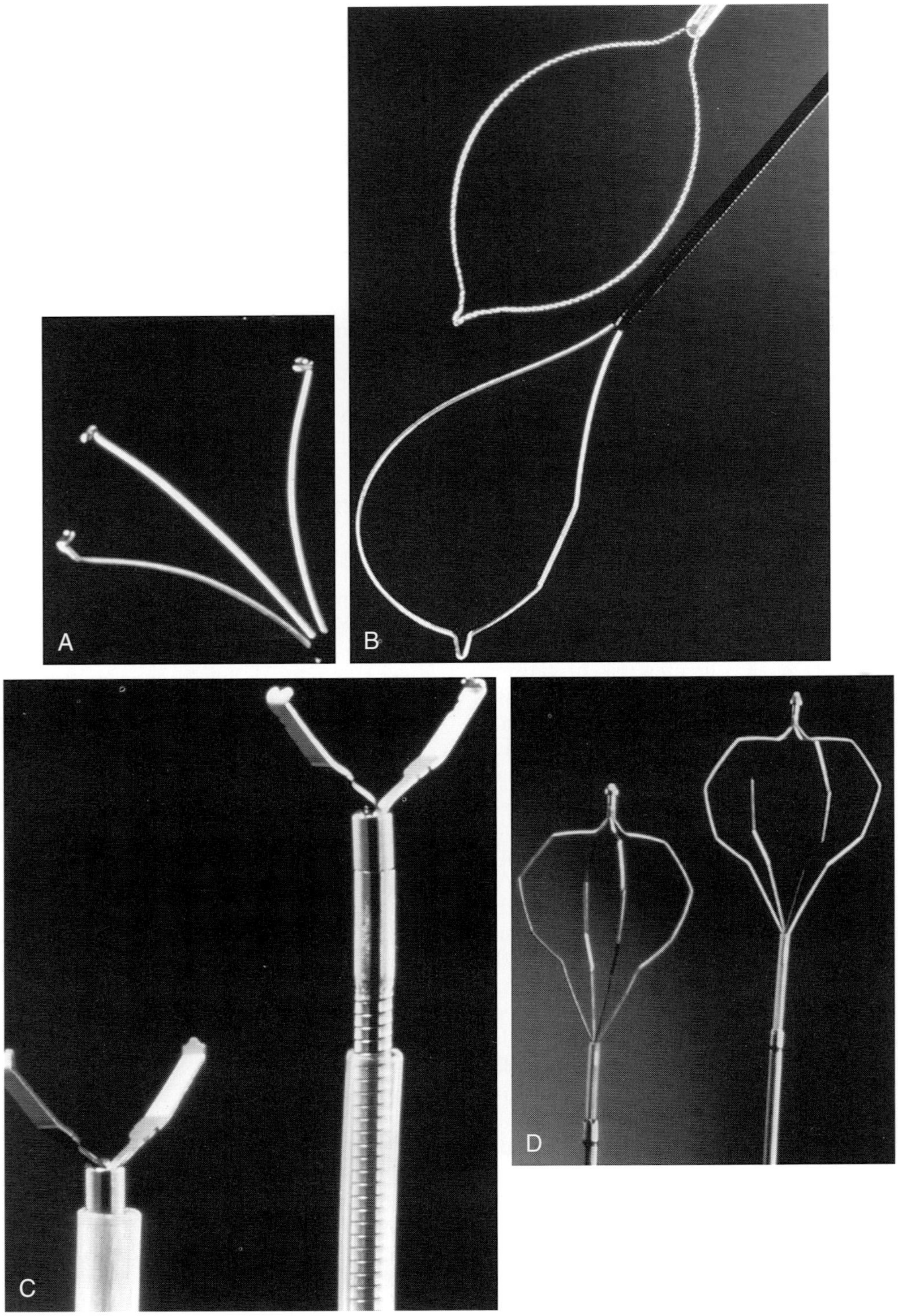

Figure 43–6 Devices available for the removal of foreign bodies. **A.** Rat-tooth forceps for grasping food or other soft objects. **B.** Basket device for grasping coins or other round objects. **C.**Three-pronged grasper used for grasping soft or irregularly shaped objects. **D.** Single snare device used to grasp soft or irregularly shaped objects. (Courtesy of Olympus America, Inc.)

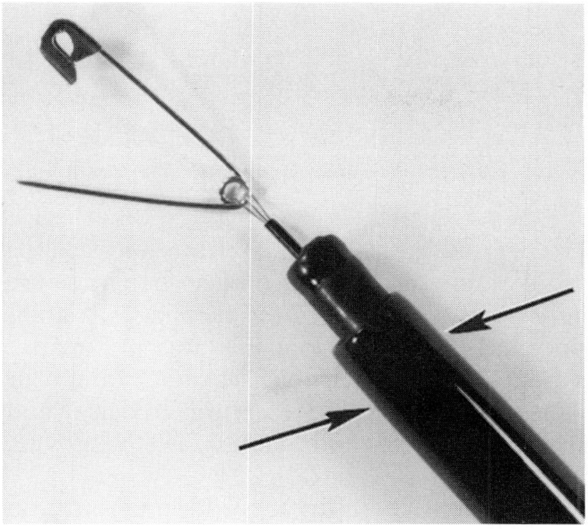

Figure 43–7 Sharp objects should be securely grasped and pulled into the overtube *(arrows),* which has been passed over the endoscope. The entire apparatus is then withdrawn. (From Wyllie R, Hyams JS: *Pediatric Gastrointestinal Disease: Pathophysiology, Diagnosis, Management.* Philadelphia, WB Saunders, 1993.)

advanced toward the foreign body. The mucosa around the object is examined for injury.

3. The object is grasped and the retrieval device is withdrawn through the endoscopic channel until the object rests against the distal end of the endoscope. If the object is sharp or irregularly shaped, it is drawn back into an overtube or modified condom catheter before being retrieved.

If the procedure is being performed with the patient under conscious sedation, a Kelly or McGill forceps and laryngoscope should be within reach. Once the object is securely grasped, the patient is placed prone and the procedure table is placed in a reverse Trendelenburg position. Then the endoscope and object are withdrawn. This way, the object is unlikely to fall into the trachea during removal if it is lost in the hypopharynx.

Occasionally, a child must have a foreign body removed from his/her colon or rectum. Depending on its size, shape, and location, the object may be removed via speculum, rigid anoscope, sigmoidoscope, colonoscope, or upper endoscope with an overtube or modified condom catheter.

Other procedures have successfully removed foreign bodies from the esophagus. Coins have been removed under fluoroscopy using a Foley catheter. The distal end of the catheter is introduced beyond the coin and the balloon is insufflated with barium. If the procedure is performed when the airway is unprotected (i.e., under conscious sedation), the patient is placed prone, in the reverse Trendelenburg position, before the catheter and coin are retrieved. Again, Kelly or McGill forceps and a laryngoscope should be on hand. Sometimes, the object cannot be easily pulled out with the catheter and a dose of glucagon is required to relax the esophageal musculature. If this fails, endoscopic removal is necessary. Fluoroscopy should not be used to remove disk batteries. Mucosal inspection is necessary because of the caustic potential of these batteries and the consequent risk of mucosal burns and perforation.

POST-PROCEDURE CARE

Recovery is similar to recovery from upper endoscopy and colonoscopy. Further management is determined by whether mucosal injury or perforation was identified. If perforation is suspected, the procedure should be followed by a contrast study, surgical consultation, placement of a nasogastric tube for gastric decompression, and the administration of broad-spectrum antibiotics: The patient should be maintained on intravenous fluids. If a significant mucosal burn resulting from disk battery ingestion was found, a contrast study of the esophagus should be performed in 3 to 4 weeks to rule out esophageal stricture formation.

COMPLICATIONS

In addition to the complications for routine upper endoscopy, foreign body removal carries an increased risk of mucosal trauma, perforation, or aspiration of all or part of the foreign body if the object becomes dislodged in an unprotected airway during retrieval through the hypopharynx.

Upper Endoscopy: Caustic Ingestion

Small children, especially children between the ages of 1 and 3 years, are at particular risk of significant injury to the oropharynx, upper airway, and especially the esophagus from the accidental ingestion of caustic substances (Fig. 43–8) (Adams and Birck, 1982). Alkali ingestion leads to liquefaction necrosis, which rapidly destroys the mucosal barrier and causes injury to the deeper muscle layers, possibly leading to perforation, especially in the thin-walled esophagus. Coagulation necrosis results from acid ingestion. Sometimes, acids cause only limited injury to the relatively alkaline esophageal mucosa but significantly harm the stomach and duodenum (Friedman, 1989).

The button battery, used in watches, toys, and calculators, is another potentially corrosive agent. Smaller batteries may pass uneventfully through the gastrointestinal tract and can be traced radiographically. Larger batteries are more likely to remain in the esophagus. Significant burns have been demonstrated in a matter of hours due to electrolyte leakage (sodium or potassium hydroxide), mercury toxicity, and current flow (Kost and Shapiro, 1987; Litovitz, 1985).

The extent of injury depends not only on the form of the caustic substance (liquid, crystalline, powdered) but also on the pH, the volume ingested, and contact time with the mucosa. Crystalline lye, for example, adheres to the oral and esophageal mucosa and often leads to severe damage. Vomiting can increase injury because the corrosive agent comes in contact a second time with an already compromised mucosa. Gastric and duodenal injury

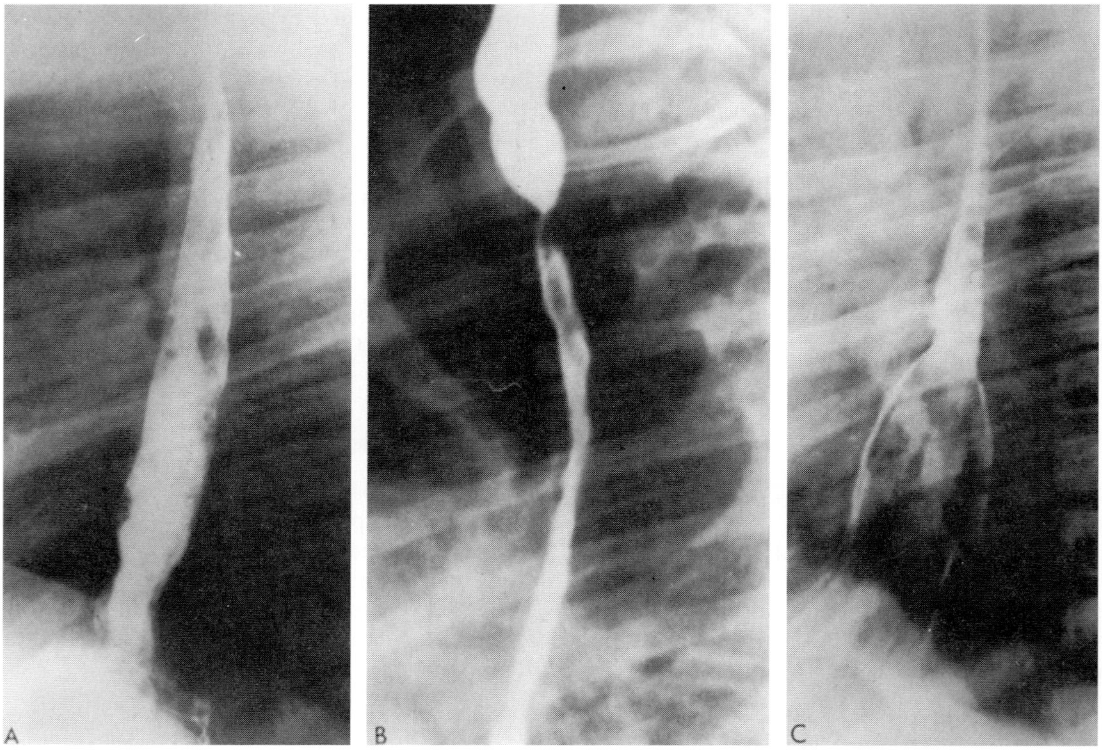

Figure 43–8 Ingestion of Drano in a 2-year-old child. **A.** Initial esophagogram made several hours after ingestion of the caustic agent shows ill-defined mucosa probably resulting from edema and mucus. **B.** Repeated esophagogram 3 weeks later shows constriction of the thoracic portion of the esophagus with more severe stricture in the proximal portion and dilatation of the cervical esophagus. **C.** Repeated esophagogram 3 months later shows esophageal stricture with retraction of the gastric cardia into the chest. (From Singleton EB, Wagner ML, Dutton RV [eds]: *Radiology of the Alimentary Tract in Infants and Children.* Philadelphia, WB Saunders, 1977, p 86.)

with later scarring may lead to gastric outlet obstruction or perforation (Friedman, 1989; Hodgson, 1959).

Powdered caustic agents, which are inhaled as well as ingested, or acids, whose bad taste increases gagging and choking, may cause additional injury, including epiglottitis, to the upper airway. Some children with concomitant airway edema and stridor require intubation or tracheostomy (Einhorn et al, 1989).

It is not possible to correlate the extent of esophageal injury to the clinical presentation of the child with a caustic ingestion. (Gaudrealt et al, 1983). Some patients with significant symptoms, such as drooling, dysphagia, pain, vomiting, and hematemesis, have been found to be free of severe injury. Conversely, esophageal burns were noted in more than half of the children with minimal symptoms (e.g., drooling only) and no oral lesions in a meta-analysis of several small series by Wason (1985).

The most significant late complication of caustic ingestion is stricture formation. Therefore, a thorough and timely evaluation must be carried out. The role of flexible upper endoscopy has become increasingly important in the diagnosis and management of these children.

INDICATIONS

Because symptoms do not always correlate with the extent of injury, many pediatric gastroenterologists use endoscopy to evaluate all children with a suspected history of caustic ingestion. Others may observe a child with no obvious signs or symptoms of injury and with a questionable history. The patient is allowed to ingest liquids and is monitored for evidence of dysphagia. Radiographic studies are too insensitive in the acute evaluation of caustic injury but may be used later to identify stricture formation (Ferguson et al, 1989).

Upper endoscopy is essential in identifying the location and extent of injury after caustic ingestion. Some endoscopists prefer to examine the patient within 12 hours. Upper endoscopy performed too soon after alkali ingestion may underestimate the extent of injury because liquefaction necrosis is a slow process; therefore, it may be better to examine the patient after 24 hours. Earlier intervention, however, may assist with the decision to use corticosteroids and antibiotics (Friedman, 1989). Most endoscopies are performed within 24 to 48 hours after injury. Compared with rigid endoscopy (which was the standard of care and is still used in some centers), the flexible endoscope carries less risk of perforation and can safely pass into the stomach and duodenum, in most cases, for more thorough inspection (Moore, 1986). The local poison control center should be contacted for product information regarding chemical content, pH, and toxicity of a suspected caustic substance.

PRECAUTIONS AND CONTRAINDICATIONS

Initial intervention for caustic ingestions is to prevent vomiting, choking, and aspiration. Usually, the child is given nothing by mouth, and intravenous fluids are administered. The use of ipecac, neutralizing agents (which may cause additional heat injury), diluting agents (which may further contribute to esophageal or airway edema), or the manual introduction of a nasogastric tube for gastric lavage (which increases risk of perforation) should be avoided (Maull et al, 1985; Wason, 1985).

Performing upper endoscopy increases the risk of perforation, especially when attempted with the patient under conscious sedation. Sudden patient movement can be hazardous. Nevertheless, upper endoscopy can be successfully carried out in selected circumstances, even in outpatients at some centers (Moore, 1986). Many pediatric gastroenterologists insist that endoscopy for caustic ingestion be performed only under general anesthesia.

The absolute and relative contraindications to performing upper endoscopy for caustic ingestion are similar to those described for routine upper endoscopy.

MEDICATIONS

The role of corticosteroids in decreasing the incidence and severity of stricture formation is debatable (Hawkins et al, 1980; Postlethwait, 1983). An initial dose of steroids is sometimes given before endoscopy. If upper endoscopy fails to show significant injury, the steroids are discontinued. Other times, steroids are given after esophageal burns have been identified endoscopically. When given, steroids are provided at 1 to 2 mg/kg/d (maximum 60 mg) for 3 to 4 weeks (Wason, 1985). Broad-spectrum antibiotics given during steroid therapy reduce the risk of infection. Bacteria quickly colonize and invade compromised esophageal tissue, and there is a risk that mediastinitis will develop.

Corticosteroids are contraindicated under certain circumstances. Stricture formation results from third-degree esophageal burns (circumferential injury with sloughing of the mucosa), and if perforation occurs, it may be masked by steroid therapy. Mediastinitis and infection may also be concealed. Furthermore, gastric necrosis and perforation can occur with acid ingestion. Once again, steroids may mask symptoms (Hawkins et al, 1980).

EQUIPMENT

The equipment used for endoscopy in caustic ingestion is the same as that used for routine upper endoscopy, although the smallest available endoscope is usually preferred when navigating a potentially compromised esophageal mucosa. In severe esophageal injury with circumferential burns or perforation, a nasogastric tube may be placed endoscopically to act as a stent to maintain luminal patency and to provide a means for enteral nutritional support. Suture material or string and a soft, small-caliber (5–10 French polyurethane or silicone) feeding tube are also required.

PROCEDURE

Upper endoscopy for caustic ingestion generally follows the same technique described for routine upper endoscopic procedures with the following qualifications:

1. The endoscope must be introduced slowly and carefully under direct visualization to minimize the risk of causing additional trauma or perforation. Generally, when an area of significant burn is encountered, the endoscope is passed no further.
2. If the lumen is obliterated from severe edema, marked tissue destruction, and perforation, the procedure is abandoned. A chest radiograph is obtained immediately to identify mediastinal air and the surgical team is consulted.
3. In a severely injured esophagus with circumferential burns, indicating that stricture formation is likely to occur, a soft, small-caliber nasogastric tube (silicone or polyurethane) may be safely introduced over an endoscopically placed guidewire and checked fluoroscopically.

When the esophagus has undergone severe and extensive injury, a fluoroscopically guided or surgically placed gastrostomy is usually indicated (a PEG cannot be placed because it must be pulled through the esophagus). A string is placed through the gastrostomy, grasped with endoscopic forceps, and pulled through the mouth as the endoscope is removed. One end of the string is taped to the abdomen, the other to the cheek. The string acts as a stent, helping to prevent obliteration of the esophageal lumen. The string is used later for repeated retrograde esophageal dilatation with Tucker dilators (Hawkins, 1988). (Refer to the section on dilation of the esophagus.) Meanwhile, the patient can be supported nutritionally via the gastrostomy tube.

POST-PROCEDURE CARE

Post-procedure recovery depends on the endoscopic findings, the overall condition of the patient, and whether conscious sedation or general anesthesia was used. Refer to the section on sedation for a discussion of post-procedure monitoring following conscious sedation. Patients who received general anesthesia are monitored in the recovery room.

If there is no evidence of esophageal burn, the child can be discharged when stable. Children with first-degree burns (hyperemia, edema, occasional superficial desquamation) are usually kept under observation for 24 to 48 hours and are slowly advanced to a soft diet. The use of antibiotics and corticosteroids in children with first-degree burns is not universally accepted; some centers provide no additional treatment (Estrera et al, 1986). When second-degree burns (mucosal sloughing, hemorrhagic exudates, pseudomembranes, and ulcerations) or third-degree burns (full-thickness burns, mediastinal or peritoneal involvement with total obliteration of the lumen) are present, antibiotics and steroids are administered (Anderson et al, 1990).

Patients with severe injury usually require close monitoring in an intensive care setting. The risk of mortality is high with deep circumferential second- and third-degree burns. Early, aggressive surgical intervention may be necessary (Estrera et al, 1986; Oakes et al, 1982). Three to 4 weeks after injury in any child with circumferential esophageal burns, an upper gastrointestinal series is performed to evaluate for stricture formation.

COMPLICATIONS

The complications associated with performing endoscopy for caustic ingestion are essentially the same as those for routine upper endoscopy, although the risk for perforation increases with the extent and severity of injury. There is also the additional risk attributable to the use of general anesthesia.

Endoscopic Retrograde Cholangiopancreatography

Endoscopic retrograde cholangiopancreatography (ERCP) is both a diagnostic and therapeutic technique that was developed to evaluate the pancreatobiliary tree in adult patients with choledocholithiasis or suspected pancreatitis. Visualization of the pancreas was previously possible via intraoperative pancreatography. With the development of a pediatric-sized duodenoscope (Olympus Corp., Lake Success, NY) this procedure can safely be performed in infants weighing as little as 2.5 kg, although the adult duodenoscope has been used in infants older than 6 months of age (Buckley and Connon, 1990; Guelrud, 1987).

ERCP is performed with a side-viewing endoscope (duodenoscope) that requires considerable skill to use. The technique is significantly more difficult to perform compared with the method used for front-viewing upper endoscopes. The operator must have an excellent sense of spatial orientation and an acquired technique for maneuvering through the pancreatobiliary tree. This section provides an overview of ERCP.

INDICATIONS

The main causes of pancreatitis in infants and children differ from those of adults (i.e., mainly gallstones or alcohol-related pancreatitis). Pancreatitis in children results from ductal malformations, infections, medications, or trauma (Ament et al, 1988). Indications for ERCP in infants and children include recurrent, acute, or chronic unexplained pancreatitis, cholestatic (obstructive) jaundice of unknown cause, and visualization and definition of pancreatobiliary tract anatomy before surgery (e.g., after blunt abdominal trauma while looking for ductal leakage or fistulas, or to identify a choledochal cyst) (Allendorph et al, 1987; Blustein et al, 1981; Marshall and Halpin, 1982; Waye, 1976). Biochemical evidence supporting the need for ERCP may include abnormalities in amylase, lipase, alkaline phosphatase, and liver function tests. Likewise, in the absence of biochemical abnormalities, ERCP is unlikely to reveal a pathological finding.

ERCP can be a valuable diagnostic or therapeutic tool for an array of diseases in the liver and pancreas. ERCP can identify both intrahepatic and extrahepatic ductular abnormalities, and the site and extent of obstruction in the liver or pancreas can be readily defined. Entities that may be identified or treated with ERCP in infants and children include the following:

1. Biliary atresia (ERCP is diagnostic and is faster compared with other imaging methods and biopsy) (Ament, 1987)
2. Caroli's disease (congenital cystic dilatation of intrahepatic ducts with cylindrical or saccular dilatations) (Perisic, 1987)
3. Alagille's syndrome (arteriohepatic dysplasia; syndromic paucity of intrahepatic ducts with characteristic facies, cardiac murmur, vertebral anomalies, and posterior embryotoxin) (Goerlick et al, 1982)
4. Nonsyndromic paucity of intrahepatic ducts (Evans, 1993):
    - Idiopathic
    - Infectious (e.g., CMV, rubella)
    - Genetic (e.g., Down, Zellweger, Ivemark's syndromes)
    - Metabolic (e.g., α1-antitrypsin deficiency, cystic fibrosis)
    - Immunologic (e.g., graft-versus-host disease, hepatic allograft rejection)
    - Endocrinologic (e.g., panhypopituitarism)
    - Sclerosing cholangitis (seen with inflammatory bowel disease)
    - Advanced cases of biliary cirrhosis
5. Cystic dilatation of biliary tree, focal biliary cirrhosis, obstructive jaundice from stones or debris, and recurrent pancreatitis in patients with cystic fibrosis (Bass et al, 1983)
6. Congenital hepatic fibrosis (irregular intrahepatic ducts with multiple small cysts in the liver)
7. Intrinsic versus extrinsic compression of pancreatobiliary tree (benign or malignant masses)
8. Hemobilia (rare; biliary tract hemorrhage) (Howdle et al, 1976)
9. Stent placement for benign or malignant

strictures (e.g., metastatic neuroblastoma) (Bickerstaff, 1989)
10. Hydatid disease (*Echinococcus granulosus* can be identified and, if indicated, treated with sphincterotomy for decompression) (Vignote et al, 1990)
11. Ascariasis (may present with obstructive jaundice; worms can be identified and retrieved) (van de Spuy, 1978)
12. *Clonorchis sinensis* (freshwater fluke; identified in biliary tree via ERCP; dilatation of distal intrahepatic bile ducts is seen) (Lin, 1987)
13. Choledocholithiasis (biliary tract stones are identifiable and retrievable)
14. Choledochal cyst (congenital malformation of biliary tree; jaundice, right upper quadrant mass, and pain inconsistent with clinical findings)
15. Pancreas divisum (may present as recurrent pancreatitis; ERCP is the only method of diagnosis)
16. Chronic relapsing pancreatitis due to anomalies and abnormalities of the pancreatobiliary ducts (ERCP can identify and localize a surgically correctable lesion)
17. Fibrosing pancreatitis (idiopathic; recurrent abdominal pain, jaundice due to biliary tract obstruction from extrinsic compression by the head of the pancreas) (Atkinson et al, 1988; McNeely et al, 1981)
18. Placement of nasobiliary or nasopancreatic drains to relieve obstruction as alternatives to surgery (Huibregtse et al, 1988; Wurbs et al, 1980)
19. Defining location of pancreatic pseudocysts before surgery (Cooney and Grosfeld, 1975; O'Neill et al, 1985)
20. Identification of ductular disruption secondary to trauma (may not be apparent at initial presentation) (Taxier et al, 1980)

CONTRAINDICATIONS

Contraindications for ERCP in pediatric patients are similar to those for adult patients, corresponding with the contraindications for upper endoscopy, with a few additional considerations. They can be categorized as absolute or relative:

Absolute

1. Shock
2. Suspected hollow viscus perforation
3. Cervical spine injury
4. Atlantoaxial subluxation (may be seen in Down syndrome)
5. Esophageal (e.g., stricture), gastric, or intestinal obstruction
6. Fever in the presence of biliary obstruction (unless performed with the immediate intent to provide ductal drainage) (Lai et al, 1989)
7. Inadequately trained personnel

Relative

1. Coagulopathy
2. Coma
3. Cardiac or pulmonary conditions further compromised by conscious sedation
4. Presence of pancreatitis or cholangitis (unless ERCP is performed as a therapeutic intervention)
5. Uncooperative or combative patient

ERCP is generally performed only in major medical centers that encounter large numbers of infants and children with suspected pancreatobiliary disease. Other imaging modalities are useful diagnostic tools in other centers. Ultrasound is a sensitive, noninvasive method to screen pediatric patients for pancreatobiliary stones or ductal dilatation. Parenchymal lesions of the liver and pancreas may be defined by computed tomography or magnetic resonance imaging but these methods are less sensitive than ERCP in defining ductal abnormalities. Radionuclide scan, ultrasound, and percutaneous liver biopsy are more accessible alternatives to ERCP and can be used to readily identify the cause of cholestatic jaundice such as in the infant with suspected biliary atresia (Riddlesberger, 1984).

Performing ERCP may not always be possible because of structural alterations that occur after surgery or anatomical abnormalities (e.g., malrotation of the small intestine). Percutaneous transhepatic cholangiography (PTC) is an alternative radiological procedure when bile ducts are of sufficient diameter to allow cannulation. PTC is limited in application because it cannot define the pancreatic duct and often poorly opacifies the distal common bile duct. There have been no controlled, randomized trials performed in pediatric patients to evaluate effectiveness. Since the introduction of the thinner Chiba needle, the efficacy and rate of complications of PTC are similar to those of

ERCP (Elias et al, 1976). In some instances, imaging modalities fail to adequately identify a pathological process, but a high level of suspicion remains for pancreatobiliary disease. An intraoperative cholangiogram or pancreatogram becomes the procedure of choice performed at laparotomy.

PREPARATION

Patient preparation is essentially the same as for upper endoscopy. No residual contrast material from previous studies should remain in the gastrointestinal tract because it may interfere with proper visualization during ERCP. Any patient undergoing ERCP must be an operative candidate as well. Generally, the surgical team is informed when ERCP is being performed because surgical back-up may later be required.

The guidelines previously described in the section on antimicrobial prophylaxis apply to ERCP. Antibiotic coverage in these circumstances should provide synergistic coverage for enteric organisms likely to cause cholangitis, usually an aminoglycoside and a third-generation cephalosporin with adequate *Pseudomonas* coverage (e.g., gentamicin and ceftazidime) (Dutta et al, 1983).

Conscious sedation such as that used for upper endoscopy is routinely used for ERCP, although general anesthesia provides better control of respiratory status and diaphragmatic excursion. In particular, small infants or children with chronic underlying disease may require general anesthesia.

Duodenal peristaltic activity can interfere with the successful cannulation of the ampulla of Vater. Glucagon, which causes smooth muscle relaxation of the gastrointestinal tract, can be administered in 0.2-mg increments to inhibit duodenal motility. It is preferred over atropine because it has fewer side effects (*Physicians' Desk Reference*, 1994).

EQUIPMENT

ERCP is routinely performed in the radiology suite because fluoroscopic visualization is an essential part of the procedure. Portable fluoroscopic units may be used in the operating room and, occasionally, in the endoscopy unit. The endoscopy unit or fluoroscopy suite should be adequately prepared with cardiopulmonary monitoring and resuscitation medications and equipment. The patient's reproductive organs should be shielded with a lead apron, and lead aprons and thyroid collars should be worn by the staff to limit radiation exposure. Needed equipment is as follows:

1. Adult- and pediatric-sized duodenoscopes (Putnam et al, 1991; Waye, 1976).
2. Cannulas (catheters)—standard, ball tip, and metal tip devices for injection of contrast material. A tapered tip cannula is useful for smaller pediatric patients. The cannula should be primed with diluted (15%–30%) Renografin before the procedure and any air bubbles (which may simulate stones under fluoroscopy) should be removed. A cannula can also be useful to obtain a bile sample for culture when cholangitis is suspected.
3. Papillotome or sphincterotome–a cannula that cuts via an electric current when therapeutic sphincterotomy is indicated (e.g., in stone removal, stent placement, or papillary stenosis).
4. Guidewires—often used to facilitate cannula placement and maintain access to the common bile duct and pancreatic duct.
5. Occlusion balloons and basket catheters—assist with retrieval of biliary tree stones and debris.
6. Cytology brushes—uncommonly used in the pediatric patient because malignancy is rare.

PROCEDURE

The following is a brief description of how diagnostic ERCP is performed:

1. An intravenous line is placed preferably in the right arm because the patient begins the procedure in the left lateral decubitus position with the left arm placed behind his/her back.
2. A pulse oximeter is attached to the patient and vital signs are recorded.
3. A local anesthetic agent is administered to anesthetize the hypopharynx (as described in the section on upper endoscopy), and a protective bite block is secured between the teeth.
4. After adequate conscious sedation is obtained, the esophagus is blindly intubated with the duodenoscope.
5. The distal esophagus is inspected for varices and the stomach is quickly examined (with minimal insufflation to minimize discomfort) because the duodenoscope is advanced through the pylorus. If prior upper endoscopy has not been performed, the stomach may be more carefully examined.

6. The duodenal bulb is briefly examined and the endoscope is then maneuvered into the descending portion of the duodenum. The ampulla of Vater is typically found on the medial wall of the duodenum and brought into close proximity to the side-viewing "window" of the duodenoscope to facilitate cannulation.
7. The patient is placed in the prone position to provide better access to the ampulla. Glucagon is usually administered to decrease peristalsis through the duodenum.
8. With proper positioning, the cannula is advanced a few millimeters into the ampulla and a small amount of contrast material is injected (1–2 ml renografin). Fluoroscopy identifies whether the pancreatic or common bile duct is being filled. Films are obtained as each duct is identified fluoroscopically.
9. With the patient (prone) placed in a reverse Trendelenburg position, the proximal hepatic ducts are more easily filled with contrast (Waye, 1976).
10. The duodenoscope is removed after films are obtained and the patient is placed supine to better visualize the distal common bile duct and the right hepatic ductular system.

In brief, the ampulla is cannulated in a similar fashion to diagnostic ERCP, except that a papillotome (a modified cannula for cutting) is used and is usually powered by the same electrocautery equipment used for colonoscopic polypectomy. Sphincterotomy or papillotomy is necessary for stone removal with balloon or basket devices, or stent placement over a guidewire is required to improve drainage as with benign pancreatic strictures. The use of stents to manage benign disease (which require regular replacement over the years) must be weighed against performing a corrective surgical procedure.

Fluoroscopy is a technique with high radiation exposure, so actual fluoroscopic view time should be kept to a minimum. In addition to the radiation risk to the patient and staff, fluoroscopy shortens the life of the fiberoptic bundles in the duodenoscope.

POST-PROCEDURE CARE

Patient recovery after ERCP is similar to that of other endoscopic procedures, with continuous cardiorespiratory monitoring via pulse oximetry provided until the patient is awake and alert. Post-procedure vital signs are recorded. In the presence of obstruction to the common bile duct or pancreatic duct, contrast material does not adequately drain, increasing the risk of cholangitis, so antibiotics should be administered.

COMPLICATIONS

Complications associated with ERCP, although uncommon, may not be insignificant. The most common complication of diagnostic ERCP in adults is pancreatitis (LaFerla et al, 1986). Amylase and lipase levels are often elevated after cannulation and injection of the pancreatic duct, but biochemical abnormalities rarely translate into clinical evidence of pancreatitis (Brandes et al, 1981; Okuno et al, 1985). In a large, multicenter retrospective analysis of adults who had undergone ERCP, a correlation existed between the level of experience of the endoscopist and the complication rate (Bilbao et al, 1976). The amount and force with which contrast is injected, and the degree of ductular manipulation each increase the risk of complications (Roszler and Campbell, 1985).

Few studies in children have attempted to define the incidence of complications associated with ERCP. In a study by Guelrud et al (1987), the most common complication was respiratory depression, probably secondary to oversedation and compression of the trachea reported in 10% of infants. Another series reported an 8% incidence of mild pancreatitis from 42 ERCPs performed in 37 children, but these three children did not have a prior history of pancreatitis (Putnam et al, 1991).

Cholangitis is also a reported serious complication of ERCP in adults, especially in the presence of biliary obstruction (Lai, 1989). This warrants the administration of prophylactic antimicrobial coverage or, when unsuspected obstruction is identified at the time of ERCP, antibiotics are subsequently provided. There are no reports of death following ERCP in the pediatric population, which is probably because pediatric candidates for ERCP are generally not as ill (malignancy is rare) and, overall, had less invasive therapeutic ERCPs performed compared with adults.

Other complications reported with ERCP include perforation or hemorrhage associated with sphincterotomy, stone retrieval, traumatic use of guidewires, and stent placement or removal (Nebel et al, 1975). Perforation can occur into the peritoneal cavity, which is readily identified radiographically. If a perforation is suspected, the procedure is immediately abandoned, nasogastric suction, intravenous fluids, and antibiotics are administered, and a surgical consult is obtained. Retroperitoneal perforation may be insidious and may be overlooked during ERCP (Martin and Tweedle, 1990). In the patient who develops increasing abdominal pain, fever, and an elevated white blood cell count in the absence of significantly elevated amylase and lipase levels over several days following ERCP, a retroperitoneal perforation should be suspected.

ERCP cannot be performed using sterile technique because the duodenoscope passes through a contaminated oropharynx, transferring potential pathogens into the biliary tree. Careful consideration must be given to all patients who may benefit from antimicrobial prophylaxis, even if they fall outside the guidelines put forth by the American Heart Association (see section on antimicrobial prophylaxis). Previously, infections due to *Pseudomonas aeruginosa* were shown to be associated with improperly sterilized equipment and contaminated water bottles, so proper cleaning and disinfection of equipment and accessories is imperative (Classen et al, 1988).

Finally, ERCP is an expensive, invasive procedure with limited availability for infants and children. Nevertheless, it should be considered when other, less invasive and conventional modalities are untimely or have failed. In certain situations, such as attempting to make the diagnosis of biliary atresia in a 2-month-old infant, it is the procedure of choice (when available). A 5- to 7-day period is needed to obtain an appropriate radionuclide scan (HIDA or DSIDA scan) because the infant must be "primed" with phenobarbital to promote bile flow. With an adjunctive percutaneous liver biopsy, diagnosis can be delayed for up to 2 weeks. Performing the Kasai procedure (hepatoportoenterostomy) after 2 months of age, which has been shown to decrease morbidity and mortality in these infants, has a significantly less favorable outcome (Mowat et al, 1976).

Endoscopic Control of Gastrointestinal Bleeding in Children: Variceal Bleeding

Injection sclerotherapy has been used successfully in children for many years (Howard et al, 1984). It can be an effective technique for the control of acute esophageal variceal bleeding, and, when performed prophylactically, it can decrease the frequency of recurrent variceal bleeding (Hill and Bowie, 1991). Sclerotherapy may be tried first, before vasoactive agents such as vasopressin and somatostatin infusions. Long-term outcome for the control of variceal hemorrhage with sclerotherapy appears to be comparable with the outcome achieved with portocaval shunting (Korula et al, 1985; Planas et al, 1991).

Sclerotherapy has several advantages over surgical shunting procedures. It can be performed at the bedside in the pediatric intensive care unit (PICU) and has a lower incidence of hepatic encephalopathy after the procedure. It eliminates the risk of shunt thrombosis, which is more likely to occur in young children with smaller-caliber blood vessels than in older children and adults. It can be used repeatedly, allowing time for collateral vessels to develop that can act as natural shunts, decreasing portal pressure and lowering the risk of bleeding. This may also give the child time to grow until he/she becomes a more appropriate candidate for a surgical shunt (Ament and Vargas, 1991).

INDICATIONS

Sclerotherapy is indicated in those patients with portal hypertension who (1) have acute esophageal variceal hemorrhage, (2) have recurrent variceal bleeding, (3) have variceal bleeding and are poor surgical candidates, and (4) have decompensated liver disease. Sclerotherapy may also be performed prophylactically in children with a history of variceal bleeding to prevent further bleeding episodes.

The source of bleeding must be determined endoscopically in any patient with known or suspected variceal hemorrhage; up to 50% of bleeding episodes in these patients occur from nonvariceal sources such as erosive esophagitis and peptic ulceration (Dagradi et al, 1970).

CONTRAINDICATIONS

Endoscopic injection of esophageal varices under conscious sedation should not be attempted in uncooperative, combative patients. If adequate conscious sedation or general anesthesia cannot be safely provided, sclerotherapy should not be attempted. Any coagulopathy must be corrected before performing injection sclerotherapy. Otherwise, the same contraindications as for routine upper endoscopy apply.

ANTIBIOTIC PROPHYLAXIS

The recommendations outlined in the section on antimicrobial prophylaxis for gastrointestinal procedures apply to patients requiring sclerotherapy. In addition, some gastroenterologists prefer prophylaxis in those patients with decompensated liver disease or hepatic failure. There is a five- to seven-times greater incidence of bacteremia in patients with chronic liver disease than in other hospitalized patients, due to their impaired ability to remove bacteria from the blood stream, their impaired reticuloendothelial system phagocytosis, and their defective serum bacteriocidal and opsonic activity (Fieror and Finley, 1979; Graudal et al, 1986; Rimola et al, 1984; Ruttenberg et al, 1959; Wycke et al, 1983). Gram-positive organisms such as *Streptococcus pneumoniae*, *Staphylococcus aureus*, and group A beta-hemolytic streptococcus are the most common in children and adults with fulminant hepatic failure. *Escherichia coli* is the most commonly encountered gram-negative organism in this group of patients (Larcher et al, 1982). Broad-spectrum antibiotic coverage with a second-generation cephalosporin or vancomycin and an aminoglycoside should be administered.

SEDATION AND MEDICATIONS

In the cooperative patient without liver failure, routine conscious sedation has been safely used. In the uncooperative or combative patient, general anesthesia is necessary. General anesthesia may also be more appropriate when there is uncontrolled, massive bleeding and the airway must be protected against possible aspiration.

Atropine is often given before the procedure to decrease secretions, and glucagon is administered to inhibit esophageal peristalsis for better isolation of the varices.

PATIENT PREPARATION

In emergent sclerotherapy, gastric lavage using a large-bore orogastric tube (e.g., a Salem sump) should be performed to remove blood, clots, and any food debris that might clog the working channel of the endoscope. When sclerotherapy is being performed electively as prophylaxis for rebleeding, the patient is given nothing by mouth as described in the section on routine upper endoscopy. Laboratory tests should include a complete blood count and coagulation studies, and in emergent procedures, blood should be typed and crossmatched. A large-caliber intravenous line should be placed in those patients requiring emergent sclerotherapy in case cardiovascular resuscitation or blood products are required.

EQUIPMENT

Standard pediatric upper endoscopes are used for sclerotherapy. A disposable 23-gauge, 4-mm sheathed sclerotherapy needle is inspected, tested, and loaded with sclerosant before it is introduced into the endoscope.

A variety of sclerosing agents are used: sodium morrhuate, tetradecylsulfate, hypertonic glucose or saline, ethanolamine oleate, ethanol, or combinations of these solutions (Kochhar et al, 1990). The procedure can be performed under fluoroscopy with contrast material added to the sclerosant to assess more accurately whether a varix has been injected. Or, a pressure gauge can be connected to the sclerotherapy needle to detect intravariceal pressure when the varix is entered. An endoscopic overtube with a "window" at its distal end may be used to isolate each varix for injection.

The water stream dispensed via the control button of the endoscope is insufficient in force and volume to effectively clear large amounts of blood from the field of view. Therefore, a large-volume (50-ml) syringe connected to a blunt needle and filled with sterile water should be available. Some gastroenterologists use a pressurized water system that, like the syringe, operates through the working channel of the endoscope.

A Sengstaken-Blakemore, Minnesota, or Nicolas-Linton tube should be pretested and available in case emergent sclerotherapy or vasoactive medications fail to control variceal hemorrhage (see section on use of balloon tamponade). Protective eyewear should be worn by all endoscopy personnel and eye covers should be provided for the patient because accidental spraying of sclerosant may occur during injection. Whenever sclerosant is being injected, the syringe should be pointed away from the patient and personnel.

PROCEDURE

1. If sclerotherapy is performed with the patient under conscious sedation, a topical anesthetic is applied to the patient's oropharynx to reduce the risk of gagging and retching, which may increase the risk of bleeding. Conscious sedation is typically used for prophylactic procedures; general anesthesia is administered for most acute variceal bleeding in order to protect the airway.
2. The endoscope (with or without the overtube) is passed under direct visualization; the esophageal mucosa is carefully inspected for sources of bleeding.
3. The stomach and proximal duodenum are similarly examined. If no other source of bleeding is found, the endoscope is withdrawn into the distal portion of the esophagus and positioned just proximal to the bleeding varix or varices. When prophylactic sclerotherapy is being done, the endoscope is positioned just proximal to the most distal varix.
4. The "windowed" overtube is advanced beyond the distal end of the endoscope to cover the varices. It is slowly rotated until a varix protrudes into the lumen through the "window" or slot in the wall of the overtube.
5. The pretested, preloaded sheathed injection needle is advanced to the varix. Abutting the sheath against the distal end of the varix, causing a slight indentation, reduces the risk of a mucosal tear. A protruding, misguided injection needle can cause significant bleeding.
6. The needle is pushed into the most distal portion of the varix (usually less than 5 mm to minimize local and systemic complications). Because blood flows cephalad in esophageal varices, it is more effective to inject sclerosant at the base of the varix. One to 3 ml of sclerosant is injected. The needle is held in place for 30 to 60 seconds. Blanching or discoloration commonly occur after injection of sclerosant. Although it is not always possible, variceal rather than paravariceal injection is preferred because it causes less stricture formation.
7. The overtube can be rotated to provide tamponade to the varix that was just injected as the next varix appears through the window. The procedure is repeated until all varices are sclerosed or until the maximum volume of sclerosant safely allowable in one session has been administered.

As a rule of thumb, the total volume of sclerosant used during one procedure should not exceed 10 ml in infants, 20 ml in small children, and 30 ml in older children and adolescents.

If bleeding continues after injection when no overtube is used, the endoscope can be advanced beyond the varix and held in place for 1 to 2 minutes to tamponade the lesion. An additional injection of sclerosant below the bleeding site may be required if bleeding persists.

If varices are not prophylactically obliterated after 5 or 6 sessions, sclerotherapy is unlikely to be effective. Gastric varices do not respond to sclerotherapy. In an acutely bleeding gastric varix, a Sengstaken-Blakemore, Minnesota, or Nicolas-Linton tube may be required to provide tamponade. If gastric varices appear after esophageal sclerotherapy, further sclerotherapy will be ineffective and may actually increase the risk of gastric bleeding. When this occurs, surgical intervention (e.g., portocaval shunting) for decompression is the procedure of choice.

Balloon tamponade is rarely required. Whether injection sclerotherapy succeeds depends on several factors: the severity of portal hypertension, the degree of decompensated liver disease, and the ability of the endoscopist to identify, isolate, and treat the source of bleeding.

POST-PROCEDURE CARE

Vital signs and evidence of gastrointestinal bleeding are monitored. In the stable patient, clear liquids only are given for 24 hours, followed by a soft diet for 24 to 48 hours. If the soft diet is tolerated, the patient may return to a regular diet. The unstable patient is given nothing by mouth and is closely monitored in an intensive care setting; a surgical team is consulted.

At 6 and 24 hours after the procedure, a

hematocrit is obtained. Antacids or a sucralfate slurry (which adheres to ulcerated, eroded, sloughed, or abraded areas in the esophagus), and an H_2-antagonist are administered for 5 days to promote healing.

COMPLICATIONS

Sclerotherapeutic injection of esophageal varices carries a considerable risk of complication, including hemorrhage at the injection site from a needle-induced mucosal tear (common), esophageal ulceration (2%), esophageal stricture (2%), left pleural effusion (1.5%), mucosal sloughing (0.5%), and esophageal perforation (0.7%) (Donovan et al, 1986; Vane et al, 1985).

Many patients have retrosternal chest pain that lasts for several days after the procedure. An early post-procedure complaint of dysphagia may indicate altered esophageal peristalsis due to procedure-related inflammation; late-onset dysphagia, although rare, may indicate stricture formation (Cohen et al, 1985).

Colonoscopy

INDICATIONS

Colonoscopy in the pediatric patient is useful in differentiating a diffuse inflammatory process (e.g., colitis) from a focal lesion (e.g., juvenile polyp). In infants and children, the most common indications for colonoscopy are rectal bleeding (hematochezia, melena, or occult bleeding), chronic diarrhea of unknown cause, and suspected inflammatory bowel disease (e.g., abdominal pain, decreased weight, or decreased height velocity) (Kawamitsu et al, 1989; Williams et al, 1982). The major cause of rectal bleeding in children is juvenile polyps, which typically present with asymptomatic hematochezia and, in one third of cases, evidence of microcytic, hypochromic anemia secondary to chronic blood loss (Harris, 1967; Silverberg, 1970). These polyps generally do not become malignant but, rarely, adenomatous polyps have been reported in children (Cynamon et al, 1989). Children with more than five colonic polyps should be evaluated for hereditary gastrointestinal polyposis syndromes (Haggitt and Reed, 1986).

Nodular lymphoid hyperplasia is another common cause of rectal bleeding in infants and children who complain of mild, intermittent abdominal pain. Lymphoid nodules are readily identified either endoscopically in the colon or by barium enema (Kaplan et al, 1984). Bleeding from vascular lesions is more commonly found in adults. Nevertheless, when it does occur in children, colonoscopy is a sensitive method to detect and ablate the lesions (Trudel et al, 1988). In infants (usually younger than 6 months of age), allergic colitis (cow's milk or soy milk allergy) should be considered when rectal bleeding, with or without diarrhea, occurs (Jenkins et al, 1984). Uncommonly, allergic colitis occurs in breast-fed infants (Lake et al, 1982).

Infants and small children with upper gastrointestinal bleeding often present with rectal bleeding. Upper gastrointestinal sources of bleeding should be ruled out before proceeding with colonoscopy. Also, before performing colonoscopy in children with rectal bleeding or diarrhea of unknown origin, infectious causes should be ruled out by microscopic examination of the stool for white cells, stool bacterial culture, ova and parasite examination, and assay for *Clostridium difficile* toxin. In the immunocompromised host, a number of pathogenic organisms may be involved, including *Candida*, atypical mycobacteria, cryptosporidia, adenovirus, and CMV (Cello, 1988; Meyers, 1990).

Chronic diarrhea in a child with associated weight loss and no infection or immunocompromised state should be investigated for inflammatory bowel disease. Colonoscopy with biopsy is a good way to detect the type and extent of disease in the colon and terminal ileum. It can also be used to observe entities that carry a malignant potential, such as ulcerative colitis or familial polyposis coli (Deschner and Lipkin, 1975; Lashner et al, 1990). Surveillance colonoscopy is recommended every 1 to 2 years for patients who have had pancolitis for more than 7 years or left-sided colitis for longer than 15 years, owing to increased risk of malignant change (Nugent et al, 1991).

Gastrointestinal tuberculosis, like Crohn's disease, is often localized to the ileocecal area and can be distinguished by colonoscopy with biopsy. Characteristic caseating granulomas and acid-fast bacilli are readily identifiable histologically (Bretholz et al, 1987; Rossi, 1988).

Other diagnostic indications for colonoscopy in children include severe abdominal pain of unknown cause, follow-up of abnormality identified by barium enema, family history of hereditary polyposis syndromes, and intraoperative localization of a lesion not identifiable by palpation or gross inspection.

Therapeutic procedures done by colonoscopy include the following: (1) polypectomy, (2) control of bleeding (e.g., in vascular anomalies, ulcerations, polypectomy sites) by electrocautery, heater probe, laser, or injection sclerotherapy, (3) foreign body removal, (4) decompression of acute, nontoxic megacolon, and (5) balloon dilation of stenotic lesions (e.g., anastomotic strictures) (Bines and Winter, 1991).

Colonoscopy is rarely diagnostic and is not generally indicated in children with chronic abdominal pain who have normal clinical findings, radiographic examinations, and laboratory parameters (Hassal et al, 1984).

Colonoscopy is not always initially the procedure of choice. In children with ongoing, moderate to severe gastrointestinal bleeding (when the rate of bleeding is suspected to be greater than 0.1 ml/min), a ^{99m}Tc sulfur colloid radionuclide scan or labeled red cell scan should be considered first (Winzelberg et al, 1983). Barium enema or hyperemia and bowel inflammation due to bowel preparation and colonoscopy may obscure the ability of the radionuclide test to localize the lesion (Rossi, 1988). Barium enema or upper gastrointestinal series with small bowel follow-through may complement colonoscopy when the terminal ileum is not visualized and inflammatory bowel disease is suspected. If scintigraphy or a barium study is not being considered, whole bowel irrigation with an ethylene glycol solution can be used to prepare a patient with active lower gastrointestinal bleeding for emergent colonoscopy (Caos et al, 1986).

Indications for flexible proctosigmoidoscopy are virtually the same as for colonoscopy. Colonoscopy is technically more difficult to perform than proctosigmoidoscopy, however. Rigid sigmoidoscopes are available for use in infants and children but have been used rarely since the introduction of flexible pediatric endoscopy.

CONTRAINDICATIONS

Although colonoscopy is safe in infants and children when performed by an experienced pediatric gastroenterologist, there are risks of bleeding and perforation. Contraindications are listed below as absolute and relative:

Absolute

1. Possible perforated viscus
2. Peritonitis or marked abdominal tenderness
3. Toxic or fulminant colitis
4. Inadequately trained personnel

Relative

1. Bowel inadequately prepared (prevents proper visualization and maneuvering: pathologic condition is easily missed; lengthens procedure time owing to removal of stool; stool adherent to the lens of the colonoscope requires insufflation of additional air and water; retained stool and liquid in the colon during polypectomy increases the risk of adjacent mucosal damage during electrocautery and risks igniting flammable colonic gases) (Taylor et al, 1981)
2. Massive gastrointestinal bleeding (visualization difficult and risk of perforation greater with potentially compromised bowel integrity)
3. History of recent bowel surgery (weak anastomotic site)
4. Abnormalities in adjacent organs, such as aneurysm of the abdominal or ileac aorta, splenomegaly (maneuvering of colonoscope may lead to trauma and bleeding in these organs)
5. Partial or complete intestinal obstruction
6. Coagulopathy
7. Neutropenia
8. Patients with connective tissue disorders (e.g., Ehlers-Danlos syndrome, Marfan's syndrome) have greater risk of bowel perforation
9. Severe or unstable medical conditions (e.g., cardiovascular or pulmonary disease)
10. Uncooperative/combative patient

BOWEL PREPARATION

Colonoscopy is usually performed as an outpatient procedure, and most children are prepared at home. However, some children (e.g., patients with severe mental retardation or chronic underlying disease) may require hospitalization for safe and effective cleanout (i.e., bowel cleansing). Several bowel preparation regimens are available. The age and condition of the patient and his/her preference often determine the method. The child with chronic constipation requires more extensive preparation, whereas the child with diarrhea may need only minimal preparation.

Infants who are exclusively breast-fed or formula-fed can be adequately prepared by substituting clear liquids for 12 to 24 hours before the procedure. Administration of one or two pediatric-sized saline enemas before the procedure is usually necessary to evacuate any residual stool, especially in older infants whose diet includes solid foods. By giving the infant nothing by mouth for 3 to 4 hours before the procedure, the risk of reflux and aspiration is avoided; intravenous glucose may be administered in sick newborns or premature infants to avoid hypoglycemia.

In children and adolescents, a liquid and clear, soft (gelatin) diet is instituted for 48 to 72 hours before the procedure, and magnesium citrate (1 ounce per age in years to a maximum of 10 ounces) is taken the night before. Some children find magnesium citrate distasteful and experience considerable crampy abdominal pain. Bisacodyl tablets (Dulcolax, Boehringer Ingleheim Pharmaceuticals, Ridgefield, CT) are better tolerated and can be given as follows: 5 mg for children younger than 4 years, 10 mg for 4- to 10-year-olds, and 20 mg for children older than 10 years. The child should be fasted for 6 to 8 hours and given an enema the morning of the colonoscopy.

In children older than 5 years of age and in adolescents, colonic lavage solutions made with nonabsorbable macromolecule polyethylene glycol are sometimes preferred because they provide excellent cleanout and visualization. The solutions—GoLytely and NuLytely (Braintree Laboratories, Inc., Braintree, MA) and Colyte and Colyte-Flavored (Reed & Carnick, Inc., Jersey City, NJ)—differ slightly in composition (NuLytely contains no sulfate), but all have an osmolality of about 280 mOsm/L. These solutions cause an osmotic diarrhea without risking significant loss of fluids or electrolytes (dehydration) or causing fluid overload (Lee et al, 1987; Vila et al, 1987).

The drawbacks to using these solutions are that a large volume is required (as much as 3 to 4 L for an adult-sized adolescent), the solutions must be ingested over a relatively short period of time, and they are significantly more costly than the previously mentioned methods. The total volume required for children is based on weight as follows (Bines and Winter, 1991):

1. < 10 kg: 1100 ml (480 ml/h)
2. 10–20 kg: 1600 ml (600 ml/h)
3. 20–30 kg: 2200 ml (840 ml/h)
4. 30–40 kg: 2900 ml (1080 ml/h)
5. 40–50 kg: 3200 ml (1200 ml/h)
6. > 50 kg: 4000 ml (2240 ml/h)

If the solution is taken orally, the child should drink one fourth of the hourly volume every 10 to 15 minutes. Many children find the solution unpalatable even when it is chilled, but flavoring should not be added because it alters the electrolyte composition and can lead to dehydration. The solution may also be instilled via nasogastric tube. Nausea, vomiting, abdominal distention, and cramping are commonly reported in children during infusion; these can be alleviated with a prior dose of metoclopramide (Tolia et al, 1984). The infusion is sometimes better tolerated if started at a slightly lower hourly rate, which is increased every half hour until the desired rate is achieved. Cleanout is complete when clear, watery effluent is seen.

The infusion of large volumes of ethylene glycol solutions is contraindicated when bowel obstruction is suspected. Purgatives, such as magnesium citrate, and saline enemas should be used with caution in patients with congestive heart failure or renal insufficiency. Enemas should be avoided in infants and children suspected to have colitis because hyperemia, edema, petechiae, mucus depletion, and nonspecific inflammatory changes may make diagnosis difficult (Vanderhoof and Ament, 1976).

Before the procedure (and sedation), it is important to assess cleanout by digital rectal examination. Viscous lidocaine (2%) may be used as lubricant to lessen discomfort in children with perianal disease. If liquid stool is present, an enema should be administered and the patient reevaluated. If solid stool is present, the preparation should be considered incomplete and the procedure rescheduled. As discussed, performing colonoscopy in an inadequately prepared colon carries risks and may not provide needed diagnostic information.

BIOPSY, CYTOLOGY, AND CULTURE

Important histopathological information can be obtained by biopsy or culture through the colonoscope, even when the endoscopist does not visualize an apparent abnormality. Infection, inflammation, and malignancy can be differentiated, although colonic malignancy is rare in pediatric patients. Grasp biopsy usually provides sufficient tissue for evaluation of mucosal pathology.

Acute, self-limited infectious colitis can be distinguished from chronic or recurrent ulcerative colitis or idiopathic inflammatory bowel disease by biopsy (Nostrant et al, 1987; Surawicz and Belie, 1984). A sputum trap placed temporarily in line with the suction tubing attached near the endoscopic control panel enables collection of bacterial cultures, which can identify *Yersinia enterocolitica* or *Mycobacterium tuberculosis*, for example, in the ileocecal area (Aoki et al, 1975; Matsumoto et al, 1990).

Dysplastic changes can be readily identified by biopsy (Collins et al, 1987).

It is sometimes necessary to collect biopsy samples of grossly normal-appearing mucosa. Certain disease entities such as early inflammatory bowel disease, collagenous colitis, and amyloidosis may be identified in this manner (Geboes and Vantrappen, 1975; Gilat et al, 1969; Salt and Llaneza, 1986; Sanderson et al, 1986). Schistosomiasis can be identified by rectal biopsy specimen, which is pressed immediately between two glass slides (not fixed in formalin) for examination under the microscope at low power (Mahmoud and Wahab, 1990).

PROCEDURE

1. Adequacy of cleanout should be assessed by digital rectal examination before sedation is given. This serves also to prepare the patient for insertion of the colonoscope, to provide lubrication, and to assess the presence of any pathological condition such as an anal fissure or rectal polyp.
2. The patient is placed in the left lateral position, with his/her head at the foot of the procedure table. The endoscopist is at the left side of the table. As with upper endoscopy, infants and young children should be wrapped in a sheet or blanket for security and comfort, and to lessen risk of injury during the procedure.
3. While the assistant holds the control end of the colonoscope, the lubricated tip of the colonoscope is inserted. One hand is used to separate the buttocks and the other to insert the instrument. The patient should be asked to bear down, as in the act of defecation, to make introduction of the colonoscope easier. This step should be explained to the child beforehand, and at the time of insertion. Slight resistance is encountered when passing the instrument through the internal anal sphincter. The external portion of the colonoscope adjacent to the anal verge is lubricated throughout the procedure to decrease resistance and patient discomfort.
4. With air insufflation, the rectal mucosa is visualized. It normally has semicircular folds (valves of Houston, more easily appreciated on scope withdrawal) unlike the circular muscle rings seen in the ascending or descending colon, and the triangular pattern in the transverse colon. The normal rectal mucosa is translucent and submucosal, bluish vessels are apparent.
5. The patient often experiences discomfort as the sigmoid colon is negotiated because of its redundancy and because, like the transverse colon, the sigmoid colon is attached to mesentery and is freely movable. In general, the colonoscope is advanced under direct visualization with the judicious use of air insufflation (the bowel, however, is less rigid and, thus, more easily transversed). Less patient discomfort occurs when less air is used during endoscopic travel toward the cecum.
6. The colonoscope has a tendency to loop in the sigmoid and, sometimes, in the transverse colon; it sometimes gets stalled at the splenic and hepatic flexures. Experienced endoscopists use a variety of maneuvers to unloop and advance their instruments. The endoscopy assistant can apply abdominal pressure to the left pelvic area to assist passage through the sigmoid or left upper quadrant pressure to help negotiate the splenic flexure.
7. The descending colon appears narrow and tubular near its proximal end where an occasional bluish mucosa identifies the spleen.
8. The transverse colon is entered after an abrupt, difficult angulation requiring considerable endoscopic torquing and maneuvering. It is usually readily negotiated unless a more distal portion of colon (e.g., sigmoid) is looped and distended with the colonoscope.

9. The hepatic flexure is recognized by a widening of the lumen and a typical bluish discoloration from the adjacent liver.
10. By aspirating air and taking a deep breath, the patient can assist passage of the colonoscope into the ascending colon, which characteristically has a large lumen and asymmetric folds. In small or thin pediatric patients, light emitted from the distal tip of the colonoscope can be seen in the right lower quadrant (just above the right inguinal ligament) signifying arrival at the cecum, which sometimes is difficult to recognize endoscopically.
11. Appendiceal and ileocecal valve orifices are recognized when angulation of the colonoscope and slight air insufflation separates mucosal folds that may obscure their openings. Cannulation of the ileum can be difficult and requires operator experience. In pediatric patients, the ileum typically has a fine, stippled appearance due to lymphoid follicles. This should not be mistaken for the larger "cobblestoning" seen with small bowel involvement in Crohn's disease.
12. The endoscopist can evaluate the colon and rectum more thoroughly on withdrawal of the colonoscope, although polypectomy may be carried out as the polyps are encountered. Specimens are obtained by grasp biopsy, brush biopsy, or culture (by aspiration). The colon is slowly and thoroughly examined as the colonoscope is carefully withdrawn. Removal of the colonoscope must be controlled in order to prevent mucosa from rushing through the field of view and limiting the evaluation.
13. Retroflexion of the colonoscope in the rectum allows the endoscopist to examine the rectal mucosa more thoroughly for evidence of hemorrhoids, fissures, inflammation, and other lesions that may have been overlooked.
14. Therapeutic colonoscopic procedures such as foreign body removal (similar to esophageal foreign body removal), polypectomy, electrocautery, or thermocautery for lower gastrointestinal bleeding (Wyllie and Kay, 1993) are discussed elsewhere.

POST-PROCEDURE CARE

Post-procedure care is similar to that for upper endoscopy, but the patient usually requires a longer post-procedure period of monitoring due to the greater total dosage of sedative medications. Intravenous fluids can be continued during recovery. Post-procedure vital signs are recorded and the patient remains connected to a pulse oximeter for cardiorespiratory monitoring. Written discharge instructions and an emergency telephone number are provided. A follow-up appointment (in writing) for discussion of the biopsy results should be arranged. If colonoscopy was performed as an outpatient procedure, the child should be given nothing by mouth until he/she arrives home because meperidine frequently causes post-procedure nausea and vomiting.

COMPLICATIONS

Complications associated with colonoscopy in children are related to bowel preparation, sedation, and the procedure itself (similar to those described in adults) as follows:

Bowel Preparation

1. Nausea and vomiting (especially with large volume, ethylene glycol lavage solutions)
2. Abdominal distention and cramping
3. Fluid and electrolyte imbalance (especially in smaller children or with prolonged fasting and repeated saline enemas)

Sedation

1. Respiratory depression (transient respiratory arrest) (Hassal et al, 1984)
2. Thrombophlebitis (minimized by dilution of midazolam and meperidine before administration)
3. Nausea and vomiting (post-procedure)

Procedure

1. Bleeding (usually minimal with diagnostic colonoscopy and biopsy; more common following polypectomy; may occur immediately or 5 to 14 days later when the fibrin clot dislodges; on rare occasions, requires cautery or surgical intervention to control) (Macrae et al, 1983)
2. Perforation (four reported cases in pediatric patients, usually related to polypectomy) (Gans et al, 1975; Holgersen et al, 1978; Overholt et al, 1976)

3. Abdominal cramping and distention
4. Infection (bacterial endocarditis)
5. Diastatic mucosal tears (without perforation) (Livstone et al, 1974)
6. "Post-polypectomy syndrome" or "colon coagulation syndrome" (fever, localized abdominal pain, and leukocytosis occurring 12 to 24 hours after polypectomy; no evidence of perforation; due to peritoneal inflammation secondary to mucosal coagulation burn; treated conservatively with intravenous antibiotics and fluids) (Hunt, 1983)
7. Explosion (due to ignition of colonic gas produced by bacteria in the colon; may occur during polypectomy or coagulation; proper bowel preparation eliminates risk) (DiPalma et al, 1984)

Colonoscopic Polypectomy

INDICATION

Most polyps in children are juvenile polyps with no malignant potential (Fig. 43–9). However, in a report by Cynamon et al (1989), adenomatous polyps and iron-deficiency anemia were noted in a subset of pediatric patients undergoing colonoscopic polypectomy. Some pediatric gastroenterologists may, then, be more likely to recommend removal, although many polyps autoamputate. Colonoscopy is also helpful in ruling out other potential sources of bleeding.

CONTRAINDICATIONS

Contraindications are the same as for diagnostic colonoscopy. When performing polypectomy, surgical back-up must be available (especially if a large polyp is encountered), and adequate bowel preparation is required because residual debris makes polyp removal technically more difficult and increases the risk of complication. Potentially combustible colonic gases may be present if there is incomplete bowel preparation or if a lavage solution containing mannitol has been used. These gases place the patient at undue risk of explosion when the electrocautery snare is activated (Bigard et al, 1979).

For this reason, carbohydrates should be removed from the patient's diet on the day before the procedure. Finally, the coagulation status of the patient should be verified.

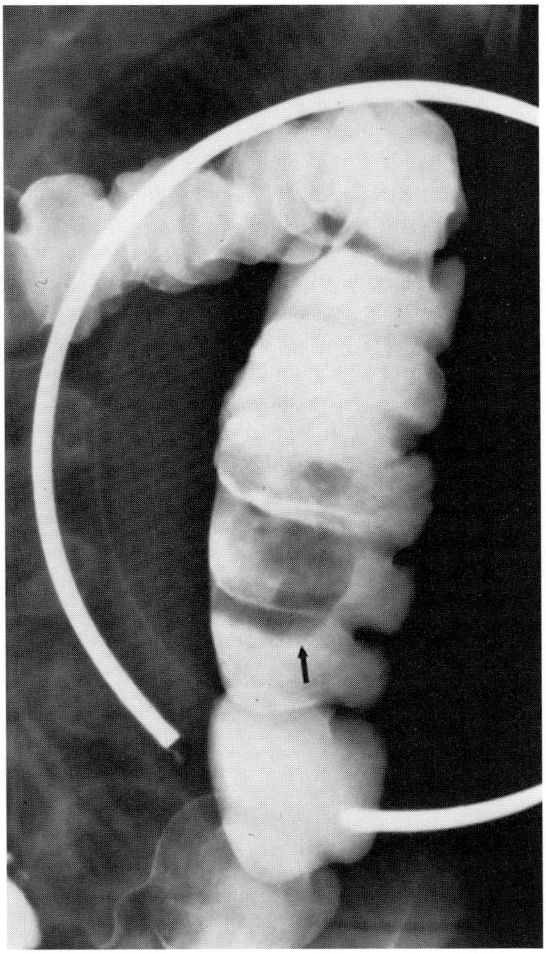

Figure 43–9 This barium enema spot film of the distal colon demonstrates a large juvenile polyp *(arrow)*. (From Wyllie R, Hyams JS: *Pediatric Gastrointestinal Disease: Pathophysiology, Diagnosis, Management.* Philadelphia, WB Saunders, 1993.)

PATIENT PREPARATION

See previous sections on colonoscopy, sedation, and antimicrobial prophylaxis. Preferably, an intravenous line is placed before the child enters the procedure area.

EQUIPMENT AND SUPPLIES

In addition to the routine endoscopic equipment for colonoscopy, the following items are necessary:

1. An electrocautery unit
2. Disposable, plastic-sheathed wire snare
3. Ground plate (disposable or reusable)
4. Retrieval forceps (rat tooth and tripod forceps)
5. Suction trap
6. 1 : 10,000 dilution of epinephrine
7. An endoscopic catheter (for instilling epinephrine in case bleeding occurs; the sheath from a cytology brush can be used)

PROCEDURE

1. The electrocautery unit should be tested according to the manufacturer's recommendations.
2. The ground plate is connected to the patient's thigh.
3. Colonoscopy is performed as previously described. Polyps are removed as the colonoscope is retrieved.
4. Most polyps in children are pedunculated with an easily identifiable stalk. Infrequently, a large sessile polyp is encountered and may be removed in pieces (more than one session might be required for complete eradication, or, if the polyp is too large, surgical removal may be warranted). If multiple polyps are encountered, the most proximal polyp is removed first so that the colonoscope does not pass over a previously cauterized stalk, increasing the risk of hemorrhage. If there are too many polyps for safe removal in one session, as might be encountered in cases of hereditary polyposis syndromes, representative polyps are removed for histological evaluation.
5. The polyp is brought into direct view just beyond the tip of the colonoscope.
6. The assistant advances the sheathed wire snare (snare remains inside the sheath) until it is visualized exiting the distal end of the colonoscope.
7. The wire snare is advanced out of the distal end of the plastic sheath (triggered by the handle at the proximal end of the snare).
8. A typical pedunculated polyp is lassoed halfway along the length of the stalk.
9. The plastic sheath is advanced until it contacts the stalk. The snare is then lightly closed around the stalk. Whether the polyp head or mucosa is caught in the snare can be determined by gently moving the snare in and out. If the snare is not positioned properly or the polyp cannot be adequately visualized, the snare is removed, the colonoscope is repositioned, and the steps are repeated. Tightening the snare too snugly around the polyp will sever it and result in bleeding.
10. A short burst of air inflates the adjacent bowel and, if necessary, the polyp can be aligned in the middle of the lumen, directly in front of the colonoscope. To avoid transmural burn or perforation, it is important to keep the polyp off adjacent mucosa and the snare out of a pool of fluid, stool, or blood.
11. The head of the polyp usually becomes cyanotic as blood supply is compromised when the snare is closed.
12. A short, 1- to 5-second burst of current is passed through the snare as the loop around the polyp is gently and gradually tightened. The polyp becomes whitish and a small amount of vaporization occurs as the stalk is coagulated. This step should be repeated if the polyp has not been severed from the stalk. If the polyp fails to change color, operation of the cautery equipment should be verified before repeated attempts to coagulate the stalk are made.
13. If the polyp inadvertently contacts the mucosa during coagulation, the snare can be gently moved back and forth to minimize the contact with the mucosal surface.
14. Once the polyp is removed, the stalk is observed. If bleeding is noted, the snare can be tightened around the remaining polyp stalk (no current applied) for several minutes to provide tamponade. If this fails or it is not possible to snare the stalk, the 1 : 10,000 solution of epinephrine is flushed through a catheter that is firmly pushed against the stalk. This promotes vasoconstriction of the vessels in the surrounding mucosa. Rarely, surgical intervention is required.
15. Polyps can be removed either with suction (using an in-line trap) or retrieval forceps, depending on polyp size. Occasionally, it is not possible to extract the polyp after cauterization. A parent should strain the

child's stool for the polyp, then return the polyp for analysis.

POST-PROCEDURE CARE

The polyp is stored in formalin or a formalin-equivalent fixative for histological interpretation. The patient should be monitored until he/she is awake and alert. Areas of localized abdominal tenderness should be sought. The family should contact the physician if bleeding, pain, or fever occurs. It is helpful when written instructions and telephone numbers are provided. Later, the patient can resume a normal diet.

COMPLICATIONS

In addition to the routine complications associated with colonoscopy, there are further risks related to polyp removal. These include the following:

1. Hemorrhage (a small amount of rectal bleeding commonly occurs after polypectomy; the risk of hemorrhage is 40 to 60 times greater with polypectomy than with colonoscopy alone) (Hunt, 1983)
2. Late hemorrhage (can occur 5 to 14 days after polypectomy when the fibrin clot falls off; may require repeat colonoscopy or surgery and blood transfusion) (MacRae et al, 1983)
3. Perforation (estimated at 0% to 5% in children) (Hassal et al, 1984; Liebman, 1977; Williams et al, 1982)
4. Mucosal burn resulting in abdominal pain, fever, and a leukocytosis 12 to 24 hours after the procedure with no evidence of free abdominal air on radiograph. This is also referred to as the "post-polypectomy" or "colon coagulation syndrome." Bowel rest, intravenous fluids and antibiotics, and observation are required (Hunt, 1983).

Studies have demonstrated a correlation between the experience of the endoscopist and the frequency of complications (MacRae et al, 1983).

Percutaneous Endoscopic Gastrostomy Tube Placement

The technique for percutaneous endoscopic gastrostomy (PEG) tube placement in pediatric patients (Fig. 43–10) was first described by Gauderer and colleagues in 1980. In infants and children whose gastrointestinal tract is intact, PEG is the procedure of choice to provide nutritional support when oral intake is inadequate or impossible. The PEG tube can be placed without general anesthesia, which is an advantage for those patients at increased risk for surgery. The use of a PEG tube eliminates the cost associated with the use of general anesthesia, feedings can be initiated earlier, and discharge from the hospital occurs sooner than for patients with a surgically placed gastrostomy tube.

INDICATIONS

It is important to identify those patients who may develop or recover their ability to eat and drink before gastrostomy tube placement is considered. Usually, a gastrostomy tube is advisable when the patient requires more than 3 months of enteral nutritional support. Alternatively, a soft, inert, small-caliber nasogastric tube (polyurethane or silicone) can be used for short-term use.

Pediatric patients who benefit from gastrostomy tube placement include the following:

1. Former premature infants with sucking and swallowing disturbances (oropharyngeal incoordination)
2. Infants and children who are neurologically compromised due to congenital or genetic defects, infections, tumors, or trauma and who cannot safely or adequately swallow to support themselves nutritionally
3. Infants and children with severe cardiac or pulmonary disease who have increased metabolic requirements and are often too weak to eat
4. Patients with cystic fibrosis (increased metabolic demands due to work of breathing

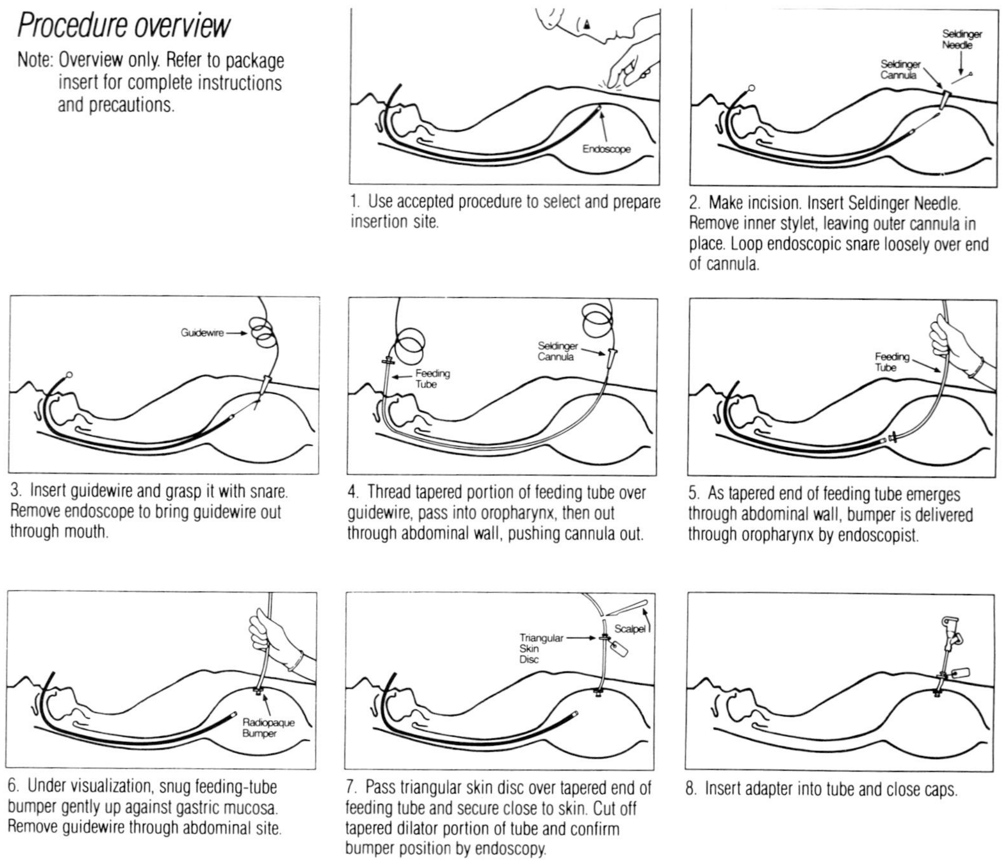

Figure 43–10 Procedure overview for percutaneous endoscopic gastrostomy (PEG) tube placement. (From Gastrostomy Feeding Devices. October 1990. Courtesy of Ross Laboratories, Division of Abbott Laboratories, Columbus, OH.)

and chronic infection) in whom, by providing sufficient supplemental calories, the patient may approach optimal growth and development and possibly attenuate infectious pulmonary complications (Levy et al, 1985)

5. Patients with inflammatory bowel disease in whom an elemental diet would be beneficial, and in some cases, even steroid-sparing (Morin et al, 1982; Sanderson et al, 1987)
6. Patients with AIDS-related malnutrition (Bentler and Stanish, 1987; Fennoy and Leung, 1990)

PEG tube placement allows the child to be given bolus feeds through a syringe or pump. Infants and children with failure to thrive can also be given continuous overnight infusions. Feedings can be delivered more conveniently, frequently being provided while the whole family dines together or while the child sleeps. PEG tube placement does not necessarily prevent oral intake but the child no longer depends on it.

CONTRAINDICATIONS

The contraindications for routine upper endoscopy apply to PEG tube placement. Sometimes, a Stamm gastrostomy rather than insertion of a PEG tube is indicated. In a Stamm gastrostomy, the serosal layer of the stomach is sutured to the anterior abdominal wall, creating a stronger stomal opening than a PEG. It is less likely to leak or for the tube to become dislodged, and it is more likely to heal. The type of incision enables the surgeon to lyse adhesions, allows visualization of alterations in anatomy, and avoids instrumentation of the esophagus. The following situations usually require a Stamm gastrostomy:

1. Previous abdominal surgery that may have altered abdominal anatomy or caused adhesions
2. Stenosis or stricture of the esophagus (the endoscope or gastrostomy tube may not

safely pass through the stenosis or stricture; retrograde stricture dilation through a PEG tube places excessive traction on the stoma leading to disruption of the tract); infants and children with congenital (e.g., tracheoesophageal fistula), posttraumatic (e.g., burns, caustic ingestion), or tumor-related (e.g., nasopharyngeal craniopharyngioma) lesions or abnormalities of the oropharynx or esophagus; a surgically placed Stamm gastrostomy is indicated in these conditions
3. High-dose steroid or immunosuppressive therapy (their ability to form adhesions between the stomach and anterior abdominal wall may be compromised, increasing the risk of tube dislodgement or leakage of gastric contents into the peritoneal cavity)
4. Severe malnourishment
5. Esophageal varices

These conditions require surgical intervention at which time a Stamm gastrostomy tube is also installed. Placement of a PEG tube is contraindicated in the patients with gastric outlet obstruction, intestinal malrotation, or gastroesophageal reflux, which may require a Nissen fundoplication.

Medical management of ascites, peritonitis, and gastric conditions (e.g., an ulcer) at the tube site must precede gastrostomy tube placement. In patients with chronic ascites, a Stamm gastrostomy is the procedure of choice.

Absolute contraindications to PEG or Stamm gastrostomy tube placement include malignant infiltration of the abdominal or stomach wall (tumor may infiltrate the stomal tract) and a rapidly deteriorating medical condition.

PATIENT PREPARATION

The preparation for PEG tube placement is the same as for routine upper endoscopy.

SEDATION

Sedation such as that used for routine upper endoscopy may be used. Or, the patient may be given deep sedation (e.g., using ketamine instead of meperidine) and the airway is monitored (in the intensive care unit setting or endoscopy suite). The procedure may also be performed in the operating theater with the patient under general anesthesia.

ANTIMICROBIAL PROPHYLAXIS

All patients requiring PEG tube placement should receive antibiotic coverage with a cephalosporin such as cefazolin before and after the procedure to cover skin flora that may contaminate the peristomal area. Patients already receiving antibiotics need no further coverage or change in coverage (Jain et al, 1987). In those patients at risk for bacterial endocarditis or in the immunocompromised patient, additional antibiotic coverage is indicated (see the section on antimicrobial prophylaxis). Some endoscopists prefer to wash or swab the mouth and oropharynx with an antibacterial iodine solution to minimize the risk of oral flora contaminating the gastrostomy tube as it is drawn through the mouth and oropharynx. This is recommended in the immunocompromised patient.

EQUIPMENT AND SUPPLIES

Standard pediatric upper endoscopes, accessories, and supplies for performing routine endoscopy are used for this procedure. A PEG "kit," which is most commonly used for the "pull-through" method, includes the following:

- Gastrostomy tube
- Sterile drapes
- Iodine swabs
- Sterile gauze
- Lidocaine
- Syringe and 25-gauge needle
- 16-gauge medicut needle
- No. 11 scalpel
- Suture material
- Guidewire

Alternatively, a prepackaged PEG "kit" for the "introducer" method includes the following:

- Peel-away sheath
- J-tipped guidewire
- Obturators (dilators) in increasing sizes
- 18-gauge needle
- Foley catheter
- Suture material with needle

There is a wide assortment of commercially available PEG kits. The contents and method of placement may vary slightly but they use the same basic principles.

Some gastrostomy tubes can be removed through the skin tract without requiring an additional endoscopic procedure to remove the internal bolster or bumper. This is the most cost-effective and least invasive PEG design.

PROCEDURE

PEG tube placement is usually performed by two physicians—one performing the endoscopy while the other makes the abdominal incision and later maneuvers the gastrostomy tube into position. PEGs are generally placed by either the "pull-through" method (simpler and more popular), or the push, or "introducer," method.

Pull-Through Method (Gauderer et al, 1980)

1. The abdominal incision site is identified and a sterile skin preparation is performed. The site for the gastrostomy tube is approximately one third the distance from the mid-left costal margin to the umbilicus.
2. The upper endoscopy is performed with the patient lying supine.
3. The stomach is distended with air, which brings the anterior gastric wall in proximity to the anterior abdominal wall while the liver, spleen, and bowel are displaced away from the area.
4. The room is darkened and the stomach is transilluminated from within using the light at the tip of the endoscope to verify location of the gastric antrum in the left upper quadrant. The light usually appears as a distinctive glow on the anterior abdominal wall.
5. The endoscopist directs the other physician to make an impression with a sterile gloved finger or blunt instrument on the proposed incision site, which should be readily visualized endoscopically as a well-defined indentation on the gastric wall. Uncommonly, transillumination is unsuccessful or the indentation is not sharply defined. This is most likely due to viscera lying between the stomach and anterior abdominal wall. In an obese patient, transillumination is not always reliable, but a clearly demarcated indentation should be identifiable in most cases. The patient can be rotated from supine to the left lateral or right lateral decubitus position, and the head of the bed can be raised 10 or 15 degrees to displace interfering viscera. The patient is then repositioned on his/her back and identification of a distinct light source is attempted again. If the light source is present, an indentation is again made on the external abdominal wall. If a sharp, well-defined impression is not seen, the procedure is abandoned because the risk of visceral perforation is significant. This complication occurs rarely but is more likely in patients with morbid obesity, a history of abdominal distention unrelated to endoscopic insufflation, or previous abdominal surgery.
6. The skin site is infiltrated with 1% lidocaine using a 25-gauge needle and a small incision (about 1/4 to 1/3 inch) is made with a No. 11 scalpel.
7. The medicut catheter is held perpendicular to the abdominal wall and thrusted (not slowly pushed) through the incision, piercing the stomach.
8. A snare is passed through the endoscope and placed over the medicut needle, seen endoscopically to protrude into the gastric lumen. A flexible guidewire or suture is passed through the hollow medicut needle and grasped with the endoscopic snare forceps.
9. The endoscope, snare, and guidewire or suture are withdrawn in tandem from the stomach and out through the mouth.
10. The medicut needle is removed while the guidewire or suture is held in place.
11. Depending on the type of PEG kit chosen, the gastrostomy tube may be tied to the suture, lubricated, and pulled into place, or its tapered tip is introduced over a guidewire and pulled through the abdominal incision.
12. The endoscope is reinserted into the stomach as the gastrostomy tube is sliding into place to verify proper positioning of the internal portion of the tube. Sometimes, the abdominal incision must be widened to avoid tissue necrosis and necrotizing fasciitis when there is resistance when pulling the gastrostomy through the abdominal wall
13. An external bumper is positioned over the gastrostomy tube to prevent eventual tube migration due to gastric peristalsis.

Introducer Method (Miller et al, 1988)

The introducer method is used more commonly in adults. A peel-away sheath with obturators (dilators), guidewire, and a Foley catheter (serving as a gastrostomy tube) are used as follows:

1. An upper endoscopy is performed as described.
2. An 18-gauge needle is inserted through the gastrostomy tube site into the stomach.

3. A flexible guidewire is inserted through the needle into the stomach and the needle is removed.
4. With a No. 11 scalpel blade, the incision is widened to accommodate the sheath and dilator (obturator).
5. The lubricated peel-away sheath with obturator positioned inside of it is passed through the abdominal incision, using a clockwise motion to facilitate passage. Another physician observes endoscopically.
6. The initial dilator is removed and replaced with dilators of increasing size until the desired Foley catheter (gastrostomy tube) diameter is attained (the size of the catheter depends on the size of the patient).
7. The Foley catheter (gastrostomy tube) is lubricated and inserted into the stomach under endoscopic view.
8. The Foley catheter is inflated, pulled against the anterior wall of the stomach, and observed for leaks. If intact, the sheath is peeled away and removed.
9. The Foley catheter can either be sutured to the anterior abdominal wall, or, before insertion, a bolster (crossbar) can be slipped over the catheter to prevent catheter travel.

This introducer method is more likely to result in complications, especially in infants and small children in whom forceful manipulation of the abdominal wall (avoided with the pull-through method) can lead to injury of adjacent viscera. Furthermore, the larger incision tract required for the introducer method compared to the pull-through technique can more easily be disrupted, causing leakage into the peritoneal cavity or displacement of the gastrostomy tube. The pull-through method, then, is generally preferred for PEG tube placement. Nevertheless, the introducer method is performed routinely in many hospitals.

POST-PROCEDURE CARE

The length of post-procedure monitoring depends on whether conscious sedation or general anesthesia was used. The gastrostomy tube can be placed to low intermittent suction if prolonged anesthesia was requred or if a large gastric residual was encountered intraoperatively despite sufficient null per os status. Otherwise, low-volume continuous feeds can be initiated once the patient is awake and alert, and these feeds can be advanced as tolerated. Intravenous fluids should be provided until full feedings are attained. The patient should be closely monitored for evidence of gastroesophageal reflux because some patients may have increased reflux episodes after PEG tube placement. By fixing the stomach to the anterior abdominal wall, traction is placed on the gastroesophageal junction which may result in lower esophageal sphincter incompetence (Grunow et al, 1989).

The gastrostomy tube should be flushed with water before and after every feeding or whenever medications are administered through it to avoid clogging. If residual formula contacts an acidic medication (most are slightly acidic), the acid will precipitate the protein in the formula, leading to a plugged gastrostomy tube. The skin site should be cleansed with mild soap and water or 1/2-strength peroxide to minimize the risk of infection at the skin site.

COMPLICATIONS

It is not uncommon to incidentally note radiographically benign subcutaneous emphysema or pneumoperitoneum for up to 1 week after gastrostomy tube insertion (Larson et al, 1987; Orchard and Barlow, 1987). These generally occur as a result of the procedure itself and do not imply that leakage into the peritoneal cavity has occurred. Other, more serious complications reported include the following:

1. Peristomal infection (erythema, induration, purulent discharge, tenderness at the skin site, and possibly fever) (Larson et al, 1987)
2. Tissue necrosis due to excessive traction at the skin site (incision may have been too small or the tube was too tightly secured) (Larson et al, 1987)
3. Abscess or necrotizing fasciitis due to excessive skin traction and bacterial wound contamination) (Cave et al, 1986)
4. Gastrostomy tube displacement into the abdominal wall (the "buried bumper" syndrome) (Shaldman et al, 1988)
5. Gastrocolic fistula (a late complication) (Stefan et al, 1989)
6. Esophageal bleeding (due to pulling the gastrostomy tube and bumper through the esophagus during placement) (Cappell, 1988)
7. Chemical peritonitis from delayed identification of tube displacement into the peritoneal cavity (Ditesheim et al, 1989)
8. Small bowel obstruction due to unidentified tube migration into the duodenum or jejunum (Kaplan and Fried, 1989)

9. Increased incidence of gastroesophageal reflux (Grunow et al, 1989)

In general, patients with severe, underlying medical conditions and poor nutritional status who would most benefit from gastrostomy tube placement are probably at greatest risk for complications. A Stamm gastrostomy should be considered in patients who are candidates for PEG if they can tolerate general anesthesia.

Wound infection, the most common complication, can best be avoided by using prophylactic antibiotics and making a generous skin incision. Neurologically compromised pediatric patients who cannot be restrained from pulling at their gastrostomy tube are at increased risk for complications. If the tube is dislodged before the stomal tract forms sufficient adhesions, gastric contents can leak into the peritoneal cavity. Signs and symptoms of peritonitis are not necessarily readily identifiable in a neurologically compromised patient. If this complication occurs, the gastrostomy should be surgically closed to prevent any additional spillage of gastric contents intraperitoneally.

Esophagogastric Balloon Tamponade

Esophageal variceal bleeding is an uncommon but often life-threatening occurrence in children. Sengstaken and Blakemore (1950) first described the use of balloon tamponade for acute control of massive bleeding due to esophageal varices. Since the advent of endoscopic sclerotherapy for esophageal variceal bleeding, the role of balloon tamponade has been used as a temporizing measure.

The smaller diameter pediatric upper endoscope has only one channel (which contains the sclerosant injection needle). Sclerotherapy is significantly more difficult in infants and children because the field of view cannot be cleared using suction or washing while sclerotherapy is performed as is done with a double-channel endoscope in adults. Balloon tamponade may sometimes control bleeding emergently so that sclerotherapy can be performed later under more controlled conditions.

Balloon tamponade acutely controls bleeding in more than 90% of patients, but rebleeding occurs in approximately 60% immediately after removal of the tube (Panes et al, 1988). The risk of rebleeding, although decreased by the additional use of sclerotherapy, remains significant (Paquet and Feussner, 1985). Long-term patient outcome somewhat depends on the severity of the liver disease.

INDICATIONS

In infants and children, variceal bleeding can occur for a number of reasons secondary to increased portal venous pressure. Portal hypertension can be classified as presinusoidal, sinusoidal, or postsinusoidal obstruction (intrahepatic or extrahepatic) (Pasquale and Cerra, 1992):

1. Massive splenomegaly (increased inflow)
2. Extrahepatic portal vein obstruction due to
    - Developmental defect of portal vein
    - Portal vein thrombosis
    - Omphalitis
    - Sepsis
    - Trauma
    - Enterocolitis
    - Severe dehydration
    - Blood dyscrasias
    - Benign tumor or neoplasm
    - Idiopathic origin
3. Intrahepatic portal vein obstruction due to
    - Congenital hepatic fibrosis
    - Schistosomiasis (main cause of variceal bleeding outside the U.S.)
    - Benign tumor or neoplasm
    - Myeloproliferative disease
    - Wilson's disease
    - Constrictive pericarditis
    - Right-sided heart failure
    - Congenital obstruction of suprahepatic inferior vena cava
    - Trauma
    - Sepsis
    - Benign tumor/neoplasm

After gastric lavage and while clotting abnormalities are being assessed and corrected (if necessary), balloon tamponade can play an important role in the control of esophageal or gastric variceal hemorrhage when (1) bleeding is massive and the patient remains hemodynamically unstable despite ongoing resuscitative efforts, (2) an infusion of intravenous vasopressin, longer-acting terlipressin (triglyceryl-vasopressin), or somatostatin is unsuccessful, (3) sclerotherapy fails to control bleeding or rebleeding occurs after sclerotherapy, (4) sclerotherapy is not readily available, (5) awaiting surgical intervention, or (6) surgery is contraindicated or ill-advised. Balloon tamponade has been used successfully for persistently bleeding Mallory-Weiss tears (Berry and Perrault, 1991).

CONTRAINDICATIONS

If variceal bleeding has stopped or if there is history of recent surgery at the esophagogastric junction, balloon tamponade should not be attempted. Because this procedure carries a significant risk of complication (20% to 35%), there are several additional relative contraindications that must be considered (Berry and Perrault, 1991; Conn and Simpson, 1967):

1. Inadequately trained ancillary staff
2. Defective equipment (the tube should be pretested)
3. Underlying medical condition (congestive heart failure, arrhythmia, respiratory failure)
4. Incomplete gastric lavage
5. Inability to confirm variceal bleeding by angiography or endoscopic means
6. Bleeding due to esophageal ulceration (the gastric balloon may still be used)

PATIENT PREPARATION

The patient should be hemodynamically resuscitated, the stomach lavaged, and blood products or whole blood transfused, as indicated. Endoscopy or angiography should precede balloon placement to positively identify variceal bleeding. Patients with liver disease and a history of variceal bleeding can still bleed from nonvariceal sources such as gastric or duodenal peptic ulcer or erosive esophagitis.

The procedure should be explained to older children before balloon insertion. The pediatric patient should receive adequate sedation for both safety and comfort. It is often necessary to intubate the patient to protect the airway from aspiration, especially when the patient is stuporous or comatose due to hepatic encephalopathy. If coughing is present, a cough suppressant should be used to prevent recurrent, sudden increases in intra-abdominal pressure that could dislodge a variceal clot or the balloon. Antibiotic prophylaxis is generally unnecessary.

EQUIPMENT AND SUPPLIES

Three tube designs are generally used for variceal tamponade, which come in adult and pediatric sizes. The Sengstaken-Blakemore tube is a triple-lumen tube with a gastric balloon (200 to 400 ml capacity), a sausage-shaped esophageal balloon, and a gastric aspiration port. Esophageal aspiration is performed via a nasogastric tube placed just proximal to the esophageal balloon. The Minnesota tube is a modified Sengstaken-Blakemore tube. The spherical gastric balloon has an increased capacity (500 ml); the esophageal balloon is identical to that of the SB tube; the tube has separate ports for suctioning of the esophagus and stomach. The Linton-Nachlas tube has only a gastric balloon (600 ml) but has aspiration ports for the esophagus and stomach; it is used primarily for bleeding gastric varices, although it does interrupt esophageal submucosal venous blood flow. However, it is markedly less effective for esophageal varices than the Minnesota or Sengstaken-Blakemore tube, so it is no longer recommended for this purpose (Nachlas, 1955).

The esophageal and gastric port each has a dedicated pressure bulb for balloon insufflation with an in-line manometer to measure and monitor individual balloon inflation pressures (Fig. 43–11).

The tube should be carefully inspected and pretested. Inflation of each balloon should be pretested using the manometer to correlate a given volume of air with a specific pressure reading. For example, 100 ml of air is added to the gastric balloon and the pressure attained is recorded. This pressure should be reproducible later with the gastric balloon in the patient. If the pressure is more than 15 mm Hg higher than the pretest value, the gastric balloon is probably in the esophagus.

The ancillary staff should be prepared for potential complications and emergent removal of the tube. A pair of scissors should be taped to the head of the bed in case immediate release of balloon pressure is necessary. Plastic plugs are provided for both air inlet (balloon) ports, and both the air inlet and pressure ports

GASTROENTEROLOGIC PROCEDURES

Minnesota Four-Lumen Tube

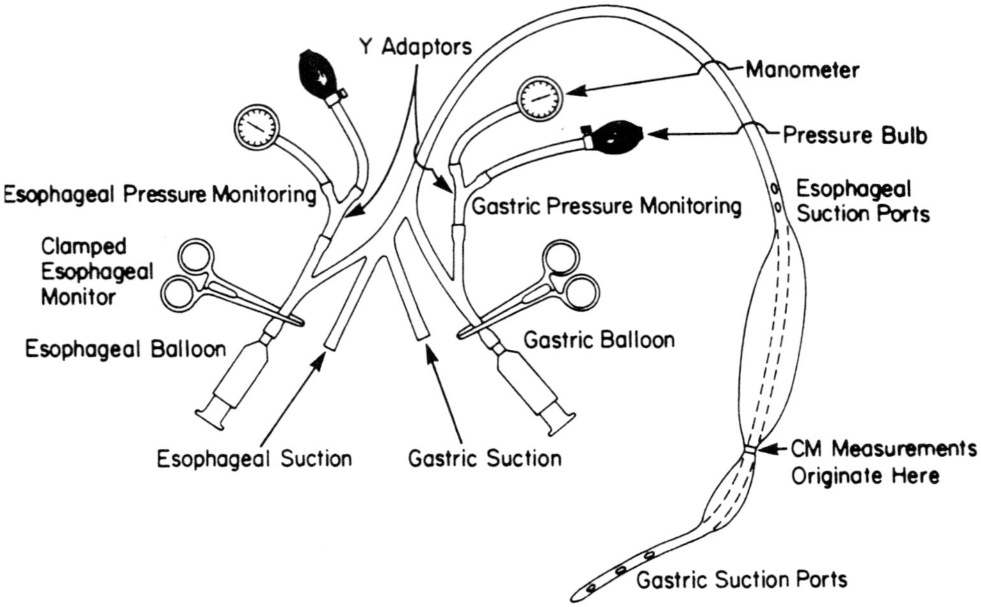

Figure 43–11 Minnesota four-lumen tube. (From Drussman DA: *Manual of Gastroenterologic Procedures,* 2nd ed. New York, Raven Press, 1987).

have rubber or padded clamps (total of four) as an extra safety feature. Each port may be double clamped. A football helmet with a facemask or a baseball catcher's mask to which the esophagogastric balloon device will later be attached should be fitted over the patient's face. A 2.2-kg weight is suspended by over-the-head traction to determine the proper amount of traction required for adequate gastric tamponade before the device is secured to the facemask, Alternatively, the suspended weight can be used without the facemask, but doing so risks balloon dislodgement whenever the patient is repositioned.

PROCEDURE

Children usually require sedation for the Minnesota tube to be safely placed and most also require intubation. The use of sedation may mask symptoms of discomfort and increase the risk of serious complications. Without sedation, however, there is increased agitation and coughing, which also increases the risk of aspiration. The Minnesota tube is inserted as follows:

1. The oropharynx is anesthetized with a topical anesthetic.
2. The patient is placed with his/her left side down and rechecked for gastric residuals. (Incomplete evacuation of gastric contents increases risk of aspiration during tube insertion.)
3. All air is squeezed from the balloons and plastic plugs are reinserted. A clamp is secured to each pressure port after the manometers are removed and the tube is lubricated.
4. The distance from the lower incisors to the earlobe to the sternal notch is measured. This measurement approximates the distance from the proximal end of the gastric balloon to the mouth.
5. The tube is inserted into the stomach and the clamps and plastic plugs are removed. (Nasogastric intubation may be attempted in larger children or adolescents.)
6. The manometers are inserted, and the gastric balloon is insufflated by syringe with 100 ml of air. (It is helpful to auscultate the epigastric area during inflation.) This value should correlate with the pretest reading within 15 mm Hg. If not, the tube should be removed and reinserted. If the patient experiences pain, the balloon should be deflated immediately.

7. Based on the patient's size, the gastric balloon can be slowly inflated with 250 to 500 ml of air in increments of 50 to 100 ml.
8. The balloon inlet and manometer ports are clamped. The tube is pulled gently until resistance is felt as the balloon presses against the gastroesophageal junction. The tube is marked with tape where it crosses the lower incisors. This serves as a reference point in case tube movement is suspected. (The tube may stretch or the diaphragm may relax, so some tube travel is expected.)
9. The esophageal and gastric drainage ports are connected to intermittent wall suction and observed for bleeding.
10. If bleeding is apparent from the esophageal port, 25 to 45 mm Hg of pressure is additionally insufflated into the esophageal balloon, using the lowest pressure possible to control the bleeding. Once insufflated, the tube is clamped. The esophageal balloon should never be inflated before the gastric balloon.
11. The head of the bed should be elevated about 30 degrees.

Placement of the Sengstaken-Blakemore or Linton-Nachlas tube is similar to that of the Minnesota tube. The former requires a nasogastric tube to aspirate the esophagus, and the latter is efficacious only for gastric variceal bleeding.

POST-PROCEDURE CARE

1. A portable chest radiograph is obtained immediately; the gastric balloon should be just beneath the diaphragm.
2. The esophageal balloon must be deflated for 10 minutes every 2 to 3 hours to prevent tissue ischemia and necrosis.
3. Traction is checked every 3 hours.
4. The patient should be given nothing by mouth, but medications can be provided through the gastric port.
5. Oral hygiene should be provided.
6. The suction ports should be checked regularly and flushed if clogging is suspected. This reduces the risk of aspiration.
7. The nonintubated patient is observed for respiratory distress, which can occur owing to proximal migration of the esophageal balloon into the oropharynx, occluding the airway.
8. The patient is observed for chest pain due to migration of the gastric balloon into the chest. If this occurs, the tube must be cut immediately.
9. If bleeding has been controlled for 24 hours, the esophageal balloon is deflated and traction is released.
10. If hemostasis continues for the next 6 to 12 hours, the gastric balloon is deflated but the tube is kept in place.
11. If rebleeding occurs, the gastric, and, if necessary, the esophageal balloon can be inflated for another 24 hours. Sclerotherapy may be performed at this point and has been shown to be more effective than tamponade alone (Barsoum et al, 1982; Paquet and Fuessner, 1985).
12. If no rebleeding occurs, the tube is removed and cut to prevent reuse.

COMPLICATIONS

Significant complications occur approximately 20% to 35% of the time and are often directly related to the level of experience of the medical staff or the severity of the underlying liver disease of the patient (Conn and Simpson, 1967; Pitcher, 1971). Complications include the following:

1. Pulmonary aspiration and pneumonia (more common with the Sengstaken-Blakemore tube; occurs most commonly during tube placement or when the esophageal suction port becomes clogged)
2. Esophageal erosion or rupture
3. Respiratory obstruction (due to proximal migration of the esophageal balloon with deflation of the gastric balloon)
4. Alar necrosis in nasogastric intubation
5. Arrhythmias
6. Pulmonary edema
7. Nasopharyngeal bleeding
8. Chest pain
9. Hiccups (diaphragmatic irritation)
10. Agitation (especially with excessive traction)
11. Balloon impaction
12. Gastric erosion
13. Tube malfunction
14. Death

Esophageal Dilatation

Several widely used techniques are used to dilate esophageal strictures in children. The indications, advantages, and drawbacks for each method as well as studies to assist in defining anatomy or abnormal motility are discussed in this section.

INDICATIONS

Esophageal strictures in children are rarely due to carcinoma. Most commonly, strictures in children occur after (1) chronic, severe gastroesophageal reflux disease, (2) caustic ingestions, (3) congenital webs, rings (Schatzki's rings), or tracheobronchial remnants, (4) stricture at the anastomotic site after surgery for tracheoesophageal fistula or esophageal atresia, or (5) achalasia (a functional "stricture" of the lower esophageal sphincter) (Ament and Vargas, 1991; Berquist et al, 1983).

Children with esophageal strictures often present with difficulty swallowing, the sensation of food getting stuck, pain, or regurgitation of undigested food. A barium study can define structural abnormalities that are difficult to assess endoscopically such as tracheoesophageal fistulas, webs, or rings. If the lower esophageal sphincter fails to relax and a proximal dilated esophageal segment is identified on barium swallow, then esophageal manometry can help identify achalasia. If tracheobronchial remnants are suspected, a computed tomography (CT) scan or magnetic resonance imaging (MRI) scan may be obtained to define the extent of the extrinsic masses causing the obstruction.

Upper endoscopy can be used for diagnostic and therapeutic intervention, providing direct visualization and biopsy of the esophageal mucosa. It also allows assessment of the stomach and duodenum to rule out other diffuse upper tract inflammation that may predispose the patient to reflux esophagitis and stricture. It can also obtain samples for culture if esophagitis is due to moniliasis as occurs with dysmotility (e.g., achalasia) or in immunocompromised patients. In some instances, the stricture may be too narrow to allow passage of the endoscope. In this situation, dilatation may be performed over a guidewire, usually under fluoroscopic guidance.

CONTRAINDICATIONS

Dilatation should not be performed in children who have (1) a significant, uncorrectable bleeding disorder, (2) had esophageal biopsies within the last 10 to 14 days, (3) food impaction in the esophagus, (4) an esophageal ulcer, (5) esophageal varices, or (6) recent esophageal or upper gastrointestinal tract surgery.

PATIENT PREPARATION

Most children require conscious sedation, and, in some cases, general anesthesia may be necessary to eliminate the risk of movement during the procedure. Infants should be given nothing by mouth for only 4 hours, whereas children and adolescents should be fasted overnight. The procedure should be explained to older children beforehand. Patient preparation and comfort during the procedure is especially important in the child who may require repeated dilatations. Antibiotic prophylaxis should be given (refer to the section on antibiotic prophylaxis).

DILATATION WITH MERCURY-FILLED BOUGIES

Peptic esophageal stricture secondary to chronic, severe dilatation reflux often requires repeated dilatations. Mercury-filled bougies, either the blunt-tipped Hurst dilators or the tapered-tipped Maloney dilators, are used (Fig. 43–12A). These are manufactured in many sizes (French) to accommodate most strictures and allow for gradual, stepwise dilatation. Even though this technique is probably the least expensive to perform, it requires a physician who is experienced in the technique, that is, one who can feel when the dilator engages the stricture and who avoids excessive force when resistance is met. Fluoroscopy is sometimes used to verify position of the dilator.

Prior radiographic or endoscopic assessment of the stricture should be obtained. If significant dilation of the esophagus proximal to the stricture is identified, manual bougienage should not be attempted because there is an increased risk of esophageal perforation or rupture. The bougie can falsely track into the di-

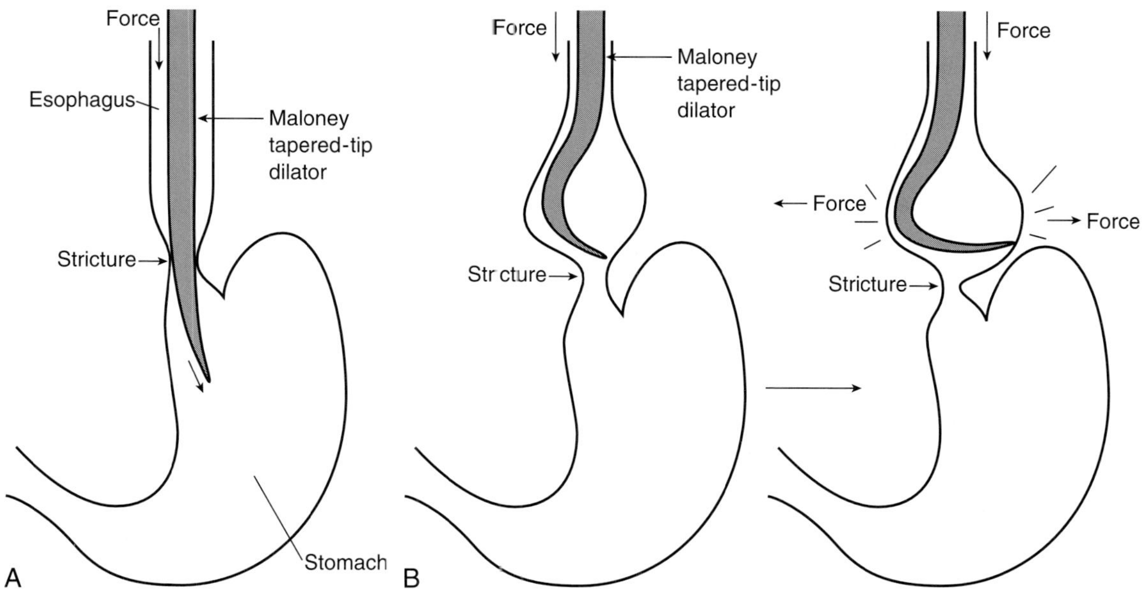

Figure 43–12 **A.** Maloney mercury-filled dilator useful for uncomplicated strictures (e.g., absence of esophageal diverticulum). **B.** Risk of unguided esophageal dilation: false tracking increases the risk of perforation.

lated proximal sac while it is being negotiated through the stricture, even under fluoroscopic guidance (Fig. 43–12B).

Although blunt-tipped Hurst dilators can be used for most esophageal strictures, the tapered-tip Maloney dilator is more easily negotiated in the stricture and is preferred by many physicians.

Procedure

1. The oropharynx is anesthetized with a topical anesthetic.
2. After sedation (or general anesthesia), the patient is placed in the lateral decubitus position to reduce the risk of aspiration. In an unusually cooperative adolescent, the procedure can be performed with only topical anesthetic with the child in the seated position.
3. The approximate diameter of the stricture and the distance from the lower incisors to the stricture and to the esophagogastric junction should have been determined during prior endoscopy. These measurements enable the physician to choose an appropriately sized bougie and to estimate the distance that the bougie should be introduced.
4. An index finger guides the tip of a well-lubricated dilator as it is introduced into the posterior pharynx.
5. Either the patient may swallow or the dilator can be gently introduced until resistance is met (when it has contacted the stricture).
6. The dilator is held lightly between the thumb and fingers to avoid excessive force and is slowly advanced until resistance is reduced. Resistance is also felt as the dilator is pulled back through the stricture.
7. To reduce the risk of perforation, no more than three dilators of increasing diameter (following the initial dilator that meets resistance) should be used during one procedure.
8. A dilator should not be forcibly passed if substantial resistance is encountered.
9. Dilation should be stopped when either blood is seen on the bougie or the patient complains of chest pain.
10. A second dilatation should be scheduled for a few days later.

Dilatation with Wire-Guided Bougies

Dilatation of tight strictures or strictures associated with a tortuous or significantly dilated esophagus makes attempts at passage of mercury-filled bougies difficult and increases the risk of perforation. In this situation dilatation is preferably performed using a bougie designed with a central lumen or channel that can be introduced over an endoscopically placed

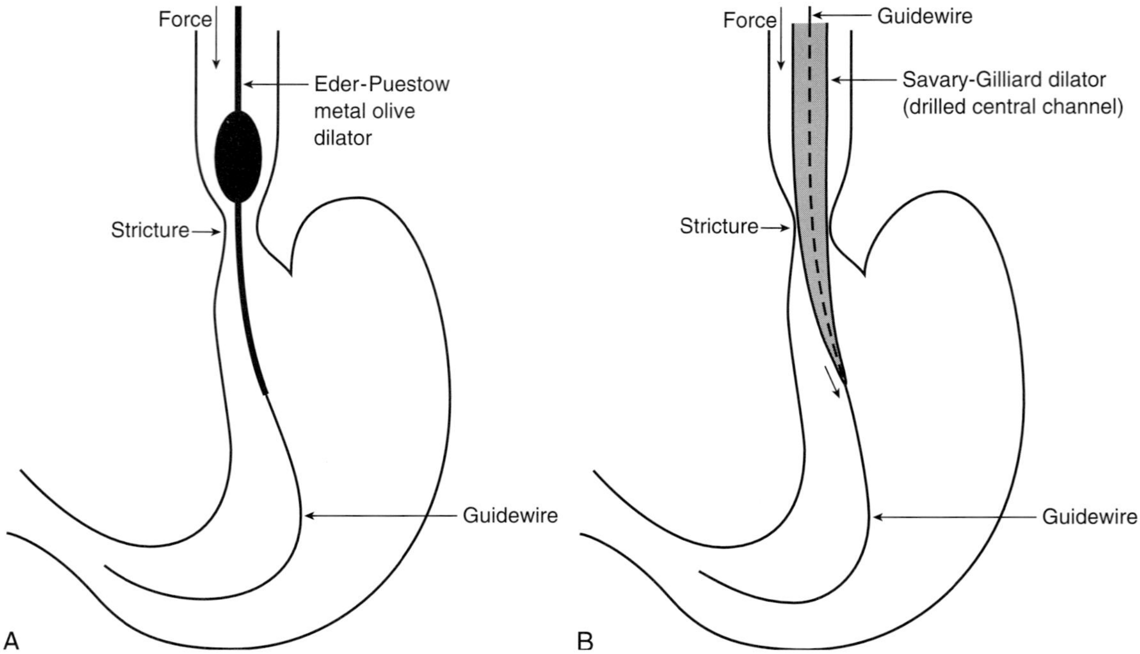

Figure 43–13 **A.** Eder-Puestow metal olive dilator. **B.** Savary-Gilliard dilator passed over a guidewire avoids false tracking.

guidewire previously positioned through the stricture (aided by fluoroscopy, if necessary). Two types of wire-guided bougies are available: the Eder-Puestow metal olive dilators (Fig. 43–13A) and the more popular Savary-Gilliard (Fig. 43–13B). Savary-Gilliard dilators are easier to use than the Eder-Puestow, which require interchanging metal olives and two people to perform the procedure (Dumon et al, 1985).

The Eder-Puestow dilator set consists of (1) a flexible wire with a coiled spring tip that passes through the biopsy channel of the endoscope (but not through the smaller pediatric endoscopes), (2) a set of graded metal olives, and (3) a flexible stainless steel rod to which various-sized olives can be threaded (one at a time). This setup is then passed over the flexible wire.

The Savary-Gilliard dilator set resembles a mercury-filled Maloney dilator in shape and size but is actually a plastic-coated polyvinyl bougie with a centrally drilled channel to accommodate a guidewire. The tip is tapered and flexible and the shaft is more rigid.

PROCEDURE

1. The patient is prepared for upper endoscopy as previously described.
2. The endoscope is advanced up to the stricture and the guidewire is passed through the stricture under direct visualization.
3. The endoscope is withdrawn in 5- to 10-cm increments (marked on the outside of the endoscope) as the flexible wire (Eder-Puestow) or guidewire (Savary-Gilliard) is simultaneously advanced by the same increments. Fluoroscopy can verify that the tip of the guidewire is safely positioned in the stomach.
4. The smallest olive or bougie is passed over the wire while the wire is held taught.
5. The dilator is advanced until resistance is felt (location of the stricture can be confirmed fluoroscopically).
6. With slightly additional force, the dilator is advanced carefully through the stricture. Resistance may suddenly or gradually be felt to decrease (passage through the stricture can be confirmed by fluoroscopy). Uncommonly, this is accompanied by significant, unremitting chest or back pain, indicating that perforation has likely occurred. In such a case, the procedure should be abandoned and an immediate esophogram and a surgical consultation should be obtained.
7. Resistance can be felt as the dilator passes back through the stricture during removal.
8. As with the mercury-filled bougie technique, to reduce the risk of perforation, it

is best to limit dilatation to three sizes above the initial size that encountered resistance.

9. The procedure should be stopped if blood is seen on withdrawal of the bougie or olive.
10. The flexible wire or guidewire is carefully withdrawn.

BALLOON DILATATION

In recent years, the Gruentzig balloon catheter has been used for esophageal dilatation. Its design is based on that of cardiac catheters used for angioplasty (London et al, 1981). It can be directly introduced through the biopsy channel of the endoscope or inserted over an endoscopically placed guidewire. The smaller pediatric endoscope does not permit passage of the catheter but it can be safely introduced alongside the endoscope. Alternatively, it can be introduced using only fluoroscopy.

The Gruentzig balloon consists of a flexible catheter to which a low-compliance (nonelastic) polyvinyl balloon is attached. Balloon catheters range in size from 19 to 60 French (9 to 19 mm) in diameter. There is a maximum diameter and pressure, above which the balloon breaks. This reduces the risk of esophageal rupture from overinflation of the balloon.

The balloon dilator exerts only a radial force to the wall of the esophagus rather than the shearing longitudinal force applied with bougienage, theoretically lessening the risk of tear or rupture. Randomized, controlled studies remain to be carried out in children to demonstrate this advantage.

Procedure (Endoscopically Guided Technique)

1. The patient is prepared for upper endoscopy as previously described.
2. The endoscope is introduced into the esophagus until the stricture is identified. The guidewire or the lubricated balloon catheter is passed through the stricture under direct visualization and the endoscope is removed.
3. A small amount of contrast material (Gastrografin) is instilled into the balloon, which is then positioned, under fluoroscopic guidance, halfway across the stricture (Fig. 43–14A).
4. The balloon is fully inflated with Gastrografin and held in place for, typically, 10 to 15 seconds. The initial thin-waisted, hourglass appearance of the balloon across the stricture slowly expands as the stricture stretches (Fig. 43–14B). This can be observed with short bursts of fluoroscopy. This step is repeated only two or three

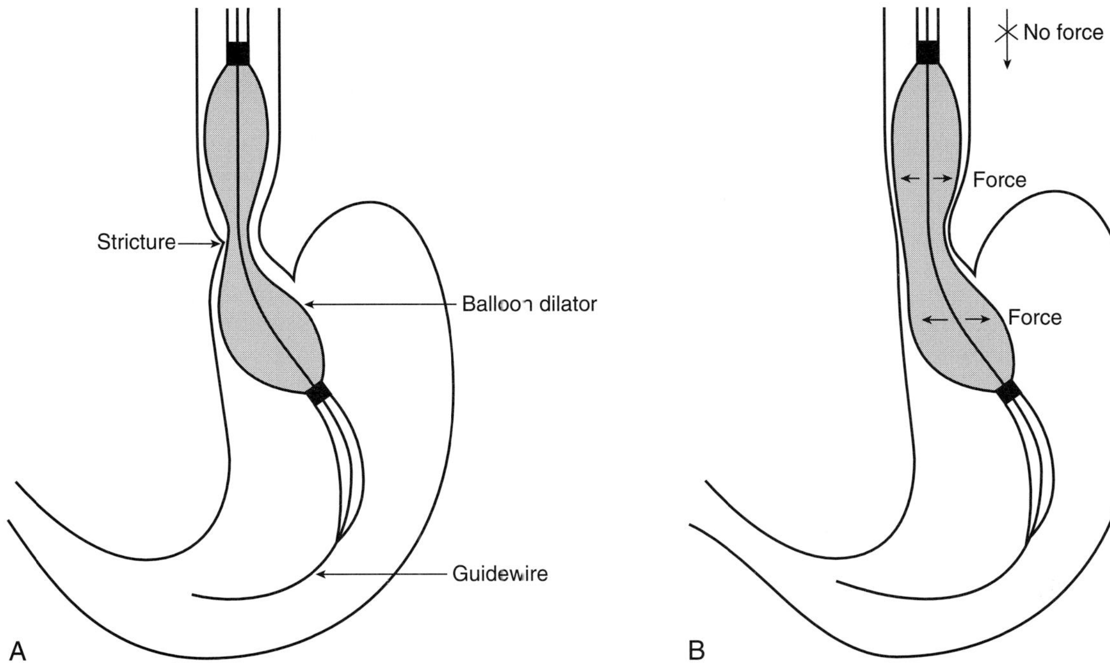

Figure 43–14 **A.** Before dilatation, the balloon is positioned to straddle the esophageal stricture, giving the balloon an hourglass appearance. **B.** As the balloon is inflated, the stricture expands, losing the hourglass appearance.

times per dilatation session. The amount of pressure and the length of inflation time should be based on patient comfort, appearance of the stricture, and previous experience with a given patient.

5. If the patient complains of pain, the procedure should be stopped.
6. Most physicians do not use more than one balloon diameter per session. Larger diameter balloons may be used in subsequent dilatations.
7. The balloon is deflated and removed.

PNEUMATIC DILATATION

Pneumatic dilatation was developed for the treatment of achalasia because more conventional bougienage had complications and disappointing results (Azizkan et al, 1980; Yon and Christensen, 1975). The Brown-McHardy pneumatic dilator uses a balloon inside a nylon bag (which limits the balloon diameter) located near the end of a mercury-filled bougie. The proximal end contains two ports: one for a pressure pump and the other for a manometer.

Recently, the Gruentzig balloon (nonelastic, polyvinyl) technique has been used for patients with a variety of esophageal strictures due to peptic disease, anastomotic strictures, restrictive Nissen fundoplication, as well as achalasia (Sato et al, 1988). This technique may eventually replace the use of the Brown-McHardy pneumatic dilator altogether.

Procedure

1. The esophagus should be inspected (radiographically with a small amount of contrast) for any debris as is commonly present in achalasia. It can be removed with a large-bore Ewald tube.
2. The Brown-McHardy dilator is passed in a similar fashion to that of the Hurst or Maloney mercury-filled dilators as described.
3. The position of the balloon across the lower esophageal sphincter is confirmed fluoroscopically (the hourglass effect).
4. Usually, filling pressure is approximately 9 to 12 lb/in^2, lasting for 5 to 10 seconds. The balloon is filled slowly and observed with intermittent bursts of fluoroscopy. If the walls of the hourglass expand before 10 to 12 lb/in^2 of pressure is attained, then the pressure should be held at that level. Likewise, if the patient experiences pain, dilatation should be stopped.
5. The device is removed and the balloon inspected for blood, which is not an uncommon finding after dilatation for achalasia.
6. Some centers routinely perform a post-procedure esophagram because perforations may not be initially symptomatic (Ott et al, 1987).
7. Most centers admit the patient for overnight observation after pneumatic dilatation for achalasia because the risk of perforation is significant.

POST-PROCEDURE CARE

1. Vital signs and oxygen saturation via pulse oximeter should be monitored until the patient is awake and alert.
2. The patient should not receive anything by mouth until the anesthetic has worn off.
3. Antacids or sucralfate, with or without an H_2-antagonist, is usually provided for 4 to 5 days after dilatation.
4. Liquid diet for 12 to 24 hours followed by a soft diet for 24 to 48 hours should be given before a regular diet is resumed. (This regimen varies from center to center.)
5. The patient or family should inform the physician if chest pain, back pain, abdominal pain, fever, vomiting of blood, or the appearance of melanotic stool occurs.
6. A patient who is symptomatic should be observed overnight.

COMPLICATIONS

The most feared complication of dilatation is esophageal perforation, the incidence of which varies according to physician experience, the technique, and the type of stricture. Peptic strictures are less likely to perforate than caustic strictures in which a full-thickness scar may have weakened the esophageal wall. The lower esophageal sphincters in patients with achalasia are at greater risk for perforation because higher pressures are required to dilate them. Overall, the risk of perforation varies from approximately 0.3 to 2.5%, but an incidence as high as 9.5% was reported in one study that performed an early post-procedure esophagram (Okike et al, 1979; Ott et al, 1987; Vantrappen and Hellemans, 1980). This suggests that asymptomatic esophageal perforations are more common after dilatation for achalasia than previously thought.

Esophageal perforation requires immediate intervention and carries a mortality risk ranging up to 50% (Miller and Tiszenkel, 1988; Okike et al, 1979; Vantrappen and Hellemans,

1980). In some cases, total parenteral nutrition and broad-spectrum antibiotics are used for 2 weeks; in others, aggressive surgical intervention is used (Miller and Tiszenkel, 1988; Vantrappen and Hellemans, 1980).

Other complications of esophageal dilatation include bleeding, aspiration, fever, pain, bacteremia, late development of dilatation reflux, and allergic reaction to contrast media (Nurko, 1991).

Percutaneous Liver Biopsy

Percutaneous liver biopsy has been safely performed in children since the 1950s (Walker et al, 1967). Following the introduction of the Menghini suction/aspiration technique (described in subsequent paragraphs), morbidity and mortality rates were significantly decreased; consequently, the incidence of complications is low (Cohen et al, 1992). Pediatric liver disease often manifests in infants. Percutaneous liver biopsy can be performed in newborn infants, even premature infants, using conscious sedation and local analgesia only.

Percutaneous liver biopsy has a high diagnostic yield for diffuse parenchymal disease as well as for focal, but extensive lesions. When the technique is guided by CT or ultrasonography, isolated lesions can be diagnosed as well. A sampling of representative liver architecture is not usually accurate because the biopsy specimen obtained by this technique is thin. In this case, an open (surgically obtained) wedge biopsy is indicated.

Inborn errors of metabolism (e.g., glycogen storage disease, type IV) or quantitative analysis of specific trace minerals such as iron (e.g., hemochromatosis) or copper (e.g., Wilson's disease) may be diagnosed from percutaneously obtained specimens. Tissue samples for electron microscopy may also be obtained in this manner.

INDICATIONS

Percutaneous live biopsy is indicated in the following conditions or for the following reasons:

1. Hepatomegaly of unknown cause
2. Unexplained, persistent conjugated (direct) hyperbilirubinemia
3. Elevated hepatic enzymes
4. Pyrexia of unknown origin (biopsy can also be cultured)
5. Systemic or infiltrative diseases affecting liver parenchyma (e.g., sarcoidosis, miliary tuberculosis, or hemochromatosis)
6. Primary or metastatic tumors of the liver (e.g., hepatocellular carcinoma; neuroblastoma or Wilms' tumor, which may metastasize to the liver)
7. Allograft dysfunction (to determine rejection versus lymphoproliferative disease or infectious hepatitis after liver transplantation)
8. To distinguish graft versus host disease from drug toxicity or infectious hepatitis after bone marrow transplantation
9. To follow the progression of known liver disease or response to therapy (e.g., autoimmune hepatitis)
10. To monitor hepatotoxic drug therapy (e.g., methotrexate for psoriasis or dermatomyositis)

Tests that might be worthwhile to perform before liver biopsy in cases of persistent jaundice include hepatobiliary ultrasonography, which can identify a choledochal cyst, absence of the gallbladder (commonly associated with biliary atresia in full-term infants), or hepatic masses. A technetium ^{99m}Tc hepatobiliary scan is also useful in identifying biliary patency.

CONTRAINDICATIONS

The only absolute contraindication is an uncooperative patient. Several relative contraindications to performing percutaneous liver biopsy may be amenable to corrective therapy:

1. Prothrombin time greater than 4 seconds over control
2. Platelet count less than 50,000/mm
3. Bleeding time greater than 10 minutes
4. Hematocrit less than 30
5. Local infection (e.g., infected pleural effu-

sion or peritonitis; ascites should be cultured before biopsy)
6. Massive ascites

Pediatric patients with underlying malignancy or after bone marrow or organ transplantation may be at increased risk to bleed after percutaneous liver biopsy, despite relatively normal clotting parameters (McGill et al, 1990). Obtaining a biopsy sample of tissue other than that of liver may be a safer alternative when attempting to determine graft versus host disease (e.g., esophageal, rectal, or skin biopsy). If liver biopsy is necessary, an open or laparoscopic biopsy should be considered.

PATIENT PREPARATION

Routine laboratory work before biopsy (within 48 hours) should include a complete blood count and differential, prothrombin/partial thromboplastin time, and a blood type and screen. Bleeding time may also be obtained especially in patients with platelet dysfunction syndromes, vascular defects, or a family history of von Willebrand's disease. If intervention is required to correct a potential bleeding problem, parameters should be repeated before the biopsy is obtained.

If pulmonary or gastrointestinal condition is suspected, a chest radiograph or abdominal plain film should be obtained to determine whether there is pleural effusion or bowel overlying the liver, respectively.

The patient should take nothing by mouth before the procedure, that is, 4 to 6 hours for infants and 8 hours for children or adolescents. An intravenous line is necessary for sedation and in case resuscitation is required. The full-term newborn or premature infant, especially if ill, may require intravenous glucose to prevent hypoglycemia during the preprocedure fasting period.

The older, cooperative patient can be coached to hold his/her breath at end-expiration. This is the point at which the biopsy is most safely obtained (lessening the chance of pneumothorax). The physician can simulate the timing and action of the liver biopsy needle using an index finger. In this way, when under conscious sedation, the patient can usually follow a familiar, rehearsed simple command.

SEDATION

In most cases, a combination of conscious sedation using midazolam (Versed) and meperidine (Demerol) and local analgesia (1% lidocaine) is all that is required. If the patient is uncooperative (despite maximum doses of sedation) or if the child suffers from severe anxiety and stress associated with chronic illness or repeated hospitalizations and procedures, a percutaneous liver biopsy can be performed under general anesthesia.

ANTIMICROBIAL PROPHYLAXIS

The guidelines discussed for antimicrobial prophylaxis apply to patients undergoing percutaneous liver biopsy because transient bacteremia may occur (Le Frock et al, 1975). Immunocompromised patients (e.g., from cancer, organ or marrow transplantation, or AIDS) should receive broad-spectrum coverage before and after the procedure because bacteremia in these patients can lead to sepsis, disseminated intravascular coagulation, and death (Cohen et al, 1992).

EQUIPMENT AND SUPPLIES

A sterile, prepackaged, disposable biopsy tray is most commonly used. Equipment and supplies necessary to perform a percutaneous liver biopsy should consist of the following:

1. A 16- or 18-gauge Jamshidi needle (Pharmaseal, Baxter Healthcare Corp., Valencia, CA) with locking syringe, or either a 16T-gauge Klatskin (Becton-Dickenson, Scientific Supply, Schiller Park, IL) or a Tru-Cut needle (20 mm, 11.4-cm cannula, Travenol Laboratories, Inc., Deerfield, IL) are the most commonly used needles. A newly designed, spring-loaded disposable liver biopsy needle (Monopty) is also available (C.R. Bard, Inc., Tewksbury, MA). A 16- versus an 18-gauge needle provides a larger, more representative specimen and is safe to use even in infants; easier specimen retrieval is possible with the larger diameter Klatskin or Tru-Cut needle if the liver is cirrhotic, but risk of bleeding is greater.
2. No. 11 scalpel blade
3. Vial of 1% lidocaine
4. A 10- to 25-ml vial of sterile saline
5. Syringes (2 to 5 ml)
6. Needles (25- and 22-gauge)
7. Sterile towels or disposable drapes
8. Betadine and alcohol swabs
9. Sterile gauze
10. Fixative solutions (for histology, electron microscopy, and iced saline for fresh tissue evaluation)

11. Media for bacterial, fungal, and viral cultures

In addition, a sphygmomanometer and a pulse oximeter are connected to the patient for monitoring before, during, and after the procedure. Mask, gown, sterile gloves, and 2- or 3-inch wide surgical tape and sterile gauze for a pressure bandage are also required.

PROCEDURE

The procedure may be performed in the endoscopy suite or treatment room, or at the bedside, but only when the child cannot be moved (e.g., ICU setting). It is best performed with two assistants: one nurse who is experienced in assisting with a percutaneous liver biopsy, and another nurse to obtain vital signs and monitor the patient before, during, and after the procedure.

1. The patient is positioned supine with the right arm held above or under the head. It may be best to place the intravenous line in the left arm or hand.
2. After obtaining adequate conscious sedation, the liver biopsy site is percussed. The usual site for biopsy is identified as being slightly below the right midaxillary line and midway between the borders of hepatic dullness. This landmark is usually in the vicinity of the ninth or 10th rib, although it may be below the costal margin if hepatomegaly is significant.
3. The biopsy site is prepared in standard sterile fashion with Betadine and alcohol. The patient's chest and abdomen are covered with sterile drapes.
4. Using a 25-gauge needle, a subcutaneous bleb is created with 1% lidocaine. The biopsy tract is infiltrated down to the level of the diaphragm with a 22-gauge needle and 1% lidocaine. A small incision is made with the No. 11 scalpel blade to ease the passage of the biopsy needle.
5. The liver biopsy needle is attached to a specially designed, locking 10-ml syringe filled with 4 to 5 ml of sterile saline. The needle is flushed to remove air. It is inserted horizontally and perpendicular to the midline of the body to the depth of the diaphragm, a point at which some resistance is usually felt (distance varies based on the size of the child). When this procedure is performed in an intercostal space, the needle must be carefully positioned just over the rib to avoid blood vessels and nerve that lie just inferior to (beneath) the adjacent rib.
6. The diaphragm may be identified by slowly inserting the needle and following the patient's respirations. The head of the needle moves caudally when positioned at the diaphragm as the patient inhales. Likewise, the needle is located in the liver if, upon inspiration, the head of the needle moves cephalad.
7. Once the needle passes through the diaphragm, it is directed toward the xiphoid and flushed with 1 ml of saline to clear tissue and fat from the cannula. Negative pressure is then created in the syringe by pulling back the plunger 1 to 2 ml and turning it into the locking position.
8. A 2- to 2.5-cm length of tissue is needed for evaluation. This is the length of needle that is inserted into the liver added to the distance to the diaphragm. The left hand marks the needle at the predetermined distance; the right hand inserts and retrieves the needle (opposite for a left-handed person).
9. The needle is inserted in a swift, 1-second "in-and-out" motion at end-expiration. The negative pressure enables the specimen to be aspirated into the syringe. If bleeding occurs, direct pressure can be applied with sterile gauze.
10. If the sample appears inadequate or fragmented, or if additional tissue is required for testing, the procedure can be repeated a second or third time, although the risk of complication increases with each passage of the needle. Also, the needle may be quickly dulled, especially in a cirrhotic liver, making it difficult to obtain an adequate specimen with subsequent attempts. The larger diameter Klatskin or Tru-Cut needle is generally preferred for obtaining a biopsy from a cirrhotic liver.
11. If a spring-loaded disposable liver biopsy needle is used, e.g., Monopty, the procedure is essentially performed in the same manner except there is no need to "cock" the needle to create negative pressure before insertion.
12. The liver biopsy specimen is placed in an appropriate medium depending on the patient's condition. The fluid surrounding the specimen ("liver juice") may be sent for culture, too.

POST-PROCEDURE CARE

Pressure is applied to the skin site with 2- or 4-inch sterile gauze pads, depending on the patient's size. A pressure bandage is applied with long strips of 2- or 3-inch surgical tape (crossing the midline anteriorly and posteriorly). The patient is positioned with the right side down for at least 2 hours. In most cases, the medications used for conscious sedation usually cause the patient to sleep for a couple of hours after the procedure. Nevertheless, a parent or caregiver should remain with the patient for the first few hours to ensure that the child remains on his/her right side.

In most cases, vital signs are monitored every 15 minutes for 2 hours, every 30 minutes for 2 hours, and every 1 hour for 4 hours. Thereafter, they are followed every 4 hours until discharge. Complications are most likely to occur within the first 8 hours after biopsy, with the greatest incidence occurring within 2 hours of the procedure (Gonzalez-Vallina et al, 1993).

A hematocrit is obtained at 6 hours and again at 24 hours, or at any time the patient appears unstable. Post-procedure orders should include pulse (tachycardia) and blood pressure (hypotension) parameters for which a physician should be immediately notified. Patients may be allowed to eat or drink 2 hours after the biopsy, if they are awake and alert. The patient is restricted to bed rest for the first 8 to 12 hours, after which he or she may have bathroom privileges. Activity is restricted for 24 hours.

Some hepatology referral centers selectively perform percutaneous liver biopsy on an outpatient basis, with the rate of complications comparable with those of patients admitted for a 24-hour period of observation (Gonzalez-Vallina et al, 1993). Medically complicated, high-risk patients or infants younger than 4 weeks of age should not have a percutaneous liver biopsy performed as an outpatient.

COMPLICATIONS

Percutaneous liver biopsy can have complications, although most studies report a low incidence (Cohen et al, 1992; Lichtman et al, 1987). Cohen and colleagues (1992) concluded that the rate of complications in children is greater than that reported in adults and is highest in children with cancer or those having undergone bone marrow transplantation. The rate of complications in adults and children who have undergone percutaneous liver biopsy on an outpatient basis does not differ significantly from that of those performed in inpatients. Furthermore, the complications identified in these outpatients almost always occurred within the 6- to 8-hour observation period (most commonly within 1 hour), which does not differ from the inpatient time frame for complications to be identified. Late complications were rare and occurred after 24 hours in either case (Knauer, 1987).

The risk of bleeding following percutaneous liver biopsy has not been predictable based on preoperative assessment of coagulation parameters. Normal studies do not preclude postoperative bleeding because the procedure is performed without visualization, so there is always a small risk of severing a blood vessel, regardless of the patient's coagulation status (McGill, 1981). Conversely, patients with minor bleeding abnormalities did not demonstrate a higher incidence of bleeding after biopsy in a recent study by McVay and Toy (1990).

Complications associated with percutaneous liver biopsy include (Cohen et al, 1992; Gonzalez-Vallina et al, 1993; McGill et al, 1990):

1. Bleeding (may require transfusion; can be delayed in onset; may occur externally as a hematoma, within the liver capsule or liver parenchyma, or intraperitoneally)
2. Pain
3. Hypotension and shock
4. Bowel perforation (with potential peritoneal abscess)
5. Gallbladder perforation
6. Pneumothorax
7. Bile leak, hemobilia, bile peritonitis, pulmonary bile embolism
8. Ascitic fluid leak
9. Sepsis (immunocompromised patients)
10. Disseminated intravascular coagulation (immunocompromised patients)
11. Death

Hydrogen Breath Analysis

The hydrogen breath test (HBT) is a simple, noninvasive investigation initially used to determine carbohydrate malabsorption in infants, children, and adults (Nose et al, 1979). Gastrointestinal tract metabolism of a substrate such as lactose, when given orally, produces hydrogen due to fermentation by gut bacteria. The hydrogen gas is then excreted by the lungs. This can be collected from the expired air for analysis.

INDICATIONS

The HBT is useful in the detection of carbohydrate intolerance due most commonly to lactose, but also to sucrose and other carbohydrate substrates such as fructose or sorbitol (Barr et al, 1981; Nelis et al, 1990; Perman et al, 1978). HBT is a valuable, noninvasive test for determining bacterial overgrowth of the small intestine, and transit time can be measured using the HBT with a nonabsorbable substrate such as lactulose or sorbitol in small doses (Davidson et al, 1984; King and Toskes, 1986; Read, 1984).

Children complaining of recurrent abdominal pain, cramping, gaseous distention, flatulence, or diarrhea may be suffering from lactase deficiency, which can be identified by HBT (Barr et al, 1979). The HBT has also been used to determine that there is a high incidence of secondary lactose malabsorption in children with acute gastroenteritis and a low incidence of secondary sucrose malabsorption (Davidson et al, 1984). An HBT can be performed to estimate which infants will tolerate milk without causing diarrhea or whether infants and children with diarrhea will tolerate bolus versus continuous feedings (lactose, glucose, or glucose polymers can be used as substrates) (Lifschitz et al, 1983).

Although a sucrose breath test does not replace small bowel biopsy for definitive enzymatic analysis, primary sucrase-isomaltase deficiency can be tentatively diagnosed by performing an HBT as a screening measure (Ford and Barnes, 1983). In some children with symptoms of irritable bowel syndrome, malabsorption of fructose or sorbitol may be suspected as contributing factors based on a dietary history. These sugars can be administered as substrate for an HBT (King and Toskes, 1986). Small bowel bacterial overgrowth may be suspected in children with chronic diarrhea, immune deficiency syndromes, blind or stagnant loop syndrome (as sometimes is seen in short bowel syndrome), or leukemia (Davidson et al, 1984; Nose et al, 1984; Piquata et al, 1990; Smith et al, 1990).

Transit time of a test meal from the mouth to the cecum may be associated with certain disease states (Read, 1984). Slow transit may indicate an intestinal obstruction or chronic intestinal pseudo-obstruction (constipation does not slow transit through the small intestine), whereas rapid transit may correspond with malabsorption and diarrhea.

CONTRAINDICATIONS

There are no contraindications to performing the HBT.

PATIENT PREPARATION

Infants should be given nothing by mouth for 4 to 6 hours, and children or adolescents should be fasted overnight. In addition, if there is a possibility of bacterial overgrowth, the pretest dinner meal should consist of red meat and rice only (no other carbohydrates).

Patients should have completed any antibiotic therapy at least 7 days before the test because such therapy adversely affects the population of bacterial gut flora (Murphy and Calloway, 1972). The patient may not smoke before or during the test.

EQUIPMENT

1. Hydrogen breath analyzer (e.g., Model 12i MicroLyzer, Quintron, Menomonee Falls, WI (Fig. 43–15). This instrument has an internal gas chromatograph column through which the sample is flushed. Hydrogen content is determined as parts per million (ppm). The sample value appears as a digital readout, and it can be connected to a strip recorder.
2. Breath collection devices. The highest breath hydrogen content is present in the end-tidal air. Samples are collected from cooperative patients in a variety of ways, for example, using a balloon or Teflon bag fitted with a low-resistance valve that permits

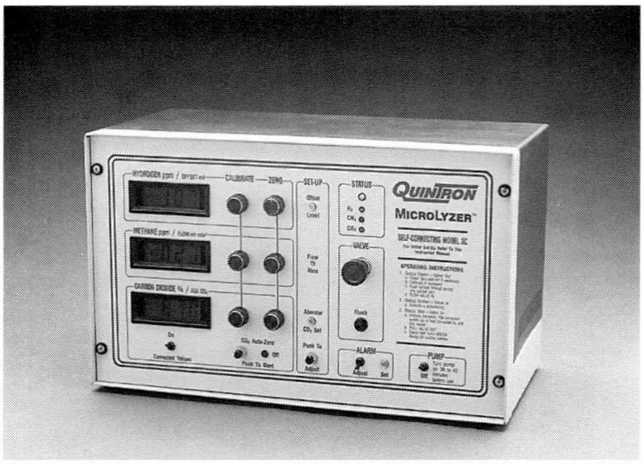

Figure 43–15 A hydrogen breath analyzer: Model 12i MicroLyzer. (Courtesy of Quintron, Menomonee Falls, WI.)

the technician to collect that portion of expired air near the end of expiration. Infants or young children are generally uncooperative, breathe quickly, and their tidal volumes are small. Nasal prongs or a nasopharyngeal catheter may be used, but this method may produce lower than expected breath hydrogen values (MacClean and Fink, 1980; Perman et al, 1978). An automatic sampling device has recently been developed that relies on end-tidal carbon dioxide (Young et al, 1991). Expired air approaches the temperature of alveolar air. A sensor detects this critical point and triggers the sampling device to withdraw the sample, which contains 87% of the end-tidal volume in small infants.

PROCEDURE

1. A baseline breath sample is collected and analyzed before the test dose of carbohydrate is given. Hydrogen excretion in expired air tends to decline with fasting, so the baseline sample should reflect the lowest value in a given sampling period. This is usually in the range of a few parts per million (a value greater than 10 to 12 ppm is considered abnormal). A high baseline value suggests small bowel bacterial overgrowth (Perman et al, 1984). Alternatively, anaerobic mouth flora may produce hydrogen, causing an elevated baseline value (Mastrapaola and Rees, 1987). This is more common in patients with poor oral hygiene. Having the patient gargle with an antiseptic mouthwash often brings the repeat baseline sample value down to the expected range.
2. Patients older than 6 years of age are given a 20% solution of carbohydrate; patients younger than 6 years of age receive a 10% solution to minimize osmotic diarrhea. For example, lactose is provided as 2 g/kg or 1 g/kg, respectively, with a maximum dose of 50 g.
3. Breath samples are collected every 30 minutes for 3 hours when carbohydrate intolerance or bacterial overgrowth is suspected (Fig. 43–16). Transit time studies should be sampled every 10 to 15 minutes after the first test sample is taken at 30 minutes, until a rise in hydrogen is detected.
4. Samples from patients with suspected carbohydrate intolerance or bacterial overgrowth can be analyzed directly or stored in syringes or Mylar-coated foil bags. Glass syringes are better than plastic ones. Refrigerating the syringes at −20°C increases the storage time. Storage allows samples to be collected in a physician's office or at home.
5. Transit time samples should be analyzed as the test proceeds to determine an end point to the study.

POST-PROCEDURE CARE

The infant or child can resume normal activity. If test results demonstrate carbohydrate intolerance, parents should watch for evidence of abdominal discomfort or diarrhea, which is due to the sugar solution, and symptoms soon resolve. These symptoms do not indicate that the child is "sick."

COMPLICATIONS

Patients with carbohydrate intolerance may develop transient abdominal discomfort, cramping, distention, flatulence, or diarrhea.

INTERPRETATION

Carbohydrate intolerance is defined as an increase in hydrogen excretion greater than 10 ppm from baseline, although most clinicians feel that a change of 10 to 20 ppm is equivocal and that greater than 20 ppm is diagnostic (Barr et al, 1981; Solomons and Barillas, 1986). This increase or peak usually occurs when the unabsorbed carbohydrate reaches the colonic bacteria for fermentation at about 120 to 180 minutes.

An early increase in hydrogen excretion (usually in the first 30 minutes) may indicate small bowel overgrowth, especially if a second peak appears later when the carbohydrate is fermented by the colonic bacteria (Rhodes et al, 1979).

A single elevated fasting (baseline) hydrogen breath sample has also been correlated to bacterial overgrowth of the small intestine in

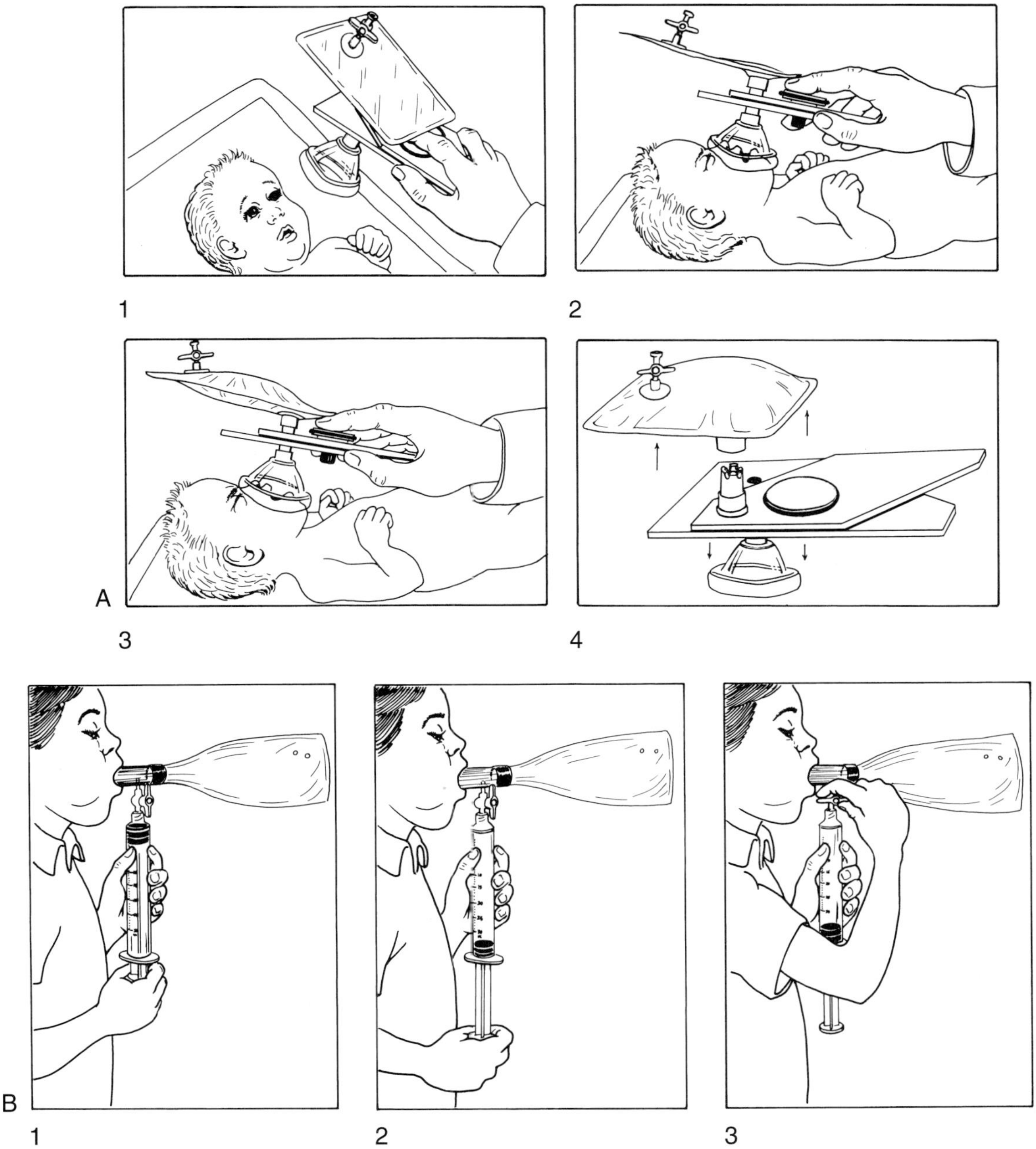

Figure 43–16 **A.** Masked device with a one-way valve and a removable collection bag fitted with a stopcock, used to obtain breath samples from infants or younger children The mask is placed over the nose and mouth to create an airtight seal. As the infant exhales, the collection bag slowly insufflates (1 to 3). The bag can then be removed and a test sample withdrawn for analysis of hydrogen content (4). **B.** Breath sampling device for the older, cooperative child, fitted with a one-way breathing valve, stopcock, sampling syringe, and collection bag. The child seals his/her lips around the mouthpiece and is asked to exhale into the bag (1). The child (or technician) then withdraws the exhaled air sample into the syringe (2). The child (or technician) closes the stopcock to prevent loss of the sample from the syringe before it is removed (3). The contents of the syringe are then analyzed for hydrogen content. (Courtesy of Quintron; Menomonee Falls, WI.)

a study by Perman and colleagues (1984), in which healthy control subjects had an average fasting hydrogen value of 2 ppm and those with bacterial overgrowth had an average baseline of 42 ppm.

Mouth-to-cecum transit time is measured using a non-absorbable sugar, lactulose (expensive) or sorbitol (inexpensive). When the increase in breath hydrogen is 10 to 15 ppm over the baseline value, the sugar has reached the cecum (Korth et al, 1984; Staniforth, 1989). If lactulose is provided in a test meal with protein and fat, transit is not hastened, making the test results more reliable (Read, 1984).

Esophageal Manometry

Manometry is commonly used in the evaluation of motor disorders of the esophagus in infants and children. The technique uses a catheter with radially distributed pressure sensors along its length. It is introduced nasally or orally into the stomach and then withdrawn into the esophagus. Function of the lower and upper esophageal sphincters (LES and UES, respectively) as well as esophageal peristalsis can be examined when the patient swallows (Fig. 43–17A).

INDICATIONS

The transport of food from the mouth to the stomach and the prevention of gastroesophageal reflux are the main functions of the esophagus. Thus, infants and children may exhibit feeding difficulties that might include dysphagia, odynophagia, feeding refusal, weight loss, failure to thrive, or regurgitation and emesis. Although isolated esophageal disorders do occur, they are often associated with other medical conditions that are anatomical, myopathic, or neurological in origin. Chest pain is rare in children. When it does occur, it is usually described as substernal or retrosternal, and may be induced by eating or drinking.

Esophageal manometry may be indicated in infants and children for the following reasons:

1. To evaluate complaints of dysphagia, odynophagia, or chest pain (uncommon in pediatric patients) (Fig. 43–17B)
2. To localize the LES for pH probe placement (Scott, 1991)
3. To follow up an unexplained motility abnormality identified radiologically or by radionuclide scanning
4. To assess esophageal and LES function before an antireflux procedure, and later to assess the effectiveness of the procedure in increasing LES pressure (Vantrappen, 1987)
5. To diagnose achalasia (Fig. 43–17C) or diffuse esophageal spasm (Gelfand and Botoman, 1987)
6. As follow-up to pneumatic dilatation or myotomy of the LES in patients with achalasia to assess treatment efficacy
7. To evaluate esophageal function in patients with a history of cerebral palsy, head trauma, or intracranial hemorrhage, thrombosis, tumor, or cyst who are experiencing swallowing difficulties, gastroesophageal reflux, or recurrent aspiration
8. To evaluate esophageal dysfunction in patients with esophageal atresia (Fig. 43–17D) or tracheoesophageal fistula repair (Biller et al, 1987)
9. To evaluate esophageal dysfunction in patients with history of caustic ingestion (Cadrenel et al, 1990)

Esophageal manometry may be used to aid in the diagnosis or help to identify the extent of disease in disorders such as the following:

1. Chronic intestinal pseudo-obstruction (Vargas et al, 1988)
2. Scleroderma (progressive systemic sclerosis) (Flick et al, 1988)

Figure 43–17 **A.** Normal esophageal manometry. Schematic representation of the peristaltic pressure sequence associated with a wet swallow (WS). The dotted lines indicate the pressure rise rate slope. UES, upper esophageal sphincter; LES, lower esophageal sphincter. (From Dodds WJ, Stef JJ, Hogan WJ: Factors determining pressure measurement accuracy by intraluminal esophageal manometry. *Gastroenterology,* 70:117–123, 1976.) **B.** Spontaneous gastroesophageal reflux associated with inappropriate lower esophageal sphincter (LES) relaxation. A micro pH probe exits the manometry assembly 3 cm above the LES. The LES pressure is continuously monitored with a Dent sleeve. Basal LES pressure is in the normal range but undergoes a transient relaxation lasting 25 seconds. Acid reflux occurred during the interval of LES relaxation. (From Werlin SL, Dodds WJ, Hogan WJ, et al: Mechanisms of gastroesophageal reflux in children. *J Pediatr,* 97:244–249, 1980.) **C.** Achalasia. Manometric recording of a peristaltic sequence and lower esophageal sphincter (LES) pressure. Six manometric recording sites spaced 3 cm apart span the entire esophagus. A Dent sleeve spans the LES for continuous recording of LES pressure. A low pressure simultaneous contraction occurs after each wet swallow (WS). Normal peristalsis is not seen. The LES fails to relax with swallowing. Basal LES pressure is high. (From Wyllie R, Hyams JS: *Pediatric Gastrointestinal Disease: Pathophysiology, Diagnosis, Management.* Philadelphia, WB Saunders, 1993. Courtesy of Walter Hogan, MD.) **D.** Esophageal atresia. Manometric recording of a peristaltic sequence. Six manometric recording sites spaced at 3-cm intervals span the entire esophagus. After swallowing (WS), a peristaltic pressure wave 80 mm Hg in amplitude is seen at the most proximal recording site, disappears at the aortic arch level, but reappears in the distal half of the esophagus. The LES functions normally. (From Werlin SJ, Dodds WJ, Hogan WJ, et al: Esophageal function in esophageal atresia *Dig Dis Sci,* 26:796–800, 1981.)

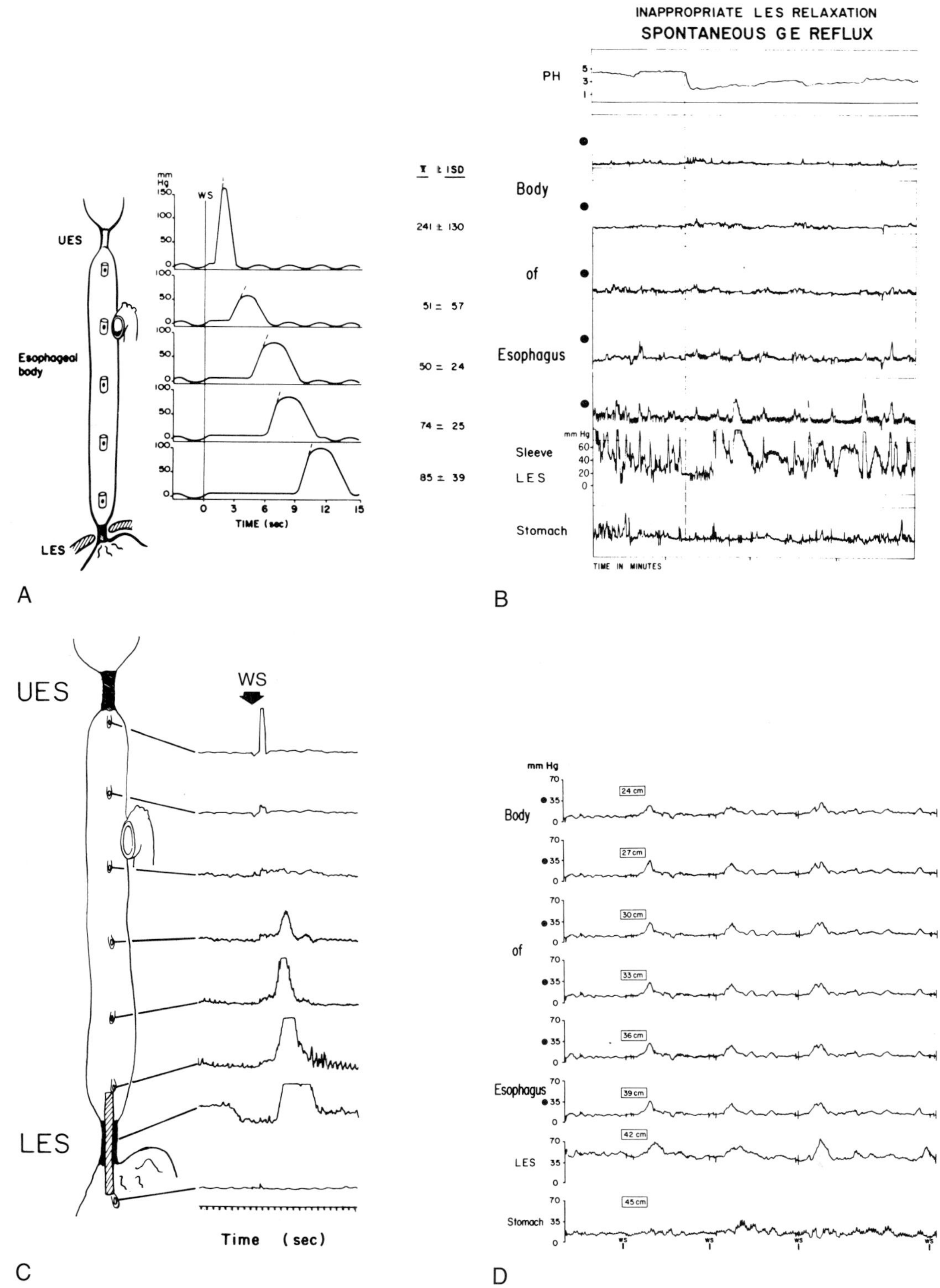

3. Mixed connective tissue disease (Flick et al, 1988)
4. Muscular dystrophies (Eckardt et al, 1986; Kilman and Goyal, 1976; Sack and Sleisenger, 1989)
5. Myasthenia gravis (Kilman and Goyal, 1976)
6. Multiple sclerosis (Kilman and Goyal, 1976)
7. Infantile botulism (Cannon, 1985)

Studies that may precede or complement esophageal manometry include (1) a barium swallow to define anatomy and act as a screening test for transit, peristaltic, or sphincteric abnormalities; (2) cinefluoroscopy, which can record in real time the activity in the cervical esophagus associated with swallowing and then be replayed in slow motion to detect occult nasal or tracheal aspiration or other oropharyngeal abnormalities; (3) an esophageal scintiscan, which provides less radiation exposure than radiologic studies and helps determine the rate of emptying of the esophagus, immediate tracheal or pulmonary aspiration, or delayed aspiration secondary to gastroesophageal reflux; and (4) 24-hour esophageal pH probe to detect pathological gastroesophageal reflux.

CONTRAINDICATIONS

Esophageal manometry can generally be performed safely and successfully in infants and children, but contraindications include an uncooperative or combative patient; recent oropharyngeal, esophageal, or gastric surgery; recent history of caustic ingestion; presence of an esophageal foreign body or food bolus; or cardiopulmonary instability.

PATIENT PREPARATION

Infants should be fasted for 4 hours, and children and adolescents should be given nothing by mouth overnight (at least 8 hours). Many medications as well as beverages, candy, and smoking affect LES pressure and esophageal motor function. These should be withheld before the study. Common culprits include metoclopramide (Reglan), cisapride, anticholinergics (e.g., Levsin, Robinul), theophylline, caffeine, alcohol, chocolate, and peppermint.

Antibiotic coverage is not indicated. Sedation is usually required, especially for infants and young children. Chloral hydrate can be given orally at 50 mg/kg (maximum 1 g) because it does not interfere with esophageal motility, but sleeping infants and children may not swallow when required. Recently, midazolam (0.25 mg/kg) was successfully used to sedate infants for esophageal manometry. Unlike other benzodiazepines (e.g., diazepam), midazolam does not lower LES pressure or affect esophageal motility (Fung et al, 1992). One infant did develop transient apnea requiring resuscitation with a bag and mask and administration of a benzodiazepine antagonist after a second dose of midazolam. A pulse oximeter and flumazenil are necessary if this drug is to be used. The dose of midazolam used in this study was slightly higher than recommended for endoscopy (0.1 to 0.2 mg/kg). The optimal dose for esophageal manometry remains to be determined.

EQUIPMENT AND SUPPLIES

There are two systems available to conduct esophageal motility studies. One, the microtransducer method, consists of a solid catheter with embedded transducers that directly sense pressure; it has not been extensively used because of its greater cost (Humphries and Castell, 1977). The second and most widely available, well-validated technique for evaluating esophageal motor activity is the infused, multilumen manometry catheter with radially distributed distal side holes through which water is continuously infused by a low-compliance pump (Vanderhoof et al, 1978). The infused manometric catheter system is described here. Equipment includes the following:

1. Multilumen polyvinyl catheter. These are manufactured in various diameters and sizes to accommodate infants, children, and adults and can be custom made. Catheters for infants are made with fewer ports, enabling the tube to be thinner. The perfusion ports are spaced 2 to 5 cm apart.
2. Pneumohydraulic capillary infusion system (e.g., Arndorfer Medical Specialties Company, Greendale, WI) with an infusion rate of 0.5 ml/min/port.
3. Multichannel strip recorder (Hewlett Packard Co., Palo Alto, CA, or Beckman Instruments Inc., Schiller Park, IL), which is run at a chart speed of 1.0 or 2.5 mm/sec.
4. Alternatively, a completely computerized motility (manometric) analysis system is available (Sandhill Scientific, Littleton, CO). It includes an infusion system and a strip recorder, which are integrated with a computer program for rapid data analysis.
5. A 10-ml syringe with a short piece of soft tubing, or a cup and sipping straw for wet swallows.

PROCEDURE

1. The multichannel strip recorder is calibrated before each study according to manufacturer's specifications; the catheter is checked for cracks or obstructed ports. The pressure of the transducers (one for each port) is checked for accuracy using a sphygmomanometer. The pressure response rate of the system is checked by perfusing the catheter and occluding each orifice with a finger.
2. The patient is sedated and placed in the supine position.
3. The nares are anesthetized with a local anesthetic (e.g., 1% viscous lidocaine) on a cotton swab.
4. The well-lubricated catheter is introduced through the nose and esophagus into the stomach. All channels should be recording gastric pressure, that is, higher pressure

waves than in the esophagus that are increased by deep inspiration but are unaffected by swallowing.

5. The catheter is pulled back until the most proximal port is in the LES, which is seen as a high-pressure zone between stomach and esophagus. Normal LES pressure is age dependent: 40 to 45 mm Hg in infants younger than 1 year old, 28 to 33 mm Hg after 1 year of age; 10 to 35 mm Hg in adults (Werlin and Brown, 1993). Because the LES is not symmetric, the LES pressure is computed as the average of the port readings as it is withdrawn through the LES in 0.5 cm-increments (the station pull-through technique). Several wet and dry swallows are then initiated and recorded.
6. At least one port is left in the LES initially to verify LES relaxation as the catheter is withdrawn into the esophagus. The primary peristaltic wave (after a swallow) propagates caudally at 3 to 4 cm/sec and lasts less than 7 seconds (Diamant, 1987). The LES relaxes immediately after the onset of a swallow and remains relaxed until the peristaltic wave passes (approximately 10 seconds). This is normally followed by a brief rebound LES contraction of higher amplitude than resting LES pressure. Secondary peristaltic waves may also occur due to an intraluminal stimulus such as a food bolus or gastric acid reflux (Milla, 1988). Tertiary contractions are the result of spontaneous depolarization of the smooth muscle cells of the esophagus when the swallowing center in the brain stem is disrupted (Clouse, 1989). These are always considered pathological. Five to 10 wet swallows should be recorded while examining the LES in conjunction with lower esophageal contractions. An additional 5 to 10 swallows should be recorded in the esophageal body as the catheter is pulled back in 1-cm increments. This helps assess motility through the entire esophagus.
7. The first port of the catheter is withdrawn into the high-pressure zone of the UES (normal UES pressure in adults is 27 to 37 mm Hg and 14 to 29 mm Hg in children) (Sondheimer, 1983). The UES normally relaxes with a food or fluid bolus initiating primary peristaltic activity in the esophagus. Like the LES, the UES demonstrates a transient rebound higher amplitude contraction after relaxation.
8. The catheter is withdrawn so that the most proximal port lies in the pharynx (perfusion is stopped through this port), leaving a port in the UES and remaining ports in the upper esophageal body. Five to 10 wet swallows are initiated with the chart speed increased to 2.5 mm/sec for better delineation of the coordination between pharyngeal contractions, UES relaxation, and esophageal peristalsis. As ports enter the posterior pharynx, they should be turned off because the continuous perfusion of water not only initiates continued swallowing but also may cause a sedated infant or child to choke, cough, or aspirate.
9. Perfusion is shut off to all ports and the catheter is removed.

POST-PROCEDURE CARE

Vital signs are monitored using pulse oximetry until the patient is awake and alert. The patient can then resume normal activities.

COMPLICATIONS

Esophageal manometry is considered a safe procedure; esophageal perforation has not been reported. There is a theoretical risk of causing trauma and bleeding in the nasopharynx, which can usually be avoided or minimized with proper technique. Choking and aspiration in a sedated infant or child is a potential serious complication that must be monitored closely. A long study may lead to accumulation of water in the stomach, which may later be aspirated if emesis occurs. Oversedation and allergic reactions to sedative medications must be considered.

INTERPRETATION

Abnormal events associated with swallowing might include lack of peristalsis, failure of a peristaltic wave to propagate the entire length of the esophagus, or failure of swallowing to consistently initiate peristalsis. Quantitative abnormalities in amplitude, velocity, and duration of contractions are also identifiable.

For a discussion of the pathophysiology, diagnosis, and management of achalasia and other esophageal motility disorders in infants and children, refer to *Pediatric Gastrointestinal Disease: Pathophysiology, Diagnosis, Management*, which details diseases and disorders of the upper (striated muscle) esophagus and the lower (smooth muscle) esophagus (Herbst, 1993).

Anorectal Manometry

Anorectal manometry is performed routinely in infants and children using a variety of equipment, including pressure transducers, nonperfused multiple balloons, and a single balloon attached to an infusion catheter (Rosenberg and Vela, 1983; Tobon et al, 1968). There is no standard method for performing anorectal manometry. The versatile, single balloon/infusion catheter device is practical because it works on the same principle as esophageal manometry in which the catheter is connected to pressure transducers, a pneumohydraulic pump, and a recording device. In this case, a rectal distending balloon is attached to the distal end of the catheter. The size of the balloon and catheter must accommodate premature infants, full-term newborns, children, and adolescent patients (Rosenberg and Vela, 1983).

INDICATIONS

Anorectal manometry in pediatric patients has the following clinical applications:

1. To rule out Hirschsprung's disease in a newborn or in the older child with atypical constipation (Tobon et al, 1968).
2. To evaluate anal sphincter function in anorectal malformations, or after surgery or trauma (including sexual abuse)
3. To evaluate anal sphincter function in neuromuscular disease such as spina bifida or chronic intestinal pseudo-obstruction syndrome
4. To provide biofeedback training for children with functional fecal retention resulting in overflow incontinence associated with decreased sensitivity of the rectal vault to distention by stool or for children with-neuromuscular disease, or following surgery or trauma

CONTRAINDICATIONS

Anorectal manometry is generally considered safe and simple to perform even in premature infants, but it should not be performed in an uncooperative patient or in an infant or child who has had recent anorectal surgery. If a painful anal fissure is detected during the rectal examination just prior to catheter insertion, anorectal manometry should be postponed until the fissure has healed. The emotionally traumatized child (as a result of anal sexual abuse) may have evidence of functional fecal retention and stool incontinence. Such patients may fail to respond to conventional clean-out/lubricant treatment. These children often require intensive, long-term psychological counseling before they can be approached with the option of biofeedback training for their fecal incontinence. Until then, the procedure should be postponed.

PATIENT PREPARATION

Anorectal manometry is usually performed without a full bowel preparation or enema. Sometimes, a large amount of stool is identified on rectal examination when the test is about to be performed. A Fleet enema may then be given. Under many circumstances (e.g., functional fecal retention or neuromuscular disease), it may be necessary to postpone the test until the child has been adequately cleaned out at home.

Although anorectal manometry is not particularly painful, many children regard it as an invasive, unwanted intervention (like an enema); this is especially true in a child who is already experiencing loss of control of body function. Sedation is usually avoided because the child must be alert to give adequate information to the physician. Sedation may be necessary for comfort, however, in the infant or very young child in whom Hirschsprung's disease is being considered. Sedation is effective in this circumstance because it does not alter internal anal sphincter relaxation in response to anorectal balloon distention (Rosenberg and Vela, 1983). Anorectal procedures cause bacteremia. Refer to the section on antimicrobial prophylaxis.

The child with a disorder of defecation, regardless of its cause, requires emotional understanding, support, and thoughtful preparation regarding interventional testing. A collaborative effort between the physician, the pediatric gastrointestinal nurse, a child-life therapist (who can engage the child in play therapy), and a pediatric psychologist, is often essential for the emotional well-being of the child and to ensure a successful study. Soft music playing in the background, a video playing on the television, or a parent reading a story to the child during the procedure are helpful anxiety-reducing interventions.

EQUIPMENT AND SUPPLIES

The following list of equipment and supplies is based on the perfused catheter system, the technique most commonly used in pediatric patients.

1. A multilumen catheter with a distal latex balloon (manufactured in various sizes by a number of medical supply companies, including Arndorfer Medical Specialists, Inc., Greendale, WI). The catheter usually contains 3 or 4 distal ports spaced radially 0.5 cm apart for infants and 1.0 cm apart for larger children and adolescents.
2. Pressure transducers (one for each port)
3. Pneumohydraulic pump
4. Chart (strip) recorder
5. Four 50-ml syringes
6. Lubricant
7. Gauze pads (4 × 4 inch)
8. Sterile disposable needle

PROCEDURE: EVALUATION OF RECTAL AND ANAL SPHINCTER FUNCTION

The technique for anorectal manometry is similar to that used for performing esophageal manometry. It is important to communicate with the child, if possible, throughout the procedure. Because the patient cannot see what is being done, each step should be described. It is helpful to know which expressions are used in the patient's home to refer to defecation and the anal area so that communication is in familiar terms.

1. The recording system is calibrated according to manufacturer's specifications. The catheter is inspected for cracks or obstructed ports. The pressure transducers (one for each port) are tested for accuracy using a sphygmomanometer. The pressure response rate of the system is checked by perfusing the catheter and occluding each orifice with a finger.
2. The rectal balloon is tested by distending it with 50 ml of air or water for 30 seconds. An air-filled balloon can be tested for leaks by holding it under water and observing it for bubbles. A water-filled balloon should be dried, then inspected for seepage.
3. The balloon is lubricated.
4. The patient is positioned with the left side down and the knees flexed.
5. The external anal sphincter and perianal area are examined by gently separating the buttocks with both hands. Soiling or anal fissure is sought.
6. Anal wink is sought using a pinprick test with a sterile disposable needle. The child is asked to contract the external anal sphincter.
7. A careful rectal examination is performed. Anal tone is noted. If a painful fissure is present on examination, manometry should be rescheduled and the fissure treated. A hard stool in the rectum may interfere with results. Either a Fleet enema should be administered or the test should be rescheduled until after clean-out at home has taken place.
8. The balloon/catheter assembly is inserted through the anus until all of the ports are inside (Fig. 43–18).
9. The internal and external anal sphincters (IAS and EAS, respectively) are then located by slowly withdrawing the catheter 0.5 to 1.0 cm at a time (visualized in real time on the chart recorder). This is the same "station pull-through" technique as is used for esophageal manometry. A cooperative child can squeeze the external sphincter or cough at each station. Normally, both the IAS and EAS are tonically contracted. The location of the IAS high-pressure zone is usually 3 to 7 cm from the anal verge and is 2 to 5.5 cm long. Normal IAS basal pressure ranges from 25 to 85 cm H_2O with an average of 60 cm H_2O. The EAS has a lower basal pressure than

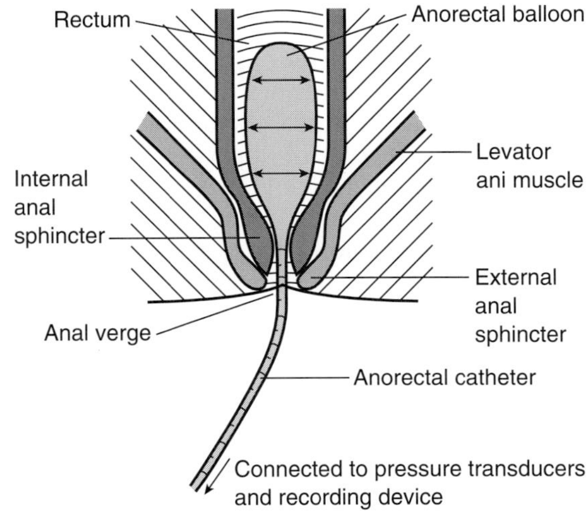

Figure 43–18 Anorectal manometry (water-perfused system).

the IAS (about 30 cm H_2O). Lower atmospheric pressure is reached as the ports are pulled past the anal sphincters (Werlin and Brown, 1991).

10. The station pull-through procedure is repeated several times to confirm location and pressure readings.
11. The balloon is reinserted in the rectum and at least one port of the catheter is inserted into the IAS high-pressure zone. The balloon is distended with 30 to 50 ml air or water (a water-filled balloon more closely resembles actual stool in the rectum). Without telling the child that the balloon is being insufflated, the physician should ask if the patient can sense the distended balloon inside the rectum. The balloon is deflated and reinflated with incremental boluses of air or water (about 10 ml at a time) until the patient senses the balloon. This maneuver provides three important pieces of information regarding anorectal functioning. First, it establishes a threshold for rectal sensitivity. Normal range in children is 10 to 25 ml (Arhan et al, 1983). This threshold is sometimes increased in children with chronic constipation or neuromuscular disorders that may contribute to inadvertent soiling. Second, the IAS should relax after this procedure. Third, the rectoanal inhibitory response is established (normally, rectal distention should induce IAS relaxation and EAS contraction). This response is present in patients with constipation but absent in patients with Hirsch-sprung's disease (Werlin and Brown, 1991).
12. Maximum squeeze pressure of the EAS can be determined by the patient's squeezing down (normally, the maximum squeeze pressure exceeds the resting EAS pressure by twofold to threefold in adults) (Schiller et al, 1982). In some neuromuscular disorders, little increment in pressure over baseline is identified, which may contribute to incontinence.
13. The balloon and catheter assembly are removed. The perianal area is cleaned with soft gauze or tissue.

PROCEDURE: BIOFEEDBACK THERAPY FOR FECAL INCONTINENCE

Chronic constipation and encopresis are common in infants and children. Some reports indicate that 10% to 25% of patients are referred to pediatric gastroenterology services for this problem (Fleisher, 1976; Monar et al, 1983). The preferred approach to management in these infants and children is to eliminate soiling, establish a regular bowel pattern, restore the urge to defecate, and prevent constipation that leads to impaction. This is accomplished with a combination of behavioral training and lubricant (mineral oil) treatment (Hatch, 1988).

Some children are unresponsive to conventional treatment and require further evaluation with anorectal manometry. Paradoxical closure of the external anal sphincter occurs in response to the urge to defecate in a subset of these children. It is an unconscious function that is probably self-conditioned. Children in this group who are old enough to cooperate (usually aged 4 to 5 years) may be treated using biofeedback therapy (Arhan et al, 1983; Wald et al, 1987). Biofeedback is the conscious attempt by the patient to gain control of an unconscious function.

Another subset of children or adolescents who might benefit from biofeedback training for fecal incontinence include those with a history of anorectal surgery, spinal surgery, trauma, or neuromuscular disease. Anorectal dysfunction in these children may include either a decreased sensitivity threshold or altered innervation and function of the EAS, or both. Children with relatively intact EAS innervation may benefit from learning to contract or strengthen the contraction of the EAS in response to progressively lower volumes of rectal distention. The long-term effectiveness of biofeedback training in this group remains controversial (Loening-Boecke et al, 1988; Miner et al, 1990; Whitehead, 1986).

1. Routine anorectal manometry is performed as previously described.
2. Using the rectal balloon volume at which the sensitivity threshold was determined, the patient is asked to either relax (children with paradoxical EAS contraction) or contract the EAS (children with low EAS tone such as in neuromuscular disease) in response to balloon distention. Some children have significantly higher sensitivity threshold values than normal. In these children, the volume of air or water in the rectal balloon is decreased in a stepwise fashion (by 5 to 10 ml) so that the patient senses smaller and smaller volumes over time. This may require several biofeedback sessions.
3. The patient is allowed to see the tracing of the external anal sphincter on the chart recorder as he/she is asked to voluntarily relax or squeeze down. It may be helpful to draw the desired response on the chart paper beforehand.

4. The technique is repeated without visually cuing the patient, that is, the patient is not allowed to see the chart recorder or the act of balloon distention. The patient is asked to duplicate the EAS response that he/she previously produced while viewing the chart recorder. Several attempts may be required before the child responds appropriately.
5. The catheter is removed and the perianal area is cleaned with tissue or soft gauze.

POST-PROCEDURE CARE

The child can resume normal activities. Based on findings of the test, the child may continue lubricant therapy, require a rectal suction biopsy to confirm Hirschsprung's disease, or return for biofeedback training. Children undergoing biofeedback training should be instructed to practice the new technique (relaxation or contraction of the EAS) whenever the sensation of rectal distention is felt. The next session should be scheduled in 1 to 2 weeks, depending on the child's motivation and ability to successfully perform the maneuver. Some regression is expected, especially in times of emotional stress.

COMPLICATIONS

Rectal trauma or bleeding can occur if the catheter assembly is improperly inserted or withdrawn, although no serious complications have been reported in this regard. Several children, especially those with spina bifida, have had an allergic reaction to latex. Most cases have been mild but anaphylactic reactions have also been reported (Nguyen et al, 1991). Silicone balloons are available.

INTERPRETATION

Basal anal sphincter pressures in children with chronic constipation may be high, low, or normal (Loening-Baucke, 1982; Monar et al, 1983). In children with chronic constipation and encopresis, the IAS often relaxes at stool volumes below conscious perception, that is, below the sensation threshold, which may contribute to leakage and soiling in these children (Arhan et al, 1983). Some children with chronic constipation and encopresis have been noted to contract rather than relax the pelvic musculature with attempts to defecate. These children may benefit from biofeedback training (Arhan et al, 1983).

Patients with Hirschsprung's disease are unable to relax the IAS after transient rectal distention. (This differentiates Hirschsprung's disease from chronic constipation.) A falsely abnormal response may result, however, if the rectal balloon is not adequately distended (especially in premature or newborn infants), if the patient has a large amount of stool in the rectum, or if the patient moves causing the catheter to move away from the high-pressure zone of the IAS (Boston et al, 1977; Bowes and Kling, 1979). When Hirschsprung's disease is suspected, a rectal biopsy must be performed to confirm the diagnosis demonstrated histologically by the absence of ganglion cells (Weinberg, 1986). Anorectal manometry, however, may be the only method to determine short-segment Hirschsprung's disease, which can easily be missed on rectal biopsy as a result of sampling error (Tobon et al, 1968).

Intubation of the Gastrointestinal Tract in Infants and Children

Tube placement into the gastrointestinal tract of infants and children has been routinely performed for many years. Gastrointestinal tubes (Fig. 43–19) are manufactured from a variety of materials: polyvinyl chloride (PVC), polyurethane, rubber (latex), and silicone (and silicone elastomers). Although inexpensive (per unit cost), PVC tubes should be limited to short-term use such as decompression, drainage, lavage, or diagnostic sampling because of their tendency to stiffen, become brittle, and split after exposure to gastric or duodenal contents (Hafner et al, 1961). PVC and latex rubber tubing have a higher incidence of tissue irritation, necrosis, and gastrointestinal bleeding (Fegerman and Lysen, 1987). Long-

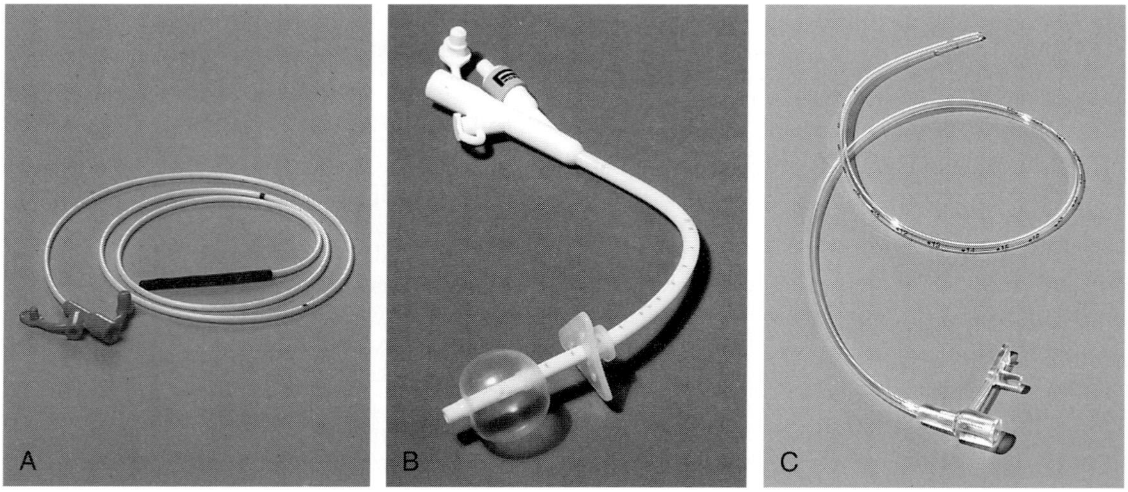

Figure 43–19 A. Dobhoff catheter for nasojejunal feeds. **B.** Gastrostomy tube. **C.** Nasogastric tube. (Courtesy of Ross Laboratories, Division of Abbott Laboratories, Columbus, OH.)

term tube placement is best tolerated with small-bore, flexible, inert tubes made from polyurethane or silicone (the softest and most comfortable material) (Hermann et al, 1989).

The risk of complications, including pharyngeal, esophageal, and intestinal perforation, is greater when placing a tube in a small infant (Johnson et al, 1982; MacAlister et al, 1985; Per-Rodriguez et al, 1978). This is likely due to weaker pharyngeal, esophageal, and gastrointestinal musculature as well as to comparatively smaller anatomical structures, large tube size, and the forces exerted during tube introduction (Vandenplas et al, 1989). Long-term placement of enteric feeding tubes in young infants without concomitant oral stimulation and feedings may lead to the development of a significant aversion to oral activities and may delay the development of speech and gross motor skills (Kennedy-Caldwell et al, 1990).

DIAGNOSTIC/THERAPEUTIC INDICATIONS FOR GASTROINTESTINAL INTUBATION

Esophageal Intubation

1. For newborn resuscitation (suctioning)
2. To aid radiological identification of anatomical anomalies in newborn infant (e.g., choanal or esophageal atresia, or tracheoesophageal fistula [non–H-type]) (Davies, 1990)
3. For esophageal lavage
4. For esophageal manometry
5. For esophageal pH probe placement
6. For acid provocation test (Bernstein test)

Gastric Intubation

1. For newborn resuscitation (e.g., removal of meconium)
2. For gastric emptying before endotracheal intubation to decrease the risk of aspiration
3. For gastric decompression for gastric atony, paralytic ileus, obstruction, or postoperative protection of suture lines
4. For gastric lavage to detect the presence of blood, drugs (overdose), or toxic substances
5. For gastric lavage to evacuate blood, drugs, or toxic substances
6. To administer charcoal infusion for drug overdose or toxic ingestion
7. To measure volume of gastric secretions, acid, pH sampling, or the production of intrinsic factor
8. For administration of medications when oral route is unavailable or impractical
9. To deliver balanced electrolyte solutions for whole bowel irrigation (e.g., for constipation or acute iron ingestion) (Tenebein, 1987; Tolia et al, 1984).
10. For rehydration or nutritional support when the oral route is inadequate

(e.g., in central nervous system disease or coma) or uncomfortable/inaccessible (e.g., in herpetic stomatitis, oral surgery, or trauma)

11. To obtain mycobacteria culture specimens

Intestinal Intubation

1. To sample pH or to detect the presence of bile in the duodenum
2. For nutritional support when gastric feeds are not tolerated or contraindicated when there is
   a. Risk or history of aspiration (e.g., in altered mental status, uncontrolled seizure disorder, unconscious patient with impaired gag reflex)
   b. Gastric atony
   c. Delayed gastric emptying
   d. Gastric or duodenal surgery
   e. Superior mesenteric artery syndrome (duodenal obstruction)
3. For decompression in obstruction or paralytic ileus
4. For Crosby-Kugler or Watson jejunal capsule biopsy (nonendoscopic)
5. For antroduodenal motility study

CONTRAINDICATIONS TO TUBE PLACEMENT IN THE UPPER GASTROINTESTINAL TRACT

1. Known obstruction of naso-oropharynx or esophagus (e.g., atresia or mass lesion)
2. Maxillofacial anomalies, surgery, or trauma that cause structural defects that disrupt internal anatomy (e.g., basilar skull fracture) (Adler et al, 1992)
3. Uncontrolled coagulopathy or thrombocytopenia
4. Epidermolysis bullosa of the esophagus (Gryboski et al, 1988)
5. Prolonged use when varices or severe esophagitis is present (especially with PVC or latex tubing) (Lopez-Torres and Waye, 1973)
6. Caustic ingestion or burn injury to the esophagus or upper gastrointestinal tract
7. Presence of a foreign body in the esophagus

COMPLICATIONS RELATED TO UPPER GASTROINTESTINAL INTUBATION

Complications can occur during placement, use, and removal of enteric tubes. The premature infant has weaker pharyngeal musculature, placing these infants at greater risk for injury and perforation. Injury can occur with silicone as well as PVC tubing (Koehane et al, 1983)

Placement

1. Nasopharyngeal trauma (e.g., bleeding)
2. Laryngeal, tracheobronchial trauma
3. Esophageal, gastric trauma
4. Perforation of the pharynx, tracheobronchial/pleuropulmonary areas, esophagus, and upper gastrointestinal tract (Hermann et al, 1989; Johnson et al, 1982; Miller et al, 1985; Wells et al, 1969)
5. Intracranial placement (Adler et al, 1992)
6. Bradycardia, apnea, hypoxia in premature infants (Herrill et al, 1980)
7. Pseudodiverticulum formation (especially in premature infants and full-term newborns during resuscitation) (Girdamy et al, 1969)

During Use

1. Pulmonary aspiration (most common complication) leads to the following (Schwartz et al, 1980; Wolfson et al, 1989):
   a. Bacterial pneumonia
   b. Chemical pneumonitis (if pH is less than 2.5 or food particles are present in aspirate)
   c. Lipoid pneumonia
   d. Tracheobronchitis
   e. Severe hypoxia due to increased pulmonary shunting
   f. Bacterial contamination (an indwelling gastrointestinal tube may act as a reservoir for multiple antibiotic-resistant microorganisms) (Bussy et al, 1992)
2. Tube displacement due to coughing or emesis (especially with fine-bore, soft tubes) (Metheny et al, 1986)
3. Gastrointestinal complications including nausea, vomiting, gastroesophageal

reflux, bloating, delayed gastric emptying, cramping, diarrhea, constipation, duodenal perforation, and tracheoesophageal fistula (Siegle et al, 1976; Silk and Payne-James, 1990)

4. Tube obstruction due to (Cataldi-Betcher et al, 1982; Kohn and Keithley, 1989) the following:
   a. High viscosity of formula or medication
   b. Coagulation of formula/medication mixture (common with acidic medications reacting with formula proteins)
   c. Pill or food fragments
   d. Slow infusion rate through small-bore tubing
   e. Knotting
5. Tube malfunction due to cracking and splitting (especially with PVC and latex tubes) (Cappell et al, 1992)
6. Long-term placement is associated with the following:
   a. Sinusitis (Bos et al, 1989; Desmond et al, 1991)
   b. Otitis media (Berman et al, 1978)
   c. Eustachian tube dysfunction (Wake et al, 1990)
   d. Pharyngitis
   e. Erosions, ulcerations (more common with PVC/latex tubes) (Hafner et al, 1961)
   f. Vocal cord paralysis, the "nasogastric tube syndrome" (rare; not due to inadvertent tracheal intubation but rather due to chronic pressure applied to the posterior pharynx/cervical esophagus by the tube). The patient may initially complain of dysphonia or aphonia; this is a medical emergency requiring immediate nasogastric tube removal and intubation (Sofferman et al, 1990).

Removal

1. Damage to the mucosal surfaces that have been in prolonged contact with the tube
2. Knotted tubing causing trauma and bleeding to the esophagus or nasopharynx (Cappell et al, 1992)

NASAL VERSUS ORAL GASTROINTESTINAL INTUBATION

Nasogastric/naso-enteric tube placement has several advantages over the orogastric/oroenteric route. Gagging is decreased by minimizing the foreign body sensation in the hypopharynx, contact with the teeth and palate is avoided, and concomitant oral intake of nutrients is facilitated. Nevertheless, there are multiple complications associated with the location of a naso-enteric tube, including sinusitis, otitis media, and eustachian tube dysfunction (Berman et al, 1978; Bos et al, 1989; Wake et al, 1990). In infants weighing less than 2 kg, nasally placed tubes lead to compromised pulmonary function (Herrill et al, 1980). Some neonates are obligate nose breathers, so the presence of a nasal tube can interfere with respiration as a result of nasal airway restriction, increasing the work of breathing. It can also lead to ulceration or erosion of the nasal septum and mucosa (Benda, 1979). Nevertheless, nasogastric or nasojejunal feedings using soft, small-bore tubes in premature and full-term newborn infants have been successful (Beddis and McKenzie, 1979; Cheek and Staub, 1973; Wells and Zachman, 1975).

Orogastric/oroenteric tubes avoid nasal trauma and are advantageous for short-term use such as in gastric lavage when a large-bore catheter is required. They are not associated with sinusitis and are commonly used in infants weighing less than 2 kg to avoid the adverse affect on pulmonary functioning. Orally placed tubes eliminate the risk of tube-induced epistaxis, which can occur in a child with thrombocytopenia or a bleeding disorder. Prolonged use of oral tubes in premature infants may lead to a grooved palate, and oral tubes are more difficult to secure than nasal tubes (Arens and Reichman, 1992).

TUBE PLACEMENT FOR NUTRITIONAL SUPPORT

Selection of tube size is based on the child's weight (Table 43–1). Large-bore tubes are uncomfortable, interfere with coughing and spontaneous respiration, and reduce the competency of the lower esophageal sphincter, which increases the risk of gastroesophageal reflux and aspiration (James, 1975; Hayhurst and Wyman, 1975). Using the smallest bore tube possible reduces the chance of tube dislodge-

Table 43-1 French Size Considerations

Determine appropriate diameter (Fr) based on weight of child:

Size (Fr)	5	8	10	12	14	16
Weight (kg)	2	3–9	10–20	20–30	30–50	50+

ment or removal by minimizing the child's discomfort.

When a gastric or enteric tube is placed for nutritional support, the infant or child should be given nothing by mouth for several hours to decrease the risk of aspiration in case vomiting occurs during introduction. The stomach should be empty to decrease the chance of abdominal distention, gastroesophageal reflux, or emesis during feedings. Small infants may require intravenous glucose support during prolonged fasting before tube placement. The procedure should be explained to the child if appropriate (a child-life specialist can provide valuable assistance).

MEDICAL CONDITIONS IN WHICH NUTRITIONAL SUPPORT VIA TUBE FEEDING MAY BE BENEFICIAL (Moore and Greene, 1985; Skale, 1992)

Gastrointestinal

1. Short bowel syndrome
2. Inflammatory bowel disease
3. Chronic liver disease
4. Inborn errors of metabolism (e.g., glycogen storage disease types I and III)
5. Chronic nonspecific diarrhea
6. Superior mesenteric artery syndrome
7. Surgery of the gastrointestinal tract
8. Pancreatic insufficiency (e.g., cystic fibrosis)

Neurological

1. Altered mental status or coma
2. Severe mental motor retardation, cerebral palsy, or stroke, in which it is impossible or unsafe for the child to suck or swallow without risk of aspiration

Metabolic/Hypermetabolic Status

1. Burns
2. Sepsis
3. Severe head trauma or multiple trauma
4. Cardiac disease
5. Respiratory disease

Congenital Anomalies

1. Cleft lip
2. Esophageal atresia
3. Tracheoesophageal fistula

Other

1. Anorexia nervosa or weight loss
2. Growth failure
3. Malnutrition—acute or chronic; hypoproteinemia
4. Cancer with associated surgery, radiation, or chemotherapy
5. Prematurity
6. AIDS

Long-term nutritional support (longer than 3 months) is usually accomplished by gastrostomy tube placement. Initial placement of a nasogastric tube, nevertheless, is useful because it helps to establish whether gastric feedings will be tolerated before a gastrostomy tube is inserted. If uncontrolled gastroesophageal reflux and/or aspiration occurs with nasogastric feeds, antireflux surgery along with gastrostomy tube placement is generally necessary.

COMPLICATIONS ASSOCIATED WITH ENTERAL TUBE FEEDING (LeLeiko et al, 1993)

1. Overhydration (more likely when parenteral fluids are also given)
2. Hyperglycemia
3. Azotemia (with excessively increased protein intake)
4. Hypovitaminosis K

5. Dehydration due to diarrhea
6. Electrolyte and mineral disorders (increased when vomiting or diarrhea is present)
7. Failure to gain weight (secondary to inadequate energy intake)
8. Aspiration
9. Nutrient deficiency (secondary to formula error)

PREPARATION AND INSERTION OF NASOGASTRIC TUBES

1. The tube should be checked for manufacturing defects, such as cracks and occluded entry or exit ports. If the tube uses a guidewire for insertion, it should be lubricated with silicone or mineral oil (both are more effective than a water-soluble gel). Some stylets have a water-activated hygromer lubricant coating; others are coated with Teflon (polytetrafluoroethylene). The guidewire should be inserted and removed before the tube is inserted to assess whether the guidewire can easily be withdrawn once it is placed in the patient.
2. Tube length is measured. For example, nasogastric tube placement is as follows (Burrows et al, 1992):
   a. The distal opening (not always the tip on weighted tubes) is placed at the end of the child's nose.
   b. The tubing is extended to the child's earlobe and down to the xiphoid process. In infants, the endpoint lies half way between the xiphoid process and umbilicus.
   c. This approximates the distance from the nares to the stomach. Underestimation of the distance may place the tube in the esophagus.
   d. The tube is marked at this point with a piece of tape.
3. If the child is conscious, he/she should sit upright or the head of the bed should be raised at least 45 degrees. Otherwise, the child is placed in the left lateral position to lessen the risk of aspiration.
4. In infants or children with neurological compromise or altered mental status, the presence of a gag reflex should be sought. If the gag reflex is diminished or absent, a postpyloric tube (preferably nasojejunal) is indicated to decrease the risk of aspiration (Rombeau, 1981).
5. The most patent nasal passage can be determined when the child "sniffs" through each nostril while occluding the other.
6. Before tube insertion, the infant should be given a pacifier. The older child can swallow or take small sips of water through a straw. The apprehensive child may tolerate the procedure better if given some sense of control. For example, the child may take a small sip of water into his/her mouth and swallow it "on the count of three," as the tube is inserted.
7. Discomfort and apprehension can be reduced when the nose is anesthetized with a small amount of 2% viscous lidocaine, instilled via a 1-ml syringe. The emotional state and developmental stage of the child may preclude additional manipulation of the nose and throat, and the least overall trauma may result from swift and efficient placement of the tube. Premedication of a child with a conscious-altering medication such as chloral hydrate increases the risk of aspiration so should be discouraged.
8. The distal 5 to 10 cm of the tube is lubricated with water or water-soluble gel (some brands of enteric tubes have a water activated lubricant).
9. With the head aimed in an anatomically neutral position and slightly flexed forward, the tip of the tube is gently inserted posteriorly into the nostril, following the floor of the nasal cavity (this avoids trauma to the turbinates). Then, the tube is aimed toward the ear on that side. At this point, the child should swallow. With a slight twist of the wrist, the tube is advanced to the tape mark. (Mild resistance is expected at the posterior pharynx but only gentle pressure should be needed to pass the tube into the oropharynx. Once the oropharynx is reached, a brief pause in the procedure allows the child to regain composure.)
10. If the tube does not pass readily, it should not be forced. The tube should then be passed in the other nostril, and it should be withdrawn immediately if vomiting or any change in respiratory status (due to inadvertent tracheal intubation) occurs. Cyanosis, tachypnea, tachycardia, flaring, retracting, grunting, wheezing, coughing, and choking are warning signs.
11. If the enteric tube has a guidewire, it should be carefully removed. The guidewire should never be reinserted into the tubing while the tube is in the patient.
    This can result in the wire's inadvertently exiting through a distal feeding

port, leading to trauma or perforation of a viscus. This caution applies to both partially and completely removed guidewires.

VERIFICATION OF TUBE POSITION

Several methods to localize tube placement in the stomach have been used.

1. pH testing. A syringe is attached and aspirated. If the tube is in the stomach, fluid should return into the tubing or syringe. Retrieval of fluid is difficult and not always possible through the soft, fine-bore tubing often used in the small infant or child. When the aspirate is obtained, the pH can be checked. If the aspirate is acidic (pH less than 3), it likely originated from the stomach. No study provides a reliable threshold that identifies gastric pH; acidic pH assumed to be gastric may originate from the pleural space. False-negative results may occur if the child is taking antacids or H_2 antagonists, or if the tube has inadvertently entered the duodenum (Metheny et al, 1989). Although this method is worthwhile, it is not exact.
2. Auscultation. One to 5 ml (infant) or 10 to 20 ml (child) of air is quickly injected while the physician auscultates over the left upper quadrant. If the tube is in the stomach, the air is heard as a "swoosh" or gurgling sound. The inaccuracy of this method has resulted in serious pulmonary complications. It is possible to mistake peristalsis for air insufflation (Metheny et al, 1990).

   Auscultation in infants and small children can be particularly misleading owing to the increased transmission of sound through a relatively thin chest wall and diaphragm. This can make localization difficult.
3. Bubble test. The proximal end of the tube can be placed in a container of water. Theoretically, when the patient exhales, few bubbles should be seen if the tube is in the stomach, whereas a steady stream of bubbles should be present if the tube is in the airway. This is not always true, however (Metheny, 1988).
4. Radiological confirmation. It is safest to confirm tube placement by radiograph before use, especially with small-bore tubes, because none of the methods previously discussed is 100% sensitive. Radiological confirmation is not routinely practiced with insertion of PVC tubing, however (Metheny, 1988).

Unconscious patients may not be able to respond adversely to tube placement in the trachea (especially with small-bore catheters). Cyanosis and increasing respiratory rate or effort are adverse indicators. The bubble test should be performed using a small container of water when being performed emergently. Otherwise, it is best to confirm placement radiologically.

A nasogastric tube can easily pass by even a cuffed endotracheal tube. There is a tendency for endotracheal and nasogastric tube materials to attract and adhere to one another, making passage of a nasogastric tube into the respiratory tract more likely in the intubated patient (Lopez-Torres and Waye, 1973).

SECURING THE TUBE

1. The most practical and comfortable way to secure the tube is to tape it to the upper lip and across the cheek (and over the ear in infants). The upper lip is prepared with tincture of benzoin and a hypoallergenic or semipermeable plastic tape is applied to the upper lip and cheek. Alternatively, a clear plastic, hypoallergenic bandage can be placed across the cheek and the tube taped onto it for less skin irritation. The tube is tolerated better when positioned out of the child's visual field. The tubing is secured with a continuous strip of tape from the nose (minimizing contact with the nostril) to the ear. If any segment of tubing is exposed on the patient's face, one could purposely or inadvertently grasp the tube and dislodge or remove it.
2. Enterically placed feeding tubes can inadvertently be dislodged or removed with surprising frequency. The infant or child in the intensive care unit is particularly susceptible to tube displacement. Altered mental status, the need for passive positioning for nursing care, portable radiographs, and other tests and procedures are contributing factors.
3. The tube is labeled with the date and time of placement. PVC tubing should be used for short-term use only to reduce the risk of tissue necrosis and bleeding. It is best to use silicone or polyurethane tubes for enteral feeds because they can remain in place for up to 4 weeks (Keoshian and Nelson, 1969).
4. When removing a nasogastric or nasoen-

teric tube, one must first clamp the tube to reduce the risk of causing the patient to aspirate the tube contents.

MANUAL TUBE PLACEMENT BEYOND THE PYLORUS (WITHOUT ENDOSCOPIC OR FLUOROSCOPIC ASSISTANCE)

A technique originally developed to facilitate the passage of antroduodenal motility catheters beyond the pylorus has been adapted for introducing naso-enteric feeding tubes into the small intestine in the vicinity of the ligament of Treitz (DiLorenzo et al, 1990).

Erythromycin, a motilin agonist, stimulates propagating gastric and duodenal contractions at a dose of 1 to 3 mg/kg intravenously infused over 30 minutes. This technique has been used in premature infants as well as older children and adolescents with only an occasional complaint of mild abdominal cramping and no serious side effects (DiLorenzo et al, 1990).

It is recommended that electrocardiographical monitoring be carried out during drug infusion because there is potential for cardiotoxic reactions (Benoit et al, 1991). The cardiotoxic effects described in the case report on two premature infants occurred at doses 6 to 20 times greater (antimicrobial doses) than the doses recommended for duodenal intubation, however. Erythromycin is thought to be a safe alternative to metoclopramide, which may cause dystonic reactions, especially in smaller infants and children (Casteele-Van Daele et al, 1970; Low and Gael, 1980). Tube placement beyond the pylorus is as follows:

1. Tube insertion length is measured.
2. After the tube is introduced into the stomach, a radiograph can be useful in verifying that the tip of the tube is in the gastric antrum (if the tip is in the fundus or curled in the stomach, it is unlikely to pass beyond the pylorus).
3. Erythromycin is infused at 1 to 3 mg/kg intravenously over 30 minutes.
4. The patient is placed in the right lateral decubitus position to promote passage from the antrum through the pylorus.
5. Erythromycin is infused for 10 to 15 minutes before any additional tubing is advanced.
6. The tube is advanced 1 cm every 20 to 30 seconds until an additional 10 cm has been introduced (in older children and adolescents, an additional 20 to 30 cm may be required).
7. Aspiration of bile indicates transpyloric passage has probably occurred (this assumes that there has been no bile reflux into the stomach). If the fluid is nonbilious in appearance, pH should be tested. If pH is at least 6.5, then the aspirate is likely from the duodenum (Metheny, 1988).
8. Verification of tip placement can be made by the following:
   a. Radiograph. An abdominal flat plate is normally sufficient to demonstrate that the tube has crossed the midline (tip at or near the ligament of Treitz). If the presence of an overlying gastric air bubble makes tube location uncertain, a cross-table lateral film will show that a tube correctly positioned in the duodenum lies posterior to the stomach, i.e., closer to the spine. A few milliliters of diluted barium injected through the tube enhances visualization of the small intestinal lumen.
   b. Fluoroscopy. Fluoroscopy is accurate but exposes the infant or child to a significantly greater amount of radiation compared with routine radiography.
9. To further advance a tube that has entered the proximal duodenum only, the patient is placed supine for several hours. This promotes tube travel through the duodenum. This should be followed by placing the patient's left side down to encourage tube travel toward the ligament of Treitz. An additional dose of erythromycin may be beneficial.
10. If the first attempt fails, the technique should be tried again (if clinically appropriate) because endoscopy and fluoroscopy are not only more invasive but also are not available at every institution. Several hours should pass before an additional infusion of intravenous erythromycin is used in infants to reduce the risk of cardiotoxicity due to multiple, closely spaced doses of erythromycin.
11. Alternatively, the method just outlined without facilitating tube passage with erythromycin, has been used successfully but takes considerably more time (24 to 48 hours) (Whatley et al, 1983). In patients with altered upper gastrointestinal motility who fail to respond to a prokinetic agent such as erythromycin, tube placement with endoscopic or fluoroscopic assistance is indicated.

PLACEMENT OF A NASO-ENTERIC FEEDING TUBE VIA ENDOSCOPY

(Mitchell et al, 1992; Rives et al, 1989)

When nasojejunal intubation fails despite a non-invasive trial (with or without intravenous erythromycin) or when anatomical considerations such as an esophageal diverticulum or stricture, large hiatal hernia, previous upper gastrointestinal tract surgical alterations, or pyloric outlet obstruction prevent manual passage, endoscopically guided tube placement is possible.

A number of tube placement methods have been described. A commonly used technique involves grasping successive loops of suture or umbilical tape that have been attached to the distal half of the tubing at short intervals with endoscopic forceps. The stylet, catheter, and endoscope should be lubricated with silicone spray to minimize sticking and potential dislodgement of the catheter with the eventual removal of the endoscope.

1. After introducing the endoscope into the distal third of the esophagus, a polyurethane or silicone naso-enteric catheter is advanced manually through the nasopharynx and down the esophagus until it enters the visual field of the endoscope. The most distal loop of suture or umbilical tape is grasped with the endoscopic grasping forceps.
2. In tandem, the endoscope and tube are passed into the stomach, through the pylorus, and beyond the second portion of the duodenum.
3. The forceps and tubing are advanced through the endoscope until the next loop of suture or umbilical tape is visualized.
4. The forceps are released and withdrawn toward the endoscope until they are aligned with the next most distal loop of suture or tape, which is grasped. This sequence is repeated until the tube is advanced to the desired location.
5. This procedure has a higher success rate when performed in conjunction with fluoroscopy to verify tube placement and that tube position has been maintained during removal of the endoscope.
6. Once the endoscope is removed, the stylet is gently removed. If the stylet does not easily slide out of the catheter, dislodgement may occur. Tube location may be verified by an abdominal radiograph or fluoroscopy.

References

Adam JS, Birck HG: Pediatric caustic ingestion. *Ann Otol Rhinol Laryngol*, 91:656–658, 1982.

Adler JS, Graeb DA, Nugent RA: Inadvertent intracranial placement of a nasogastric tube in a patient with severe head trauma. *Can Med Assoc J*, 147:668–669, 1992.

Allendorph M, Werlin SL, et al: Endoscopic cholangiopancreatography in children. *J Pediatr*, 110:206–211, 1987.

Ament M: Is endoscopic cholangiopancreatography needed for the jaundiced infant? *Gastrointest Endosc*, 33:49–52, 1987.

Ament ME, Berquist WE, et al: Fiberoptic upper intestinal endoscopy in infants and children. *Pediatr Clin North Am*, 35:141–155, 1988.

Ament ME, Vargas J: Fiberoptic upper intestinal endoscopy. In Walker WA, Durie PR, et al (eds): *Pediatric Gastrointestinal Disease: Pathophysiology, Diagnosis, Management.* Philadelphia, BC Decker, 1991, p 1250.

American Society for Gastrointestinal Endoscopy: *Infection Control During Gastrointestinal Endoscopy.* Manchester, MA, ASGE Publications, 1988. Booklet.

Anderson KD, Rouse TM, Randolph JG: A controlled trial of corticosteroids in children with corrosive injury of the esophagus. *N Engl J Med*, 323:637–640, 1990.

Aoki G, Nagasako K, et al: The fiberendoscopic diagnosis of intestinal tuberculosis. *Endoscopy*, 7:113, 1975.

Arens R, Reichman B: Grooved palate associated with prolonged use of orogastric feeding tubes in premature infants. *J Oral Maxillofac Surg*, 50: 64–65, 1992.

Arhan P, Devroede G, et al: Idiopathic disorders of fecal incontinence in children. *Pediatrics* 71: 774–779, 1983.

Atkinson GO, Wyly JB, et al: Idiopathic fibrosing pancreatitis: a cause of obstructive jaundice in childhood. *Pediatr Radiol*, 18:28–31, 1988.

Azizkan RG, Tapper D, Eraklis A: Achalasia in childhood: a 20 year experience. *J Pediatr Surg*, 15:452–456, 1980.

Baillie J: *Gastrointestinal Endoscopy: Basic Principles and Practice.* Oxford, Butterworth-Heinemann, 1992, p 18.

Barr RG, Levine MD, Watkins JB: Recurrent abdominal pain of childhood due to lactose intolerance. *N Engl J Med*, 300:1449–1452, 1979.

Barr RG, Watkins JB, Perman JA: Mucosal function and breath hydrogen excretion: comparative studies in the clinical evaluation of children with non-specific abdominal complaints. *Pediatrics* 68:526–533, 1981.

Barsoum MS, Bolous FI, et al: Tamponade and injection sclerotherapy in the management of bleeding oesophageal varices. *Br J Surg*, 69: 766–768, 1982.

Bass S, Connon JJ, Ho CS: Biliary tree in cystic fibrosis: biliary tract abnormalities in cystic fibrosis demonstrated by endoscopic retrograde cholangiography. *Gastroenterology*, 84:1592–1596, 1983.

Beddis I, McKenzie S: Transpyloric feeding in the very low birthweight (1500 g and below) infant. One year's experience in an intensive care neonatal unit. *Arch Dis Child*, 54:213, 1979.

Benda GIM: Modes of feeding low–birth-weight infants. *Semin Perinatol*, 3:407–415, 1979.

Benoit A, Bodiou C, et al: QT long et arret circulatoire apres eure injection d'erythromycine chez un nouvea-ne. *Arch Fr Pediatr*, 48:39–41, 1991.

Bentler M, Stanish M: Nutrition support for the pediatric patient with AIDS. *J Am Diet Assoc*, 488–491, 1987.

Berman SA, Balkany TJ, Simmons MA: Otitis media in the neonatal intensive care unit. *Pediatrics* 62:198, 1978.

Berquist WE, Byrne WJ, et al: Achalasia: diagnosis, management, and clinical course in 16 children. *Pediatrics*, 71:798–805, 1983.

Berry R, Perrault J: Gastrointestinal bleeding. In Walker WA, Durie PR, et al (eds): *Pediatric Gastrointestinal Disease: Pathophysiology, Diagnosis, Management.* Philadelphia, BC Decker, 1991, p 125.

Bickerstaff KI, Britton BJ, Gough MH: Endoscopic palliation of malignant biliary obstruction in a child. *Br J Surg*, 766:1092–1093, 1989.

Bigard MA, Gaucher P, Lassalle C: Fatal colonic explosion during colonoscopic polypectomy. *Gastroenterology*, 177:1307–1310, 1979.

Bilbao MK, Dotter CT, et al: Complications of endoscopic retrograde cholangiopancreatography (ERCP). *Gastroenterology*, 70:314–320, 1976.

Biller JA, Allen JL, et al: Long-term evaluation of esophageal and pulmonary function in patients with repaired esophageal atresia and tracheoesophageal fistula. *Dig Dis Sci,* 32:985–990, 1987.

Bines JE, Winter HS: Lower endoscopy. In Walker WA, Durie PR, et al (eds): *Pediatric Gastrointestinal Disease: Pathophysiology, Diagnosis, Management.* Philadelphia, BC Decker, 1991, pp 1257–1260.

Blustein PK, Gaskin K, et al: Endoscopic cholangiopancreatography in pancreatitis in children and adolescents. *Pediatrics*, 68:387–393, 1981.

Bos AP, Tibboel D, et al: Sinusitis: hidden source of sepsis in post-operative pediatric intensive care patients. *Crit Care Med*, 17:886–888, 1989.

Boston VE, Cywes S, Davies MRQ: Qualitative and quantitative evaluation of internal and external anal sphincter function in the newborn. *Gut*, 18:1036–1044, 1977.

Bowes KS, Kling KS: Anorectal manometry in premature infants. *J Pediatr Surg*, 14:533–535, 1979.

Brandes JW, Scheffer B, et al: Complications and prophylaxis, a controlled study. *Endoscopy*, 133: 27–30, 1981.

Bretholz A, Strasser H, Knoblauch M: Endoscopic diagnosis of ileocecal tuberculosis. *Gastrointest Endosc*, 24:250, 1987.

Buckley A, Connon JJ: The role of ERCP in children and adolescents. *Gastrointest Endosc*, 36:360–372, 1990.

Burrows C, Geggie J, et al: *Feeding by Tube—Eating by Mouth. A Handbook for Parents.* Calgary, Alberta, Alberta Children's Hospital Foundation, 1992, p 5.

Buss DH, Scharyj M: Herpes virus infection of the esophagus and other visceral organs in adults. Incidence and clinical significance. *Am J Med*, 66:457–462, 1979.

Bussy V, Marechal F, Nasca S: Microbial contamination of enteral feeding tubes occurring during nutritional treatment. *J Parent Enter Nutr*, 16: 552–557, 1992.

Byrne WJ: Foreign bodies and bezoars. In Wyllie R, Hyams JS (eds): *Pediatric Gastrointestinal Disease: Pathophysiology, Diagnosis, Management.* Philadelphia, WB Saunders, 1993, p 172.

Byrne WJ, Euler AR, et al: Bacteremia in children following upper endoscopy or colonoscopy. *J Pediatr Gastroenterol Nutr*, 1:551–553, 1982.

Cadranel S, Lorenzo D, Rodesch P: Caustic ingestion and esophageal function. *J Pediatr Gastroenterol Nutr*, 10:164–168, 1990.

Cannon RA: Differential effect of botulina toxin on esophageal motor function in infants. *J Pediatr Gastroenterol Nutr*, 4:563–567, 1985.

Caos A, Benner KG, et al: Colonoscopy after GoLytely preparation in acute rectal bleeding. *J Clin Gastroenterol*, 8:46–49, 1986.

Cappell NJ: Esophageal bleeding after percutaneous endoscopic gastrostomy. *J Clin Gastroenterol*, 10:383–385, 1988.

Cappell MS, Scarpa PJ, et al: Complications of nasoenteral tubes. Intragastric tube knotting and intragastric splitting. *J Clin Gastroenterol*, 14:144–147, 1992.

Caravati EM, Bennett DL, McElwee NE: Pediatric coin ingestion. *Am J Dis Child*, 143:549–551, 1989.

Casteels-Van Daele M, Jackson J, et al: Dystonic reactions in children caused by metoclopramide. *Arch Dis Child*, 45:130–133, 1970.

Cataldi-Betcher EL, Seltzer MH, et al: Complications occurring during enteral nutritional support. A prospective study. *JEPN J Parenter Enter Nutr*, 7:546–552, 1982.

Cave DR, Robinson WR, Brotschi EA: Necrotizing fasciitis following percutaneous endoscopic gastrostomy. *Gastrointest Endosc*, 32:294–296, 1986.

Cello JP: Gastrointestinal manifestations of HIV infection. *Infect Dis Clin North Am*, 2:387–396, 1988.

Cheek JA, Staub GF: Nasojejunal alimentation for premature and full-term newborn infants. *J Pediatr*, 82:955, 1973.

Classen DC, Jacobson JA, et al: Serious *Pseudomonas* infections associated with endoscopic retrograde cholangiopancreatography. *Am J Med*, 84:590–596, 1988.

Clouse RE: Motor disorders. In Sleisenger MH, Fordtran JS (eds): *Gastrointestinal Disease*, 4th ed. Philadelphia, WB Saunders, 1989, pp 561–562.

Cohen LB, Simon C, et al: Esophageal motility and symptoms after endoscopic injection sclerotherapy. *Dig Dis Sci*, 30:29–32, 1985.

Cohen MB, A-Kader HH, et al: Complications of percutaneous liver biopsy in children. *Gastroenterology*, 102:629–832, 1992.

Collins R, Feldman M, Fordtran J: Colon cancer, dysplasia and surveillance in patients with ulcerative colitis. *N Engl J Med*, 316:1654–1658, 1987.

Conn HO, Simpson J: Excessive mortality associated with balloon tamponade of bleeding varices. *JAMA*, 202:587–591, 1967.

Cooney DR, Grosfeld JL: Operative management of pseudocysts in infants and children: a review of 75 cases. *Ann Surg*, 182:590–596, 1975.

Cronan J, Burrell M, Trepeta R: Aphthoid ulcerations in gastric candidiasis. *Radiology*, 134: 607–611, 1980.

Cynamon HA, Milov DE, Andres JM: Diagnosis and management of colonic polyps in children. *J Pediatr*, 114:593–596, 1989.

Czinn SJ, Carr H: Rapid diagnosis of *Campylobacter pyloridis*–associated gastritis. *J Pediatr*, 110: 569–570, 1987.

Dagradi A, Mehler R, et al: Sources of upper gastrointestinal bleeding in patients with liver cirrhosis and large esophageal varices. *Am J Gastroenterol*, 54:458–463, 1970.

Dahms BB, Rothstein FC: Barrett's esophagitis in children: a consequence of chronic gastroesophageal reflux. *Gastroenterology*, 86:318–323, 1984.

Dajani AS, Bisno AL, et al: Prevention of bacterial endocarditis: recommendations by the American Heart Association. *JAMA*, 264:2919–2922, 1990.

Davidson GP, Goodwin D, Robb TA: Incidence and duration of lactose malabsorption in children hospitalized with acute enteritis: study in a well-nourished urban population. *J Pediatr*, 105: 587–590, 1984.

Davidson GP, Robb TA, Kirubakaran CP: Bacterial contamination of the small intestine as an important cause of chronic diarrhea and abdominal pain: diagnosis by breath hydrogen test. *Pediatrics*, 74:229–235, 1984.

Davies MR: The use of nasogastric intubation in the radiological diagnosis of esophageal atresia. *S Afr Med J*, 78:670–672, 1990.

Deschner EE, Lipkin M: Proliferative patterns in colonic mucosa in familial polyposis. *Cancer*, 35: 413–418, 1975.

Desmond P, Raman R, Idikulu J: Effect of nasogastric tubes on the nose and maxillary sinus. *Crit Care Med*, 19:509–511, 1991.

Diamant NE: Physiology of the esophagus. In Champion MC, McCallum RW (eds): *Physiology, Diagnosis, and Therapy in GI Motility Disorders*. Philadelphia, The Medicine Publishing Foundation, 1987, pp 1–14.

DiLorenzo C, Lachman R, Hyman PE: Erythromycin for post-pyloric intubation. *J Pediatr Gastroenterol Nutr*, 11:45–47, 1990.

DiPalma JA, Brady CE, et al: Comparison of colon cleansing methods in preparation for colonoscopy. *Gastroenterology*, 86:856–860, 1984.

Ditesheim JA, Richards W, Sharp K: Fatal and disastrous complications following percutaneous endoscopic gastrostomy. *Am Surg*, 55:92–96, 1989.

Donovan T, Ward M, Shephard R: Evaluation of endoscopic sclerotherapy of esophageal varices in children. *J Pediatr Gastroenterol Nutr*, 5:696–700, 1986.

Drumm B, Sherman P: Gastritis in childhood. In Walker WA, Durie PR, et al (eds): *Pediatric Gastrointestinal Disease: Pathophysiology, Diagnosis, Management*. Philadelphia, BC Decker, 1991, pp 426–437.

Dumon JF, Meric B, et al: A new method of esophageal dilation using Savary-Gilliard bougies. *Gastrointest Endosc*, 31:379–382, 1985.

Durack DT, Kaplan EL, Bisno AL: Apparent failures of endocarditis prophylaxis: analysis of 52 cases submitted to a national registry. *JAMA*, 250: 2318–2322, 1983.

Dutta SK, Cox M, et al: Prospective evaluation of the risk of bacteremia and the role of antibiotics in ERCP. *J Clin Gastroenterol*, 5:325–329, 1983.

Eckardt VF, Nix W, et al: Esophageal motor function in patients with muscular dystrophy. *Gastroenterology*, 90:628–635, 1986.

Einhorn A, Horton L, et al: Serious respiratory consequences of detergent ingestions in children. *Pediatrics*, 84:472–474, 1989.

Elias E, Hamlyn AN, et al: A randomized trial of percutaneous transhepatic cholangiography with the Chiba needle versus endoscopic retrograde cholangiography for bile duct visualization in jaundice. *Gastroenterology*, 71:439–443, 1976.

Estrera A, Taylor W, et al: Corrosive burns of the esophagus and stomach: a recommendation on an aggressive surgical approach. *Ann Thorac Surg*, 41:276–283, 1986.

Evans JS: Abnormalities of the bile ducts. In Wyllie R, Hyams JS (eds): *Pediatric Gastrointestinal Disease: Pathophysiology, Diagnosis, Management*. Philadelphia, WB Saunders, 1993, pp 922–923.

Fegerman KE, Lysen LK: Enteral feeding tubes: a comparison and history. *Nutr Supp Serv*, 7: 10–14, 1987.

Fennoy I, Leung J: Refeeding and subsequent growth in the child with AIDS. *Nutr Clin Pract*, 5:54–58, 1990.

Ferguson MK, Migliore M, et al: Early evaluation and therapy for caustic esophageal injury. *Am J Surg*, 157:116–120, 1989.

Fernbach SK, Tucker GF: Coin ingestion: unusual

appearance of the penny in a child. *Radiology*, 158:512–514, 1986.

Fieror J, Finley F: Deficient serum bacteriocidal activity against *Escherichia coli* in patients with cirrhosis of the liver. *J Clin Invest*, 63:912–921, 1979.

Fleischer D: Recommendations for antibiotic prophylaxis before endoscopy. *Am J Gastroenterol*, 84:1489–1491, 1989.

Fleischer DR: Diagnosis and treatment of disorders of defecation in children. *Pediatr Ann*, 5: 71–101, 1976.

Flick JA, Boyle JT, Tuchman DN: Esophageal motor abnormalities in children and adolescents with scleroderma and mixed connective tissue disease. *Pediatrics*, 82:107–111, 1988.

Ford RPK, Barnes GL: Breath hydrogen test and sucrase-isomaltase deficiency. *Arch Dis Child*, 58:595–597, 1983.

Freedman PG, Weiner BC, Balthazar EJ: Cytomegalovirus esophagitis in a patient with acquired immune deficiency syndrome. *Am J Gastroenterol*, 80:434–437, 1985.

Friedman EM: Caustic ingestions and foreign bodies in the aerodigestive tract of children. *Pediatr Clin North Am*, 36:1403–1410, 1989.

Fung KP, Math MV, et al: Midazolam as a sedative in esophageal manometry: a study of the effect on esophageal motility. *J Pediatr Gastroenterol Nutr*, 15:85–88, 1992.

Gans SL, Ament M, Cristie DL: Pediatric endoscopy with flexible fiberscopes. *J Pediatr Surg*, 10: 375–380, 1975.

Gauderer MW, Ponsky JL, Izant RJ Jr: Gastrostomy without laparotomy: a percutaneous endoscopic technique. *J Pediatr Surg*, 15:872–875, 1980.

Gaudreault P, Parent M, et al: Predictability of esophageal injury from signs and symptoms: a study of caustic ingestion in 378 children. *Pediatrics*, 71:767–770, 1983.

Geboes K, Vantrappen G: The value of colonoscopy in the diagnosis of Crohn's disease. *Gastrointest Endosc*, 22:18–23, 1975.

Gelfand MD, Botoman VA: Esophageal motility disorders: a clinical overview. *Am J Gastroenterol*, 82:181–186, 1987.

Gilat T, Revach M, Sohar E: Deposition of amyloid in the gastrointestinal tract. *Gut*, 10:98–104, 1969.

Girdamy B, Sieber W, Osman M: Traumatic pseudodiverticulas of the pharynx in newborn infants. *N Engl J Med*, 280:237–240, 1969.

Glucagon for injection. *Physicians' Desk Reference*. Midvale, NJ, Medical Economics Data Production, 1994, pp 1225–1226.

Goerlick FS, Dobbins JW, et al: Biliary tract abnormalities in patients with arteriohepatic dysplasia. *Dig Dis Sci*, 25:815–820, 1982.

Gonzalez-Vallina R, Alonso EM, et al: Outpatient percutaneous liver biopsy in children. *J Pediatr Gastroenterol Nutr*, 17:370–375, 1993.

Graudal N, Milman N, et al: Bacteremia in cirrhosis of the liver. *Liver*, 66:297–301, 1986.

Grunow JE, Al-Hafidh AS, Tunnell WP: Gastroesophageal reflux following percutaneous endoscopic gastrostomy in children. *J Pediatr Surg*, 24:42–45, 1989.

Gryboski JD, Touloukian R, Camponella RA: Gastrointestinal manifestations of epidermolysis bullosa in children. *Arch Dermatol*, 124:746–752, 1988.

Guelrud M, Jaen D, et al: Endoscopic cholangiopancreatography in the infant: evaluation of a new prototype pediatric duodenoscope. *Gastrointest Endosc*, 33:4–8, 1987.

Hafner CD, Wylie JH Jr, Brush BE: Complications of gastrointestinal intubation. *Arch Surg*, 83: 147–160, 1961.

Haggitt RC, Reed BJ: Hereditary gastrointestinal polyposis syndromes. *Am J Surg Pathol*, 10:871–887, 1986.

Harris JW: Polyps of the colon and rectum in children. *Dis Colon Rectum*, 10:267–272, 1967.

Hassall E, Barclay GN, Ament ME: Colonoscopy in childhood. *Pediatrics*, 73:594–599, 1984.

Hassall E, Dimmidk JE: Unique features of *Helicobacter pylori* infection in children. *Dig Dis Sci*, 36:417–423, 1991.

Hatch TF: Encopresis and constipation in children. *Pediatr Clin North Am*, 35:2, 1988.

Hawkins DB: Dilation in esophageal strictures: comparative morbidity of antegrade and retrograde methods. *Ann Otol Rhinol Laryngol*, 97: 460–465, 1988.

Hawkins DB, DeMeter MJ, Barnett TE: Caustic ingestion: controversies in management: a review of 214 cases. *Laryngoscope*, 90:98–109, 1980.

Hayhurst E, Wyman M: Morbidity associated with prolonged use of polyvinyl chloride feeding tubes. *Am J Dis Child*, 129:72–74, 1975.

Healy GB: Foreign bodies of the air and food passages in children. *Am J Dis Child*, 141:239, 1987.

Henson D: Cytomegalovirus inclusion bodies in the gastrointestinal tract. *Arch Pathol*, 93:477–482, 1972.

Herbst JJ: Achalasia and other motor disorders. In Wyllie R, Hyams JS (eds): *Pediatric Gastrointestinal Disease: Pathophysiology, Diagnosis, Management*. Philadelphia, WB Saunders, 1993, pp 391–401.

Hermann M-E, Liehr R-M, et al: Subjective distress during continuous enteral alimentation: superiority of silicone rubber to polyurethane. *J Parenter Enter Nutr*, 13:281–285, 1989.

Herrill N, Martin RJ, Fanaroff A: Arterial oxygen tension during nasogastric feedings in the premature infant. *J Pediatr*, 96:914–916, 1980.

Hill ID, Bowie MD: Endoscopic sclerotherapy for control of bleeding varices in children. *Am J Gastroenterol*, 86:472–476, 1991.

Hodgson JH: Corrosive stricture of the stomach. Case report and review of the literature. *Br J Surg*, 46:358–361, 1959.

Holgersen LO, Mossberg SM, Miller RE: Colonoscopy for rectal bleeding in childhood. *J Pediatr Surg*, 13:83–85, 1978.

Holt H: Candida infection of the esophagus. *Gut*, 9:227, 1986.

Howard E, Stamatakis J, Mowat A: Management of esophageal varices in children by injection sclerotherapy. *J Pediatr Surg*, 19:2–5, 1984.

Howdle P, Miloszewski K, et al: Diagnosis of biliary tract hemorrhage (hemobilia) by endoscopy. *Gastrointest Endosc*, 23:94–95, 1976.

Howiler W, Goldberg HI: Gastroesophageal involvement in herpes simplex. *Gastroenterology*, 70:775–778, 1976.

Huibregtse K, Schneider B, et al: Endoscopic pancreatic drainage in chronic pancreatitis. *Gastrointest Endosc*, 344:9–15, 1988.

Humphries TJ, Castell DO: Pressure profile of esophageal peristalsis in normal humans as measured by direct intraesophageal transducers. *Dig Dis Sci*, 22:641–644, 1977.

Hunt R: Toward safer colonoscopy. *Gut*, 24: 371–375, 1983.

Hyams JS, Ricci A Jr, Leichtner AM: Clinical and laboratory correlates of esophagitis in young children. *J Pediatr Gastroenterol Nutr*, 7:52–56, 1988.

Infection control during gastrointestinal endoscopy: guidelines for clinical application. *Gastrointest Endosc*, 34:37S–40S, 1988.

Jain NK, Larson DE, et al: Antibiotic prophylaxis for percutaneous endoscopic gastrostomy: a prospective, randomized, double-blind clinical trial. *Ann Intern Med*, 107:824–828, 1987.

James RH: An unusual complication of passing a narrow bore nasogastric tube. *Anesthesia*, 33: 716–718, 1975.

Jenkins HR, Pincott JR, et al: Food allergy: the major cause of infantile colitis. *Arch Dis Child*, 59:326–329, 1984.

Johnson DE, Fokes J, Munson DP: Management of esophageal and pharyngeal perforation in the newborn infant. *Pediatrics* 70:592–596, 1982.

Kaplan B, Benson J, et al: Lymphonodular hyperplasia of the colon as a pathologic finding in children with lower gastrointestinal bleeding. *J Pediatr Gastroenterol Nutr*, 3:704–708, 1984.

Kaplan DS, Fried MW: Migration of PEG tubes. *Am J Gastroenterol*, 84:1590–1591, 1989.

Kawamitsu T, Nagashima K, et al: Pediatric total colonoscopy. *J Pediatr Surg*, 24:371–374, 1989.

Kennedy-Caldwell C, Caldwell MD, Zitarelli ME: Pediatric enteral nutrition. In Rombeau JL, Caldwell MD (eds): *Clinical Nutrition: Enteral and Tube Feeding*. Philadelphia, WB Saunders, 1990, p 341.

Keoshian LA, Nelson TS: A new design for a feeding tube. *Plast Reconstr Surg*, 44:508–509, 1969.

Killbridge PM, Dahms BB, Czinn SJ: *Campylobacter pylori*–associated gastritis and peptic ulcer disease in children. *Am J Dis Child*, 142:1149–1152, 1988.

Kilman WJ, Goyal RK: Disorders of pharyngeal and upper esophageal sphincter motor function. *Arch Intern Med*, 136:592–601, 1976.

King CE, Toskes PP: Comparison of the 1-gram [^{14}C]xylose, 10-gram lactulose-H_2 and 80-gram glucose H_2 breath tests in patients with small intestine bacterial overgrowth. *Gastroenterology*, 91:1447–1451, 1986.

Klein S, Heare BR, Soloway RD: The "buried bumper" syndrome: A complication of percutaneous endoscopic gastrostomy. *Am J Gastroenterol*, 85:448, 1990.

Knauer CM: Percutaneous biopsy of the liver as a procedure for outpatients. *Gastroenterology*, 74:101–102, 1987.

Koch H: Operative endoscopy. *Gastrointest Endosc*, 24:65–68, 1977.

Kochhar R, Goenka MK, et al: A comparative evaluation of sclerosants for esophageal varices: a prospective randomized controlled study. *Gastrointest Endosc*, 36:127–130, 1990.

Koehane PP, Attrill H, et al: Limitations and drawbacks of fine-bore nasogastric feeding tubes. *Clin Nutr*, 2:85–86, 1983.

Kohn CL, Keithley JK: Enteral nutrition: potential complications and patient monitoring. *Nurs Clin North Am*, 24:339–340, 1989.

Korth H, Muller I, Erckenbrecht WM: Breath hydrogen as a test for intestinal transit. *Hepatogastroenterology*, 31:282–284, 1984.

Korula J, Balart L, et al: A prospective, randomized controlled trial of chronic esophageal variceal sclerotherapy. *Hepatology*, 5:584–589, 1985.

Kost KM, Shapiro RS: Button battery ingestion: a case report and review of the literature. *J Otolaryngol*, 16:252–257, 1987.

LaFerla G, Gordon S, et al: Hyperamylasaemia and acute pancreatitis following endoscopic retrograde cholangiopancreatography. *Pancreas*, 1: 160–163, 1986.

Lai ECS, Lo C, et al: Urgent biliary decompression after endoscopic retrograde cholangiopancreatography. *Am J Surg*, 157:121–125, 1989.

Lake AM, Whitington PF, Hamilton SR: Dietary protein-induced colitis in breast-fed infants. *J Pediatr*, 101:906–910, 1982.

Larcher VF, Wyke RJ, et al: Bacterial and fungal infection in children with fulminant hepatic failure: possible role of opsonisation and complement deficiency. *Gut*, 23:1037–1043, 1982.

Larson DE, Burton DD, et al: Percutaneous endoscopic gastrostomy: indications, success, complications, and mortality in 314 consecutive patients. *Gastroenterology*, 93:48–52, 1987.

Lashner BA, Kane SV, Hanauer SB: Colon cancer surveillance in chronic ulcerative colitis: historical cohort study. *Am J Gastroenterol*, 85:1083–1087, 1990.

Lee JMH, Tam PKH, Saing H: Whole gut irrigation in infants and young children. *Dis Colon Rectum*, 29:252–254, 1987.

LeFrock JL, Ellis CA, et al: Transient bacteremia with percutaneous liver biopsy. *J Infect Dis*, 131: S104–S107, 1975.

LeLeiko NS, Burke P, Cewin-Chao L: Enteral nutrition. In Wyllie R, Hyams JS (eds): *Pediatric Gastrointestinal Disease: Pathology, Diagnosis, Management.* Philadelphia, WB Saunders, 1993, p 1135.

Levy LD, Durie PR, et al: Effects of long-term nutritional rehabilitation on body composition and clinical status in malnourished children and adolescents with cystic fibrosis. *J Pediatr*, 107: 225–230, 1985.

Lichtman S, Guzman C, et al: Morbidity after percutaneous liver biopsy. *Arch Dis Child*, 62: 901–904, 1987.

Liebman WM: Fiberoptic endoscopy of the gastrointestinal tract in infants and children. *Am J Gastroenterol*, 68:452–455, 1977.

Lifschitz CH, Irving CS, Gopalakrishna GS: Carbohydrate malabsorption in infants with diarrhea studies with the breath hydrogen test. *J Pediatr*, 102:371–375, 1983.

Lin AC, Chapman SW, et al: Clonorchiasis: an update. *South Med J*, 80:919–923, 1987.

Litovitz TL: Battery ingestions: product accessibility and clinical course. *Pediatrics*, 75:469–476, 1985.

Livstone EM, Cohen GM, et al: Diastatic serosal lacerations: an unrecognized complication of colonoscopy. *Gastroenterology*, 67:1245–1247, 1974.

Loening-Baucke VA: Sensitivity of the sigmoid colon and rectum in children treated for chronic constipation. *J Pediatr Gastroenterol Nutr*, 3:454–459, 1984.

Loening-Baucke V, Desch L, Wolraich M: Biofeedback training for patients with meningomyelocele and fecal incontinence. *Dev Med Child Neurol*, 30:781–790, 1988.

Loening-Baucke V, Yonoszai MK: Abnormal anal sphincter response in chronically constipated children. *J Pediatr*, 100:213–218, 1982.

Logan RF, Hastings JGM: Bacterial endocarditis: a complication of gastroscopy. *BMJ*, 296:1107, 1988.

London RL, Trotman BW, et al: Dilation of severe esophageal strictures by an inflatable balloon catheter. *Gastroenterology*, 80:173–175, 1981.

Lopez-Torres A, Waye JD: The safety of intubation in patients with esophageal varices. *Am J Dig Dis*, 18:1032, 1973.

Low DE, Shoenut JP, et al: Prospective assessment of risk of bacteremia with colonoscopy and polypectomy. *Dig Dis Sci*, 32:12339–12343, 1987.

Low LCK, Gael KM: Metoclopramide poisoning in children. *Arch Dis Child*, 55:310–312, 1980.

MacAlister WH, Siegel MJ, Shakelford GD: Intestinal perforations by tube feedings in small infants. *Am J Radiol*, 145:687–689, 1985.

MacClean WC, Fink BB: Lactose malabsorption by premature infants: magnitude and clinical significance. *J Pediatr*, 97:383–388, 1980.

MacRae FA, Tan KG, Williams CB: Towards safer colonoscopy: a report on the complications of 5000 diagnostic or therapeutic colonoscopies. *Gut*, 24:376–383, 1983.

Madsen R, Skibba R, Galvan A: Gastric bezoars. A technique of endoscopic removal. *Dig Dis Sci*, 23:717–720, 1978.

Mahmoud AAF, Wahab MFA: Schistosomiasis. In Warren KS, Mahmoud AAF (eds): *Tropical and Geographic Medicine.* New York, McGraw-Hill, 1990, pp 458–473.

Maleki M, Evan WE: Foreign body perforation of the intestinal tract. *Arch Surg*, 101:475–477, 1970.

Marshall JB, Halpin TC: Choledochocele as the cause of recurrent obstructive jaundice in childhood: diagnosis by ERCP. *Gastrointest Endosc*, 28:88–90, 1982.

Martin DF, Tweedle DEF: Retroperitoneal perforation during ERCP and endoscopic sphincterotomy: causes, clinical feature and management. *Endoscopy*, 22:174–175, 1990.

Mastropaola G, Rees WDW: Evaluation of the hydrogen breath test in man: Definition and elimination of the early hydrogen peak. *Gut*, 28: 721–725, 1987.

Matsumoto T, Iida M, et al: Endoscopic findings in *Yersinia enterocolitica* enterocolitis. *Gastrointest Endosc* 36:583–587, 1990.

Maull KI, Osmand AP, Maull CD: Liquid caustic ingestions: An in vitro study of the effects of buffer, neutralization, and dilution. *Ann Emerg Med*, 14:1160–1162, 1985.

McGill DB: Predicting hemorrhage after liver biopsy. *Dig Dis Sci*, 26:385–387, 1981.

McGill DB, Rakela J, et al: A 21-year experience with major hemorrhage after percutaneous liver biopsy. *Gastroenterology*, 99:1396–1400, 1990.

McNeely RL, O'Neill JA, Ghishan FK: Fibrosing pancreatitis—an obscure cause of painless obstructive jaundice: a case report and review of the literature. *Pediatrics*, 67:136–139, 1981.

McVay PA, Toy PTCY: Lack of increased bleeding after liver biopsy in patients with mild hemostatic abnormalities. *Am J Clin Pathol*, 94: 747–753, 1990.

Metheny NA: Measures to test placement of nasogastric and nasointestinal feeding tubes: a review. *Nurs Res*, 37:324–329, 1988.

Metheny NA, McSweeney M, et al: Effectiveness of the auscultative method in predicting feeding tube location. *Nurs Res*, 39:262–267, 1990.

Metheny NA, Spies M, Eisenberg P: Frequency of enteral tube displacement and associated risk factors. *Res Nurs Health*, 9:241–247, 1986.

Metheny NA, Williams P, et al: Effectiveness of pH measurements in predicting feeding tube placement. *Nurs Res*, 38:280–285, 1989.

Meyers JD: Infections in bone marrow transplant recipients. In Mandell GL, Douglas RG, Bennett JE (eds): *Principles and Practice of Infectious Diseases.* New York, Churchill-Livingstone, 1990, p 2291.

Milla PJ: Gastrointestinal motility disorders in children. *Pediatr Clin North Am*, 35:311–330, 1988.

Miller K, Tomlinson J, Sahn S: Pleuropulmonary complications of enteral tube feeding. *Chest*, 88: 230–233, 1985.

Miller RE, Tiszenkel HI: Esophageal perforation due to pneumatic dilatation for achalasia. *Surg Gynecol Obstet*, 166:458–460, 1988.

Miller RE, Winkler WP, Kotler DP: The Russell percutaneous endoscopic gastrostomy: key technical steps. *Gastrointest Endosc*, 34:339–342, 1988.

Miner PB, Donnelly TC, Read NW: Investigation of mode of action of biodfeedback in treatment of fecal incontinence. *Dig Dis Sci*, 35:1291–1298, 1990.

Mitchell RG, Kerr RM, et al: Transnasal endoscopic technique for feeding tube placement. *Gastrointest Endosc*, 38:596–597, 1992.

Monar D, Taitz LS, et al: Anorectal manometry results in defecation disorders. *Arch Dis Child*, 58: 257–261, 1983.

Moore MC, Greene HL: Tube feeding of infants and children. *Pediatr Clin North Am*, 32:402, 1985.

Moore WR: Caustic ingestions: pathophysiology, diagnosis, and treatment. *Clin Pediatr*, 25:192–196, 1986.

Morin CL, Roulet M, et al: Continuous elemental alimentation in the treatment of children and adolescents with Crohn's disease. *J Parenter Enter Nutr*, 6:194–199, 1982.

Mowat AP, Psacharopoulos HT, Williams R. Extrahepatic biliary atresia versus neonatal hepatitis. Review of 137 prospectively investigated infants. *Arch Dis Child*, 51:763–770, 1976.

Murphy EL, Calloway DH: The effect of antibiotic drugs on the volume and composition of intestinal gas from beans. *Am J Dig Dis* 17:639–642, 1972.

Nachlas MM: A new triple lumen tube for the diagnosis and treatment of upper gastro-intestinal hemorrhage. *N Engl J Med*, 252:720–721, 1955.

Nebel OT, Silvis SE, et al: Complications associated with endoscopic retrograde cholangiopancreatography. *Gastrointest Endosc*, 22:34–39, 1975.

Nelis GF, Vermeeren MA, Jasen W: Role of fructose-sorbitol malabsorption in the irritable bowel syndrome. *Gastroenterology*, 99:1016–1020, 1990.

Neu HC: Recommendations for antibiotic prophylaxis before endoscopy. *Am J Gastroenterol*, 84:1488–1489, 1989.

Nguyen DH, Burns MW, et al: Intraoperative cardiovascular collapse secondary to latex allergy. *J Urol*, 146:571–574, 1991.

Niv Y, Batt L, Motro M: Bacterial endocarditis after Hurst bougienage in a patient with benign esophageal stricture and mitral valve prolapse. *Gastrointest Endosc*, 31:265–267, 1985.

Nose O, Iada Y, et al: Breath hydrogen test for detecting lactose malabsorption in infants and children. Prevalence of lactose malabsorption in Japanese children and adults. *Arch Dis Child*, 54:436–440, 1979.

Nose O, Kai H, et al: Breath hydrogen test in infants and children with blind loop syndrome. *J Pediatr Gastroenterol Nutr*, 3:364–367, 1984.

Nostrant TT, Kumar NB, Appelman HD: Histopathology differentiates acute self-limited colitis from ulcerative colitis. *Gastroenterology*, 92: 318–328, 1987.

Nugent FW, Haggitt RC, Gilpin PA: Cancer surveillance in ulcerative colitis. *Gastroenterology*, 100: 1241–1248, 1991.

Nurko S: Motor disorders. In Walker WA, Durie PR, et al (eds): *Pediatric Gastrointestinal Disease: Pathophysiology, Diagnosis, Management.* Philadelphia, BC Decker, 1991, p 405.

Nussbaum E, Fleming DG, et al: Stridor due to radiotransparent esophageal foreign body. *Am J Dis Child*, 138:1081–1083, 1984.

Oakes DD, Sherck JP, Mark JB: Lye ingestion: clinical patterns and therapeutic implications. *J Thorac Cardiovasc Surg*, 83:194–204, 1982.

Okike N, Payne SW, et al: Esophagomyotomy versus forceful dilatation for achalasia of the esophagus: results in 899 patients. *Ann Thorac Surg*, 28:119–125, 1979.

Okuno M, Himeno S, et al: Changes in serum levels of pancreatic isoamylase, lipase, trypsin, and elastase 1 after endoscopic retrograde pancreatography. *Hepatogastroenterology*, 32:87–90, 1985.

O'Neill JA, Greene H, Ghishan FK: Surgical implications of chronic pancreatitis. *J Pediatr Surg*, 20:58–60, 1985.

Orchard JL, Barlow J: Benign subcutaneous emphysema after percutaneous gastrostomy. *Gastrointest Endosc*, 33:51, 1987.

Ott DJ, Richter JE, et al: Radiographic evaluation of esophagus immediately after pneumatic dilatation for achalasia. *Dig Dis Sci*, 32:962–967, 1987.

Overholt BF, Hargrove RL, et al: Colonoscopic polypectomy: silent perforation. *Gastroenterology*, 70:112–113, 1976.

Panes J, Teres J, et al: Efficacy of balloon tamponade in treatment of bleeding gastric and esophageal varices: results in 151 consecutive episodes. *Dig Dis Sci*, 33:454–459, 1988.

Paquet K-J, Feussner H: Endoscopic sclerosis and esophageal balloon tamponade in acute hemorrhage from esophagogastric varices: a prospective controlled randomized trial. *Hepatology*, 5:580–583, 1985.

Pasquale MD, Cerra FB: Sengstaken-Blakemore tube placement. Use of balloon tamponade to control bleeding varices. *Crit Care Clin*, 8:743–753, 1992.

Perisic V: Role of PTC and ERCP in diagnostic imaging of the hepatobiliary tree: Caroli's disease in two siblings. *J Pediatr Gastroenterol Nutr*, 6: 647–648, 1987.

Perman JA, Barr RG, Watkins JB: Sucrose malabsorption in children: noninvasive diagnosis by interval breath hydrogen determination. *J Pediatr*, 93:17–22, 1978.

Perman JA, Modler S, et al: Fasting breath hydrogen concentration: normal values and clinical application. *Gastroenterology*, 87:1358–1363, 1984.

Per-Rodriquez J, Quiro J, Frias E: Duodenorenal perforation in a neonate by a tube of silicone rubber during transpyloric feeding. *J Pediatr*, 92: 1113–1116, 1978.

Piquata C, Budillon G, et al: Jejunal bacterial overgrowth and intestinal permeability in children with immune deficiency syndrome. *Gut*, 31: 879–882, 1990.

Pitcher JL: Safety and effectiveness of the modified Sengstaken-Blakemore tube: a prospective study. *Gastroenterology*, 61:291–298, 1971.

Planas R, Boix J, et al: Portocaval shunt versus endoscopic sclerotherapy in the elective treatment of variceal hemorrhage. *Gastroenterology*, 100: 1078–1086, 1991.

Postlethwait RW: Chemical burns of the esophagus. *Surg Clin North Am*, 63:915–924, 1983.

Putnam PE, Kocoshis SA, et al: Pediatric endoscopic retrograde cholangiopancreatography. *Am J Gastroenterol*, 86:824–830, 1991.

Read NW: Small bowel transit time of food in man: measurement, regulation, and possible importance. *Scand J Gastroenterol*, 19(suppl 96): 77–85, 1984.

Rhodes JM, Middleton P, Jewell DP: The lactulose hydrogen breath test as a diagnostic test for small-bowel bacterial overgrowth. *Scand J Gastroenterol*, 14:333–336, 1979.

Riddlesberger MM: Diagnostic imaging of the hepatobiliary system in infants and children. *J Pediatr Gastroenterol*, 3:353–364, 1984.

Rimola A, Soto R, et al: Reticuloendothelial system phagocytic activity in cirrhosis and its relationship to bacterial infections and prognosis. *Hepatology*, 4:53–58, 1984.

Rives DA, LeRoy JL, et al: Endoscopically assisted nasojejunal feeding tube placement. *Am Surg*, 55:88–91, 1989.

Rodriguez W, Levine JS: Enterococcal endocarditis following flexible sigmoidoscopy. *West J Med*, 140:951–953, 1984.

Rombeau JL: Enteral nutritional therapy. *Surg Clin North Am*, 61:605–620, 1981.

Rosenberg AJ, Vela AR: A new simplified technique for pediatric anorectal manometry. *Pediatrics*, 71:240–245, 1983.

Rossi T: Endoscopic examination of the colon in infancy and childhood. *Pediatr Clin North Am*, 35:331–356, 1988.

Roszler MH, Campbell WL: Post-ERCP pancreatitis: association with urographic visualization during ERCP. *Radiology*, 157:595–598, 1985.

Ruttenberg AM, Sonnenblick E, et al: Comparative response of normal and cirrhotic rats to intravenously injected bacteria. *Proc Soc Exp Biol Med*, 101:279–281, 1959.

Sack TL, Sleisenger MH: Myotonic dystrophy (myotonia dystrophica). In Sleisinger MH, Fordtran JS (eds): *Gastrointestinal Disease*, 4th ed. Philadelphia, WB Saunders, 1989, pp 516–517.

Salt WB, Llaneza PP: Collagenous colitis: a cause of chronic diarrhea diagnosed only by biopsy of normal appearing colonic mucosa. *Gastrointest Endosc*, 32:421–423, 1986.

Sanderson IR, Boyle S, et al: Histologic abnormalities in biopsies from macroscopically normal colonoscopies. *Arch Dis Child*, 61:274–277, 1986.

Sanderson IR, Udeen S, et al: Remission induced by an elemental diet in small bowel Crohn's disease. *Arch Dis Child*, 61:123–127, 1987.

Sartor RB: Upper gastrointestinal endoscopy. In Drossman DA (ed): *Manual of Gastroenterologic Procedures*, 2nd ed. New York, Raven Press, 1987, p 97.

Sato Y, Frey EE, et al: Balloon dilatation of esophageal stenosis in children. *AJR*, 150:639–642, 1988.

Schiller LR, Santa Ana CA, et al: Pathogenesis of fecal incontinence in diabetes mellitus: evidence for internal anal sphincter dysfunction. *N Engl J Med*, 307:1666–1671, 1982.

Schlang H: Acetylcysteine in removal of bezoar. *JAMA*, 214:1329, 1970.

Schwartz DJ, Wynne JW, et al: The pulmonary consequences of aspiration of gastric contents at pH values greater than 2.5. *Am Rev Respir Dis*, 121: 119–126, 1980.

Schwartz GF, Polsky HS: Ingested foreign bodies of the gastrointestinal tract. *Am Surg*, 51:173–179, 1985.

Schunk JE, Cornele H, Bolt R: Pediatric coin ingestions. *Am J Dis Child*, 143:546–548, 1989.

Scott B: Motility studies. In Walker WA, Durie PR, et al (eds): *Pediatric Gastrointestinal Disease: Pathophysiology, Diagnosis, Management*. Philadelphia, BC Decker, 1991, pp 1324–1330.

Sengstaken R, Blakemore A: Balloon tamponage for the control of hemorrhage from esophageal varices. *Ann Surg*, 131:781–789, 1950.

Shorron PJ, Eykyn SJ, Cotton PB: Gastrointestinal instrumentation, bacteremia, and endocarditis. *Gut*, 24:1078–1093, 1983.

Siegle RL, Rabinowitz JG, Sarasohn C: Intestinal perforation secondary to nasojejunal feeding tubes. *AJR*, 126:196–197, 1976.

Silk DBA, Payne-James JT: Complications of enteral nutrition. In Rombeau JL, Caldwell MD (eds): *Clinical Nutrition: Enteral and Tube Feeding*, 2nd ed. Philadelphia, WB Saunders, 1990, p 513.

Silverberg SG: Juvenile retention polyps of the colon and rectum. *Dig Dis Sci*, 15:617–619, 1970.

Skale N: Nasogastric tube insertion. *Manual of Pediatric Nursing Procedures*. Philadelphia, JB Lippincott, 1992, p 406.

Smith GM, Chester IM, et al: Small intestinal bacterial overgrowth in patients with lymphocytic leukemia. *J Clin Pathol*, 43:57–59, 1990.

Sofferman RA, Hirsch CE, et al: The nasogastric tube syndrome. *Laryngoscope*, 100:962–968, 1990.

Solomons NW, Barillas C: The cut-off criterion for a

positive hydrogen breath test in children: a reappraisal. *J Pediatr Gastroenterol Nutr*, 5:920–925, 1986.

Sondheimer JM: Upper esophageal sphincter and pharyngoesophageal motor function in infants with and without gastroesophageal reflux. *Gastroenterology*, 85:301–305, 1983.

Staniforth DH: Comparison of orocaecal transit times assessed by the lactulose/breath hydrogen and the sulpha-salazine/sulphapyridine methods. *Gut*, 30:978–982, 1989.

Stanten A, Peters H: Enzymatic dissolution of phytobezoars. *Am J Surg*, 130:259–261, 1975.

Stefan MM, Holcomb GW, Ross AJ: Cologastric fistula as a complication of percutaneous endoscopic gastrostomy. *JEPN J Parenter Enter Nutr*, 13:554–556, 1989.

Sullam PM, Drake TA, Sande MA: Pathogenesis of endocarditis. *Am J Med* 78(suppl 6B):110–115, 1985.

Surawicz CM, Belic L: Rectal biopsy helps to distinguish acute self-limited colitis from idiopathic inflammatory bowel disease. *Gastroenterology*, 866:104–113, 1984.

Taxier M, Sivak MV, et al: Endoscopic retrograde pancreatography in the evaluation of trauma to the pancreas. *Surg Gynecol Obstet*, 150:65–68, 1980.

Taylor EW, Bentley S, et al: Bowel preparation and the safety of colonoscopic polypectomy. *Gastroenterology*, 81:1–4, 1981.

Taylor RB: Esophageal foreign bodies. *Emerg Med Clin North Am*, 301–311, 1987.

Tenebein M: Whole bowel irrigation in iron poisoning. *J Pediatr*, 111:142–145, 1987.

Tobon F, Reid NC, et al: Nonsurgical test for the diagnosis of Hirschsprung's disease. *N Engl J Med*, 278:188–193, 1968.

Tolia V, Fleming S, Dubois RS: Use of GoLytely in children and adolescents. *J Pediatr Gastroenterol Nutr*, 3:468–470, 1984.

Trudel JL, Fazio VW, Sivak MV: Colonoscopic diagnosis and treatment of arteriovenous malformations in chronic lower gastrointestinal bleeding. *Dis Colon Rectum*, 31:107–110, 1988.

Vandenplas Y, Delree M, et al: Cervical esophageal perforation diagnosed by endoscopy in a premature infant: review of recent literature. *J Pediatr Gastroenterol Nutr*, 8:390–393, 1989.

Vanderhoof JA, Ament ME: Proctosigmoidoscopy and rectal biopsy in infants and children. *J Pediatr*, 89:911–915, 1976.

Vanderhoof JA, Rappaport PJ, Paxson CL: Manometric diagnosis of lower esophageal sphincter incompetence in infants: use of a small, single lumen perfused catheter. *Pediatrics*, 62:805–808, 1978.

van de Spuy S: Endoscopic retrograde cholangiopancreatography (ERCP) in children. *Endoscopy*, 10:173–175, 1978.

Vane D, Boles E, Clatworthy H: Esophageal sclerotherapy: An effective modality in children. *J Pediatr Surg*, 20:703–707, 1985.

Vantrappen G: Diagnostic methodology of esophageal problems. In Champion MC, McCallum RW (eds): *Physiology, Diagnosis, and Therapy in GI Motility Disorders*. Philadelphia, The Medicine Publishing Foundation, 1987, pp 51–60.

Vantrappen G, Hellemans J: Treatment of achalasia and related motor disorders. *Gastroenterology*, 79:144–154, 1980.

Vargas JH, Sachs P, Ament ME: Chronic intestinal pseudo-obstruction syndrome in pediatrics. *J Pediatr Gastroenterol Nutr*, 7:323–332, 1988.

Vignote ML, Mino G, et al: Endoscopic sphincterotomy in hepatic hydatid disease open to the biliary tree. *Br J Surg*, 77:30–31, 1990.

Vila JJ, Gutierrez C, et al: Whole bowel irrigation: experience in pediatric patients. *J Pediatr Surg*, 55:447–450, 1987.

Wake M, McCullough DE, Bennington JD: Effect of nasogastric tubes in eustachian tube function. *J Laryngol Otol*, 104:17–19, 1990.

Wald A, Chandra R, et al: Evaluation of biofeedback in childhood encopresis. *J Pediatr Gastroenterol Nutr*, 6:554–558, 1987.

Walker WA, Krivit W, Sharp HL: Needle biopsy of the liver in infancy and childhood. A safe diagnostic aid in liver disease. *Pediatrics*, 40:946–950, 1967.

Walker-Smith JA, Phillips AD, Richman PI: Intestinal biopsy. In Walker WA, Durie PR, et al (eds): *Pediatric Gastrointestinal Disease: Pathophysiology, Diagnosis, Management*. Philadelphia, BC Decker, 1991, pp 1307–1323.

Wason S: The emergency management of caustic ingestions. *J Emerg Med*, 2:175–182, 1985.

Waye JD: Endoscopic cholangiopancreatography in the infant. *Am J Gastroenterol*, 65:461–463, 1976.

Weinberg AG: Acetylcholinesterase and Hirschsprung's disease. *J Pediatr Gastroenterol Nutr*, 5:837–843, 1986.

Wells DH, Zachman RD: Nasojejunal feedings in low birthweight infants. *Pediatrics*, 87:276, 1975.

Wells S, Leonidas J, Conkle D: Traumatic prevertebral pharyngoesophageal pseudodiverticulum in the newborn infant. *J Pediatr Surg*, 9:217–222, 1969.

Werlin SL, Brown CW: Gastrointestinal motility. In Wyllie R, Hyams JS (eds): *Pediatric Gastrointestinal Disease: Pathophysiology, Diagnosis, Management*. Philadelphia, WB Saunders, 1993, pp 1018–1024.

Whatley K, Turner WW, et al: Transpyloric passage of feeding tubes. *Nutr Supp Serv*, 3:18–21, 1983.

Whitehead WE, Parker L, et al: Treatment of fecal incontinence in children with spina bifida: comparison of biofeedback and behavioral modification. *Arch Phys Med Rehab*, 67:218–223, 1986.

Williams CB, Laage NJ, et al: Total colonoscopy in children. *Arch Dis Child*, 57:49–53, 1982.

Winzelberg GG, Froelich JW, et al: Scintigraphic detection of gastrointestinal bleeding: a review of current methods. *Am J Gastroenterol*, 78:324–327, 1983.

Wolfson BJ, Allen JL, et al: Lipid aspiration pneumonia due to gastroesophageal reflux. A complication of nasogastric lipid feedings. *Pediatric Radiol*, 19:545–547, 1989.

Wurbs D, Phillip J, Classen M: Experiences with the long standing nasobiliary tube in biliary diseases. *Endoscopy*, 12:219–223, 1980.

Wyke RJ, Rajkovic IA, Williams R: Impaired opsonisation by serum from patients with chronic liver disease. *Clin Exp Immunol*, 51:91–98, 1983.

Wyllie R, Hyams JS: *Pediatric Gastrointestinal Disease: Pathophysiology, Diagnosis, Management.* Philadelphia, WB Saunders, 1993.

Wyllie R, Kay M: Esophagogastroduodenoscopy, colonoscopy, and related techniques. In Wyllie R, Hyams JS (eds). *Pediatric Gastrointestinal Disease: Pathophysiology, Diagnosis, Management.* Philadelphia; WB Saunders, 1993.

Yin PP, Dellipiani AW: Bacterial endocarditis after Hurst bougienage in a patient with a benign esophageal stricture. *Endoscopy*, 15:27–28, 1983.

Yon J, Christensen J: An uncontrolled comparison of treatments of achalasia. *Ann Surg*, 182:672–676, 1975.

Young CY, Ma YP, et al: Automatic end-expiratory air sampling device for breath hydrogen test in infants. *Lancet*, 337:90–93, 1991.

Young JA, Hughes HE, Lee FD: Evaluation of endoscopic brush and biopsy touch smear cytology and biopsy histology in the diagnosis of carcinoma of the lower esophagus and cardia. *J Clin Pathol*, 33:811–814, 1980.

Section K

Endocrine

Chapter 44

Pediatric Endocrine Procedures

Robert O. Christiansen

Within the past several years the number and accuracy of endocrine assays as well as the determination of metabolic intermediates, antibodies, and other substances have made the use of procedures in which the endocrine system is manipulated (usually by stimulation or suppression) somewhat less common. As the reliability of the tropic hormone assays has improved, for example, specific diagnoses often can be made without manipulating the endocrine system. Nevertheless, there are certain times when there is a need for such procedures to clarify or ascertain a diagnosis. This is particularly true in the areas of growth hormone testing, the diagnosis of hypoglycemia, and uncovering of the more cryptic forms of congenital adrenal hyperplasia. This chapter is concerned mainly with procedures that manipulate the endocrine system.

PREPARATION FOR ENDOCRINE PROCEDURES

Several preparatory actions should be taken before the procedures are employed. It is essential to get to know the laboratory and to inform it that you plan to carry out a special procedure. In many hospitals special determinations are referred to specialty labs, and in such cases, familiarity with the reference laboratory is essential. Such issues as how much blood per sample is required, what kind of tube the blood sample should be placed in, whether the samples need to be kept on ice, or whether the samples need to be separated and the plasma or serum need to be frozen are critical to carrying out testing in a meaningful way. Because many of these tests are time consuming and difficult for both the patient and physician, adequate preparation and performance of the test will ensure that the procedure will not have to be repeated.

Before performing the procedure, a tray should be assembled with all of the tubes, labels, syringes, alcohol swabs, arm boards (if needed), and such items as heparin locks. It is essential that all tubes and laboratory slips be labeled with both the date and time of the sample and that the laboratory transfer such data to computer records for each sample. Medications to be administered during the procedure should be ordered in advance and be present on the tray so that time is not lost procuring drugs. Likewise, if there are potential complications with the procedure, medications (such as adrenal steroids or glucose solutions) should be ordered in advance and be present on the tray.

Many physicians find it useful to place an indwelling venous catheter for sampling. This can be kept open by using a heparin lock system. Heparin is diluted 1:10 and is used to keep the intravenous access open. In this case blood must be withdrawn to clear the line before the sample is taken; the introduction of a three-way stopcock into the system may facilitate blood drawing, and the blood withdrawn to clear the line can be replaced in a sterile fashion. It is also essential to calculate the total amount of blood to be withdrawn during the tests to be sure that the test is feasible. With the advent of the anesthetic eutectic mixture of local anesthetics (EMLA) patches, establishing an intravenous line may be done in a painless fashion. If a procedure has a high potential for complications, a second access line with normal saline running at a "keep open" rate may be used as well; this is particularly to be recommended when procedures are done on infants and very young children. In addition, when performing tests on infants and small children, the availability of a colleague to assist in case of need is highly recommended.

Many of the tests require an overnight fast. In such cases, especially with small children, it is important to allow the child access to a bedtime snack at the latest possible hour and to perform the test as early in the morning as possible.

The preparation of both the patient and parents is likewise essential to good testing. The need for the procedure, what one hopes to learn from it, what the potential results might show and what would then be done therapeutically, what the potential complications are, and the mechanics of testing should all be discussed in detail. It is also important that the parents be allowed adequate time to ask questions. In some cases, it may be important to query the parents to ensure that they understand exactly what is to be done to have truly informed consent. Many patients and parents are concerned about multiple venipunctures and the attendant distress. The painless establishment of intravenous access, as described earlier, can do a great deal to alleviate this cause for anxiety. Whether the parents should be allowed to stay with the child during testing is a decision that must be made on an individual basis; in most cases, the presence of the parents can exercise a calming effect on the child. It is, of course, possible that parental anxiety will be conveyed to the child, but proper preparation of the family should do much to alleviate this.

HUMAN GROWTH HORMONE

Growth hormone (GH) secretion is controlled by two hormones, growth hormone–releasing hormone (GHRH) and somatostatin (SS), which is inhibitory. Growth hormone negatively feeds back to decrease GHRH secretion, and GH and insulin-like growth factors (IGF-I and IGF-II) positively feed back to increase SS production (Devusa et al, 1992; Harel and Tannenbaum, 1992). SS has a predominant effect on GH secretion, which will override the effects of other controlling substances. The secretion of GH is modulated by hormonal, metabolic, and neurotransmitter mechanisms. Thyroxine, glucocorticoids, and sex steroids are responsible for hormonal mediation (Giustina and Wehrenberg, 1992; Kerrigan and Rogol, 1992; Wehrenberg and Giustina, 1992).

Thyroxine is required for GHRH synthesis, and decreased GH secretion is seen in hypothyroidism; glucocorticoids normally stimulate GH synthesis and GHRH receptors at physiological concentrations, but at pharmacological concentrations they inhibit the stimulating effect of GHRH by increasing the sensitivity of the pituitary to SS; sex steroids are responsible for the increased GH production that is seen with puberty, most likely by modulating both GHRH and SS secretion. Metabolic control is exerted through glucose, amino acids, and free fatty acids. The effect of glucose appears to be mediated by changes in sensitivity to SS; hypoglycemia stimulates GH release and hyperglycemia inhibits both basal and GHRH-stimulated GH secretion. Arginine is the main amino acid stimulator of GH release, and this seems to occur by decreasing the sensitivity of the pituitary to SS. Free fatty acids inhibit the GH response of the pituitary to GHRH, most probably by increasing the sensitivity to SS.

Neural control is exerted by α_2-adrenergic, β-adrenergic, dopaminergic, and cholinergic pathways. GH release is stimulated by α-adrenergic mechanisms by decreasing SS release, while β-adrenergics stimulate SS release and inhibit GH release. The effects of dopaminergic stimulation are somewhat confusing; bromocriptine, a central acting dopamine agonist, results in increased secretion of both GHRH and GH. Cholinergic agents enhance GH secretion, seemingly by decreasing the sensitivity to SS. To further complicate the picture, it appears that GHRH and SS may exert reciprocal effects on one another at the level of the hypothalamus, each diminishing the secretion of the other.

GH is secreted in a pulsatile fashion at night mainly during rapid eye movement (REM) sleep, but also may be secreted with stress, exercise, and nutrient intake (Brabant et al, 1992). For this reason, GH secretion needs to be stimulated in order to be assessed as concentrations in awake individuals are quite low and non-indicative of the patient's GH status.

GH testing is not indicated in the growth-deficient child until adequate screening has been carried out. Initial assessment should include the patient's actual height, its relationship to the patient's chronological age and midparental height, and determination of growth velocity. GH deficiency is to be distinguished from constitutional shortness of stature. Most patients with constitutional shortness of stature will grow below but parallel to the fifth centile; their growth velocity will thus be normal until the normal time of puberty. A progressive deceleration in the rate of growth will suggest GH deficiency, as will a height of > 3 SD below the mean, but other conditions, such as renal tubular acidosis, psychosocial growth delay, gastrointestinal disorders such as inflammatory bowel disease, celiac disease, and cystic fibrosis, can be responsible for the growth changes.

Initial evaluation should include a complete blood count (CBC) with red cell indices and erythrocyte sedimentation rate (ESR), measurement of serum electrolytes, blood urea nitrogen (BUN) and creatinine, serum calcium, phosphorus, and alkaline phosphatase, total protein and albumin, urinalysis, thyroid function tests (including thyroid stimulating hormone [TSH]), IGF-I level, a karyotype in significantly short girls, and a radiograph of the left wrist to determine bone age. The bone age radiograph should be read by a person experienced in this procedure, comparing the patient's wrist to those in a bone-age atlas. A variance of greater than 2 standard deviations (SD) from normal is usually seen in patients with GH deficiency or hypothyroidism, although radiographs in the very young may be less reliable. A normal bone age in a child 4 years of age or older essentially rules out GH deficiency and suggests a diagnosis of familial shortness of stature. In interpreting the IGF-I (or somatomedin C) concentration, several factors need to be taken into consideration: normal values as a function of age, the nutritional status of the patient, the degree of sexual maturation, and the thyroid status. As the concentration of IGF-I rises sharply with puberty, patients who have absent or delayed sexual maturation will have values in the prepubertal range.

There are a variety of stimuli that can be used to provoke GH release. Most authorities suggest that two different stimuli be used to evaluate a potentially GH-deficient patient. The most commonly used stimuli include both physiological (exercise, sleep) and pharmacological (L-dopa, clonidine, glucagon, and insulin and arginine) modalities. Vigorous exercise, such as running or riding a bicycle for 20 minutes, is the usual exercise stimulus (Seip et al, 1990). The patient is fasted for at least 4 hours prior to performing the test, and samples are drawn at 20 and 40 minutes after the onset of the exercise. About 80% of those capable of responding will respond by 20 minutes, with an additional 10% responding at the 40-minute sample. There is a difference of opinion as to what constitutes a positive response. For a long time a single value of greater than 7 ng/ml was considered a positive response, but many authorities now consider a value of greater than 10 ng/ml required to declare a positive response.

There are several ways to perform an overnight sleep study (Ginsberg, 1990). No preparation is required (except for the placement of a heparin lock), and no medications are given. Blood is withdrawn either continuously or at specific intervals (every 20 to 30 minutes), either over the course of the night (8 P.M. to 8 A.M.) or for part of the night (10 P.M. to 6 A.M. or 4 A.M. to 8 A.M.). The schedule selected must take into account the child's age and the amount of blood to be withdrawn. Normal values would include at least three values of greater than 5 ng/ml in addition to at least one value of greater than 10 ng/ml. The mean concentration is about 3 ng/ml.

Simple outpatient tests of GH secretion involve the use of clonidine or L-dopa (Ginsberg, 1990; Lanes et al, 1985; Nichols Institute, 1994; Weldon et al, 1973). The patient is fasted for at least 4 hours and should not be taking any medications. The patient should be lying down and resting during the test because clonidine may cause drowsiness. Water may be taken. Blood pressure determinations should be performed during the test because clonidine may cause mild hypotension. Clonidine in a dose of 5 μg/kg (maximum dose, 250 μg) or 150 $\mu g/m^2$ is given orally with water. Samples are drawn at 30, 60, 90, and 120 minutes. Blood cortisol level may be obtained at 90 minutes as well. A positive test response requires a single value of greater than 7 or greater than 10 ng/ml, as noted before. The L-dopa test is performed after at least 4 hours of fasting. Oral L-dopa is given in doses of 125 mg (for the child weighing less than 30 lb), 250 mg (for the child weighing 30 to 70 lb), or 500 mg (for the child weighing more than 70 lb). GH measurements are made at 30, 60, 90, and 120 minutes. Interpretation is the same as for the clonidine test. Patients may have water during the test but should remain lying down. Nausea and vomiting may occur an hour or so into the test.

The glucagon stimulation test may be used when the physician does not wish to perform the insulin and arginine test, especially if both GH and cortisol deficiencies are suspected (Ginsberg, 1990). Preparation for the glucagon stimulation test requires an adequate diet for at least 3 days prior to testing and at least 4 hours of fasting. Glucagon in a dose of 0.03 mg/kg (maximum dose 1 mg) is given either intramuscularly or subcutaneously after the baseline sample is drawn. Blood samples for GH are drawn at 0, 60, 120, 150, and 180 minutes. As with other tests, water may be taken during the test; the patient may be allowed to ambulate. Nausea and vomiting may occur. Interpretation is the same as in other tests.

The arginine and insulin test (Penny et al, 1969) is useful if one suspects adrenocorticotropic hormone (ACTH) or cortisol deficiency but carries with it the hazard of potential symptomatic hypoglycemia. If this test is to be done, it is essential that bedside methods be available for monitoring blood glucose, that adequate intravenous access is available, and that glucose and hydrocortisone are available at the bedside to terminate the test if necessary. There are several variants of this test. The patient should be fasted for at least 4 hours prior to testing. L-Arginine hydrochloride is administered in a dose of 0.5 g/kg (maximum dose 30 g) by intravenous infusion over 30 minutes. Samples for GH are obtained at 0, 30, 60, 90, and 120 minutes. After the 120-minute sample is taken, insulin in a dose of 0.075 U/kg is given by intravenous bolus. GH levels are obtained every 15 minutes for a 2-hour period. During the second part of the test, glucose and cortisol levels are drawn at 0 and 60 minutes.

In order for the test to be acceptable, the blood glucose concentration during the second part of the test should fall to a value less than 50% of the value obtained before the insulin was given. If the glucose does not fall to acceptable levels, the insulin portion of the test may be performed again using 0.1 U/kg of insulin. GH values are interpreted as with previous studies. A rise in the cortisol concentration to 15 μg/dl or greater indicates intactness of the hypothalamic-pituitary-adrenal axis. Some authors recommend priming with estrogen and/or administering propranolol in conjunction with GH stimulation tests, although there is a great deal of difference of opinion about the use of these agents.

Once GH deficiency has been documented, it is possible to determine the site of the deficiency. This is done by performing the GHRH stimulation test (Chalew et al, 1985; Ginsberg, 1990; Nichols Institute, 1994). In this test GHRH is administered and the GH response is measured. In patients who have GH deficiency but respond normally to GHRH, the defect would be in the anterior hypothalamus, presumably as a deficiency of GHRH or an imbalance with SS. This test should not be used to diagnose GH deficiency.

After at least a 4 hour fast, GHRH in a dose of 1 to 1.5 μg/kg is administered intravenously. The patient should be lying down during the test. GH samples are determined at 30, 60, 90, and 120 minutes. Normal GH release generally indicates that the lesion is in the hypothalamus, but failure of GH release does not rule out hypothalamic disease, especially in the patient with long-standing GH deficiency.

If hypersecretion of GH is suspected (acromegaly, gigantism, excessive tall stature), then the glucose suppression of GH test is performed (Ginsberg, 1990; Nichols Institute, 1994). The patient should fast from midnight and have had an adequate dietary intake for at least 3 days prior to the test. A baseline sample for GH and glucose is drawn, and oral glucose in a dose of 1.75 g/kg (maximum dose 75 g) is administered. Samples for GH and glucose are drawn at 0, 30, 60, 90, and 120 minutes. A normal response is the suppression of GH values to 5 ng/ml or less. Values between 5 and 10 ng/ml are not interpretable, but values of 10 ng/ml or greater suggest the presence of a pituitary adenoma. Water is allowed during the test.

THE PITUITARY-ADRENAL AXIS

Regulation of adrenocortical steroid biosynthesis and secretion is a complex process regulated by central and feedback mechanisms. Corticotropin-releasing hormone (CRH) is a 41 amino acid peptide produced from a much larger peptide. ACTH is a 39–amino acid peptide (of which only the first 24 amino acids are required for activity) derived from a more complex molecule called pro-opiomelanocortin (POMC), which is cleaved in corticotropes to give rise to both ACTH and β-lipotropin (which is further metabolized to β-endorphin).

ACTH undergoes diurnal variation, with the highest secretion occurring in the early morning hours. ACTH secretion is stimulated by CRH and inhibited by cortisol (Won and Orth, 1990). In addition, vasopressin acts in concert with CRH to stimulate the secretion of ACTH (Won and Orth, 1990). Oxytocin and angiotensin II also enhance the effect of CRH on ACTH secretion. The effect of ACTH on the adrenal gland is to stimulate adrenocortical hormone production and release. This effect is greatest as regards the secretion of glucocorticoids, although it also has some stimulating effects on androgen secretion. ACTH has essentially very little effect on the secretion of mineralocorticoids, which is regulated by the renin-angiotensin mechanism and the serum potassium concentration.

A procedure that can help to dissect this mechanism is the ovine corticotropic releasing hormone (oCRH) stimulation test (Nichols Institute, 1994). This test is useful both in the diagnosis of adrenal insufficiency due to ACTH deficiency and in the diagnosis of central Cushing's disease. A diagnosis of pituitary ACTH deficiency is suggested when symptoms of adrenal insufficiency (weakness, easy fatiguability, anorexia, weight loss, gastrointestinal symptoms such as diarrhea and nausea, hypotension, and dizziness associated with change in posture) are present, with or without other pituitary deficiencies; such patients often have CNS symptoms but do not have increased pigmentation or vitiligo.

A diagnosis of Cushing's disease is suggested by growth arrest during a period of rapid weight gain, weakness, hirsutism, and pubertal arrest or menstrual changes and hypertension; such well-known signs as purple striae, bruising, and increased pigmentation are rather less common in children. Laboratory findings include an increased 24-hour urinary free cortisol excretion, increased 24-hour urinary 17-hydroxysteroid excretion, and an absence of the normal diurnal variation in plasma cortisol concentrations.

The CRH stimulation test is usually performed in the morning but may be performed at any time of day, after a minimum of a 4 hour fast. Baseline samples are drawn and synthetic oCRH is administered as an intravenous bolus in a dose of 1 to 1.5 μg/kg (maximum dose is 100 μg). ACTH and cortisol are measured at 30, 60, 90, and 120 minutes. Some authorities suggest earlier samples for ACTH at 5, 10, and 15 minutes (Nichols Institute, 1994). Normal values include a two- to four-fold rise in plasma ACTH concentration (especially if the earlier samples are taken at 5–15 minutes) and a rise in plasma cortisol to greater than 20 μg/dl in the later samples. The baseline and peak values will vary with the time of day, but the incremental changes will be as previously described. In primary adrenal insufficiency, normal to exaggerated ACTH responses will be accompanied by no cortisol responses. In pituitary ACTH deficiency, there will be sluggish to absent ACTH responses, also accompanied by subnormal cortisol responses. Patients with Cushing's disease (central Cushing's) will have normal ACTH incremental responses, whereas those with adrenal Cushing's syndrome or the syndrome of ectopic ACTH will not respond. For this test to be useful, the ACTH assay used must be reliable.

Another test that may be helpful in the diagnosis of Cushing's syndrome is the dexamethasone suppression test (Ginsberg, 1990; Nichols Institute, 1994). This test depends of the suppression of CRH, ACTH, and plasma cortisol by exogenously administered dexamethasone. For this test to be valid, patients should not be receiving exogenous adrenal steroids. A simple screening test is the overnight dexamethasone test, in which the patient receives 15 to 20 μg/kg of dexamethasone (maximum dose 1 mg) at 11:00 P.M., and plasma cortisol (and ACTH if desired) is measured at 8:00 A.M. on the following morning. A normal response is a plasma cortisol of 5 μg/kg or less and an ACTH of 5 pg/ml or less.

A normal response excludes a diagnosis of Cushing's syndrome, but equivocal responses can be seen in situations of stress, in obesity, and in patients receiving the commonly used anticonvulsants phenobarbital, phenytoin, and carbamazipine. In such cases it is necessary to perform the standard dexamethasone suppression test (Ginsberg, 1990; Nichols Institute, 1994). This test is carried out in a 6-day period. The first 2 days are for baseline determinations. Low-dose dexamethasone is administered orally for the next 2 days in a dosage of 5 μg/kg/dose (maximum 0.5 mg/dose) every 6 hours. During the last 2 days of the test, dexamethasone is administered in a dosage of 20 μg/kg/dose (maximum 2 mg/dose) every 6 hours. Daily 24-hour urine values are obtained during the performance of the test and determinations of 17-hydroxycorticosteroids, urinary free cortisol, and creatinine are made.

Plasma cortisol (and ACTH if desired) is measured on the morning of a baseline day, and on the mornings following the completion of the low and high doses. The patient is allowed to ambulate and have free access to food and water but must be cautioned about the importance of complete 24-hour urine collections; the adequacy of the collections are assessed by comparing creatinine excretion values per day. Normal values indicate suppression of plasma cortisol to 5 μg/dl or less, suppression of ACTH to 5 pg/ml or less, and a greater than 50% fall in urinary free cortisol excretion. Blood androgen determinations may be followed as well; a fall of 50% or greater is regarded as a normal response. Failure to suppress may suggest ovarian origin of androgens. Normal and obese individuals will suppress on day 4. Patients with pituitary hypersecretion of ACTH will not suppress on day 4 (low dose) but will suppress on day 6 (high dose). Patients with adrenal adenomas, adrenal carcinomas, micronodular adrenal disease, and the syndrome of ectopic ACTH production will not suppress at any time during the test.

In patients suspected of having adrenocortical malfunction, such as primary adrenal insufficiency, adrenal steroid biosynthetic defects, or adrenocortical unresponsiveness, the ACTH stimulation test (Ginsberg, 1990; Nichols Institute, 1994) may be useful. In many cases, however, accurate diagnosis can be achieved by history, physical examination, and hormone levels alone. Collection of two 24-hour urine samples for free cortisol and creatine assessment should be done prior to the use of this test. This test exists in a short and long version as well. In the short version, synthetic 1-24 amino acid ACTH (cosyntropin) is administered in a dose of 250 μg by intravenous bolus after initial samples have been drawn; additional samples are drawn at 30 and 60 minutes. The test is usually performed at 8:00 A.M. but may be performed at any time, as is necessary. Plasma cortisol is measured routinely, but other adrenal steroids may be measured if a defect in adrenal steroid biosynthesis is suspected. A normal response is achieved when the baseline value of cortisol has doubled. A maximal plasma cortisol value of 18 μg/dl or less suggests a diagnosis of adrenal insufficiency. If other steroids are measured, a normal response would consist of the doubling of the cortisol response and the preservation of the precursor-product ratio observed in the baseline sample. In cases where partial defects in adrenal steroid biosynthesis are present, the incremental change in the plasma cortisol is less than the change in the precursor as a general rule. In ACTH unresponsiveness a negative result will occur.

The long ACTH stimulation test is performed by administering cosyntropin by continuous intravenous infusion in a dose of 250 μg/12 hours for 2 to 4 days. Plasma cortisol values are determined daily and 24-hour urine collections are analyzed for 17-hydroxycorticosteroids, urinary free cortisol, and creatinine. Normal values would be at least a doubling in the urinary steroids and a rise in the plasma cortisol to 30 μg/dl or greater. In primary adrenal insufficiency there is no increase in glucocorticoids by the end of the test. In ACTH deficiency a positive result is usually obtained by the end of the second or third day. While it would be optimal to remove all patients undergoing ACTH stimulation tests from adrenal steroids, this could be very hazardous in certain situations, particularly in significant primary adrenal insufficiency (Addison's disease). In such cases, the patients should be placed on maintenance doses of dexamethasone (20 μg/kg/day) to prevent adrenal crisis. Some authorities suggest this for all patients subjected to the long ACTH stimulation test.

Assessment of pituitary ACTH activity in response to absence of adrenal feedback may be performed by using the metyrapone test (Ginsberg, 1990; Nichols Institute, 1994). Metyrapone inhibits 11-β hydroxylase, which converts 11-deoxycortisol to cortisol; the decreased cortisol then stimulates ACTH release, which increases the precursor, 11-deoxycortisol. It has been used to assess patients after prolonged treatment with corticosteroids. It is rarely used today because reliable ACTH and cortisol assays are now available. It should not be used in patients with primary adrenal insufficiency. Patients should not be receiving glucocorticoids and should be off of drugs such as phenytoin, which enhances the action of metyrapone. Mild activity or bed rest should be observed on the day the metyrapone is administered. Glucocorticoids should be kept at the bedside.

The patient is administered 300 mg/m^2 (15 mg/kg) of metyrapone orally every 4 hours for 24 hours. A baseline 24-hour urine is collected on the day before the metyrapone is given and for the next 2 days, and creatinine 17-hydroxycorticosteroids and 17-ketogenic steroids are measured. Plasma cortisol, 11-deoxycortisol, and ACTH are measured 4 hours after the last dose of metyrapone is given. A positive response would be marked by at least a doubling of the urinary 17-ketogenic steroids, a fall in plasma cortisol to 5 μg/dl or less, a rise in 11-deoxycortisol to greater than 5 μg/dl, and a rise in the ACTH level to 100 pg/ml or greater. The 11-deoxycortisol level should be greater than the plasma cortisol level. A failure of ACTH and 11-deoxycortisol levels to rise indicates inadequate pituitary reserve or an inadequate test result. Adrenal reserve may, of course, be assessed by the ACTH stimulation test. Complications include hypotension and vomiting, and vertigo, which may be diminished by giving food at the same time as the metyrapone. Because of the complications and the variability in the response to metyrapone, this procedure is not performed often.

A shortened form of the test (Ginsberg, 1990; Nichols Institute, 1994) may be performed by giving 30 mg/kg of metyrapone at midnight (maximum dose 1 g in children) and measuring plasma cortisol, 11-deoxycortisol, and ACTH at 8:00 A.M. Interpretation is the same as the long form of the test, and the problems and caveats are also the same.

PITUITARY THYROID AXIS

With the development of modern tests of thyroid function, perturbation tests to evaluate the pituitary-thyroid axis have been used less frequently. For example, if a diagnosis of primary hypothyroidism is suspected, measurements of both total and free thyroxine (T_4) and triiodothyronine (T_3) will show subnormal values for age and TSH values will be elevated. T_3 resin uptake values will generally be subnormal. Further delineation may be achieved by measuring thyroid autoantibody titers, such as antithyroglobulin antibody, antimicrosomal antibody (antithyroid peroxidase or anti-TPO), thyrotropin binding inhibiting immunoglobulin (TBII), and thyrotropin blocking antibody (TBA). In cases of hypothyroidism due to dyshormonogenesis, the autoantibodies will not be present; thyroid scan and uptake are useful in the diagnosis of this group of disorders (see nuclear medicine section for particulars). In cases of pituitary or hypothalamic hypothyroidism, the autoantibody titers will also be normal, but TSH values will be normal to low in the presence of low T_3 and T_4 levels. In selected cases, the use of the thyrotropin-releasing hormone (TRH) test may be useful.

Hashimoto's thyroiditis presents a special case because patients may be euthyroid, hypothyroid, or thyrotoxic at the time of presentation. Most patients (80–90%) have an enlarged, slightly irregular, and rather firm thyroid gland. Antithyroid autoantibodies such as anti-TPO are present in 90% to 95% of cases; antithyroglobulin and anti-TSH receptor antibodies may be present as well.

In cases of Graves' disease, patients will usually present with a gradual onset of symptoms, up to 100% will have prominence of the eyes, and some 95% will have goiter; other typical symptoms are usually present. The most accurate laboratory value supporting the diagnosis will be complete suppression of TSH to values of < 0.03 mIU/L in the third-generation assay. Laboratory values also include elevations in total and free T_3, frequent elevations in total and free T_4, and the presence of antithyroid antibodies such as TBII and thyroid-stimulating immunoglobulin (TSIG); antithyroid antibodies, such as antithyroglobulin and anti-TPO, may also be present. In the rare event of TSH-driven hyperthyroidism, elevated TSH concentrations will be found in the presence of elevated T_3 and T_4 values (and clinical indications of hyperthyroidism); in such cases, evidence of antithyroid antibody production is not found, but this condition must be differentiated from the syndromes of TSH insensitivity.

As was mentioned earlier, the TRH test (Ginsberg, 1990; Nichols Institute, 1994; Spencer et al, 1993) may be useful in evaluating the hypothalamic-pituitary axis for potential dysfunction. In addition, this test may be used to evaluate prolactin production because TRH is generally regarded as a prolactin stimulator.

Patients are prepared for the test by being taken off all thyroid medications, iodine-containing medications, and chronic aspirin therapy for at least a week prior to the performance of the test. In addition, prolactin response may be diminished or suppressed by glucocorticoids, L-dopa, or dopamine. Most patients should fast from midnight if the test is to be performed in the morning because of the side effects of TRH administration. Because prolactin values increase during sleep, the patient should be awake for a significant period of time prior to the test. As TRH may cause an elevation in blood pressure, this test is contraindicated in patients with hypertension or evidence of cerebrovascular disease. The main side effects of TRH administration include transient flushing, nausea, emesis, and the urge to urinate; these symptoms usually last only for a short period (up to a minute) during TRH administration. It is a good idea to prepare the patient by explaining both the potential side effects and their short duration. Some authors have suggested diluting the TRH in an equal volume of normal saline may lessen the side effects.

After drawing baseline samples for TSH and prolactin, TRH (7 μg/kg up to a maximum dosage of 400 μg) is administered intravenously over 30 to 90 seconds. Further samples for both TSH and prolactin are drawn at 15, 30, and 60 minutes. Increases in TSH of 5 to 30 mIU/L over baseline are regarded as normal for children. Prolactin increases of three- to five-fold at

15 to 30 minutes are considered normal in children and adult males; postpubertal females will normally show a 5- to 20-fold increase in prolactin response. An absent response of TSH to TRH stimulation suggests either primary pituitary disease (for which the patient should be evaluated) or suppression by elevated thyroid hormones, such as is seen in hyperthyroidism or exogenous thyroid hormone administration. Patients with hypothyroidism show an exaggerated response of both TSH and prolactin to TRH stimulation. A failure of TSH levels to return to normal at the end of the test may suggest hypothalamic dysfunction.

PITUITARY-GONADAL AXIS

The control of the secretion of gonadotropins is mediated by the pulsatile secretion of gonadotropin-releasing hormone (GnRH) in both older children and adults. Following birth there is a surge in luteinizing hormone (LH) secretion followed by an increase in testosterone (for up to 12 hours) in males. As placental steroids are cleared from the circulation, both follicle stimulating hormone (FSH) and LH rise in a pulsatile fashion. Males have increases in testosterone concentration (due to higher levels of LH secretion), which fall to low levels by about 6 months of age. In females, estradiol concentrations rise in response to higher concentrations of FSH and fall to low levels sometime before 2 years of age. Pulsatile secretion of GnRH is low during childhood and is associated with low FSH and LH levels. The response of the pituitary to exogenous GnRH is low at this time. Further, the gonadotropins exert increased feedback inhibition on GnRH secretion. The onset of puberty is heralded by the slow reactivation of the pulsatile secretion of GnRH as well as a decrease in the feedback inhibition sensitivity of GnRH to gonado-tropins (Grumbach and Styne, 1992). GnRH surges occur initially at night and slowly increase in frequency; they then begin to occur during the day as puberty progresses. Accompanying these changes are corresponding changes in FSH and LH. As puberty is completed, pulses of FSH and LH occur every 1-1/2 to 2 hours. The development of the midcycle LH surge completes pubertal development in girls.

Helpful in assessing these changes is the GnRH test (Ginsberg, 1990; Kelch et al, 1976; Nichols Institute, 1994), which measures the maturing of the GnRH-gonadotropin axis. This test is therefore useful in cases of delayed puberty, hypopituitarism, and Kallmann's syndrome. It also may be useful in cases of precocious puberty in which a positive test indicates maturing gonadotropin secretion. There is no special patient preparation required. The patient may eat and/or ambulate during the test. Blood samples for FSH and LH are obtained, and GnRH in a dose of 2.5 μg/kg (up to a maximal dose of 100 μg) is administered intravenously. Further blood samples for FSH and LH are drawn at 30, 45, 60, and 90 minutes. If a longer test is desired, GnRH in a dose of 100 $\mu g/m^2$ may be infused over 4 to 6 hours, with gonadotropin samples obtained at time 0 and at the end of the infusion. The new immunochemiluminometric assays (ICMAs) are reported to be more sensitive than the currently used assays (Neely et al, 1995). Following the administration of GnRH, an LH response of > 5 IU/L would appear to be indicative of maturation of gonadotropin secretion (Neely et al, 1995).

As stated earlier, normal prepubertal children have a minimal to absent response to GnRH infusion. It must be remembered, however, that infants may respond during the period when the gonadotropins are elevated. As puberty occurs the response becomes more pronounced. The response of LH to GnRH almost always exceeds that of FSH once puberty has begun in both males and females. The usual positive LH response to GnRH is a 4- to 10-fold increase. Lesions in the area of the arcuate nucleus should produce GnRH deficiency with resultant hypogonadotrophic hypogonadism. A special case is Kallmann's syndrome, characterized by hypogonadotrophic hypogonadism and anosmia (or hyposmia); such patients may also have cryptorchidism and/or microphallus as well as GnRH deficiency, although not all patients have identical responses to GnRH. Secondary hypogonadotrophism may be differentiated from tertiary (GnRH deficiency) in that the former usually will not have a positive GnRH test, while the latter may, although, as noted earlier, a prolonged test may be required. This test will not distinguish delayed puberty from hypogonadotrophic hypogonadism.

Another test which may have some usefulness is the human chorionic gonadotrophin (HCG) stimulation test (Forest, 1979; Ginsberg, 1990; Nichols Institute, 1994). This test is performed by injecting HCG and measuring resultant testosterone levels and is useful in differentiating the vanishing testes syndrome from bilateral cryptorchidism, in cases where the hormonal functional capacity of the testis is in question and in diagnosing 5α-reductase deficiency. The syndrome of the vanishing testes, otherwise known as congenital anorchia, is a situation in which the testes can not be identified in an otherwise male infant. Because there is male internal and external genital development, it stands to reason that there must have been testes at some time during sexual differentiation and that something has caused them to disappear; such patients will have a negative HCG stimulation test. On the other hand, the patient with bilateral cryptorchidism should have a positive HCG test. 5α-reductase deficiency is characterized by the inability during gestation, infancy, and childhood to convert testosterone to dihydrotestosterone.

There are a variety of methods proposed for performing this test, consisting of a single injection of HCG (5000 IU/m^2), with samples at the onset and on day 3; the daily injection of 1500 to 3000 IU/m^2 for 4 days, with samples at the beginning and end of the test; and the injection of 1500 to 3000 IU/m^2 of HCG every other day for three or four doses, with sampling at the onset and at the end of the test. Samples are collected for testosterone (and dihydrotestosterone if 5α-reductase deficiency is suspected), and some authors suggest measuring FSH and LH as well. In general, the amount of the rise in testosterone concentration is proportionate to amount and duration of HCG administered. Acceptable increases are from about threefold to values of about one half of adult male normals in prepubertal children. The normal T-DHT ratio at the end of the test is 5 to 15 (Pang et al, 1979). The test may produce testicular hyalinization. There is no equivalent test for use in females.

PROLACTIN SECRETION: DOPAMINE AGONIST TEST

Prolactin is a single chain polypeptide synthesized in the lactotropes; it shares a great deal of common sequence with GH. Serum prolactin values are high in the neonatal period and in infancy and then become associated with sleep. Physiological stimulators of prolactin include, in addition to sleep and the normal rises in infancy, stress, estrogens, and exercise. Pharmacological stimulators include opiates, dopamine antagonists (such as phenothiazines, reserpine, cimetidine, and methyldopa), cholinergic agonists, and serotonin agonists. Nevertheless, prolactin secretion, under normal circumstances, is suppressed by dopamine under the control of the anterior hypothalamus. Water loading, obesity, dopamine dopamine agonists (such as L-dopa), and thyroxine also will inhibit prolactin secretion.

Patients suspected of having abnormally elevated secretion of prolactin may be evaluated by the L-dopa suppression test (Buckman et al, 1973; Ginsberg, 1990). Patients are prepared by allowing them to have a bedtime snack and then placing them on nothing by mouth (NPO). The test is done the following morning. A baseline prolactin level is drawn and the patient is given L-dopa by mouth (125 mg for those weighing less than 30 lb, 250 mg for those weighing between 30 and 70 lb, and 500 mg for those weighing more than 70 lb). Blood samples for prolactin are drawn at 30, 60, 90, 120, and 180 minutes. The side effects of L-dopa administration are the same as during the GH stimulation test. The patient may be given small amounts of water during the test. A normal response is a fall of prolactin values to 50% of baseline at 1 to 3 hours. The lack of such a fall indicates abnormal secretion of prolactin. Prolactin secreting tumors in children are characterized by growth failure, obesity, abnormalities in timing of sexual maturation (delayed or precocious puberty), and breast development with or without galactorrhea. Postpubertal females will often have menstrual irregularities and infertility; postpubertal males will often have gynecomastia (with or without galactorrhea) and report decreased libido. Other causes of hyperprolactinemia include hypothyroidism, hypothalamic dysfunction, surgical interference with the pituitary stalk, and drug ingestion; it is also seen following head trauma.

ANTERIOR HYPOTHALAMUS: COMBINED ANTERIOR PITUITARY OR MULTIPLE HORMONE STIMULATION TEST

This test (Nichols Institute, 1994; Sheldon et al, 1985) was designed to allow for assessment of pituitary function within a 2-hour period on a single morning. It is a compilation of several of the pituitary function tests previously described. The test is generally used as a screening test for those at high risk for hypothalamic or pituitary dysfunction, such as following surgery in the area of the hypothalamus or pituitary, following hypothalamic or pituitary radiation, or following significant head trauma. Side effects, complications, and caveats are given under the individual function tests and will not be repeated here.

The patient is given a bedtime snack and then is placed on NPO. The test is performed the following morning. Intravenous access is established using either a heparin lock or by slow infusion of normal saline. Patient monitoring is as previously described. Baseline samples are drawn (see later). The patient is administered TRH (7 μg/kg to a maximum of 500 μg), oCRH (1.5 μg/kg or 100 μg/1.73 m^2 to a maximum dose of 100 mg), GnRH (2.5 μg/kg to a maximum dose of 100 μg), and GHRH (1.5 μg/kg or 100 μg/1.73 m^2); these hormones are given over a period of 30 seconds from separate syringes. It is possible to give the TRH last and over a longer period of time to minimize side effects. Samples to be drawn include GH, FSH, LH, ACTH, cortisol, TSH, and prolactin. Samples are drawn a time 0, and then at 15, 30, 60, 90, and 120 minutes following the infusion. Normal values and interpretation are listed under the descriptions of the individual tests.

Radiation to the area of the hypothalamus/pituitary is most likely to cause GH deficiency and precocious puberty. GH deficiency increases both with the amount of radiation administered above 1800 cGy and with time following irradiation. Precocious puberty is seen in patients given greater than 1800 cGy for leukemia and greater than 3000 cGy given for brain tumors. Deficiencies of FSH, LH, ACTH, and TSH are much less common and are generally associated with doses of radiation exceeding 3500 cGy. Hyperprolactinemia requires even more irradiation and is rarely seen in patients given less than 4500 cGy.

POSTERIOR PITUITARY: DIABETES INSIPIDUS AND RELATED DISORDERS

Disorders of water balance are characterized by polydipsia, polyuria, and the elaboration of a dilute urine. Polyuria is usually defined as a urine volume of greater than 30 ml/kg/24 hr (or 1500 ml/m^2/24 hr), and a dilute urine has an osmolality of less than 250 mOsm/kg water or a specific gravity of less than 1.005. Three conditions need to be distinguished: (1) complete or partial deficiency of vasopressin secretion, called central, hypothalamic, or neurogenic diabetes insipidus; (2) decreased or absent renal response to the action of vasopressin, called nephrogenic diabetes insipidus; and (3) suppression of vasopressin secretion caused by excessive fluid intake, called primary polydipsia. These conditions can be differentiated by the water deprivation test (Ginsberg, 1990; Nichols Institute, 1994).

The water deprivation test asks the physiological question of whether, when deprived of water, the patient will concentrate the urine (a normal response) or the plasma (an abnormal response). No special preparation is required, but the patient should be off of all medications that influence vasopressin secretion or action for a period of 24 hours prior to the test. Medications that enhance arginine vasopressin (AVP) release include amitryptyline, carbamazepine, chlorpropamide, clofibrate, narcotics, nicotine (including smoking), phenothiazines, and vincristine. Medications that enhance the action of AVP include chlorpropamide, cyclophosphamide, and prostaglandin inhibitors. Medications that inhibit the release of AVP include ethanol, narcotic antagonists, and phenytoin. Medications that inhibit the action of vasopressin include acetohexamide, demeclocycline, lithium, and propoxyphene.

Prior to the test the child is allowed free access to water. The test begins by having the child empty the bladder and measuring baseline vital signs, body weight, serum electrolytes and osmolality, urine specific gravity and osmolality, and plasma (and urine) AVP levels. At this point, all fluid intake is restricted. It is important that the child be observed constantly during the test and not allowed to use the bathroom unaccompanied. Serial measurements are now made: urine volume, specific gravity, and osmolality are measured hourly; serum osmolality is measured every 2 hours; the patient is weighed every 4 hours. The test is continued until either the urine osmolality rises above 600 mOsm/kg or the plasma osmolality rises to 300 mOsm/kg or more. The test is usually not carried out for more than 24 hours.

If there has been no decrease in the urine volume by 4 to 6 hours into the test, it is important to consider that either the patient has severe neurogenic diabetes insipidus and requires closer monitoring or that the patient has had access to water. If the urine osmolality rises above 600 mOsm/kg, the test is terminated by measuring plasma (and urine) AVP levels and serum electrolytes. If the serum osmolality rises to or above 300 mOsm/kg, then measurements are made of plasma (and urine) AVP levels and serum electrolytes. At this point intranasal desmopressin acetate (DDAVP) is administered (10 μg in infants and 20 μg in children), and urine osmolality is measured at 30 and 60 minutes. It is important to understand that small children with severe forms of neurogenic diabetes insipidus can develop significant degrees of dehydration during the water deprivation test and may require intravenous hydration; in patients in whom such a diagnosis is suspected, more frequent measurements of body weight and serum osmolality are recommended. Further, patients with partial defects of vasopressin secretion may be missed unless an elevation in serum osmolality is allowed to occur before the test is terminated.

The normal child will not become dehydrated and will demonstrate a continuous rise in urine osmolality to greater than 600 mOsm/kg; at the end of the test, the plasma (and urine) AVP levels will be elevated.

The child with severe neurogenic diabetes insipidus will fail to decrease the urine volume significantly, will develop dehydration early in the test (5 to 8 hours), will have only a very minimal rise in the urine osmolality (less than 30 mOsm in consecutive samples), will have a rise in serum osmolality to above 300 mOsm/kg and/or a rise in serum Na^+ of > 10 mEq/L in less than 12 hours, and will fail to increase plasma (and urine) AVP levels.

The patient with partial neurogenic diabetes insipidus will show a less dramatic response but will still fail to increase the urine osmolality to above 600 mOsm/kg at a time when the serum osmolality is at or above 300 mOsm/kg. These patients may or may not become dehydrated but show low AVP levels at the end of the test (less than 2 pg/ml).

The patient with nephrogenic diabetes insipidus will continue to elaborate a dilute urine while developing early dehydration; by the end of the test the urine osmolality will be less than that of serum, the plasma AVP will be elevated (usually greater than 5 pg/ml), and desmopressin administration will fail to effect a significant rise in the urine osmolality and a fall in the urine volume. There are milder forms of nephrogenic diabetes insipidus in which dehydration may fail to occur and urine osmolality may rise above that of plasma. Such patients still show a rise in AVP levels at the end of the test (greater than 5 pg/ml when the serum osmolality is 300 mOsm/kg or greater).

Patients with primary polydipsia may have a normal test or may have partial suppression of AVP responsiveness and ability to concentrate the urine due to chronic, excessive hydration. In such patients the urine volume decreases during the first 4 to 6 hours of the test and urine osmolality exceeds 200 mOsm/kg. When the serum osmolality reaches 300 mOsm/kg, AVP levels will be in the 2 to 6 pg/ml range; urinary AVP levels will also be elevated. There is usually a blunted response to desmopressin administration.

PARATHYROID HORMONE

Hypoparathyroidism is characterized by low serum Ca^{++}, elevated serum phosphate, and low intact PTH levels.

Hypoparathyroidism may be caused either by inadequate synthesis and release of parathormone or by peripheral resistance to the hormone. Recent advances in the ability to measure parathyroid hormone (PTH) in plasma in its multiple forms have improved diagnostic abilities. The C-terminal and M-terminal fragments tend to be most abundant in plasma but do not reflect the rapid turnover of the active forms of PTH. The N-terminal fragments are more biologically active and thus tend to give a better picture of acute changes but are not always detected in the plasma of normal persons. The development of a highly sensitive radioimmunoassay for intact PTH has solved this problem in that now not only is it possible to measure PTH in all normal persons, but diurnal variations and pulsatile release have been demonstrated as well. The ready availability of assays for 25-hydroxyvitamin D and 1,25-dihydroxyvitamin D have been useful in differentiating cases of the various forms of rickets from hypoparathyroidism.

The two main forms of peripheral resistance to PTH are magnesium deficiency and pseudohypoparathyroidism. It is very important to recognize significant hypomagnesemia in a patient with hypocalcemia because the disease process may not be reversed until magnesium is administered; magnesium is required for both the synthesis and the action of PTH, so such patients may have low measurable PTH levels and mimic hypoparathyroidism. The diagnosis of pseudohypoparathyroidism (PHP) is rather more complicated. The disorder has been subgrouped into types I and II, with further division of type I into types Ia and Ib. Most patients with type I disease are characterized by hypocalcemia, hyperphosphatemia, short stature, round facies, brachymetacarpy, obesity, and mild to moderate mental retardation. Patients with type I PHP have hypophosphaturia and decreased urinary cyclic AMP generation in response to PTH administration; patients with type Ia have the body habitus described earlier due to deficient function of the receptor guanine nucleotide regulatory protein (Gs); and patients with type Ib generally have normal appearance and normal Gs activity. Type II is quite rare; patients rarely have the body habitus and do generate urinary cyclic AMP in response to PTH; Gs activity is normal. The diagnosis of PHP used to be made by the EDTA infusion test and the Ellsworth-Howard test, but neither of these tests is used presently. Currently the diagnosis can be made by the administration of synthetic human PTH fragments 1 to 24 (Parathar) and the measurement of subsequent urinary or plasma cyclic AMP and creatinine levels. A normal response is a rise of 10- to 20-fold in the CAMP:creatinine ratio. In type I PHP, the rise is no more than 2- to 3-fold. Results are interpreted on the basis of the information give earlier.

Medullary carcinoma of the thyroid occurs in childhood as part of the multiple endocrine neoplasia (MEN) type 2 syndromes, currently subdivided into types 2a and 2b; both are inherited as autosomal dominant conditions. MEN 2a consists of medullary carcinoma of the thyroid, hyperparathyroidism, and pheochromocytoma. MEN 2b consists of medullary carcinoma of the thyroid and pheochromocytoma with a marfanoid habitus and multiple mucosal neuromas. In any family in which there is a history of MEN type 2, all children should be studied by measuring baseline and stimulated calcitonin levels. This is done by performing the calcium-pentagastrin test (Ginsberg, 1990; Nichols Institute, 1994). This test should be repeated on a yearly basis until the patient is an adult. The identification of the genetic abnormalities responsible for MEN type 2a, MEN type 2b, and familial medullary carcinoma of the thyroid (Mulligan et al, 1994; Hofstra et al, 1994) and the ability to detect their presence will probably make this test obsolete.

The patient is placed on NPO after midnight or a bedtime snack; the patient may have small amounts of water. The patient is supine while the test is performed. It is important to establish adequate intravenous access (such as with an intravenous catheter) because calcium is to be infused; infiltration of significant amounts of calcium into the subcutaneous tissues causes tissue necrosis. Baseline measurement of calcitonin is drawn, and the test is begun by the intravenous infusion of 2 mg of elemental calcium over 1 minute followed by pentagastrin (0.5 μg/kg) over 5 seconds. Calcium gluconate contains 10% elemental calcium, calcium lactate contains 13% elemental calcium, and calcium chloride contains 27% elemental calcium. Blood samples for calcitonin are drawn at 2, 3, 5, and 10 minutes into the test.

Calcium infusions produce flushing, a feeling of warmth, the urge to urinate, and a sense of gastric fullness; these symptoms last less than 5 minutes. Pentagastrin infusion produces substernal, retrosternal, and pharyngeal discomfort; a sensation of gastric fullness and abdominal pain; and nausea. These symptoms last less than 2 minutes. Either calcium alone or pentagastrin alone may also be used; pentagastrin gives the better diagnostic response when administered alone. Values of calcitonin rise in the first 5 minutes; a fivefold increase in calcitonin levels is generally regarded as diagnostic for medullary carcinoma of the thyroid.

ADRENAL MEDULLA: PHEOCHROMOCYTOMA

Pheochromocytoma is rare in childhood and usually presents with signs of catecholamine excess (hypertension, sweating, palpitations, nervousness, headache, polydipsia, polyuria, orthostatic hypotension, and gastroenterological complaints, such as nausea and vomiting), which may either be sustained or paroxysmal. More than half of children will have sustained hypertension. The tumor develops from chromaffin cells wherever they are located, but most tumors are found in the adrenal medulla, although bilateral or multifocal tumors are recognized to occur, especially in children.

Most pheochrocytomas in childhood are benign and occur maximally from 9 to 12 years of age, but have been reported at all ages. Predisposing causes include MEN-2a, MEN-2b, neurofibromatosis, Cushing's syndrome, and von Hippel–Lindau disease. The diagnosis is most easily made by measuring norepinephrine, epinephrine, and the metanephrines in a 24-hour urine collection. Plasma catecholamine determinations also may be measured. If the patient is having intermittent symptoms, the measurements must be performed while the symptoms are present. Urinary vanillylmandelic acid (VMA) analysis is a less reliable diagnostic test. Catecholamine excretion patterns are not useful in sorting out the 10% or so that are malignant. Once the tumor catecholamine determinations typical of pheochromocytoma are reached, localization studies (computed tomography, magnetic resonance imaging, or MIBG scintigraphy) are next used. Although arteriography was used in the past, it is no longer utilized because it can cause significant hypertension and has been replaced by less invasive methods. In very rare cases in which the diagnosis cannot be established with certainty, stimulation tests (glucagon, histamine) and suppression tests (clonidine) have been used in the past. These tests are potentially dangerous and rarely definitive and are not recommended (Taylor et al, 1986).

CARBOHYDRATE METABOLISM PROCEDURES

A diagnosis of diabetes mellitus in the child or adolescent is suggested by the history of polydipsia, polyphagia, polyuria, weight loss, and fatigue associated with glucosuria (and often ketonuria) and with a blood glucose of greater than 200 mg/dl. Such patients may, of course, present in frank diabetic ketoacidosis. The oral glucose tolerance test is rarely performed at present and is rarely required for diagnosis; it is generally thought of as a research tool. In certain asymptomatic individuals with equivocal glucose values, the test may be of use, although recent advances indicating the fact that the HLA antigens DR3 and/or DR4 are present in some 90% of individuals with insulin-dependent diabetes mellitus (IDDM) lessens the need for the test. Prior to testing, the patient's weight should have been stable and the patient should be free of disease for the previous 10 days or so, and patients are prepared with a diet that contains at least 50% of calories from carbohydrate for 3 days prior to the performance of the test. The patient is fasted except for water from midnight and the test is performed in the morning (Ginsberg, 1990; Nichols Institute, 1994). A glucose solution is administered orally in a dose of 1.75 g/kg (maximum dosage 75 g) after the baseline samples have been drawn. Samples for glucose and insulin are drawn at time 0 and at 1, 2, and 3 hours. Interpretation is based on the criteria established by the National Diabetes Data Group in 1979 (National Diabetes Data Group, 1979). These criteria include *both* an elevated fasting glucose concentration *and* a sustained elevated glucose concentration during the test on more than one occasion. Fasting values for venous plasma of 140 mg/dl or higher and a 2 hour sample, and at least one other sample of 200 mg/dl, are required for the diagnosis of diabetes mellitus. Normal insulin values are 8, 40, 35, and 18 μU/ml for children from 1 to 6 years of age and 15, 60, 55, and 20 μU/ml for children from 6 to 11 years of age for the four sampling times listed earlier. The intravenous glucose tolerance test is not indicated for the diagnosis of diabetes mellitus.

A diagnosis of hypoglycemia is suggested when symptoms attributable to either decreased central nervous system glucose (headache, visual disturbances, confusion, difficulty with speech, restlessness, irritability, coma, convulsions, and loss of intellectual functions) or to the autonomic response to hypoglycemia (diaphoresis, tachycardia, hunger, nausea, vomiting, tremulousness, weakness, and a feeling of anxiety) occur. The diagnosis is based upon the demonstration of a blood glucose of 40 mg/dl or less. Glucose is best measured after the blood has been drawn into tubes containing fluoride. The causes of this syndrome complex are numerous. Generally diagnosis is assisted by the measurements of blood insulin, cortisol, ACTH, growth hormone, glucagon, free fatty acids, lactate, and carnitine at a time when the child is hypoglycemic; urinary ketones must also be measured because they are not present in insulin-induced hypoglycemia. Liver function tests should also be performed. In some cases, prolonged fasting is required to bring about the hypoglycemia. Baseline measurement of serum and plasma glucose, insulin, growth hormone, glucagon, cortisol, ACTH, catecholamines, alanine, lactate, and pyruvate and urinary ketones are obtained, and a fast is carried out. When hypoglycemia occurs, these determinations are made again. A "keep open" line with normal saline is established, and glucose and hydrocortisone are kept at the bedside. Absence of ketones in the urine at the time of the hypoglycemia suggests insulin-induced hypoglycemia. This may be due to islet cell hyperplasia, insulinoma, or mesidioblastosis. In a child older than age 5 presenting with hypoglycemia, islet cell adenoma should be ruled out. Factitious hyperinsulinoma may be investigated by measuring C-peptide. Ketotic hypoglycemia that occurs in the 1- to 5-year age range is characterized by the presence of urinary ketones, low insulin levels, and low blood alanine levels.

Certain procedures may be useful in elucidating the etiology of the hypoglycemia. If hyperinsulinemia is suspected, the C-peptide suppression test (Nichols Institute, 1994) is performed. In this test, regular insulin in a dose of 0.1 U/kg in infused over 1 hour and blood is sampled every 10 minutes for glucose and C-peptide. Adequate venous access is essential for the performance of this test. Strips for testing blood glucose must be available and glucose (and hydrocortisone) should be available at the bedside to terminate the test if necessary. Normal individuals will suppress C-peptide levels to 1.6 ng/ml or less when the glucose concentration is below 50 mg/dl. The failure to suppress C-peptide indicates continued insulin secretion in the face of hypoglycemia and suggests the diagnosis of beta cell hyperplasia, insulinoma, or nesidioblastosis. Another test that was utilized in the past to document insulin hypersecretion was the tolbutamide tolerance test (Ginsberg, 1990). Because intravenous tolbutamide is no longer available, it would be pointless to describe this procedure. Because the differential diagnosis of hypoglycemia is extensive, the reader is directed to a review of this complex process (Kappy, 1994).

References

Brabant G, Prank K, Schofl C: Pulsatile patterns in hormone secretion. *Trends Endocrinol Metab*, 2:183, 1992.

Buckman M, Kaminsky N, Conway M, et al: Utility of L-dopa and water loading in evaluation of hyperprolactinemia. *J Clin Endocrinol Metab*, 36:911, 1973.

Chalew SA, Armour KM, Levin PA, et al: Growth hormone (GH) responses to GH-releasing hormone in children with subnormal integrated concentrations of GH. *J Clin Endocrinol Metab*, 62:1110, 1985.

Devusa J, Lima L, Tresguerres JAF: Neuroendocrine control of growth hormone secretion in humans. *Trends Endocrinol Metab*, 3:175, 1992.

Forest M: Pattern of the response of testosterone and its precursors to human chorionic gonadotropin stimulation in relation to age in infants and children. *J Clin Endocrinol Metab*, 49:132, 1979.

Ginsberg LJ: A practical approach to tolerance testing in children. In Lifshitz F (ed): *Pediatric Endocrinology*, 2nd ed. New York, Marcel Dekker, p 953, 1990.

Giustina A, Wehrenberg WB: The role of glucocorticoids in the regulation of growth hormone secretion. *Trends Endocrinol Metab*, 8:306,1992.

Grumbach MM, Styne DM: Puberty: Ontogeny, neuroendocrinology, physiology, and disorders. In Wilson JD, Foster DW (eds): *Williams Textbook of Endocrinology*. Philadelphia, WB Saunders, p 1139, 1992.

Harel Z, Tannenbaum GS: Synergistic interaction between ICF-I and -II in central regulation of pulsatile GH secretion. *Endocrinology*, 131:758, 1992.

Hofstra RMW, Landsvater RM, Ceccherine I, et al: A mutation in the RET proto-onchogene associated with multiple endocrine neoplasia type 2B and sporadic medullary thyroid carcinoma. *Nature*, 367:375, 1994.

Kappy MS: Carbohydrate metabolism and hypoglycemia. In Kappy MS, Blizzard RM, Migeon CT (eds): *The Diagnosis and Treatment of Endocrine Disorders in Childhood and Adolescence*, Springfield, IL, Charles C Thomas, 1994, pp 919–959

Kelch RP, Markovs M, Huss J: LH and FSH responsiveness to gonadotropin releasing hormone (GnRH) in children with hypothalamic or pituitary disorders. Lack of effect of replacement therapy with human growth hormone. *J Clin Endocrinol Metab*, 42:1104, 1976.

Kerrigan JR, Rogol AD: The impact of gonadal steroid hormone action on growth hormone secretion during childhood and adolescence. *Endocr Rev*, 13:281, 1992.

Lanes R, Becker B, Fort P, et al: Low dose oral clonidine: A simple and reliable growth hormone screening test for children. *Am J Dis Child*, 139:87, 1985.

Mulligan LM, Eng C, Healy CS, et al: Specific mutations of the RET proto-oncogene are related to disease phenotype in MEN-2A and FMTC. *Nature Genet*, 6:70, 1994.

National Diabetes Data Group: Classification and diagnosis of diabetes mellitus and other categories of glucose intolerance. *Diabetes*, 28:1039, 1979.

Neely EK, Hintz RL, Wilson DM, et al: Normal ranges for immunochemiluminometric gonadotropin assays. *J Pediatrics*, 127:40, 1995.

Nichols Institute: *Pediatric Endocrine Testing*. Endocrine Function Testing, Nichols Institute, San Juan Capistrano, California, 1994.

Pang S, Levine LS, Chow D, et al: Dihydrotestosterone and its relationship to testosterone in infancy and childhood. *J Clin Endocrinol Metab*, 48:821, 1979.

Penny R, Blizzard RM, Davis WD: Sequential arginine and insulin tolerance tests on the same day. *J Clin Endocrinol Metab*, 29:1499, 1969.

Seip RC, Weltman A, Goodman D, et al: Clinical utility of cycle exercise for the physiological assessment of growth hormone release in children. *Am J Dis Child*, 144:998, 1990.

Sheldon WR, Jr, DeBold CR, Evans WS, et al: Rapid sequential intravenous administration of four hypothalamic releasing hormones as a combined anterior pituitary function test in normal subjects. *J Clin Endocrinol Metab*, 10:623, 1985.

Spencer CA, Schwarzbein D, Guttler RB, et al: Thyrotropin (TSH)-releasing hormone stimulation test responses employing third and fourth generation TSH assays. *J Clin Endocrinol Metab*, 76:494, 1993.

Taylor HC, Mayes D, Anton AH: Clonidine suppression test for pheochromocytoma: Examples of misleading results. *J Clin Endocrinol Metab*, 63:238, 1986.

Wehrenberg WB, Giustina A: Mechanisms and pathways of gonadal steroid modulation of growth hormone secretion. *Endocr Rev*, 13:299, 1992.

Weldon VV, Gupta SK, Haymond MW et al: The use of L-dopa in the diagnosis of hyposomatotropism in children. *J Clin Endocrinol Metab*, 36:42, 1973.

Won JGS, Orth DN: Roles of intracellular and extracellular calcium in the kinetic profile of adrenocorticotropin secretion by perfused rat anterior pituitary cells. I. Corticotropin releasing factor stimulation. *Endocrinology*, 126:849, 1990.

Bibliography

Aksnes L, Aarskog D: Effect of parathyroid hormone on 1,25-dihydroxyvitamin D formation in type I pseudohypoparathyroidism. *J Clin Endocrinol Metab*, 51:1223, 1980.

Kruse K, Kracht U: A simplified diagnostic test in hypoparathyroidism and pseudohypoparathyroidism type I with synthetic 1-38 fragment of human parathyroid hormone. *Eur J Pediatr* 146: 373, 1987.

Chapter 45

Diagnostic Nuclear Medicine Imaging in Pediatric Endocrinology

Panukorn Vasinrapee, Michael E. Spieth, Azizullah N. Ansari, and Julie A. Ressler

Nuclear medicine uses tracer doses (small amounts that do not disturb normal physiology) of radiopharmaceuticals to image and to perform quantitative measurements. The radiopharmaceutical may be a simple compound (^{99m}Tc sodium pertechnetate [$^{99m}TcO_4^-$], ^{123}I sodium iodide, and ^{201}Tl thallous chloride) or may be combined with a chemical that directs it to a specific location (^{123}I- or ^{131}I-labeled metaiodobenzylguanidine [MIBG] for neuroendocrine tissue imaging, ^{131}I-labeled 1–6ß-iodomethyl-19-norcholesterol [NP-59] for adrenal cortex imaging, and ^{99m}Tc-sestamibi [MIBI] for myocardial imaging). Diagnostic doses of radiopharmaceuticals do not usually expose the patient to as much whole-body radiation as routine radiographs although they may deposit more radiation in an individual organ (Coffey et al, 1987; Conway et al, 1972; Society of Nuclear Medicine, 1988). In some examinations, such as voiding cystourethrograms (VCUGs), the radionuclide study may deliver as much as 100 times less radiation to the patient than a standard roentgenographic examination (Conway et al, 1972). There is no significant hazard to the patient, family, or health care workers when tracer doses of radionuclide are used. For pediatric patients, the dose is scaled down by age, height, weight, or body surface area. See Table 45–1 for methods of pediatric dose calculation (Chilton and Witcofski, 1986; Shore and Hendee, 1986).

The nuclear medicine physician is best able to select the most appropriate study and agent for a particular use. The supporting history, physical examination, laboratory findings, and results from other imaging modalities, as well as a specific question, are necessary for optimal interpretation. If radionuclide imaging cannot resolve the question, another imaging modality may be suggested. Some nuclear medicine studies require patient preparation such as premedication with phenobarbital for biliary atresia or urinary catheterization to demonstrate vesicoureteral reflux. Without appropriate preparation the examination may be suboptimal or invalid. The nuclear medicine department can provide information on how to prepare a patient for a specific examination.

Table 45-1 Methods of Pediatric Dose Calculation

1. Clark's Rule (Parameter: Weight)

$$\frac{\text{Weight (in lb)} \times \text{adult dose}}{\text{150 lb}}$$

2. Webster's Rule (Parameter: Age; Modified Young's Rule)

$$\frac{\text{Age (in years)} + 1}{\text{Age (in years)} + 7} \text{ times the adult dose}$$

3. Young's Rule (Parameter: Age)

$$\frac{\text{Age (in years)}}{\text{Age (in years)} +} \text{ times the adult dose}$$

4. Method 1 (Parameter: Height)

$$\frac{\text{Height}}{\text{174 cm}}$$

5. Method 2 (Parameter: Body Surface Area)

$$\frac{\text{Body Surface Area}}{1.73 \text{ m}^2}$$

6. Body Surface Area

Weight		Surface Area	Fraction of
(kg)	(lb)	(m^2)	Adult Dose
2	4.4	0.15	0.09
4	8.8	0.25	0.14
6	13.2	0.33	0.19
8	17.6	0.40	0.23
10	22.0	0.46	0.27
15	33.0	0.63	0.36
20	44.0	0.83	0.48
25	55.0	0.95	0.55
30	66.0	1.08	0.62
35	77.0	1.20	0.69
40	88.0	1.30	0.75
45	99.0	1.40	0.81
50	110.0	1.51	0.87
55	121.0	1.58	0.91

Thyroid Uptake and Imaging

The first clinical application of nuclear medicine was to evaluate thyroid function (Beierwaltes, 1979). Thyroid imaging allows the visualization and functional evaluation of thyroid tissue, which may be found from the level of the foramen cecum at the base of the tongue to the mediastinum. Although thyroid uptake studies and thyroid scans may be performed independently, they are usually done together because they are complementary.

THYROID UPTAKE

Thyroid uptake is an index of the ability of the thyroid gland to trap and organify iodine. It is a measure of the percentage of the total dose of administered iodine taken up by the gland. The normal uptake value is dependent on iodine intake from both diet and other sources, oral and topical medications, and diagnostic agents. Thus, in the United States, the value has decreased since the initiation of iodine supplementation (Boyett et al, 1974; Halpern et al, 1973).

Indications

Thyroid uptake studies are used to evaluate patients with thyrotoxicosis, for following patients on antithyroid medication, in the dose calculation for the therapeutic ^{131}I treatment of hyperthyroidism, to evaluate thyroiditis, and to identify organification defects.

Patient Preparation

Before a thyroid uptake study, the patient must fast overnight. This facilitates transit of the administered radioiodine through the stomach to the gastrointestinal tract, where it is absorbed, helping obtain a more consistent early (2-, 4-, or 6-hour) uptake value. Eating does not affect the 24-hour uptake value. Recent exposure to large amounts of iodine such as from radiographic contrast media, iodinated medications (amiodarone), a diet high in iodine (kelp and multivitamins containing iodine), and surgery using betadine on the mucosa (cervical cone biopsy) interferes with the thyroid radioiodine uptake, resulting in low uptake values. Thyroid medications—liothyronine (T_3 or Cytomel), levothyroxine sodium (T_4 or Synthroid), propylthiouracil (PTU), and methimazole (Tapazole)—must be discontinued for days to weeks before the examination.

Procedure

After the oral administration of 20 to 100 μCi of radioiodine (^{123}I), 2-, 4-, or 6- and 24-hour uptake values are obtained. Although performing only the 24-hour uptake is easier for the patient, a single 24-hour uptake provides less information than is provided when both early and late uptakes are obtained (Werner, 1979).

Pertechnetate can be used to estimate iodine uptake. Multiple quantitative methods have been used with minimal general acceptance (Preston et al, 1974). Many practitioners visually compare the thyroid activity with the salivary activity. Normal thyroid uptake shows equal thyroid and salivary gland activity. Increased and decreased thyroid gland activity correspond with more and less salivary gland activity, respectively.

Interpretation

Uptake values vary by technique, patient population, and diet. Therefore, each laboratory must establish its own normal range. By itself, the uptake can be increased, normal, or decreased. Thus, the uptake must be correlated with a thyroid scan and the appropriate laboratory values for proper interpretation. The normal uptake values at 2, 4, 6, and 24 hours are 5% to 12%, 6% to 18%, 8% to 25%, and 10% to 35%, respectively. The 24-hour value should be about twice the earlier uptake. There is no relationship between the 2- or 24-hour thyroid uptake and iodine half-life ($T_{1/2}$) (Banerji and Spencer, 1974).

Elevated 24-hour uptake values have been reported in hyperthyroidism (Graves' disease, toxic adenoma, toxic multinodular goiter), secondary to pituitary overactivity, in iodine deficiency, in the recovery phase of subacute thyroiditis, after the withdrawal of antithyroid medication, and with thyroid hormone use.

Decreased 24-hour uptake values occur in hypothyroidism (congenital, spontaneous, post-thyroidectomy, postradiation), Hashimoto's thyroiditis, the acute phase of subacute thyroiditis, thyroid and antithyroid medication, iodine contamination, factitious thyrotoxicosis, and toxic struma ovarii (Shafer et al, 1974; Teixeira et al, 1985; Werner et al, 1950).

Two- to 6-hour uptake values greater than the 24-hour uptake value occur in patients with organification defects and in patients with hyperthyroidism and a rapid iodine turnover.

THYROID SCANNING

Indications

Since the advent of ultrasound, computed tomography (CT), and magnetic resonance imaging (MRI), the indications for radionuclide thyroid scans have become fewer. The size and location of the thyroid gland can be determined by all these methods. However, the radionuclide thyroid scan is the method of choice for determining the functional status of the thyroid gland or a thyroid nodule.

Patient Preparation

Thyroid scans may be done using either radioiodine or pertechnetate. The patient preparation for a thyroid scan is the same as the preparation for thyroid uptake if radioiodine is used. No special preparation is required if pertechnetate is used.

Procedure

The patient lies in a supine position with his/her neck extended with a neck support. The pertechnetate thyroid scan is performed after the intravenous administration of 75 μCi/kg (with a minimum dose of 1 mCi to a maximum of 6 mCi adult dose) of ^{99m}Tc pertechnetate. An anterior view of the thyroid, which includes the salivary glands, is obtained 20 minutes after injection. It is used to visually estimate the uptake. The anterior view usually includes one image with and one image without markers on the suprasternal notch and thyroid cartilage to determine the position and size of the thyroid gland. Three pinhole images of the thyroid are then obtained (anterior and right and left anterior oblique views).

The ^{123}I thyroid scan is performed 2 to 6 hours after the oral administration of 30 μCi/kg (or a minimum of 30 μCi to a maximum of 100 μCi) of ^{123}I sodium iodide. ^{123}I is expensive and has limited availability. It is no longer commercially produced in the United States and is obtained from Canada. Previously, there were problems with ^{124}I contamination of ^{123}I, but this is no longer a problem.

Because ^{123}I and pertechnetate are available, routine thyroid scanning with ^{131}I is no longer advised. Both ^{123}I and pertechnetate deliver a lower radiation dose to the patient and produce superior images. All forms of commercially available radioiodine are administered by mouth.

Table 45–2 Thyroid Size By Age

Age	Newborn	1 y	5 y	10 y	15 y	STD
Size (g)	1.9	2.5	6.1	8.7	15.8	20

Interpretation

Most thyroid glands are located between the thyroid cartilage and the suprasternal notch. In a normal thyroid scan, both lobes of the thyroid are seen. The right lobe is usually slightly larger than the left lobe (Spencer and Banever, 1970). There should be uniform distribution of activity throughout the thyroid gland. Each adult lobe measures approximately 5 by 2 cm and weighs approximately 10 g. The newborn thyroid gland is about 1.7 cm long and grows 1.8 mm/year (Spencer and Banever, 1970). Table 45–2 shows pediatric thyroid weights (Spector, 1956). The pyramidal lobe, which lies superior to the isthmus and between the right and left lobes of the thyroid, is visualized in 15% of patients and usually shows less activity than the rest of the thyroid. The isthmus varies in appearance and is usually too thin to be visualized well (Fig. 45–1).

A radioiodine scan shows almost no soft-tissue or vascular blood pool activity, and the salivary glands are seldom seen after 2 hours. Pertechnetate scans, on the other hand, almost always demonstrate the salivary glands and a high soft-tissue and vascular blood pool background. Activity may also be seen in the mouth, nasopharynx, and, occasionally, the esophagus because pertechnetate is secreted by the salivary glands and then swallowed.

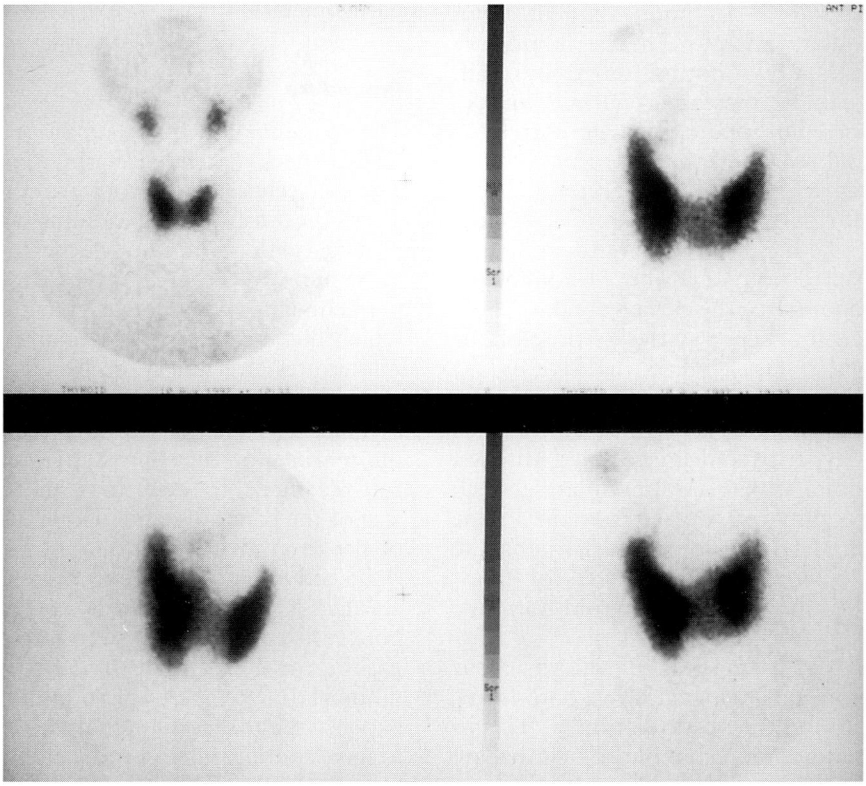

Figure 45–1 Normal thyroid gland.

DISEASE STATES PRESENTING WITH ABNORMAL FINDINGS

CONGENITAL HYPOTHYROIDISM: Congenital hypothyroidism may occur with lingual thyroid tissue, ectopic gland position (sporadic) (Fig. 45–2), or a normally positioned gland. It is often associated with increased trapping from organification defects (hereditary) (Fig. 45–3) or thyroid agenesis (Fig. 45–4).

DIFFUSELY ENLARGED THYROID: Diffusely enlarged thyroid with increased trapping and organification occurs in Graves' disease (Fig. 45–5), the recovery phase of subacute thyroiditis (Fig. 45–6), rebound after withdrawal of antithyroid medication or thyroid hormone use, iodine deficiency, and lithium use. Increased trapping with pertechnetate and a low iodine uptake value may occur in organification defects.

THYROID NODULES: Thyroid nodules occur in 4% of the general population, and their incidence increases with age. They are four times more common in females than males, and they may be cold (or cool), warm, or hot; single or multiple; concordant (similar on pertechnetate and ^{123}I scans) or discordant (hot on pertechnetate and cold on ^{123}I scans). Most thyroid nodules are benign; however, discordant and cold nodules have an increased risk for thyroid carcinoma.

Cold (or cool) nodules (Fig. 45–7) have no activity (or much less activity) in relation to the surrounding thyroid tissue. Approximately 80% to 85% of cold nodules are benign. The most common causes of cold nodules are colloid cysts and adenomas. Less common causes of benign cold nodules include parathyroid cysts, parathyroid adenomas, extrinsic neck masses, thyroiditis, hematomas, abscesses, and branchial cysts (Lisbona et al, 1973). Fifteen percent to 20% of cold nodules are malignant primary thyroid neoplasms, which may be papillary, follicular, mixed papillary–follicular, Hürthle cell, undifferentiated anaplastic, or medullary carcinoma. Papillary, follicular, and mixed papillary–follicular carcinomas occur in the pediatric age group. Anaplastic, medullary (MTC), and Hürthle cell carcinomas usually occur in the middle-aged to elderly population and are seldom a pediatric problem. Metastatic neoplasms occur infrequently.

Many agents have been used to distinguish benign from malignant nodules; however, none of them have received wide acceptance. For differentiating benign from malignant nodules, ^{67}Ga gallium citrate has a 100% negative predictive value (NPV) but only a 31% positive predictive value (PPV); ^{67}Ga citrate has a 100% NPV and PPV for identifying undifferentiated or anaplastic carcinoma (Heidendal et al, 1975; Senga et al, 1982). Thallium, which

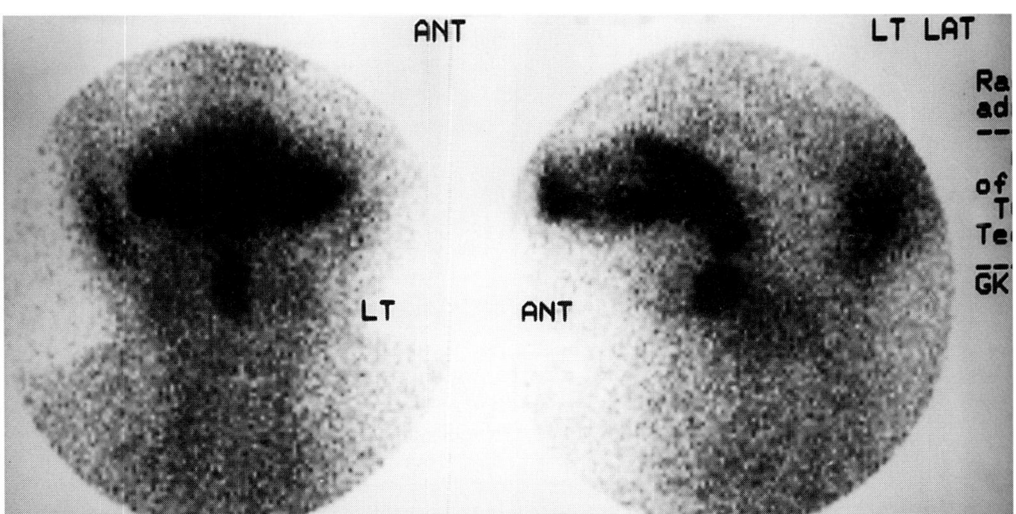

Figure 45–2 Lingual thyroid gland.

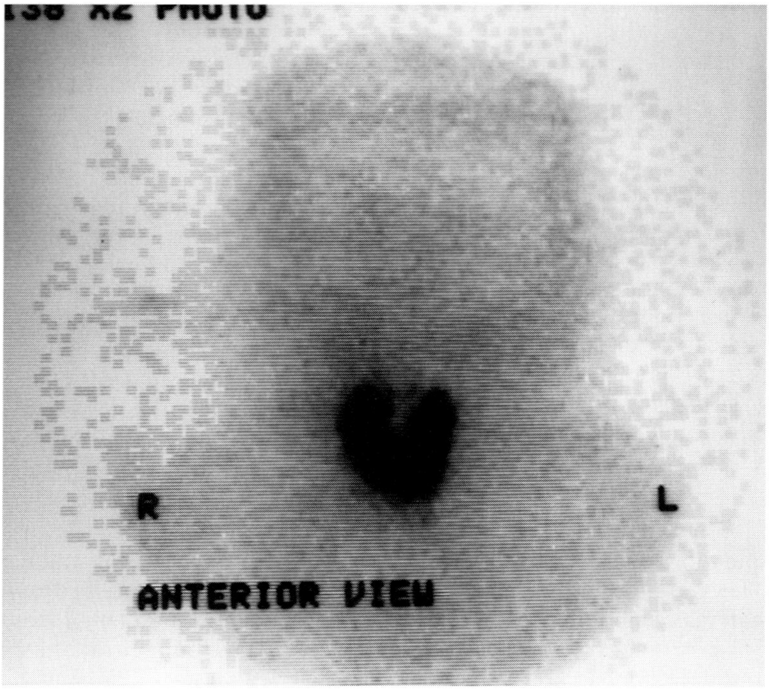

Figure 45–3 Organification defect.

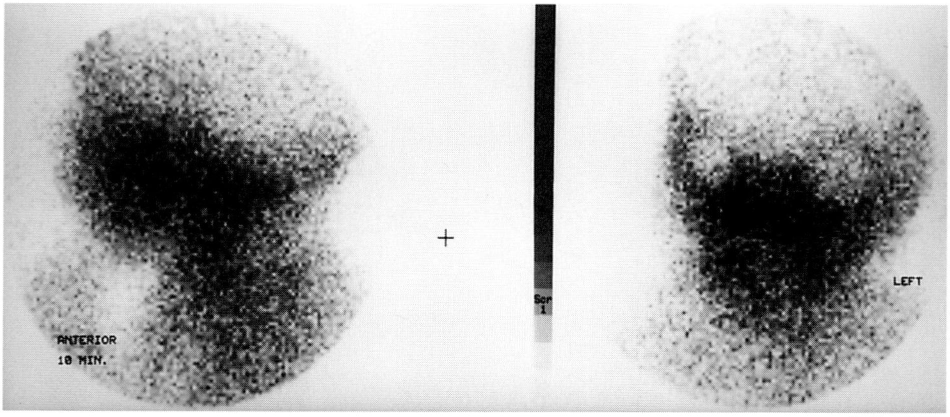

Figure 45–4 Thyroid agenesis.

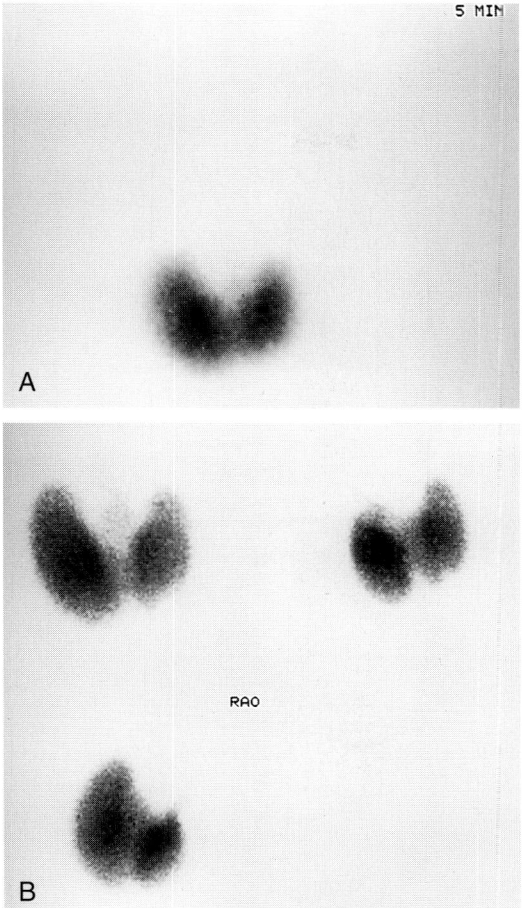

Figure 45–5 Graves' disease. **A.** Five-minute parallel hole image. **B.** Twenty-minute pinhole images. RAO, right anterior oblique.

is the best-characterized radionuclide, has a 60% to 67% PPV, a 90% to 93% NPV, and a sensitivity of 80% in identifying well-differentiated carcinoma (Henze et al, 1986; Hoschl et al, 1984; Senga et al, 1982). MIBI imaging has not been well studied but usually has results similar to thallium's. Even ^{99m}Tc medronate (bone agent) flow studies have been used to help distinguish solid from cystic lesions, but they cannot differentiate benign from malignant lesions. OctreoScan, a newly released agent, may help identify MTC, but results are also positive in benign conditions such as Graves' disease (Krenning et al, 1993a; Kwekkeboom et al, 1993).

Warm nodules are palpable nodules with the same activity as the surrounding thyroid tissue. They may be nonfunctioning nodules located deeply within the thyroid gland. They are seldom malignant. The term "warm nodule" is seldom used.

Hot nodules (Fig. 45–8) have increased activity compared with the surrounding tissue. They are rarely malignant (less than 1% of cases) (Miller and Hamburger, 1965). Autonomous hyperfunctioning adenomas are the most common cause of hot nodules.

Multinodular goiters (Fig. 45–9) may have multiple cold or a mixture of hot and cold nodules. Only 4% to 17% of them contain malignant tissue.

Discordant nodules are warm or hot on pertechnetate study and cold on ^{123}I scans. These nodules have the same risk for thyroid carcinoma as cold nodules.

The term "toxic" nodule is reserved for those nodules occurring with thyrotoxicosis. They cannot be reliably diagnosed from the thyroid scan alone. However, a greatly elevated uptake is strongly suggestive of a toxic state.

DISTRIBUTION: Nonuniform distribution of activity in the thyroid gland may occur in Hashimoto's thyroiditis, nodular Graves' disease, and postradioactive iodine therapy (Charkes, 1972).

CHRONIC THYROIDITIS: Chronic thyroiditis usually affects the thyroid gland diffusely; however, it may occur as a diffuse goiter, a multinodular goiter, or a solitary hot or cold nodule (Paull et al, 1974). In the acute phase of subacute thyroiditis, the uptake is decreased and the thyroid function test (TFT) results are increased. This helps distinguish thyroiditis from Graves' disease. In the recovery phase, the uptake may be increased with normal TFTs.

ANATOMICAL VARIANTS

A gland that is asymmetrical may be normal. The right lobe is larger than the left in 48% of cases; the left lobe is larger than the right in 15% of cases; they are equal in size in the rest. Asymmetrical glands also occur with intrathyroidal lesions, in unilateral thyroid hypoplasia, and in patients after a partial thyroidectomy.

Poor visualization or absence of one lobe of the thyroid occurs in patients with a prior hemithyroidectomy (Fig. 45–10), with replacement of an entire lobe by a cold intrathyroidal lesion (Fig. 45–11), in hemiagenesis, which involves the left lobe more often than the right

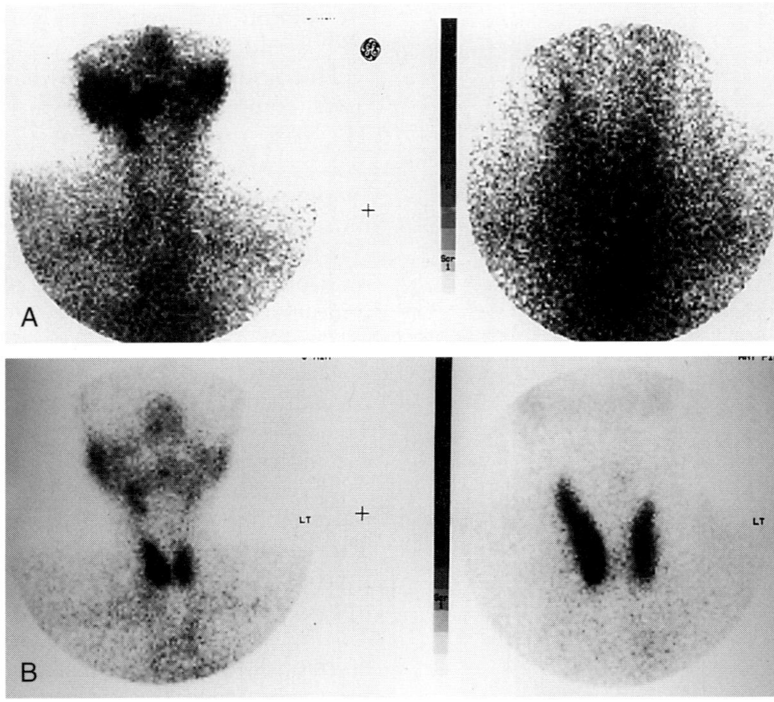

Figure 45–6 Thyroiditis in the same patient as in Figure 45–5. **A.** Acute phase. **B.** Recovery phase (2 months later).

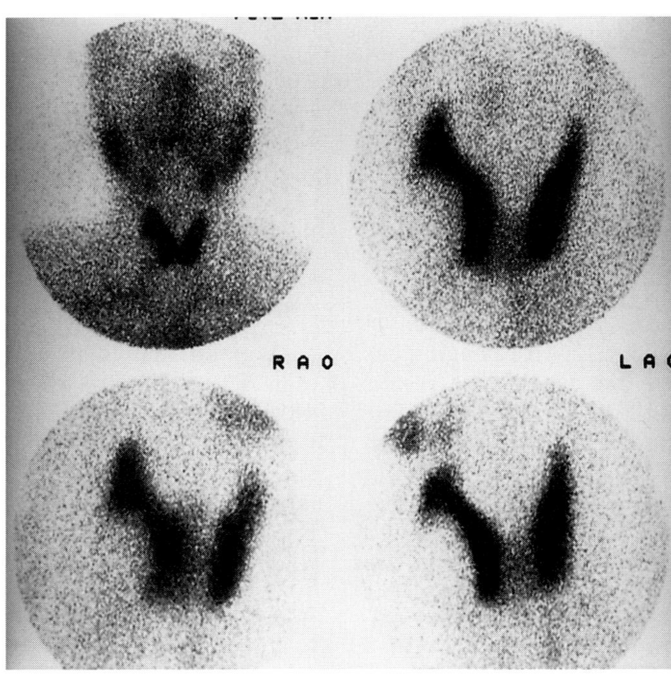

Figure 45–7 Cold nodule in the right lobe. RAO and LAO, right and left anterior oblique.

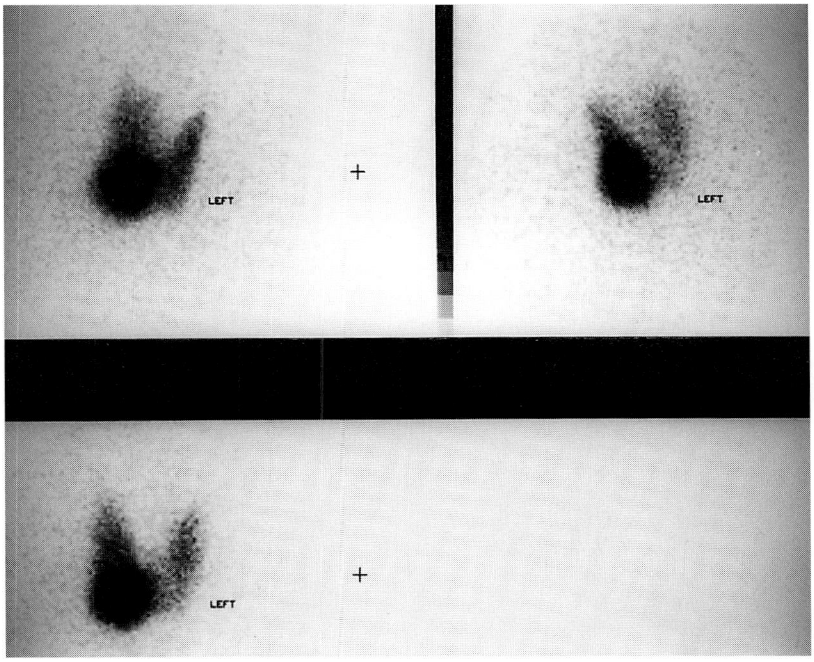

Figure 45–8 Hot nodule in the inferior right lobe.

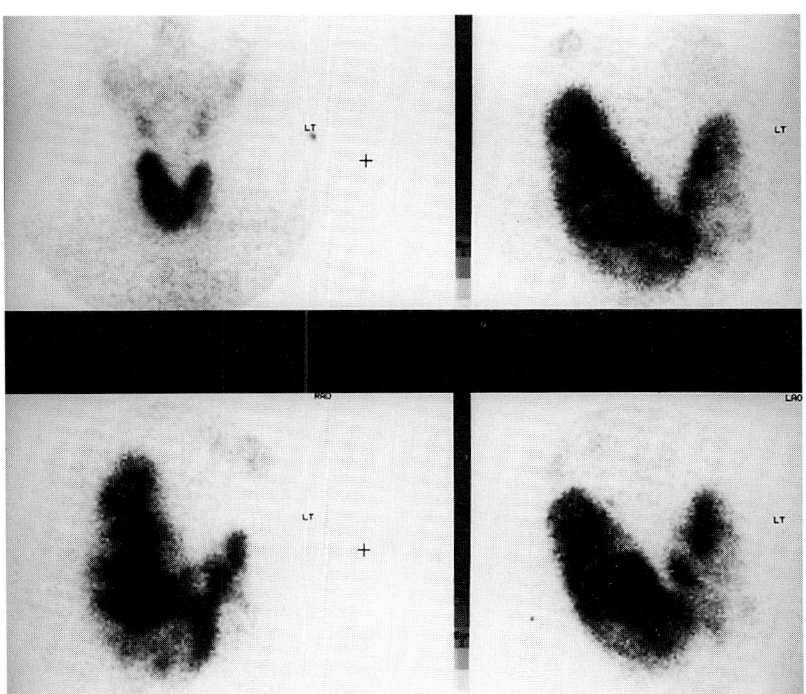

Figure 45–9 Multinodular goiter.

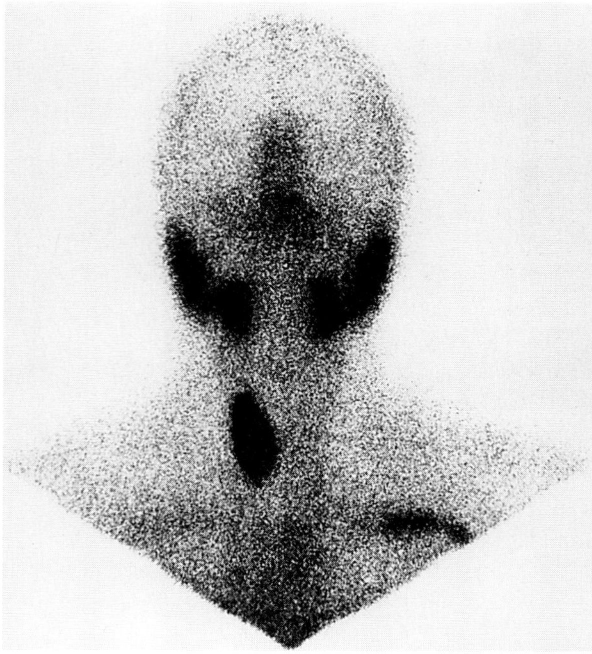

Figure 45–10 Left hemithyroidectomy.

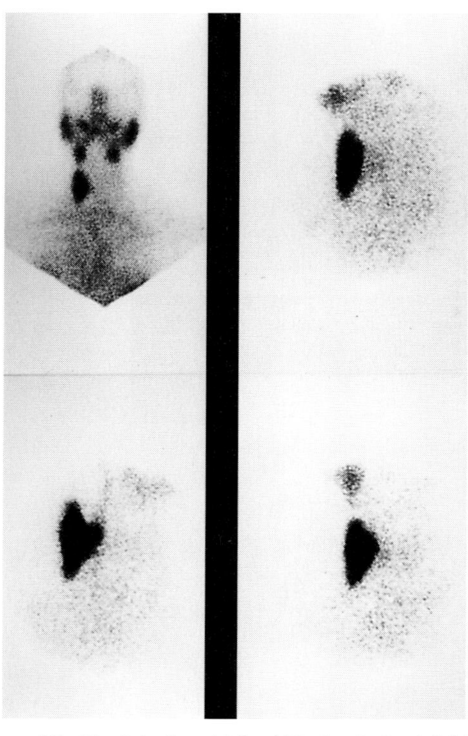

Figure 45–11 Intrathyroidal cold lesion in the left lobe.

lobe, and in suppression of the normal thyroid tissue by an autonomous nodule on the contralateral side (Fig. 45–12).

The pyramidal lobe is a remnant left from the embryological migration of the thyroid gland. Sometimes, it contains functional thyroid tissue. It is a linear structure lying between the right and left lobes of the thyroid. Activity within the pyramidal lobe can be differentiated from swallowed saliva within the esophagus on the oblique pertechnetate scans. Saliva remains in a relatively unchanged position because it is within the esophagus, a posterior structure. Activity within the pyramidal lobe appears to move laterally on oblique images because it is a more anterior structure. If there is any question, most of the pertechnetate retained in the esophagus is removed when the patient drinks a glass of water.

Ectopic thyroid tissue is seen in mediastinal goiters, lingual thyroids, and accessory thyroid tissue in the mediastinum.

An isthmus that is not visualized may be a normal variant; however, it could also be an intrathyroidal lesion.

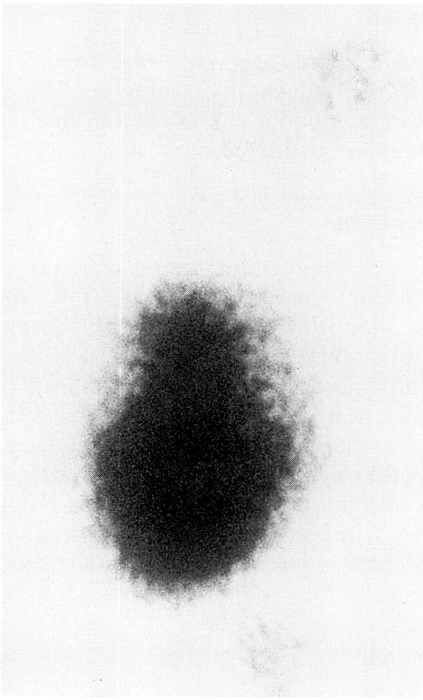

Figure 45–12 Autonomous functioning nodule.

THYROID HORMONE (T_3 SUPPRESSION) TEST (Jackson and Cobb, 1986)

Indications

The T_3 suppression test was used before the advent of the ultrasensitive thyroid stimulating hormone (sTSH) test for the determination of hyperthyroidism.

Principle

The T_3 suppression test determines the gland suppressibility using the physiological negative feedback system.

Procedure

A baseline uptake value and scan are obtained. The patient is then given T_3, 25 μg three times a day for 7 days, which suppresses the normal thyroid tissue. A repeat uptake value and thyroid scan are performed on the eighth day.

Alternatively, suppression may be performed using L-thyroxine, 0.3 mg/d for 10 days, or a single 3-mg dose given 1 week before the scan.

Interpretation

The normal thyroid response to suppression is for the uptake to decrease to less than 20% of the initial uptake when the baseline is 40% or greater. If the baseline uptake is less than 40%, the normal thyroid response to suppression is for the uptake to decline to less than 50% of the baseline uptake. An elevated uptake on a compensatory basis, that is, a rebound phenomenon or iodine deficiency, decreases sharply after suppression. The gland does not suppress in hyperthyroidism due to Graves' disease, and autonomous nodules do not suppress.

TSH STIMULATION TEST (Jackson and Cobb, 1986)

Indications

The TSH stimulation test is used to demonstrate normal, TSH-dependent thyroid tissue that has been suppressed by autonomous thyroid tissue.

Procedure

A baseline ^{123}I scan is performed and an uptake value is obtained. The patient is given human recombinant (or bovine) TSH, 10 U intramuscularly for 3 days, after which a repeat uptake value or thyroid scan is obtained.

Interpretation

The response of normal thyroid to TSH stimulation is an increase in uptake of 10% or more over the baseline uptake. A normal response occurs when there is autonomous thyroid tissue suppressing the normal thyroid tissue, in patients taking thyroid hormones, and in secondary hypothyroidism.

An alternative method of demonstrating suppressed thyroid tissue is to give the patient ^{201}Tl chloride, 2 to 3 mCi, or ^{99m}Tc MIBI, 10 to 30 mCi, and then obtain images of the neck (Fig. 45–13) (Corstens et al, 1988). Thallium and ^{99m}Tc MIBI are taken up by normal thyroid tissue whether or not that tissue is being suppressed by autonomous thyroid tissue and in situations with decreased TSH.

PERCHLORATE DISCHARGE TEST (Jackson and Cobb, 1986)

Indications

The perchlorate discharge test is used to demonstrate iodine organification defects.

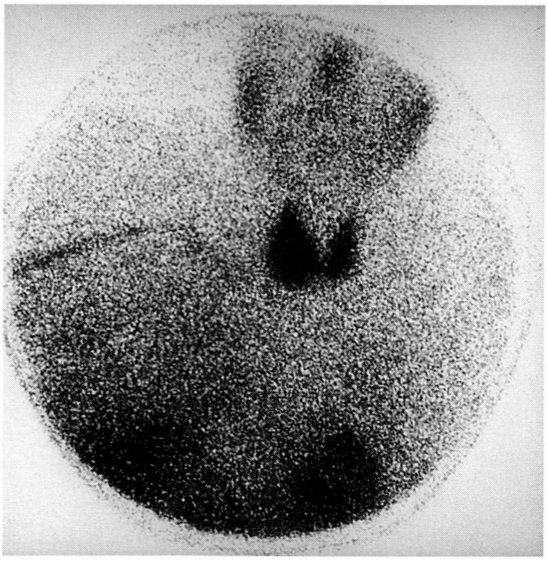

Figure 45–13 Thyroid imaging in the same patient as in Figure 45–12 using Tl-201, which helps visualize suppressed thyroid tissue through a non-TSH–dependent mechanism.

Procedure

A baseline 2-hour uptake is measured. The patient is then given potassium perchlorate by mouth, and uptake values are obtained at 30-minute intervals for 2 hours.

Interpretation

In the normally functioning thyroid gland, the uptake remains the same or decreases by less than 10% compared with the baseline after potassium perchlorate is administered. If the uptake decreases by more than 10%, an organification defect is present. The causes of diffuse organification defects include Hashimoto's thyroiditis, anti-thyroid medication use, and congenital hypothyroidism due to a peroxidase or "coupling" defect. Thyroid carcinoma may occur as a focal organification defect.

Management of Well-Differentiated Thyroid Carcinoma

Radioiodine plays an integral part in the management of well-differentiated thyroid carcinoma. ^{131}I can be used to ablate the remnant thyroid tissue after surgical thyroidectomy and to identify and treat metastases or recurrent functioning thyroid carcinoma.

As cited by Sisson (1983) and Goolden (1985), there are multiple reasons to ablate thyroid remnants with ^{131}I radioiodine after a surgical thyroidectomy. Papillary carcinomas are multifocal in 20% to 30% of cases. Residual thyroid tissue is a source of thyroglobulin, which diminishes the specificity of thyroglobulin as a tumor marker in screening for recurrent carcinoma. Residual thyroid tissue is also a source of thyroid hormone, which inhibits pituitary thyroid stimulating hormone (TSH) secretion. A high TSH level is necessary in the identification and treatment of thyroid carcinoma because much less radioiodine is taken up when the TSH level is normal. Residual thyroid tissue also competes with recurrent or metastatic thyroid cancer for radioiodine uptake, making the cancer more difficult to identify and treat.

The value of postsurgical ablation of the residual thyroid tissue is somewhat controversial. DeGroot and colleagues (1990) retrospectively demonstrated that the postoperative ablation of residual thyroid tissue with ^{131}I in patients with intrathyroid papillary carcinomas larger than 1 cm in diameter, with or without cervical metastases, was associated with a significant increased risk of recurrence or death. Mazzaferri (1991) evaluated a different population and found that ablation of remnant thyroid tissue in patients without known residual carcinoma after their initial thyroidectomy resulted in significantly fewer recurrences than occurred with surgical treatment alone.

Functional metastasis from thyroid carcinoma or recurrence of thyroid carcinoma can be identified by a number of methods, and perhaps a combination of tests should be considered. These include thyroglobulin (Tg) level, radioiodine (sodium ^{131}I) whole-body imaging, ^{201}Tl chloride and ^{99m}Tc MIBI tumor imaging agents, chest radiographs, chest CT scans, and positron emission tomography

(PET). Plain film bone surveys and head CT scans add little additional information unless there is a high clinical suspicion of bony and cerebral metastasis.

By combining data from 10 large surveys, Maxon and Smith (1990) found that cervical node metastases were present at the time of the initial diagnosis in 36% of patients with papillary carcinoma and 13% of patients with follicular carcinoma. Distant metastases were found at the initial work-up in 4% of patients with papillary carcinoma and 16% of patients with follicular carcinoma. They also evaluated the subsequent development of recurrent or metastatic well-differentiated thyroid carcinoma in patients who were considered disease free after their initial surgical treatment. Six percent of patients with papillary carcinoma and 8% of patients with follicular carcinoma experienced local cancer recurrence in or adjacent to the thyroid bed. Cervical node metastases developed in 9% of patients with papillary carcinoma and 7% of patients with follicular carcinoma. Distant metastases developed in 4% of patients with papillary carcinoma and 13% of patients with follicular carcinoma.

When distant metastases occurred, just the lung was involved in 29% of cases; both the lung and bone were involved in 10% of cases; other sites such as the mediastinum and the brain were involved in 16% of cases. ^{131}I was found to concentrate in sites of recurrent or metastatic well-differentiated carcinoma in approximately 73% of patients with such lesions.

Ashcroft and Van Herle (1981) reviewed 1323 reported cases of well-differentiated thyroid cancer in patients who had undergone both whole-body ^{131}I radionuclide scans and serum Tg measurement tests. Metastases were documented in 22% of patients (284 of 1323). ^{131}I scans were normal in 13% of patients (37 of 284) with known metastasis, and Tg values were within the normal range in 4% of patients (12 of 284) with positive ^{131}I scans. Black and colleagues (1987) analyzed serial serum Tg levels in 416 patients after initial therapy for well-differentiated thyroid cancer. Only 2.3% of patients (7 of 298) with serum Tg levels less than 5 μg/L after initial treatment developed evidence of recurrent or metastatic disease within a mean follow-up time of 3.1 years. In 42% of patients (8 of 19) with serum Tg levels greater than 5 μg/L but without evidence of residual disease initially, recurrent or metastatic disease became evident within 0.8 to 3.5 years.

Pacini and colleagues (1987) found that, postoperatively, 13% of patients with well-differentiated thyroid cancer had positive serum Tg levels and negative nuclear scans obtained 48 to 72 hours after a 5-mCi dose of sodium ^{131}I.

These data suggest that there is a subgroup of patients in whom an abnormal serum Tg level may be the only indicator of residual or recurrent disease after the initial therapy.

Schlumberger and colleagues (1986) evaluated 238 patients with pulmonary metastases from well-differentiated thyroid carcinoma. Standard chest radiographs were normal in 30% of these patients, 33% had a micronodular pattern (nodules less than 1 cm) on chest radiograph, and 37% had a macronodular pattern (nodules more than or equal to 1 cm) on chest radiograph. In the patients who had normal standard chest radiographs, CT examination of the chest was abnormal in approximately one half. Thus, when pulmonary metastases became evident by ^{131}I scanning or by an elevation in Tg level, 85% of patients had demonstrable pulmonary lesions by standard chest radiographs or CT scan and no discernible disease elsewhere. When pulmonary metastases were seen on ^{131}I images only, two thirds of the time they were seen on 2-mCi diagnostic scans, and in one third of cases they were seen only on scans obtained after the much larger therapeutic doses of ^{131}I were administered. It is thought that lesions seen on ^{131}I scans only after treatment doses may not respond to radioiodine therapy. When micronodular disease was present on the chest radiograph, the relative risk of death tripled; when macronodular disease was present on the chest radiogaph, the relative risk of death increased sixfold. Also, higher diagnostic doses may "stun" the gland, decreasing the efficiency of future treatment. Thus, low-dose diagnostic scans may still be the best choice. More research is needed.

The distribution of skeletal metastases from well-differentiated thyroid cancer has been evaluated by several groups (Castillo et al, 1980; Schlumberger et al, 1986). The combined data indicate that, at the time of diagnosis, 70% of patients have multiple skeletal metastases and 30% of patients have solitary skeletal metastasis. The most common sites (in decreasing order of frequency) are the spine, pelvis, skull, ribs, and sternum. Skeletal metastases from well-differentiated thyroid cancer are almost always lytic on standard bone radiographs. Schlumberger and colleagues (1986) pointed out that only 6% of skeletal metastases are seen only on ^{131}I scans and not on standard radiographs. DeGroot and Reilly (1984) found that ^{131}I whole-body scans resulted in the identification of skeletal metastases in only 14% of patients (4 of 29) who had them. They also showed that standard ^{99m}Tc diphosphonate bone imaging was of little value. Maxon and colleagues (1992) subsequently evaluated 382 standard bone scans in 85 patients with well-differentiated thyroid cancers during a span of 0.8 to 8.5 years after their initial diagnosis. They found that none of the bone scans identified the skeletal metastases correctly.

Parathyroid Imaging

INDICATIONS

Parathyroid imaging is indicated primarily in a patient with hypercalcemia and an elevated parathyroid hormone (PTH) level, with suspected parathyroid adenoma after surgical failure to locate the glands (Mullan and Brown, 1990). Experienced surgeons can locate the diseased glands in 90% to 95% of cases (Hartshorne, 1991; Petti, 1990). However, preoperative localization may decrease the operative time. Parathyroid imaging is not reliable for identifying hyperplastic glands and is of questionable value in localization of functional parathyroid carcinoma (Burckhardt et al, 1976).

PATIENT PREPARATION

No specific patient preparation is required; however, the patient must be able to hold still for at least 30 minutes if the thallium/pertechnetate subtraction technique is used.

TECHNIQUE

There are several techniques of parathyroid imaging. Although the thallium/technetium subtraction technique is the most established method, it has drawbacks (motion artifacts, misregistration, the need for prolonged patient cooperation). A newer method is the sestamibi washout technique. Sestamibi washout is easier to perform and better suited for SPECT (single photon emission computed tomography) imaging.

^{201}Tl/Pertechnetate Subtraction

Twenty minutes after the injection of thallium, images of the patient's neck and mediastinum are obtained. Without moving the patient, pertechnetate is administered, and the patient's neck and mediastinum are imaged 10 minutes later. Thallium goes to the thyroid and the parathyroid glands. Pertechnetate is taken up by the thyroid tissue only. Thus, when the technetium image is subtracted from the thallium image, activity is seen only in the parathyroid tissue. The pertechnetate may be administered before the thallium if image background subtraction is performed. Using dual isotope acquisition decreases the time required for the study and decreases motion artifacts (Moskowitz et al, 1995; Neumann, 1992).

Alternative techniques include $^{201}Tl/^{123}I$ subtraction and ^{99m}Tc pertechnetate/^{131}I toluidine blue subtraction. The last technique can be used for intraoperative localization because it stains the parathyroid glands blue but it is seldom used.

^{99m}TC Sestamibi (Cardiolite)

MIBI (Cardiolite) is administered intravenously (Burke et al, 1993), and images of the anterior and right and left anterior oblique neck are obtained at 10, 30, 60, and 120 minutes. If abnormal parathyroid tissue is seen, SPECT is performed 2 hours after injection to better localize the abnormal parathyroid tissue.

NORMAL IMAGE

Both thallium and pertechnetate go to salivary and thyroid glands. Thallium localizes in the glandular tissue according to regional blood flow and ATP-ase-dependent Na/K pump function. Enlarged parathyroid glands take up thallium and not pertechnetate. The subtraction technique removes the normal thyroid gland and shows the parathyroid activity. Normal parathyroid glands are not visualized because of their small size and minimal mitotic activity. The normal subtraction image leaves a negative image (Fig. 45–14A).

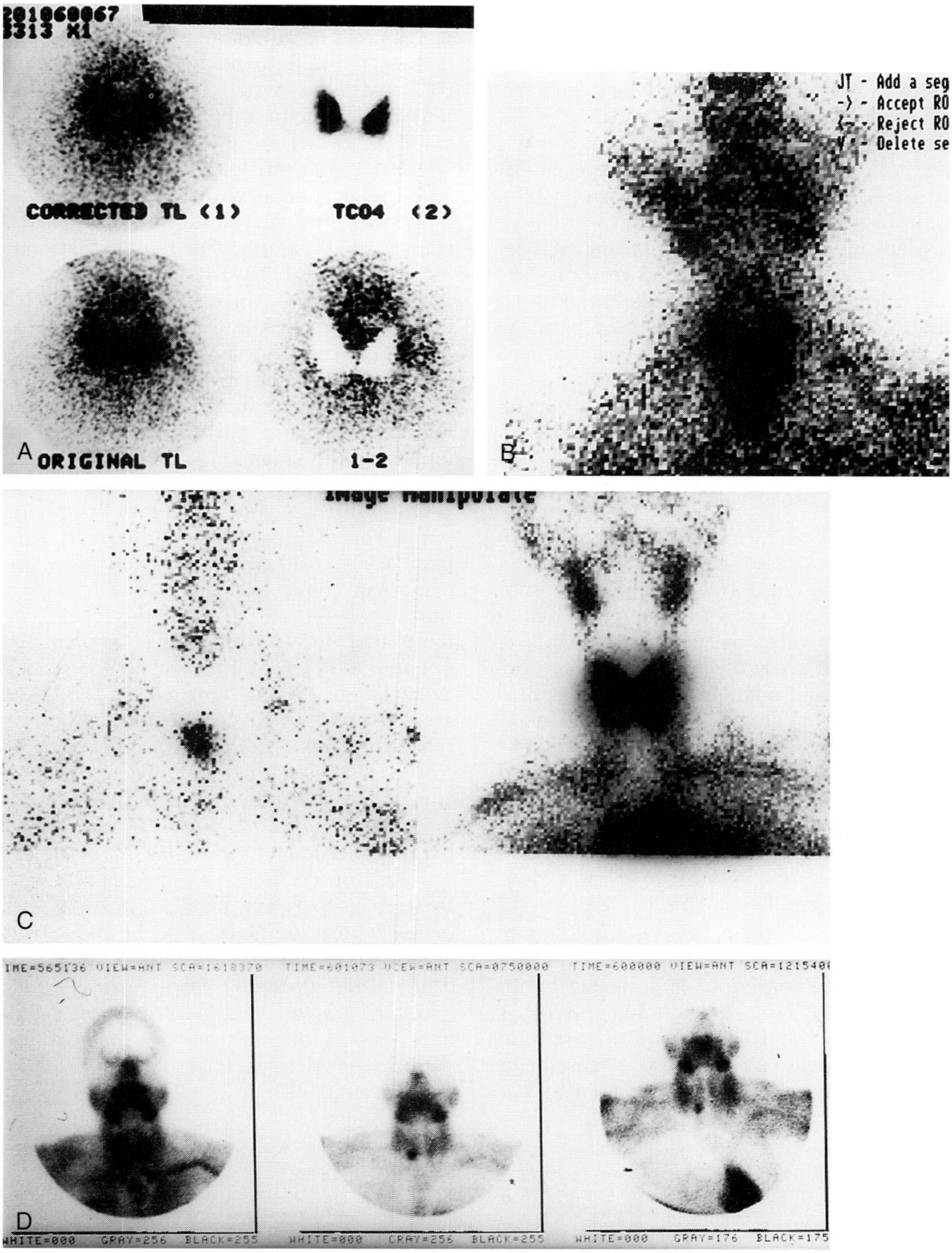

Figure 45–14 **A.** Normal thallium/technetium subtraction parathyroid examination. **B.** Normal thallium image without subtraction. **C.** Positive thallium/technetium subtraction image for an inferior thyroid parathyroid adenoma on the left and normal pertechnetate image on the right. **D.** Sestamibi-positive image shown over time.

The parathyroid glands are located in their usual anatomical sites in 75% of cases and in ectopic sites in 25%. Supernumerary (more than four) glands occur in 5% of cases. Ectopic glands may be found lateral to the thyroid gland, in the mediastinum, in the thymus, or posterior to the esophagus or pharynx (Mullan and Brown, 1990).

Parathyroid glands, thyroid, and salivary glands take up thallium so it is nonspecific for parathyroid tissue (Mullan and Brown, 1990). Visualization of parathyroid glands with thallium depends more on their mitotic activity than their size. Glands in the lower poles are visualized more often than glands in the upper poles. Noncervical, nonmediastinal parathyroid tissue is sometimes autotransplanted into the forearm. There it can easily be followed by thallium imaging alone (Takebayashi et al, 1990).

DIFFERENTIAL DIAGNOSIS

Motion artifact or misregistration will invalidate most studies.

Multiple large focal areas of uptake on subtraction images may represent benign or malignant nodules in the same patient (Veluvolu et al, 1991). Focal areas of increased activity occur in parathyroid adenomas (Fig. 45–15B to D) and primary hyperparathyroidism. Primary hyperparathyroidism occurs in a solitary parathyroid gland in 80% to 90% of cases and in multiple glands in 2% (Winzelberg, 1987a). Many adenomas are apparent from the thallium scan without subtraction, but subtraction imaging increases the sensitivity of the examination (Mullan and Brown, 1990).

Parathyroid adenomas are visualized more commonly than hyperplasia (Mullan and Brown, 1990). Parathyroid hyperplasia is not visualized in 50% of cases. It may occur as multiple hot foci in 10% to 15% of cases and as a single focus in the rest (Winzelberg, 1987b). Parathyroid carcinoma is seen in 2% of cases. It must be functional to be visualized (Sandrock et al, 1990).

Focal areas of increased thallium activity within the mediastinum may represent ectopic parathyroid or supernumerary parathyroid adenomas, multiple gland hyperplasia, squamous cell carcinoma of the lung, mediastinal lymphoma, ectopic parathyroid carcinoma, or sarcoidosis (Lossef et al, 1993; Statz and Oates, 1988; Tonami and Hisada, 1977; Winzelberg, 1987c). Focal areas of increased thallium activity in the forearm are seen in patients with transplanted parathyroid glands that will be hyperplastic (Takebayashi et al, 1990).

Focal areas of increased thallium activity within the mediastinum have also been seen due to patient motion artifacts, Hodgkin's disease, ectopic retrosternal thyroid tissue, brown tumors in the sternum, oxyphilic-cell adenomas, cervical osteoporosis, large vessel accumulation, lipoadenomas, solitary hypofunctioning thyroid nodules, multinodular goiter, Graves' disease associated with lymphadenopathy, chronic thyroiditis, undifferentiated and papillary thyroid carcinomas, and fetal adenomas (Asp et al, 1987; Bleiweiss et al, 1989; Burckhardt et al, 1976; Ferlin et al, 1983; Krubsack, 1987; Mullan and Brown, 1990; Tonami and Hisada 1977; Tonami et al, 1978; Winzelberg, 1987a; Yang et al, 1989). Focal areas of decreased technetium activity may represent thyroid adenomas, enlarged parathyroid glands, lymph nodes involved with sarcoidosis, primary thyroid carcinomas, metastatic carcinoma, Hodgkin's lymphoma, and parathyroid adenomas (Shimshak et al, 1979).

A diffuse decrease in pertechnetate activity is seen in patients ingesting excess dietary or exogenous iodine, thyroid hormone administration, thyroiditis, prior thyroidectomy, recently administered intravenous contrast, lymph nodes with sarcoid infiltration, metastatic disease, Hodgkin's disease, and lymphoma with hypercalcemia (Gelfand, 1993; Mullan and Brown, 1990).

Adrenal Gland Imaging

The adrenal gland is unique among those imaged in nuclear medicine in that anatomically there are two glands, one above each kidney, and each is physiologically separated into two glands. By using agents designed to identify its different functions, each portion of the adrenal gland can be looked at separately. Thus, the cortical and medullary portions of the gland are discussed separately.

Table 45–3 Thyroid-Blocking Dosage By Age

Agent	Daily Dosing	0–1 y	1–4 y	4+ y
Lugol's solution (6 mg iodine/drop)	2 gtt-bid-tid	6 mg	12 mg	18 mg
SSKI (50 mg iodine/drop)	3 gtt qd	50 mg	50 mg	50 mg
Potassium perchlorate (1 g for adults and 10 mg/kg by weight for children)	b d	150 mg	300 mg	450 mg

bid, twice a day; gtt, drops; tid, three times a day; qd, every day; SSKI, supersaturated potassium iodide.

PATIENT PREPARATION

Pregnancy is the only absolute contraindication to adrenal imaging. Before administration of radioiodine-based agents, thyroid uptake–blocking drugs are given to block free iodine uptake by the thyroid. This permits imaging of the neck region and reduces the radiation dose to the thyroid (Gelfand, 1993). Any of the thyroid blocking agents may be used, beginning 1 to 2 days before injection of radioiodinated agents and continued for 5 days afterward (Kazerooni et al, 1990; Munkner, 1985). Each agent provides the patient with about 300 mg of iodine (see Table 45–3 for dosages) (Horne et al, 1991; Paltiel et al, 1994).

BACKGROUND

^{131}I norcholesterol (NP-52, then NP-59), a cholesterol analogue, has been used for adrenal cortical imaging since 1970 (Bierwaltes et al, 1971; Counsell et al, 1970; Lieberman et al, 1971).

Approximately 10 years after NP-59 was developed, Wieland and colleagues (1979) first described MIBG for adrenal medullary imaging. MIBG was further refined over the next several years (Wieland et al, 1980a, 1980b, 1981). ^{131}I MIBG is concentrated in the adrenal medulla as early as 2 hours and continuing for as long as 8 days after injection (Wieland et al, 1980a). Approximately 95% of the total is excreted by the kidneys within 24 hours. This background activity interferes with adrenal visualization (Sarkar et al, 1975). Thus, the best images of the adrenal gland are seen at 3 days after injection because there is better target-to-background ratio (Wieland, 1980a). MIBG and OctreoScan can be used to identify adrenal and extra-adrenal tumors, which are discussed subsequently under Neuroendocrine Imaging.

Adrenal Cortical Imaging

INDICATIONS

Adrenal cortical imaging with NP-59, a cholesterol analogue, has been used for the scintigraphic identification of adrenal cortical adenomas, primary aldosterone adenomas, adrenal tumors, or CT "incidentalomas," to find the etiology of Cushing's syndrome and hyperandrogenism, to identify residual adrenal cortical tissue postoperatively, and to identify bilateral adrenal micronodular or macronodular hyperplasia (Ikeda et al, 1989; Kazerooni et al, 1990). NP-59 is used at few institutions because it is investigational and better laboratory and anatomical imaging modalities have replaced it. It is available only from a noncommercial source (Nuclear Pharmacy, Division of Nuclear Medicine, Department of Medicine, University of Michigan Medical Center, Ann Arbor, MI).

^{75}Se is used for adrenal cortical imaging in Europe but is not used in the United States because of the high radiation exposure to the patient.

PATIENT PREPARATION

NP-59 is a radioiodine-labeled agent, so precautions must be taken to prevent thyroid uptake. (See Patient Preparation under Adrenal Gland Imaging.) Glucocorticoids may interfere with the adrenal uptake of NP-59. Dexamethasone suppression, 1 mg by mouth four times per day, needs to be started 7 days before the intravenous administration of NP-59 and continued for 5 days afterwards to rule out autonomous adrenal adenomas (primary aldosteronism or testosterone producing tumors) (Kazerooni et al, 1990). Laxatives are given to reduce bowel activity, which could hide an abnormal site of activity in the abdomen. Adverse reactions to NP-59 occur in less than 1% of cases, and none have been life threatening (Kazerooni et al, 1990).

TECHNIQUE

To image the adrenal cortex, 1 mCi of ^{131}I-labeled NP-59 is given intravenously and images are obtained 3 to 5 days later (Gross et al, 1988, Kazerooni et al, 1990). In the case of hyperaldosteronism, imaging is performed no later than 5 days after injection because the adenoma may "escape" suppression and give indeterminant results (Kazerooni et al, 1990). Posterior and lateral abdomen images are obtained; markers on the skin surfaces are used as landmarks (Gross et al, 1988).

NORMAL IMAGES

The normal percent uptake can be measured as 0.16% (0.07 to 0.26%) (Freitas et al, 1977). After NP-59 administration, activity is normally seen in the bowel, bladder, liver, gallbladder, and adrenal glands. The adrenal glands are not visualized if dexamethasone is given for suppression. The right adrenal gland is higher than the left in 90% of cases and is round or has a truncated appearance. The left adrenal gland is typically oval with the vertical diameter being greater than the horizontal diameter (Thrall et al, 1978).

DIFFERENTIAL DIAGNOSIS

Euadrenal tumors may cause the adrenal gland to have a distorted appearance, with increased, decreased, or equal activity when the right and left glands are compared (Kazerooni et al, 1990). Increased activity occurs with adrenal cortical or primary aldosterone adenomas (Kazerooni et al, 1990). Glucocorticoid-producing adenomas result in contralateral nonvisualization due to suppression of the normal adrenal cortical tissue (Fig. 45–15), (Thrall et al, 1978). Cushing's syndrome (adrenal cortical hyperplasia) usually appears as bilateral and symmetrical adrenal visualization with laboratory evidence of glucocorticoid excess (Kazerooni et al, 1990; Thrall et al, 1978). Failure of suppression with high-dose dexamethasone indicates that there is an autonomous lesion. Unilateral uptake, bilateral uptake, or bilateral nonvisualization may occur in hyperandrogenism. Residual adrenal cortical tissue post operatively shows activity when present (Kazerooni, 1990). Carcinomas show bilateral nonvisualization because they are nonfunctional when there is adrenal glucocorticoid excess (Thrall et al, 1978). Aldosteronomas are seen as early unilateral visualization on the side of the lesion with nonvisualization of the contralateral gland (Thrall et al, 1978). Micronodular and macronodular hyperplasia cause bilateral adrenal gland visualization prior to the fifth day after injection (Thrall et al, 1978). Further imaging with ^{67}Ga can be used to help to identify metastatic adrenal cortical carcinoma.

Pediatric patients rarely have adrenal disorders, so experience is limited. Congenital virilizing hyperplasia, which is seen with bilateral symmetrical adrenal visualization after suppression, is the most common adrenocortical abnormality. Adrenal calcification secondary to infarction can produce nonfunctioning tissue in the region of the calcification (Thrall et al, 1978).

Percent uptake measurements are done in-

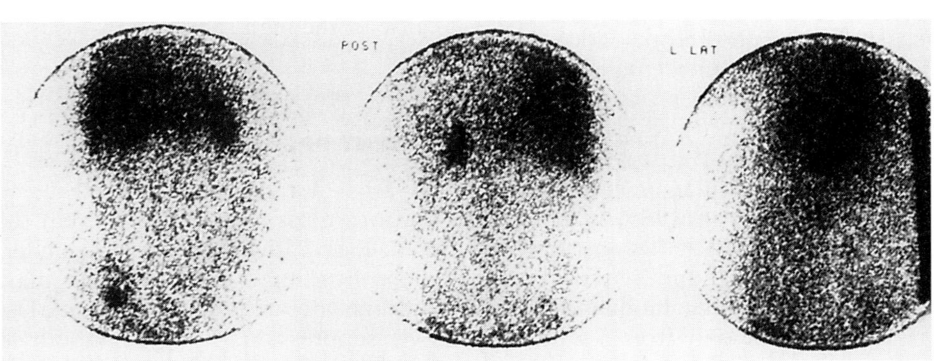

Figure 45–15 Left adrenal adenoma suppressing the right adrenal gland.

frequently, and less than 0.5% uptake per gland is seen in Cushing's disease (Moses et al, 1974).

The adrenal uptake is increased by an elevated adrenocorticotropic hormone (ACTH) level and suppressed by elevated serum cholesterol, exogenous glucocorticoids, and spironolactone. Bilateral increased uptake is caused by pituitary hyperfunctioning or ectopic etiology.

ACCURACY

There is no significant difference between CT and NP-59 scintigraphy in the identification of adrenal cortical adenomas. Sensitivity for CT is 88%; sensitivity for NP-59 is 100%. Specificity of CT is 83% and of NP-59 is 50%. Accuracy of both CT and NP-59 is 82% (Ikeda et al, 1989). However, CT is far better than NP-59 in detecting adrenal hyperplasia. Sensitivity is 80% to 83% versus 50% to 56%, respectively; specificity is 88% versus 100%, respectively; accuracy is 82% versus 82%, respectively (Gleason et al, 1993; Ikeda et al, 1989). NP-59 is 100% sensitive in the diagnosis of Cushing's syndrome, 73% sensitive in primary aldosteronism, and 73% sensitive in the differential diagnosis of euadrenal incidentalomas (Kazerooni et al, 1988).

Adrenal Medullary Imaging

INDICATIONS

MIBG imaging has long been established in localizing sympathetic nervous system tissue and tumors. It is most commonly used to locate pheochromocytomas. Pheochromocytomas occur predominantly in adults but occasionally occur in teen-agers. Approximately 10% of pheochromocytomas are bilateral, 10% are extra-adrenal, and 10% are malignant. The incidence of malignancy in extra-adrenal tumors is higher than 10%. The problems with using MIBG to search for pheochromocytomas include expense, lack of experience by clinicians in performing and interpreting the study, and limited availability of MIBG because its use was only recently approved by the Food and Drug Administration (FDA).

Another agent recently approved by the FDA (June 1994) for imaging neuroendocrine tumors is ^{111}In octreotide (OctreoScan). Octreotide is a long-acting analogue of somatostatin. OctreoScan is discussed in the subsequent section entitled Neuroendocrine Imaging.

PATIENT PREPARATION

Because MIBG is a radioiodine-based agent, the same thyroid-blocking precautions must be taken as with the radioiodine used for adrenal cortical imaging (see Patient Preparation under Adrenal Gland Imaging). MIBG uptake is suppressed by numerous prescription and over-the-counter medications (Khafagi et al, 1989). The imaging physician must be aware of all medications that the patient is taking to ensure a valid study. Elevated plasma and urinary catecholamine levels obtained before imaging may help distinguish adrenal medullary hyperplasia from pheochromocytoma (Valk et al, 1981).

TECHNIQUE

^{131}I MIBG

A total of 500 μCi/1.73 m^2 body surface area (BSA) or about 7 μCi/kg of ^{131}I MIBG is given by slow intravenous injection, and images are obtained at 48 and 72 hours (Englaro et al, 1992; Gelfand, 1993; Paltiel et al, 1994). SPECT imaging cannot be used with ^{131}I MIBG imaging because too few counts are obtained (Paltiel et al, 1994). Images of the anterior head and neck and the anterior and posterior thorax, abdomen, and pelvis are obtained.

^{123}I MIBG

A total of 70 μCi/kg of ^{123}I MIBG is given by slow intravenous injection and images are obtained at 24 and 48 hours, if necessary (Englaro et al, 1992; Paltiel et al, 1994). SPECT can be used with ^{123}I MIBG imaging in the localization of neuroendocrine tumors (Paltiel et al, 1994). Images of the anterior head and neck, thorax, abdomen, and pelvis, with and without skin markers for landmarks, are obtained.

NORMAL IMAGES

^{131}I MIBG

In adults, activity is normally seen with ^{131}I MIBG in the salivary glands, heart, lower lung fields, liver, bladder, and, less often, colon (Fig. 45–16). There is faint or no activity seen in the normal adrenal glands (17% at 48 hours) (Fig. 45–17) (Munkner, 1985). Failure to see activity in the salivary glands indicates suppression, usually by a medication that the patient is taking, which invalidates the study. Inadequate suppression of the thyroid gland results in thyroid visualization. Normally, there are no intense foci of extra-adrenal activity. Heart intensity is much higher in patients without pheochromocytoma than with pheochromocytoma (Nakajo et al, 1983).

The normal pediatric distribution of uptake differs somewhat from the normal adult distribution (Nakajo et al, 1983). In pediatric patients, the salivary glands, liver, spleen, and urinary bladder are usually visualized, and visualization of the neck muscles has been reported. The heart and lower lung fields are seen 50% of the time. The adrenal glands are seen in 2% of cases at 24 hours and in 16% of cases at 48 hours. Approximately 20% of adrenal glands that are not seen at 24 hours are seen at 48 hours. The thyroid is visualized only 7% to 8% of the time with adequate iodine blockade. Occasionally, the colon and kidneys are visualized.

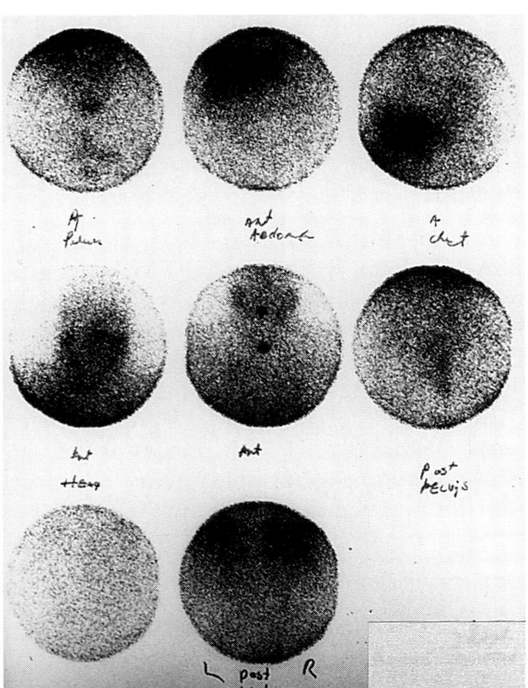

Figure 45–16 Normal ^{131}I MIBG adrenal imaging without adrenal visualization.

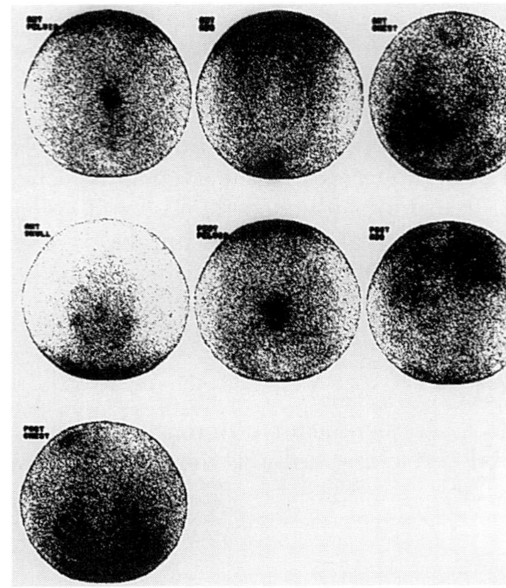

Figure 45–17 Normal ^{131}I MIBG adrenal imaging with adrenal visualization.

^{123}I MIBG

In the pediatric population, as in adults, ^{123}I MIBG activity is normally seen in the salivary glands, liver, and urinary bladder 100% of the time. In children, such activity is seen in the gastrointestinal tract and the heart more than 90% of the time, in the lungs 75% of the time, and in the normal adrenal medulla 49% of the time (Gelfand, 1993). However, activity in the neck (trapezius) muscles is seen only in the pediatric age group 26% of the time. The adequately blocked thyroid gland is seen 17% of the time (Paltiel et al, 1994). The spleen is not visualized (Gelfand, 1993). The left adrenal gland is seen more often than the right when both are present (Paltiel et al,

1994). In patients with normal adrenal glands, 35% are seen at 48 hours and not at 24 hours, and 12% of those seen at 24 hours are better visualized at 48 hours. Less than 5% are seen at 24 hours and not at 48 hours (Paltiel et al, 1994).

DIFFERENTIAL DIAGNOSIS

^{131}I MIBG

Pheochromocytomas as small as 1 cm^3 can be identified with ^{131}I MIBG. They are usually unilateral and focal, and the tumor gives the adrenal glands a rounded configuration (Fig. 45–18) (Thrall et al, 1978). Pheochromocytomas are multifocal 10% of the time and malignant 17% of the time. Necrotic pheochromocytomas also show increased activity. Both primary and metastatic tumors can be identified (Fig. 45–19). Adrenal medullary hyperplasia is the other main consideration in the differential diagnosis. It can be differentiated from pheochromocytoma in that it is usually bilateral and the adrenal glands are triangular (Valk et al, 1981). Both adrenal hyperplasia and pheochromocytoma usually present with elevated plasma and urinary catecholamine levels (Valk et al, 1981). Normal adrenal medullary tissue may progress from microndular to diffuse macronodular adrenal medullary hyperplasia to pheochromocytoma.

Infrequently, focal ^{131}I MIBG activity is seen in patients with hepatic cavernous hemangiomas, adrenal cortical nodules, ischemic kidneys with renal artery stenosis, and adrenocortical carcinomas (Horne et al, 1991; Houghton et al, 1990).

In patients taking many prescribed and over-the-counter medications, pheochromocytomas may not be identified because MIBG uptake is suppressed by the medications (Fig. 45–20). Small pheochromocytomas may also be obscured by overlying organs, such as the liver, that normally show activity.

Extra-adrenal activity is seen in paragangliomas, carcinoids, medullary thyroid carcinoma, neuroblastomas, and metastases from pheochromocytomas.

^{123}I MIBG

The findings on ^{123}I MIBG imaging are similar to those for ^{131}I MIBG imaging. However, the adrenal glands are almost always visualized with ^{123}I, so normal adrenal activity cannot be differentiated from very small intra-adrenal tumors or adrenal hyperplasia (Paltiel et al, 1994).

SENSITIVITY

CT and magnetic resonance imaging (MRI) are more accurate than both ^{123}I MIBG and ^{131}I MIBG imaging in the detection of pheochromocytomas but are inferior to MIBG in the detection of extra-adrenal tumors and metastases. MIBG can also be used to identify skeletal metastases. However, bone scans are more sensitive (Gelfand, 1993) in some studies, and MIBG is more sensitive in others (Hadj-Djilani et al, 1994).

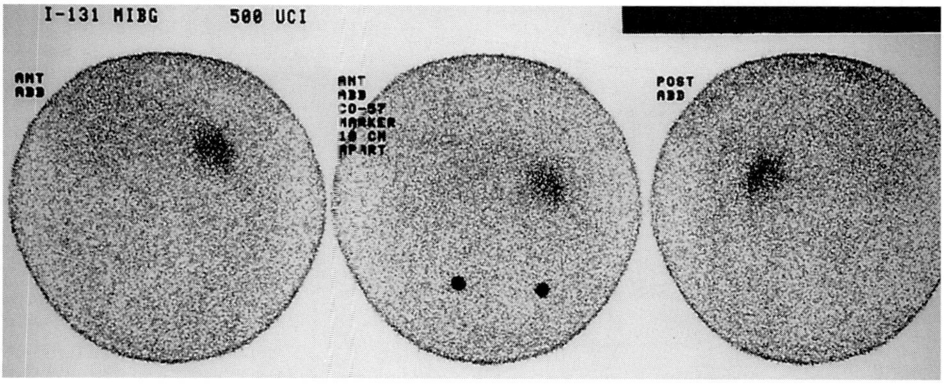

Figure 45–18 Surgically proven left pheochromocytoma.

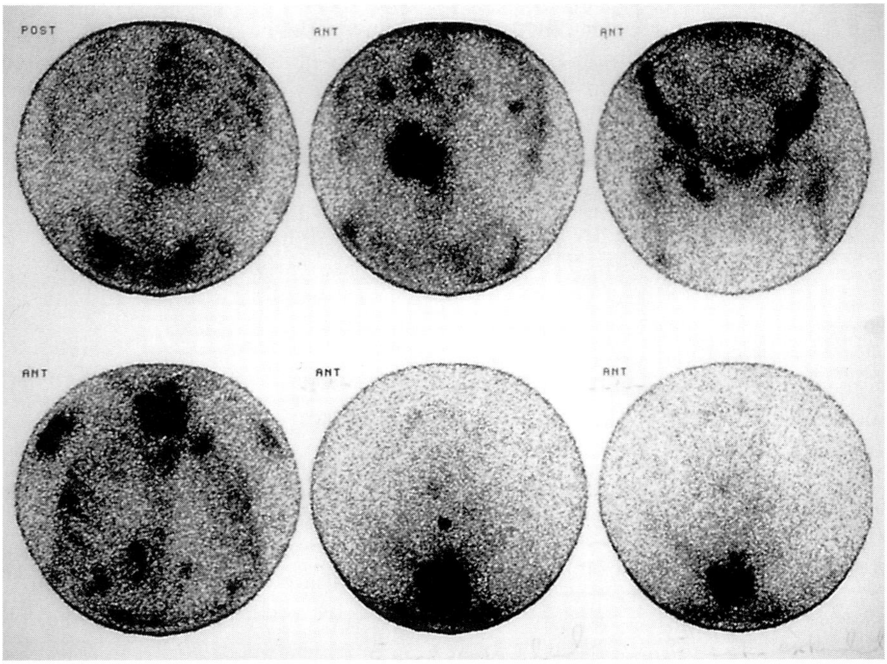

Figure 45–19 Metastatic pheochromocytoma visualized using ^{131}I MIBG .

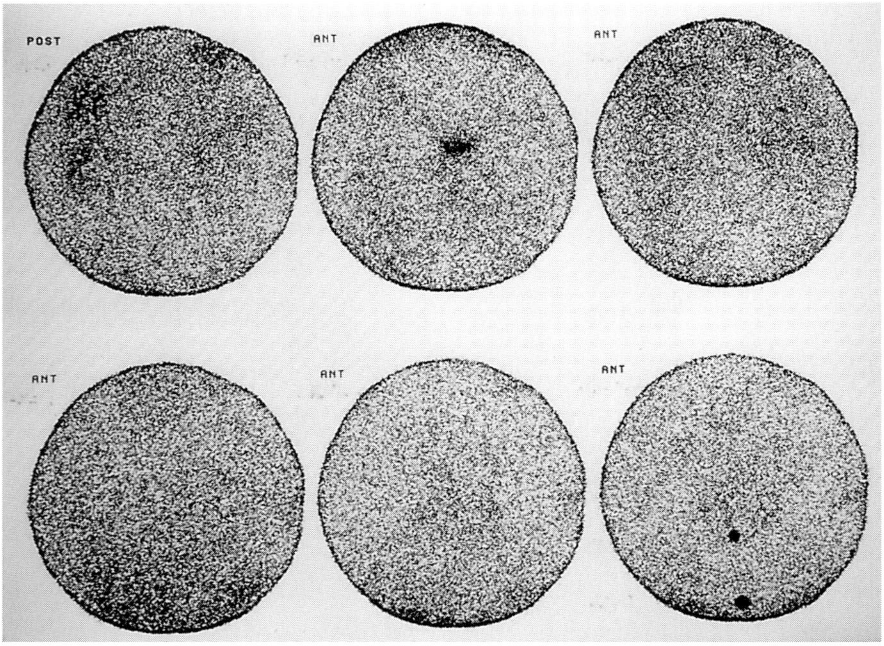

Figure 45–20 ^{131}I MIBG with over-the-counter medication suppression in a large, surgically proven pheochromocytoma.

Neuroendocrine Imaging

MIBG is used for imaging neuroendocrine tumors including neuroblastomas. Recently, indium ^{111}In pentetreotide (OctreoScan) was released for use in the United States. It has similar but broader indications than MIBG, including nonneuroendocrine tumors and benign disease imaging.

^{123}I/^{131}I MIBG

Indications

MIBG imaging has long been established for localizing sympathetic nervous system tissue and tumors, including pheochromocytomas, chemodectomas, functional paragangliomas, carcinoid tumors, medullary carcinoma of the thyroid, and Merkel's cell cancer of the skin (Campeau and Graves, 1991; McEwan et al, 1985). It has also been used to screen patients in families with multiple endocrine neoplasia (MEN) II (4% of metabolically unscreened patients) and von Hippel-Lindau disease (19%) (Neumann et al, 1993). The problems with MIBG include expense, lack of expertise by the clinician in performing and interpreting the examinations, and limited availability because its use was only recently approved by the FDA.

Patient Preparation

Thyroid-blocking agents must be administered before radioiodinated MIBG administration, just as with adrenal medullary imaging.

Technique

^{131}I MIBG

The imaging technique for identifying neuroendocrine tumors with ^{131}I MIBG is the same as that used for adrenal medullary imaging.

^{123}I MIBG

Except for the imaging of advanced neuroblastoma, ^{123}I MIBG, 70 μCi/kg, is given intravenously and images are obtained at 24 and 48 hours. For the imaging of advanced neuroblastoma, 140 μCi/kg is required (Englaro et al, 1992; Gelfand, 1993; Paltiel et al, 1994). SPECT is often useful to better localize the pathological condition (Paltiel et al, 1994). Planar images are obtained of the anterior head and neck, thorax, abdomen, and pelvis, with and without ^{123}I skin markers on the sternum and pelvis for anatomical localization.

Normal Images

The normal distribution of MIBG is described under Adrenal Medullary Imaging.

Differential Diagnosis

MIBG can be used to image pheochromocytomas, chemodectomas in the carotid body, adrenal rests or paragangliomas from the pelvis to base of skull, medullary thyroid carcinoma, neuroblastomas, and carcinoids (in the appendix, small intestine [66%], stomach, rectum, and, infrequently, biliary tree, pancreas, and bronchi) (McEwan et al, 1985; Toney et al, 1992). Small-cell lung carcinoma has similar amine precursor uptake and decarboxylation properties but does not take up MIBG (see Fig. 45–20) (Vincent et al, 1987).

Sensitivity

^{123}I MIBG provides superior images to those provided by ^{131}I MIBG (Edeling et al, 1987). ^{131}I MIBG imaging has a sensitivity of 90% to 100% in neuroblastoma. Lesions smaller than 3 cm in diameter may be missed. Liver metastases are difficult to detect due to normal background activity within the liver. There have been several reports of missed bone lesions that were detected by bone scan. Imaging with ^{131}I MIBG after therapy detects more metastatic foci than pretherapy diagnostic scans do.

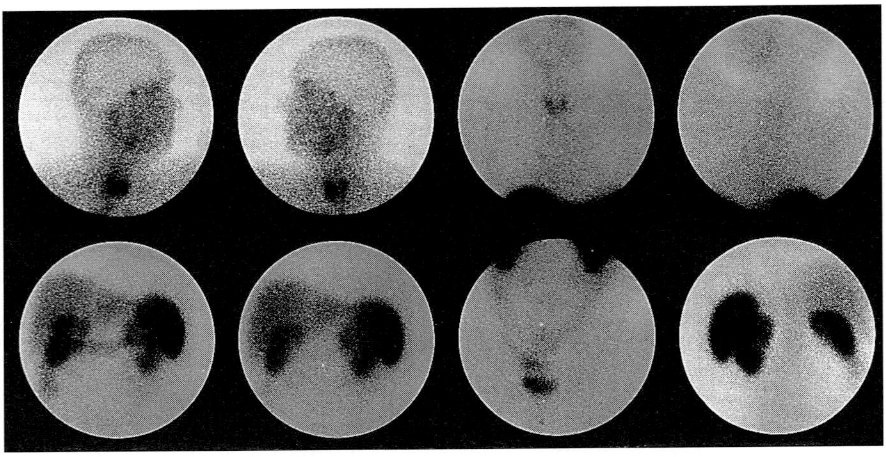

Figure 45–21 Normal OctreoScan distribution at 24 hours.

OCTREOSCAN

Indications

OctreoScan, a somatostatin analogue, has been shown in multiple European studies to be useful in the imaging of pituitary tumors, endocrine pancreatic tumors (gastrinomas, insulinomas, glucagonomas, and undifferentiated tumors), somatostatinomas, paragangliomas, medullary carcinoma of the thyroid, carcinoid, Merkel's cell tumors, and lung neoplasms (small-cell primary and metastases, and adenocarcinoma primary tumor sites). It also shows activity in a number of benign diseases such as granulomatous disease (tuberculosis, Wegener's granulomatosis, sarcoidosis) and nonneuroendocrine neoplasms such as those occurring in the breast and lymphoma (Krenning et al, 1989; Krenning et al, 1993a; Lamberts et al, 1990; Weinel et al, 1993).

Patient Preparation

Therapeutic injections of octreotide must be stopped 3 days before imaging with OctreoScan. Otherwise, receptor site blockade may produce a falsely normal examination.

Technique

Planar images are obtained at 4, 24, and, in some cases, 48 hours after the injection of 1 to 6 mCi of OctreoScan. SPECT images are taken at 24 and if necessary 48 hours after injection (Lamberts et al, 1990). A laxative should be given before imaging the abdomen because 2% of the tracer is excreted in the bowel.

Normal Images

With OctreoScan imaging, normal activity is seen in the kidneys, liver, spleen, urinary bladder, pituitary, and colon starting 24 hours after injection (Fig. 45–21).

Differential Diagnosis

Somatostatin receptors occur in neuroendocrine tumors such as pheochromocytomas, carcinoids, chemodectomas, paragangliomas, and neuroblastomas, which can also be imaged with MIBG (Figs. 45–22 and 45–23), as well as in nonneuroendocrine diseases such as granulomatous disease (sarcoidosis, tuberculosis, Wegener's granulomatosis), aspergillosis, Graves' disease, meningiomas, lymphomas, and gastrointestinal endocrine tumors because they also have somatostatin receptors (Krenning et al, 1989; Krenning et al, 1993b).

Acknowledgements

We wish to thank Lawrence B. Givens for his assistance in preparing the photographs, Erik P. Krenning, M.D., for copies of his personal OctreoScan images, Edgar Surprenant, M.D., for his perchlorate washout cases, and Isaac C. Reese, Ph.D., for his computer graphics assistance.

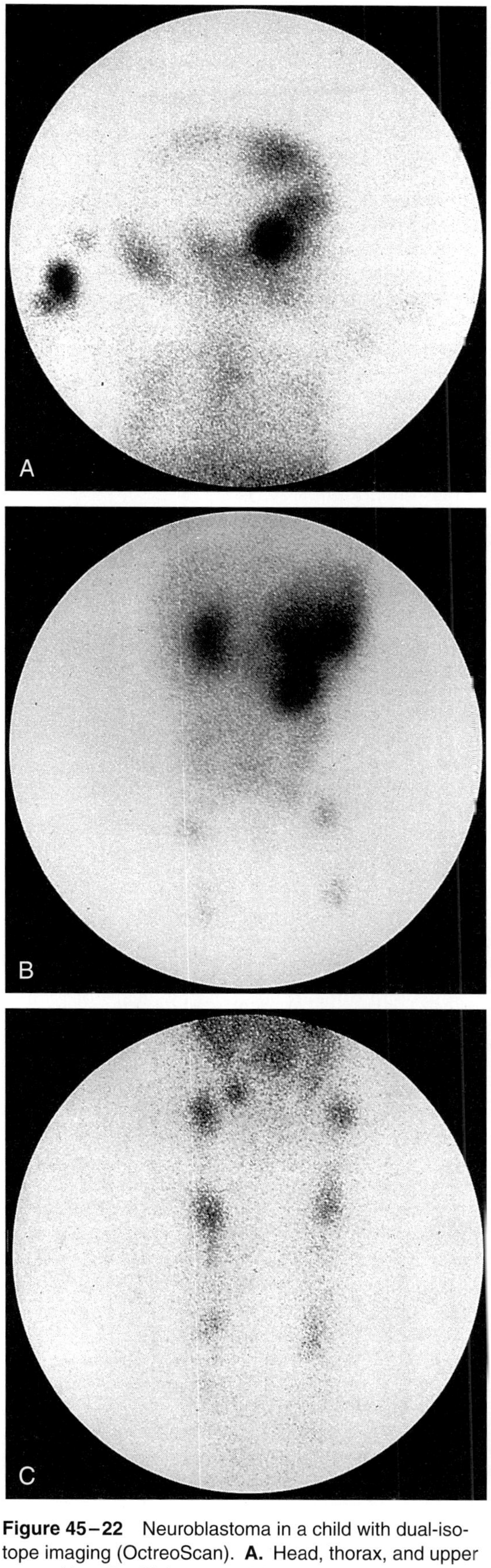

Figure 45–22 Neuroblastoma in a child with dual-isotope imaging (OctreoScan). **A.** Head, thorax, and upper extremities. **B.** Abdomen, pelvis, and proximal lower extremities. **C.** Pelvis and lower extremities.

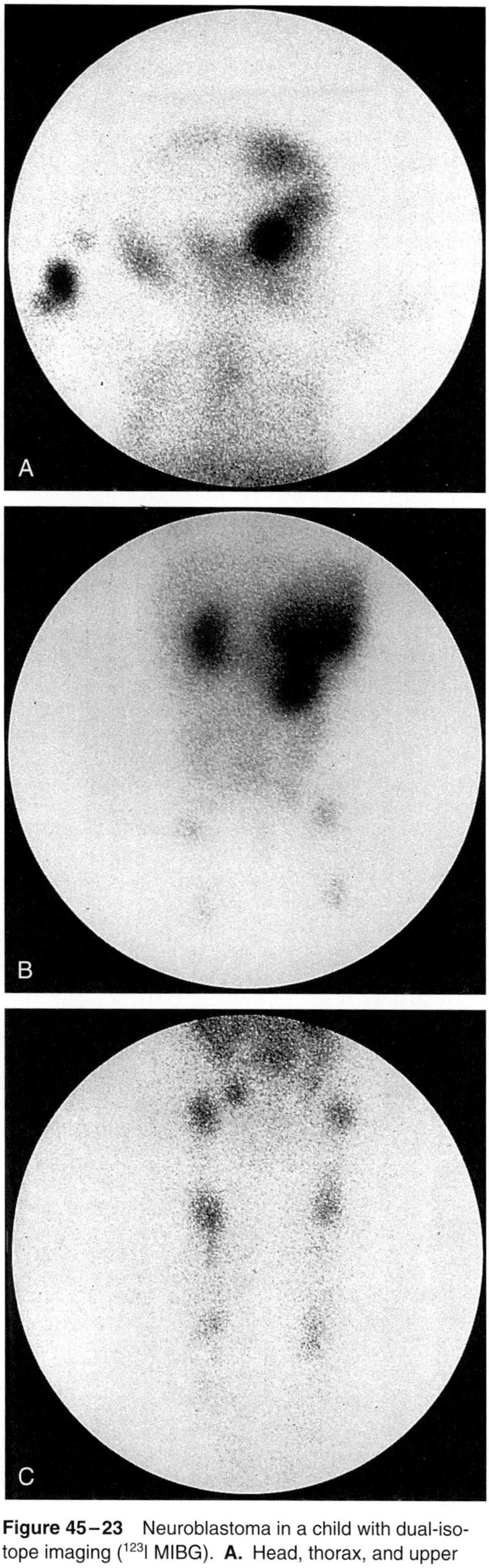

Figure 45–23 Neuroblastoma in a child with dual-isotope imaging (^{123}I MIBG). **A.** Head, thorax, and upper extremities. **B.** Abdomen, pelvis, and proximal lower extremities. **C.** Pelvis and lower extremities.

References

Ashcroft MW, Van Herle AJ: The comparative value of serum thyroglobulin in the follow-up of patients with treated differentiated thyroid cancer. *Am J Med*, 71:806–814, 1981.

Asp A, Hasbargen J, et al: Ectopic thyroid tissue on thallium/technetium parathyroid scan. *Arch Intern Med*, 147:595–596, 1987.

Banerji H, Spencer RP. Thyroidal radioiodine "turnover" in hyperthyroidism. *J Nucl Med*, 15:476, 1974.

Beierwaltes WH: The history of the use of radioactive iodine. *Semin Nucl Med*, 9:151–155, 1979.

Beierwaltes WH, Lieberman LM, et al: Visualization of human adrenal glands in vivo by scintillation scanning. *JAMA* 216:275–277, 1971.

Black EG, Sheppard MC, Hoffenberg R: Serial serum thyroglobulin measurements in the management of differentiated thyroid carcinoma. *Clin Endocrinol*, 27:115–120, 1987.

Bleiweiss IJ, Harpaz N, et al: Functional lipoadenoma of the parathyroid: case report and literature review. *Mt Sinai J Med*, 56:114–117, 1989.

Boyett JD, Mahler DJ, Jansen A: Thyroid uptake of ^{131}I. *J Nucl Med*, 15:213, 1974. Letter.

Burckhardt P, Bischof-Delaloye A, et al. Preoperative localization of hyperfunctioning parathyroid tissue by parathyroid scintigraphy. *Acta Endocrinol*, S1:298–309, 1976.

Burke GJ, Wei JP, Binet EF: Parathyroid scintigraphy with iodine-123 and Tc-99m-sestamibi: imaging findings. *Am J Roentgenol* 161: 1265–1268, 1993.

Campeau RJ, Graves C: Pheochromocytoma associated with prior carotid body tumors (chemodectomas): detection with I-131 MIBG. *Clin Nucl Med,* 16:511–512, 1991.

Castillo LA, Yeh SD, et al: Bone scans in bone metastases from functioning thyroid carcinoma. *Clin Nucl Med*, 5:200–209, 1980.

Charkes ND: Graves' disease with functioning nodules (Marine-Lenhart syndrome). *J Nucl Med*, 13:885–892, 1972.

Chilton HM, Witcofski RL: Radiation dose and risks. In *Nuclear Pharmacy: An Introduction to the Clinical Application of Radiopharmaceuticals*. Philadelphia, Lea & Febiger, 1986, p 47.

Coffey JL, Watson EE, et al: Radiopharmaceutical absorbed dose considerations. In Hladik WB III, Saha GB, Study KT (eds): *Essentials of Nuclear Medicine Science*. Baltimore, Williams & Wilkins, 1987, p 52.

Conway JJ: Considerations for the performance of radionuclide procedures in children. *Semin Nucl Med,* 2:305–315, 1972

Conway JJ, King LR, et al: Detection of vesicoureteral reflux with radionuclide cystography: a comparative study with roentgenographic cystography. *Am J Roentgenol*, 115:720–727, 1972.

Corstens F, Huysmans D, Kloppenborg P: Thyroid scintigraphy with thallium, an alternative for scanning after TSH. *J Nucl Med* 29:860, 1988. Abstract.

Counsell RE, Ranade VV, et al: Tumor localizing agents XI radioiodinated cholesterol. *Steroids*, 16:317–328, 1970.

DeGroot LJ, Kaplan EL, et al: Natural history, treatment and course of papillary thyroid carcinoma. *J Clin Endocrinol Metab*, 71:414–424, 1990.

DeGroot LJ, Reilly M: Use of isotope bone scans and skeletal survey x-rays in follow-up of patients with thyroid carcinoma. *J Endocrinol Invest,* 7:175–179, 1984.

Edeling C-J, Frederiksen PB, et al: Diagnosis and treatment of neuroblastoma using metaiodobenzylguanidine. *Clin Nucl Med*, 12:632–637, 1987.

Englaro EE, Gelfand MJ, et al: I-131 MIBG imaging after bone marrow transplantation for neuroblastoma. *Radiology*, 182:515–520, 1992.

Ferlin G, Borsato N, et al: New perspectives in localizing enlarged parathyroids by technetium-thallium subtraction scan. *J Nucl Med*, 24: 438–441, 1983.

Freitas JE, Thrall JH, et al. Normal adrenal imaging. *J Nucl Med,* 18:599, 1977. Abstract.

Gelfand MJ: Meta-iodobenzylguanidine. *Semin Nucl Med*, 23:231–242, 1993.

Gleason PE, Weinberger MH, et al: Evaluation of diagnostic tests in the differential diagnosis of primary aldosteronism: unilateral adenoma versus bilateral micronodular hyperplasia. *J Urol,* 150:1365–1368, 1993.

Goolden AW: The indications for ablating normal thyroid tissue with I-131 in differentiated thyroid cancer. *Clin Endocrinol,* 23:81–86, 1985.

Gross MD, Shapiro B, et al. Distinguishing benign from malignant euadrenal masses. *Ann Intern Med*, 109:613–618, 1988.

Hadj-Djilani NL, Lebtahi N-E, et al: Diagnosis and follow-up of neuroblastoma by means of iodine-123 metaiodobenzylgnanidine scintigraphy and bone scan, and the influence of histology. *Eur J Nucl Med,* 22:322–329, 1995.

Halpern S, Alazraki N, et al: ^{131}I thyroid uptakes: capsule versus liquid. *J Nucl Med*, 14:507–510, 1973.

Hartshorne MF: Parathyroid scintigraphy. In Eisenberg B (ed): *Imaging of the Thyroid and Parathyroid Glands: A Practical Guide*. New York, Churchill Livingstone, 1991, pp 161–175.

Heidendal GAK, Roos P, et al: Evaluation of cold areas on the thyroid scan with ^{67}Ga-citrate. *J Nucl Med*, 16:793–794, 1975.

Henze E, Roth J, et al: Diagnostic value of early and delayed ^{201}Tl thyroid scintigraphy in the evaluation of cold nodules for malignancy. *Eur J Nucl Med*, 11:413–416, 1986.

Horne T, Glasser B, et al: Unusual causes of I-131 metaiodobenzylguanidine uptake in non-neural crest tissue. *Clin Nucl Med*, 16:239–242, 1991.

Hoschl R, Murray IPC, et al: Radiothallium scintigraphy in solitary nonfunctioning thyroid nodules. *World J Surg*, 8:956–962, 1984.

Houghton A, Clarke S, Jourdan M: False-positive diagnosis of adrenal phaeochromocytoma on metaiodobenzylguanidine (MIBG) scan. *Br J Clin Pract*, 44:411–412, 1990.

Ikeda DM, Francis IR, et al: The detection of adrenal tumors and hyperplasia in patients with primary aldosteronism: comparison of scintigraphy, CT, and MR imaging. *Am J Roentgenol*, 153:301–306, 1989.

Jackson IMD, Cobb WE: Disorder of the thyroid. In Kohler PO, Jordan RM. (eds): *Clinical Endocrinology*, New York, Wiley & Sons, 1986, pp. 73–165.

Kazerooni E, Shapiro B, et al: How accurate and useful is NP-59 scintigraphy in the diagnosis of adrenal diseases? *J Nucl Med*, 29:859, 1988. Abstract.

Kazerooni LA, Sisson JC, et al: Diagnostic accuracy and pitfalls of [iodine-131] 6-beta-iodomethyl-19-norcholesterol (NP-59) imaging. *J Nucl Med*, 31:526–534, 1990.

Khafagi FA, Shapiro B, et al: Labetalol reduces iodine-131 MIBG uptake by pheochromocytoma and normal tissue. *J Nucl Med*, 30:481–489, 1989.

Krenning EP, Bakker WH, et al: Localisation of endocrine-related tumours with radioiodinated analogue of somatostatin. *Lancet*, 1:242–244, 1989.

Krenning EP, Kwekkeboom DJ, et al: Somatostatin receptor scintigraphy with [^{111}In-DTPA-D-Phe^{1}] and [^{123}I-Tyr^{3}]: the Rotterdam experience with more than 1000 patients. *Eur J Nucl Med*, 20: 716–731, 1993a.

Krenning EP, Kwekkeboom DJ, et al: Octreotide agent shows peptide imaging potential. *Diagn Imag*, 15:88–91, 1993b.

Krubsack AJ: Fetal adenoma of the thyroid. A common source for false-positive thallium-201/technetium pertechnetate subtraction parathyroid scintigraphy. *Clin Nucl Med*, 12:539–542, 1987.

Kwekkeboom DJ, Reubi JC, et al: In vivo somatostatin receptor imaging in medullary thyroid carcinoma. *J Clin Endocrinol Metab*, 76:1413-1417, 1993.

Lamberts SWJ, Bakker WH, et al: Somatostatin-receptor imaging in the localization of endocrine tumors. *N Engl J Med*, 323:1246–1249, 1990.

Lieberman LM, Beierwaltes WH, et al: Diagnosis of adrenal disease by visualization of human adrenal glands with ^{131}I-19-iodocholesterol. *N Engl J Med*, 285:1387–1393, 1971.

Linde R, Basso L: Hodgkin's disease with hypercalcemia detected by thallium-201 scintigraphy. *J Nucl Med*, 28:112–115, 1987.

Lisbona R, Lacourciere Y, Rosenthall L: Aspergillomatous abscess of the brain and thyroid. *J Nucl Med*, 14:541–542, 1973.

Lossef SV, Zeissman HA, et al: Multiple hyperfunctioning mediastinal parathyroid glands in a patient with tertiary hyperparathyroidism. *Am J Roentgenol*, 161:285–286, 1993.

Maxon HR III, Enlaro EE, et al: Radioiodine-131 therapy for well differentiated thyroid cancer—A qualitative radiation dosimetric approach: outcome and validation in 85 patients. *J Nucl Med*, 33:1132–1136, 1992.

Maxon HR III, Smith HS: Radioiodine-131 in the diagnosis and treatment of metastatic well differentiated thyroid cancer. *Endocrinol Metab Clin North Am*, 19:685–718, 1990.

Mazzaferri EL: Treating differentiated thyroid carcinomas; where do we draw the line? *Mayo Clin Proc*, 66:105–111, 1991.

McEwan AJ, Shapiro B, et al: Radio-iodobenzylguanidine for the scintigraphic location and therapy of adrenergic tumors. *Semin Nucl Med*, 15: 132–153, 1985.

Miller JM, Hamburger JI: The thyroid scintigram. I. The hot nodule. *Radiology*, 84:66–73, 1965.

Moses DC, Schteingart DE, et al: Efficacy of radiocholesterol imaging of the adrenal glands in Cushing's disease. *Surg Gynecol Obstet*, 139:201–204, 1974.

Moskowitz GW, Attie JN, et al: Parathyroid adenomas: a retrospective analysis of 102 patients studied with technetium–thallium scintigraphy. *J Nucl Med*, 31:935, 1990. Abstract.

Mullan BP, Brown ML: Case 12: mediastinal parathyroid adenoma. In Thrall JH (ed): *Nuclear Radiology (Fourth Series) Test and Syllabus*, Vol 30. Reston, VA: American College of Radiology, 1990, pp 248–261.

Munkner T: I-131-meta-iodobenzylguanidine scintigraphy of neuroblastomas. *Semin Nucl Med*, 15:154–160, 1985.

Nakajo M, Shapiro B, et al: Inverse relationship between cardiac accumulation of meta-[^{131}I] iodobenzylguanidine (I-131 MIBG) and circulating catecholamines in suspected pheochromocytoma. *J Nucl Med*, 24:1127–1134, 1983.

Neumann DR: Simultaneous dual-isotope SPECT imaging for the detection and characterization of parathyroid pathology. *J Nucl Med*, 33: 131–134, 1992.

Neumann HPH, Berger DP, et al: Pheochromocytomas, multiple endocrine neoplasia type 2, and von Hippel-Lindau disease. *N Engl J Med*, 329: 1531–1538, 1993.

Pacini F, Lippi F, et al: Therapeutic dose of iodine-131 reveals undiagnosed metastases in thyroid cancer patients with detectable serum thyroglobulin levels. *J Nucl Med*, 28:1888–1891, 1987.

Paltiel HJ, Gelfand MJ, et al: Neural crest tumors: I-123 MIBG imaging in children. *Radiology*, 190:117–121, 1994.

Paull BR, Alderson PO, et al: Thyroid scan in lymphocytic thyroiditis. *J Nucl Med*, 15:522, 1974. Abstract.

Petti GH Jr: Hyperparathyroidism. *Otolaryngol Clin North Am*, 23:339–355, 1990.

Preston DF, Winternitz WW, Kopp J: Detection of hyperthyroidism by neck uptake of pertechnetate. *J Nucl Med*, 15:525, 1974. Abstract.

Sandrock D, Merino MJ, et al: Parathyroid imaging by Tc/Tl scintigraphy. *Eur J Nucl Med*, 16:607–613, 1990.

Sarkar SD, Beierwaltes WH, et al: A new and superior adrenal scanning agent. *J Nucl Med*, 16: 1038–1042, 1975.

Schlumberger M, Tubiana M, et al: Long term results of treatment of 283 patients with lung and bone metastases from differentiated thyroid carcinoma. *J Clin Endocrinol Metab*, 63:960–967, 1986.

Senga O, Miyakawa M, et al: Comparison of Tl-201 chloride and Ga-67 citrate scintigraphy in the diagnosis of thyroid tumor: concise communication. *J Nucl Med*, 23:225–228, 1982.

Shafer RB, Nuttall FQ, et al: Thyroid function following radiation and surgery in patients with head and neck cancer. *J Nucl Med*, 15:531, 1974. Abstract.

Shimshak RR, Schoenrock GJ, et al: Case report: preoperative localization of a parathyroid adenoma using computed tomography and thyroid scanning. *J Comput Assist Tomogr*, 3:117–119, 1979.

Shore RM, Hendee WR: Radiopharmaceutical dosage selection for pediatric nuclear medicine. *J Nucl Med*, 27:287–298, 1986.

Sisson JC: Applying the radioactive eraser: I-131 to ablate normal thyroid tissue in patients from whom thyroid cancer has been resected. *J Nucl Med*, 24:743–745, 1983. Teaching Editorial.

Society of Nuclear Medicine: Radiobiology and radiation protection. In Siegel BA, Kirchner PT (eds): *Nuclear Medicine: Self-Study Program I. Part I Syllabus and Multiple Choice Questions*. New York, Society of Nuclear Medicine, 1988, p 5.

Spector W (ed): *Handbook of Biological Data*. Philadelphia, WB Saunders, 1956, p 162.

Spencer RP, Banever C: Human thyroid growth: a scan study. (preliminary report). *Invest Radiol*, 5:111–116, 1970.

Statz E, Oates E: Scintigraphic demonstration of an ectopic parathyroid adenoma. *Clin Nucl Med*, 13:130, 1988.

Takebayashi S, Matsui K, et al: Hyperplasia of autotransplanted parathyroid in the forearm. *Clin Nucl Med*, 15:354–355, 1990.

Teixeira VL, Romaldini JH, et al: Thyroid function during the spontaneous course of subacute thyroiditis. *J Nucl Med*, 26:457–460, 1985.

Thrall JH, Freitas JE, Beierwaltes WH: Adrenal scintigraphy. *Semin Nucl Med*, 8:23–41, 1978.

Tonami N, Bunko H, et al: Clinical applications of Tl-201 scintigraphy in patients with cold thyroid nodules. *Clin Nucl Med*, 3:217–221, 1978.

Tonami N, Hisada K: Clinical experience of tumor imaging with Tl-201. *Clin Nucl Med*, 2:75–81, 1977.

Toney MO, Brown JW Jr, et al: Correlative imaging in a patient with a necrotic adrenal pheochromocytoma. *Clin Nucl Med*, 17:67–68, 1992.

Valk TW, Frager MS, et al: Spectrum of pheochromocytoma in multiple endocrine neoplasia: a scintigraphic portrayal using ^{131}I-metaiodobenzylguanidine. *Ann Intern Med,* 94:762–767, 1981.

Veluvolu P, Kransow AZ, et al: Abnormal parathyroid can (thallium-technetium mismatch) with benign and malignant thyroid nodules in the same patient. *Clin Nucl Med*, 16:784–785, 1991.

Vincent MD, Babich J, et al: Failure of iodine-131 MIBG imaging in small cell lung carcinoma. *J Nucl Med*, 28:1230, 1987. Letter.

Weinel RJ, Neuhaus C, et al: Preoperative localization of gastrointestinal endocrine tumors using somatostatin-receptor scintigraphy. *Ann Surg,* 218:640–645, 1993.

Werner SC: The 24-hour thyroidal uptake test. *Semin Nucl Med*, 9:156–158, 1979.

Werner SC, Goodwin LD, et al: Some results from the use of radioactive iodine, I^{131}, in the diagnosis and treatment of toxic goiter. *Am J Roentgenol*, 63:889–894, 1950.

Wieland DM, Brown LW, et al: Imaging primate adrenal medulla with [^{123}I] and [^{131}I] metaiodobenzylguanidine: concise communication. *J Nucl Med,* 22:358–364, 1981.

Wieland DM, Brown LE, et al: Structural and mechanistic studies of adrenomedullary radiopharmaceuticals. *J Nucl Med* 21:P13, 1980b. Abstract.

Wieland DM, Swanson DP, et al: Imaging the adrenal medulla with an I-131-labeled antiadrenergic agent. *J Nucl Med*, 20:155–158, 1979.

Wieland DM, Wu J-L, et al: Radiolabeled adrenergic neuron-blocking agents: adrenomedullary imaging with (^{131}I) iodobenzylguanidine. *J Nucl Med*, 21:349–353, 1980a.

Winzelberg GG: Thallium-201/Tc-99m parathyroid subtraction scintigraphy of the neck: single area of increased thallium uptake. *Semin Nucl Med*, 17:273–275, 1987a.

Winzelberg GG: Thallium-201/Tc-99m parathyroid subtraction scintigraphy of the neck: multiple areas of increased thallium uptake. *Semin Nucl Med*, 17:276–277, 1987b.

Winzelberg GG: Thallium-201/Tc-99m parathyroid subtraction scintigraphy of the mediastinum. *Semin Nucl Med*, 17:278–279, 1987c.

Yang CJC, Seabold JE, Gurll NJ: Brown tumor of bone: a potential source of false-positive thallium-201 localization. *J Nucl Med*, 30:1264–1267, 1989.

Section L

Hematological

Chapter 46

Hematological Tests and Procedures

H. William Taeusch

Blood Drawing Techniques

Blood drawing from children and infants is an art. The goal is to obtain the specimen with minimal trauma to the child. Therefore, preparation of the child (and parents), when possible, and pain control are critical. Pain control is achieved by

1. Determination of real need for the test
2. Consideration of whether individual tests could be "batched" in a single blood letting
3. Dermal anesthetic (e.g., EMLA)
4. Judicious selection of the vessel; for example an artery should not be used for obtaining blood for other than blood gas analysis
5. Skill in the person doing the blood drawing
6. Knowledge of the type of anticoagulant and the amount of blood needed
7. Careful handling of the specimen after obtaining it so that repeated blood letting is avoided by "QNS" or "lost" samples
8. Discussion with the child after the procedure for the child to air concerns

SELECTION OF A SITE FOR VENIPUNCTURE

The site for venipuncture should be safe, easily accessible, and of sufficient size to contain a volume of blood adequate for the specimen sought. Veins that are visible or palpable are generally easier and safer venipuncture sites than are veins located solely by anatomical relationships. The following are the more commonly used sites, listed in order of preference:

1. Veins of the forearm and antecubital fossa. The usual sites of choice in children older than 2 or 3 years, these vessels are often of adequate size for a satisfactory venipuncture in smaller infants. They are usually both visible and palpable.

2. Veins on the dorsum of the hand and foot. More easily accessible in children older than 2 years, these veins are usually both visible and palpable.
3. External jugular vein. This vein is used in infants younger than 1 year. It is usually visible, occasionally palpable, and best seen when the patient cries.
4. Scalp veins. The scalp veins can be used for collection of a small aliquot of blood in infants younger than 1 year. They are always visible but rarely palpable. At times, one may palpate these veins as a "negative space."
5. Femoral vein. This vein can be used at any age. However, in children older than 2 or 3 years, smaller and more superficial veins are recommended. It is neither visible nor palpable.
6. Internal jugular vein. This vein is readily accessible in infants and older children but should be used only in infants younger than 1 year. It is neither visible nor palpable.

The following factors may be of aid in locating a specific vein:

- Knowledge of the normal anatomical course of the vein and its relationship to other structures is paramount to a successful venipuncture.
- Visualization of superficial vessels is possible. However, in some instances, a visible vein may be more difficult to puncture than a more deeply situated vessel that can be felt but not seen. Red goggles used by radiologists for fluoroscopic work may be useful in locating veins near the skin surface.
- Distention of the vein aids location by palpation. This may be accomplished in one or more ways:

1. Application of a tourniquet proximal to the selected site
2. By gravity, holding the limb dependent and below the horizontal level of the body
3. Heating the area by application of warm packs
4. Gently rapping or flicking the vein with the hand or fingers
5. Applying a blood pressure cuff as a tourniquet. The cuff should be inflated to just above the systolic pressure and left at this pressure for 30 to 60 seconds, then deflated to just above diastolic pressure; venous distention distal to the cuff is usually marked and prompt.
6. Swabbing the area over the vein with wet alcohol gauze or a cotton sponge, leaving a wet film of alcohol. The resulting transient sheen may make vessels more visible.

Veins of the Forearm and Antecubital Fossa

Veins of the proximal forearm and antecubital fossa are those most frequently used for venipuncture. This area is the site of choice for collection of blood if the vessels are of sufficient size and condition for the procedure.

Anatomy

The anatomical relationship of the veins on the volar aspect of the forearm and antecubital fossa is illustrated in Figure 46–1. The vessels are superficial and may be easily visible and palpable through the skin. An anastomosis at the antecubital fossa with the deep veins of the arm tends to fix the basilic vein in position and prevent movement as the needle enters the vein. Veins in that area include the following:

CEPHALIC VEIN: On the radial side of the limb.

BASILIC VEIN: On the ulnar side of the extremity.

MEDIAN VEIN: In the midportion of the volar aspect of the forearm. It bifurcates into the median basilic and median cephalic veins 1 cm

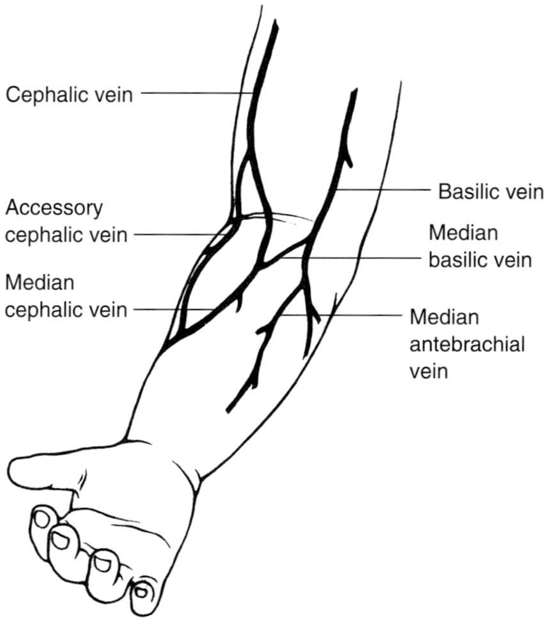

Figure 46–1 Veins of the antecubital fossa. (Redrawn from Hughes WT, Buescher ES: *Pediatric Procedures*. Philadelphia, WB Saunders, 1980.)

distal to the middle of the bend of the elbow. Opposite the same point, but beneath the deep fascia, is the bifurcation of the brachial artery. In some cases, the median vein is not present. In its absence will be found a *median cubital vein* passing from the cephalic to the basilic vein.

MEDIAN BASILIC AND MEDIAN CEPHALIC VEINS: Diverge as they ascend one on each side of the biceps tendon.

Common sources of error

1. Improper position
2. Inadequate restraint
3. Needle with too long a bevel
4. Obstructed needle lumen or loose connection between the needle and syringe
5. Too great an angle between the skin surface and needle
6. Too forceful aspiration, causing vasospasm, collapse of the vessel, or attachment of the vein wall to the needle opening
7. Use of alcohol sponge on the puncture site after the needle is removed. This is painful; a dry sponge is not.
8. Failure to remove the tourniquet before the needle is withdrawn
9. Failure to release suction in the syringe before withdrawing the needle. This negative pressure permits a sudden inflow of air, which may hemolyze red blood cells.

Hazards

INFECTION: Cellulitis and abscess formation may occur at the venipuncture site if an unsterile technique is used. Osteomyelitis rarely occurs.

HEMATOMA: Some degree of hematoma frequently forms. If a large tear in the vessel occurs, extramural bleeding may be excessive. This can be minimized by keeping pressure on the puncture site until bleeding stops.

FAILURE TO REMOVE TOURNIQUET: If the tourniquet is inadvertently left in place for a long time, serious ischemia may develop.

VIRAL HEPATITIS: Contaminated equipment may be responsible for introduction of hepatitis B virus. This infection can be prevented by the use of equipment prepared in one of the following ways:

New, disposable syringes and needles (recommended)

Autoclaving at 121°C (15 pounds pressure) for 15 minutes

Boiling in water for 30 minutes

ARTERIAL TRAUMA: An aberrant artery in the antecubital area, found in 10% of persons, can, because of its proximity, be mistaken for a vein.

Veins on the Dorsum of the Hand and Foot

Veins on the dorsum of the hand or foot are safe and readily accessible vessels for the collection of blood. The technique is similar for venipuncture at either of these sites.

HAND: Tributaries of the cephalic and basilic veins along with the dorsal venous arch are visible or palpable beneath the skin surface (Fig 46–2).

FOOT: The median and lateral marginal veins on the dorsum of the foot are usually identifiable by palpation or visually after a tourniquet has been applied (Fig. 46–3).

Common sources of error

Common sources of error are the same as those described for the forearm and antecubital fossa. On occasion, insertion of the needle into the vein opposite the direction of blood flow, although awkward, yields better

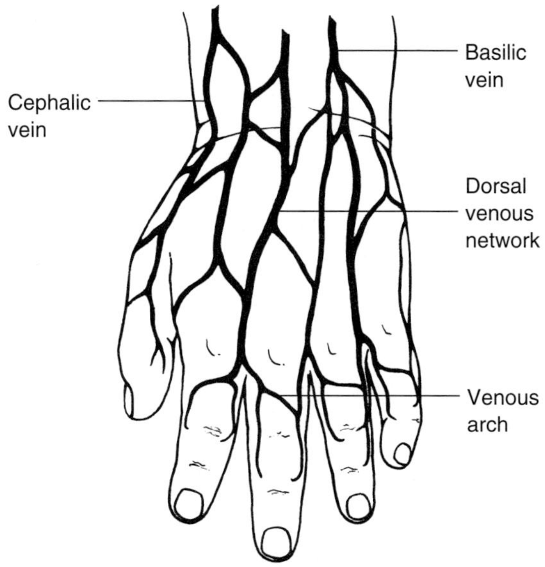

Figure 46–2 Venous anatomy of the dorsum of the hand. (Redrawn from Hughes WT, Buescher ES: *Pediatric Procedures.* Philadelphia, WB Saunders, 1980.)

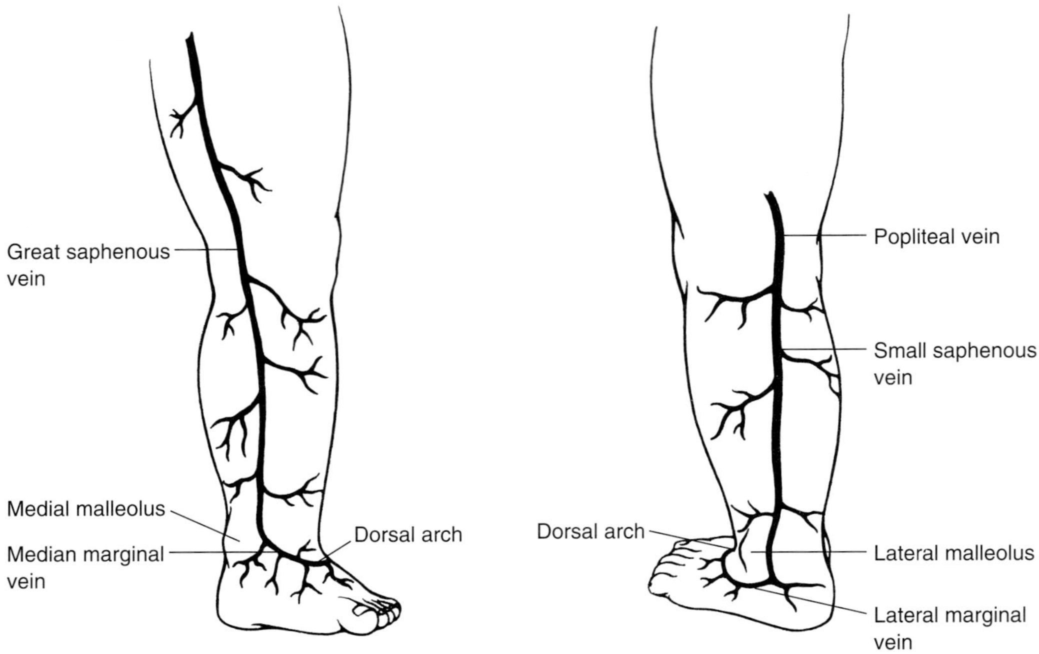

Figure 46–3 Venous anatomy of the leg and foot. (Redrawn from Hughes WT, Buescher ES: *Pediatric Procedures.* Philadelphia, WB Saunders, 1980.)

results. This is because blood is drawn into the syringe, in the same direction as the blood flow in the vein, and the vein will not collapse.

External Jugular Vein

The external jugular vein (Fig. 46–4) is easily accessible in infants and children who are not obese or whose necks are not too short. This vein, usually visible through the skin, courses in a line from the angle of the mandible to the middle of the clavicle. It is formed on the superficial surface of the sternocleidomastoid muscle, immediately below and posterior to the angle of the mandible, by junction of the posterior auricular vein with a branch from the posterior facial vein. The external jugular vein descends in a slightly posterior direction to the anterior part of the subclavian portion of the posterior triangle of the neck, where it pierces the deep fascia and terminates in the subclavian vein.

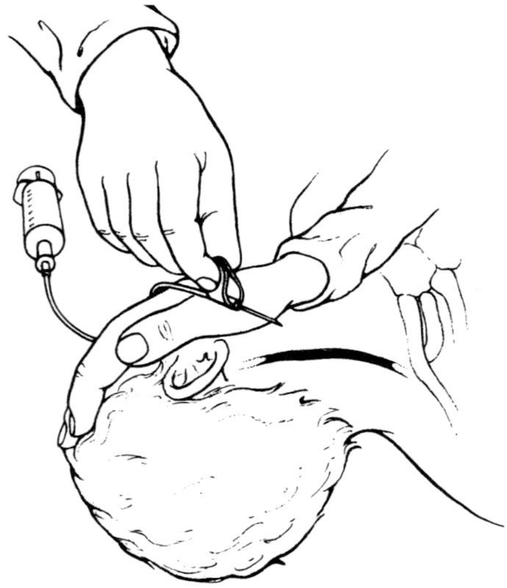

Figure 46–4 The external jugular vein. (Redrawn from Hughes WT, Buescher ES: *Pediatric Procedures.* Philadelphia, WB Saunders, 1980.)

Common sources of error

1. Failure to rotate the infant's head adequately to stretch the vein
2. Movement of the infant's head after the needle has been inserted into the vein
3. Overpenetration of the vessel and hematoma formation
4. Failure to stimulate the infant to cry

Scalp Veins

In infants younger than 1 year, it is often possible to obtain blood specimens from the scalp veins with small-gauge scalp vein needles (Fig. 46–5). Any of the superficial veins of the scalp can be used: the superficial temporal vein, the supraorbital vein, the frontal vein, or the occipital vein. These veins can usually be visualized, but at times, areas of hair overlying the veins must be shaved for them to be seen clearly.

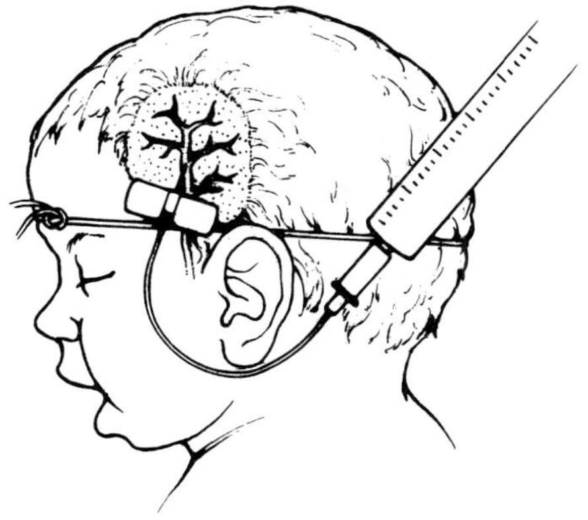

Figure 46–5 Venipuncture of the scalp veins. Site of the superficial temporal vein. (Redrawn from Hughes WT, Buescher ES: *Pediatric Procedures.* Philadelphia, WB Saunders, 1980.)

Common sources of error

1. Failure to place traction on the skin around the vein to partially immobilize it
2. With use of small-gauge needles, advancing the bevel too quickly and not waiting to see the blood appear in the clear plastic tubing attached to the needle
3. Failure to introduce the needle against the flow of blood

Femoral Vein

The femoral vein is an undesirable and less safe site for venipuncture in infants when more superficial veins are accessible. This vein courses through an anatomical triangle in the proximal portion of the thigh (Fig. 46–6). The femoral triangle is bounded by the inguinal ligament, laterally by the sartorius muscle, and medially by the adductor longus muscle. The femoral vein enters the distal part of the triangle posterior to the femoral artery; but in the proximal half of the triangle, it is on the medial side of the artery.

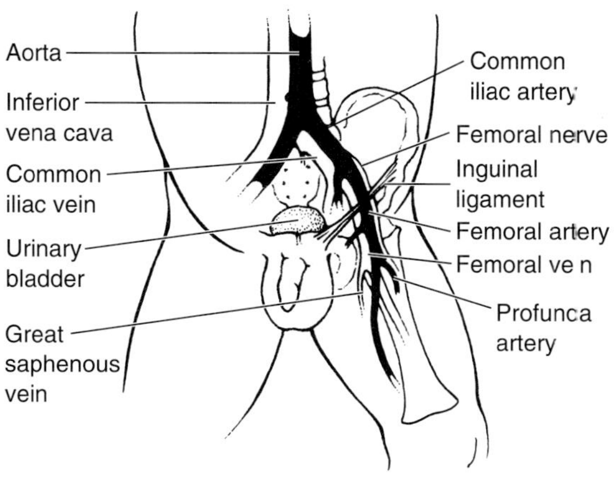

Figure 46–6 Anatomy of the femoral triangle. (Redrawn from Hughes WT, Buescher ES: *Pediatric Procedures.* Philadelphia, WB Saunders, 1980.)

Common sources of error

1. Improper position
2. Movement of the patient during the procedure
3. Making the puncture too far distal to the femoral triangle
4. Failure to maintain location of the femoral artery by digital palpation. This is a landmark for identifying the position of the femoral vein.

Hazards

INFECTION: Infection is relatively uncommon:

1. Subcutaneous cellulitis or abscess
2. Osteomyelitis of the femur
3. Abscess of the hip joint

HEMATOMA: If a tear of the vessel wall occurs at the puncture site, a massive hematoma may develop. Because of the loose tissue planes adjacent to the site, a large quantity of blood can be extravasated before it is easily recognized.

ARTERIAL SPASM: Spasm of the femoral artery may occur from two mechanisms:

1. Reflex arteriospasm from puncture of the vein possibly mediated by sympathetic nerves. The leg becomes pale and pulseless, but this is usually transitory. Prolonged arteriospasm may be relieved by application of heat or infiltration of 2% procaine hydrochloride in the proximity of the vessel. Gangrene of the leg has been reported after femoral puncture.
2. Mechanical trauma to the artery. Inadvertent puncture of the femoral artery usually causes no serious complication. Occasionally, an intramural or extramural hematoma may occlude the lumen, resulting in more serious ischemia of the extremity.

PENETRATION OF THE PERITONEAL CAVITY: A long needle inserted underneath the inguinal ligament can reach the peritoneal cavity.

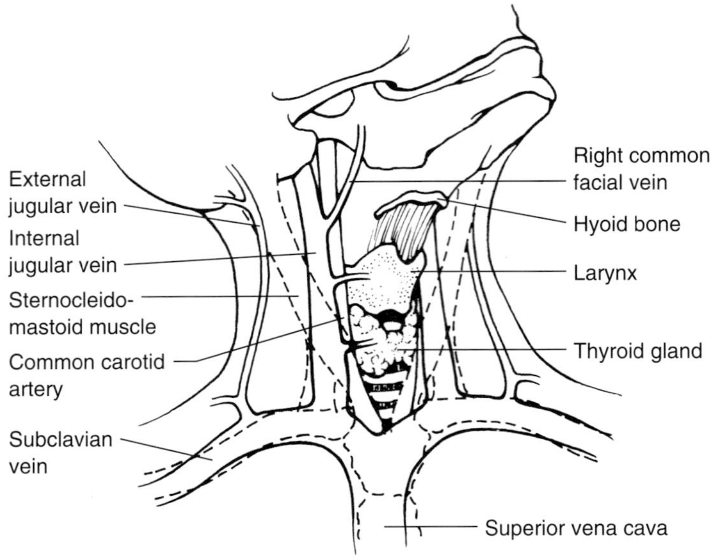

Figure 46–7 Vascular anatomy of the neck. (Redrawn from Hughes WT, Buescher ES: *Pediatric Procedures.* Philadelphia, WB Saunders, 1980.)

Internal Jugular Vein

The internal jugular vein should be reserved for venipuncture in infants in whom more superficial veins, such as those of the antecubital fossa, those on the dorsum of the hand or foot, or the femoral vein, are inaccessible (Fig. 46–7 and 45–8). This vein is formed superiorly at the base of the skull as the continuation of the cerebral sinuses that receive blood from the brain. Inferiorly, the internal jugular vein unites with the subclavian vein to form the innominate vein. The inferior portion courses alongside and superficial to the common carotid arteries. Therefore, it passes on the underside of the inferior two thirds of the sternocleidomastoid muscle.

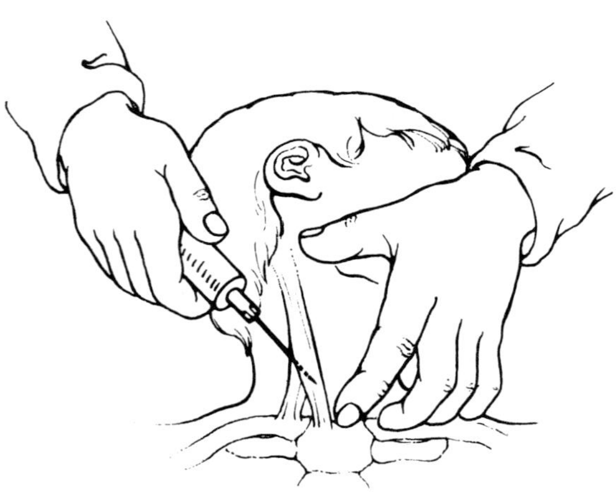

Figure 46–8 Internal jugular venipuncture. (Redrawn from Hughes WT, Buescher ES: *Pediatric Procedures.* Philadelphia, WB Saunders, 1980.)

Hazards

1. The airway and respiration may be impaired by position or restraint.
2. This procedure is contraindicated in infants with respiratory distress and central nervous system hemorrhage.
3. With deep probing, the adjacent arteries, trachea, vagus nerve, or pleura can be injured. Hemorrhage, pneumothorax, and subcutaneous emphysema can occur.
4. Parents witnessing the procedure are always frightened. To avoid emotional reaction, they should not be permitted to observe.

CAPILLARY PUNCTURE

Site

Sites most adaptable to the collection of capillary blood are the heel for infants younger than 2 years; the finger for the infant or older child; and the great toe for the older child, if the heel and finger are inaccessible.

Heel puncture

The heel is the site of choice for infants, especially the premature baby.

Because the course of the plantar arteries and veins is on the medial aspect of the plantar surface of the heel, this is the preferred site for puncture. However, almost any place on the fleshy, uncalloused heel of the infant is suitable for blood collection. The more medial surface of the heel pad should be avoided as a precaution against scar formation that might be a nidus of pain when the infant begins to walk.

The heel is easily restrained with the operator's free hand. No other restraint is usually required. If, in large infants, considerable movement of body and extremities will interfere with the procedure, body restraint can be used.

Procedure

1. If more than a few drops of blood are to be obtained, especially if the patient is a small or premature infant, the entire foot can be wrapped in a warm (not hot) wet towel for 5 to 10 minutes to produce hyperemia.
2. The site is prepared with a warm antiseptic, such as 70% alcohol, and permitted to dry.
3. The heel is encircled with the thumb and index finger, and blood is "milked" centrally by gentle squeezing with the rest of the hand. The heel appears "flushed" when ready for capillary puncture.
4. The lancet or No. 11 Bard-Parker blade is grasped firmly, and the point is forcefully introduced through the skin into the subcutaneous tissue and quickly removed from the incision.
5. The first drop of blood is blotted off with gauze, which may be smeared with sterile petroleum jelly or bacitracin ointment so that the blood beads on the oily skin surface. Extreme haste in beginning collection of the specimen is contraindicated. If free flow of blood does not immediately appear at the incision site, wait a minute or so and then massage the lower portion of the extremity and foot. Brief pauses between squeezing of the site will allow the capillaries to refill. Excessive squeezing of the area should be avoided, because this may dilute the specimen with serum. If an adequate volume of blood is not forthcoming, a deeper incision can be made or a new site selected. Occasionally, an oblique or X-shaped puncture is more effective for collecting large amounts of blood.
6. When an adequate volume of blood appears on the skin surface, the tip of the collecting apparatus (capillary tube or micropipet, for example) is introduced into the blood droplet, permitting it to flow into the container. Care should be taken not to allow large drops of blood to accumulate on the surface; this tends to increase hemolysis. Some pipets may require suction created by attachment of a rubber tube from the opposite end of the pipet to the operator's mouth. Under this circumstance, the free tip of the pipet must remain submerged in the drops of blood while negative pressure is being exerted.
7. If a blood smear is to be made, allow a small bead of blood to appear, then touch the surface of a slide or coverslip to the top of the drop and remove and smear.
8. When collection is completed, a dry, sterile gauze pad is pressed over the incision and held firmly for 2 to 3 minutes or until there is no evidence of bleeding.

ARTERIAL PUNCTURE

Under certain circumstances, it may be necessary to obtain a sample of arterial blood for studies such as oxygen concentration, hemoglobin saturation, blood cultures, and some types of blood chemistries.

Site

The preferred sites for arterial puncture are the radial and brachial arteries in older children. In small infants, the radial, brachial, dorsalis pedis, posterior tibial, or even temporal artery can be used for arterial blood sampling.

The radial artery is the continuation of the brachial artery after it bifurcates below the elbow into the ulnar and radial arteries. It is located on the lateral side of the forearm and wrist, becoming most superficial at the wrist before it enters the hand and unites with the ulnar artery through the palmar arch (Fig. 46–9).

The brachial artery is the continuation of the axillary artery and follows the medial as-

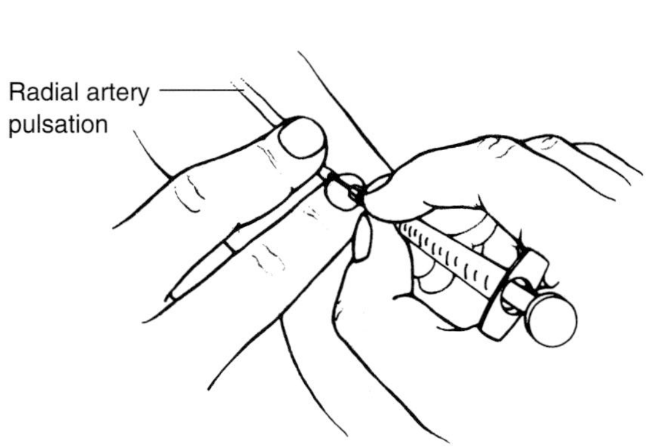

Figure 46–9 Arterial puncture of the radial artery. (Redrawn from Hughes WT, Buescher ES: *Pediatric Procedures.* Philadelphia, WB Saunders, 1980.)

pect of the arm until it divides into the radial and ulnar arteries. It is most superficial at the level of the antecubital fossa, on the medial side. When possible, the radial artery should be used in preference to the brachial artery, because it has an open anastomosis through the palmar arch with the ulnar artery, and puncture-induced arteriospasm of the radial artery does not usually cause ischemia distal to it.

Procedure

1. Clean the site with tincture of iodine, let it dry, then remove it with 70% alcohol.
2. With antiseptic, sterilize the fingertip that palpates the artery. In small infants, only one finger at a time is able to palpate the artery.
3. Check the syringe and needle for proper function.
4. Visualization of the artery is possible during the procedure in small infants by holding the dorsum of the wrist on a fiberoptic transilluminator.
5. The skin should be entered with the needle bevel down at a flat angle (approximately 10 degrees), directly over the artery but approximately 1 cm below the intended needle-artery intersection point.
6. After the needle has entered the skin, negative pressure should be applied with the syringe, and the needle should be advanced toward the palpable arterial pulsation. Arteriopuncture is signaled by the appearance of bright red blood in the needle hub. These arteries are usually easily palpable and occasionally visible. A flat skin entry and approach are necessary for success.

Hazards

A tear or large puncture of the vessel wall may result in a massive hematoma. This can be avoided by using small-gauge needles. Clots or debris inadvertently injected into the artery may produce embolic obstruction to the distal portion of the vessel. Blind probing for an artery can cause damage to surrounding structures (i.e., nerves and veins). Visualization of the radial artery may be aided by holding the wrist over a transilluminator. This reveals the artery as a pulsatile shadow and greatly aids in the arteriopuncture.

ARTERIAL CATHETER PLACEMENT

When frequent arterial blood gas studies or intra-arterial blood pressure monitoring is required for a patient, an indwelling arterial catheter is indicated. Percutaneous placement of peripheral arterial lines using the radial artery is a common pediatric procedure in all ages.

Site

The catheter is placed in the radial artery just proximal to the wrist.

Equipment

Teflon (polytetrafluoroethylene) or Silastic (polymeric silicone, not polypropylene) 20-

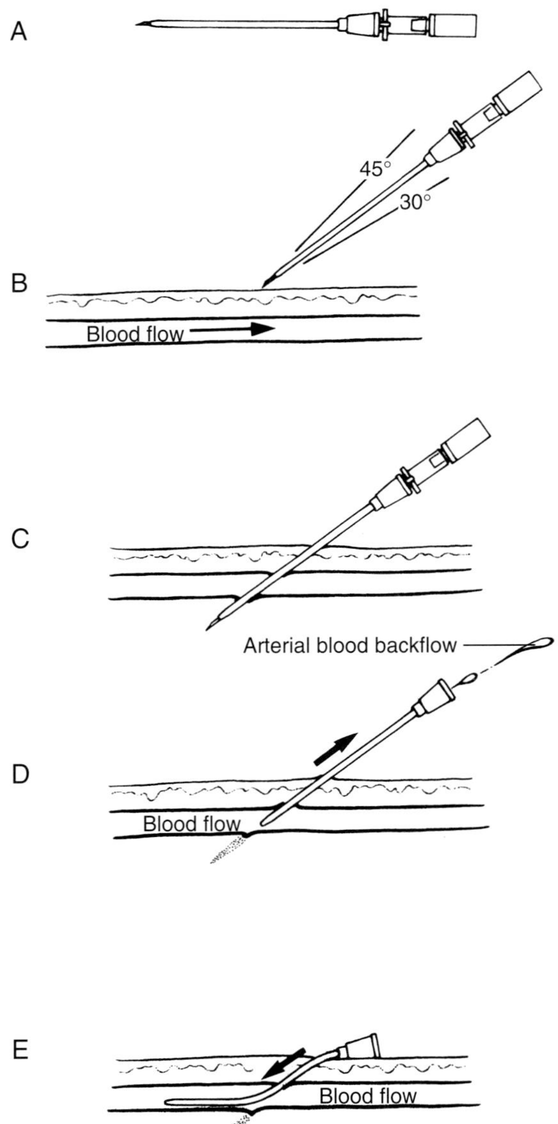

Figure 46–10 Percutaneous insertion of arterial catheter. (Redrawn from Hughes WT, Buescher ES: *Pediatric Procedures.* Philadelphia, WB Saunders, 1980.)

to 22-gauge nontapered, 3- to 4-cm catheter (catheter-over-the-needle type)
70% alcohol and tincture of iodine
Dry, sterile gauze pads
Armboard
Adhesive tape (4-cm wide)

Procedure

1. The ulnar artery is identified and is checked for collateral flow (anastomosis) with the radial artery.
2. The wrist is hyperextended to approximately 45 degrees over a soft gauze pad and fastened securely to an armboard. The hand should be secured in such a way that the thumb and fingertips are exposed to check for skin color.
3. The radial artery is found by palpation over the carpal tunnel, and the overlying skin is sterilized with antiseptic. The index fingertip of the operator's free hand should also be sterilized so that it can be placed within the sterile area.
4. The artery is aggressively punctured, both anterior and posterior walls, at an angle of 30 to 45 degrees, and the stylet is removed. There should be no blood backflow (Fig. 46–10).
5. The catheter is slowly pulled back until pulsatile blood issues from it, signaling entry of the catheter tip into the arterial lumen.
6. The catheter is then advanced up the arterial lumen to its hub.
7. The catheter is sutured to the skin with 4–0 silk suture.
8. A "T-piece" tubing or three-way stopcock is attached to the catheter, and a flush solution of 0.9% sodium chloride with 5 units of heparin per milliliter is run through the catheter at a slow continuous rate.
9. Blood specimens should be obtained through the T-piece or stopcock with a new sterile syringe each time; 2 to 3 ml of blood should be removed first in a separate syringe, the blood specimen taken, then the "wash" 2 to 3 ml returned to the patient through the arterial line. This eliminates intravenous fluid contamination of blood specimens and prevents excessive iatrogenic blood loss.
10. The catheter should be irrigated at least every 3 to 4 hours.
11. The catheter site should be inspected daily for signs of inflammation.
12. When the catheter is discontinued, pressure should be applied to the site for a full 10 minutes.

Hazards and Complications

1. Arterial thrombosis
2. Arterial embolism—proximal or distal
3. Skin ischemia *proximal* to catheter site
4. Arteriospasm with vascular insufficiency
5. Hematoma formation
6. Gangrene of the hand and forearm

Common Laboratory Tests

COMPLETE BLOOD COUNT

Complete blood counts are now nearly always carried out by use of automated impedance as the means of red blood cell, white blood cell, or platelet counting. The principle is illustrated in Figure 46–11.

On occasion, the need may arise for manual blood counts. A solution of 2% acetic acid, to which gentian violet has been added until a pale color is obtained, is used as a diluting solution for anticoagulated blood. A Thoma white cell pipet is used to aspirate blood to the 0.5 mark (Fig. 46–12). The pipet tip is wiped, and the acetic acid diluent is aspirated until fluid volume reaches the 11 mark above the missing bulb. The diluent-blood sample is mixed for 2 minutes. Three drops are then discarded, and the next is used to charge an improved Neubauer counting chamber by taking the pipet tip to the lower edge of the coverslip and allowing the chamber to fill by capillary action. The dilution is 1 volume blood to 20 volumes diluent.

The Neubauer chamber (Fig. 46–13) has a volume depth of 0.1 mm. Each of the nine large

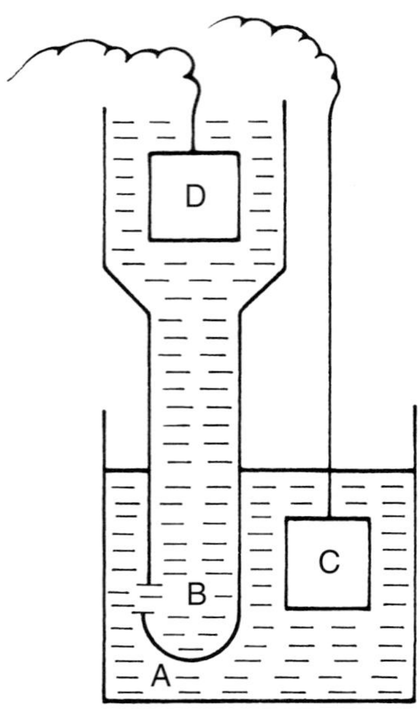

Figure 46–11 Principle of impedance counting. A, electrolyte in counting vial. B, The 100-μ aperture—fluid and cells are drawn through for a preset time. C, External electrode. D, Internal electrode. The electrical resistance between C and D as a cell is drawn through aperture B registers as a voltage pulse on the counter. (Redrawn from Raphael SS: *Lynch's Medical Laboratory Technology*, 4th ed. Philadelphia, WB Saunders, 1983.)

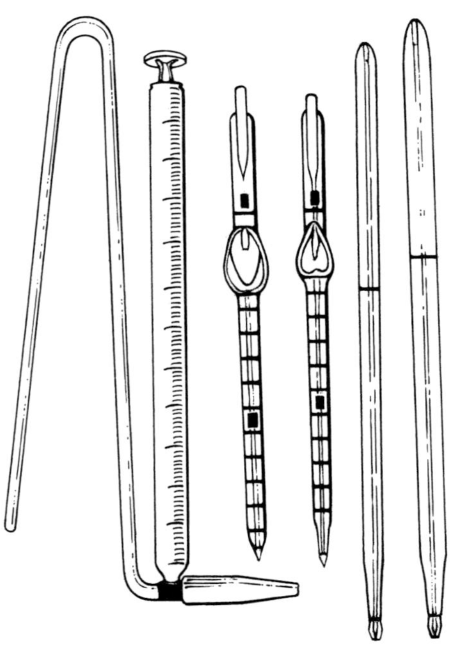

Figure 46–12 *Left to right:* Suction cleaner and Wintrobe hematocrit tube; red cell pipet; white cell pipet; 50-μL pipet; 20-μL pipet. (Redrawn from Raphael SS: *Lynch's Medical Laboratory Technology*, 4th ed. Philadelphia, WB Saunders, 1983.)

squares has sides of 1 mm. Therefore, when the white blood cells in the four corner large squares are counted, they represent the cells in a volume of 0.4 mm^3 that have been diluted 1:20. To correct for both volume and dilution, the white blood cells counted in the four large squares are multiplied by 50 to give the number of white blood cells per mm^3 of blood.

Manual counts of platelets are carried out in a similar manner. The diluent is a fresh aqueous solution of 1% ammonium oxalate. Blood is drawn into the Thoma pipet as described for white blood cell counting. Mixing is for 2 minutes. The Neubauer chamber is filled. The chamber is placed on moist gauze in a covered Petri dish for 20 minutes to allow the platelets to settle. Platelets are counted in the five squares marked R under reduced light. The number of platelets counted in the five R squares (each with a volume of 0.004 mm^3) is multiplied by 1000 to give the number of platelets per mm^3.

MICROHEMATOCRIT

Blood is drawn up in heparinized microhematocrit tubes by capillary action, and one end is sealed. In the good old days, the end of the glass microtube was sealed by melting the tip of the tube in a flame from a Bunsen burner (ask a clinician older than 40 if you do not know what

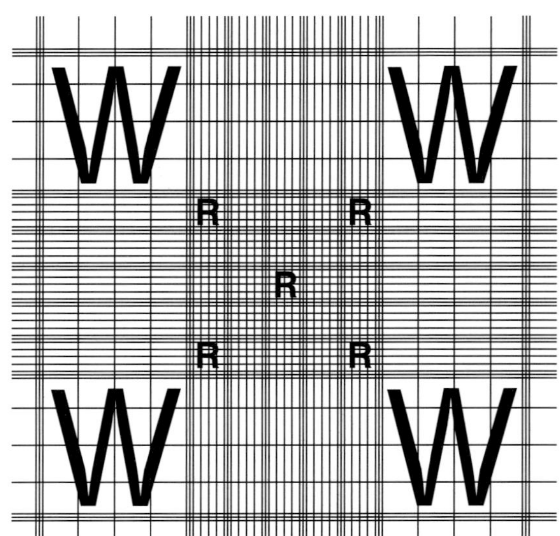

Figure 46–13 Rulings for an improved Neubauer counting chamber. The areas counted for the leukocyte count are marked W. The platelet areas are marked R. (Redrawn from Raphael SS: *Lynch's Medical Laboratory Technology*, 4th ed. Philadelphia, WB Saunders, 1983.)

that is). These days, the end is sealed with clay. The capillary tubes are centrifuged for 5 minutes. The height of the packed red blood cell column divided by the height of the total (red blood cell plus plasma) column multiplied by 100 is the hematocrit in percentage units. The white blood cells usually pack at the top of the red blood cell column in the microhematocrit tube. To create a slide of this white blood cell "buffy coat," a three-sided file can be used to nick the microhematocrit tube just below the buffy coat in the red blood cell column. The tube is snapped at this site, and plasma and white blood cells are prepared as described for the white blood cell differential (see following). The buffy coat smear is evaluated for white blood cell types and detection of bacteria.

DIFFERENTIAL BLOOD COUNTS

Preparation of Blood Films

A blood film or smear can be satisfactorily prepared on either coverslips or glass microscope slides. Whichever method is used, it is important to have meticulously clean, greaseless, and dry equipment.

Coverglass Method

This method produces a better distribution of leukocytes than the slide method does. It is the method of choice for making smears for differential white blood cell counts.

Equipment

Two No. 2 coverglasses, 22-mm^2, for each set of smears

Procedure (Fig. 46–14)

1. One coverglass is picked up in the left hand and held by its edges with the index finger and thumb. Another coverglass is held in the right hand in a similar manner.
2. The bottom of the coverglass in the right hand is touched to a small bead of blood on the skin at the site of capillary puncture. The glass must not touch the skin.
3. The bottom of the coverglass with the drop of blood in the center is placed on the top of the coverglass in the left hand.
4. With the two coverglasses in contact, the drop of blood is allowed to spread toward the edges. Air bubbles must be avoided. The coverglasses should not be pressed together.

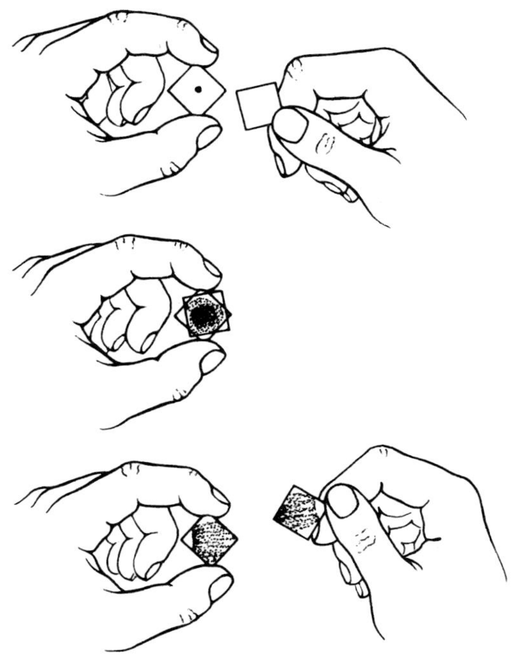

Figure 46–14 Preparation of coverglass smears. (Redrawn from Hughes WT, Buescher ES: *Pediatric Procedures.* Philadelphia, WB Saunders, 1980.)

5. Just before the blood reaches the edges of the coverglasses, they are briskly pulled apart in the absolutely horizontal axis. Any tendency to a vertical pull ruins the preparation, because holes in the smear result.
6. The preparations are allowed to dry in the air. Rapid fanning of the smears immediately after they are pulled apart helps to preserve morphological features of the cells by drying them quickly.

Microscope Slide Method

This method produces a good distribution of erythrocytes. However, large leukocytes may be pushed to the sides, which makes the differential white blood cell count less satisfactory (Fig. 46–15).

Equipment

Clean, dry microscope slides (two for each smear to be made)

Procedure

1. One slide is picked up by the edges between the thumb and index finger.
2. The flat surface of the slide is touched to a bead of blood at the site of capillary punc-

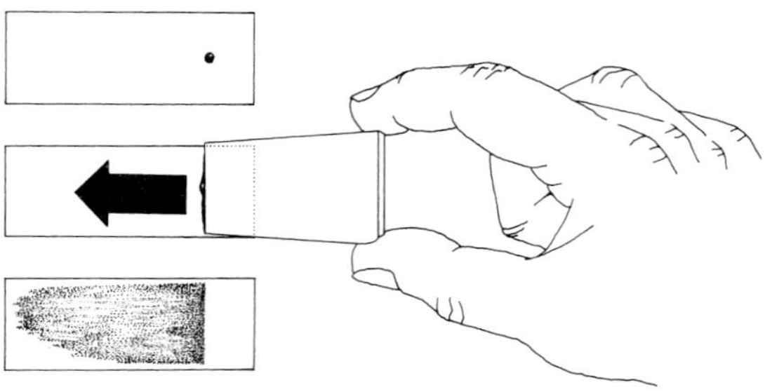

Figure 46–15 Preparation of blood smear on microscopic slide. (From Hughes WT, Buescher ES: *Pediatric Procedures.* Philadelphia, WB Saunders, 1980.)

ture. The blood should touch the slide in the midline and about 5 mm from one end.

3. Place the slide on a flat surface with the blood drop on the top side.
4. Grasp a second slide between the thumb and index finger of the right hand and place at a 30-degree angle on the slide with the drop of blood.
5. Pull back the upper slide until it touches the drop. Allow the blood to spread along the end of the slide until it almost reaches the edges.
6. Holding the bottom slide firmly with the left hand, push the upper slide smoothly and steadily forward toward the opposite end of the bottom slide. The slower the movement is carried out, the thicker the film; the greater the angle between the two slides, the thicker the film.
7. Allow to dry in the air.
8. A good preparation should have a smooth, homogeneous film without streaks or holes, and the edges of the smear should not extend to the edges of the slide.

Staining of Blood Films

The air-dried slide or coverslip is fixed by flooding with Wright-Giemsa stain for more than 3 minutes. Add drops of acid phosphate buffer to the slide or coverslip, taking care that the mixture does not drain off. Allow the stain and buffer to remain for 10 minutes. (Old-timers blow on the dye to induce mixing, which is a swirling metallic sheen on the surface.) Then wash the slide with distilled water. Wipe the dye off the unstained surface and place vertically to dry in room air.

A complete histological description of blood cells is beyond our scope. The slide is examined for red blood cells, platelets, and white blood cells. Five white blood cells per low-power field in a site where red blood cells are just touching approximate a white blood cell count of 1000 cells/mm^3 (Linne and Ringsrud, 1979). Morphological characterization of red blood cells, identification and counting of white blood cells, and evaluation of platelets is done under oil immersion high power.

Techniques for automation of white blood cell identification ("the differential") are becoming available with use of combinations of impedance, cytochemistry, and light scattering.

COAGULATION STUDIES

History, examination of a blood smear, bleeding time, prothrombin time, platelet count, activated

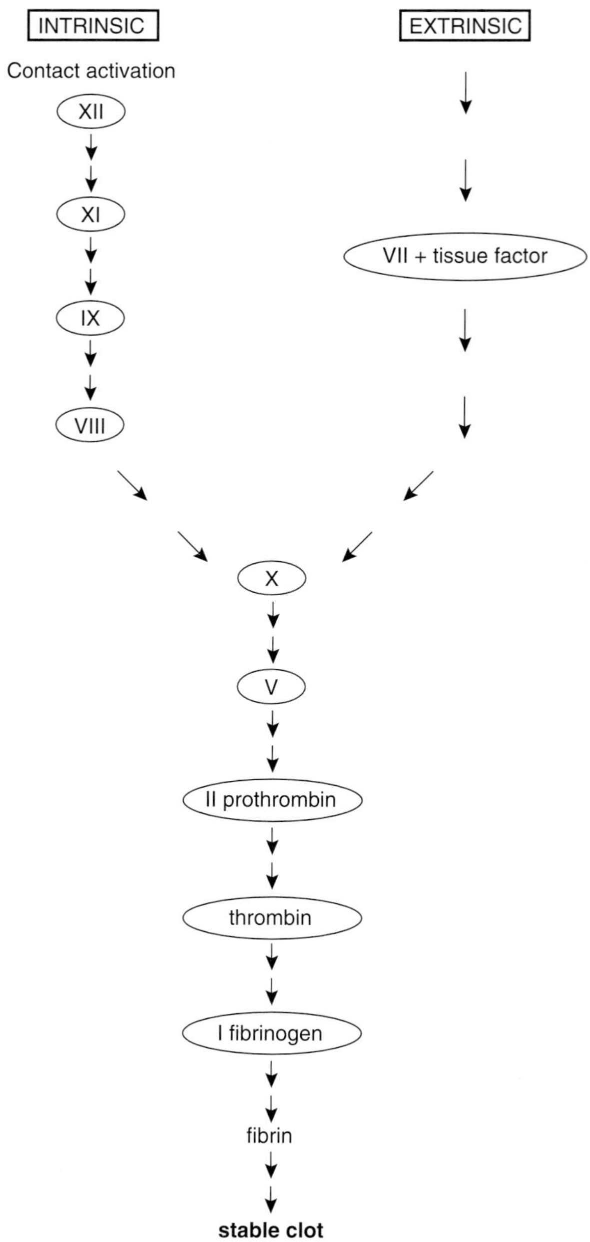

Figure 46–16 The extrinsic clotting cascade.

Table 46-1 Clotting Factors

I	Fibrinogen
II	Prothrombin
III	Thromboplastin
IV	Calcium
V	Proaccelerin
VII	Proconvertin
VIII	Antihemophilic factor
IX	Plasma thromboplastin component
X	Stuart factor
XI	Plasma thromboplastin antecedent
XII	Hageman factor (glass or contact factor)

Table 46-2 Abnormalities of Prothrombin Time, Activated Prothrombin Time, and Thrombin Time

Prothrombin time

Vitamin K and factor II, V, VII, and X deficiency
Affected by a long list of drugs

Activated prothrombin time

Common use—heparin monitoring
Factor II, V, VIII, IX, X, XI, XII, and fibrinogen deficiency

Thrombin time

Fibrinogen deficiency
Thrombin/fibrinogen

partial thromboplastin time, and thrombin time are the first-line studies for evaluating bleeding disorders. The bleeding time starts with a blood pressure cuff on the upper arm at a pressure of 40 mm. With a blade, make two 1 × 10-mm incisions in the forearm, starting a stopwatch. Blot the bleeding sites on filter paper every 10 seconds. Note the time when the bleeding stops. Less than 8 minutes is normal (Cohr, 1991).

The prothrombin time (one-step, Quick's test) is carried out by adding extrinsic factor to the patient's plasma. Plasma is anticoagulated with citrate. After the plasma samples are mixed, the time to appearance of the first fibrin strand is the prothrombin time (Raphael, 1983). In rough terms, the prothrombin time measures clotting factors in the extrinsic clotting cascade (Fig. 46-16).

The activated prothrombin time measures the intrinsic pathway. It is carried out in a fashion similar to the prothrombin time, using Koalin (traditionally) and partial thromboplastin added to the patient's plasma. The end point is the same as for prothrombin time.

Thrombin time, as the name suggests, involves adding thrombin to the patient's plasma and observing the time for fibrin formation. Names of the clotting factors are given in Table 46-1. Abnormalities of prothrombin time, activated prothrombin time, and thrombin time are indicated in Table 46-2. Normal coagulation values are listed in Table 46-3 (Corrigan, 1985).

Table 46-3 Comparison of Coagulation Data Between Normal Newborns and Older Children/Adults*

	Term	Preterm	Normal
Partial thromboplastin time (sec)	25–45	35–50	25–40
Prothrombin time (sec)	12–17	14–22	12–14
Thrombin time (sec)	12–16	14–18	12–14
Platelet count (× 10^9/L)	150–400	150–400	150–400
Assays			
Fibrinogen (mg/dl)	150–300	150–300	175–450
Factor II (units/dl)	23–74	21–54	60–150
Factor V (units/dl)	50–150	50–150	50–150
Factor VII (units/dl)	20–70	20–45	50–150
Factor VIII (units/dl)	50–250	50–180	50–150
Factor IX (units/dl)	20–60	10–25	50–150
Factor X (units/dl)	20–55	10–45	50–150
Factor XI (units/dl)	15–70	5–20	70–120
Factor XII (units/dl)	25–70	15–45	70–120
Factor XIII (h)	> 24	> 24	> 24
Prekallikrein	Reduced	Reduced	—
High-molecular-weight kininogen	Reduced	Reduced	—

*Data from the author's laboratory and from published reports.

Bone Marrow Puncture

Marrow is a soft tissue that fills the medullary cavity of the long bones, the large haversian canals, and all spaces between the trabeculae of spongy bone. It is an organ roughly the size of the liver and produces approximately 10^{10} red blood cells and half that number of granulocytes and platelets per hour. It consists of a framework of reticular tissue in which large numbers of either fat cells or blood and blood-forming cells are supported. In infants, the marrow is contained in the medullary cavity of long bones, where it persists in diminishing quantity until puberty. During the first few years of life, marrow in the long bones is gradually replaced by fat until hematopoiesis takes place only in the sternum, pelvis, cranium, vertebrae, ribs, and epiphysis of long bones.

The technique for bone marrow aspiration is similar to that used for intraosseous infusions (Chapter 29). The iliac crest is used for children, the sternum for young adults, and the tibia for infants younger than 2 years. After discussion with the child and the family, written consent, and adequate conscious sedation (Chapter 21) in all cases, 2% lidocaine is injected into the subcutaneous space and onto the periosteum. (Table 46–4).

ANTERIOR ILIAC CREST

Position

The patient is placed on a firm table in either the lateral recumbent or supine position.

Table 46–4 Sites for Bone Marrow Puncture

Site	Age to Which Adaptable
Anterior iliac crest	Any age
Posterior iliac crest	Any age
Femur	Birth to 2 years
Spinous vertebral process	2 years and older
Sternum	6 years and older
Tibia	Birth to 2 years

Restraint

If physical restraint is required, it is best maintained by two assistants positioning the patient as dictated by the operator.

Site

The anterior superior iliac spine and iliac crest are located and outlined by palpation. The site for puncture is one-fourth the distance from the anterior superior iliac spine. The point of puncture is approximately 2.5 cm below the superior margin of the crest (Fig. 46–17).

Insertion of Needle

The needle is inserted through the skin at an angle approximately 90 degrees to the long axis of the body until the bone is reached.

POSTERIOR ILIAC CREST

Position

The patient is placed in a lateral recumbent position on a firm table. The head is flexed, and the knees are drawn up to the abdomen.

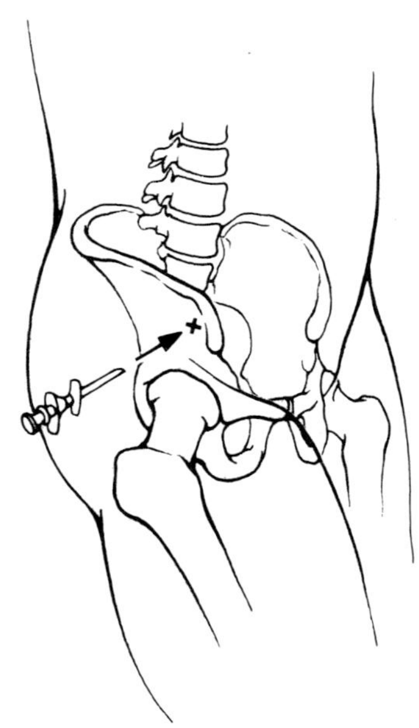

Figure 46–17 Puncture site at the anterior iliac spine. (Redrawn from Hughes WT, Buescher ES: *Pediatric Procedures.* Philadelphia, WB Saunders, 1980.)

Alternatively, the patient can be placed prone, with a pillow under the pelvis to elevate it slightly.

Restraint

Manual assistance is required. One arm of an assistant restrains the lower extremities at the knees, and the other maintains flexion of the neck in the same manner as for lumbar spinal puncture.

Site

The posterior superior iliac spine is located as a visible and palpable bone prominence superior and lateral to the intergluteal cleft (Fig. 46–18). It is inferior and medial to the crest of the ilium. The posterior iliac spinous process area is the thickest marrow-containing site in the child.

Insertion of Needle

The needle is introduced at the midpoint of the posterior iliac crest just superior to the posterior superior iliac spine. The needle is advanced into the marrow cavity in a line toward the anterior superior iliac spine, which may be palpated through the drapes with the operator's free hand. Subsequent procedure depends on the type of needle used.

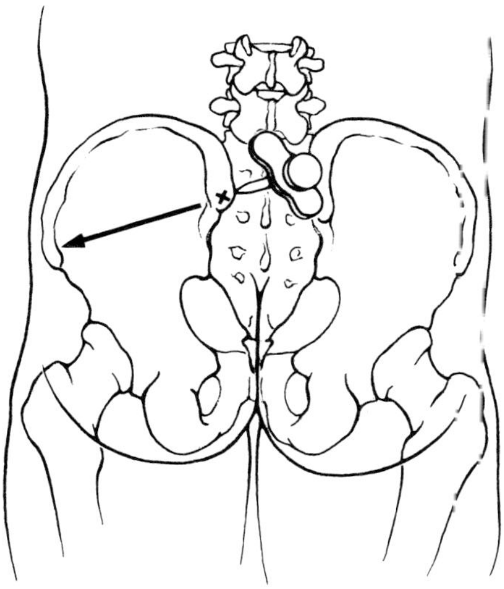

Figure 46–18 Puncture site at the posterior iliac crest. (Redrawn from Hughes WT, Buescher ES: *Pediatric Procedures.* Philadelphia, WB Saunders, 1980.)

STERNUM

Position

The patient is placed on a firm table in a supine position with upper extremities alongside the trunk and feet together.

Restraint

The patient is restrained manually, one assistant securing the upper extremities at the shoulders and another the lower extremities at the pelvis.

Site

In small children, only the manubrium can be used for sternal puncture, and it should be used only when other sites are not available. The site for puncture is opposite the first interspace (Fig. 46–19). In the older child and adult, either the manubrium or the body of the sternum may be used (Fig. 46–20). If the manubrium is to be used, the puncture should be made opposite the first interspace or approximately 2 cm from the manubriosternal junction. If the body of the sternum is chosen, the puncture is made approximately 3 cm inferior to the manubriosternal junction.

Insertion of Needle

At either of the sites for sternal puncture, the needle is always directed cephalad and advanced through the skin, subcutaneous tissue, and bony cortex at an angle 50 to 60 degrees to the sternal axis. The bevel of the needle is nearly parallel to the sternal plate.

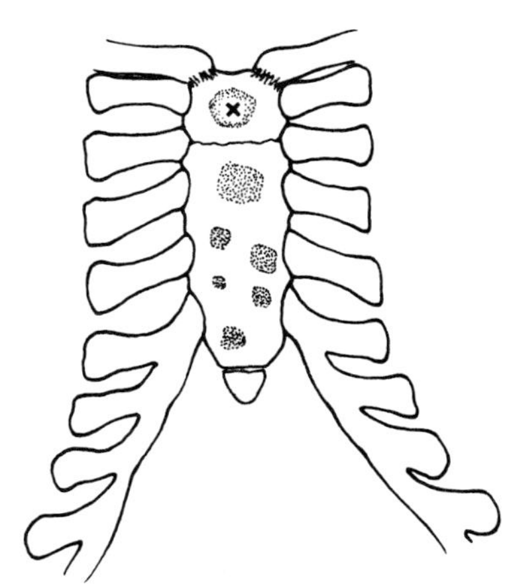

Figure 46–19 Puncture site at the manubrium in the infant. (Redrawn from Hughes WT, Buescher ES: *Pediatric Procedures.* Philadelphia, WB Saunders, 1980.)

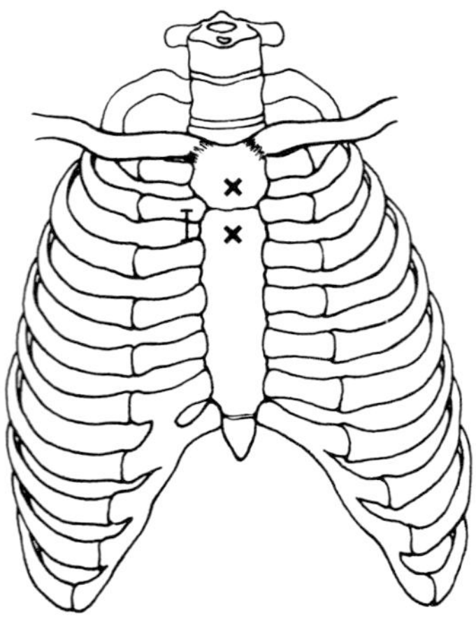

Figure 46–20 Puncture sites at the manubrium and body of the sternum in the older child. (Redrawn from Hughes WT, Buescher ES: *Pediatric Procedures.* Philadelphia, WB Saunders, 1980.)

TIBIA

Position and Restraint

The infant is placed in a supine position and restrained with body restraint. A small sandbag is placed underneath the proximal third of the lower leg directly beneath the puncture point. The leg is restrained in this position manually by an assistant.

Site

The anterior surface of the tibia is palpated in a cephalad direction until the metaphysis is reached. The tibial tuberosity is palpated in the metaphyseal end of the bone. The site for puncture is about 1 cm medial and 1 cm distal to the tibial tubercle (Fig. 46–21).

Insertion of Needle

The needle should be introduced in a slightly caudal direction at an angle approximately 45 to 60 degrees from the tibia. The sandbag must be directly beneath the puncture site to prevent trauma, which may accrue from levered pressure on the tibia. Subsequent procedure depends on the type of needle used (see description of bone marrow needles).

Several needles are available for performance of a bone marrow aspiration or biopsy. (Fig. 46–22). Certain requirements are basic to a satisfactory needle. The needle should be no smaller than 19-gauge and should have an obturator fitted to the lumen and bevel. The bevel must be short and sharp. The needle should be no more than 1 to 2 cm longer than the distance between the center of the marrow cavity and the skin surface.

The needle with stylus is inserted perpendicular to the bone surface. If insufficient pain control is evident, more lidocaine should be used or more time taken for its effects to optimize. A screwing motion with downward pressure is used until a startling "pop" is felt as the needle traverses the outer bony cortex and enters the marrow cavity. The needle is well fixed when it is in proper position (as with intraosseous infusions). The stylet is removed, and repeated strong negative pressures are applied by aspirating with a 10-ml heparin-rinsed syringe.

1. Only 0.1 to 0.2 ml of marrow should be aspirated as a suitable specimen for cytological study. A larger volume will be diluted with peripheral blood. If a larger specimen is required for culture or other studies, a second syringe is used to remove another sample of marrow for this purpose. Removal of additional marrow makes it possible to concentrate the cells if they are sparse

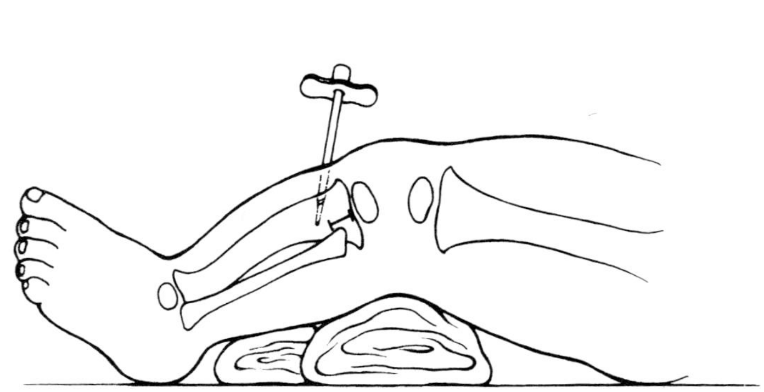

Figure 46–21 Puncture site at the tibia. (Redrawn from Hughes WT, Buescher ES: *Pediatric Procedures.* Philadelphia, WB Saunders, 1980.)

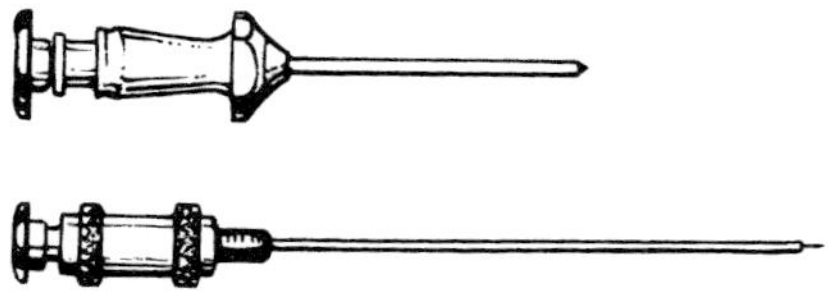

Figure 46–22 Turkel trephine needle. (Redrawn from Hughes WT, Buescher ES: *Pediatric Procedures.* Philadelphia, WB Saunders, 1980.)

and to select particles for special examination.

2. A more satisfactory specimen will be obtained if suction in the syringe is released before the syringe is removed from the intramedullary needle. This maneuver avoids spreading the aspirate along the walls of the syringe.
3. The glass microscope slides to be used for smears should be meticulously cleaned with 70% to 95% alcohol and dried with a soft, clean, lint-free cloth or lens paper.

Immediately after aspiration of a specimen, the syringe is removed from the needle and a drop of marrow expelled onto each of several (six to ten) clean slides. It is preferable to have an assistant take the syringe immediately after the specimen is collected and to prepare the specimen.

From the drop of marrow placed on the end of a slide, a smooth, even smear is made (see Figs. 46–14 and 46–15).

The marrow particles can be concentrated by placing several drops on glass slides and removing most of the blood and serum with a capillary pipet or allowing it to drain off. The particles adhere to the glass and may be picked up with a spreader and smeared onto a clean slide.

An "imprint" of the specimen can be made by picking up one or more gross bone marrow particles with the cut end of a wooden applicator and, holding this vertically to the slide surface, touching the tissue to the glass with a slight smearing motion. The slide is allowed to air dry before staining.

At times, little or no marrow may be obtained with the aspiration technique. This may result from faulty technique or from hypoplasia of the marrow, but the importance of further investigation of such circumstances must be emphasized.

HAZARDS OF BONE MARROW PUNCTURE

1. Hemorrhage. Bone marrow puncture is contraindicated in hemophilia.
2. Cardiac tamponade from sternal puncture
3. Osteomyelitis
4. Paraplegia from vertebral abscess after spinous process puncture
5. Fracture of tibia
6. Pneumothorax may result from inadvertent entrance into the pleural cavity during either injection of local anesthetic or sternal puncture when landmarks are lost and puncture is made lateral to the sternal border.
7. Infection in the mediastinum and mediastinal tissues

Exchange Transfusion

HISTORY

In 1924, before the cause of hemolytic disease of the newborn was known, Hart and MacDonald successfully performed the first exsanguination transfusion on an infant with "familial" icterus gravis of the newborn, hoping to remove toxins from the blood that might perhaps be responsible for the malady. During this historic operation, 300 ml of blood were removed from the infant's anterior fontanel while 335 ml of donor blood were simultaneously transfused into the saphenous vein at the ankle.

It was not until 1946 that the technique was developed more fully. Wiener and Wexler (1946) removed blood into the saphenous vein at the ankle. In 1948, Diamond described a method of cannulating the umbilical vein and alternately withdrawing and infusing volumes of blood.

Another variation on this theme was described by Gairdner (1966), who used the umbilical vein for blood infusion and the umbilical artery for blood removal. (The advantage to these "isovolumic" exchange transfusion methods is that hemodynamic shifts within the vascular system are minimized, possibly diminishing complication risks.)

PREPARATION

Exchange transfusions have become something of a lost art with the widespread use of anti–Rh antibody for prevention of isoimmune hemolysis and of phototherapy. In large pediatric teaching programs, residents are now lucky to have carried out such procedures.

Infants should not be fed for 3 to 4 hours before the procedure to minimize risk of aspiration. The procedure is usually done with the infant in a servocontrolled overhead warmer. Monitoring is carried out with a heart rate monitor and intravascular or external blood pressure monitoring. End-tidal carbon dioxide monitoring is useful if the infant is on a ventilator. A peripheral intravenous line with maintenance glucose is ideal.

Written informed consent is obtained from the parents.

The volume of donor blood to be given is 160 to 180 ml/kg of the infant's weight. This represents a two-volume exchange transfusion.

The physician in charge checks the blood for confirmation of proper type and crossmatch. Serial number, patient's name, donor's name, and blood types recorded on laboratory reports must correlate with the label on the blood. This is noted on the operative record.

Fresh heparinized blood has the advantages of low potassium level and adequate amounts of labile clotting factors; it is not diluted with a large amount of anticoagulant, as is acid citrate dextrose (ACD) blood. On the negative side, it cannot be stored; and it requires postexchange administration of protamine sulfate and determinations of clotting time. Additionally, heparin increases the plasma concentration of nonesterified fatty acids, which may cause redistribution of bilirubin. In most instances, ACD or citrate phosphate dextrose (CPD) anticoagulated blood is used. It should be as fresh as possible (never more than 3 to 4 days old) and warmed as near to body temperature as possible. As ACD blood ages, the plasma potassium rises and can attain dangerous levels. In addition, the pH of 2-day-old ACD blood ranges from 6.4 to 6.8.

A second problem with ACD blood for exchange transfusion is that the citrate anticoagulant continues to bind both calcium and magnesium ions after transfusion and can cause low ionized calcium and magnesium levels.

Most blood banks crossmatch donor blood against both the mother and the infant (at least for the first exchange) and use washed red blood cells reconstituted in fresh frozen plasma with a hematocrit of approximately 45%. Blood should be negative for cytomegalovirus and irradiated where possible (unless reconstituted white cell–free red blood cells are used).

The blood for exchange should be warmed to a temperature between room temperature and body temperature, and a delivery coil run through a blood warmer (the temperature of which is 32 to 34°C) is monitored throughout the procedure. (A malfunction of one of these devices "baked" the donor blood on at least one occasion, with predictably adverse effects in the recipient.)

The exchange apparatus can be assembled and connected to the umbilical vein catheter already in place. If available, a four-way stopcock is used (Fig. 46–23). (These are contained in some of the commercially available exchange transfusion kits.) If only three-way stopcocks are available, aseptically attach two in tandem (Fig. 46–24); one side port is connected to the blood administration set, and the other side port is connected securely to tubing that empties into the waste blood receptacle. A metal weight attached to the end of the waste blood tubing keeps it in the waste blood recep-

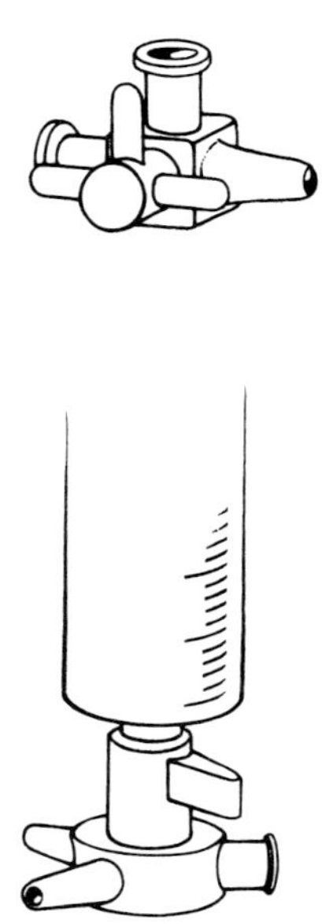

Figure 46–23 Stopcocks. (Redrawn from Hughes WT, Buescher ES: *Pediatric Procedures.* Philadelphia, WB Saunders, 1980.)

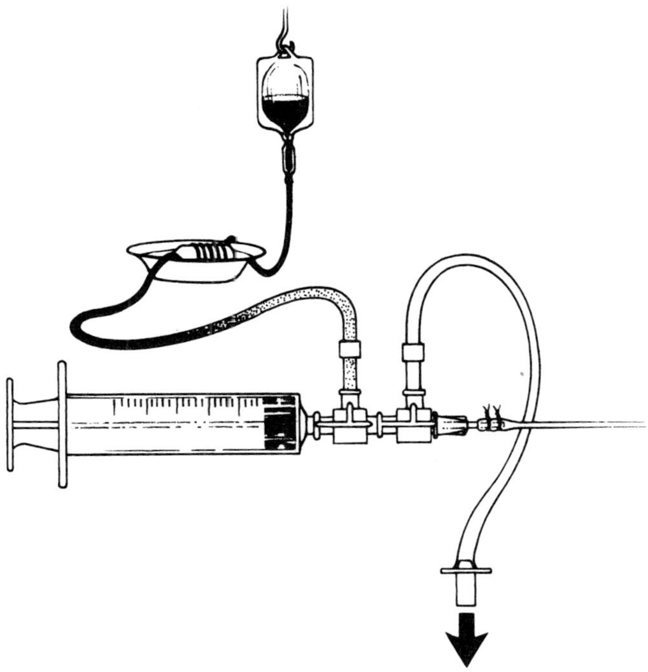

Figure 46–24 Exchange transfusion apparatus with stopcocks in tandem. (Redrawn from Hughes WT, Buescher ES: *Pediatric Procedures.* Philadelphia, WB Saunders, 1980.)

tacle when blood is injected throughout the tubing. The forward port of the tandem stopcocks is attached securely to the hub of the umbilical vein catheter, and a 20-ml syringe is attached to the rear port.

When the exchange transfusion is being done for removal of substances that bind to albumin (characteristically bilirubin), some clinicians administer albumin approximately 1 hour before or during the exchange. Probably because of the efficacy of phototherapy in obviating the need for repeated exchange transfusion, this practice is now uncommon.

Remove the donor blood from the blood warmer and attach the administration set. Fill the tubing of the blood administration set with blood and attach it to the appropriate side port of the stopcocks. If the blood has not yet warmed adequately, an empty intravenous fluid bottle can be filled with water at 32°C and stoppered. Wind the slack blood administration set tubing around the bottle and lay the bottle on the side in a warm water bath. If the water bath begins to cool during the procedure, the temperature can easily be adjusted by adding small amounts of warm water.

Before beginning the exchange transfusion procedure, attach the heparinized saline syringe to the rear stopcock port and flush 5 to 30 ml of solution through the system and out the waste blood tube into the waste receptacle. Check for leaks at the stopcock and tubing joints. If all is intact, detach the heparinized saline syringe and replace it with an empty 20-ml syringe.

The infant should be restrained gently at the hands and feet while the umbilical vein catheter is in place.

PROCEDURE

1. The initial increment of blood after clearing the dead space of the catheter should be sent for pre-exchange laboratory studies (e.g., culture; hematocrit; bilirubin and electrolyte determinations).

   It is prudent to keep tubes of pre-exchange blood for future unanticipated studies that would otherwise be "contaminated" by donor blood. For similar reasons, it is a good idea to keep a tube of donor blood if questions need to be addressed after the exchange transfusion.
2. Replace the syringe containing the first blood increment with a fresh syringe. Place the first increment blood in the appropriate blood containers. Draw donor blood into the new syringe after appropriate positioning of the stopcock valves; thus, the volume of blood to be exchanged per pass should

be approximately 3 to 5 ml/kg. Transfuse this blood into the patient slowly, reverse the stopcock valves, and aspirate into the syringe the same volume of blood as was transfused. Again adjust the stopcock valves and empty this blood into the waste container; readjust the stopcock valves, draw blood into the syringe, adjust the stopcock valves again, and transfuse the blood into the patient. This cycle is repeated over and over until the appropriate blood volume has been exchange transfused. The exchange should last about an hour.

3. The operator instructs an associate to record each volume of blood removed and each volume replaced (Fig. 46–25).
4. As the procedure goes on, the operator may note "sticking" of the stopcock valves or syringe plunger that will slow blood passes. When this occurs, close the valve to the syringe, remove the blood syringe, replace it with a heparinized saline syringe, and gently flush several milliliters of solution through the system. This, along with a fresh blood syringe, usually clears the sticking and improves the smoothness of the blood passes.
5. During the exchange, the donor blood unit should be regularly agitated to keep the red blood cells from settling. If the donor blood is not agitated during the exchange transfusion, the baby's hematocrit will be lower at the end of the exchange.

RECORD OF EXCHANGE TRANSFUSION

Louisville Children's Hospital
Department of Pediatrics, University of Louisville, School of Medicine

Patient's Name ______________ Date ________ Hosp. # ______

INFANT'S BLOOD: Type ________ Coombs' test ______________

Rh ________ Bilirubin: pre-exchange ____________

post-exchange ____________

MOTHER'S BLOOD: Type ________ Hemoglobin: pre-exchange ____________

Rh ________ post-exchange ____________

DONOR'S BLOOD: Type ________ Date collected ______________

Number ________
Correct correlation between laboratory report and bottle label.

EXCHANGE TRANSFUSION: First ___ Second ___ Third ___ Fourth ___ Etc ___

Time	Total Blood Out	Total Blood In	Drugs and Other Fluids	Comments

Condition at completion of operation ______________

Physician (sign) ______________

Assistants ______________

TOTAL IN ____________ TOTAL OUT ____________

Figure 46–25 Record of volume of blood removed and volume of blood replaced. (Redrawn from Hughes WT, Buescher ES: *Pediatric Procedures.* Philadelphia, WB Saunders, 1980.)

6. At termination of the exchange transfusion, when the final volume of blood is removed, a portion is placed in tubes for post-exchange electrolyte, calcium, and bilirubin determinations and complete blood count. The first 2 or 3 ml of this aliquot must be discarded, because it is donor blood filling the catheter. The subsequent withdrawal is then a true sample of the infant's blood.
7. No rigid rule can be given regarding leaving a deficit, replacing an equal volume of blood for that withdrawn, or infusing a small amount of donor blood in excess of that removed. Such decisions should be based on the complete evaluation of the infant. MacLaurin et al (1975) found that during exchange transfusion, blood volume increases a mean of 19 ml per kilogram of body weight, the rise being largely due to an increase in the red blood cell mass, with the plasma volume remaining the same. However, they also found a slight increase in the serum albumin level and an increase in the serum sodium concentration during exchange (probably owing to the use of ACD blood) and thought that all these factors increased the oncotic pressure. This leads to the increase in blood volume, and they warned that the 10- to 20-ml deficit incurred by removing a large initial increment may not be enough to maintain pre-transfusion blood volumes.
8. If no further exchange transfusions are anticipated, the umbilical vein catheter can be removed gently.

Difficulty in Withdrawing Blood

Withdrawal of blood may be difficult owing to

1. Obstruction of the catheter by venospasm, kinking, or clot.
2. Improperly fitted stopcocks, which permit entrance of air into the system.
3. Failure to frequently flush the system with heparinized saline. A sticky syringe may give a false impression that the catheter is no longer at an adequate source of blood.

Difficulty in Injecting Blood

Difficulty in injection of blood may result from clot formation in the system. Force should never be exerted to inject. Clots may be dislodged and produce fatal embolism.

After disconnection from the umbilical catheter, the system is first cleared with heparinized saline flushing out through the open stopcock. If obstruction still exists, the catheter must be replaced.

Incorrect Positioning of the Stopcock

An incorrect stopcock position can conceivably cause donor blood to be inadvertently injected back into the donor flask or the waste basin rather than into the infant. Also, blood may be withdrawn from either of these sources rather than from the infant, and the mistake may go unnoticed.

Improper Collection of Blood Specimen

If blood for hemoglobin and bilirubin determinations is withdrawn from the infant after an aliquot of donor blood has been injected, the portion of blood filling the catheter is donor blood. This amount must be withdrawn and discarded before the proper specimen of the infant's blood can be collected.

Inaccurate Measurement of Blood Volumes Infused and Withdrawn

Unless care is taken to prevent air in the syringe and to observe carefully the increment markings on the barrel, an error of 1 ml or so can easily be made with a 20-ml syringe. Conceivably, if errors of a 1-ml deficit of the infant's blood are made with each 20-ml volume exchanged, the infant's circulation would be overloaded with 100 ml during an exchange of 500 ml of donor blood.

A frequent complication is confusion over how much blood has been introduced and how much has been removed. Commonly, after the initial stress and enthusiasm associated with the start of the procedure, levity ensues at the expense of care in recording amounts of blood in and blood out. To avoid this, a clear statement, "10 ml in," repeated by the associate who records the datum is ponderous but effective.

HAZARDS OF EXCHANGE TRANSFUSION

CARDIAC DECOMPENSATION: Causative factors are

1. Anemia
2. Excessive blood volume and increased venous pressure
3. Sudden surge of cold blood into the right atrium and ventricle

HYPERKALEMIA: A toxic concentration of potassium accumulates in blood stored for longer than 1 week. Transfusing such blood produces a marked—and sometimes fatal—increase in the infant's serum potassium concentration.

HYPOCALCEMIA: The citrate of donor blood can depress the calcium ion concentration sufficiently to produce hypocalcemic tetany, although this has been shown to be uncommon.

SHOCK: Hypovolemic shock may follow inadequate replacement of blood removed from the infant or accidental catheter disconnections.

AIR EMBOLISM: Air embolism may arise from

1. Air in the system
2. Measuring venous pressure

If the venous pressure is being measured with an umbilical catheter, care should be taken to prevent sucking of air into the cardiovascular system by sudden negative pressure. Clamping of the umbilical catheter may be lifesaving when this situation is encountered. Normal pressure in the vena cava at birth is 4 to 8 cm and is decreased 2 to 4 cm by inspiration. Because of the risk of air embolism and because of improvements in other maintaining techniques, venous pressure is no longer routinely measured during exchange transfusion.

COMPLICATIONS AFTER EXCHANGE TRANSFUSION

Infarcts in a variety of tissues may follow exchange transfusion. Blood (and clots or emboli) may easily bypass the filtration of the pulmonary capillary bed, traverse the foramen ovale in the atria, and enter the left ventricle and arterial circulation. Major central nervous system infarcts are possible but extremely rare. More commonly, hematuria or blood in the stool may be detectable.

Sepsis is possible during a long sweaty procedure on a squirming infant under an overhead warmer. Nonbacterial infections may also ensue from the use of blood products. Rarely, in premature infants for whom nonirradiated blood is used, graft-versus-host disease has been reported.

Hypoglycemia should be prevented. CPD or ACD blood constitutes a sugar load with resulting hyperglycemia followed by hypoglycemia because of the induced hyperinsulinemia. More commonly, one forgets to run an intravenous line with dextrose during an exchange with heparinized (often low-glucose) blood.

Hypocalcemia may occur in association with the chelation by citrate containing anticoagulated donor blood. Many gave calcium boluses during the exchange as prophylaxis or when the infant showed clinical signs of hypocalcemia during the exchange—irritability and tachycardia. Admixture of calcium with citrated blood may lead to clotting, and this practice is now uncommon.

AFTERCARE

After an exchange transfusion, the most important issue is assessment of blood volume and perfusion. Disconnects with blood loss, accidental large deficits, and finishing the exchange with low-hematocrit plasma because of improper mixing of donor blood are common errors.

After it is ascertained that the infant is well, a talk with the parents, a procedure note on the chart, and follow-up on the pre- and post-exchange laboratory values are important. Antibiotic levels may be reduced by as much as 30% by an exchange transfusion, so doses or blood levels need to be considered. Follow-up of (usually) bilirubin and consideration of need for a second exchange are addressed (cross-match blood, maintain the catheter). If the catheter is removed, careful observation for bleeding should occur for at least the next 6 hours.

Infants may be fed when hungry if they are not distended and if bowel sounds are normal.

ALTERNATIVES TO PUSH-PULL EXCHANGES THROUGH AN UMBILICAL VENOUS CATHETER

A continuous exchange withdrawing through an umbilical artery catheter and infusing through an umbilical venous catheter is probably ideal in minimizing perturbations of blood volume. Therefore, this technique is optimal and most feasible in small premature infants at risk of intracranial hemorrhage. It requires two operators and a recorder and thereby is technically somewhat more difficult. Care should be taken that the time for the exchange be sufficient to allow bilirubin equilibration and to minimize risks of vascular "steals" from rapid withdrawal on the arterial catheter. Blood should not be instilled into the umbilical artery because of the possibility of arterial infarcts. (At least one infant has been made paraplegic because of a vertebral artery infarct during a push-pull umbilical artery exchange.) Use of a radial artery for withdrawal and the umbilical venous line for infusion is also feasible.

PARTIAL EXCHANGE TRANSFUSION

For polycythemia, partial exchanges are carried out to lower the hematocrit to less than 65% to reduce risk of cerebral hypoperfusion due to hyperviscosity. Blood is removed in aliquots similar to those for exchange transfusion and replaced with fresh frozen plasma, 5% albumin, lactated Ringer's solution, or normal saline. In a term infant, a total of approximately 70 ml (or approximately one-fourth of the blood volume) is effective.

References

Diamond LK: Replacement transfusion as a treatment for erythroblastosis fetalis. *Pediatrics*, 2:520, 1948.

Gairdner D: Exchange transfusion techniques. *Lancet*, 2:545, 1966.

Linne JJ, Ringsrud KM: *Basic Techniques for the Medical Laboratory*, 2nd ed. New York, McGraw-Hill, 1979.

MacLaurin JC, Coulter JBS, Hoby AM: Changes in blood volume associated with exchange transfusion. *Arch Dis Child*, 50:404, 1975.

Pochedly C: How to perform bone marrow puncture in small children. *Clin Pediatr*, 8:705, 1969.

Raphael SS: *Lynch's Medical Laboratory Technology.* Philadelphia, WB Saunders, 1983.

Wiener AS, Wexler LB: The use of heparin when performing exchange blood transfusions in newborn infants. *J Lab Clin Med*, 31:1016, 1946.

Bibliography

Aranda JV, Sweet AY: Alterations in blood pressure during exchange transfusion. *Arch Dis Child,* 52:545, 1977.

Baumgart S, Kim HC: Exchange transfusion in the neonate. In Stockman JA III, Pochedly C (eds): *Developmental and Neonatal Hematology.* New York, Raven Press, 1988, pp 199–212.

Cohr JA: *Pediatric Outpatient Procedures.* Philadelphia, JB Lippincott, 1991.

Comely A, Wood BEN: Albumin administration in exchange transfusion for hyperbilirubinemia. *Arch Dis Child,* 43:151, 1968.

Corrigan JJ Jr: *Hemorrhagic and Thrombotic Diseases in Childhood and Adolescence.* University of Arizona, 1985.

Cremer RJ, Perryman PW, Richards DH: Influences of light on hyperbilirubinemia of infants. *Lancet,* 1:1094, 1958.

Hann IM, Lake BD, et al: *Colour Atlas of Paediatric Haematology*, 2nd ed. Oxford, Oxford University Press, 1990.

Lanskowsky P: *Manual of Pediatric Hematology and Oncology.* New York, Churchill Livingstone, 1989.

Lilleyman JS, Hann IM (eds): *Paediatric Haematology.* New York, Churchill Livingstone, 1992.

McClatchey KD: *Clinical Laboratory Medicine.* Baltimore, Williams & Wilkins, 1994.

Mentzer WC Jr, Matthay K: Hematology and oncology. *Curr Opin Pediatr*, 6:43–45, 1994. Editorial.

Miller DR, Baehner RL, et al: *Blood diseases of Infancy and Childhood: In the Tradition of C.H. Smith,* 6th ed. St Louis, CV Mosby, 1989.

Nathan DG, Oski FA: *Hematology of Infancy and Childhood*, 4th ed. Philadelphia, WB Saunders, 1993.

Ravel R: *Clinical Laboratory Medicine,* 5th ed. Chicago, Year Book Medical Publishers, 1989.

Woods RR: An exchange transfusion formula. *Am J Dis Child*, 98:692, 1959.

Zachman RD: Alternate photography in neonatal hyperbilirubinemia. *Biol Neonate*, 25:283, 1974.

Section M

Immunology/ Infectious Disease

Chapter 47

Immunology and Infectious Diseases Procedures and Tests

E. Stephen Buescher

The frequency with which the pediatrician must deal with the ill, febrile child clearly indicates that infectious diseases are common in children. This prevalence of infectious diseases in children necessitates the use of many types of tests but relatively few procedures for the diagnosis and management of their infections. The frequency with which these tests and procedures are used varies somewhat with the age of the child. In the newborn, whose host defenses are poor, the significant morbidity and mortality related to infection prompt the aggressive use of diagnostic tests, cultures, and procedures. In the toddler and older child, in whom immune defenses are good and infection-related morbidity and mortality are less, the same tests, cultures, and procedures are used less aggressively, and more attention is paid to the history and physical findings. Regardless of age, a number of points about procedures and tests for the diagnosis of infectious diseases in children are worth making.

COMMENTS ON CULTURES

Three general points about the specimens obtained for the diagnosis of infection are important (Washington, 1979). First, the specimen collected should be representative of the disease process. Second, the quantity of specimen should be adequate to allow complete examination. Third, great attention should be paid to minimizing the risk of contaminating the specimen with indigenous local flora. If these points are followed, the pediatrician maximizes the likelihood that the microbiology laboratory will be able to isolate and identify the responsible infectious agent.

Blood Cultures

The effectiveness with which blood culture identifies an agent causing infection is dependent on a number of factors, including the type and location of the infection, the number of cultures obtained, and the volume of blood cultured. Only the last two can be modified by the pediatrician. In adults, bacteremia is quantitatively small, with 10^1 to 10^2 colony-forming units (CFU)/ml of blood being typical. With this level of bacteremia, three blood culture specimens of 20 to 30 ml are adequate for diagnosis of bacteremia in greater than 97% of untreated infective endocarditis cases (Shanson, 1990; Washington, 1982). In children, the magnitude of bacteremia is variable and is related to age and severity of illness (severely ill infants and younger children can have 10^4 to 10^6 CFU/ml). It has been assumed that this quantitative difference between adult and pediatric bacteremias allows the diagnosis of bacteremias in pediatric patients to be made accurately with use of smaller volumes of blood per culture (1–5 ml) and fewer cultures. In some instances, this may be true (Neal et al, 1986); but because not all children have high-grade bacteremias, this approach risks missing the 30% to 40% (Sullivan et al, 1982) of children who have bacteremias quantitatively similar to those seen in adults. To maximize the likelihood of recovering the causative organism in a bacteremic child, multiple culture specimens with as large a blood volume as is reasonable (Shanson, 1990) should be obtained. This approach identifies children with all grades of bacteremia, as opposed to only those with high-grade bacteremia.

Unlike in the past, when a pair of liquid media, one aerobic and the other anaerobic, were the standard for use in blood cultures, a number of different blood culture media and systems are now commercially available and in use. Media for aerobic and anaerobic cultures are still available. These have been supplemented, however, with a wide variety of other specialized media. Biphasic media (with both liquid and solid growth media incorporated into the same container) optimize the recovery of fungi. Media containing particulates or detergents to lyse blood cells, liquid media that are directly subcultured to plates to allow quantitation of bacteremia, and media containing resinous materials that remove antibiotics from the patient's blood sample are routinely available. In addition, the systems used to screen and monitor blood cultures have advanced significantly beyond visual screening and manual subculture. Systems that automatically monitor cultures for the appearance of microbial metabolic byproducts, such as carbon dioxide, and notify the laboratory personnel when they are detected are in routine use in many medical facilities. With these systems, the criteria for a culture to be positive are ultimately the same (i.e., growth of the organism), but the ability to detect growth more rapidly is typically much enhanced.

Despite changes in culture monitoring systems, the procedure for obtaining blood culture specimens has changed little. The skin is prepared with an iodinated antiseptic (tincture of iodine, povidone-iodine solution), which is allowed to sit 1 to 2 minutes and dry before it is removed with 70% alcohol. Failure to effectively prepare the skin often results in blood culture specimens that are contaminated by skin flora. Although these organisms are usually opportunists as opposed to pathogens, they can behave as true pathogens in small infants and other patients with compromised host defenses, making interpretation of the culture difficult. To avoid this situation, proper preparation of the skin before the venipuncture cannot be overemphasized. Optimally, the vein for venipuncture will be visible after the site is prepared, and the venipuncture can be done without further palpation (and potential contamination) of the skin at the puncture site. After the venipuncture, the blood is obtained and placed in containers holding the proper type of growth media. In situations in which the vessel for venipuncture must be palpated, the operator's palpating fingertip (either gloved or natural) is also aseptically prepared. Each culture specimen is typically obtained at a different puncture site and can use blood that is either venous or arterial. If blood is obtained from an intravascular device rather than by venipuncture, an additional complexity, the question of whether positive cultures indicate catheter "colonization" or true bacteremia, is sometimes raised. While this question may or may not be valid, it almost always makes for lively debate, but there is usually no dependable way to decide the answer. It is therefore advisable to avoid raising the question by using venipuncture-obtained blood for culture whenever possible.

Urine Cultures

In children, the techniques by which urine specimens are obtained for culture are determined largely by the age of the patient. Infants and small children who are not yet toilet trained usually have a urine collection bag placed after the skin of the perineum is cleaned. Alternatively, they can be catheterized to obtain the specimen, or urine can be obtained by suprapubic puncture (Fig. 47–1). The urine collection bag method is limited by the invariable contamination of the specimen by "skin" flora, which on the perineum includes the enteric flora. Because of this, only colony counts of greater than 10^5 organisms/ml of bag-collected urine may be interpreted as suggestive of infection. If the child is old

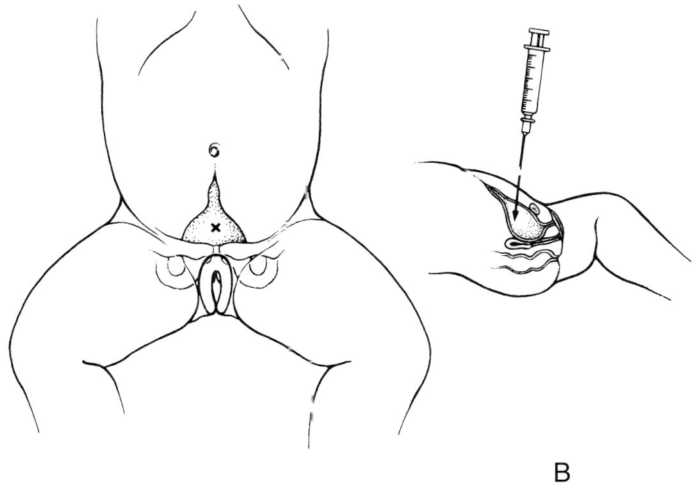

Figure 47–1 **A.** The site for suprapubic bladder aspiration, denoted by an "X." **B.** The general direction for passage of the needle.

enough to cooperate with obtaining a midstream clean catch urine specimen, the presence of greater than 10^5 organisms/ml correlates well with infection.

Catheterization of the bladder is less susceptible to contamination, but factors such as the sex of the child (girls are usually easier to catheterize) or whether a boy has been circumcised alter the effectiveness with which the urethral meatus can be cleaned and hence the likelihood of culture contamination by superficial flora. For culture specimens obtained by catheterization, colony counts of greater than 10^3 organisms/ml are usually taken as indicative of infection. Obtaining a urine specimen for culture from a child with an indwelling urinary catheter is best done by aseptically preparing the surface of the catheter and then using a fine-gauge needle to pierce the wall and aspirate urine from the catheter lumen. This procedure minimizes the risks of introducing infection that accompany repeatedly breaking the continuity of the urine drainage system. Suprapubic bladder aspiration after effective aseptic preparation of the skin carries the least risk of contamination by superficial flora, making cultures obtained by this method the least susceptible to errors of interpretation. In general, the presence of any organisms grown in urine obtained by suprapubic bladder aspiration is considered significant.

Wound and Body Site Cultures

Although obtaining appropriate culture specimens from wounds seems almost too simple to mention, a problem frequently encountered in the microbiology laboratory is that of an inadequate specimen, typically a blood-tinged swab of the infected site. For purposes of culturing, the general rules "more is better" and "tissue, not tinge" are well worth remembering when the specimen for culture is being obtained. In addition, when solid pieces of tissue are to be obtained, if the specimen is not being placed directly into culture media, the fluid used to transport the specimen should not contain preservative (e.g., "bacteriostatic" saline should not be used).

Selective and Special Media

In some situations, the objective of culturing is to determine whether a specific organism is present at a particular site. At sites where a normal bacterial flora exists (the female genitourinary tract, the gastrointestinal tract, the upper respiratory tract), this flora may interfere with the recovery of the organism of interest if routine culturing methods are used. In these situations, use of selective media or a specific culture procedure can optimize the growth or survival of the organism of interest. Table 47–1 lists several of the selective media used to help identify specific organisms.

For some diseases, the responsible infectious agents are difficult to recover by routine culture methods because of their nutritional requirements. When these diseases (Table 47–2) are suspected, it is prudent to notify the microbiology laboratory ahead of time so that the specimens can be collected and handled properly.

Table 47–1 Clinically Useful Selective Growth Media and the Agents They Are Used to Isolate

Organism	Selective Medium	Mechanism
Neisseria sp.	Thayer-Martin	Selective growth
Shigella sp. and *Salmonella* sp.	Hektoen enteric agar	Selective growth
Gram-negative rods and non–lactose-fermenting organisms	MacConkey agar	Selective growth and color
Legionella sp. and *Nocardia* sp.	Charcoal-yeast extract agar	Selective growth
Gram-positive organisms	Colistin/nalidixic acid agar	Selective growth
Listeria sp.	Cold enrichment*	Selective growth
Streptococci and staphylococci	Phenylethyl alcohol	Selective growth
Mycobacterium tuberculosis	Löwenstein-Jensen	Selective growth

*A portion of the specimen is stored at 4°C for up to 4 weeks and subcultured weekly.

ANTIOBIOTIC LEVELS AND SENSITIVITIES

For antibiotics that have relatively narrow therapeutic margins, blood levels are routinely measured to ensure that the doses being administered are effective but not toxic. These antibiotics include the aminoglycoside agents gentamicin, tobramycin, and amikacin; the glycopeptide antibiotic vancomycin; and chloramphenicol. On the basis of intensive studies of the pharmacokinetics of the aminoglycosides, two types of blood level determinations are useful for guiding adjustments to both the dose and the interval between doses: peak levels and trough levels. Peak levels are typically obtained 30 to 60 minutes after completion of an intravenous dose, and trough levels are usually obtained 5 to 15 minutes before an intravenous dose is given. The timing for peak and trough antibiotic level determinations is based on the observation that both peak and trough antibiotic levels in blood achieve steady-state (plateau) levels after about five doses in the absence of an initial loading dose. (If a loading dose is given, plateau levels are theoretically achieved after this dose). After two and four doses, approximately 75% and 94%, respectively, of the plateau levels are achieved. In most instances, it is therefore reasonable to measure peak and trough levels after three or four antibiotic doses, which will be 85% to 90% of the plateau levels for that dose and interval. An additional utility of determining the peak level is that it can help maximize the therapeutic effectiveness of the antibiotic. A strong relationship exists between the peak aminoglycoside level, the aminoglycoside's minimal inhibitory concentration (MIC) for the organism being treated, and the probability of a response to therapy. For aminoglycosides, a ratio of peak antibiotic level to MIC greater than 6 is associated with a treatment response rate of more than 80% (Moore et al, 1987). Whereas persistent, excessively high peak levels can be associated with some toxic effects, elevated trough levels correlate better with the development of toxic injury. Therefore, keeping these levels as low as possible while maintaining maximal peak levels is the ultimate objective of monitoring blood levels.

Chloramphenicol is an exception to these rules in that measurements of peak and trough levels are not appropriate. Because of the complex distribution and redistribution of this antibiotic in tissues, pharmacokinetic peaks and troughs do not really occur. A chloramphenicol

Table 47–2 Diseases and Agents That Require Prior Consultation with the Microbiology Laboratory for Isolation and Diagnosis

Disease	Causative Agent
Granuloma inguinale	*Calymmatobacterium granulomatis*
Leptospirosis	*Leptospira* sp.
Oroya fever	*Bartonella bacilliformis*
Rat-bite fever	*Streptobacillus moniliformis*
Lyme disease	*Borrelia burgdorferi*
Relapsing fever	*Borrelia* sp.
Tularemia	*Francisella tularensis*
Whooping cough	*Bordetella pertussis*
Brucellosis	*Brucella* sp.
Plague	*Yersinia pestis*

blood level, usually measured after the third or fourth dose at a midpoint between doses, is used to guide the dose being administered.

In the clinical microbiology laboratory, several types of susceptibility testing may be available to help guide the choice of antibiotics. Susceptibility testing based on diffusion of antibiotic from a disk of filter paper placed on a Petri dish inoculated with the isolate of interest is an older method. Because the size (diameter) of the zone of inhibition of the organism's growth around the disk approximates the $\log_2$ of the MIC for the organism, this size can be used to predict the sensitivity or resistance of the organism when the testing is performed under standardized conditions. Although this method is at best only semiquantitative, when done carefully, it can provide useful information for antibiotic selection. More recently, growth of standard inocula of bacteria in liquid cultures containing serial dilutions of antibiotic has gained popularity because this method allows the direct estimation of the MIC of the antibiotic. Under standardized conditions, the last antibiotic dilution with no visible bacterial growth is taken as the MIC. If aliquots of each antibiotic dilution at which no visible bacterial growth was observed are taken and subcultured in media without antibiotic for an additional 24 hours, the last dilution at which no bacterial regrowth appears is taken as the minimal bactericidal concentration (MBC). Typically, the ratio of the MIC to the MBC is less than 8 (within three dilutions of one another). The situation in which this ratio is greater than 32 (greater than five dilutions) is termed "antibiotic tolerance," which may negatively influence the clinical effectiveness of a specific antibiotic.

The MIC and MBC are used to estimate in vitro microbial susceptibility to antibiotics, but they do not necessarily predict the effectiveness of therapy. In some situations, the serum inhibitory titer (SIT) and serum bactericidal titer (SBT) are used to try to better predict therapy effectiveness. In contrast to the MIC and MBC, which measure only antibiotic effects, the SIT and SBT measure the cumulative effectiveness of the antibiotic plus other endogenous serum factors (e.g., complement and antibody) at inhibiting and killing the organism. Typically, SIT and SBT measurements are done with serum obtained 1 to 2 hours after an antibiotic dose. The serum is diluted serially, and each dilution is inoculated with a standard amount of the patient's isolate. The lowest serum titer at which no visible bacterial growth is observed is taken as the SIT; after subculture of nongrowth serum dilutions into serum-free growth media, the lowest serum titer at which no growth occurs is taken as the SBT. Depending on the organism being treated, SBT values of 1:8 or greater are recommended (Nelson, 1978).

SEROLOGICAL TESTS

Identification of an infectious agent by demonstration of a specific humoral immune response (specific antibody formation) is an alternative to the recovery of the agent by culture. Despite continued improvement of laboratory methods for propagation of a wide variety of infectious agents, diagnosis of many common infectious diseases remains based on demonstration of specific serological responses. For serological testing, the patient's serum is usually used. Whole blood is obtained and allowed to clot; the serum is separated and tested at regular dilutions for the presence of antibody. Historically, results of these tests have been reported as either the presence/absence of antibody or the titer of antibody activity in serum. With the application of more modern and rapid laboratory methods (e.g., enzyme immunoassays and Western blot) to serodiagnosis, results in optical density units (a measure of color in enzyme-linked immunoassays) or specific antigen reactivities (a measure of serum antibody reactivity with individual antigens first separated by their size or charge, blotted onto a solid-phase background, and then reacted with the serum specimen) are sometimes reported. Understanding which unit of measure is used and how it correlates with more classical results becomes an important part of test interpretation. The utility of the paired sera specimen, with one specimen obtained during the acute illness and a second obtained during convalescence, remains unchanged. It optimizes the diagnostic accuracy of serological testing (regardless of the laboratory method used for testing): by testing both specimens at the same time, the contribution of day-to-day variability inherent to every laboratory procedure is minimized.

Table 47–3 is a partial list of the infectious diseases diagnosed primarily by serology.

"CLASSICAL" DIAGNOSTIC METHODS

Gram's Stain

When a body fluid or tissue is obtained for diagnosis of infection, the first information that returns to the pediatrician results from exami-

Table 47–3 Infectious Diseases Diagnosed Serologically in Children

Epstein-Barr virus infection	Trichinosis	Ehrlichiosis
Tularemia	Brucellosis	Echinococcosis
Lyme disease	Syphilis	Leptospirosis
Toxocariasis	Rocky Mountain spotted fever	Toxoplasmosis
Human immunodeficiency virus infection	Hepatitis C	Mycoplasmosis
		Coccidioidomycosis
Psittacosis	Hepatitis B	Blastomycosis

nation of the Gram's stained material. By use of two clean glass slides, the specimen is applied to the surface of one slide and, with the second slide, compressed between them. Briskly pulling one slide over the other to separate them usually results in an appropriately thin smear of the specimen. The specimen is then air dried and heat fixed (by passing the slide through a flame to fix it to the glass). The fixed specimen is flooded with 2% crystal violet in methanol for 10 to 15 seconds, rinsed with tap water, flooded with iodine solution (0.33% iodine crystal, 0.66% potassium iodide in water) for 10 to 15 seconds, rinsed again with tap water, and then decolorized.

Decolorization is the step that poses the most problem for the inexperienced because too much or too little makes interpretation of the results difficult. With the slide held at an angle to allow rapid draining of applied decolorizer, the decolorizing solution (25% acetone in 95% ethanol) is applied in a continuous stream. The draining decolorizer is initially tinted dark blue, but with continued application, this color rapidly pales to clear. As soon as decolorizer draining from thin areas of the specimen is colorless, this step is complete, and the specimen is immediately rinsed in tap water. The slide is then flooded with counterstain (1% safranin O in water) for 10 to 15 seconds followed by rinsing in tap water and is then air dried and examined microscopically. In properly stained areas, polymorphonuclear leukocyte nuclei are red (blue nuclei represent under-decolorization), and gram-positive and gram-negative organisms are blue and red, respectively. In over-decolorized areas, gram-positive organisms appear gram-negative.

Stool for Ova and Parasites

To diagnose the causative agents for parasite-induced gastroenteritis or unexplained eosinophilia, stool is collected for ova and parasite examination. This examination should be done promptly because some agents, such as *Giardia lamblia* and *Entamoeba histolytica*, may be missed if fresh stool is not used. If the stool is not to be examined immediately, it should be fixed in 10% formalin. Initially, the stool specimen is examined grossly for the presence of adult worms or proglottids, followed by concentration and microscopic examination for ova. Microscopic examination typically involves examination of both wet mount specimens and permanent specimens stained with trichrome or iron hematoxylin.

Cellophane Tape Test

This test is used to diagnose infestation with pinworms (*Enterobius vermicularis*) and is based on the fact that gravid female worms move from the rectum to the skin of the anus at night to lay their eggs (Fig. 47–2). The best time to perform the test is first thing in the morning without the patient's bathing. With use of a tongue depressor as an applicator, the end of a length of cellophane tape is attached just proximal to one end of the tongue blade, and the free length of tape is folded back over the end of the tongue blade and down the other side (to expose the sticky surface). The free length is held in place by a clean microscope slide on the opposite side of the tongue depressor. With the patient recumbent on the side in the knee-chest position, the sticky surface of the tape at the end of the tongue blade is pressed against the skin all around the anus; the tape is removed from the tongue blade and attached to a glass slide for microscopic examination. The presence of pinworm ova attached to the tape is evidence of pinworm infestation.

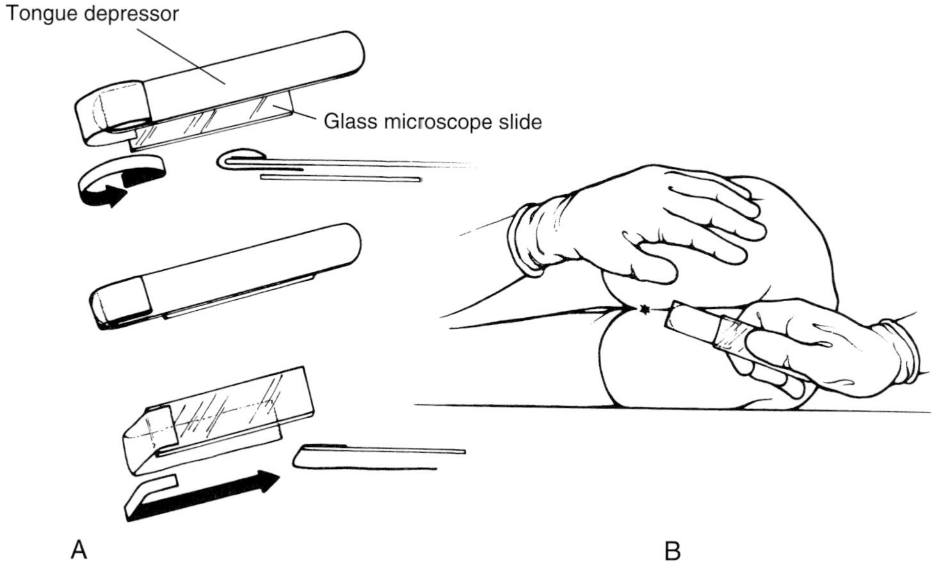

Figure 47–2 The cellophane tape test is used to diagnose infestation with pinworms and is based on the fact that gravid female worms move from the rectum to the skin of the anus at night to lay their eggs. **A.** Assembly of the cellophane tape tool. **B.** The use of the tool to collect perianal pinworm eggs. (Redrawn from Hughes WT, Buescher ES: *Pediatric Procedures.* Philadelphia, WB Saunders, 1980.)

Test for Fecal Leukocytes

This test examines the feces for the presence of leukocytes, whose presence implies lower gastrointestinal tract inflammation as is seen with diarrheal illnesses caused by *Shigella, Campylobacter, Salmonella*, or *Yersinia* organisms. A small amount of fresh stool is smeared on a glass slide and stained with several drops of 0.5% methylene blue in saline. After 2 to 3 minutes, a coverslip is placed over the preparation, and it is examined microscopically with low power. As a vital dye, the methylene blue accentuates the leukocyte nuclei without staining the cytoplasm, making the leukocytes easy to see. The number of fecal leukocytes present is graded 1+ to 4+.

RAPID DIAGNOSTIC METHODS

Although cultures, or in some cases paired serological samples, have been the "gold standard" for diagnosis of most infectious diseases, these tests are difficult to perform rapidly enough to provide useful clinical information. For situations in which the causative agent is difficult to isolate, in which isolation is slow, or in which serological responses can be deceptive (e.g., transplacentally acquired maternal antibody), rapid diagnostic tests have been developed (and are continuing to be developed) to supply information that can help in diagnosis and management. Rapid diagnostic tests are not available for every infectious agent. Most of these tests are currently based on the detection of a specific antigen, but in the future, many will likely be based on the detection of characteristic gene sequences by polymerase chain reaction (PCR) methods. As rapid diagnostic tests, these methods are *not* alternatives to culture; they are supplemental to culture methods and are intended only to provide information that may help guide initial treatment. They are difficult to interpret and of limited use when performed in lieu of a culture.

Latex agglutination assays for the detection of *Streptococcus pneumoniae*, *Streptococcus agalactiae*, *Neisseria meningitidis*, *Haemophilus influenzae* type B, and *Cryptococcus neoformans* are widely available. Cross-reactivity between *Neisseria gonorrhoeae* capsular antigen and some *Escherichia coli* K1 antigens leads to false-positive test results in some instances of infection with *E. coli.* With these assays, beads of latex coated with specific antibody are mixed with the fluid for examination (cerebrospinal fluid, urine). The presence of antigen in the fluid causes cross-linking between latex particles, and the suspension macroscopically agglutinates. In the absence of antigen, the mixture remains homogeneous and milky. Application of latex agglutination rapid diagnostic tests to biological fluids is not universal. In general, fluids with high protein contents (plasma and exudate fluids) give unreliable results. Counterimmunoelectrophoresis (CIE), which is about a tenth as sensitive as latex agglutination tests, can be applied to fluids containing significant amounts of protein. CIE uses an electrical field to move a biological fluid specimen and specific antibody toward one another from opposite ends of a gel matrix. When the antibody and biological fluid pass through each other, specific antibody cross-links the antigen, and a visible band of precipitated immune complexes forms.

Enzyme immunoassays for a number of infectious agents (particularly viral agents) are also available. As a group, these assays detect antigen with either specific antibody directly conjugated with an enzyme or specific antibody detected with a second enzyme-conjugated antibody. After treatment with antibody, addition of a chromogenic substrate for the conjugated enzyme results in color development proportional to the amount of antigen present. Enzyme immunoassays for rotavirus, herpes simplex virus, *G. lamblia*, respiratory syncytial virus, cytomegalovirus, influenza A virus, chlamydia, human immunodeficiency virus, and hepatitis C virus are available, and many are in wide use in microbiology laboratories.

Fluorescence assays used to detect antigen microscopically in biological specimens use either specific antibody directly labeled with fluorochrome (direct fluorescence assay, DFA) or unlabeled specific antibody that is detected with a second fluorochrome-labeled antibody (indirect fluorescence assay, IFA). DFA and IFA for the rapid diagnosis of some viruses (e.g., respiratory syncytial virus) and a number of difficult to grow agents (e.g., *Ehrlichia, Legionella, Pneumocystis*) are in use. An important point about DFAs and IFAs is that their interpretation involves a large degree of subjectivity (as opposed to objective spectrophotometric measurement of color in enzyme immunoassays). Both inclusion of appropriate positive and negative controls and experience with assay interpretation are critically important if assays of these types are to be clinically dependable.

The PCR is a molecular biology method that is being applied to the diagnosis of many agents, even some (such as hepatitis C virus) that cannot yet be isolated. To apply PCR methods, information on the molecular genetic make-up of the organism (preferably a unique genetic sequence) is necessary. On the basis of this information, short nucleic sequences (PCR primers) complementary to the organism's sequence are synthesized in vitro and then used to initiate and support repeated rounds of organism-specific nucleic acid synthesis. The presence of amplified amounts of organism-specific nucleic acid sequences after repeated rounds of PCR is then taken as evidence that organism-specific nucleic acid was present in the initial sample. Because of the stable nature of many types of nucleic acids and the requirement (theoretically) for only one template nucleic acid sequence to be present for a positive PCR, the broad application for PCR-based testing for diagnosis of infectious diseases in the future is almost ensured. However, in most instances, PCR is a qualitative (not quantitative) method, and PCR-based testing should usually be interpreted as such. In addition, because of the extreme sensitivity of the method, false-positive results can occur and must be considered when results are interpreted. At present, PCR-based diagnostic testing for human immunodeficiency virus, *Borrelia burgdorferi*, mycobacteria, and herpes simplex virus is available.

IMMUNOLOGICAL TESTING

In some situations, the immunocompetence of a child may come into question and it is necessary to examine various aspects of the immunological defenses. As with childhood infectious diseases, more tests than specific procedures are used in such an evaluation. The dramatic expansion of knowledge regarding human immunology and host defenses that has occurred in the past 20 years has resulted in the availability of a large number of tests for assessing immunocompetence and diagnosing specific immunodeficiency states.

Immunoglobulin Tests

Tests for quantitation of individual immunoglobulin isotypes (IgM, IgG, IgA, IgE), for quantitation of IgG subclasses (IgG1–4), and for assessing specific antibody responses to defined antigens (tetanus toxoid, diptheria toxoid, *H. influenzae* type B polyribose phosphate, mumps virus, poliovirus) are available. These tests are usually done by either radial immunodiffusion assay or enzyme immunoassay. In a radial diffusion assay, a small quantity of serum is placed into a well cut into a gel matrix that contains isotype-specific anti-immunoglobulin. As the immunoglobulin in the serum sample diffuses into the gel, it complexes with anti-immunoglobulin to form a circle of precipitated immune complexes whose diameter correlates with the immunoglobulin content of the serum specimen. In enzyme immunoassays, a series of serum dilutions are placed in wells that have anti-immunoglobulin bound to their surface. The immunoglobulin in the serum dilution is the antigen that is captured by the solid-phase anti-immunoglobulin, and the captured immunoglobulin is detected with a second anti-immunoglobulin that is enzyme linked.

Leukocyte Surface Antigen Expression

Flow cytometry–based quantitation of specific surface antigen expression has become the standard for determining the types and subtypes of leukocytes present in blood. Fluorochrome-labeled monoclonal antibodies directed against specific surface antigens are used to label particular cell types, and the flow cytometer is used to rapidly count the numbers of labeled and unlabeled cells in the blood. From these counts, the cytometer then calculates an estimate of the percentage of cells bearing the antigen of interest. To determine the absolute number of a particular type of cell, a complete blood count must also be done. The product of the percentage of total cells that a particular cell type represents multiplied by the total cell number yields the absolute number. The nomenclature for the surface antigens used to identify cell types is based on "clusters of differentiation" (CDs) as defined by the International Workshop and Conference on Human Leukocyte Differentiation Antigens (Knapp et al, 1989). The presence/absence of individual or groups of CD antigens on a leukocyte allows its identification. The most commonly used CD antigens and the cell types they identify are given in Table 47–4.

Table 47–4 CD Antigens Commonly Used in Flow Cytometry to Quantitate the Percentages of Specific Blood Leukocytes

Cluster of Differentiation	Leukocyte Type
CD3	All T cells
CD4	Helper T cells
CD8	Suppressor T cells
CD9	All B cells
CD14	Monocytes
CD15	Granulocytes

The absence of particular CD antigens on a cell type can be diagnostic for a few specific conditions. The diagnosis of leukocyte adhesive protein deficiency is made by demonstrating that CD11b and CD18 antigens are missing from monocytes and granulocytes. Paroxysmal nocturnal hemoglobinuria is characterized by the absence of phosphoinositol-linked surface antigens on blood cells, including the absence of CD16 from blood monocytes.

Skin Tests

Administration of antigen into the skin to test either immediate or delayed-type hypersensitivity is used frequently in pediatrics. Prick testing, in which a sterile needle tip is coated with antigen and then used to prick the skin for delivery of a minute amount of the antigen, is commonly used to identify immediate-type hypersensitivity responses to allergens. The use of tiny amounts of material is intended to minimize the magnitude of the allergic response should an allergen be identified. Because anaphylactic reactions can occur even in the presence of tiny allergen exposures, the operator applying prick tests for diagnostic purposes should always be prepared to treat anaphylaxis. Rapid access to and familiarity with the use of emergency equipment and medications are necessary whenever testing for allergens is being done. Intradermal administration of antigen preparations can also be used to test immediate-type hypersensitivity, but more typically this method is used to assess delayed-type hypersensitivity responses. The validity and interpretation of skin test responses observed when intradermal tests are inadvertently administered subcutaneously are unknown. It is therefore important to be certain that intradermal skin tests be applied correctly to allow their correct interpretation.

Despite the many in vitro tests available for assessment for cell-mediated immunity, the intradermal skin test is still one of the best and simplest ways to determine whether these responses are intact. Failure to develop induration at an intradermal injection site 48 to 72 hours after antigen administration can be due to either lack of a previous exposure to the antigen or an inability to express delayed-type hypersensitivity (cutaneous anergy) to the applied antigen. To decide between these two possibilities, a control skin test that gives a positive response under normal conditions is usually administered at the same time as the test antigen, but at a different site. The choice of this control test is obviously important, because it must be an antigen that the patient has had sure contact with in the past. If the control response is positive and the test response is negative, previous exposure to the test antigen is unlikely. If the control response is negative and the test response is negative, the patient is anergic (i.e., unable to mount a delayed-type hypersensitivity response). If both control and test responses are positive, the interpretation is that the patient has had previous exposure to the test antigen.

Phagocyte Function Tests

In some instances, examination of phagocyte cell function is indicated. Phagocyte cell function is complex and highly integrated and requires considerable laboratory sophistication for analysis and interpretation. Because of the high levels of integration among specific phagocyte functions (e.g., phagocytosis and bactericidal activity, adherence and locomotion), a relatively minor abnormality in a selected in vitro function may reflect major clinical derangements of host defenses, and so testing of phagocyte function is usually done in dedicated research laboratories. The clinically relevant phagocyte function tests and the disease syndromes that they are used to diagnose are listed in Table 47–5.

Complement Tests

In humans, complement is a complex system in which the sequential assembly and activation of multimolecular convertases serve as a biological amplification system within the inflammatory response. Recognizable disorders of complement underlie less than 5% of inherited immunodeficiency diseases, but its participation in the inflammatory response makes testing of certain aspects of complement function common. In many laboratories, three complement-related tests are available: quantitation of serum C3 levels and C4 levels and estimation of total hemolytic complement activity. In dedicated research laboratories, methods exist for the quantitation and functional analysis of nearly every complement protein.

Blood specimens for complement tests must be handled carefully; several complement components are labile, and unrecognized loss of complement activity due to inappropriate specimen handling can be easily misinterpreted. Whole blood should be obtained by venipuncture, placed in a glass tube at room temperature for no longer than 30 minutes, and allowed to clot. After clot formation, the tube should be "rimmed" and the specimen held at 4°C for an additional 30 to 40 minutes to allow clot retraction. After clot retraction, the clot should be separated from serum by centrifugation; the serum is collected and either assayed immediately or frozen at −70°C until tested. Both C3 and C4 are acute phase reactants, meaning that acute inflammation usually increases their blood levels. Consumption of C3 and C4, diminished production in the liver, or inappropriate specimen handling may explain low levels. Total hemolytic complement activity is estimated on the basis of the CH_{50} determination (the titer of the patient's fresh serum that causes 50% hemolysis of sensitized erythrocytes). Terminal complement component deficiencies (C5–C9), because they interfere with the formation of the porin (membrane attack complex), are usually associated with low CH_{50} values.

Table 47–5 Clinically Useful Phagocyte Function Tests and Their Interpretation

Phagocyte Function Test	Interpretation
Nitroblue tetrazolium reduction	Absent/abnormal in chronic granulomatous disease
CD11/CD18 surface expression	Absent or diminished in leukocyte glycoprotein deficiency
Leukocyte peroxidase activity	Absent in myeloperoxidase deficiency
Examination of peripheral blood smear	Giant granules in nucleated cells in Chédiak-Higashi syndrome

References

Knapp W, Dörken B, et al: *Leukocyte Typing IV. White Cell Differentiation Antigens.* Oxford, Oxford University Press, 1989.

Moore RD, Lietman PS, Smith CR: Clinical response to aminoglycoside therapy: importance of the ratio of peak concentration to minimal inhibitory concentration. *J Infect Dis*, 155:93–99, 1987.

Neal PR, Kleiman MB, et al: Volume of blood submitted for culture from neonates. *J Clin Microbiol*, 24:353–356, 1986.

Nelson JD: Oral antibiotic therapy for serious infections in hospitalized patients. *J Pediatr*, 92: 175–176, 1978.

Shanson DC: Blood culture technique: current controversies. *J Antimicrob Chemother*, 25 (suppl C):17–29, 1990.

Sullivan TD, LaScolea LJ, Neter E: Relationship between the magnitude of bacteremia in children and the clinical disease. *Pediatrics*, 69:699–702, 1982.

Washington JA: The clinician and the microbiology laboratory: bacteria, fungi and parasites. In Mandell GL, Douglas RG, Bennett JE (eds): *Principles and Practice of Infectious Diseases*, 2nd ed. New York, John Wiley & Sons, 1979, p 108.

Washington JA: The role of the microbiology laboratory in the diagnosis and antimicrobial treatment of infective endocarditis. *Mayo Clin Proc*, 57:22–32, 1982.

Section N

Developmental Assessments

Chapter 48

Developmental and Psychological Assessment Procedures and Instruments

Kathleen E. Gilbride and Michael G. Regalado

Child health care providers have early and frequent contact with children and their families. This enables them to promote healthy developmental environments, identify children at risk for disabling conditions, and serve as advocates for children with special needs as part of their professional roles. Assessment of the child's developmental and psychological capabilities is an important aspect of these activities.

Assessment refers to the comprehensive evaluation of children to determine specific areas of cognitive, adaptive, and social-emotional strengths and deficits. *Developmental assessment* refers to the process of evaluating infants and preschool children who may have (1) relatively normal lags in development (e.g., late onset of speech); (2) difficulty adjusting at various developmental time periods (e.g., weaning, toilet training, birth of a sibling, entrance to kindergarten); or (3) significant developmental delays or disorders (e.g., mental retardation, autism, sensory impairments). Developmental assessment activities include surveillance, screening, and diagnostic evaluation. Psychological evaluations are comprehensive evaluations of preschool children, school-age children, and adolescents that include measures of cognition, academic achievement, adaptive skills, and personality or emotional functioning.

Both developmental and psychological assessments should involve integration of information obtained from observations, interviews, and tests across multiple settings (e.g., home, school, office) and from several sources (e.g., parents, teacher, day care provider, physician). The results of this evaluation process can be critical to making an accurate diagnosis and developing an effective intervention plan. Developmental and psychological assessments may be conducted by a single professional (e.g., child clinical psychologist) or may involve a team of professionals (e.g., physician, child psychologist, speech pathologist, physical therapist).

This chapter presents an overview of developmental and psychological procedures and instruments. The goal is to familiarize the reader with activities and instruments involved in evaluating child development and behavior in the context of routine health care delivery and in more thorough diagnostic evaluations when the need arises. Child health care clinicians are consulted frequently to give parenting advice, to evaluate problematic behavior, and to assess developmental achievement. The clinician should be able to evaluate the child's behavior to determine whether further assessment is required and should be familiar with resources and professional activities that are available to aid in evaluation.

PROPERTIES OF PSYCHOMETRIC INSTRUMENTS

Before continuing to an overview of specific testing procedures and instruments, we present a brief discussion of psychometric test properties useful in understanding and evaluating the strengths and weaknesses of a particular instrument. Psychometric tests vary in format and focus. Some instruments are questionnaires, whereas others require the examiner to elicit an observable response from the child. Psychometric tests may be either norm-referenced or criterion-referenced. Norm-referenced tests compare a child's performance relative to a specific group of children, which aids in interpreting the individual child's performance. A normative test score provides an indication of the average performance for the group, and how the individual child performs in comparison to this norm. The normative group is usually representative of the population as a whole (e.g., based on U.S. census data for race, age, geographic location, and socioeconomic level). Norm-referenced tests are preferred when measuring individual differences between children and assessing levels of proficiency. In contrast, criterion-referenced tests compare an individual child's performance to some predetermined criterion or established standard of performance. Thus, they measure the child's level of mastery and achievement of the criterion (e.g., able to spell 90% of words on a spelling test), not how the child compares with other children.

All psychometric tests, including screening tests, are judged based upon various test properties, particularly reliability and validity. *Reliability* refers to the amount of test measurement error between different observers (interobserver reliability), over time (test-retest reliability), or within the test itself (internal reliability or consistency), and is determined usually by correlating results of evaluations between observers, between different evaluations over time, or between different test items that measure the same psychological construct, respectively. Reliable instruments yield similar results over time regardless of who performs the test. *Validity* refers to whether the test measures what it purports to measure (content and construct validity) and whether the test predicts future outcome (predictive validity). Validity is evaluated by comparing a test with some "gold standard" concurrently or at some later age.

A useful way of evaluating the validity of a particular screening test is to determine the instrument's capability for identifying children who truly have developmental disability and excluding those who do not have a disability. This is accomplished most frequently using classificational analysis (Sackett et al, 1985), in which the occurrence of true-positives (TP), true-negatives (TN), false-positives (FP), and false-negatives (FN) is used to derive clinical indexes for evaluating the performance of a particular test. These indexes include *sensitivity* [TP/(TP + FN)], the proportion of individuals who are truly at risk and correctly classified as at risk; *specificity* [TN/(TN + FP)], the proportion of individuals truly not at risk and correctly classified as without risk; *false-negative fraction* [FP/(TP + FN)], the proportion incorrectly classified by the screening test to be without risk; and *predictive value of a positive test* [TP/(TP + FP)], the proportion of individuals classified as at risk who indeed are at risk (Meisels, 1989).

With regard to screening tests, there are some additional considerations. In evaluating a screening instrument it is important to know the two types of error rates, that is, false-positives and false-negatives. The ideal screening instrument would have a 100% sensitivity, that is, no false-negatives, and 100% specificity (or 0% false-negative fraction), that is, no false-positives. When a test uses a cut-off point or criterion score performance, that is, a certain number of failures to define classification as being at risk, then changing the cut-off score reduces one error rate and necessarily increases the other. For example, if a cut-off score of five failures is changed to four failures, it is likely to increase the number of children identified as at risk, thereby increasing its sensitivity, but also would likely increase the number of children falsely identified as at risk, thereby reducing the specificity. The choice of criterion score for a screening test is based upon a decision regarding which type of error one prefers to make.

Another consideration is the effect of the base rate of the particular condition for which one is screening. A condition's prevalence in the population being screened will affect the significance of a positive or negative test classification. A condition with an extremely low prevalence, as is the case for many of the developmental disabilities, will inflate the significance of the false-negative fraction. For example, a screening test that has a specificity of 99% (false-negative fraction of 1%) will falsely classify 90% of individuals identified to be at risk for a condition that has a prevalence of 1:1000, even with a sensitivity of 99%.

DEVELOPMENTAL ASSESSMENT

Developmental Screening

Selection of a screening test depends on individual circumstances, including time constraints, population served, and personal style but should also consider the test's psychometric properties. It has been suggested that conservative requirements for both test sensitivity and specificity be at least .80 (Meisels, 1989).

Denver Developmental Screening Test (DDST; DDST-R; Denver II)

The DDST is the most widely used developmental screening tool in this country. Standardized on a Denver area sample and first published in 1967, it originally consisted of 105 test items selected from other existing developmental and psychometric instruments on the basis of ease of administration and time span across which most children could accomplish an item (Frankenburg and Dodds, 1967). The test has been revised twice and restandardized (Frankenburg and Dodds, 1975, 1992), and it now has 125 test items, including more language items and a behavior rating scale. The items are arranged in one of four functional categories: gross motor, fine motor–adaptive, language, and personal-social. The categories yield pass, fail, or questionable scores using parental interview and observation of spontaneous and elicited responses. The test covers ages 2 weeks through 6 years and takes 10 to 20 minutes to administer. The Denver test has been criticized for its poor sensitivity, that is, *underidentifying* children who have a developmental disability (Meisels, 1989).

Denver Prescreening Developmental Questionnaire (PDQ and R-PDQ)

Because of the time required to routinely perform screening tests, most health professionals use them primarily to confirm their clinical impressions (Smith, 1978). The Denver group recommends a two-stage approach to developmental screening. The first step uses the PDQ (Frankenburg et al, 1976, 1987), which includes 97 of the 105 DDST items formulated into questions answered by the parent in 10 minutes. Poor performance on the prescreening questionnaire indicates the need for thorough screening evaluation using the DDST. Caution must be used in using the PDQ because it has the same sensitivity problems as the DDST has from which it was derived.

Home Screening Questionnaire (HSQ)

The HSQ was designed for use with *high-risk* infants to measure the quality of home environmental factors demonstrated to correlate with cognitive development (Frankenburg and Coons, 1986). It is not appropriate for use with low-risk children or to measure emotional climates or other environmental aspects of the home. The HSQ consists of two forms completed by parents, one for birth to 3 years and one for 3 to 6 years, and does not require a home visit. Questionnaires have 30 and 34 multiple choice questions, respectively, formulated at a third to sixth grade reading level. The questionnaire takes 15 to 20 minutes to complete with 5 minutes to score. Using the HSQ may raise parental consciousness about the importance of the learning environment at home.

Batelle Developmental Inventory

The Batelle Developmental Inventory (Newborg et al, 1984) combines historical, observational, and structured test items into categories of adaptive, gross motor, fine motor, receptive language, expressive language, cognitive, and personal-social skills. The screening test uses 96 out of the 341 items in the full battery. It uses a basal-ceiling scoring system, with raw scores converted into either T scores or deviation quotients (mean = 100, SD = 15). It covers ages birth to 8 years and takes about 30 minutes to administer. Standardization is satisfactory, based on the 1981 U.S. census data, with high reliability (test-retest and inter-rater) and acceptable validity. Guidelines for referral are provided based upon subtest scores. As with other interview screening instruments, reliability of the informant's report also determines how valid the results are.

Child Development Inventory (CDI)

The CDI is a questionnaire completed by the parent containing 270 empirically derived, short "yes and no" questions that describe children's development and behavior (Ireton, 1992). It is designed for children ages 1 to 6½ years and takes about 30 minutes to complete. Eight categorical scales are derived from the questionnaire: gross motor, fine motor, expressive language, comprehension-conceptual, situation comprehension, self-help, personal-social, and a general development scale composed of the most discriminating items from the seven other scales.

Early Language Milestone scale (ELM)

There may be occasions when a more specific focus on language development is desirable. The ELM is an inventory of 41 language items intended for use in the first 3 years of life (Coplan, 1984). It broadly assesses communication by evaluating receptive and expressive communicative abilities expressed visually and auditorily. The ELM was standardized on a sample of 191 children representing a demographic cross section of the Syracuse, New York area. A study of the instrument's concurrent validity using a clinically referred sample of 119 children showed a sensitivity of .97 and a specificity of .93 in determining the presence of developmental disabilities (Coplan, 1984).

Pediatric Symptom Checklist (PSC)

Few screening measures exist for behavioral and emotional problems. One reason for this is the difficulty inherent in the conceptualization and diagnostic classification of behavioral and emotional problems in young children, particularly in infants. For instance, behavioral problems in infants cannot be conceptualized outside the context of the parent-infant-family relationship, and an accepted classification system for relationship disorders does not yet exist (Sameroff and Emde, 1989). In spite of the difficulties inherent in screening for emotional and behavioral problems, mental health screening is an important health surveillance activity (Dailard and Melden, 1992).

The PSC is an example of a mental health screening tool for school-age children. It is a 35-item questionnaire completed by parents of 6- to 12-year-old children. It takes 3 to 5 minutes to complete and evaluates the parent's view of the child's psychosocial functioning in different contexts as well as the child's general mood (Jellinek et al, 1986). The PSC has been cross-validated against multiple measures to test its effectiveness for determining the need for further evaluation of possible psychosocial disturbance using a small, limited sample of 300 English-speaking 6- to 12-year-olds in the Boston area. Compared with the Children's Global Assessment Scale, the PSC has a sensitivity of .95 and a specificity of .68 (Jellinek et al, 1988).

For a more comprehensive inventory of instruments, see Mitchell (1985).

Screening tests were intended for testing whole populations for conditions that were not clinically evident based on assumptions of available early treatment and cost-effectiveness (Frankenburg, 1973; Whitby, 1974). However, developmental screening tests in general do not meet these assumptions, are too lengthy to be administered routinely, and suffer from reliability and validity problems (Dworkin, 1989b). Furthermore, the efficiency of a screening test is influenced greatly by the prevalence of the disorder in question, as noted previously. The early identification of developmentally disabling conditions has become a major focus of developmental monitoring, particularly since the passage of Public Law 99-457, the Amendments to the Education for All Handicapped Children Act. That law mandated services for children with special needs from birth (Blackman et al, 1992). Clinicians are confronted with the problem that public policy is far ahead of the system's ability to meet the legal mandate, particularly as far as infants and toddlers are concerned. While many developmental screening tests are available to aid the clinician in determining an individual child's risk for later disability and/or need of diagnostic evaluation, no single test can be recommended with confidence for mass screening purposes at this time.

Developmental Surveillance

Because screening instruments for developmental disabilities are inaccurate, their use should remain part of a more general surveillance strategy. The breadth of clinical problems that a pediatrician is likely to encounter in practice is wide and includes mental retardation, neuromuscular conditions such as cerebral palsy, speech and language disorders, school-related learning problems, and emotional-behavioral problems. Within any clinical picture, individual motor, cognitive, linguistic, and social influences may dominate and/or interact with each other. Adding to the complexity of clinical assessment of developmental and behavioral problems is the transactional nature of development (Sameroff and Chandler, 1975). Biological and environmental factors are in dynamic flux, each influencing change in the other over time. This makes developmental assessment particularly challenging.

Anticipatory guidance, early identification of developmental disabilities, and advocacy can be subsumed under the concept of developmental surveillance. All of these activities involve some ongoing appraisal of a child's development and behavior as part of the larger picture of child health care maintenance (Dworkin, 1989a; Hutchison and Nicoll, 1988). Developmental surveillance requires a solid knowledge base of child development and developmental processes. It assumes accessibility to the health care system and health care provider, continuity of care, and participation of both clinician and family. In the well-child care setting, appraisals of development and behavior include a determination of a child's abilities as well as the ability of the caregiving environment to foster developmental achievement. Parental concerns and perspectives are elicited and considered carefully in the assessment process. This process creates a cumulative database that enables the clinician to individualize health care advice, foster adaptive parenting, and determine whether behavior in a particular context is problematic and warrants further investigation. If developmental progress is not proceeding appropriately, it may signal the existence of a developmentally disabling condition. The administration of a screening test then can be useful within the larger process of developmental assessment. Additionally, as a semistructured play opportunity, it can be an important educational and therapeutic modality beyond its screening intent (Parker and Zuckerman, 1990).

When to Refer

Referral to a specialist or multidisciplinary group should be done when behavior or developmental progress is worrisome to the clinician and/or parent. Referral for a comprehensive evaluation is appropriate when a problem is identified but the specific diagnosis is unclear and additional information is needed. For example, an evaluation is appropriate when the clinician is trying to differentiate among borderline or mild intellectual impairment versus specific learning disabilities versus depression resulting in cognitive impairment. Comprehensive evaluation is also appropriate when an initial diagnosis has been made (e.g., mental retardation, learning disability, depression, autism) but more information is needed to develop an intervention program. For example, is the mental retardation mild or moderate? Is the learning disability limited to reading or does it include spelling and math? How severe is the depression and is it related to an acute event or might it be more enduring? Is the child with autism mildly or moderately retarded? Comprehensive evaluation is needed in follow-up to identify progress or change in status and to update the intervention plan. Referrals should be made sensitively and discretely so as not to alarm parents needlessly, and diagnoses should not be proffered (Meisels, 1985).

Diagnostic Developmental Assessment of Children 0 to 3

Once a concern has been raised and the need for further testing determined, an in-depth developmental assessment can accurately determine the nature of any suspected delays, delineate areas for intervention, and assess progress following intervention. Standardized measures of developmental assessment provide information regarding the current functioning of an infant but do not have good predictive validity. In part, this is because assessment of early infancy focuses on sensorimotor functions, whereas language becomes more important after 18 months. Also, development is a dynamic process that often occurs in spurts and lags, and thus changes dramatically in the first few years of life. The exception appears to be children identified as moderately to severely retarded in infancy (Dubose, 1976; Vander Veer and Schweid, 1974). These children remain retarded, although early intervention is important for optimizing their developmental outcome. Overall, repeated measures over time are needed to accurately monitor developmental progress.

Gesell developmental schedules

The Gesell schedules are designed for infants aged 4 weeks to 36 months and divide behavior into five areas: Language, Adaptive, Personal-Social, Fine Motor, and Gross Motor skills (Knobloch and Pasamanick, 1974). The instrument was not designed as a measure of intelligence but to identify normal developmental patterns and deviations from normal expected development (Gesell and Amatruda, 1945). They provide age scores in each domain, and a developmental quotient can be calculated. The scale is particularly useful for its clinical assessment of intra-infant variability. However, it has been criticized for its lack of rigorous standardization, which is based upon a small sample drawn from a limited geographic area and is not stratified by race, parental education, or socioeconomic level.

Bayley Scales of Infant Development (BSIDII)

The BSID is the most psychometrically sound infant measure developed to date and thus is widely used in clinical and research settings (Bayley, 1969, 1993). The BSID draws many of its items from the Gesell, but is organized strictly by percentage of passes at each age level. It was restandardized as the BSIDII on 1700 infants 1 to 42 months of age, and stratified by geographic area, sex, race, and education of parent. It consists of the Mental Scale, the Motor Scale, and the Behavior Rating Scale. Standardized scores (mean = 100, SD = 15) are computed for the Mental and Motor Scales. Items are grouped into one of four facets (Cognitive, Language, Personal/Social, Motor) to aid in interpretation. It has very good internal reliability and moderate predictive validity for children 24 to 30 months of age. The Behavior Rating Scale provides ratings of the child's behavioral style during the evaluation.

PSYCHOLOGICAL ASSESSMENT

A complete diagnostic assessment battery for preschool and school-age children should include a detailed developmental history, a clinical interview with the child, and measures of overall cognitive functioning, visual-motor skills, expressive and receptive language, adaptive skills, behavior problems, and emotional functioning. Additional tests exist for further specifying particular areas of difficulty (e.g., for determining the specific nature of a reading disability).

There are several test instruments available for evaluating cognition, language, visual-motor skills, etc. The task of the psychologist is to determine which test is best suited for evaluating an individual child's capabilities. This decision should be based on the specific referral question, the characteristics of the child, and the qualities of the test. The most commonly used test instruments for each area are reviewed here.

Cognitive Assessment of Children

A measure of cognitive ability is essential in determining whether a child is developmentally delayed, has learning problems, or is cognitively affected by emotional or environmental events. Interest in standardized cognitive assessment began as a result of Alfred Binet's work in the area of mental deficiency, as he devised ways of identifying retarded children in need of special education (Binet and Simon, 1916). Definitions of intelligence vary widely but generally include the ability to learn, adapt, and solve problems (Sattler, 1988). Tests of intelligence, or cognitive functioning, have evolved significantly since Binet's time but continue to be most useful for predicting school achievement.

Stanford-Binet

The Stanford-Binet was one of the earliest measures designed for assessing intelligence. It has been revised several times, with the current version, the fourth edition, published in 1986 (Thorndike et al, 1986). It is designed for ages 2 years to adulthood. It consists of four areas: Verbal Reasoning, Abstract/Visual Reasoning, Quantitative Reasoning, and Short-Term Memory. A Standardized Area Score is computed for each area (mean = 100, SD = 16), and a Test Composite Score is computed from the four area scores (mean = 100, SD = 16). Within each area, individual subtests are administered, and these provide Standard Age Scores (mean = 50, SD = 10). Comparisons across area scores allow one to identify strengths and deficits and to separate verbal from nonverbal skills. The test is well standardized on 5013 people ranging from 2 to 23 years, stratified by geographic region, age, gender, ethnicity, and socioeconomic status, based on 1980 census data. It has excellent reliability (internal consistency and test-retest reliability) and satisfactory concurrent and predictive validity. The primary drawback to this test is that it is lengthy to administer, which may be taxing for younger children, and it has a limited number of items at the 2- and 3-year levels, providing less information for these ages.

Wechsler tests of intelligence

The Wechsler tests were designed initially as alternative measures of intelligence, and they separate intelligence into verbal and nonverbal abilities, employing deviation intelligence quotients (IQs) (Wechsler, 1949). Previously, IQs were derived by dividing mental age by chronological age, and multiplying by 100.

Wechsler maintained that IQs should be obtained by comparing scores to those earned by same-aged peers in a standardization sample. Deviation IQs are standardized scores that are more psychometrically sound and allow comparison across ages.

The Wechsler Preschool and Primary Scale of Intelligence–Revised (WPPSI-R) assesses children 3 years to 7 years, 3 months (Wechsler, 1989), and the Wechsler Intelligence Scale for Children III (WISC III) is for children 6 years to 16 years, 11 months (Wechsler, 1991). Both tests provide a Full Scale IQ, a Verbal IQ, and a Performance IQ (mean = 100, SD = 15). Subtests within the Verbal and Performance Scales provide information about a variety of skills within each domain, and a scaled score is achieved for each subtest (mean = 10, SD = 3). Profiles of scaled scores in each area allow for pattern analysis of strengths and weaknesses, as do factor scores that are available for Verbal Comprehension, Perceptual Organization, Freedom From Distractibility, and Processing Speed. Both tests are well standardized with updated norms and adequate reliability and validity. Separate verbal and nonverbal IQs make these tests useful for assessing children with limited language skills or learning problems.

The WPPSI-R is lengthy to administer and is not as useful with children who have visual, auditory, or motor impairments. Also, IQ norms for both tests extend down to only 40 or 41, so that they are not able to provide scores for retarded children below this point (the Stanford-Binet extends down to a score of 36).

McCarthy scales of children's abilities

The McCarthy scales are designed for children 2½ to 8½ years of age (McCarthy, 1972). They provide a General Cognitive Index (mean = 100, SD = 16), which is comprised of Verbal, Perceptual, and Quantitative Scales (mean = 50, SD = 10). In addition, they have a Memory and a Motor Scale (mean = 50, SD = 10). The profile of scale scores allows one to identify specific strengths and weaknesses. The items at the lower ages are especially appealing to younger children, and the gross motor component is a useful feature not included on other preschool measures. The test is well standardized, based on the 1970 census data. The standardization group consists of 1032 children, stratified by age, sex, race, geographic region, and father's occupation. The internal reliability is extremely good for the general cognitive index and satisfactory for the five scales. The test-retest reliability indicates appropriate stability over time. Concurrent validity with the Stanford-Binet, Wechsler Intelligence Scale for Children–Revised (WISC-R), and WPPSI is acceptable, although the McCarthy is noted to produce lower global scores than these other measures. Predictive validity is satisfactory using correlations with later achievement measures (Kaufman and Kaufman, 1977).

Leiter International Performance Scale

The Leiter scale is a nonverbal measure of intelligence that is useful for children with language difficulties or hearing impairments (Leiter, 1948). It requires no verbal instructions on the examiner's part, only pointing, and no verbal response from the child. The child's task is to match a series of blocks to a legend (mounted on a frame) based on color, shape, number, pattern, or abstract concept. The tasks become progressively more difficult at each age level, between 2 and 18 years. The test provides an IQ score using the ratio method (mental age divided by chronological age, multiplied by 100). This test has significant limitations in that the norms are dated, the standardization was inadequate, and little information is available regarding reliability. It appears to have adequate validity, as it correlates significantly with other intelligence tests, although IQ scores are lower on the Leiter than on other measures (Ratcliffe and Ratcliffe, 1980). It is best used as an adjunct to other tests for clinical diagnosis, especially when language-impaired children are evaluated.

Tests of Language

Many cognitive instruments contain measures of language (e.g., the WISC III has measures of vocabulary and verbal similarities); however, additional language measures may be needed to further delineate language deficits and strengths. Any assessment of language should include measures of receptive and expressive skills.

Peabody Picture Vocabulary Test–Revised (PPVT-R)

The PPVT-R is a measure of receptive vocabulary designed for ages 2 ½ years to adulthood (Dunn and Dunn, 1981). The child is shown a group of four pictures and asked to point to the one that is named by the examiner (e.g., doll, chair). No expressive language is required on the child's part. The test provides a standardized score (mean = 100, SD = 15), percentile rank, and age equivalent. Reliability and validity are adequate, although standard scores are lower for ethnic minority children than with other measures of verbal cognition (e.g., WISC-R). Thus, the test is primarily useful for assessing the language comprehension of children who have expressive difficulties and should not be used as a measure of general cognitive ability (Sattler, 1988).

Reynell developmental language scales

The Reynell Scales (Reynell, 1969) assess verbal comprehension and expressive language in children from 1 to 6 years of age. They consist of 134 items that can be administered in less than 30 minutes. They provide standard scores, percentile ranks, and age equivalents. The standardization, based on 600 children stratified by geographic region, ethnicity, and parental education, is somewhat limited. The test appears most useful for young or developmentally delayed children with language difficulties, especially if used in conjunction with other language and cognitive measures.

Tests of Visual-Motor and Visual-Perceptual Skills

Assessment of visual-motor and visual-perceptual skills is necessary, given their relevance to academic success. For example, these skills are essential to learning how to read, write, spell, and understand mathematical relationships. Tests of intelligence usually contain subtests assessing aspects of these abilities; however, additional tests are useful for detection of deficits or strengths in these areas.

Bender Visual-Motor Gestalt Test

The Bender-Gestalt test (Bender, 1938) is widely used as a developmental measure of visual-motor maturation in children. Nine geometric forms are shown individually to the child, who is asked to copy them on a blank, unlined sheet of paper. Designs are scored according to the Koppitz Developmental Bender Scoring System (Koppitz, 1975). Scores are based on number of errors made, with errors including distortion of shape, rotation, integration difficulties, and perseveration; certain kinds of errors at upper age levels are used as indicators of brain injury. Standard scores (mean = 100, SD = 15) and age equivalents are available for children 5 years to 11 years, 11 months. The test-retest reliability and validity are not high enough to use it for diagnostic decisions, so it should be included as one measure in a battery of tests.

Beery Test of Visual-Motor Integration (VMI)

The VMI is designed for children 4 to 13 years of age (Beery, 1989). The child copies up to 24 designs, or until three consecutive failures are reached. It provides a standardized score (mean = 100, SD = 15), percentile rank, and age equivalent. Reliability and validity studies are based on the original 1964 norms; thus with this test, as with the Bender-Gestalt, diagnostic decisions should be made in conjunction with other test data.

Adaptive Measures

Measures of adaptive or self-help skills provide information about how children actually function in their world. In addition, when making an assessment of mental retardation, a measure of adaptive behavior is critical, as a child must be significantly delayed in adaptive functioning as well as in cognitive functioning to be classified as retarded (Grossman, 1983).

Vineland adaptive behavior scales

The Vineland scales (Sparrow et al, 1984) are the most commonly used measure of adaptive functioning. They can be used from birth to age 19 years. They are administered by interviewing a respondent familiar with the child (usually the parents) about behavior in four domains: communication, daily living skills, socialization, and motor skills. A score is given in each area and for the adaptive behavior composite (mean = 100, SD = 15). The instrument has been well standardized; however, there are great fluctuations in mean scores from age group to age group. Thus, caution is recommended for relying solely on this measure for diagnostic purposes (Silverstein, 1986). Also, because it is based on the respondent's perceptions, the reliability of his or her perceptions must be taken into account.

Achievement Tests

Assessment of academic achievement is essential in school-age children when a question of learning problems arises. For children who are referred for evaluation of emotional or behavior problems, a measure of academic achievement helps determine how these problems affect school performance, or even how learning difficulties may result in behavior or emotional problems.

Wide Range Achievement Test–3 (WRAT-3)

The WRAT-3 (Wilkinson, 1993) is the best-known achievement test because it is a brief, easily administered test of reading, spelling, and arithmetic. The Reading subtest assesses the ability to recognize letters and pronounce words but does not include reading comprehension. The Spelling subtest requires children to copy designs resembling letters, write their names, and write words from dictation. The arithmetic subtest includes counting, verbal math problem solving, and completing written math problems. It is designed for ages 5 years to adulthood and provides standardized scores (mean = 100, SD = 15), percentile ranks, and grade equivalents. It is standardized on a large sample, stratified for age, sex, race, geographical region, and metropolitan/nonmetropolitan residence. Reliability and validity are adequate. Because it is a brief measure, it is best used as a general assessment of academic functioning, but it should not be used alone for academic planning.

Behavior Rating Scales

In addition to standardized tests administered to children, behavior rating scales are often used to gain information about a child's behavior in the home, school, and day care or afterschool care. Standardized behavior rating scales allow one to compare a child's behavior with that of same-aged and even same-sexed peers, providing an indication of how common particular behaviors are for a given age or sex (e.g., hyperactivity, fearfulness, stealing).

Child Behavior Checklist (CBCL)

The CBCL is one of the best-standardized scales available (Achenbach, 1991). There are several versions available, including one for ages 2 to 3 years and one for ages 4 to 16 years, both of which are to be completed by the parent or caregiver. There is also a teacher report form for ages 4 to 16 years and a self-report form for ages 11 to 18 years. The checklist contains a list of behaviors, which are rated on a 0 to 2 point scale for being not true, somewhat true, or very often true. Items are separated into different scales based on factor analysis (e.g., social withdrawal, somatic complaints, hyperactive, aggressive, depressed), and the scales are grouped into two broad factors, internalizing and externalizing. Standardized T scores are available (mean = 50, SD = 10), based on age and gender. Reliability and validity are adequate, though interpretation must bear in mind that scores are based on the perceptions of the respondent.

Connors behavior rating scale

The Connors scale is also a popular measure, especially for assessing hyperactive behaviors (Connors, 1989). It can be completed by parents or teachers, and there are long and short versions for each. It is designed for children 3 to 17 years of age. A list of behaviors is rated from 0 to 3 for occurring not at all, just a little, pretty much, and very much. Items are divided into factors (e.g., conduct problem, learning problem, psychosomatic, impulsive-hyperactive, and anxiety). Age by sex normative data are available, using standardized T scores (mean = 50, SD = 10). T scores above 70 (two or more standard deviations above the mean) are considered significant. Reliability and validity data are satisfactory, and, as with the CBCL, interpretation should consider that data are based on perceptions of behavior.

Measures of Emotional Functioning

Assessment of children's emotional functioning, or personality characteristics, is often completed by means of objective measures of personality or subjective measures of personality, usually referred to as projective techniques. Objective measures, which are usually paper and pencil inventories describing personality characteristics, have gained popularity because they are quantifiable and can be used to obtain norm-referenced scores. As a result, they are often more reliable and valid than less structured projective techniques. They are also easy to administer and score in a relatively brief period of time. In contrast, projective techniques can offer indirect ways of assessing emotional factors or personality characteristics that may not be so apparent on objective tests. This may be the case with children who are guarded, are defensive, or desire to be socially appropriate on objective measures. In terms of projective techniques, the underlying rationale is that when presented with an ambiguous, unstructured task or set of stimuli (e.g., pictures of family scenes), children will project onto the stimulus their own perceptions of the world, including how they view themselves and their relationships with others. These responses can then be interpreted in terms of how accurately the child views the world, how emotionally distressed he/she is, what his/her coping mechanisms are, and how at risk for emotional disturbance he/she is. Both kinds of measures can be useful in a comprehensive assessment battery.

Personality Inventory for Children (PIC)

The PIC is an example of an objective measure of personality for children (Wirt et al, 1977). It consists of 600 true-false questions completed by parents. The items are designed to describe personality or emotional characteristics for children aged 6 to 16 years. It has three validity scales to assess distortions or defensiveness, and 13 clinical scales, which identify personality traits and adjustment patterns. T scores are available for each scale (mean = 50, SD = 10) based on age norms, with scores over 70 indicating disturbance. While providing quantitative data on emotional functioning, it is unclear that the PIC yields significantly more useful information than a clinical interview with the parents. More research is needed to determine its long-term usefulness in diagnosis.

Apperception Tests

The most common projective techniques used with children include apperception tests, such as the Thematic Apperception Test (TAT) (Murray, 1943) or the Roberts Apperception Test (McArthur and Roberts, 1982). The latter tool is gaining in popularity because it consists of pencil drawings of children in commonly occurring situations (e.g., pictured with peers, with parents, with a new sibling) that are more up to date and child oriented than the older TAT, with its darker, more dated settings (e.g., a boy staring at a violin). Also, the Roberts has an objective scoring system for quantifying responses, whereas the TAT has no accepted scoring system or normative data. This may lend the Roberts to being a more reliable and valid measure of emotional functioning; however, to date few research studies have been reported on this instrument.

Sentence Completion Tests

The Incomplete Sentence technique (Rotter and Rafferty, 1958) is also often used to assess a child's projection of relationships, self-esteem, fears, needs, and strengths. The child is asked to complete a series of sentences, such as "My mother . . . " and "At school . . . ." Responses can be scored for degree of conflict, but usually, general themes are abstracted from the responses. Like other projective techniques, it has limited reliability and validity. The information obtained is integrated with other sources of information about the child to create a picture of the child's overall emotional functioning.

Children's Drawings

Human figure drawings (e.g., Draw A Man, House-Tree-Person, Kinetic Family Drawing) can be useful in looking at both developmental factors (e.g., age-appropriate details) and emotional factors. They can provide clues as to a child's view of his or her own body image, family relationships, and self-esteem. They can be especially useful with children who have verbal difficulties, with shy or withdrawn children, or to break the ice with children in the beginning of an assessment. While various methods of interpreting drawings have been presented (Di Leo, 1973), none have been shown to have good reliability or validity. Thus, as with all projective techniques, the information obtained can be used to develop hypotheses regarding the child's emotional functioning and specific issues of concern, but it should never be used alone as the basis of a diagnosis.

Limitations of Testing

When interpreting test results, one must be aware of how the characteristics of the child, the test, and the context all affect the outcome obtained. These characteristics may limit the reliability or validity of the information produced, and the clinician must make decisions within the constraints imposed by these limits.

Common characteristics of children that affect test performance include age, temperament, and physical and emotional states. Older children tend to produce more stable performances, as they are able to attend for longer periods of time, and their experience with school has prepared them for the testing situation (i.e., they are familiar with paper and pencil tasks, and responding to questions). Younger children may need several sessions to complete a test battery given their shorter attention span. The temperamental style of an individual child, regardless of age, may make the evaluation process easy or difficult and can affect the pace at which the testing proceeds. For example, quiet, inhibited children may need more time to adjust and thus may not respond to test questions initially. Talkative, hyperactive children may have impaired performance because of their impulsivity. The time of day the tests are administered may determine the child's performance, as fatigue or hunger can be interfering factors. Also, children who are evaluated at stressful times in their life (e.g., following a separation from parents or a prolonged illness) may not perform at an optimal level. All of these conditions should be qualified in the test report, so that the clinician can make a judgment about the usefulness of the results obtained.

Environmental factors determine the context in which the results are obtained. For example, the socioeconomic status of the family, the ethnicity and culture of the family, and the primary language spoken in the home should all be taken into consideration when interpreting test results. Minority children from low socioeconomic status backgrounds traditionally score lower on standardized tests, especially those in which language skills are heavily weighted. In such cases, nonverbal measures of ability should be included in the assessment battery, or tests with standardized norms for minorities should be used. Some tests are designed to be "culture free"; however, the extent to which these tests are truly culturally unbiased is controversial (Sattler, 1988).

The clinician should also be aware of the limits of the specific tests used in the evaluation, in terms of their reliability and construct, content, and predictive validity. Developmental tests in infancy, for example, have low predictive validity for school performance because of the major developmental changes that occur in cognition over the first 5 years of life. Thus, the results of a test could be used to develop an infant stimulation program for current functioning but should not be used for informing parents about their child's future functioning.

The clinician should not make a diagnosis based on test data alone. The assessment process should lead to decision making based on the integration of several sources of information, and the assessment should be periodically repeated, with diagnoses and interventions updated. Only with repeated measures over time of multiple areas can accurate diagnoses and effective interventions be made.

SUMMARY AND CONCLUDING REMARKS

Comprehensive health care maintenance for children includes addressing developmental and behavioral issues. The health care clinician can play an active role as advisor and advocate, and must play a central role in the early identification of children at risk for developmental disabilities. This entails ongoing developmental surveillance supplemented by developmental screening instruments when an objective measure is needed. If a child is determined to be at risk for developmental problems, a referral should be made for a comprehensive developmental or psychological evaluation to determine an appropriate diagnosis and treatment plan.

The process of assessment should be a comprehensive one, integrating multiple sources of information across multiple settings. This requires a sound knowledge of child development and behavior, experience in observing children's behavior, informed use of screening tests, and knowledge of the roles and activities of other professionals who evaluate and treat children's developmental and psychological problems.

References

Achenbach T: *Manual for the Child Behavior Checklist.* Burlington, VT, University of Vermont, 1991.

Bayley N: *Manual for the Bayley Scales of Infant Development.* Berkeley, CA, Psychological Corporation, 1969.

Bayley N: *Bayley Scores of Infant Development,* 2nd ed. The Psychological Corporation, San Antonio, TX, 1993.

Beery K: *The Development Test of Visual-Motor Integration.* Cleveland, OH, Modern Curriculum Press, 1989.

Bender L: A visual-motor Gestalt test and its clinical use. *American Orthopsychiatric Association Research Monograph,* 3, 1938.

Binet A, Simon T: *The Development of Intelligence in Children.* Baltimore, MD, Williams & Wilkins, 1916.

Blackman J, Healy A, Ruppert E: Impetus from public law 99–457. *Pediatrics,* 89:98–102, 1992.

Connors K: *Connors Rating Scales.* New York, Multi-Health Systems, 1989.

Coplan J: *ELM (Early Language Milestone Scale)-Revised.* Tulsa, OK, Modern Education Corporation, 1984.

Dailard C, Melden M: Screening for mental health problems in children. *Clearing House Rev* 26:898–905, 1992.

Di Leo J: *Children's Drawings as Diagnostic Aids.* New York, Brunner/Mazel, 1973.

Dubose R: Predictive value of infant intelligence scales with muiltipli-handicapped children. *Am J Ment Defic,* 81:388–390, 1976.

Dunn L, Dunn L: *Peabody Picture Vocabulary Test-*

Revised. Circle Pines, MN, American Guidance Service, 1981.

Dworkin P: British and American recommendations for developmental monitoring: The role of surveillance. *Pediatrics*, 84:1000–1010, 1989a.

Dworkin P: Developmental screening—Expecting the impossible? *Pediatrics*, 83:619–622, 1989b.

Frankenburg W: Pediatric screening. *Adv Pediatr*, 20:149–175, 1973.

Frankenburg W, Coons C: Home screening questionnaire: Its validity in assessing home environment. *J Pediatr*, 108:624–626, 1986.

Frankenburg W, Dodds J: *Denver Developmental Screening Test-Revised (DDST)*. Denver, CO, DDM, Inc., 1975.

Frankenburg W, Dodds J: The Denver Developmental Screening Test. *J Pediatr*, 71:181–191, 1967.

Frankenburg W, Dodds J: The Denver II: a major revision and restandardization of the Denver Developmental Screening Test. *Pediatrics*, 89: 91–97, 1992.

Frankenburg W, Fandal A, Thornton S: Revision of Denver Prescreening Developmental Questionnaire. *J Pediatr*, 110:653–657, 1987.

Frankenburg W, van Doornick W, Liddell T: *The Denver Prescreening Developmental Questionnaire (PDQ)*. Denver, CO, DDM, Inc., 1976.

Gesell A, Amatruda C: *The Embryology of Behavior*. New York, Harper & Brothers, 1945.

Grossman H: *Classification in Mental Retardation*. Washington, DC, American Association on Mental Deficiency, 1983.

Hutchison T, Nicoll A: Developmental screening and surveillance. *Br J Hosp Med*, 39:22–29, 1988.

Ireton H: *The Child Development Inventory Manual*. Minneapolis, MN, Behavioral Science Systems, 1992.

Jellinek M, Murphy J, Burns B: Brief psychosocial screening in outpatient pediatric practice. *J Pediatr*, 109:371–378, 1986.

Jellinek M, Murphy J, Robinson J, et al: Pediatric symptom checklist: Screening school-age children for psychosocial dysfunction. *J Pediatr*, 112: 201–209, 1988.

Kaufman A, Kaufman N: *Clinical Evaluation of Young Children With the McCarthy Scales*. New York, Grune & Stratton, 1977.

Knobloch H, Pasamanick B: *Gesell and Amatruda's Developmental Diagnosis: The Evaluation and Management of Normal and Abnormal Neuropsychologic Development in Infancy and Early Childhood*. New York, Harper & Row, 1974.

Koppitz E: *The Bender Gestalt Test for Young Children*, Vol 2: *Research and Application. 1963–73*. New York, Grune & Stratton, 1975.

Leiter R: *Leiter International Performance Scale*. Chicago, Stoeling Co., 1948.

McArthur D, Roberts G: *Roberts Apperception Test for Children Manual*. Los Angeles, CA, Western Psychological Services, 1982.

McCarthy D: *Manual for the McCarthy Scales of Children's Abilities*. New York, Psychological Corporation, 1972.

Meisels S: *Developmental Screening in Early Childhood: A Guide. Revised Edition*. Washington, DC, National Association for the Education of Young Children, 1985.

Meisels S: Can developmental screening tests identify children who are developmentally at risk? *Pediatrics*, 83:578–585, 1989.

Mitchell JJ: *The Ninth Mental Measurements Yearbook*, Vols 1–2. Lincoln, NE, The Buros Institute of Mental Measurements of the University of Nebraska-Lincoln, 1985.

Murray H: *Thematic Apperception Test: Pictures and Manual*. Cambridge, MA, Harvard University Press, 1943.

Newborg J, Stock J, Guidubaldi J, et al: *Batelle Developmental Inventory Screening Test*. Allen, TX, DLM-Teaching Resources, 1984.

Parker S, Zuckerman B: Therapeutic aspects of the assessment process. In Meisels S, Shonkoff J (eds): *Handbook of Early Childhood Intervention*. New York, Cambridge University Press, 1990.

Ratcliffe M, Ratcliffe K: A comparison of the Wechsler Intelligence Scale for Children-Revised and the Leiter International Performance Scale for a group of educationally handicapped adolescents. *J Clin Psychol*, 36:310–312, 1980.

Reynell J: *Reynell Development Language Scales*. Buckinghamshire, NFER, Slough, 1969.

Rotter J, Rafferty J: *Manual for the Rotter Incomplete Sentence Blank*. New York, Psychological Corporation, 1958.

Sackett D, Haynes R, Tugwell P: *Clinical Epidemiology: A Basic Science for Clinical Medicine*. Boston, Little Brown & Co, 1985.

Sameroff A, Chandler M: Reproductive risk and the continuum of caretaking casualty. In Horowitz F, Hetherington M, et al (eds): *Review of Child Development Research*. Chicago, University of Chicago Press, 1975, pp 187–244.

Sameroff A, Emde R: *Relationship Disturbances in Early Childhood*. New York, Basic Books, 1989.

Sattler J: *Assessment of Children*. San Diego, CA, Jerome M. Sattler, 1988.

Silverstein A: Nonstandard scores on the Vineland Adaptive Behavior Scales: A cautionary note. *Am J Ment Defic*, 91:1–4, 1986.

Smith R: The use of developmental screening tests by primary-care pediatricians. *J Pediatr*, 93: 524–527, 1978.

Sparrow S, Balla D, Cicchetti D: *Vineland Adaptive Behavior Scales*. Circle Pines, MN, American Guidance Service, 1984.

Thorndike R, Hagen E, Sattler J: *The Stanford-Binet Intelligence Scale: Fourth Edition*. Chicago, IL, Riverside Publishing, 1986.

Vander Veer B, Schweid E: Infant assessment: Stability of mental functioning in young retarded children. *Am J Ment Defic*, 79:1–4, 1974.

Wechsler D: *Manual for the Wechsler Intelligence Scale for Children*. New York, Psychological Corporation, 1949.

Wechsler D: *Manual for the Wechsler Preschool and Primary Scale of Intelligence-Revised*. San Antonio, TX, The Psychological Corporation, 1989.
Wechsler D: *Manual for the Wechsler Intelligence Scale for Children III*. San Antonio, TX, The Psychological Corporation, 1991.
Whitby L: Screening for disease: Definitions and criteria. *Lancet*, 11:819–821, 1974.
Wilkinson G: *Wide Range Achievement Test–3 Administration Manual*. Wilmington, DE, Jastak Associates, 1993.
Wirt R, Lachar D, et al: *Multidimensional Description of Personality*. Los Angeles, CA, Western Psychological Services, 1977.

Index

Note: Page numbers in *italics* refer to illustrations; page numbers followed by t refer to tables.

ISBN 0-7216-5159-3

90038

9 780721 651590